Pediatric Inflammatory Bowel Disease

Petar Mamula • Andrew B. Grossman
Robert N. Baldassano • Judith R. Kelsen
Jonathan E. Markowitz
Editors

Pediatric Inflammatory Bowel Disease

Third Edition

Springer

Editors
Petar Mamula
Division of GI, Hepatology and Nutrition
The Children's Hospital of Philadelphia
Philadelphia, PA
USA

Andrew B. Grossman
Division of GI, Hepatology and Nutrition
The Children's Hospital of Philadelphia
Philadelphia, PA
USA

Robert N. Baldassano
Division of GI, Hepatology and Nutrition
The Children's Hospital of Philadelphia
Philadelphia, PA
USA

Judith R. Kelsen
Division of GI, Hepatology and Nutrition
The Children's Hospital of Philadelphia
Philadelphia, PA
USA

Jonathan E. Markowitz
Division of Pediatric Gastroenterology
and Nutrition
University of South Carolina School
of Medicine - Greenville
Greenville, SC
USA

ISBN 978-3-319-49213-1   ISBN 978-3-319-49215-5   (eBook)
DOI 10.1007/978-3-319-49215-5

Library of Congress Control Number: 2017935021

Printed on acid-free paper

This Springer imprint is published by Springer Nature
The registered company is Springer International Publishing AG
The registered company address is: Gewerbestrasse 11, 6330 Cham, Switzerland

We dedicate this book...

To our families.

To Gordana-Dana, to Melissa, to Joanne, and to Kay. For their love, understanding, and encouragement.

To Niko; to Alex and Matthew; to Julie, Steven, Chris, Linda, William, and Andrew; and to Jack, Leo, and Benjamin. For helping us believe the best is yet to come.

To our colleagues everywhere, past and present. For working hard each day to make a difference.

To our patients. For constantly inspiring us.

Petar, Andrew, Bob, Judith, and Jon

Foreword

Pediatric inflammatory bowel diseases (IBD) are the most common and most significant chronic disorders in pediatric gastroenterology. The onset of Crohn disease and ulcerative colitis in the first two decades of life presents a number of diagnostic and therapeutic challenges that are unique to pediatric patients. Although the studies available for pediatric diagnosis have improved dramatically in the past three decades, the improvement in technology alone cannot account for the increased frequency of IBD recognized in early childhood. While therapy for older patients has improved dramatically with the use of immunomodulators and the development of exciting biologic strategies, rarely if ever have comprehensive studies of the pharmacokinetics, safety, and efficacy of any of the IBD medications been performed in pediatric patients. A number of excellent medications are not available in liquid preparations that can be swallowed by children, and others, such as timed-release formulations, are developed for delivery to an adult gastrointestinal tract. It is unfortunate that the care we provide to children is often an extrapolation of what is known about and available for adults with IBD.

Pediatric patients with IBD face a number of unique challenges. The onset of disease before puberty can be devastating. Growth failure is a particularly difficult problem with potentially permanent consequences. Much of the pediatric specific research has focused on the role of nutritional therapy to treat growth failure and induce remission. Strategies such as nocturnal nasogastric administration of supplements are widespread in most pediatric centers and are surprisingly well tolerated even by the youngest patients, particularly when the value of nutritional therapy is presented in advance to both the family and the child. Nutrition must be strongly advocated for pediatric patients, as it has great therapeutic value and it is the only therapy for which there are no serious potential complications.

The long-term consequences of medical and surgical therapy are particularly troubling for pediatric patients. The complications of corticosteroids in childhood and adolescence can seem worse than the disease itself. While most of the cosmetic side effects are reversible, the psychological trauma to an adolescent can be overwhelming. We are only beginning to understand and address the long-term consequences of therapy given at an early age. Bone mass accumulation and linear growth are critical processes that are age dependent, with peaks in early adolescence. Failure of therapy at this stage will have permanent and possibly debilitating consequences. In order to spare cumulative steroid exposure, there has been a marked shift in the last two decades to immunomodulator and biologic therapies, often initiated in the first decade of life. Most recently, biologic therapies have resulted in a dramatic shift in therapeutic armamentarium and the sequence of its administration. In adults, the "therapeutic pyramid" has been turned on all of its sides, with a resulting dramatic improvement in quality of life and a decrease in overall corticosteroid exposure, but with a new set of adverse events from therapy. While pediatric patients undoubtedly benefit from the adult data supporting the "top-down" strategies, the data in adults does not necessarily predict the optimal strategies for children. The effects of more "aggressive" therapy are being recognized for their positives and negatives, and the risks and benefits are undoubtedly different in children and adolescents. Whether it is the state of the immature immune system, the effect of rapid growth, or the background susceptibility to different malignancies at different ages, the incidence of profound problems such as hepatosplenic T-cell lymphomas reminds all practitioners that we do not understand the unique aspects of the younger patient that may confer increased susceptibility.

The rate of advance in the science and the understanding of the causes of and the therapies for IBD are truly astounding and fully warrant a third edition of this book. In the decades since the first IBD gene association was discovered, another 200 loci have been identified, and the individual characteristics and functions of these sites are increasingly understood. This is only the beginning of the synergy that can be achieved from the combination of the human genome project results and the availability of genome-wide arrays. The increased focus on the unique aspects and causes of very early onset IBD has led to an exciting and new group of diseases that are more likely to be monogenic and are unlikely to be identified by genome-wide array analysis. These high-impact variants can cause devastating disease in infancy, and some will have entirely novel causes and therapies. Whole exome sequencing will provide a better understanding of the role of individual genes at important loci, and the potential for the "thousand-dollar genome sequencing" is actually within reach, providing not only a true potential for "personalized medicine" but also for predictive identification of "at-risk" children who then might be enrolled in "prevention" studies (as are ongoing in GI allergic diseases and celiac disease) rather than merely treatment protocols. To complement these advances, there is incredible progress in the technology available to study the microbiome, its role in immunomodulation, and the effects of prebiotic, probiotic, antibiotic, and nutritional therapy for gastrointestinal diseases. This work has given insight into the complex relationship between the human immune system and the enteric inhabitants that reside within us. This work will likely identify one important group of environmental triggers that comprise part of the cause of IBD, and through that understanding, we may have one more route for the prevention of IBD in genetically susceptible individuals. A better understanding of the resident microbiota will undoubtedly inform better enteric therapy for IBD.

There is no better care than that given by a well-educated and experienced practitioner who considers all aspects of a patient's problems. This book is designed for those practitioners who care for children. IBD therapy must be customized for each individual patient. There is no more ultimate "individual" patient than a child or adolescent with IBD. The many challenges of growth, nutrition, psychology, and adaptation weigh heavily upon the profound challenges of pediatric Crohn disease and ulcerative colitis. In addition to the need for induction and maintenance of remission, the pediatric gastroenterologist must be obsessed not only with the benefits of early achievement of mucosal healing but also with the long-term consequences of therapy, not just a decade away, but hopefully a half century or more hence. Although these patients will move on to adult gastroenterologists, the problems may only accumulate and multiply. "Above all else, do no harm" is a wise admonition for pediatric IBD, where therapies are rapidly improving and there is a great potential for a cure of these devastating illnesses. These therapies and ultimate cures for Crohn disease and ulcerative colitis will come from the extraordinary advances in immunology and immunogenetics that are well detailed in this book. Until that time, we must rely on the conventional approaches developed in adults, but with the conviction to verify their efficacy for children with IBD.

This book is a landmark step toward better understanding of pediatric IBD and the challenges of IBD therapy in children. The editors are highly respected clinical scientists who have each contributed substantially to the knowledge about pediatric IBD. In addition, the knowledge gained from their extensive clinical experience is reflected in this book. They have assembled a truly extraordinary group of authoritative leaders whose contributions to this volume will guarantee that this will be a reference for all who care for pediatric IBD. The book is a tribute to those authors, but is dedicated to the children and adolescents with Crohn disease and ulcerative colitis. It is remarkable how far we have come since the first edition, yet sobering how far the journey is yet to go. It is a sign of the times that increased focus at every level is directed toward children, and this book is one significant step along that road toward improving care for the hundreds of thousands of children and adolescents with inflammatory bowel diseases. It should be a required reading for all those who care for these children.

David A. Piccoli, MD
Chief, Division of Gastroenterology, Hepatology and Nutrition,
The Children's Hospital of Philadelphia,
Raymond and Ruth Perelman School of Medicine at the University of Pennsylvania,
Philadelphia, PA, USA

Preface

We are pleased to present the third edition of *Pediatric Inflammatory Bowel Disease*. Since the publication of the last edition, there has continued to be an explosion of discoveries and advances in the areas of genetics, immunology, pharmacogenomics, microbiome, optimization of therapeutic delivery, and epidemiologic knowledge, particularly regarding our youngest pediatric patients afflicted with inflammatory bowel disease. These advances have resulted in improved understanding of the etiology and pathogenesis of inflammatory bowel disease and have provided mechanisms to optimize therapeutic management of our patients.

The focus of the textbook remains unchanged. We hope to provide a reference that assists clinicians from multiple disciplines, including primary care, pediatric, and internal medicine gastroenterology – all healthcare providers who care for children with inflammatory bowel disease. This textbook will augment other utilized references, focusing on pediatrics while also incorporating the adult evidence and experience that has informed and influenced the care of children.

The format of the textbook is similar to the last edition, with sections dedicated to etiology and pathogenesis, epidemiology and clinical features, diagnosis, medical and nutritional therapy, surgical therapy, research, and special considerations – a section that includes topics which have become increasingly important and challenging for the experienced clinician, including addressing the psychological aspects of pediatric inflammatory bowel disease, legislative advocacy, transition from pediatric to adult care, and quality improvement. We are pleased to offer topical new chapters regarding immune dysregulation in very early onset pediatric inflammatory bowel disease, fecal markers of disease activity, therapeutic drug monitoring, dietary therapies, complementary and alternative therapies, management of intra-abdominal complications, postoperative surveillance, and fostering self-management and patient activation, coauthored by two parents of patients with pediatric inflammatory bowel disease.

As with the previous two editions, we are indebted to the internationally recognized experts who contributed to this book, inculcating the latest research- and evidence-based clinical opinion to the updated chapters. This edition would not have been possible if not for their generous contributions and dedication.

Philadelphia, PA, USA
Petar Mamula, MD
Andrew B. Grossman, MD
Robert N. Baldassano, MD
Judith R. Kelsen, MD
Greenville, SC, USA
Jonathan E. Markowitz, MD

Contents

Part VII   Special Considerations

Contributors

Jeremy Adler Department of Pediatrics and Communicable Diseases, Pediatric Inflammatory Bowel Disease Program, C.S. Mott Children's Hospital, University of Michigan Health System, Ann Arbor, MI, USA

Lindsey Albenberg Perelman School of Medicine, The University of Pennsylvania, Philadelphia, PA, USA

Division of Pediatric Gastroenterology, Hepatology, and Nutrition, The Children's Hospital of Philadelphia, Philadelphia, PA, USA

Marina Aloi Pediatric Gastroenterology and Liver Unit, Department of Pediatrics, University of Rome "La Sapienza", Rome, Italy

Tara Altepeter Division of Gastroenterology and Inborn Errors Products, US Food and Drug Administration, Silver Spring, MD, USA

Ana Catalina Arce-Clachar Division of Gastroenterology, Hepatology and Nutrition, Cincinnati Children's Hospital Medical Center, Cincinnati, OH, USA

Monica I. Ardura Division of Infectious Diseases and Immunology, Host Defense Program, Nationwide Children's Hospital, 700 Children's Hospital, Columbus, OH, USA

Janis Arnold IBD Center, Children's Hospital Boston, Boston, MA, USA

Robert N. Baldassano Department of Pediatrics, The Children's Hospital of Philadelphia, Philadelphia, PA, USA

Perelman School of Medicine at the University of Pennsylvania, Philadelphia, PA, USA

Division of Gastroenterology, Hepatology, and Nutrition, The Children's Hospital of Philadelphia, Philadelphia, PA, USA

Arthur M. Barrie Division of Gastroenterology, Hepatology, and Nutrition, University of Pittsburgh Medical Center, Pittsburgh, PA, USA

Eric I. Benchimol Division of Gastroenterology, Hepatology and Nutrition, Children's Hospital of Eastern Ontario, Department of Pediatrics and School of Epidemiology, Public Health and Preventive Medicine, University of Ottawa, Ottawa, ON, Canada

Athos Bousvaros IBD Center, Children's Hospital Boston, Boston, USA

Kurt Brown Immuno-Inflammation Therapy Area Unit, Research and Development, GlaxoSmithKline, Collegeville, PA, USA

Sarah Buchanan Crohn's and Colitis Foundation of America, New York, NY, USA

Christopher J. Cardinale Center for Applied Genomics, Children's Hospital of Philadelphia, Philadelphia, PA, USA

Che Yung Chao Advanced Clinical Fellow in IBD, Division of Gastroenterology, Faculty of Medicine, McGill University, Montreal, QC, Canada

Richard B. Colletti Department of Pediatrics, University of Vermont College of Medicine, Burlington, VT, USA

ImproveCareNow, Burlington, VT, USA

Máire A. Conrad Division of Gastroenterology, Hepatology and Nutrition, The Children's Hospital of Philadelphia, Philadelphia, PA, USA

Wallace V. Crandall Department of Pediatrics, The Ohio State University College of Medicine, Center for Pediatric and Adolescent Inflammatory Bowel Disease, Nationwide Children's Hospital, Columbus, OH, USA

Salvatore Cucchiara Pediatric Gastroenterology and Liver Unit, Department of Pediatrics, University of Rome "La Sapienza", Rome, Italy

Carmen Cuffari Division of Pediatric Gastroenterology and Nutrition, Department of Pediatrics, The Johns Hopkins University School of Medicine, Baltimore, MD, USA

The Johns Hopkins Hospital, Department of Pediatrics, Division of Gastroenterology, Baltimore, MD, USA

Jennifer Damman Stanford Children's Inflammatory Bowel Disease Center, Department of Pediatrics, Stanford, CA, USA

Andrew S. Day Pediatric Gastroenterology, Christchurch Hospital, Christchurch, New Zealand

Department of Pediatrics, University of Otago, Christchurch, New Zealand

Edwin F. de Zoeten Childrens Hospital Colorado, Digestive Health Institute, Denver, CO, USA

Dianne Deplewski Section of Adult and Pediatric Endocrinology, Diabetes and Metabolism, University of Chicago, Chicago, IL, USA

Stephen M. Druhan Ohio State University School of Medicine, Columbus, OH, USA

School of Medicine, University of Toledo Medical College, Toledo, OH, USA

Nationwide Children's Hospital, Columbus, OH, USA

Marla C. Dubinsky Icahn School of Medicine at Mount Sinai, New York, NY, USA

Dana MH. Dykes Division of Gastroenterology, Hepatology and Nutrition, Cincinnati Children's Hospital Medical Center, Cincinnati, OH, USA

Khalil I. El-Chammas Children's Hospital Medical Center, Cincinnati, OH, USA

Raphael Enaud Unit of Pediatric Gastroenterology and Nutrition, Children's Hospital, Bordeaux, France

Jessi Erlichman The Children's Hospital of Philadelphia, Division of Gastroenterology, Hepatology and Nutrition, Philadelphia, PA, USA

Johanna C. Escher Department of Pediatric Gastroenterology, Erasmus MC-Sophia Children's Hospital, University Medical Center, Rotterdam, The Netherlands

William A. Faubion Jr Department of Gastroenterology and Hepatology, Mayo Clinic, Rochester, MN, USA

Melissa A. Fernandes Department of Pediatrics, University of California, San Francisco, San Francisco, CA, USA

Ivan J. Fuss National Institute of Allergy Immunology and infectious Disease, Mucosal Immunity Section, National Institutes of Health, Bethesda, MD, USA

Benjamin D. Gold Pediatric Gastroenterology, Hepatology and Nutrition, Children's Center for Digestive Healthcare, LLC, Atlanta, GA, USA

Michelle Gonzalez Division of Pediatric Gastroenterology and Hepatology, Mayo Clinic Children's Center, Rochester, MN, USA

Alka Goyal Department of Gastroenterology, Hepatology and Nutrition, Children's Mercy Hospital, Kansas City, MO, USA

Amy Grant Division of Gastroenterology, Department of Pediatrics, Izaak Walton Killam Health Centre, Halifax, NS, Canada

Anne M. Griffiths Division of Gastroenterology, Hepatology and Nutrition, The Hospital for Sick Children, University of Toronto, Toronto, ON, Canada

Andrew B. Grossman Division of Gastroenterology, Hepatology, and Nutrition, The Children's Hospital of Philadelphia, Philadelphia, PA, USA

Neera Gupta Pediatric Gastroenterology and Nutrition, New York, NY, USA

Hakon Hakonarson Center for Applied Genomics, Children's Hospital of Philadelphia, Perelman School of Medicine at the University of Pennsylvania, Philadelphia, PA, USA

Melvin B. Heyman Department of Pediatrics, University of California, San Francisco, San Francisco, CA, USA

Pediatric Gastroenterology/Nutrition, University of California, San Francisco, San Francisco, CA, USA

Peter D.R. Higgins Department of Internal Medicine, Inflammatory Bowel Disease Program, University of Michigan Health System, Ann Arbor, MI, USA

David A. Hill Department of Pediatrics, Division of Allergy and Immunology, The Children's Hospital of Philadelphia, Philadelphia, PA, USA

Jeffrey S. Hyams Division of Digestive Diseases, Hepatology and Nutrition, Connecticut Children's Medical Center, Hartford, CT, USA

University of Connecticut School of Medicine, Farmington, CT, USA

Aisha Peterson Johnson Division of Gastroenterology and Inborn Errors Products, Silver Spring, MD, USA

Howard Kader Department of Pediatrics, Division of Pediatric Gastroenterology and Nutrition, University of Maryland Children's Hospital, Baltimore, MD, USA

Stacy A. Kahn Transitional IBD Clinic, The University of Chicago Medicine, Chicago, IL, USA

Binita M. Kamath Division of Gastroenterology, Hepatology and Nutrition, The Hospital for Sick Children, Toronto, Canada

University of Toronto, Toronto, Canada

Sunanda Kane Mayo Clinic, Rochester, MN, USA

Jess L. Kaplan Harvard Medical School, Pediatric Gastroenterology, MassGeneral Hospital for Children, Boston, MA, USA

Marsha Kay Cleveland Clinic Foundation, Department of Pediatric Gastroenterology, Hepatology and Nutrition, Cleveland, OH, USA

Judith R. Kelsen Division of Gastroenterology, Hepatology and Nutrition, The Children's Hospital of Philadelphia, Perelman School of Medicine at the University of Pennsylvania, Philadelphia, PA, USA

Sandra C. Kim Gastroenterology, The Ohio State University College of Medicine, Department of Pediatrics and Center for Pediatric and Adolescent IBD, Nationwide Children's Hospital, Columbus, OH, USA

Barbara S. Kirschner Section of Gastroenerology, Hepatology and Nutrition, University of Chicago, Chicago, IL, USA

Subra Kugathasan Department of Pediatrics, Emory University School of Medicine and Children's healthcare of Atlanta, Atlanta, GA, USA

Emory University School of Medicine, Division of Pediatric Gastroenterology, Emory Children's Center, Atlanta, GA, USA

Jacob Kurowski Cleveland Clinic Foundation, Department of Pediatric Gastroenterology, Hepatology and Nutrition, Cleveland, OH, USA

Thierry Lamireau Unit of Pediatric Gastroenterology and Nutrition, Children's Hospital, Bordeaux, France

Oren Ledder Juliet Keidan Institute of Pediatric Gastroenterology and Nutrition, The Hebrew University of Jerusalem, Shaare Zedek Medical Center, Jerusalem, Israel

Dale Lee Department of Pediatrics, Seattle Children's Hospital, University of Washington, Seattle, WA, USA

Gary R. Lichtenstein Inflammatory Bowel Disease Center, The University of Pennsylvania, Philadelphia, PA, USA

Ying Lu Division of Pediatric Gastroenterology, Cohen Children's Medical Center of New York, Lake Success, NY, USA

David R. Mack Department of Paediatrics, Faculty of Medicine, University of Ottawa, Ottawa, ON, Canada

CHEO IBD Centre, Ottawa, ON, Canada

Pediatric Gastroenterology, Hepatology and Nutrition, Children's Hospital of Eastern Ontario, Ottawa, ON, Canada

Laura M. Mackner Center for Biobehavioral Health, Nationwide Children's Hospital, Columbus, OH, USA

Peter A. Margolis James M. Anderson Center for Health System Excellence, Cincinnati Children's Hospital Medical Center, Cincinnati, OH, USA

James Markowitz Hofstra Northwell School of Medicine, Hempstead, NY, USA

Division of Pediatric Gastroenterology and Nutrition, Steven and Alexandra Cohen Children's Medical Center of NY, Northwell Health, New Hyde Park, NY, USA

Maria Mascarenhas The Children's Hospital of Philadelphia, Division of Gastroenterology, Hepatology and Nutrition, Philadelphia, PA, USA

Peter Mattei Division of General, Thoracic and Fetal Surgery, The Children's Hospital of Phladelphia, Philadelphia, PA, USA

Department of Surgery, Perelman School of Medicine of the University of Pennsylvania, General, Thoracic and Fetal Surgery, The Children's Hospital of Philadelphia, Philadelphia, PA, USA

Elizabeth C. Maxwell Division of Gastroenterology, Hepatology, and Nutrition, The Children's Hospital of Philadelphia, Philadelphia, USA

Philip Minar Division of Gastroenterology, Hepatology and Nutrition, Cincinnati Children's Hospital Medical Center, Cincinnati, OH, USA

Andrew E. Mulberg Gastroenterology and Inborn Errors Products, Food and Drug Administration, Silver Spring, MD, USA

Benedict C. Nwomeh Pediatric Surgery Residency Program, The Ohio State University, Columbus, OH, USA

Center for Pediatric and Adolescent IBD, Nationwide Children's Hospital, Columbus, OH, USA

Maria Oliva-Hemker Division of Pediatric Gastroenterology and Nutrition, The Johns Hopkins University School of Medicine, Baltimore, MD, USA

Mark T. Osterman Division of Gastroenterology, Department of Medicine, Penn Presbyterian Medical Center, University of Pennsylvania School of Medicine, Philadelphia, PA, USA

Anthony R. Otley Faculty of Medicine, Dalhousie University, Halifax, Canada
Division of Gastroenterology and Nutrition, IWK Health Centre, Halifax, NS, Canada

Jennifer Panganiban Division of Gastroenterology, Hepatology and Nutrition, The Children's Hospital of Philadelphia, Perelman School of Medicine, University of Pennsylvania, Philadelphia, PA, USA

K.T. Park Stanford Children's Inflammatory Bowel Disease Center, Department of Pediatrics, Stanford, CA, USA

Adam Paul Lehigh Valley Children's Hospital, Allentown, PA, USA

Shervin Rabizadeh Pediatric Inflammatory Bowel Disease Program, Department of Pediatrics, Cedars-Sinai Medical Center, Los Angeles, CA, USA

Farzana Rashid The University of Pennsylvania, Philadelphia, PA, USA

Bonney Reed-Knight Children's Healthcare of Atlanta, Atlanta, GA, USA
Department of Pediatrics, Division of Gastroenterology, Hepatology, and Nutrition, Emory University School of Medicine, Atlanta, GA, USA
GI Care for Kids, Atlanta, GA, USA

Miguel Regueiro Division of Gastroenterology, Hepatology, and Nutrition, University of Pittsburgh Medical Center, Pittsburgh, PA, USA

Amanda Ricciuto Division of Gastroenterology, Hepatology and Nutrition, The Hospital for Sick Children, University of Toronto, Toronto, Canada

Suzanne Rosenthal Crohn's and Colitis Foundation of America, New York, NY, USA

Joel R. Rosh Pediatric Gastroenterology, Clinical Development and Research Affairs, Goryeb Children's Hospital/Atlantic Health, Morristown, NJ, USA
Icahn School of Medicine at Mount Sinai, New York, NY, USA

Pierre Russo Department of Pathology and Laboratory Medicine, Perelman School of Medicine at The University of Pennsylvania, Philadelphia, PA, USA

Division of Anatomic Pathology, The Children's Hospital of Philadelphia, Philadelphia, PA, USA

Shehzad A. Saeed Division of Gastroenterology, Hepatology and Nutrition, Cincinnati Children's Hospital Medical Center, Cincinnati, OH, USA

Benjamin Sahn Hofstra Northwell School of Medicine, Hempstead, NY, USA

Division of Pediatric Gastroenterology and Nutrition, Steven and Alexandra Cohen Children's Medical Center of NY, Northwell Health, New Hyde Park, NY, USA

Charles M. Samson Gastroenterology, Hepatology and Nutrition, Department of Pediatrics, Washington University School of Medicine, St Louis, MO, USA

Ana Maria Sant'Anna Pediatric Capsule Endoscopy Lab, GI Division, Montreal Children's Hospital, McGill Faculty of Medicine, Montreal, QC, Canada

Ernest G. Seidman Division of Gastroenterology, McGill Faculty of Medicine, McGill University Health Center, Montreal, QC, Canada

Edisio Semeao Department of Pediatrics, The Children's Hospital of Philadelphia, University of Pennsylvania School of Medicine, Philadelphia, PA, USA

Shishu Sharma Sheffield Children's Hospital, Sheffield, UK

Mary E. Sherlock Division of Gastroenterology and Nutrition, Hamilton Health Sciences, McMaster Children's Hospital, Hamilton, ON, Canada

Namita Singh Pediatric IBD Center at Cedars-Sinai Medical Center, Los Angeles, CA, USA

David Geffen School of Medicine at UCLA, Los Angeles, CA, USA

Manu R. Sood Division of Pediatric Gastroenterology, Hepatology and Nutrition, Department of Pediatric, Medical College of Wisconsin, Milwaukee, WI, USA

Children's Hospital of Wisconsin, Milwaukee, WI, USA

Ronen Stein Department of Pediatrics, The Children's Hospital of Philadelphia, Philadelphia, PA, USA

Perelman School of Medicine at the University of Pennsylvania, Philadelphia, PA, USA

Division of Gastroenterology, Hepatology, and Nutrition, The Children's Hospital of Philadelphia, Philadelphia, PA, USA

Calen A. Steiner Department of Internal Medicine, University of Michigan Health System, Ann Arbor, MI, USA

Judith J. Stellar Department of Nursing and General Surgery, The Children's Hospital of Philadelphia, Philadelphia, PA, USA

Michael Stephens Division of Pediatric Gastroenterology and Hepatology, Mayo Clinic Children's Center, Rochester, MN, USA

Jennifer Strople Division of Pediatric Gastroenterology, Hepatology and Nutrition, Ann and Robert H. Lurie Children's Hospital of Chicago, Chicago, IL, USA

Kathleen Sullivan Division of Allergy and Immunology, The Children's Hospital of Philadelphia, Philadelphia, PA, USA

Francisco Sylvester The University of North Carolina at Chapel Hill, Chapel Hill, NC, USA

Mike Thomson Sheffield Children's Hospital, Sheffield, UK

Peter Townsend Division of Digestive Diseases, Hepatology, and Nutrition, Connecticut Children's Medical Center, Hartford, CT, USA

University of Connecticut School of Medicine, Farmington, CT, USA

Dan Turner Juliet Keidan Institute of Pediatric Gastroenterology and Nutrition, The Hebrew University of Jerusalem, Shaare Zedek Medical Center, Jerusalem, Israel

Thomas A. Ullman The Dr. Henry D. Janowitz Division of Gastroenterology, The Mount Sinai School of Medicine, New York, NY, USA

Justin Vandergrift Member of the Parent Working Group of the ImproveCareNow Learning Health System, Charlotte, NC, USA

Krishnappa Venkatesh Sheffield Children's Hospital, Sheffield, UK

Sofia Verstraete Department of Pediatrics, University of California, San Francisco, San Francisco, CA, USA

Daniel von Allmen Division of Pediatric General and Thoracic Surgery, Cincinnati Children's Hospital Medical Center, Cincinnati, OH, USA

Thomas D. Walters Division of Gastroenterology, Hepatology and Nutrition, The Hospital for Sick Children, University of Toronto, Toronto, ON, Canada

Emily P. Whitfield Department of Pediatrics and Communicable Diseases, Pediatric Inflammatory Bowel Disease Program C.S. Mott Children's Hospital, University of Michigan Health System, Ann Arbor, MI, USA

Harland S. Winter Harvard Medical School, Pediatric IBD Program, MassGeneral Hospital for Children, Boston, MA, USA

David Alain Wohl Member of the Parent Working Group of the ImproveCareNow Learning Health System, Chapel Hill, NC, USA

Gary D. Wu Perelman School of Medicine at the University of Pennsylvania, Hospital of University of Pennsylvania, Philadelphia, PA, USA

Robert Wyllie Cleveland Clinic Foundation, Department of Pediatric Gastroenterology, Hepatology and Nutrition, Cleveland, OH, USA

Rona Yaeger Memorial Sloan Kettering Cancer Center, New York, NY, USA

Mary Zachos Department of Pediatrics, McMaster University, McMaster Children's Hospital, Hamilton, ON, Canada

Part I

Etiology and Pathogenesis

Genetics of Inflammatory Bowel Diseases

Christopher J. Cardinale and Hakon Hakonarson

Introduction

The inflammatory bowel diseases (IBD), Crohn disease and ulcerative colitis, are immune-mediated disorders resulting in chronic, relapsing inflammation of the gastrointestinal tract. The etiology of IBD is multifactorial, influenced by both genes and environmental factors. It has been hypothesized that environmental factors and maladaptive immune responses to gastrointestinal flora generate a dysregulated inflammatory cascade creating mucosal injury in genetically susceptible individuals. Over the last two decades, considerable interest and research have focused on the genetic aspect of IBD. The identification of linkage between Crohn disease and the pericentromeric region of chromosome 16 (IBD1) by Hugot et al. in 1996 spawned a series of genome scans and linkage analyses in search of susceptibility and phenotypic modifier genes [1]. In 2001, the discovery that specific polymorphisms in the CARD15/NOD2 gene at the IBD1 locus were associated with Crohn disease introduced a new era of genotype-phenotype investigations [2, 3]. The advent of genome-wide association studies has resulted in the successful identification of new, well-replicated disease associations, now encompassing 200 independent loci [4]. This abundance of associations shows that IBD is highly polygenic with a complex mode of inheritance.

The field of IBD genetics is of special interest to pediatric gastroenterologists for both practical and investigational reasons. From a clinical practice standpoint, pediatric gastroenterologists are often faced with questions from concerned parents regarding the risk of IBD among current or future siblings, as well as the eventual offspring of the affected child. Understanding genetic associations of IBD can provide patients and their families with useful information that may help them cope with the disease. Furthermore, as our knowledge of genotype-phenotype associations grows, it is anticipated that genotyping at the onset of disease may enable physicians to predict disease course and tailor medical therapies specific for each patient. Insofar as advancing the field of gastroenterology through research, studies of pediatric IBD genetics are significant because children have been exposed to fewer environmental confounders of disease than their adult counterparts. Examining the disease in young individuals could provide us with keys to unlock intrinsic genetic mechanisms in IBD that may not otherwise be detected in adult studies. This may be especially important in individuals with very early-onset IBD (<5 years), whose disease course and phenotypes are the most discordant with those of adult-onset IBD.

Crohn Disease and Ulcerative Colitis: Genetic Epidemiology

Ethnic and Racial Variations of Disease

The genetic underpinnings of IBD are supported by ethnic and racial variations in disease prevalence. The highest rates of IBD are found in Caucasian individuals, especially those of Jewish heritage. Among Jewish subgroups, Ashkenazi Jews have a two- to ninefold greater prevalence of IBD over non-Jewish counterparts [5]. This increased occurrence has been noted to be stable over time and geographic distribution, substantiating the important role of genetics in IBD. While the vast majority of genetic investigations in IBD have been conducted in Caucasians, it is apparent that it can occur in all racial and ethnic groups. African Americans and Asians are believed to have a lower risk of IBD, although there appears to be a trend toward growing prevalence in these populations. Basu et al. reported that African Americans and whites were more likely to have Crohn disease, whereas

C.J. Cardinale, MD, PhD (✉)
Center for Applied Genomics, Children's Hospital of Philadelphia, Philadelphia, PA, USA
e-mail: CardinaleC@email.chop.edu

H. Hakonarson, MD, PhD
Center for Applied Genomics, Children's Hospital of Philadelphia, Perelman School of Medicine at the University of Pennsylvania, Philadelphia, PA, USA

© Springer International Publishing AG 2017
P. Mamula et al. (eds.), Pediatric Inflammatory Bowel Disease, DOI 10.1007/978-3-319-49215-5_1

ulcerative colitis predominated among Mexican Americans [6]. While intestinal manifestations did not appear to vary based upon race or ethnicity, there were differences in extraintestinal manifestation between groups. Among Crohn patients, African Americans were more likely to develop arthritis and uveitis than whites, whereas joint symptoms and osteoporosis were more common among whites with UC than Mexican Americans.

Family Studies

The concept that IBD may, in part, be hereditary has been well established through observations of familial disease aggregation. Family studies have demonstrated that 5–30% of probands with Crohn disease and ulcerative colitis identify the presence of IBD in a family member [5]. This association appears to be stronger for Crohn disease than ulcerative colitis. Phenotypically, relatives of probands with IBD are more likely to develop the same form of disease as the affected family member, with a concordance between family members in terms of localization of disease but not disease severity. With regard to age of disease onset, patients with a family history of IBD are thought to be more likely to develop disease at an earlier age than affected individuals lacking a family history [7]. Among family members, the risk of developing IBD is greatest among first-degree relatives, especially siblings. The relative risk (RR) for a sibling of a Crohn patient developing disease is 13–26; for ulcerative colitis patients, the RR for a sibling is 7–17 [8]. Orholm et al. reported that 6.2% of children born to a parent with ulcerative colitis developed IBD and 9.2% of children born to a parent with Crohn disease developed IBD [9]. In the rare instance that both parents have IBD, studies estimate that their children have a 33% chance of developing IBD by age 28 [8]. While second- and third-degree relatives of IBD probands have a lower likelihood of disease, their risk is still elevated compared to the background population.

Twin Studies

Investigations of monozygotic and dizygotic twins have provided strong evidence that genetics play an integral role in the etiology of IBD. Twin studies are based upon the premise that in the setting of a similar environmental milieu, rates of disease concordance between twins correlate with the influence of genetic factors. To date, three large studies of twin pairs with IBD from Scandinavia and the UK have consistently identified higher concordance rates among monozygotic twins with Crohn disease and ulcerative colitis than dizygotic twins [10–12]. The influence of genetics appears to be greater in Crohn disease than ulcerative colitis with

reported cumulative monozygotic concordance rates of 30 and 15%, respectively [13]. Concordance rates for dizygotic twins are approximately 4% in both Crohn disease and ulcerative colitis. Co-twins with IBD are more likely to develop the same disease type, although mixed pairs of dizygotic twins with ulcerative colitis and Crohn disease have been reported. With regard to disease-specific characteristics, Scandinavian twin registries demonstrated concordance of 40–77% for disease location; however, there appeared to be no association of disease behavior or extent among co-twins [10, 12]. A trend toward concordance for age at diagnosis was identified with 40–67% receiving a diagnosis of IBD within 2 years of one another. Thus, the concordance data from twin studies provide strong evidence that genetic influences are important in the development of IBD. However, monozygotic concordance is not 100%, and the low concordance between dizygotes suggests that genotype alone is not sufficient for disease evolution.

Identifiable Gene Variants in Crohn Disease

NOD2/CARD15 Gene and Crohn Disease

The *NOD2/CARD15* gene located on the *IBD1* locus of chromosome 16 is associated with an increased susceptibility to Crohn disease but not ulcerative colitis. Among the more than 30 known amino acid polymorphisms identified in the *NOD2* gene [14], the most common variants are two missense mutations, R702W and G908R, and one frameshift mutation L1007fsinsC. From a disease pathogenesis perspective, NOD proteins (NOD1 and NOD2) are mammalian pattern recognition receptors which serve the innate immune system as bacterial sensing molecules. NOD2 is a cytosolic protein found in a variety of cells including monocytes, macrophages, B and T lymphocytes, dendritic cells, and intestinal epithelial cells. Stimulation of NOD2 by its ligand, muramyl dipeptide (MDP), propagates signal transduction pathways leading to nuclear factor κB (NF-κB) and mitogen-activated protein kinase (MAPK) activation. These three polymorphisms impair activation of NF-κB, suggesting that deficiencies in innate immune cell function play a role in the development of Crohn disease [15].

Epidemiology of NOD2 Mutations

A *NOD2* risk allele confers a two- to threefold relative risk of developing Crohn disease; this risk is increased to 17-fold if two alleles are present [16]. Ten to thirty percent of patients with Crohn disease are heterozygous for one of the three mutations, while 3–15% are homozygous or compound heterozygotes [17]. Although these variants are associated with an increased risk of Crohn disease, 8–15% of the healthy population possesses at least one of these mutations, and 1% of healthy individuals are homozygous or compound heterozygotes. That genotypic variants are found in individuals without known Crohn disease suggests phenotypic expression of disease is subject to polygenic factors, variable penetrance, and other environmental mediators.

Studies of patients with Crohn disease worldwide have revealed that the association of *NOD2* polymorphisms with Crohn disease varies between different ethnic populations. North American adult Caucasian cohorts report carriage rates of 10–30% for the three common *NOD2* variants, while minority groups were found to have lower allele frequencies. A North American, multicenter study of pediatric patients with Crohn disease identified *NOD2* polymorphisms among 25% White, 1.6% African American, and 1.6% Hispanic participants [18]. Significant diversity in allele carriage has been described among Crohn patients in European countries and background control populations. *NOD2* variants are virtually absent in Japanese, Korean, Chinese, and sub-Saharan African individuals. High rates of *NOD2* mutations have been seen in the Jewish Ashkenazim with one Israeli group reporting the presence of variants in 51% of pediatric and 37.5% of adult Crohn patients studied [19].

HLA Type and IBD Susceptibility

The major histocompatibility complex (MHC) locus on chromosome 6p encodes genes in the human leukocyte antigen (HLA) family which serve an immunoregulatory function through their role in antigen presentation to T cells. Associated polymorphisms between HLA types and IBD have included HLA-B, HLA-DRB1, HLA-DQB1, HLA-DP, tumor necrosis factor (TNF), heat shock protein (HSP)-70, and MICA [20]. The polymorphic nature of the HLA region as well as its complex linkage disequilibrium has resulted in heterogeneous findings among investigators. Of the greater than 100 association studies of IBD and HLA performed to date, stronger evidence exists for an association with class II alleles than class I alleles.

Class II alleles DRB1*0103, DRB*1502, and DRB*401 have been consistently associated with ulcerative colitis [21]. Phenotypic analyses have identified DRB1*0103 to be predictive of a more aggressive form of ulcerative colitis with shorter time to colectomy than those without the allele. In Crohn patients, a particular link between DRB1*0103 and isolated colonic disease has been reported [22]. The correlation of DRB1*0103 with both colonic Crohn disease and ulcerative colitis has been postulated to provide a unifying molecular mechanism for colonic involvement in IBD. HLA associations with extraintestinal manifestations of IBD have also been evaluated. One small study of both ulcerative coli-

tis and Crohn disease identified a connection between TNF promoter variants and erythema nodosum [23]. HLA-B*27, HLA-B*35, and HLA-DRB*103 have been associated with type I peripheral arthropathy, whereas HLA-B*44 is associated with type II peripheral arthropathy [24, 25]. Symptoms of uveitis have been linked with HLA-B27 and DRB*0103.

High-density genotyping in the MHC region has reinforced the primacy of HLA-DRB1*0103 in both Crohn disease and ulcerative colitis in a study by Goyette et al. Their study genotyped 7,406 single nucleotide polymorphisms in 32,000 IBD cases and an equal number of controls [26], finding that DRB1*0103 gave by far the strongest signal. The fine resolution of mapping allowed localization to specific amino acid substitutions in the MHC molecule which revealed that the causal variants are located within the peptide-binding groove and thereby influence antigen presentation directly [26].

Genome-Wide Association Studies in IBD

A major new development in the field of complex human genetics has been the capacity to perform dense genotyping across the genome on microarrays. This technological development has made possible the performance of genome-wide association studies (GWAS). These studies have the capacity to assay a large fraction of the common human genetic variation and have the potential to markedly increase understanding of the genetic basis for complex, polygenic disorders. GWAS tests each of millions of single nucleotide polymorphisms (SNPs) for direct association with the trait of interest by comparing the population allele frequency between IBD cases and healthy controls [27]. This direct association testing approach has the advantage of greater power to detect small effects. Risch and Merikangas estimated that 17,997 affected sibling pairs would be necessary to detect a risk allele with 50% frequency and odds ratio of 1.5 by linkage analysis [28]. By contrast, direct association analysis would require only 484 cases and controls. The early GWAS studies detected only dozens of associations, but with the introduction of meta-analysis combining case-control data from many cohorts along with large-scale genotyping on the Immunochip and trans-ancestry analysis, the number of associated loci has risen to 200 [4].

Association of *IL23R* (Interleukin 23 Receptor) Polymorphisms to Crohn Disease and Ulcerative Colitis

A genome-wide association study in a North American Crohn disease cohort identified multiple new gene associations, notably including multiple polymorphisms within the

IL23R gene on chromosome 1p31 [29]. In particular, an amino acid polymorphism, Arg381Gln, located in the cytoplasmic domain of the *IL23R* protein, demonstrated highly significant evidence for association. The less common glutamine allele conferred significant protection against developing IBD in non-Jewish and Jewish Crohn disease cohorts, as well as in non-Jewish ulcerative colitis cohorts. Additional independent association signals were observed indicating the presence of multiple associations within the *IL23R* gene [29]. Since the initial report, the *IL23R* associations have been replicated in a childhood-onset IBD cohort from Scotland [30], as well as in a Belgian CD cohort [31]. The functional IL-23 heterodimeric receptor is comprised of the *IL23R* (chromosome 1p31) and *IL12RB2* (chromosome 19p13) [32] subunits, with the latter subunit shared with the functional IL-12 receptor. Similarly, the IL-23 cytokine is comprised of a unique subunit, p19 (chromosome 12q13), as well as the p40 subunit which is common to the IL-12 functional cytokine. Additional support for the role of the IL12/IL23 pathway in mediating end-organ inflammation has been generated in mouse models demonstrating requirement for IL-23 in murine colitis [33–36], experimental autoimmune encephalitis [37], and collagen-induced arthritis. Similar *IL23R* gene associations have been reported in human psoriasis [38]. Collectively, these findings would suggest that blocking the IL-23 pathway may be efficacious in the treatment of IBD. In support of this, anti-p40 antibodies (which would block both IL-12 and IL-23 pathways) [39] have been effective in the treatment of Crohn disease. Whether specific targeting of the p19 pathway to achieve IL-23-specific effects [40] will be more efficacious will be the focus of future studies.

Association of the *ATG16L1* Autophagy Gene to Crohn Disease

A GWAS focusing on coding region polymorphisms identified association of the amino acid polymorphism Thr300Ala with Crohn disease. The *ATG16L1* gene is part of the autophagosome pathway and has been implicated in the processing of intracellular bacteria [41]. *ATG16L1* is expressed in intestinal epithelial cells, as well as in CD4+, CD8+, and CD19+ primary human lymphocytes [42]. This association has been confirmed in multiple independent cohorts, including Belgian [31] and North American cohorts [42]. Of interest is that no association was observed to ulcerative colitis, suggesting that *ATG16L1*, like the NOD2/CARD15 associations, represents CD-specific risk alleles. The *ATG16L1* association suggests that autophagy and host cell responses to intracellular microbes are involved in the pathogenesis of CD. Before the discovery of this genetic association, the role of autophagy in IBD was not well appreciated, and this example demonstrates how genetic investigation can advance new treatment approaches and understanding of disease pathophysiology.

Association of *TNFRSF6B* and *IL27* to Pediatric Age of Onset IBD

Pediatric-age-onset IBD is an attractive target for GWA studies for several reasons. Early-onset IBD is characterized by unique phenotypes [43, 44], and increased severity, suggesting the possibility of loci specific to early-onset disease. Early-onset IBD also has a stronger association with family history of IBD, and the childhood population may also be less affected by exogenous factors implicated in adult-onset IBD, such as diet, smoking, and medication [45]. Therefore, GWA studies in children may provide additional power to reveal genetic risk variants with only modest effects relevant in pediatric-age- and adult-onset IBD.

Two GWAS have been performed focusing exclusively on pediatric cases. The most recent of these, conducted by Imielinski et al. in 2009 [46], built on the initial study by Kugathasan et al. in 2008[47] and involved 3,426 affected individuals and 11,963 genetically matched controls. These studies nominally replicated 29 of 32 loci previously associated with adult-onset Crohn disease, as well as 13 of 17 adult-onset ulcerative colitis loci. Further, these studies identified seven new regions associated with childhood IBD susceptibility.

Two of the newly identified loci present immediate insight regarding the pathogenic mechanisms implicated in pediatric-age-onset IBD. Kugathasan et al. found an association located on chromosome 20q13, a block which contains multiple genes, most interestingly *TNFSFR6B* [47]. This locus has since been replicated in an independent pediatric study [48]. The protein product of *TNFSFR6B*, decoy receptor 3 (DcR3), is a member of the tumor necrosis factor receptor superfamily. DcR3 binds to and neutralizes signaling by pro-inflammatory cytokines LIGHT, TL1A, and Fas ligand [49–52]. Serum DcR3 levels were elevated in pediatric cases of IBD relative to controls, most dramatically in patients harboring the 20q13 minor allelic variants [47].

The second locus of interest is in the 16p11 region, in an LD block containing several genes including *IL27*. The IL-27 cytokine regulates T-cell differentiation in adaptive immune responses, influencing the balance between pathogenic Th17 cells and inflammation-suppressing T-cell subsets. Identification of *IL27* as a candidate gene thus provides further support for involvement of the Th17 pathway in pathogenesis of Crohn disease, corroborating gene findings from other genome-wide scans (*IL23R*, *STAT3*, *JAK2*, *IL12B*) [53, 54]. Figure 1.1 shows association results for IL12/IL23 pathway genes (left panel) and IL27/TH17 pathway genes

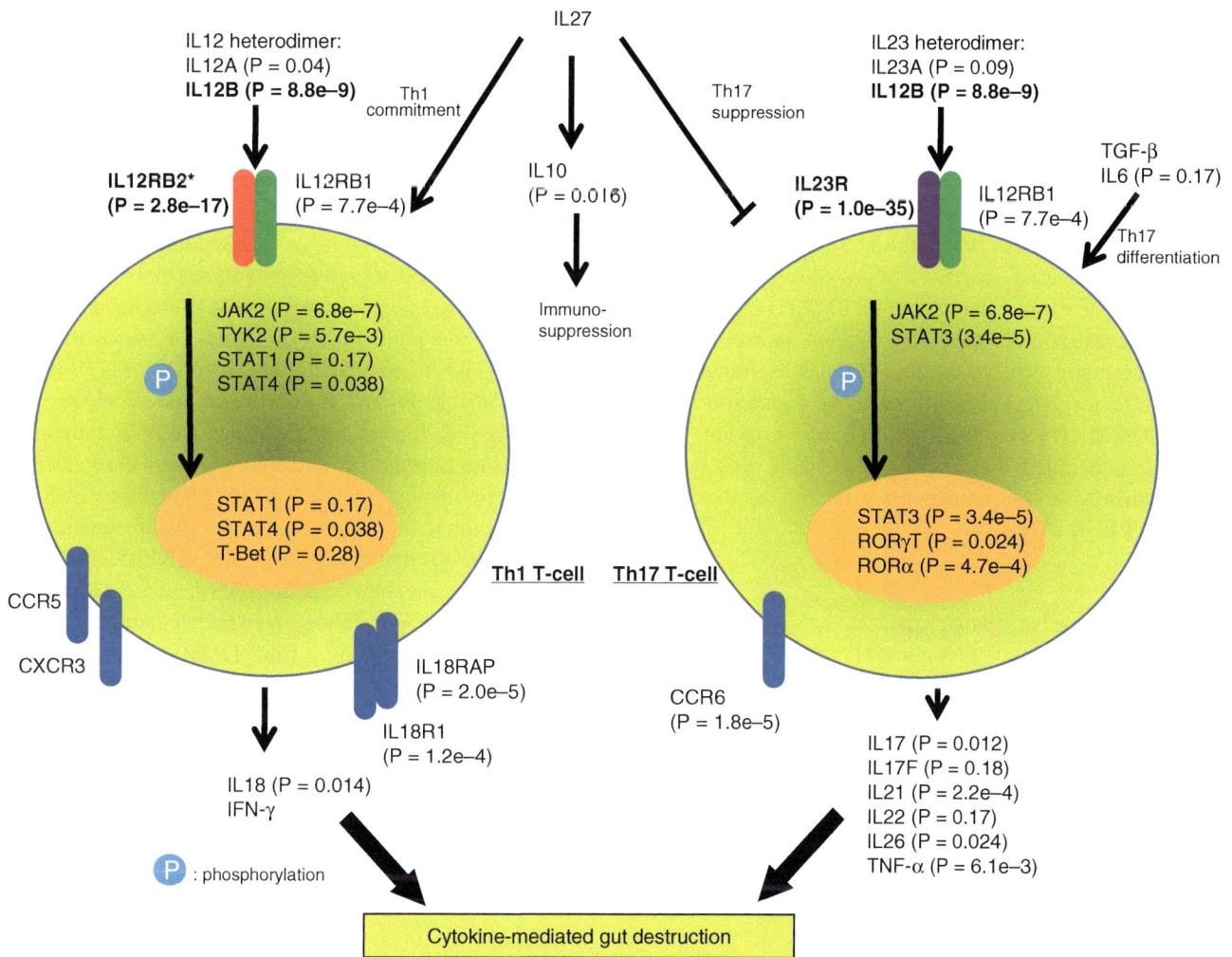

Fig. 1.1 Associations of the IL12/IL23- and IL27-regulating genes with IBD in keeping with the TH1 and TH2/TH17 theory (Wang et al. [96]). Only the main proteins in these pathways are shown. For each gene, the most significant P value among SNPs closest to the gene was annotated

(right panel) in pediatric-age-onset IBD, lending support to the relevance of these two opposing signaling pathways, with multiple associated genes, in the pathogens of IBD.

Meta-analysis

The associated common variants identified by single GWAS usually have modest individual effects, often with odds ratios of smaller than 1.2 for binary traits or with explained variance of less than 1% for quantitative traits [55]. To discover common variants with even smaller effects, a sample size larger than that of single studies is required. Meta-analysis combines large data sets and is an economical way to improve sample size. An early meta-analysis of three genome-wide Crohn scans identified 21 new Crohn susceptibility loci. It increased the number of independent loci conclusively associated with Crohn to 32, explaining approximately 20% of Crohn disease heritability [56].

Including three additional GWAS scans, a recent meta-analysis added 39 new confirmed Crohn disease susceptibility loci [57]. These 39 new loci increase the proportion of explained heritability to only 23.2%, indicating their rather modest effects. While some of these newly identified loci contain a single gene, others contain multiple genes or none at all. Some functionally interesting candidate genes in the implicated regions including *STAT3*, *JAK2*, *ICOSLG*, *ITLN1*, and *SMAD3* are briefly described below.

STAT3 (signal transducer and activator of transcription 3) and JAK2 (Janus kinase 2) both come from the JAK-STAT pathway. This major signaling pathway transmits information from cell surface receptors stimulated by cytokine and growth factors to the nucleus to regulate transcription of various genes. STATs play a central role in Th17 differentiation [58] while both contribute to IL23R signaling [32]. ICOSLG (inducible T-cell co-stimulator ligand) is a co-stimulatory molecule expressed on intestinal (and other) epithelial cells. It has been suggested that ICOSLG may have a key role in controlling the effector functions of regulatory T cells [59]. There is direct evidence showing that maturing plasmacytoid dendritic cells express different sets of molecules including ICOSLG for T-cell priming [60]. ITLN1 (intelectin-1) is known to be expressed in human small bowel and colon. It is found that the lactoferrin receptor (LFR), which is structurally identical to human ITLN1, seems critical in membrane stabilization, preventing loss of digestive enzymes and protecting the glycolipid microdomains from pathogens [61]. SMAD3 (SMAD family member 3) binds the TRE element in the promoter region of many genes that are regulated by transforming growth factor beta (TGF-β) and, on formation of the SMAD3/SMAD4 complex, activates transcription. It has been demonstrated that SMAD3 deficiency will enhance Th17 during the TGF-β-mediated induction of Foxp3+ regulatory T cells [62].

Impact of the Immunochip

Common immune disorders such as ankylosing spondylitis, celiac disease, multiple sclerosis, psoriasis, rheumatoid arthritis, systemic lupus erythematosus, and type 1 diabetes often share overlapping susceptibility loci in GWAS studies [63]. Motivated by this observation, the Immunochip Consortium was formed to produce an inexpensive genotyping array that could be used to analyze hundreds of thousands of samples in autoimmune disease. The chip interrogates approximately 200,000 SNPs at 186 loci to enable dense genotyping so that SNPs located close together in the loci of interest including those at low allele frequencies can be included in analyses [64]. The results gained from this effort played a large role in the meta-analysis of Jostins et al. which raised the tally of IBD-associated loci to 163 [65]. The Jostins study revealed that 113 of the 163 loci are shared with other complex diseases including 66 loci shared with other autoimmune diseases [63]. The economical cost of the Immunochip allowed so many samples to be genotyped that loci could be identified at a genome-wide significance level where in the previous meta-analyses they showed only marginal significance.

A further goal of the Immunochip effort is to fine-map variants so that by using Bayesian statistical analyses, the individual causal variant can be identified rather than a large ensemble of variants that are in linkage disequilibrium with each other [66]. For instance, this fine-mapping can be used to show that amino acid substitutions in *NOD2* and *IL23R* are the causal SNPs that drive the genetic association signal.

GWAS Meta-analysis in Ulcerative Colitis

Recent GWAS and candidate gene association studies have identified 18 susceptibility loci for UC, which explain approximately 11% of the heritability for this disease. A recent meta-analysis combining data from six GWAS identified 29 additional UC risk loci, increasing the number of confirmed associations to 47 [67]. Examination of the gene content of the 47 associated regions shows that three regions each contain a single gene, most (35 out of 47) contain multiple genes, and nine contain no genes. Some noteworthy candidate genes including *PRDM1, TNFRSF14, TNFRSF9, IL1R2, IL8RA*, and *IL8RB* are briefly described below.

PRDM1 (PR domain containing 1, with ZNF domain) is the master transcriptional regulator of plasma cells and acts as a transcriptional repressor of the IFN-β promoter by binding specifically to the PRDI element. It drives the maturation of B lymphocytes into Ig-secreting cells. TNFRSF14 (tumor necrosis factor receptor superfamily, member 14) has an important role in preventing intestinal inflammation in a T-cell transfer model of colitis [68]. TNFRSF9 (tumor necrosis factor receptor superfamily, member 9) is a co-stimulator in the regulation of peripheral T-cell activation, with enhanced proliferation and IL-2 secretion. This factor is expressed by dendritic cells, granulocytes, and endothelial cells at inflammation sites. IL1R2 (interleukin 1 receptor, type II) can reduce IL1B activities by competitive binding to IL1B, preventing its binding to IL1R1. It is found that IL1B production by lamina propria macrophages is increased in patients with ulcerative colitis [69]. IL8RA and IL8RB (chemokine (C-X-C motif) receptor 1/2) are two receptors for interleukin-8, which is a powerful neutrophil chemotactic factor. Binding of IL-8 to the receptor also causes activation of neutrophils. IL8RA, but not IL8RB, expression is found to be increased in macrophages, lymphocytes, and epithelium in ulcerative colitis. It has been suggested that IL8RA may help IL-8 to play a role beyond neutrophil recruitment in mediating the immune response in UC [70].

Trans-ancestry Association Studies

The vast majority of genetic studies in IBD have been conducted in European ancestry populations. However, the expansion of these studies into Asian populations has yielded some insights. In the Japanese population, the well-known *NOD2* polymorphisms are virtually absent [71]. GWAS in Japan has shown that the single largest association signal is located in the *TNFSF15* gene encoding the pro-inflammatory cytokine TL1A [72].

Liu et al. conducted a trans-ethnic meta-analysis including 86,640 individuals of European ancestry and 9,846 individuals from East Asia, India, or Iran [4]. This study implicated 38 new loci, raising the tally to 200 total loci, and determined that there were significant differences in the frequency of risk alleles in the different populations. Nevertheless, the direction and magnitude of the effect at the shared loci were very similar between ancestries, suggesting that the casual variants are likely to be common (minor allele frequency greater than 5%). Besides the large impact of TL1A in the Asian population, the HLA locus was also found to have a greater influence particularly in ulcerative colitis [4].

The Debut of Next-Generation Sequencing

The traditional method of DNA sequencing was developed by Sanger using dideoxy-nucleotides as chain terminators [73]. This technology has become quite efficient and can be run on an automated instrument to generate 700-bp sequence reads with fluorescently labeled terminators. In the last 10 years, a new generation of DNA sequencing technology has emerged which uses sequencing by synthesis on a massively parallel scale to generate hundreds of gigabases of raw sequence per day, that is, 1800 whole human genomes per year on a single instrument (Illumina Inc., San Diego, CA). This technology has revolutionized the field of Mendelian genetics, that is, rare monogenic diseases, by enabling the identification of rare variants in a family setting. Interestingly, inflammatory bowel diseases can have Mendelian mimics that can be detected by next-generation sequencing, particularly in the very early-onset (VEO) patients [74, 75]. More attention will be given to the diagnosis of these genetic phenocopies and the management of the very young patients in the chapter of this textbook on very early-onset IBD.

Sequencing in High-Risk Individuals and Families

With level of technology available as of this writing, the most cost-effective approach to massively parallel sequencing in IBD patients is to target the exome, that is, the 1% of the genome that encodes the amino acids of proteins. Congenital deficiency of the receptor for the immunomodulatory cytokine IL-10 was the first monogenic defect identified as causative of VEO-IBD in 2009. While refractory to medical therapy, these patients responded to bone marrow transplant [76]. Exome sequencing has revealed additional

patients with IL-10 receptor deficiency [75]. Since that time, multiple other monogenic defects have been identified through exome sequencing. An early example of the success of this approach was seen in a 15-month-old child who presented with perianal fistulae and failure to thrive unresponsive to standard treatments which progressed to pancolitis. The patient underwent many surgical procedures and genetic tests that did not resolve his disease. Exome sequencing revealed that this patient carried an exceedingly rare mutation on the X chromosome in the XIAP gene, a potent regulator of the inflammatory response [77]. Since this protein acts in cells of the hematopoietic lineage, he was treated by a bone marrow transplant resulting in resolution of his disease. Other monogenic cases of VEO-IBD have been identified and have resulted in lifesaving therapy.

Features that suggest a patient may be a candidate for exome sequencing include early onset of disease, unusual severity, familial pattern of transmission, and refractory response to standard therapies. It is recommended to obtain DNA samples from the parents in addition to the proband so that Mendelian errors in allele transmission can be identified since there is an error rate inherent in next-generation sequencing. The trio of exomes is also useful in identifying de novo mutations which may be pathogenic [78].

Next-Generation Sequencing as a Research Tool

It is commonly believed that some fraction of the heritability of complex genetic disorders, such as IBD and particularly VEO-IBD, is due to rare or low-frequency variants [79]. Due to their rarity, these variants are not in strong linkage disequilibrium with proxy SNPs, which is required to make the GWAS approach feasible. Therefore, discovery of additional genes and low-frequency variants will require direct sequencing of tens of thousands of genomes [80]. The cost of whole genome sequencing is still prohibitive on this scale, so some research groups have focused on the exome as discussed above. Another approach to finding rare or coding variation has been to sequence specific genes in a large cohort based on the gene's status as a GWAS candidate. Rivas et al. identified additional coding mutations in NOD2 and IL23R as well as novel coding variants in CARD9, IL18RAP, CUL2, C1orf106, PTPN22, and MUC19 [81]. Beaudoin et al. performed amplicon sequencing on 55 genes in 200 cases and 150 controls for ulcerative colitis. They confirmed the previous associations with CARD9 and IL23R, as well as a novel association in RNF186 [82].

Efforts are currently underway to extend sequencing to thousands of exomes to search for pathogenic coding variants. A difficulty to this approach is that any individual variant is so rare that there is insufficient statistical power to identify the variant at genome-wide significance. As a result, many statistical methods have been developed which aggregate all the discovered variants in a gene into a single supervariant to test the burden of rare variants between cases and controls [83]. Although the outcome of this large-scale exome sequencing in IBD is still pending, there are some early signs that there will be a low yield of novel associations based on similar studies in complex autoimmune disease. The BGI (formerly Beijing Genomics Institute) performed discovery exome sequencing of psoriasis in 781 cases and 676 controls followed by sequencing-based replication in 9,946 cases and 9,906 controls with a panel of 1,326 targeted genes [84]. They found missense SNVs in *IL23R*, *GJB2*, *LCE3D*, *ERAP1*, *CARD14*, and *ZNF816A* based on single-SNP association statistics; notably all the variants were not truly rare but ranged from low frequency to common. They analyzed their data using most of the known gene-based association tests (burden tests) and did not reveal any novel associations, leading the group to conclude that coding variants in the targeted genes account for little of the genetic risk [84]. This scenario could hold for IBD as well.

Risk Prediction in IBD

Encouraged by the notable success of GWAS in Crohn disease and ulcerative colitis, it is logical to ask if these advances can deliver sufficiently accurate predictions to make targeted intervention realistic. Several efforts have been made, but most results are generally modest or even negative. For example, in a recent study, Kang and colleagues reported the best AUC (area under the receiver operating characteristic curve) score of 0.72 in predicting CD risk using GWAS genotype data [85]. This best AUC is obtained assuming the optimal number of predictors is given. The practical AUC may be even lower because the optimal number of predictors is usually unknown and has to be inferred from data itself. However, it is noted that these early efforts usually use small or modest sample sizes. As in meta-analysis, it is possible to compile a large sample size by combining as many cohorts as possible, yielding a boost in prediction performance. Using the large sample size and wide variant spectrum of the Immunochip data set in combination with advanced machine learning methods, Wei et al. were able to achieve an AUC of 0.86 for Crohn disease and 0.83 for ulcerative colitis [86]. These statistical methods may prove to be useful in disease classification as deep whole genome sequence data becomes available.

Genotype-Phenotype Correlations in Pediatric IBD

Disease Type and Location

The discovery of genetic polymorphisms in IBD has afforded investigators with the opportunity to identify predictive correlations between specific variants and phenotypic disease characteristics. Analyses of adult populations have demonstrated that carriage of *NOD2* risk alleles predicts disease onset at an earlier age and ileal disease location in a dose-dependent manner. Subsequently, a meta-analysis of 16 case-control studies confirmed the association of *NOD2* carriage with ileal disease location and also identified a correlation with fibrostenosing behavior and family history of IBD [16].

The majority of pediatric studies have concurred with findings from adult counterparts that carriage of *NOD2* variants is associated with ileal disease. Estimates suggest that 20–65% of children with ileal Crohn disease possess at least one *NOD2* mutation; consistent phenotypic associations have not been seen for other regions of the gastrointestinal tract [43, 87–91]. In contradistinction to the adult literature, correlates of *NOD2* variants with fibrostenosing disease have demonstrated conflicting results [19, 87, 88, 90, 91]. Two large studies from the USA and Scotland found that 34–45% of Crohn patients possessing *NOD2* polymorphisms had evidence of fibrostenosing disease, especially the 1007fs and R720W variants [88, 91]. Three other pediatric studies, however, found no correlation of *NOD2* with fibrostenosing disease [19, 87, 90].

Growth Parameters

As growth failure is an important feature of pediatric IBD, several groups have investigated the relationship between anthropometric parameters and *NOD2* status. A study of 101 Crohn patients demonstrated that 44% of participants possessing a *NOD2* polymorphism were <5% for weight at the time of diagnosis, while only 15% of those without a genetic variant were <5% for weight at the time of diagnosis [87]. Although similar trends were seen for height, these results did not reach statistical significance. Another study of 93 Crohn patients, however, did not show any correlation between *NOD2* status and height or weight Z scores at disease onset or for the lowest Z score during childhood [90]. Rather, disease severity was the strongest predictor for impaired growth, and ileal involvement was associated with height retardation at disease onset and the lowest Z score during follow-up. Finally, a German group did not find any statistically significant difference in mean body mass index (BMI) or mean height percentiles at diagnosis between patients with and without *NOD2* variants [92]. The authors did note a nonsignificant trend of greater numbers of patients possessing *NOD2* polymorphisms being below the 3% for BMI. These data imply that while *NOD2* variants may be associated with poor growth, this effect may be more a reflection of malnutrition secondary to ileal location and disease severity as opposed to an inherent genetic effect.

Association with Risk of Surgery

Results of pediatric studies correlating *NOD2* status with the need for small bowel surgical resection have consistently delineated a positive association. Russell et al. estimated an odds ratio for risk of surgery among children with Crohn possessing any *NOD2* mutation to be 4.45 [91]. Pediatric Crohn patients with the 1007fsInsC variant appeared to have a greater likelihood of requiring surgery with an odds ratio of 4.8. Among US Caucasian Crohn patients, hazard ratios for surgery indicate that children possessing the 3020insC variant are at sixfold greater risk of requiring surgical intervention [88]. Furthermore, these children also showed a trend toward a need for earlier surgery at median of 14 months versus 23 months after diagnosis.

Large-Scale Phenotypic Correlations

Cleynen et al. analyzed subphenotypes of IBD in 34,819 patients who were genotyped on the Immunochip [93]. For Crohn disease, the phenotypes examined were age at diagnosis, disease location, disease behavior (penetrating, stricturing, inflammatory), and requirement for surgery. For ulcerative colitis, the phenotypes examined were age of onset, disease extent, and colectomy. Across all 186 loci on the Immunochip, only SNPs in *NOD2*, the HLA locus, and 3p21 (*MST1*) were found to have genome-wide significance, influencing all subphenotypes [93]. The disease location was essentially fixed over time and was the main independent determinant of the patient's disease process, while disease behavior and requirement for surgery were largely markers of disease progression. A composite genetic risk score based on the 163 known loci was associated all disease subphenotypes, but only the three loci named above were individually significant. The authors concluded that the binary classification of IBD into Crohn disease and ulcerative colitis is not supported by genetic data and that a ternary classification should be used: ulcerative colitis, colonic Crohn disease, and ileal Crohn disease [93].

Genetic Sharing Between Pediatric Age of Onset IBD and Other Autoimmune Diseases

As the Immunochip genotyping effort amply demonstrated, there is a shared genetic architecture for a wide variety of autoimmune diseases. Li et al. performed GWAS in 6,035 cases of ten different pediatric autoimmune diseases and 10,718 shared controls. This effort identified 27 genome-wide significant loci which had shared risk among multiple pediatric autoimmune diseases, for instance, a novel role for *CD40LG* in Crohn disease, ulcerative colitis, and celiac disease [94]. The main pathways identified as responsible for this shared risk were cytokine signaling, antigen presentation, T-cell activation, JAK-STAT signaling, and helper T-cell cytokine signaling [94]. A study of SNP-h^2, also called narrow-sense heritability, across these ten pediatric autoimmune diseases showed that the additive heritability explained by genotyped and imputable SNPs was 0.454 for Crohn disease and 0.386 for ulcerative colitis [95]. In pairwise analysis, Crohn disease and ulcerative colitis showed the strongest correlation of all pairwise combinations of the ten autoimmune diseases (0.69) [95].

Summary

Both family and twin-based studies lend strong support for a genetic basis of IBD. This is further supported by observations of racial/ethnic variations in disease prevalence. The recent advent of GWAS has markedly advanced the identification of well-replicated IBD association and has substantiated this concept at a molecular level and catapulted the field of IBD genetics into a new realm of discovery. Future sequencing studies are likely to identify rarer variants that confer greater risks at the individual level and may help uncovering new gene interactions and networks that contribute to the pathogenesis of IBD allowing for stratification of IBD patients into different therapeutic pathways and interventions in the future.

Acknowledgment We are most grateful to Dr. Judy H. Cho, Dr. Nancy McGreal, Dr. Zhi Wei, and Steve Baldassano (MD/PhD student) who wrote earlier versions of this chapter.

References

1. Hugot JP, Laurent-Puig P, Gower-Rousseau C, et al. Mapping of a susceptibility locus for Crohn's disease on chromosome 16. Nature. 1996;379:821–3.
2. Hugot JP, Chamaillard M, Zouali H, et al. Association of NOD2 leucine-rich repeat variants with susceptibility to Crohn's disease. Nature. 2001;411:599–603.

3. Ogura Y, Bonen DK, Inohara N, et al. A frameshift mutation in NOD2 associated with susceptibility to Crohn's disease. Nature. 2001;411:603–6.

4. Liu JZ, van Sommeren S, Huang H, et al. Association analyses identify 38 susceptibility loci for inflammatory bowel disease and highlight shared genetic risk across populations. Nat Genet. 2015;47:979–86.

5. Duerr RH. The genetics of inflammatory bowel disease. Gastroenterol Clin North Am. 2002;31:63–76.

6. Basu D, Lopez I, Kulkarni A, Sellin JH. Impact of race and ethnicity on inflammatory bowel disease. Am J Gastroenterol. 2005;100:2254–61.

7. Weinstein TA, Levine M, Pettei MJ, Gold DM, Kessler BH, Levine JJ. Age and family history at presentation of pediatric inflammatory bowel disease. J Pediatr Gastroenterol Nutr. 2003;37:609–13.

8. Laharie D, Debeugny S, Peeters M, et al. Inflammatory bowel disease in spouses and their offspring. Gastroenterology. 2001;120:816–9.

9. Orholm M, Fonager K, Sorensen HT. Risk of ulcerative colitis and Crohn's disease among offspring of patients with chronic inflammatory bowel disease. Am J Gastroenterol. 1999;94:3236–8.

10. Orholm M, Binder V, Sorensen TI, Rasmussen LP, Kyvik KO. Concordance of inflammatory bowel disease among Danish twins. Results of a nationwide study. Scand J Gastroenterol. 2000;35:1075–81.

11. Thompson NP, Driscoll R, Pounder RE, Wakefield AJ. Genetics versus environment in inflammatory bowel disease: results of a British twin study. BMJ. 1996;312:95–6.

12. Tysk C, Lindberg E, Jarnerot G, Floderus-Myrhed B. Ulcerative colitis and Crohn's disease in an unselected population of monozygotic and dizygotic twins. A study of heritability and the influence of smoking. Gut. 1988;29:990–6.

13. Brant S. Update on the heritability of inflammatory bowel disease: the importance of twin studies. Inflamm Bowel Dis. 2011;17:1–5.

14. Lesage S, Zouali H, Cezard JP, et al. CARD15/NOD2 mutational analysis and genotype-phenotype correlation in 612 patients with inflammatory bowel disease. Am J Hum Genet. 2002;70:845–57.

15. Li J, Moran T, Swanson E, et al. Regulation of IL-8 and IL-1beta expression in Crohn's disease associated NOD2/CARD15 mutations. Hum Mol Genet. 2004;13:1715–25.

16. Economou M, Trikalinos TA, Loizou KT, Tsianos EV, Ioannidis JP. Differential effects of NOD2 variants on Crohn's disease risk and phenotype in diverse populations: a metaanalysis. Am J Gastroenterol. 2004;99:2393–404.

17. Cummings JR, Jewell DP. Clinical implications of inflammatory bowel disease genetics on phenotype. Inflamm Bowel Dis. 2005;11:56–61.

18. Kugathasan S, Loizides A, Babusukumar U, et al. Comparative phenotypic and CARD15 mutational analysis among African American, Hispanic, and White children with Crohn's disease. Inflamm Bowel Dis. 2005;11:631–8.

19. Weiss B, Shamir R, Bujanover Y, et al. NOD2/CARD15 mutation analysis and genotype-phenotype correlation in Jewish pediatric patients compared with adults with Crohn's disease. J Pediatr. 2004;145:208–12.

20. Ahmad T, Marshall S, Jewell D. Genotype-based phenotyping heralds a new taxonomy for inflammatory bowel disease. Curr Opin Gastroenterol. 2003;19:327–35.

21. Stokkers PC, Reitsma PH, Tytgat GN, van Deventer SJ. HLA-DR and -DQ phenotypes in inflammatory bowel disease: a meta-analysis. Gut. 1999;45:395–401.

22. Silverberg MS, Mirea L, Bull SB, et al. A population- and family-based study of Canadian families reveals association of HLA DRB1*0103 with colonic involvement in inflammatory bowel disease. Inflamm Bowel Dis. 2003;9:1–9.

23. Orchard TR, Chua CN, Ahmad T, Cheng H, Welsh KI, Jewell DP. Uveitis and erythema nodosum in inflammatory bowel disease: clinical features and the role of HLA genes. Gastroenterology. 2002;123:714–8.

24. Orchard TR, Thiyagaraja S, Welsh KI, Wordsworth BP, Hill Gaston JS, Jewell DP. Clinical phenotype is related to HLA genotype in the peripheral arthropathies of inflammatory bowel disease. Gastroenterology. 2000;118:274–8.

25. Yap LM, Ahmad T, Jewell DP. The contribution of HLA genes to IBD susceptibility and phenotype. Best Pract Res Clin Gastroenterol. 2004;18:577–96.

26. Goyette P, Boucher G, Mallon D, et al. High-density mapping of the MHC identifies a shared role for HLA-DRB1*01:03 in inflammatory bowel diseases and heterozygous advantage in ulcerative colitis. Nat Genet. 2015;47:172–9.

27. Pearson TA, Manolio TA. How to interpret a genome-wide association study. JAMA. 2008;299:1335–44.

28. Risch N, Merikangas K. The future of genetic studies of complex human diseases. Science. 1996;273:1516–7.

29. Duerr RH, Taylor KD, Brant SR, et al. A genome-wide association study identifies IL23R as an inflammatory bowel disease gene. Science. 2006;314:1461–3.

30. Van Limbergen JE, Russell RK, Nimmo ER, et al. IL23R Arg381Gln is associated with childhood onset inflammatory bowel disease in Scotland. Gut. 2007;56(8):1173–4.

31. Libioulle C, Louis E, Hansoul S, et al. A novel susceptibility locus for Crohn's disease identified by whole genome association maps to a gene desert on chromosome 5p13.1 and modulates the level of expression of the prostaglandin receptor EP4. PLoS Genet. 2007;3(4):e58.

32. Parham C, Chirica M, Timans J, et al. A receptor for the heterodimeric cytokine IL-23 is composed of IL-12Rbeta1 and a novel cytokine receptor subunit, IL-23R. J Immunol. 2002;168:5699–708.

33. Hue S, Ahern P, Buonocore S, et al. Interleukin-23 drives innate and T cell-mediated intestinal inflammation. J Exp Med. 2006;203:2473–83.

34. Kullberg MC, Jankovic D, Feng CG, et al. IL-23 plays a key role in Helicobacter hepaticus-induced T cell-dependent colitis. J Exp Med. 2006;203:2485–94.

35. Uhlig HH, McKenzie BS, Hue S, et al. Differential activity of IL-12 and IL-23 in mucosal and systemic innate immune pathology. Immunity. 2006;25:309–18.

36. Yen D, Cheung J, Scheerens H, et al. IL-23 is essential for T cell-mediated colitis and promotes inflammation via IL-17 and IL-6. J Clin Invest. 2006;116:1310–6.

37. Cua DJ, Sherlock J, Chen Y, et al. Interleukin-23 rather than interleukin-12 is the critical cytokine for autoimmune inflammation of the brain. Nature. 2003;421:744–8.

38. Cargill M, Schrodi SJ, Chang M, et al. A large-scale genetic association study confirms IL12B and leads to the identification of IL23R as psoriasis-risk genes. Am J Hum Genet. 2007;80:273–90.

39. Mannon PJ, Fuss IJ, Mayer L, et al. Anti-interleukin-12 antibody for active Crohn's disease. N Engl J Med. 2004;351:2069–79.

40. McKenzie BS, Kastelein RA, Cua DJ. Understanding the IL-23-IL-17 immune pathway. Trends Immunol. 2006;27:17–23.

41. Hampe J, Franke A, Rosenstiel P, et al. A genome-wide association scan of nonsynonymous SNPs identifies a susceptibility variant for Crohn disease in ATG16L1. Nat Genet. 2007;39:207–11.

42. Rioux JD, Xavier RJ, KD T, et al. Genome-wide association study identifies new susceptibility loci for Crohn disease and implicates autophagy in disease pathogenesis. Nat Genet. 2007;39(5):596–604.

43. Meinzer U, Idestrom M, Alberti C, et al. Ileal involvement is age dependent in pediatric Crohn's disease. Inflamm Bowel Dis. 2005;11:639–44.

44. Levine A et al. Pediatric onset Crohn's colitis is characterized by genotype-dependent age-related susceptibility. Inflamm Bowel Dis. 2007;13:1509–15.

45. Henderson P. Genetics of childhood-onset inflammatory bowel disease. Inflamm Bowel Dis. 2010;17:346–61.

46. Imielinski M. Common variants at five new loci associated with early-onset inflammatory bowel disease. Nat Genet. 2009;41:1335–40.

47. Kugathasan S. Loci on 20q13 and 21q22 are associated with pediatric-onset inflammatory bowel disease. Nat Genet. 2008;40:1211–5.

48. Amre D et al. Investigation of reported associations between the 20q13 and 21q22 loci and pediatric-onset Crohn's disease in Canadian children. Am J Gastroenterol. 2009;104:2824–48.

49. Dan N, Kanai T, Totsuka T, et al. Ameliorating effect of anti-Fas ligand MAb on wasting disease in murine model of chronic colitis. Am J Physiol Gastrointest Liver Physiol. 2003;285:G754–60.

50. Jungbeck M, Daller B, Federhofer J, et al. Neutralization of LIGHT ameliorates acute dextran sodium sulphate-induced intestinal inflammation. Immunology. 2009;128:451–8.

51. Meylan F, Song YJ, Fuss I, et al. The TNF-family cytokine TL1A drives IL-13-dependent small intestinal inflammation. Mucosal Immunol. 2011;4:172–85.

52. Wang J, Anders RA, Wang Y, et al. The critical role of LIGHT in promoting intestinal inflammation and Crohn's disease. J Immunol. 2005;174:8173–82.

53. Van Limbergen J et al. The genetics of Crohn's disease. Annu Rev Genomics Hum Genet. 2009;10:89–116.

54. Cho JH. The genetics and immunopathogenesis of inflammatory bowel disease. Nat Rev Immunol. 2008;8:458–66.

55. de Bakker PI, Ferreira MA, Jia X, Neale BM, Raychaudhuri S, Voight BF. Practical aspects of imputation-driven meta-analysis of genome-wide association studies. Hum Mol Genet. 2008;17:R122–8.

56. Barrett JC, Hansoul S, Nicolae DL, et al. Genome-wide association defines more than 30 distinct susceptibility loci for Crohn's disease. Nat Genet. 2008;40:955–62.

57. Franke A, McGovern DP, Barrett JC, et al. Genome-wide meta-analysis increases to 71 the number of confirmed Crohn's disease susceptibility loci. Nat Genet. 2010;42:1118–25.

58. Mathur AN, Chang HC, Zisoulis DG, et al. Stat3 and Stat4 direct development of IL-17-secreting Th cells. J Immunol. 2007;178:4901–7.

59. Nakazawa A, Dotan I, Brimnes J, et al. The expression and function of costimulatory molecules B7H and B7-H1 on colonic epithelial cells. Gastroenterology. 2004;126:1347–57.

60. Ito T, Yang M, Wang YH, et al. Plasmacytoid dendritic cells prime IL-10-producing T regulatory cells by inducible costimulator ligand. J Exp Med. 2007;204:105–15.

61. Wrackmeyer U, Hansen GH, Seya T, Danielsen EM. Intelectin: a novel lipid raft-associated protein in the enterocyte brush border. Biochemistry. 2006;45:9188–97.

62. Lu L, Wang J, Zhang F, et al. Role of SMAD and non-SMAD signals in the development of Th17 and regulatory T cells. J Immunol. 2010;184:4295–306.

63. de Lange KM, Barrett JC. Understanding inflammatory bowel disease via immunogenetics. J Autoimmun. 2015;64:91–100.

64. Parkes M, Cortes A, van Heel DA, Brown MA. Genetic insights into common pathways and complex relationships among immune-mediated diseases. Nat Rev Genet. 2013;14:661–73.

65. Jostins L, Ripke S, Weersma RK, et al. Host-microbe interactions have shaped the genetic architecture of inflammatory bowel disease. Nature. 2012;491:119–24.

66. Wellcome Trust Case Control Consortium, Maller JB, McVean G, et al. Bayesian refinement of association signals for 14 loci in 3 common diseases. Nat Genet. 2012;44:1294–301.

67. Anderson CA, Boucher G, Lees CW, et al. Meta-analysis identifies 29 additional ulcerative colitis risk loci, increasing the number of confirmed associations to 47. Nat Genet. 2011;43:246–52.

68. Steinberg MW, Turovskaya O, Shaikh RB, et al. A crucial role for HVEM and BTLA in preventing intestinal inflammation. J Exp Med. 2008;205:1463–76.

69. Mahida YR, Wu K, Jewell DP. Enhanced production of interleukin 1-beta by mononuclear cells isolated from mucosa with active ulcerative colitis of Crohn's disease. Gut. 1989;30:835–8.

70. Williams EJ, Haque S, Banks C, Johnson P, Sarsfield P, Sheron N. Distribution of the interleukin-8 receptors, CXCR1 and CXCR2, in inflamed gut tissue. J Pathol. 2000;192:533–9.

71. Yamazaki K, Takazoe M, Tanaka T, Kazumori T, Nakamura Y. Absence of mutation in the NOD2/CARD15 gene among 483 Japanese patients with Crohn's disease. J Hum Genet. 2002;47:469–72.

72. Yamazaki K, McGovern D, Ragoussis J, et al. Single nucleotide polymorphisms in TNFSF15 confer susceptibility to Crohn's disease. Hum Mol Genet. 2005;14:3499–506.

73. Sanger F, Nicklen S, Coulson AR. DNA sequencing with chain-terminating inhibitors. Proc Natl Acad Sci U S A. 1977;74:5463–7.

74. Uhlig HH. Monogenic diseases associated with intestinal inflammation: implications for the understanding of inflammatory bowel disease. Gut. 2013;62:1795–805.

75. Kelsen JR, Dawany N, Moran CJ, et al. Exome sequencing analysis reveals variants in primary immunodeficiency genes in patients with very early onset inflammatory bowel disease. Gastroenterology. 2015;149:1415–24.

76. Glocker EO, Kotlarz D, Boztug K, et al. Inflammatory bowel disease and mutations affecting the interleukin-10 receptor. N Engl J Med. 2009;361:2033–45.

77. Worthey EA, Mayer AN, Syverson GD, et al. Making a definitive diagnosis: successful clinical application of whole exome sequencing in a child with intractable inflammatory bowel disease. Genet Med. 2011;13:255–62.

78. Cardinale CJ, Kelsen JR, Baldassano RN, Hakonarson H. Impact of exome sequencing in inflammatory bowel disease. World J Gastroenterol. 2013;19:6721–9.

79. Pritchard JK. Are rare variants responsible for susceptibility to complex diseases? Am J Hum Genet. 2001;69:124–37.

80. Zuk O, Schaffner SF, Samocha K, et al. Searching for missing heritability: designing rare variant association studies. Proc Natl Acad Sci U S A. 2014;111:E455–64.

81. Rivas MA, Beaudoin M, Gardet A, et al. Deep resequencing of GWAS loci identifies independent rare variants associated with inflammatory bowel disease. Nat Genet. 2011;43:1066–73.

82. Beaudoin M, Goyette P, Boucher G, et al. Deep resequencing of GWAS loci identifies rare variants in CARD9, IL23R and RNF186 that are associated with ulcerative colitis. PLoS Genet. 2013;9:e1003723.

83. Bansal V, Libiger O, Torkamani A, Schork NJ. Statistical analysis strategies for association studies involving rare variants. Nat Rev Genet. 2010;11:773–85.

84. Tang H, Jin X, Li Y, et al. A large-scale screen for coding variants predisposing to psoriasis. Nat Genet. 2014;46:45–50.

85. Kang J, Kugathasan S, Georges M, Zhao H, Cho JH. Improved risk prediction for Crohn's disease with a multi-locus approach. Hum Mol Genet. 2011;20:2435–42.

86. Wei Z, Wang W, Bradfield J, et al. Large sample size, wide variant spectrum, and advanced machine-learning technique boost risk prediction for inflammatory bowel disease. Am J Hum Genet. 2013;92:1008–12.

87. Tomer G, Ceballos C, Concepcion E, Benkov KJ. NOD2/CARD15 variants are associated with lower weight at diagnosis in children with Crohn's disease. Am J Gastroenterol. 2003;98:2479–84.

88. Kugathasan S, Collins N, Maresso K, et al. CARD15 gene mutations and risk for early surgery in pediatric-onset Crohn's disease.
Clin Gastroenterol Hepatol. 2004;2:1003–9.

89. Sun L, Roesler J, Rosen-Wolff A, et al. CARD15 genotype and phenotype analysis in 55 pediatric patients with Crohn disease from
Saxony, Germany. J Pediatr Gastroenterol Nutr. 2003;37:492–7.

90. Wine E, Reif SS, Leshinsky-Silver E, et al. Pediatric Crohn's disease and growth retardation: the role of genotype, phenotype, and
disease severity. Pediatrics. 2004;114:1281–6.

91. Russell RK, Drummond HE, Nimmo EE, et al. Genotype-phenotype
analysis in childhood-onset Crohn's disease: NOD2/CARD15 variants consistently predict phenotypic characteristics of severe disease. Inflamm Bowel Dis. 2005;11:955–64.

92. Roesler J, Thurigen A, Sun L, et al. Influence of CARD15 muta-
tions on disease activity and response to therapy in 65 pediatric
Crohn patients from Saxony, Germany. J Pediatr Gastroenterol
Nutr. 2005;41:27–32.

93. Cleynen I, Boucher G, Jostins L, et al. Inherited determinants of
Crohn's disease and ulcerative colitis phenotypes: a genetic association study. Lancet. 2016;387:156–67.

94. Li YR, Li J, Zhao SD, et al. Meta-analysis of shared genetic architecture across ten pediatric autoimmune diseases. Nat Med.
2015;21:1018–27.

95. Li YR, Zhao SD, Li J, et al. Genetic sharing and heritability of paediatric age of onset autoimmune diseases. Nat Commun.
2015;6:8442.

96. Wang K, et al. Diverse genome-wide association studies associate
the IL12/IL23 pathway with Crohn Disease. Am J Hum Genet.
2009;84(3):399–405.

The Intestinal Immune System During Homeostasis and Inflammatory Bowel Disease

David A. Hill and William A. Faubion Jr

Introduction

The human gastrointestinal (GI) tract is home to one of the highest densities of immune cells in the entire body [1]. This density is likely due to the fact that the GI tract is one of the two organ systems (along with the lungs) that facilitate biologic interactions with the external world, and that the surface area of the average adult GI tract is roughly equal to that of a tennis court (400 m²). The antigenic exposure of the GI tract is both immense and diverse. The GI tract is continuously exposed to foods, inert compounds, toxins, commensal organisms, and pathogens. As a result, it has the challenging task of distinguishing between these very different exposures, and errors that result in too much or two little of an inflammatory response can result in morbidity or death.

Pediatric inflammatory bowel disease (IBD) is a good example of what can occur when there is a breakdown in the normal function of the intestinal immune system. However, in order to understand what goes wrong in IBD, it is first necessary to understand the intestinal immune system's normal anatomy and function. While much is known about the intestinal immune system's anatomy [2], cellular and secretory components [3], and interactions with commensal microorganisms [4], it is important to note that a majority of our knowledge derives from studies performed in animal models or adult humans. As such, while much work is currently being performed in pediatrics, the extent to which our knowledge of the intestinal immune system applies to children is uncertain. In addition, childhood is a time of dramatic changes in both antigenic exposures (with the transition from a sterile environment to breastfeeding and ultimately to solid foods) and system characteristics (such as involution of the thymus and development of a mature humoral immune system) [5]. As such, it is reasonable to assume that there is a great deal more to be discovered about the appropriate and inappropriate intestinal inflammatory responses in children. This chapter will review currently accepted concepts surrounding the homeostatic structure and function of the intestinal immune system, with selected references to unique aspects of the pediatric immune system as well as the inappropriate inflammatory responses found in IBD.

The Anatomy of the Intestinal Immune System

The immune system of the gastrointestinal (GI) tract is segregated into anatomic and functional compartments, which act in a coordinated fashion to initiate and propagate inflammatory responses. These compartments include the epithelium and associated lamina propria, isolated lymphoid follicles, Peyer's patches, and mesenteric lymph nodes (MLNs). Each of these compartments is critical for facilitating appropriate inflammatory responses to pathogens and promoting tolerance to food antigens and commensal populations. While the majority of research has focused on the small intestine due to its large collection of immune cells, it is important to note that each section of the GI tract has specialized immune functions and can fall victim to diseases of inappropriate inflammation.

The Epithelium and Lamina Propria

The intestinal epithelium and associated lamina propria has a diverse set of functions essential to normal physiology. These include creating a physical barrier between the external environment while facilitating digestion and absorption of nutrients, promoting tolerance to food and other non-threatening

D.A. Hill, MD, PhD (✉)
Department of Pediatrics, Division of Allergy and Immunology,
The Children's Hospital of Philadelphia,
3550 Market Street, Philadelphia, PA 19104, USA
e-mail: hilld3@email.chop.edu

W.A. Faubion Jr., MD
Department of Gastroenterology and Hepatology, Mayo Clinic,
200 First Street, SW, Rochester, MN 55905, USA
e-mail: faubion.william@mayo.edu

© Springer International Publishing AG 2017
P. Mamula et al. (eds.), *Pediatric Inflammatory Bowel Disease*, DOI 10.1007/978-3-319-49215-5_2

antigens, and providing for immunologic surveillance of commensal and pathogenic microorganisms. To this end, the intestinal epithelial cell (IEC) contains actin-rich microvillar extensions creating an apical brush border that impedes microbial attachment and invasion [6]. Additionally, biochemical adaptations such as goblet cells, which produce a heavily glycosylated and mucin-rich glycocalyx, secreted immunoglobulin (Ig) A molecules, and Paneth cells which produce antimicrobial peptides, confer broad-spectrum antimicrobial properties to the epithelium [7, 8]. Despite these adaptations, the neonatal epithelium is more permeable than that of older children and adults, in part due to immature epithelial tight junctions [9].

While microbial defense is a primary function of the epithelium, the absorption of nutrients and surveillance of particulate antigens and microorganisms are constantly occurring via active transport across the epithelium to the underlying immune cell-rich lamina propria and gut-associated lymphoid tissues (GALT) [10]. Follicle-associated epithelium (FAE) overlies isolated lymphoid follicles and larger lymphoid aggregates called Peyer's patches (discussed below). The FAE is relatively deficient in goblet cells, has a lower concentration of brush border enzymes, and contains highly specialized transcytotic microfold (M) cells which facilitate sampling of luminal antigens to underlying lymphoid tissues. Sampling of luminal contents by the intestinal immune system is critical for maintaining homeostasis in the face of a diverse and immense array of antigens.

IECs are in continuous contact with beneficial and pathogenic microorganisms and as such are ideally located for immunologic surveillance of the intestinal lumen. IECs express innate pattern recognition receptors including Toll-like receptors (TLRs), NOD-like receptors (NLRs), and GPCRs that recognize microbial components and modulate immune responses [11]. Additionally, IECs express all of the molecular machinery required to process and present luminal antigens to intraepithelial lymphocytes via either major histocompatibility complex (MHC) class I or class II molecules, allowing for at least the potential for direct modulation of the adaptive immune system [12, 13]. Together, these observations paint a picture of a dynamic and functional epithelium that is essential to maintaining barrier integrity, promoting tolerance, and providing active defense against pathogenic organisms.

Evidence for Epithelial Dysfunction in IBD

Several lines of evidence suggest that the normal functions of the intestinal epithelium are disrupted in chronic intestinal inflammation. Firstly, some of the IBD-susceptibility loci have been shown to play a role in various aspects of normal epithelial function. These include hepatocyte nuclear factor 4α (*HNF4α*) which regulates epithelial tight junction formation, E-cadherin (*CDH1*) which is important for many aspects of epithelial cell function, meprin 1A (*MEP1A*) a proteinase which is associated with the brush border, and NOD2 (*CARD15*) which recognizes bacterial muramyl dipeptide [14]. There are additional lines of evidence that suggest epithelial barrier integrity is disrupted in IBD. Patients with IBD have reduced goblet cell numbers and mucus secretion as compared to healthy individuals [15]. Furthermore, abnormal intestinal permeability has been established among patients with Crohn's disease (CD) and their healthy first-degree relatives, and may represent a primary abnormality predisposing to excessive antigen uptake, continuous immune stimulation, and eventually mucosal inflammation. Finally, epithelial cell death, particularly Paneth cell dropout, has recently been demonstrated to induce terminal ileal inflammation in mice and be associated with CD in humans [16]. Interestingly, increased cell shedding with gap formation and local barrier dysfunction is observed in intestinal biopsies of patients with inflammatory bowel disease, and this dysfunction is predictive of relapse [17, 18]. In addition to the genetic factors discussed above, environmental insults may predispose to impaired intestinal barrier function in IBD. Smoking and non-steroidal anti-inflammatory drugs both negatively influence epithelial permeability and are variably associated with IBD [19]. The view that IECs are a dynamic cell type that are central to the maintenance of intestinal homeostasis is consistent with IEC dysfunction contributing to IBD pathogenesis.

Gut-Associated Lymphoid Tissues

The GALT tissues are divided into effector sights with increasing degrees of structural complexity from isolated lymphoid follicles to Peyer's patches and mesenteric lymph nodes. Each of these sites plays an important role in recognizing luminal antigens and facilitating innate and adaptive immune responses.

Isolated Lymphoid Follicles

Isolated lymphoid follicles are collections of lymphocytes that are similar to Peyer's patches, though much smaller in size. One of the best characterized roles of the isolated lymphoid follicle in maintaining intestinal homeostasis is through mediating IgA class switching and production. For example, segmented filamentous bacteria induce a robust IgA response in part through their bypassing the requirement for Peyer's patches for IgA induction by utilizing isolated lymphoid follicles and inducing tertiary lymphoid tissues in the intestine [20]. This is possible in part due to T-cell-independent induction of

B cells that can occur in isolated lymphoid follicles due to the activity of the cytokines BAFF (B-cell-activating factor) and APRIL ("a proliferation-inducing ligand") [21, 22].

Peyer's Patches

Peyer's patches are larger organized lymphoid tissues that are visible to the eye and are located along the length of the small intestine. They are formed as a result of CD3⁻CD4⁺ progenitor cells that express the chemokine receptor CXCR5, hone to the intestinal submucosa, and produce $LT\alpha_1\beta_2$. Mature Peyer's patches reside under the FAE, which contains the specialized M cell. As discussed previously, the M cell is thought to be the predominant means by which antigen is transported to the subepithelial dome. The dome is rich in dendritic cells (DCs), macrophages, B cells, and T cells as is the underlying Peyer's patch itself which contains more organized B-cell follicles with associated infiltrating T-cell areas.

Mesenteric Lymph Nodes

Mesenteric lymph nodes (MLNs) are the largest lymph nodes in the body, and they develop independently from the other GALT structures. Lymphocytes circulate to the MLNs as a result of expression of both L-selectin and $\alpha_4\beta_7$. The requirement of expression of both of these molecules is unique in that each typically directs a distinct lymphocyte migratory pattern: L-selectin-mediating lymphocyte migration into peripheral tissues and $\alpha_4\beta_7$-mediating migration of lymphocytes into the intestinal mucosa. As a result, the MLNs may act as an immunologic intersection of GI and systemic lymphocyte migration (Fig. 2.1).

The Innate Immune System and IBD

The immune system can be divided into two main branches: innate and adaptive. The innate immune system functions based on germ line-encoded recognition of microbial (and other) signals. The primary strength of the innate immune system is the rapid nature of its responses. Innate immune responses are fast because the receptor repertoire is predetermined, with specificity honed over the course of evolution. The components of the innate immune system range from pattern recognition receptors expressed by many nonimmune cell types to innate immune cell types including granulocytes,

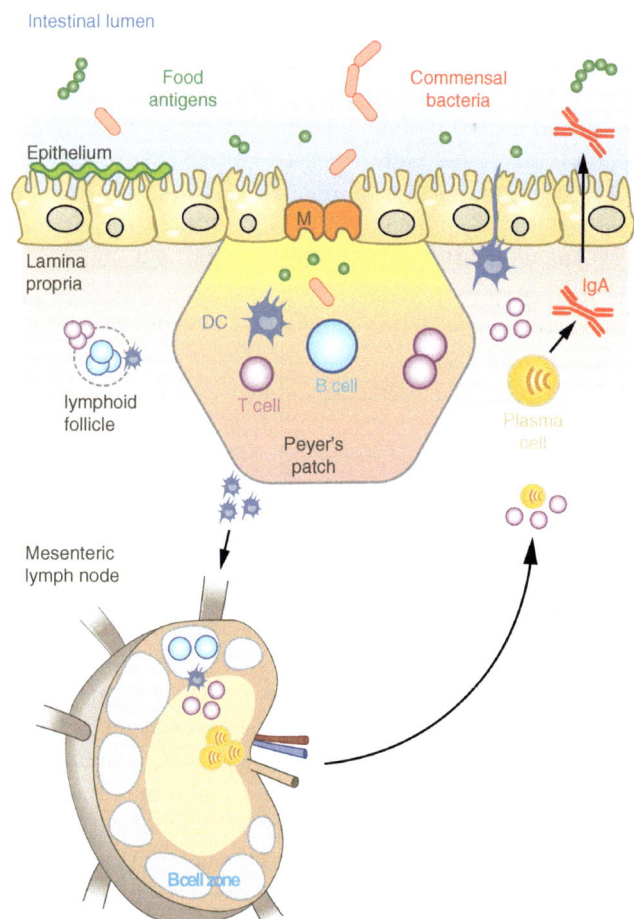

Fig. 2.1 The anatomy of the intestinal immune system. The basic organizational structure of the intestinal immune system. The follicular-associated epithelium (FAE) contains M (microfold) cells which transport antigen into the underlying subepithelial dome of Peyer's patches. Antigen is processed and presented by DCs to naïve B and T cells. A similar process can occur in smaller lymphoid follicles, or DCs can exit the lamina propria and travel to associate mesenteric lymph nodes. Activated B and T cells are targeted back to the lamina propria where they exert their respective effector functions

professional phagocytic cells (such as macrophages, dendritic cells, and neutrophils), and innate lymphocyte populations, all of which play essential antimicrobial and antineoplastic functions. The following section will review the innate immune system and its relevance to maintaining intestinal homeostasis or contributing to IBD pathogenesis.

Pattern Recognition Receptors

Pattern recognition receptors (PRRs) are germ line-encoded receptors that recognize an array of pathogen-associated molecular patterns (PAMPs). There are many families of PRRs. Two of the most well-characterized, membrane-bound Toll-like receptors (TLRs) and cytoplasmic NOD-like receptors (NLRs), will be briefly reviewed here because of their contribution to IBD pathogenesis. TLRs are a family of integral membrane proteins that are situated on the plasma membrane or on intracellular endosomes. TLRs recognize a broad array of PAMPs including bacterial lipoprotein, peptidoglycans, lipopolysaccharides, nucleic acids, and other microbial components. TLR activation results in nuclear factor kappa-light-chain enhancer of activated B-cell (NF-κB)-dependent expression of pro-inflammatory cytokines. TLRs are expressed throughout the intestine by epithelial cells and immune cells and play a central role in microbial surveillance. There are a number of lines of evidence that suggest that TLR signaling is altered in IBD. Polymorphisms that impair TLR signaling are associated with increased risk of IBD in humans [23–25]. Additionally, dysregulated TLR expression, in particular upregulation of TLR2 and TLR4, is observed in patients with IBD [26–28]. Finally, mice deficient in the TLR adaptor molecule MyD88 have a more severe disease phenotype when subjected to various models of intestinal inflammation [29].

NLRs recognize bacterial peptidoglycans that are present in the cytoplasm. NLRs signal through the CARD-containing serine-threonine kinase RIP2, which in turn activates TAK1 kinase and NEMO to cause MAPK activation and NF-κB-dependent expression of pro-inflammatory cytokines [30]. NLRs are of particular interest to the study of IBD pathogenesis because of the early observation that mutations in the NOD2 signaling pathway are significantly associated with CD, but in some cases protective from ulcerative colitis (UC) [31]. There are many theories as to why mutations in the NOD2 signaling pathway may predispose to CD. For example, NOD2 signaling inhibits cells from further TLR2 or TLR4 activation, a form of tolerance that may be lost in patients with NOD2 mutations [32, 33]. Additionally, it has been shown that mutations in an attenuator of NOD-driven cytokine responses, ATG16L1, are also associated with CD. It is not clear at this time why NOD2 mutations may be protective from UC, but this observation supports the notion that NOD2 signaling is integral to promoting immune homeostasis in the intestine.

Granulocytes: Neutrophils, Eosinophils, Mast Cells, and Basophils

Granulocytes are a group of innate immune cells that are characterized by the presence of granules in their cytoplasm. They include neutrophils, eosinophils, mast cells, and basophils. While granulocytes originate from a common myeloid precursor, they have distinct properties in their mature form. Neutrophils (PMN) are the most abundant form of granulocyte and make up the majority of peripheral circulating immune cells in humans. Unlike the other granulocytes, PMNs are primarily phagocytes (meaning they actively seek out and engulf particles, bacteria, or dead or dying cells). As a result, they play a central role in early antibacterial immunity. Eosinophils, mast cells, and basophils fall into the category of "type 2" granulocytes in that they are classically thought of as effector cells that mediate antiparasite immune responses (or allergic inflammation) downstream of T-helper (T$_H$) 2 cell differentiation. Both eosinophils and basophils are predominantly found circulating in the blood, while mature mast cells are predominantly a tissue-resident population. Eosinophils and basophils hone to sites of tissue inflammation where they, along with mast cells, exert effector functions including release of granules containing cytokines, chemokines, enzymes, and growth factors. In addition, it has more recently been appreciated that some granulocytes, most notably basophils, can circulate from sites of tissue inflammation to draining lymph nodes where they can influence the development of adaptive immune responses [34].

There is substantial evidence to support the notion that PMNs play a central role in the effector stage of IBD pathogenesis. Locally, PMNs infiltrate inflamed colonic tissue in UC as evidenced on pathology, and by measurements of fecal calprotectin (a stable by-product of neutrophilic inflammation that is tested clinically parallels intestinal inflammation and predicts relapse) [35]. It has also been shown that interfering with PMN recruitment to sites of tissue inflammation, through the use of CXCR2 antagonists, chemokine analogs, anti-CXCR2 monoclonal antibodies, or CXCR2 knockout mice, is associated with reduced colonic inflammation in animal models [36]. Additional evidence supporting a role for neutrophil dysfunction in IBD pathogenesis is the defective acute inflammatory response observed in CD patients. Impaired neutrophilic infiltration, IL-8 production, and vascular flow have all been shown in CD [37]. Furthermore, treatment of patients with GM-CSF, a growth factor that supports neutrophil development and function, has been studied as a potential therapy in CD patients [38, 39].

Macrophages

Macrophages are a phagocytic cell type that play an important role in clearance of bacteria and infected or dead cell remnants. Macrophages also circulate to associated lymphoid tissues where they help to initiate adaptive immune responses. Macrophages develop from embryonic precursors or bone marrow-derived monocytes that can be recruited to sites of tissue inflammation; however, in the steady state, mature macrophages are primarily resident in tissues such as those of the GI tract and associated lymphoid structures. So termed "tissue-resident macrophages" are highly plastic and take on unique functional characteristics specific to their resident tissue. For example, intestinal resident macrophages promote tolerance to foreign substances, food-derived proteins, and commensal bacteria [40, 41]. This unique function may be in part due to their relative hypo-responsiveness to TLR ligands and diminished ability to prime adaptive immune responses [42].

During times of infection and inflammation, however, macrophages are activated through PRRs and become effective modulators of the innate and adaptive immune systems. Activated macrophages express membrane-bound PRRs specific for opsonized particles and pathogens, complement, and bacterial proteins. Recognition of pathogens via these receptors leads to phagocytosis and intracellular degradation as well as the secretion cytokines. Activated macrophages produce large amounts of TNF-α and IL-12, two cytokines responsible for the recruitment and activation of pathogenic effector T cells. The cytokine TGF is also produced by activated macrophages and is a potent chemoattractant leading to the recruitment of monocytes and neutrophils from the blood to the site of inflammation [43]. While initially pro-inflammatory, these newly recruited monocytes can develop into an anergic state (potentially as a result TGF and IL-10 signaling) that results in profound downregulation of pro-inflammatory cytokine release resumption of mucosal homeostasis [44, 45].

The role of macrophages in IBD pathogenesis is on ongoing field of study. It is known that in IBD there is a large influx of macrophages into the intestinal mucosa, and these macrophages display a distinct phenotype and distribution as compared to tissue-resident macrophages in the steady state. For example, in UC pro-inflammatory macrophages are found throughout the epithelium and underlying lamina propria, while macrophage infiltrates observed in CD are extensive and include the underlying mesenteric muscular layer and fat tissue [42]. These infiltrating macrophages have increased expression of the CD33, the IgG receptor CD64, and the chemokine receptor CX3CR1, but express low levels of HLA-DR [46]. The infiltrating macrophages observed in IBD are likely pathogenic as they exhibit NF-κB-dependent expression of pro-inflammatory cytokines including TNF-α, IL-6, IL-8, IL-12, IL-23, IL-1β, and IFNγ

[47–49]. Consistently, the efficacy of anti-TNF-α therapy in IBD is well established [50, 51]. Furthermore, promising anti-IL-12 studies such as the use of the anti-IL-12/23p40 antibody ustekinumab have shown efficacy in Crohn disease, supporting a role for these cytokines in IBD pathogenesis [52, 53]. Finally, the ability of macrophages to enter an anergic state may be impaired in IBD [54]. Additional studies may further elucidate the role of macrophages in IBD pathogenesis.

Dendritic Cells

The dendritic cell (DC) is considered to be one of the most effective of the professional antigen-presenting cells (APCs), and intestinal DCs play an important role in determining and directing the inflammatory response to an antigen. DCs express a wide array of PRRs that detect environmental signals and modulate their expression of cytokines that promote specific lymphocyte responses [55]. DCs can encounter antigen at sites of antigen transport across the epithelium via M cells or via direct luminal sampling [56]. Upon detecting antigen, DCs activate and migrate to T-cell areas in lymphoid structures where they display major histocompatibility complex (MHC)-peptide complexes and co-stimulatory or inhibitory signals to naïve T cells. DCs and other innate cells further dictate T-effector cell polarization using membrane-bound or secreted cytokines [57]. Under homeostatic conditions, intestinal DCs express low levels of co-stimulatory molecules and cytokines and preferentially promote the differentiation of Tregs. However, under conditions of pathogen invasion or inflammation, DCs promote T-cell polarization into one of the many known inflammatory T-helper cell subtypes (T_H1, T_H2, T_H17). Through this critical role, DCs play an important role in modulating adaptive immune responses to maintain intestinal immune homeostasis (Fig. 2.2).

Recent studies have attempted to correlate murine DC subsets with those found in the intestines of humans. Through these efforts it has been found that human CD103$^+$Sirpα^- DCs express markers of cross-presentation (the ability process and present antigen via MHC class I molecules to CD8 T cells) and are most similar to mouse intestinal CD103$^+$CD11b$^-$ DCs that are protective in models of experimental colitis [58, 59]. Furthermore, human DCs that expressed both CD103 and Sirpα are most similar to murine CD103$^+$CD11b$^+$ DCs as they seem to have a prominent role in inducing Treg responses [59]. Human CD103$^+$ DC subsets induced T_H17 cells, while CD103$^-$ Sirpα^+ DCs induce T_H1 cells [59]. Finally, gut-derived DCs can cause homing of lymphocytes primed in the MLN back to the intestine by producing retinoic acid which upregulates $\alpha4\beta7$ and CCR9 on lymphocytes [60].

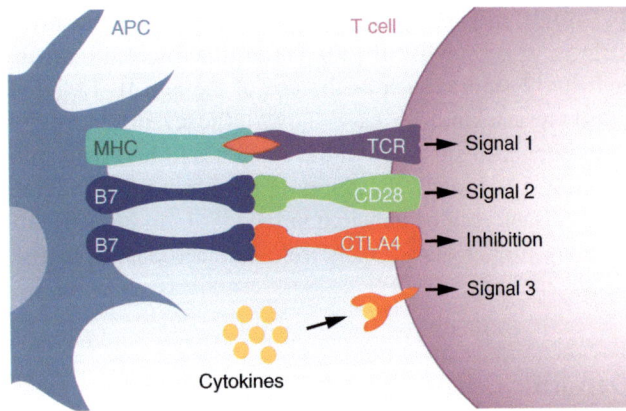

Fig. 2.2 The major molecular receptor-ligand pairs involved in antigen-specific T-cell stimulation. The initial interaction between the APC and the naïve T cell occurs between antigen bound to major histocompatibility complex (*MHC*) class II and the T-cell receptor (*TCR*) (*signal 1*). A co-stimulatory signal (*signal 2*) is required for T-cell activation. T cells become anergic when presented with signal 1 in the absence of signal 2. Many inhibitory co-stimulatory molecules have also been identified such as the cytotoxic T-lymphocyte-associated antigen 4 (*CTLA4*). Finally, cytokines (which can act in a paracrine or autocrine manner) act as third signal to help determine the T-helper cell subtype (T_H1, T_H2, T_H17, Treg) and provide for optimal activation

While the majority of our knowledge of DC function in health and disease stems from studies in mice, there have been some intriguing observations made in humans that may help us understand how this key cell type could contribute to the pathogenesis of IBD. A paradigm has emerged in experimental models where DCs promote regulatory or inflammatory responses depending on the stage of inflammation. Early in the inflammatory process, intestinal DCs seem to protect the intestinal mucosa as their depletion leads to more profound inflammatory states [58, 61]. In settings of more long-standing immune dysregulation, however, such as the constitutive absence of TGFβ signaling, DCs fail to assume a regulatory phenotype and play an active role in promoting pathologic T-cell responses [62, 63]. In light of these observations, one can envision a scenario where DCs are primarily pathogenic in human IBD. Consistent with this hypothesis, intestinal DCs from patients with CD or UC have higher baseline expression of TLR2 and TLR4 and higher expression of the activation marker CD40 [64]. Furthermore, colonic DCs from CD patients express higher levels of IL-12 and IL-6 in the steady state, suggesting that DCs from patients with IBD are constitutively active [64]. Together, these observations provide some insights into how intestinal DCs may contribute to IBD pathogenesis.

Innate Lymphoid Cells and Other Innate Lymphocytes

Innate lymphoid cells (ILCs), which lack a recombined antigen receptor, have been found to play important roles in

mouse models of infection, inflammation, and tissue repair and be dysregulated in multiple human disease states [65]. ILCs are organized into three groups, ILC1, 2, and 3, depending on the transcription factor required for their development and their functional profile. ILC1s (which include natural killer cells) are characterized by T-bet expression, are responsive to IL-12, and produce IFNγ. ILC2s are characterized by GATA3 expression; are responsive to IL-25, IL-33, and TSLP; and produce IL-4, IL-5, IL-9, and IL-13 and amphiregulin. ILC3s (which include lymphoid tissue inducer cells) are characterized by RORγt expression, are responsive to IL-1β and IL-23, and produce IL-17 and/or IL-22 [65].

NK cells, a prototypical member of the ILC1 family, are a type of cytotoxic lymphocyte that kill target cells via cytoplasmic granule toxins or through engagement of death receptors that cause caspase-dependent apoptosis [66]. NK cells are also an early source of IFNγ and can promote differentiation of T_H1 cells [67]. CD16+ NK cells have been found to be increased in the colonic lamina propria of IBD patients, and it was observed that these NK cells were reduced after azathioprine therapy [68]. As a result, NK cells may promote intestinal inflammation in some forms of IBD.

ILC3s may also be of particular relevance to human IBD, but data indicate that ILC3s can play protective or pro-inflammatory roles depending on the experimental or clinical context. On one hand, ILC3s have been shown to mediate intestinal repair in some animal models of acute injury [69–72], and their numbers are reduced (and ILC1 numbers increased) in intestinal tissue samples of some patients with IBD [73–76]. Furthermore, ILC3s can directly induce cell death of activated commensal bacteria-specific T cells, and MHCII on colonic ILC3s is reduced in pediatric IBD patients [77]. On the other hand, ILC3s seem to have a pro-inflammatory phenotype in other animal models [62, 78–80], and there are reports of both increased frequency and IL-22 production by ILC3s in IBD patients [81–83]. Part of the confusion regarding the exact role of ILC3s in IBD may stem from the heterogeneity of this group, as well as the potential for plasticity among ILCs [84, 85]. Nevertheless, further investigation of ILC3s in the context of IBD is warranted.

γδ T cells are a small subset of T lymphocytes which express a T-cell receptor (TCR) composed of the γ- and δ glycoproteins. Unlike conventional αβ T cells, γδ T cells do not require the thymus for development [86], do not recognize antigen in association with MHC class I or II [87], and do not participate in adaptive immune responses [88]. Like ILC3s, γδ T cells play protective or pro-inflammatory in IBD roles depending on the experimental or clinical context. For example, γδ T cells are recruited to inflamed tissue in CD and UC where they produce IFNγ [89, 90]. However, in two models of intestinal inflammation, γδ T cells appear to be protective [91–94], while in other models γδ T cells can take on a pathologic role [95, 96].

Invariant natural killer T cells (iNKT cells) share cell-surface proteins with conventional T cells and NK cells. iNKT cells mature in the thymus, recognize lipid antigen presented via the "MHC-like" complex CD1d, and secrete large amounts of pro-inflammatory cytokines to kill infected and neoplastic cells. Quantitative analysis has shown that iNKT cells are reduced in inflamed colonic tissue from patients with UC [97]. However, iNKT cells isolated from patients with UC produce large amounts of IL-13 and have cytotoxic activity against colonic epithelial cells [98]. As such, the exact role of iNKT cells in IBD pathogenesis is unclear.

Together, innate lymphocytes are a heterogeneous population of cells with diverse functions in health and disease. While they are almost certainly involved in IBD pathogenesis, their role seems to change with different experimental and clinical contexts. As such, more experimentation is necessary to fully understand the role of these cells in IBD pathogenesis.

The Adaptive Immune System and IBD

The adaptive immune system is made up of two subsets of lymphocytes, B and T cells. Both B and T lymphocytes develop in the bone marrow, but T lymphocytes undergo a necessary maturation process in the thymus. The primary strength of the adaptive immune system stems from the specificity of responses. In addition to mediating immunity to pathogens, the adaptive immune system provides a necessary regulatory role in controlling immune responses to self and foreign antigens. The following section will review the adaptive immune system, its relevance to maintaining intestinal homeostasis, and how it may contribute to IBD pathogenesis.

B Cells and IBD

As mentioned previously, B cells primarily develop in the bone marrow; however, B cells can also develop via extramedullary hematopoiesis. Early in embryonic development, pluripotent hematopoietic stem cells migrate to the liver where mature B cells develop and migrate to the intestine. There are several checkpoints in B-cell development directed at ensuring normal recombination of the heavy and light immunoglobulin loci and blocking cells with autoreactive B-cell receptors (BCR) from making it to maturity. The GALT and commensal microbiota of the intestine play an important role in B-cell development and tolerance. Immature transitional B cells transit through the GALT where autoreactive cells are removed from the developing

repertoire [99]. When an autoreactive BCR is detected, it causes clonal deletion, anergy, or editing of the BCR depending on the strength of the autoreactivity. Clonal deletion is the fate of approximately 85% of the newly formed immature B cells. Only cells that reach maturity are available to respond to antigen presented by follicular DCs and other APCs in the germinal center. Antigen recognition can result in activation and proliferation, but not class switching, hypermutation, or memory formation, all of which require T-cell help [100].

Class switching is a biological mechanism that changes the class of immunoglobulin produced by the B cell. Class switching occurs in the germinal center through interactions with T_H cells. Naïve mature B cells produce both IgM and IgD, which are the first two heavy chain segments in the immunoglobulin locus. The class switched molecule contains the same variable domains as generated during recombination, but possesses distinct heavy chain constant domains. After activation, B cells present antigen to cognate T cells which in turn express cell-surface co-activation molecules and cytokines. This coupling enables class switching, hypermutation, and the formation of memory cells or high-affinity antibody-producing cells which secrete IgG, IgA, or IgE molecules [101].

One of the primary roles of B cells in mucosal immunity is the production of secretory IgA, and to a lesser extent secretory IgM. IgA is a dimeric molecule in its secreted form and it plays an important role in mucosal defense. The joining or "J" chain of polymeric IgA spontaneously interacts with the polymeric Ig receptor expressed on the basolateral surface of epithelial cells facilitating exportation of the IgA to the gastrointestinal lumen [102]. In this manner, a vast quantity of IgA is secreted across the epithelium into the intestinal lumen (approximately 3 grams per day, and three-quarters of the total secreted daily immunoglobulin) where it plays an important role in regulating commensal and pathogenic bacteria [103]. However, the relationship between IgA and luminal bacterial is not unidirectional. We know from studies of germfree animals that IgA production is acutely dependent on the presence of luminal microbes (Benveniste et al. [104, 105]). The induction of IgA responses can occur in either a T-cell-dependent or T-cell-independent manner (via the cytokines BAFF and APRIL) facilitating the rapid recognition and response to commensal-derived signals [21, 22].

Despite the known roles for IgA in maintaining mucosal homeostasis, patients who lack the molecule (selective IgA deficiency) have relatively few clinical sequelae. Of those that are known to exist, the most common are recurrent sinopulmonary infections, allergies, autoimmune diseases, and progression to more significant forms of humoral immunodeficiency [106]. Associations between selective IgA deficiency and IBD have been reported (the prevalence of IBD in healthy or IgA-deficient individuals is 3.9% vs. 0.81%, respectively), suggesting that IgA provides a degree of protection from IBD [107, 108]. Under normal circumstances, the B-cell responses that result in the production of IgA are limited to the MLNs and do not occur in systemic secondary lymphoid structures. One hypothesis as to how inappropriate B-cell responses may contribute to IBD pathogenesis centers on the breakdown of this normal compartmentalization [109, 110]. In support of this hypothesis, systemic humoral responses to bacterial components, such as membrane and flagellar proteins, have been found in children with IBD [111].

T Cells and IBD

T cells play many roles in the immune system including cell-mediated immunity against tumors and virus-infected cells, providing help to stimulate B-cell activation and antibody class switching, and differentiating into key effector cell types that mediate immunity to a vast array of pathogens. Additionally, in the case of regulatory T cells (Tregs), T cells play important roles in attenuating inappropriate inflammatory responses and promoting tolerance. It is perhaps not surprising then that problems in any of these diverse functions can predispose to multiple human disease states including neoplasms, infections, allergies, and autoimmunity. T cells originate in the bone marrow but mature in the thymus. With a similar goal to the checkpoints discussed earlier for B cells, the thymus is the location where T cells undergo selection to ensure that their T-cell receptor (TCR) is both capable of interacting with MHC and not autoreactive. T lymphocytes begin to populate the lamina propria by 12 weeks of gestation, and Peyer's patches consisting of B-cell follicles and follicular CD4+ and CD8+ T cells are detected by 16–18 weeks of gestation [112]. Dendritic cells are detected at 19 weeks, representing the last of the required cellular components of an adaptive immune response [113]. The number of Peyer's patches steadily increases from 80 to 120 at birth to 250 by adolescence [114].

There are two major classes of T cells, CD4+ and CD8+. CD8+ T cells are responsible for cell-mediated immunity and provide an essential role in surveillance of tumor and virus-infected cells and are otherwise outside the scope of this chapter [115]. Naïve CD4+ T-helper (T_H) cells circulate the lymphatic tissues in search of their cognate MHC-peptide complex. Constitutive expression of the selectin CD62L (L-selectin) and the chemokine receptor 7 (CCR7) ensures that naïve T cells bind to glycosylated CD34 and the chemokine ligand 21 expressed on endothelial cells of high endothelial venules [116]. The interaction of CD62L and CD34 (among other glycosylated endothelial molecules) promotes a rolling action of the T cell across the endothelial surface. The T-cell surface adhesion molecule LFA-1 then binds to ICAM-1 and ICAM-2 promoting firm adhesion and crossing

of the endothelial lining into the lymphoid tissue. Within the underlying lymphatics await DCs loaded with antigen in variable states of activation. Naïve T cells search the DC selection for a recognizable MHC-peptide complex. If none is found, the cells exit the lymph node, return to the circulation, and reenter other nodes to repeat this process.

When a naïve T_H cell finds a suitable cognate MHC-peptide complex, it is activated via recognition of antigen via their T-cell receptor (TCR) (signal 1), as well as interactions with co-stimulatory or inhibitory molecules on the APC (signal 2) [57]. Recognition of cognate MHC-peptide complex by the TCR in the absence of co-stimulation results in anergy, defined as a lack of response upon reexposure to the same antigen in the future. A third signal, coming in the form of paracrine or autocrine cytokine signals, can enhance T-cell activation. A key consequence resulting from activation of CD4+ T cells is cytokine secretion, and the particular pattern of cytokines secreted orchestrates the type of the ensuing immune response. There are at least four commonly recognized subsets of T_H cell, each with a distinct cytokine expression profile. T_H1 cells are characterized by T-bet expression, are induced by IFNγ and IL-12, and produce IL-2, IFNγ, and TNF-α to help fight intracellular infections. T_H2 cells are characterized by GATA3 expression, are induced by IL-4 and IL-2, and produce IL-4, IL-5, IL-9, and IL-13 to help fight parasitic infections. T_H17 cells are characterized by RORγt expression; are induced by TGFβ, IL-6, and IL-21; and produce IL-17, IL-21, and IL-22 to help fight bacterial infections [65, 117]. A forth T_H subset, regulatory T cells (Tregs), will be discussed separately. Full activation of T cells takes 4–5 days and is accompanied by clonal expansion and homing of effector cells to sites of tissue inflammation (Fig. 2.3).

Within the lamina propria of the intestine, CD4+ and CD8+ T cells bearing the conventional TCR are roughly equally represented. Once activated, these effector T cells leave the lymph node and return to the circulation via the upregulation of the 47 integrin and CCR9 chemokine receptor [118]. Activated T cells produce pro-inflammatory cytokines, such as TNF, that stimulate endothelial cells to upregulate adhesion molecules such as E-selectin (which recruits monocytes and neutrophils) and VCAM-1 and ICAM-1 (both of which recruit activated T cells). TNF and IFN likewise act to alter the vascular permeability, endothelial cell shape, and blood flow, resulting in enhanced infiltration of inflammatory cells into the tissue. These inflammatory cascades set in motion by activated T cells, and the significant structural alterations they cause in the inflamed tissue, eventually trigger the signs and symptoms characteristic of active IBD.

There are multiple lines of evidence strongly supporting the notion that activated CD4+ T cells are a central feature of human IBD. First, T-cell-driven animal models of colitis

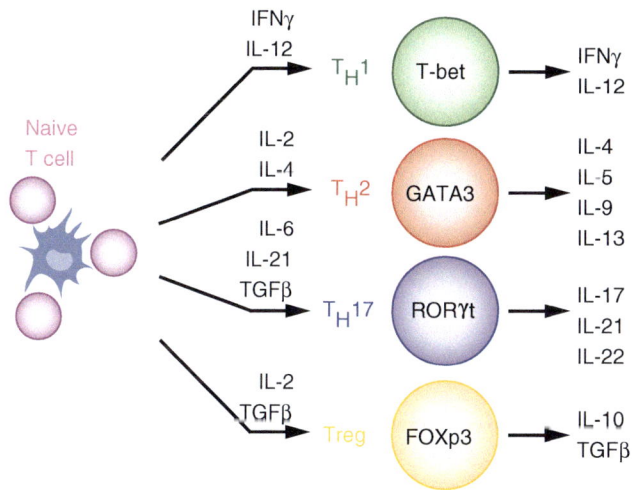

Fig. 2.3 Activation pathways, transcription factors, and effector cytokine profiles of the major T_H cell subsets. The ultimate functional phenotype of mature effector T cells depends upon the type and amount of antigen, and the cytokine milieu present at the time of activation. Activate T_H cell subsets have characteristic transcription factor and cytokine expression patterns

mimic human IBD in both histologic features and susceptibility to similar treatment regimens [84, 106, 109, 119]. In human IBD, IL-17-secreting T_H17 cells have now been an established observation in CD, while UC represents an atypical T_H2 response [98, 120, 121]. Furthermore, the IL-23 receptor variant associated with CD results in impaired IL-17 production and is a protective genetic variant [122]. Additionally, T-cell clones have been identified in patients with CD, and similar populations that specifically recognize endogenous gut bacteria promote colitis in animal models [123, 124]. Finally, there are both established and emerging therapies for IBD that are directed toward the destruction or deterrence of activated effector T cells, or blockade of Th1-driving cytokines [125].

Regulatory T Cells

Regulatory T cells (Tregs) are a subset of T lymphocytes that play an important role in the prevention and control of many autoimmune and allergic diseases [126]. Tregs are characterized by the expression of Foxp3, are induced by IL-2 and TGFβ, and produce TGFβ and IL-10. There are two generally accepted mechanisms of Treg development. So-called "naturally occurring" Tregs acquire Foxp3 expression while undergoing selection in the thymus. Alternatively, "inducible" Tregs develop in the periphery from mature CD4+ T_H cells [126]. The importance of Tregs to normal human physiology is perhaps best typified by descriptions of patients with immunodysregulation, polyendocrinopathy, enteropathy, and X-linked (IPEX) syndrome. IPEX is caused by mutations in

the *FOXP3* gene and results in the clinical phenotype of severe autoimmune phenomena including autoimmune enteropathy, dermatitis, thyroiditis, and type 1 diabetes which can result in death within the first 2 years of life if bone marrow transplant is not successful [127].

A discussion of Tregs in the context of IBD is perhaps most effective when one considers their intimate relationship with T_H17 cells. Despite their very different effector functions, Treg and Th17 cells share the requirement for TGFβ to develop from naïve T_H cells. Furthermore, naïve T_H cells will initially upregulate both Foxp3 and RORγt when stimulated by TGFβ or TGFβ and IL-6. Foxp3 can inhibit the transcriptional activity of RORγt, and as such in Treg-inducing conditions (high TGFβ), Foxp3 expression and ultimately Treg development will be favored. Alternatively, in more proinflammatory conditions (with low TGFβ and high IL-6, IL-21, or IL-1β), FoxP3 activity is inhibited and T_H17 differentiation is favored [128]. In addition to developmental competition, Tregs can directly inhibit the function of T_H17 cells via the secretion of IL-10, providing an additional layer of cross-regulation between these two T-effector-cell populations [129].

Though the importance of Tregs in suppressing mucosal inflammation in murine models has been well established, and Treg populations have been characterized in patients with IBD, specific Treg defects that may predispose to IBD in humans have not been identified [130, 131]. For example, CD4+CD25+ Tregs are present in the lamina propria of IBD patients, and they have similar in vitro T-cell suppressive activity as controls [132]. Contrary to what one might expect, Tregs are more common in inflamed bowel of patients with IBD [133]. Thus, the inflammation observed in IBD is unlikely to be due to a quantitative or functional defect in Tregs. As such, the specific contribution of Tregs to IBD pathogenesis is an ongoing area of investigation.

Commensal Bacteria and IBD

The role of commensal bacteria in IBD pathogenesis will be reviewed in detail in another chapter of this book. However, commensal bacteria play an important role in the normal development of the mucosal immune system and are required for the development of colitis in most murine models of IBD. Additionally, the presence of antibodies to bacterial antigens, and the beneficial effects of antibiotics and probiotics in most patients with IBD suggest an important role of bacteria in the instigation or perpetuation of human IBD. Thus, understanding the mechanisms by which commensal bacteria interact with the innate and adaptive immune system is highly relevant to understanding IBD pathogenesis.

As discussed previously, IECs express innate pattern recognition receptors including Toll-like receptors (TLRs),

Fig. 2.4 Potential pathways through which bacterial antigens may activate mucosal T cells. (1) Apoptosis of infected epithelial cells containing bacterial antigens by macrophages (*Mφ*) and other scavenger cell types. (2) Luminal sampling and acquisition of bacteria by mucosal dendritic cells (*DCs*). (3) Direct or indirect activation of T cells by bacterial antigens in the lamina propria via pattern recognition receptors (*PRRs*) or APCs. (4) Migration of APC-containing bacteria or bacterial components to draining mesenteric lymph nodes (*MLN*)

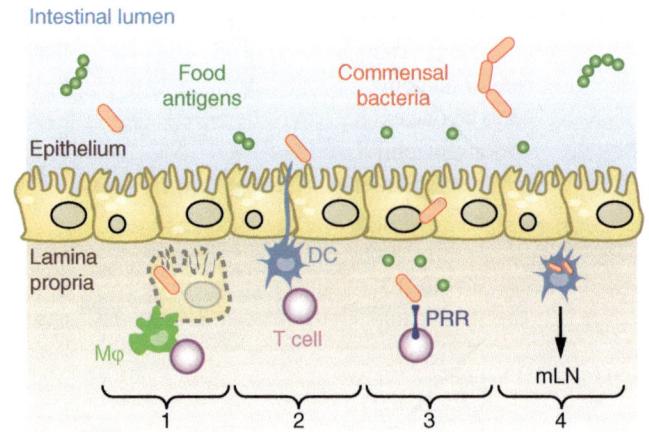

NOD-like receptors (NLRs), and GPCRs that recognize microbial components and modulate immune responses via the regulation of pro-inflammatory cytokines, chemokines, and antimicrobial peptides [11]. Experimental evidence suggests that interaction between commensal gut flora and PRRs protects against colitis and enhances the mucosal barrier [134, 135]. Furthermore, commensal bacteria play an important role in promoting B-cell development and tolerance, an important developmental checkpoint that fails in patients with autoimmunity [99].

Despite multiple mechanisms by which commensal bacteria help maintain mucosal homeostasis, there are at least four mechanisms by which commensal bacteria could be the targets of inappropriate immune responses. First, infected epithelial cells may undergo apoptosis (either spontaneously or as a result of immune-mediated cytotoxicity), and apoptotic fragments containing commensal bacteria may be cross-presented APCs via MHC class I to CD8+ T cells [136]. Second, DCs and macrophages may acquire bacteria directly, presenting bacterial antigen on MHC class II to CD4+ T cells. Third, lymphocytes may be activated by bacterial antigen in the lamina propria directly via PRRs or indirectly via APCs. Fourth, APC-containing bacteria or bacterial components may migrate to draining mesenteric lymph nodes where they could interact with lymphocytes [137]. Thus, multiple pathways exist with the potential of presenting commensal bacterial products to lymphocytes to result in inappropriate and potentially pathogenic inflammatory responses (Fig. 2.4).

The Pediatric Immune System

Maturation of the mucosal immune system is a continuum with no definitive markers defining a "mature" and "immature" status. The only evidence available from which to draw conclusions unique to the pediatric mucosal immune system is from studies of human neonates or animal studied at the time of weaning. The most noticeable difference between developing (neonatal) and established immune responses would appear to be in adaptive immunity. The rationale for this assumption is that adaptive immune responses are antigen specific and thus require postnatal exposure to dietary and microbial antigen to develop immunologic memory. In contrast, innate immune responses are for the most part germ line-encoded through recognition of microbial ligands by pathogen recognition receptors. Indeed, fetal intestinal epithelial cell lines exhibit responsiveness to inflammatory stimuli and bacterial products [138]. This section will briefly address two commonly accepted differences in the immune systems of children and adults.

Neonates are capable of some humoral and cellular immune responses at the time of birth. At birth, the gastrointestinal tract encounters microbes that are resident in the birth canal and the surrounding environment. Within hours after birth, the gastrointestinal tract begins colonization with commensal bacteria. Specific secretory IgA responses to organisms such as *Escherichia coli* are produced within the first week of life, likely via T-cell-independent mechanisms of B-cell class switching discussed earlier [139, 140]. Infants and young children are capable of generating the full spectrum of functional T_H cells and T-cell-dependent B-cell responses, though it is important to note that T-cell-independent B-cell immune responses do not reach full maturity until about 15–14 months of life [141]. This humoral deficiency is compensated to a large degree by passive transfer of antibodies and immune cells across the placenta and via breastfeeding [142]. Nonetheless, impaired B-cell responses to T-cell-independent antigens may leave young children susceptible to infection by polysaccharide-encapsulated bacteria [143].

The second major difference is the tendency of the young mucosal immune system to generate allergic immune responses to oral and environmental antigens. This is generally believed to be one explanation for the high prevalence of atopic conditions in children [144]. The evidence for this unique feature of the immature immune system exists in epidemiologic and translational studies of children with food allergy [145, 146] and animal models demonstrating impaired oral tolerance in young mice [147]. How many of the aforementioned features of the immature immune system relate to human IBD remains to be explored.

Summary

As discussed in other chapters of this book, it is obvious that all recent advances in the field of novel therapeutic approaches, notably biological therapies, are directly derived from knowledge harnessed by studies of mucosal immunity in the normal and inflamed intestine [125]. In spite of these striking advances, some aspects of gut immunity remain unclear. Perhaps the most critical one is how the mucosal immune system interacts with the endogenous commensal flora under physiological and pathological conditions, a fundamental issue considering the widely accepted notion that IBD is an abnormal immune response to the autologous enteric bacteria in genetically susceptible individuals. The characterization of the relationship between the gut microbiota and the immune system is ongoing and greatly improved through the use of shotgun metagenomic sequencing. As we understand more about the residents of the gut microbiota and the function, the interaction with the immune system provides new insights on the initiation of the inflammatory response in IBD.

Another critical aspect of gut immunity is the nature of the mucosal immune response mediating inflammation during the course of a chronic disease, as typically found in IBD. It is plausible, if not probable, that long-lasting intestinal inflammatory processes like CD and UC undergo substantial changes of the underlying biological response regardless of the initial triggering events. This point is fundamentally important for pediatric IBD, when the disease is at its earliest possible stages of detection, and there is perhaps an opportunity to change the natural history of the disease, a far more difficult goal to attain in adult IBD patients with a long clinical history. Another unique population is patients with very early-onset IBD, in whom genomics is a larger disease-driving force than older populations, including genes of immunodeficiency.

It is not a coincidence that the disease develops as the immune system and gut microbiome are in the process of maturation, largely in a codependent manner. The relationship between host genetics and developing microbiome can

be seen through germfree (GF) murine models. GF mice have underdeveloped gut-associated lymphoid tissue. In an environment with specific-defined flora, the gut microbiota elicits host-specific T-cell response and differentiation [89]. Concurrently, the aberrant T-cell development of GF mice shapes the gut microbiome, as seen by the different phylogenetic compositions of the microbiota in *Rag1*-deficient mice [125]. Zebra fish models show similar findings, in which *Rag1*-deficient zebra fish had overgrowth of *Vibrio* species [98]. Studying early events of IBD pathogenesis and following them up during disease evolution into chronicity are obviously difficult in humans and more so in children, but this can be accomplished in animal models, which are starting to generate concrete evidence of substantial changes in the gut immune response from the early to the chronic stages of inflammation. Switches from a T_H1 to a T_H2 pattern occur in at least two models of experimental IBD. In the colitis of IL-10-deficient mice and the ileitis of SAMP1/YitFc mice, both of which are Th1 mediated initially, there is a marked increase in disease-mediating Th2 cytokines in late disease, e.g., IL-4 and IL-13 in the colitis model and IL-5 and IL-13 in the ileitis model [148, 149]. The lesson here is that, even though the clinical manifestations of IBD remain constant, the underlying pathogenic immunopathology changes rather dramatically over time. Therefore, therapies that are effective in early disease may no longer be effective in chronic disease, as again exemplified by the above animal models where blockade of Th1 cytokines is therapeutically effective in early but not late inflammation, a period when blockade of Th2 cytokines ameliorates disease.

In summary, investigation of the intestinal immune system in IBD has been and still is extremely rewarding, as it has provided not only new information on the biology of its components and overall function but also practical new ways to exploit this new information for current and future therapeutic applications.

References

1. MacDonald TT, Spencer J, Viney JL, Williams CB, Walker-Smith JA. Selective biopsy of human Peyer's patches during ileal endoscopy. Gastroenterology. 1987;93:1356–62. doi: S0016508587003330 [pii]
2. Mowat AM. Anatomical basis of tolerance and immunity to intestinal antigens. Nat Rev Immunol. 2003;3:331–41. doi:10.1038/nri1057.
3. Macpherson AJ, McCoy KD, Johansen FE, Brandtzaeg P. The immune geography of IgA induction and function. Mucosal Immunol. 2008;1:11–22. doi:10.1038/mi.2007.6.
4. Hill DA, Artis D. Intestinal bacteria and the regulation of immune cell homeostasis. Annu Rev Immunol. 2010;28:623–67. doi:10.1146/annurev-immunol-030409-101330.
5. Dorshkind K, Montecino-Rodriguez E, Signer RA. The ageing immune system: is it ever too old to become young again? Nat Rev Immunol. 2009;9:57–62. doi:10.1038/nri2471.

6. Turner JR. Intestinal mucosal barrier function in health and disease. Nat Rev Immunol. 2009;9:799–809. doi:10.1038/nri2653.

7. Mukherjee S, Hooper LV. Antimicrobial defense of the intestine. Immunity. 2015;42:28–39. doi:10.1016/j.immuni.2014.12.028.

8. Pelaseyed T, Bergstrom JH, Gustafsson JK, Ermund A, Birchenough GM, Schutte A, van der Post S, Svensson F, Rodriguez-Pineiro AM, Nystrom EE, Wising C, Johansson ME, Hansson GC. The mucus and mucins of the goblet cells and enterocytes provide the first defense line of the gastrointestinal tract and interact with the immune system. Immunol Rev. 2014;260:8–20. doi:10.1111/imr.12182.

9. Udall JN, Pang K, Fritze L, Kleinman R, Walker WA. Development of gastrointestinal mucosal barrier. I. The effect of age on intestinal permeability to macromolecules. Pediatr Res. 1981;15:241–4.

10. Schulz O, Pabst O. Antigen sampling in the small intestine. Trends Immunol. 2013;34:155–61. doi:10.1016/j.it.2012.09.006.

11. Prescott D, Lee J, Philpott DJ. An epithelial armamentarium to sense the microbiota. Semin Immunol. 2013;25:323–33. doi:10.1016/j.smim.2013.09.007.

12. Hershberg RM, Mayer LF. Antigen processing and presentation by intestinal epithelial cells – polarity and complexity. Immunol Today. 2000;21:123–8.

13. Shao L, Kamalu O, Mayer L. Non-classical MHC class I molecules on intestinal epithelial cells: mediators of mucosal crosstalk. Immunol Rev. 2005;206:160–76. doi: IMR295 [pii]

14. Coskun M. Intestinal epithelium in inflammatory bowel disease. Front Med (Lausanne). 2014;1:24. doi:10.3389/fmed.2014.00024.

15. Boltin D, Perets TT, Vilkin A, Niv Y. Mucin function in inflammatory bowel disease: an update. J Clin Gastroenterol. 2013;47:106–11. doi:10.1097/MCG.0b013e3182688e73.

16. Gunther C, Martini E, Wittkopf N, Amann K, Weigmann B, Neumann H, Waldner MJ, Hedrick SM, Tenzer S, Neurath MF, Becker C. Caspase-8 regulates TNF-alpha-induced epithelial necroptosis and terminal ileitis. Nature. 2011;477:335–9. doi:10.1038/nature10400.

17. Kiesslich R, Duckworth CA, Moussata D, Gloeckner A, Lim LG, Goetz M, Pritchard DM, Galle PR, Neurath MF, Watson AJ. Local barrier dysfunction identified by confocal laser endomicroscopy predicts relapse in inflammatory bowel disease. Gut. 2012;61:1146–53. doi:10.1136/gutjnl-2011-300695.

18. Lim LG, Neumann J, Hansen T, Goetz M, Hoffman A, Neurath MF, Galle PR, Chan YH, Kiesslich R, Watson AJ. Confocal endomicroscopy identifies loss of local barrier function in the duodenum of patients with Crohn's disease and ulcerative colitis. Inflamm Bowel Dis. 2014;20:892–900. doi:10.1097/MIB.0000000000000027.

19. Ananthakrishnan AN. Epidemiology and risk factors for IBD. Nat Rev Gastroenterol Hepatol. 2015;12:205–17. doi:10.1038/nrgastro.2015.34.

20. Lecuyer E, Rakotobe S, Lengline-Garnier H, Lebreton C, Picard M, Juste C, Fritzen R, Eberl G, McCoy KD, Macpherson AJ, Reynaud CA, Cerf-Bensussan N, Gaboriau-Routhiau V. Segmented filamentous bacterium uses secondary and tertiary lymphoid tissues to induce gut IgA and specific T helper 17 cell responses. Immunity. 2014;40:608–20. doi:10.1016/j.immuni.2014.03.009.

21. He B, Xu W, Santini PA, Polydorides AD, Chiu A, Estrella J, Shan M, Chadburn A, Villanacci V, Plebani A, Knowles DM, Rescigno M, Cerutti A. Intestinal bacteria trigger T cell-independent immunoglobulin A(2) class switching by inducing epithelial-cell secretion of the cytokine APRIL. Immunity. 2007;26:812–26. doi:10.1016/j.immuni.2007.04.014.

22. Xu W, He B, Chiu A, Chadburn A, Shan M, Buldys M, Ding A, Knowles DM, Santini PA, Cerutti A. Epithelial cells trigger front-line immunoglobulin class switching through a pathway regulated by the inhibitor SLPI. Nat Immunol. 2007;8:294–303. doi:10.1038/ni1434.

23. Browning BL, Huebner C, Petermann I, Gearry RB, Barclay ML, Shelling AN, Ferguson LR. Has toll-like receptor 4 been prematurely dismissed as an inflammatory bowel disease gene? Association study combined with meta-analysis shows strong evidence for association. Am J Gastroenterol. 2007;102:2504–12. doi: AJG1463 [pii]

24. Franchimont D, Vermeire S, El Housni H, Pierik M, Van Steen K, Gustot T, Quertinmont E, Abramowicz M, Van Gossum A, Deviere J, Rutgeerts P. Deficient host-bacteria interactions in inflammatory bowel disease? The toll-like receptor (TLR)-4 Asp299gly polymorphism is associated with Crohn's disease and ulcerative colitis. Gut. 2004;53:987–92.

25. Torok HP, Glas J, Tonenchi L, Mussack T, Folwaczny C. Polymorphisms of the lipopolysaccharide-signaling complex in inflammatory bowel disease: association of a mutation in the Toll-like receptor 4 gene with ulcerative colitis. Clin Immunol. 2004;112:85–91. doi:10.1016/j.clim.2004.03.002.

26. Cario E, Podolsky DK. Differential alteration in intestinal epithelial cell expression of toll-like receptor 3 (TLR3) and TLR4 in inflammatory bowel disease. Infect Immun. 2000;68:7010–7.

27. Frolova L, Drastich P, Rossmann P, Klimesova K, Tlaskalova-Hogenova H. Expression of Toll-like receptor 2 (TLR2), TLR4, and CD14 in biopsy samples of patients with inflammatory bowel diseases: upregulated expression of TLR2 in terminal ileum of patients with ulcerative colitis. J Histochem Cytochem. 2008;56:267–74. doi: jhc.7A7303.2007 [pii]

28. Hausmann M, Kiessling S, Mestermann S, Webb G, Spottl T, Andus T, Scholmerich J, Herfarth H, Ray K, Falk W, Rogler G. Toll-like receptors 2 and 4 are up-regulated during intestinal inflammation. Gastroenterology. 2002;122:1987–2000. doi: S001650850200032X [pii]

29. Araki A, Kanai T, Ishikura T, Makita S, Uraushihara K, Iiyama R, Totsuka T, Takeda K, Akira S, Watanabe M. MyD88-deficient mice develop severe intestinal inflammation in dextran sodium sulfate colitis. J Gastroenterol. 2005;40:16–23. doi:10.1007/s00535-004-1492-9.

30. Saxena M, Yeretssian G. NOD-like receptors: master regulators of inflammation and cancer. Front Immunol. 2014;5:327. doi:10.3389/fimmu.2014.00327.

31. Jostins L, Ripke S, Weersma RK, Duerr RH, McGovern DP, Hui KY, Lee JC, Schumm LP, Sharma Y, Anderson CA, Essers J, Mitrovic M, Ning K, Cleynen I, Theatre E, Spain SL, Raychaudhuri S, Goyette P, Wei Z, Abraham C, Achkar JP, Ahmad T, Amininejad L, Ananthakrishnan AN, Andersen V, Andrews JM, Baidoo L, Balschun T, Bampton PA, Bitton A, Boucher G, Brand S, Buning C, Cohain A, Cichon S, D'Amato M, De Jong D, Devaney KL, Dubinsky M, Edwards C, Ellinghaus D, Ferguson LR, Franchimont D, Fransen K, Gearry R, Georges M, Gieger C, Glas J, Haritunians T, Hart A, Hawkey C, Hedl M, Hu X, Karlsen TH, Kupcinskas L, Kugathasan S, Latiano A, Laukens D, Lawrance IC, Lees CW, Louis E, Mahy G, Mansfield J, Morgan AR, Mowat C, Newman W, Palmieri O, Ponsioen CY, Potocnik U, Prescott NJ, Regueiro M, Rotter JI, Russell RK, Sanderson JD, Sans M, Satsangi J, Schreiber S, Simms LA, Sventoraityte J, Targan SR, Taylor KD, Tremelling M, Verspaget HW, De Vos M, Wijmenga C, Wilson DC, Winkelmann J, Xavier RJ, Zeissig S, Zhang B, Zhang CK, Zhao H, International IBD Genetics Consortium (IIBDGC), Silverberg MS, Annese V, Hakonarson H, Brant SR, Radford-Smith G, Mathew CG, Rioux JD, Schadt EE, Daly MJ, Franke A, Parkes M, Vermeire S, Barrett JC, Cho JH. Host-microbe interactions have shaped the genetic architecture of inflammatory bowel disease. Nature. 2012;491:119–24. doi:10.1038/nature11582.

32. Hedl M, Li J, Cho JH, Abraham C. Chronic stimulation of Nod2 mediates tolerance to bacterial products. Proc Natl Acad Sci U S A. 2007;104:19440–5. doi:10.1073/pnas.0706097104.

33. Kullberg BJ, Ferwerda G, de Jong DJ, Drenth JP, Joosten LA, Van der Meer JW, Netea MG. Crohn's disease patients homozygous for the 3020insC NOD2 mutation have a defective NOD2/TLR4 cross-tolerance to intestinal stimuli. Immunology. 2008;123:600–5. doi: IMM2735 [pii]

34. Hill DA, Siracusa MC, Abt MC, Kim BS, Kobuley D, Kubo M, Kambayashi T, Larosa DF, Renner ED, Orange JS, Bushman FD, Artis D. Commensal bacteria-derived signals regulate basophil hematopoiesis and allergic inflammation. Nat Med. 2012;25:18(4):538–46. doi:10.1038/nm.2657.

35. Hanai H, Takeuchi K, Iida T, Kashiwagi N, Saniabadi AR, Matsushita I, Sato Y, Kasuga N, Nakamura T. Relationship between fecal calprotectin, intestinal inflammation, and peripheral blood neutrophils in patients with active ulcerative colitis. Dig Dis Sci. 2004;49:1438–43.

36. Boppana NB, Devarajan A, Gopal K, Barathan M, Bakar SA, Shankar EM, Ebrahim AS, Farooq SM. Blockade of CXCR2 signalling: a potential therapeutic target for preventing neutrophil-mediated inflammatory diseases. Exp Biol Med (Maywood). 2014;239:509–18. doi:10.1177/1535370213520110.

37. Marks DJ, Harbord MW, MacAllister R, Rahman FZ, Young J, Al-Lazikani B, Lees W, Novelli M, Bloom S, Segal AW. Defective acute inflammation in Crohn's disease: a clinical investigation. Lancet. 2006;367:668–78. doi: S0140-6736(06)68265-2 [pii]

38. Kelsen JR, Rosh J, Heyman M, Winter HS, Ferry G, Cohen S, Mamula P, Baldassano RN. PhaseI trial of sargramostim in pediatric Crohn's disease Inflamm Bowel Dis. 2010;16(7):1203–8. doi:10.1002/ibd.21204.

39. Roth L, Macdonald JK, McDonald JW, Chande N. Sargramostim (GM-CSF) for induction of remission in Crohn's disease. Cochrane Database Syst Rev. 2011;(11):CD008538. doi:CD008538. 10.1002/14651858.CD008538.pub2.

40. Rugtveit J, Bakka A, Brandtzaeg P. Differential distribution of B7.1 (CD80) and B7.2 (CD86) costimulatory molecules on mucosal macrophage subsets in human inflammatory bowel disease (IBD). Clin Exp Immunol. 1997;110:104–13.

41. Smith PD, Smythies LE, Mosteller-Barnum M, Sibley DA, Russell MW, Merger M, Sellers MT, Orenstein JM, Shimada T, Graham MF, Kubagawa H. Intestinal macrophages lack CD14 and CD89 and consequently are down-regulated for LPS- and IgA-mediated activities. J Immunol. 2001;167:2651–6.

42. Kuhl AA, Erben U, Kredel LI, Siegmund B. Diversity of Intestinal Macrophages in Inflammatory Bowel Diseases. Front Immunol. 2015;6:613. doi:10.3389/fimmu.2015.00613.

43. Smith PD, Smythies LE, Shen R, Greenwell-Wild T, Gliozzi M, Wahl SM. Intestinal macrophages and response to microbial encroachment. Mucosal Immunol. 2011;4:31–42. doi:10.1038/mi.2010.66.

44. Schenk M, Bouchon A, Birrer S, Colonna M, Mueller C. Macrophages expressing triggering receptor expressed on myeloid cells-1 are underrepresented in the human intestine. J Immunol. 2005;174:517–24. doi: 174/1/517 [pii]

45. Smythies LE, Shen R, Bimczok D, Novak L, Clements RH, Eckhoff DE, Bouchard P, George MD, Hu WK, Dandekar S, Smith PD. Inflammation anergy in human intestinal macrophages is due to Smad-induced IkappaBalpha expression and NF-kappaB inactivation. J Biol Chem. 2010;285:19593–604. doi:10.1074/jbc.M109.069955.

46. Thiesen S, Janciauskiene S, Uronen-Hansson H, Agace W, Hogerkorp CM, Spee P, Hakansson K, Grip O. CD14(hi)HLA-DR(dim) macrophages, with a resemblance to classical blood monocytes, dominate inflamed mucosa in Crohn's disease. J Leukoc Biol. 2014;95:531–41. doi:10.1189/jlb.0113021.

47. Kamada N, Hisamatsu T, Okamoto S, Chinen H, Kobayashi T, Sato T, Sakuraba A, Kitazume MT, Sugita A, Koganei K, Akagawa KS, Hibi T. Unique CD14 intestinal macrophages contribute to the pathogenesis of Crohn disease via IL-23/IFN-gamma axis. J Clin Invest. 2008;118:2269–80. doi:10.1172/JCI34610.

48. Rogler G, Brand K, Vogl D, Page S, Hofmeister R, Andus T, Knuechel R, Baeuerle PA, Scholmerich J, Gross V. Nuclear factor kappaB is activated in macrophages and epithelial cells of inflamed intestinal mucosa. Gastroenterology. 1998;115:357–69. doi: S001650859800136X [pii]

49. Schenk M, Bouchon A, Seibold F, Mueller C. TREM-1--expressing intestinal macrophages crucially amplify chronic inflammation in experimental colitis and inflammatory bowel diseases. J Clin Invest. 2007;117:3097–106. doi:10.1172/JCI30602.

50. Kugathasan S, Werlin SL, Martinez A, Rivera MT, Heikenen JB, Binion DG. Prolonged duration of response to infliximab in early but not late pediatric Crohn's disease. Am J Gastroenterol. 2000;95(11):3189–94.

51. Lahad A, Weiss B. Current therapy of pediatric Crohn's disease. World J Gastrointest Pathophysiol. 2015;6:33–42. doi:10.4291/wjgp.v6.i2.33.

52. Khanna R, Preiss JC, MacDonald JK, Timmer A. Anti-IL-12/23p40 antibodies for induction of remission in Crohn's disease. Cochrane Database Syst Rev. 2015;5(5):CD007572. doi:10.1002/14651858.CD007572.pub2.

53. Mannon PJ, Fuss IJ, Mayer L, Elson CO, Sandborn WJ, Present D, Dolin B, Goodman N, Groden C, Hornung RL, Quezado M, Yang Z, Neurath MF, Salfeld J, Veldman GM, Schwertschlag U, Strober W, Anti-IL-12 Crohn's Disease Study Group. Anti-interleukin-12 antibody for active Crohn's disease. N Engl J Med. 2004;351:2069–79. doi: 351/20/2069 [pii]

54. Monteleone G, Boirivant M, Pallone F, MacDonald TT. TGF-beta1 and Smad7 in the regulation of IBD. Mucosal Immunol. 2008;1(Suppl 1):S50–3. doi:10.1038/mi.2008.55.

55. Schiavi E, Smolinska S, O'Mahony L. Intestinal dendritic cells. Curr Opin Gastroenterol. 2015;31:98–103. doi:10.1097/MOG.0000000000000155.

56. del Rio ML, Bernhardt G, Rodriguez-Barbosa JI, Forster R. Development and functional specialization of CD103+ dendritic cells. Immunol Rev. 2010;234:268–81. doi:10.1111/j.0105-2896.2009.00874.x.

57. Merad M, Sathe P, Helft J, Miller J, Mortha A. The dendritic cell lineage: ontogeny and function of dendritic cells and their subsets in the steady state and the inflamed setting. Annu Rev Immunol. 2013;31:563–604. doi:10.1146/annurev-immunol-020711-074950.

58. Muzaki AR, Tetlak P, Sheng J, Loh SC, Setiagani YA, Poidinger M, Zolezzi F, Karjalainen K, Ruedl C. Intestinal CD103CD11b dendritic cells restrain colitis via IFN-gamma-induced anti-inflammatory response in epithelial cells. Mucosal Immunol. 2016;9(2):336–51. doi:10.1038/mi.2015.64.

59. Watchmaker PB, Lahl K, Lee M, Baumjohann D, Morton J, Kim SJ, Zeng R, Dent A, Ansel KM, Diamond B, Hadeiba H, Butcher EC. Comparative transcriptional and functional profiling defines conserved programs of intestinal DC differentiation in humans and mice. Nat Immunol. 2014;15:98–108. doi:10.1038/ni.2768.

60. Stock A, Napolitani G, Cerundolo V. Intestinal DC in migrational imprinting of immune cells. Immunol Cell Biol. 2013;91:240–9. doi:10.1038/icb.2012.73.

61. Qualls JE, Tuna H, Kaplan AM, Cohen DA. Suppression of experimental colitis in mice by CD11c+ dendritic cells. Inflamm Bowel Dis. 2009;15:236–47. doi:10.1002/ibd.20733.

62. Ermann J, Staton T, Glickman JN, de Waal MR, Glimcher LH. Nod/Ripk2 signaling in dendritic cells activates IL-17A-secreting

innate lymphoid cells and drives colitis in T-bet-/-.Rag2-/- (TRUC) mice. Proc Natl Acad Sci U S A. 2014;111:E2559–66. doi:10.1073/pnas.1408540111.

63. Travis MA, Reizis B, Melton AC, Masteller E, Tang Q, Proctor JM, Wang Y, Bernstein X, Huang X, Reichardt LF, Bluestone JA, Sheppard D. Loss of integrin alpha(v)beta8 on dendritic cells causes autoimmunity and colitis in mice. Nature. 2007;449:361–5. doi: nature06110 [pii]

64. Hart AL, Al-Hassi HO, Rigby RJ, Bell SJ, Emmanuel AV, Knight SC, Kamm MA, Stagg AJ. Characteristics of intestinal dendritic cells in inflammatory bowel diseases. Gastroenterology. 2005;129:50–65.

65. Sonnenberg GF, Artis D. Innate lymphoid cells in the initiation, regulation and resolution of inflammation. Nat Med. 2015;21:698–708. doi:10.1038/nm.3892.

66. Yokoyama WM, Kim S, French AR. The dynamic life of natural killer cells. Annu Rev Immunol. 2004;22:405–29. doi:10.1146/annurev.immunol.22.012703.104711.

67. Martin-Fontecha A, Thomsen LL, Brett S, Gerard C, Lipp M, Lanzavecchia A, Sallusto F. Induced recruitment of NK cells to lymph nodes provides IFN-gamma for T(H)1 priming. Nat Immunol. 2004;5:1260–5. doi: ni1138 [pii]

68. Steel AW, Mela CM, Lindsay JO, Gazzard BG, Goodier MR. Increased proportion of CD16(+) NK cells in the colonic lamina propria of inflammatory bowel disease patients, but not after azathioprine treatment. Aliment Pharmacol Ther. 2011;33:115–26. doi:10.1111/j.1365-2036.2010.04499.x.

69. Hanash AM, Dudakov JA, Hua G, O'Connor MH, Young LF, Singer NV, West ML, Jenq RR, Holland AM, Kappel LW, Ghosh A, Tsai JJ, Rao UK, Yim NL, Smith OM, Velardi E, Hawryluk EB, Murphy GF, Liu C, Fouser LA, Kolesnick R, Blazar BR, van den Brink MR. Interleukin-22 protects intestinal stem cells from immune-mediated tissue damage and regulates sensitivity to graft versus host disease. Immunity. 2012;37:339–50. doi:10.1016/j.immuni.2012.05.028.

70. Mielke LA, Jones SA, Raverdeau M, Higgs R, Stefanska A, Groom JR, Misiak A, Dungan LS, Sutton CE, Streubel G, Bracken AP, Mills KH. Retinoic acid expression associates with enhanced IL-22 production by gamma delta T cells and innate lymphoid cells and attenuation of intestinal inflammation. J Exp Med. 2013;210:1117–24. doi:10.1084/jem.20121588.

71. Sawa S, Lochner M, Satoh-Takayama N, Dulauroy S, Berard M, Kleinschek M, Cua D, Di Santo JP, Eberl G. RORgammat+ innate lymphoid cells regulate intestinal homeostasis by integrating negative signals from the symbiotic microbiota. Nat Immunol. 2011;12:320–6. doi:10.1038/ni.2002.

72. Sugimoto K, Ogawa A, Mizoguchi E, Shimomura Y, Andoh A, Bhan AK, Blumberg RS, Xavier RJ, Mizoguchi A. IL-22 ameliorates intestinal inflammation in a mouse model of ulcerative colitis. J Clin Invest. 2008;118:534–44. doi:10.1172/JCI33194.

73. Bernink JH, Peters CP, Munneke M, te Velde AA, Meijer SL, Weijer K, Hreggvidsdottir HS, Heinsbroek SE, Legrand N, Buskens CJ, Bemelman WA, Mjosberg JM, Spits H. Human type 1 innate lymphoid cells accumulate in inflamed mucosal tissues. Nat Immunol. 2013;14:221–9. doi:10.1038/ni.2534.

74. Ciccia F, Accardo-Palumbo A, Alessandro R, Rizzo A, Principe S, Peralta S, Raiata F, Giardina A, De Leo G, Triolo G. Interleukin-22 and interleukin-22-producing NKp44+ natural killer cells in subclinical gut inflammation in ankylosing spondylitis. Arthritis Rheum. 2012;64:1869–78. doi:10.1002/art.34355.

75. Fuchs A, Vermi W, Lee JS, Lonardi S, Gilfillan S, Newberry RD, Cella M, Colonna M. Intraepithelial type 1 innate lymphoid cells are a unique subset of IL-12- and IL-15-responsive IFN-gamma-producing cells. Immunity. 2013;38:769–81. doi:10.1016/j.immuni.2013.02.010.

76. Takayama T, Kamada N, Chinen H, Okamoto S, Kitazume MT, Chang J, Matuzaki Y, Suzuki S, Sugita A, Koganei K, Hisamatsu T, Kanai T, Hibi T. Imbalance of NKp44(+)NKp46(−) and NKp44(−)NKp46(+) natural killer cells in the intestinal mucosa of patients with Crohn's disease. Gastroenterology. 2010;139:882–92, 892.e1–3. doi:10.1053/j.gastro.2010.05.040.

77. Hepworth MR, Fung TC, Masur SH, Kelsen JR, McConnell FM, Dubrot J, Withers DR, Hugues S, Farrar MA, Reith W, Eberl G, Baldassano RN, Laufer TM, Elson CO, Sonnenberg GF. Immune tolerance. Group 3 innate lymphoid cells mediate intestinal selection of commensal bacteria-specific CD4(+) T cells. Science. 2015;348:1031–5. doi:10.1126/science.aaa4812.

78. Buonocore S, Ahern PP, Uhlig HH, Ivanov II, Littman DR, Maloy KJ, Powrie F. Innate lymphoid cells drive interleukin-23-dependent innate intestinal pathology. Nature. 2010;464:1371–5. doi:10.1038/nature08949.

79. Munoz M, Eidenschenk C, Ota N, Wong K, Lohmann U, Kuhl AA, Wang X, Manzanillo P, Li Y, Rutz S, Zheng Y, Diehl L, Kayagaki N, van Lookeren-Campagne M, Liesenfeld O, Heimesaat M, Ouyang W. Interleukin-22 induces interleukin-18 expression from epithelial cells during intestinal infection. Immunity. 2015;42:321–31. doi:10.1016/j.immuni.2015.01.011.

80. Powell N, Walker AW, Stolarczyk E, Canavan JB, Gokmen MR, Marks E, Jackson I, Hashim A, Curtis MA, Jenner RG, Howard JK, Parkhill J, MacDonald TT, Lord GM. The transcription factor T-bet regulates intestinal inflammation mediated by interleukin-7 receptor+ innate lymphoid cells. Immunity. 2012;37:674–84. doi:10.1016/j.immuni.2012.09.008.

81. Geremia A, Arancibia-Carcamo CV, Fleming MP, Rust N, Singh B, Mortensen NJ, Travis SP, Powrie F. IL-23-responsive innate lymphoid cells are increased in inflammatory bowel disease. J Exp Med. 2011;208:1127–33. doi:10.1084/jem.20101712.

82. Longman RS, Diehl GE, Victorio DA, Huh JR, Galan C, Miraldi ER, Swaminath A, Bonneau R, Scherl EJ, Littman DR. CX(3)CR1(+) mononuclear phagocytes support colitis-associated innate lymphoid cell production of IL-22. J Exp Med. 2014;211:1571–83. doi:10.1084/jem.20140678.

83. Powell N, Lo JW, Biancheri P, Vossenkamper A, Pantazi E, Walker AW, Stolarczyk E, Ammoscato F, Goldberg R, Scott P, Canavan JB, Perucha E, Garrido-Mesa N, Irving PM, Sanderson JD, Hayee B, Howard JK, Parkhill J, MacDonald TT, Lord GM. Interleukin 6 increases production of cytokines by colonic innate lymphoid cells in mice and patients with chronic intestinal inflammation. Gastroenterology. 2015;149:456–67.e15. doi:10.1053/j.gastro.2015.04.017.

84. Klose CS, Kiss EA, Schwierzeck V, Ebert K, Hoyler T, d'Hargues Y, Goppert N, Croxford AL, Waisman A, Tanriver Y, Diefenbach A. A T-bet gradient controls the fate and function of CCR6-RORgammat+ innate lymphoid cells. Nature. 2013;494:261–5. doi:10.1038/nature11813.

85. Vonarbourg C, Mortha A, Bui VL, Hernandez PP, Kiss EA, Hoyler T, Flach M, Bengsch B, Thimme R, Holscher C, Honig M, Pannicke U, Schwarz K, Ware CF, Finke D, Diefenbach A. Regulated expression of nuclear receptor RORgammat confers distinct functional fates to NK cell receptor-expressing RORgammat(+) innate lymphocytes. Immunity. 2010;33:736–51. doi:10.1016/j.immuni.2010.10.017.

86. Kanamori Y, Ishimaru K, Nanno M, Maki K, Ikuta K, Nariuchi H, Ishikawa H. Identification of novel lymphoid tissues in murine intestinal mucosa where clusters of c-kit+ IL-7R+ Thy1+ lympho-hemopoietic progenitors develop. J Exp Med. 1996;184:1449–59.

87. Groh V, Steinle A, Bauer S, Spies T. Recognition of stress-induced MHC molecules by intestinal epithelial gammadelta T cells. Science. 1998;279:1737–40.

88. Ferreira LM. Gammadelta T cells: innately adaptive immune cells? Int Rev Immunol. 2013;32:223–48. doi:10.3109/08830185.2013.783831.

89. Fukushima K, Masuda T, Ohtani H, Sasaki I, Funayama Y, Matsuno S, Nagura H. Immunohistochemical characterization, distribution, and ultrastructure of lymphocytes bearing T-cell receptor gamma/delta in inflammatory bowel disease. Gastroenterology. 1991;101:670–8. doi: S0016508591003104 [pii]

90. McVay LD, Li B, Biancaniello R, Creighton MA, Bachwich D, Lichtenstein G, Rombeau JL, Carding SR. Changes in human mucosal gamma delta T cell repertoire and function associated with the disease process in inflammatory bowel disease. Mol Med. 1997;3:183–203.

91. Chen Y, Chou K, Fuchs E, Havran WL, Boismenu R. Protection of the intestinal mucosa by intraepithelial gamma delta T cells. Proc Natl Acad Sci U S A. 2002;99:14338–43. doi:10.1073/pnas.212290499.

92. Hoffmann JC, Peters K, Henschke S, Herrmann B, Pfister K, Westermann J, Zeitz M. Role of T lymphocytes in rat 2,4,6-trinitrobenzene sulphonic acid (TNBS) induced colitis: increased mortality after gammadelta T cell depletion and no effect of alpha beta T cell depletion. Gut. 2001;48:489–95.

93. Inagaki-Ohara K, Chinen T, Matsuzaki G, Sasaki A, Sakamoto Y, Hiromatsu K, Nakamura-Uchiyama F, Nawa Y, Yoshimura A. Mucosal T cells bearing TCR gamma delta play a protective role in intestinal inflammation. J Immunol. 2004;173:1390–8.

94. Tsuchiya T, Fukuda S, Hamada H, Nakamura A, Kohama Y, Ishikawa H, Tsujikawa K, Yamamoto H. Role of gamma delta T cells in the inflammatory response of experimental colitis mice. J Immunol. 2003;171:5507–13.

95. Kawaguchi-Miyashita M, Shimada S, Kurosu H, Kato-Nagaoka N, Matsuoka Y, Ohwaki M, Ishikawa H, Nanno M. An accessory role of TCR gamma delta (+) cells in the exacerbation of inflammatory bowel disease in TCR alpha mutant mice. Eur J Immunol. 2001;31:980–8. doi:10.1002/1521-4141(200104)31:4<980:AID-IMMU980>3.0.CO;2-U. [pii]

96. Simpson SJ, Hollander GA, Mizoguchi E, Allen D, Bhan AK, Wang B, Terhorst C. Expression of pro-inflammatory cytokines by TCR alpha beta+ and TCR gamma delta+ T cells in an experimental model of colitis. Eur J Immunol. 1997;27:17–25. doi:10.1002/eji.1830270104.

97. Shimamoto M, Ueno Y, Tanaka S, Onitake T, Hanaoka R, Yoshioka K, Hatakeyama T, Chayama K. Selective decrease in colonic CD56(+) T and CD161(+) T cells in the inflamed mucosa of patients with ulcerative colitis. World J Gastroenterol. 2007;13:5995–6002.

98. Fuss IJ, Heller F, Boirivant M, Leon F, Yoshida M, Fichtner-Feigl S, Yang Z, Exley M, Kitani A, Blumberg RS, Mannon P, Strober W. Nonclassical CD1d-restricted NK T cells that produce IL-13 characterize an atypical Th2 response in ulcerative colitis. J Clin Invest. 2004;113:1490–7. doi:10.1172/JCI19836.

99. Vossenkamper A, Blair PA, Safinia N, Fraser LD, Das L, Sanders TJ, Stagg AJ, Sanderson JD, Taylor K, Chang F, Choong LM, D'Cruz DP, Macdonald TT, Lombardi G, Spencer J. A role for gut-associated lymphoid tissue in shaping the human B cell repertoire. J Exp Med. 2013;210:1665–74. doi:10.1084/jem.20122465.

100. Melchers F. Checkpoints that control B cell development. J Clin Invest. 2015;125:2203–10. doi:10.1172/JCI78083.

101. Pieper K, Grimbacher B, Eibel H. B-cell biology and development. J Allergy Clin Immunol. 2013;131:959–71. doi:10.1016/j.jaci.2013.01.046.

102. Brandtzaeg P, Prydz H. Direct evidence for an integrated function of J chain and secretory component in epithelial transport of immunoglobulins. Nature. 1984;311:71–3.

103. Macpherson AJ, Koller Y, McCoy KD. The bilateral responsiveness between intestinal microbes and IgA. Trends Immunol. 2015;36:460–70. doi:10.1016/j.it.2015.06.006.

104. Benveniste J, Lespinats G, Adam C, Salomon JC. Immunoglobulins in intact, immunized, and contaminated axenic mice: study of serum IgA. J Immunol. 1971;107:1647–55.

105. Benveniste J, Lespinats G, Salomon J. Serum and secretory IgA in axenic and holoxenic mice. J Immunol. 1971;107:1656–62.

106. Dominguez O, Giner MT, Alsina L, Martin MA, Lozano J, Plaza AM. Clinical phenotypes associated with selective IgA deficiency: a review of 330 cases and a proposed follow-up protocol. An Pediatr (Barc). 2012;76:261–7. doi:10.1016/j.anpedi.2011.11.006.

107. Ludvigsson JF, Neovius M, Hammarstrom L. Association between IgA deficiency & other autoimmune conditions: a population-based matched cohort study. J Clin Immunol. 2014;34:444–51. doi:10.1007/s10875-014-0009-4.

108. Singh K, Chang C, Gershwin ME. IgA deficiency and autoimmunity. Autoimmun Rev. 2014;13:163–77. doi:10.1016/j.autrev.2013.10.005.

109. Konrad A, Cong Y, Duck W, Borlaza R, Elson CO. Tight mucosal compartmentation of the murine immune response to antigens of the enteric microbiota. Gastroenterology. 2006;130:2050–9. doi:10.1053/j.gastro.2006.02.055.

110. Macpherson AJ, Uhr T. Compartmentalization of the mucosal immune responses to commensal intestinal bacteria. Ann N Y Acad Sci. 2004;1029:36–43. doi:10.1196/annals.1309.005.

111. Dubinsky MC, Lin YC, Dutridge D, Picornell Y, Landers CJ, Farrior S, Wrobel I, Quiros A, Vasiliauskas EA, Grill B, Israel D, Bahar R, Christie D, Wahbeh G, Silber G, Dallazadeh S, Shah P, Thomas D, Kelts D, Hershberg RM, Elson CO, Targan SR, Taylor KD, Rotter JI, Yang H, Western Regional Pediatric IBD Research Alliance. Serum immune responses predict rapid disease progression among children with Crohn's disease: immune responses predict disease progression. Am J Gastroenterol. 2006;101:360–7. doi: AJG456 [pii]

112. Spencer J, Dillon SB, Isaacson PG, MacDonald TT. T cell subclasses in fetal human ileum. Clin Exp Immunol. 1986;65:553–8.

113. Spencer J, MacDonald TT, Isaacson PG. Heterogeneity of nonlymphoid cells expressing HLA-D region antigens in human fetal gut. Clin Exp Immunol. 1987;67:415–24.

114. Cornes JS. Peyer's patches in the human gut. Proc R Soc Med. 1965;58:716.

115. Castellino F, Germain RN. Cooperation between CD4+ and CD8+ T cells: when, where, and how. Annu Rev Immunol. 2006;24:519–40. doi:10.1146/annurev.immunol.23.021704.115825.

116. Gunn MD, Tangemann K, Tam C, Cyster JG, Rosen SD, Williams LT. A chemokine expressed in lymphoid high endothelial venules promotes the adhesion and chemotaxis of naive T lymphocytes. Proc Natl Acad Sci U S A. 1998;95:258–63.

117. Zhu J, Yamane H, Paul WE. Differentiation of effector CD4 T cell populations (*). Annu Rev Immunol. 2010;28:445–89. doi:10.1146/annurev-immunol-030409-101212.

118. Mora JR, Bono MR, Manjunath N, Weninger W, Cavanagh LL, Rosemblatt M, Von Andrian UH. Selective imprinting of gut-homing T cells by Peyer's patch dendritic cells. Nature. 2003;424:88–93. doi:10.1038/nature01726.

119. Kugathasan S, Saubermann LJ, Smith L, Kou D, Itoh J, Binion DG, Levine AD, Blumberg RS, Fiocchi C. Mucosal T-cell immunoregulation varies in early and late inflammatory bowel disease. Gut. 2007;56:1696–705. doi: gut.2006.116467 [pii]

120. Hovhannisyan Z, Treatman J, Littman DR, Mayer L. Characterization of interleukin-17-producing regulatory T cells in inflamed intestinal mucosa from patients with inflammatory bowel diseases. Gastroenterology. 2011;140:957–65. doi:10.1053/j.gastro.2010.12.002.

121. Pariente B, Mocan I, Camus M, Dutertre CA, Ettersperger J, Cattan P, Gornet JM, Dulphy N, Charron D, Lemann M, Toubert A, Allez M. Activation of the receptor NKG2D leads to production of Th17 cytokines in CD4+ T cells of patients with Crohn's disease. Gastroenterology. 2011;141:217–26, 226.e1–2. doi:10.1053/j.gastro.2011.03.061.

122. Di Meglio P, Di Cesare A, Laggner U, Chu CC, Napolitano L, Villanova F, Tosi I, Capon F, Trembath RC, Peris K, Nestle FO. The IL23R R381Q gene variant protects against immune-mediated diseases by impairing IL-23-induced Th17 effector response in humans. PLoS One. 2011;6:e17160. doi:10.1371/journal.pone.0017160.

123. Cong Y, Brandwein SL, McCabe RP, Lazenby A, Birkenmeier EH, Sundberg JP, Elson CO. CD4+ T cells reactive to enteric bacterial antigens in spontaneously colitic C3H/HeJBir mice: increased T helper cell type 1 response and ability to transfer disease. J Exp Med. 1998;187:855–64.

124. Probert CS, Chott A, Turner JR, Saubermann LJ, Stevens AC, Bodinaku K, Elson CO, Balk SP, Blumberg RS. Persistent clonal expansions of peripheral blood CD4+ lymphocytes in chronic inflammatory bowel disease. J Immunol. 1996;157:3183–91.

125. Furfaro F, Fiorino G, Allocca M, Gilardi D, Danese S. Emerging therapeutic targets and strategies in Crohn's disease. Expert Rev Gastroenterol Hepatol. 2016;10(6):735–44. doi:10.1586/174741 24.2016.1142372.

126. Feuerer M, Hill JA, Mathis D, Benoist C. Foxp3+ regulatory T cells: differentiation, specification, subphenotypes. Nat Immunol. 2009;10:689–95. doi:10.1038/ni.1760.

127. van der Vliet HJ, Nieuwenhuis EE. IPEX as a result of mutations in FOXP3. Clin Dev Immunol. 2007;2007:89017. doi:10.1155/2007/89017.

128. Lochner M, Wang Z, Sparwasser T. The special relationship in the development and function of T helper 17 and regulatory T cells. Prog Mol Biol Transl Sci. 2015;136:99–129. doi:10.1016/bs. pmbts.2015.07.013.

129. Huber S, Gagliani N, Esplugues E, O'Connor Jr W, Huber FJ, Chaudhry A, Kamanaka M, Kobayashi Y, Booth CJ, Rudensky AY, Roncarolo MG, Battaglia M, Flavell RA. Th17 cells express interleukin-10 receptor and are controlled by Foxp3(-) and Foxp3+ regulatory CD4+ T cells in an interleukin-10-dependent manner. Immunity. 2011;34:554–65. doi:10.1016/j.immuni.2011.01.020.

130. Boden EK, Snapper SB. Regulatory T cells in inflammatory bowel disease. Curr Opin Gastroenterol. 2008;24:733–41.

131. Lord JD. Promises and paradoxes of regulatory T cells in inflammatory bowel disease. World J Gastroenterol. 2015;21:11236–45. doi:10.3748/wjg.v21.i40.11236.

132. Makita S, Kanai T, Oshima S, Uraushihara K, Totsuka T, Sawada T, Nakamura T, Koganei K, Fukushima T, Watanabe M. CD4+CD25bright T cells in human intestinal lamina propria as regulatory cells. J Immunol. 2004;173:3119–30.

133. Maul J, Loddenkemper C, Mundt P, Berg E, Giese T, Stallmach A, Zeitz M, Duchmann R. Peripheral and intestinal regulatory CD4+ CD25(high) T cells in inflammatory bowel disease. Gastroenterology. 2005;128:1868–78. doi: S0016508505005664 [pii]

134. Cario E, Gerken G, Podolsky DK. Toll-like receptor 2 enhances ZO-1-associated intestinal epithelial barrier integrity via protein kinase C. Gastroenterology. 2004;127:224–38. doi: S001650850 4007103 [pii]

135. Rakoff-Nahoum S, Paglino J, Eslami-Varzaneh F, Edberg S, Medzhitov R. Recognition of commensal microflora by toll-like receptors is required for intestinal homeostasis. Cell. 2004;118:229–41. doi:10.1016/j.cell.2004.07.002.

136. Gutierrez-Martinez E, Planes R, Anselmi G, Reynolds M, Menezes S, Adiko AC, Saveanu L, Guermonprez P. Cross-presentation of cell-associated antigens by MHC class I in dendritic cell subsets. Front Immunol. 2015;6:363. doi:10.3389/fimmu.2015.00363.

137. Voedisch S, Koenecke C, David S, Herbrand H, Forster R, Rhen M, Pabst O. Mesenteric lymph nodes confine dendritic cell-mediated dissemination of Salmonella enterica serovar Typhimurium and limit systemic disease in mice. Infect Immun. 2009;77:3170–80. doi:10.1128/IAI.00272-09.

138. Nanthakumar NN, Fusunyan RD, Sanderson I, Walker WA. Inflammation in the developing human intestine: a possible pathophysiologic contribution to necrotizing enterocolitis. Proc Natl Acad Sci U S A. 2000;97:6043–8. doi: 97/11/6043 [pii]

139. Mackie RI, Sghir A, Gaskins HR. Developmental microbial ecology of the neonatal gastrointestinal tract. Am J Clin Nutr. 1999;69:1035S–45S.

140. Mellander L, Carlsson B, Jalil F, Soderstrom T, Hanson LA. Secretory IgA antibody response against *Escherichia coli* antigens in infants in relation to exposure. J Pediatr. 1985;107:430–3.

141. Fadel S, Sarzotti M. Cellular immune responses in neonates. Int Rev Immunol. 2000;19:173–93.

142. Hassiotou F, Geddes DT. Immune cell-mediated protection of the mammary gland and the infant during breastfeeding. Adv Nutr. 2015;6:267–75. doi:10.3945/an.114.007377.

143. Adderson EE. Antibody repertoires in infants and adults: effects of T-independent and T-dependent immunizations. Springer Semin Immunopathol. 2001;23:387–403.

144. Hill DA, Grundmeier RW, Ram G, Spergel JM. The epidemiologic characteristics of healthcare provider-diagnosed eczema, asthma, allergic rhinitis, and food allergy in children: a retrospective cohort study. BMC Pediatr. 2016;16:133. doi:10.1186/s12887-016-0673-z.

145. Karlsson MR, Rugtveit J, Brandtzaeg P. Allergen-responsive CD4+CD25+ regulatory T cells in children who have outgrown cow's milk allergy. J Exp Med. 2004;199:1679–88. doi:10.1084/jem.20032121.

146. Namork E, Stensby BA. Peanut sensitization pattern in Norwegian children and adults with specific IgE to peanut show age related differences. Allergy Asthma Clin Immunol. 2015;11:32-015-0095-8. doi:10.1186/s13223-015-0095-8.eCollection 2015

147. Turfkruyer M, Rekima A, Macchiaverni P, Le Bourhis L, Muncan V, van den Brink GR, Tulic MK, Verhasselt V. Oral tolerance is inefficient in neonatal mice due to a physiological vitamin A deficiency. Mucosal Immunol. 2016;9(2):479–91. doi:10.1038/mi.2015.114.

148. Bamias G, Martin C, Mishina M, Ross WG, Rivera-Nieves J, Marini M, Cominelli F. Proinflammatory effects of TH2 cytokines in a murine model of chronic small intestinal inflammation. Gastroenterology. 2005;128:654–66. doi: S0016508504021584 [pii]

149. Spencer DM, Veldman GM, Banerjee S, Willis J, Levine AD. Distinct inflammatory mechanisms mediate early versus late colitis in mice. Gastroenterology. 2002;122:94–105. doi: S0016508502653715 [pii]

Cytokines and Inflammatory Bowel Disease

Edwin F. de Zoeten and Ivan J. Fuss

Introduction

The etiology of inflammatory bowel diseases (IBD) is generally described as multifactorial including genetic predisposition, dysbiosis, and a dysregulated immune response. The immune response is the only one of these that is currently amenable to therapy. Understanding the factors that go into the activation of inflammation and those that perpetuate this effect is improving greatly. With this mastery we are able to define the cytokines that are important in the etiology of IBD. Over the past 20 years, many of the newest and arguably the most successful therapies for Crohn disease (CD) and ulcerative colitis (UC) have been due to an increased understanding of the immune response and specifically the cytokines essential to this response.

As stated above, IBD is in part due to a dysregulated or an inappropriate immune reaction, which has been thought in part to be against to the microflora of the gut. Upon activation of the immune system, cytokines and chemokines, which are proteins produced by the cells involved in the immune response, are produced and trigger a cascade of downstream reactions. These cytokines are increasingly being defined as important molecules in the pathogenesis of IBD as well as putative and known targets for the therapy of IBD.

With the advent of murine models of mucosal inflammation, a great deal of knowledge has been acquired which has advanced our understanding of inflammation in IBD. In these models, it has been initially noted that the inflamma-

tion is due either to an excessive Th1 T-cell response or an excessive Th2 T-cell responses, with the former characterized by increased IL-1, IL-2, IL-6, IL-12, IL-18, IFN-γ, and TNF-α production and the latter by increased IL-4, IL-5, IL-10, and/or IL-13 production. An example of a murine Th1 colitis is that induced by the haptenating agent TNBS [1], a colitis in which the predominant immune response is dominated by IL-12, IFN-γ, and TNF-α. This correlates with human studies, which have shown increased levels of TNF-α, IFN-γ, IL-1, and IL-6 in the intestinal tissues and the peripheral blood of CD [2]. Similar to what has been observed in UC patients [3, 4], the oxazolone model of colitis in mice, which has similar histologic features as those seen in UC, is associated with a Th2 response that is dominated by IL-13. Thus, murine models have given important insights into the IBD entities; however, questions of whether CD and UC are "true" Th1- or Th2-mediated disease processes remain. These will be discussed later in this chapter.

In the immune cascade, cytokines help to determine the nature of the immune response; they can act in a dual nature as either pro- (IL-1, IL-6, TNF-α) or anti-inflammatory (IL-4, IL-5, IL-10, TGF-β) molecules. They can affect the synthesis or secretion of reactive oxygen species, nitric oxide, leukotrienes, platelet-activating factor, and prostaglandins. In addition, they can have differing qualities depending on when they are present in the inflammatory cascade. Finally, it is important to understand that pro- and anti-inflammatory responses are required to maintain the integrity of the intestinal mucosa due to the environment in which it exists. The intestinal mucosa is constantly bombarded with antigens from food, commensal bacteria and pathogenic bacteria, and therefore it is important to be able to mount an inflammatory response to rid itself of harmful bacteria, yet, at the same time, the mucosal immune system must be able to regulate itself either by the action of specific regulatory cells or by the action of cytokines such as IL-4, IL-5, IL-10, TGF-β, IL-1RA, and TNF-α.

E.F. de Zoeten, MD, PhD
Childrens Hospital Colorado, Digestive Health Institute, Denver, CO, USA

I.J. Fuss, MD (✉)
National Institute of Allergy Immunology and infectious Disease, Mucosal Immunity Section, National Institutes of Health, Bethesda, MD, USA
e-mail: ifuss@niaid.nih.gov

© Springer International Publishing AG 2017
P. Mamula et al. (eds.), *Pediatric Inflammatory Bowel Disease*, DOI 10.1007/978-3-319-49215-5_3

Pro-inflammatory Cytokines

Tumor Necrosis Factor Alpha

For most gastroenterologists, TNF-α is the most recognized cytokine due to the increasing use of the monoclonal anti-TNF-α antibodies, infliximab, adalimumab, certolizumab, and golimumab, for the treatment of CD and UC. TNF-α is secreted by macrophages, monocytes, neutrophils, T cells, and NK cells following their stimulation by bacterial lipopolysaccharides. CD4+ T-lymphocytes secrete TNF-α, while CD8+ T cells do not. The synthesis of TNF-α is induced by many different stimuli including interferons, IL-2, and GM-CSF. The production of TNF-α is inhibited by IL-6 and TGF-β.

TNF-α is an agonist of the p38 and c-Jun N-terminal kinase (NK) cascades, two important signaling pathways of the MAP kinase family involved in the generation of the inflammatory responses [5]. It is a potent pro-inflammatory cytokine that exerts its stimulatory effect on cells that produce IFN-γ. Indeed, TNF-α in synergy with factors from non-lymphocyte lamina propria mononuclear cells can act with prostaglandin E2 to stimulate IL-12-mediated T-cell production of IFN-γ. In resting macrophages, TNF-α induces the synthesis of IL-1 and prostaglandin E2, which can act in concert to potentiate the inflammatory cascade. TNF-α can also enhance the proliferation of T cells induced by various stimuli in the absence of IL-2; in fact some subpopulations of T cells only respond to IL-2 in the presence of TNF-α. Beyond its effect on the immune response, TNF-α activates osteoclasts and thus induces bone resorption, and this effect may be associated with decreased bone mineral density in patients with CD.

Although TNF-α is required for normal host immune responses, the overexpression can have severe pathologic consequences as exemplified by mice in which the overexpression of TNF by a transgene is associated with a severe colitis [6].

In animal models, TNF-α knockout mice do not develop significant colitis [7], and as proof of principle that TNF-α is important for the pathogenesis of IBD, TNF-α-neutralizing antibodies have been shown to be effective in ameliorating intestinal inflammation. Associated human studies have reported elevated levels of TNF-α in serum, stool, and mucosal tissue [8, 9] correlating with clinical and laboratory indices of intestinal activity. Furthermore, dramatic effects have been noted in clinical studies in patients with Crohn disease treated with infliximab [10, 11]. These effects have been observed in both disease amelioration and induction of clinical remission. Important for the understanding of some of the critical side effects of infliximab, TNF-α mediates a part of the cell-mediated immunity against obligate and facultative bacteria and parasites by stimulating phagocytosis and the synthesis of superoxide dismutase in macrophages. It confers protection against *Listeria monocytogenes* infections and tuberculosis. Anti-TNF-α antibodies have been shown to weaken the ability of mice to cope with these infections. Infection with these organisms is a possible risk of using anti-TNF-α monoclonal antibody therapy in the treatment of IBD and a reason that patients are screened for tuberculosis prior to initiation of therapy with infliximab.

Interferon-Gamma

IFN-γ is produced mainly by CD4+, CD8+ T-lymphocytes, and natural killer cells activated by antigens and mitogens. IFN-γ synergizes with TNF-α and in inhibiting the proliferation of various cell types; however, the main biological activity of IFN-γ appears to be immunomodulatory in contrast to the other interferons (IFN-α or IFN-β), which are mainly antiviral. IL-2 and IFN-γ appear to be intricately interwoven in their functions. In T-helper cells, IL-2 induces the synthesis of IFN-γ and other cytokines. IFN-γ acts synergistically with IL-1 and IL-2 and appears to be required for the expression of IL-2 receptors (CD25) on the cell surface of T-lymphocytes. Blocking of the IL-2 receptor by specific antibodies inhibits the synthesis of IFN-γ. IFN-γ is a modulator of T-cell growth and functional differentiation, a growth-promoting factor for T-lymphocytes, and it potentiates the response of these cells to growth factors. Most importantly, IFN-γ can increase the expression of MHC class molecules allowing greater antigenic recognition. Furthermore, it can increase permeability at epithelial tight junction barriers, thereby allowing further antigenic exposure [12]. Finally, in concert with TNF-α, IFN-γ can cause direct tissue destruction as it increases local inflammation [12, 13].

IFN-γ secretion is one of the few cytokines that correlates with severity of disease in patients with CD. As a known pro-inflammatory cytokine, it would appear to be an obvious choice to target for treatment of IBD. IFN-γ has been targeted in CD using fontolizumab, a humanized monoclonal antibody against IFN-γ [14, 15]. In studies using these antibodies, positive results were found in patients with moderate-to-severe CD when compared to placebo. Although the studies did not reach statistical significance, the results did indicate a trend toward effect. This suggests a potential benefit of blocking IFN-γ in patients with CD.

Interleukin-1

This cytokine consists of IL-1α and IL-1β subunits, which both are produced by monocytes, macrophages, and endothelial cells. In addition to these pro-inflammatory cytokines, there is an IL-1 receptor antagonist (IL-1RA) produced by intestinal epithelial cells, which is capable of inhibiting the pro-inflammatory actions of IL-1 by binding the IL-1 receptor and competitively blocking the interaction with IL-1. IL-1RA is considered to be one intestinal mechanism for downregulation of the immune response and has been shown to be elevated in the serum of patients with CD. Stimulation of IL-1RA secretion is activated by IL-1, forming a negative feedback loop.

IL-1α and IL-1β are essentially biologically equivalent pleiotropic factors that act locally and systemically. IL-1 has a multitude of effector functions, some of which are mediated indirectly by the induction of the synthesis of other mediators including ACTH, PGE_2, IL-6, and IL-8 (a chemotactic cytokine in the chemokine family). The main biological activity of IL-1 is the stimulation of T-helper cells, which are induced to secrete IL-2 and to express IL-2 receptors. IL-1 can also act on B cells, promoting their proliferation and the synthesis of immunoglobulins. IL-1 stimulates the proliferation and activation of other immune cells such as NK cells, fibroblasts, and thymocytes. The IL-1-mediated proliferative effects can be inhibited by the suppressive cytokine, TGF-β.

The synthesis of IL-1 can be induced by other cytokines including TNF-α, IFN-α, and β or γ and also by bacterial endotoxins and viruses. Furthermore, IL-1 activity is not limited to stimulation of T cells, but it also promotes the adhesion of neutrophils, monocytes, T cells, and B cells by enhancing the expression of adhesion molecules such as ICAM-1 (intercellular adhesion molecule) and ELAM (endothelial leukocyte adhesion molecule). All of which can contribute to the pathogenesis of CD. IL-1 is also a strong chemoattractant for leukocytes, as demonstrated by the local accumulation of neutrophils at the site of injection of tissue with IL-1. Beyond activation by other cytokines, IL-1β is secreted in response to select microbial components via the NLR inflammasomes, specifically *P. mirabilis* [16]. This and other supporting data demonstrate a strong link between the microbiome and modulation of the immune response in the gut.

Finally, in combination with TNF-α, IL-1 appears to be involved in the generation of lytic bone lesions. IL-1 activates osteoclasts, thereby suppressing the formation of new bone, suggesting another etiology for decreased bone density in CD. Low concentrations of IL-1, however, can promote new bone growth.

IL-1 was one of the first cytokines targeted for therapy in animal colitis models. In these studies, administration of IL-1RA led to amelioration of colitis, in a rabbit model. Thus, it was also one of the first demonstrations that blockade of a single cytokine could be effective in therapy of colitis [17]. In patients with IBD, increased serum levels of IL-1 are seldom detected. However, in intestinal lesions in patients with both CD and UC, IL-1 levels are elevated [18]. IL-1RA is a possible intestinal mechanism for downregulation of the immune response and is elevated in the serum of patients

with CD. IL-1RA determines the biological effects of IL-1, as increased concentrations of this mediator will decrease IL-1 activity. In the inflammatory lesions of IBD patients, levels of this mediator are increased, although not as much as IL-1, leading to a disproportionate increase in IL-1 activity [19] overcoming competitive inhibition.

Interleukin-2

IL-2 is a major T-cell growth factor, secreted by activated T cells, and acts via the high-affinity IL-2 receptor (CD25) on T cells. This binding to CD25 promotes cell proliferation. Under physiological conditions, IL-2 is produced mainly by CD4+ T-lymphocytes following cell activation. Resting cells do not produce IL-2. In T-helper cells, IL-2 induces the synthesis of IFN-γ and other cytokines. IFN-γ acts synergistically with IL-1 and IL-2 and appears to be required for the expression of IL-2 receptors on the cell surface of T-lymphocytes. Blocking of the IL-2 receptor by specific antibodies also inhibits the synthesis of IFN-γ. IFN-γ in return is a modulator of T-cell growth and functional differentiation. It is a growth-promoting factor for T-lymphocytes and potentiates the response of these cells to growth factors.

IL-2 is a growth factor for all subpopulations of T-lymphocytes including importantly suppressive T regulatory (Treg) cells. It is an antigen-unspecific proliferation factor for T cells that induces cell cycle progression in resting cells and thus allows clonal expansion of activated T-lymphocytes.

In patients with CD, it has been demonstrated in many studies that IL-2 secretion from lamina propria cells is decreased as compared to normal patient samples. Daclizumab, a humanized monoclonal antibody to CD25, produced in an effort to block the binding of IL-2 to the IL-2R, was tested in patients with UC and initially appeared promising in a small open-label study [20], but upon testing in a placebo-controlled study, the therapy did not show efficacy [21]. This effect could be related to the fact that IL-2R (CD25) is also present on T regulatory cells. The inhibition of binding of IL-2 to its receptor present on Treg cells thereby inhibits the proliferation of these cells, which are important in downregulation of the immune response. This highlights a common problem in the targeting of the cytokine pathway for treatment of inflammatory diseases, in that cytokines frequently have multiple effects and can function in both a pro-inflammatory as well as an anti-inflammatory capacity.

Interleukin-6

IL-6 is a pleiotropic cytokine considered to be a major player in inflammation, regulation of T-cell responses, and apoptosis.

Many different cell types produce IL-6. The main sources in vivo are stimulated monocytes, fibroblasts, endothelial cells, macrophages, T cells, and B-lymphocytes. IL-6 is a B-cell differentiation factor in vivo and in vitro and an activation factor for T cells. In the presence of IL-2, IL-6 induces the differentiation of mature and immature T cells into cytotoxic T cells. IL-6 also induces the proliferation of thymocytes and likely plays a role in the development of thymic T cells. Most significantly IL-6 and TGF-β together can induce the development of the inflammatory T-helper-17 (Th17) cell lineage. Finally, in opposition, if IL-6 is present, there is decreased propensity to development of Foxp3-positive Treg cells.

Interestingly, IL-6 levels are increased in the serum of patients with active CD and UC compared to normal controls. A study looking at a known functional polymorphism of the IL-6 gene and the site of disease in CD patients did not demonstrate an association of IL-6 functional polymorphisms with CD or protection from CD. It did demonstrate that patients with the high-producer genotype were more likely to have ileocolonic disease, while those with the low-producer genotype had primarily colonic-type disease, whereas those with intermediate-producer genotype were more likely to have isolated ileal disease. These studies indicated an association of IL-6 production and site of disease [22]. The activity of IL-6 has made it an obvious target for clinical trials not only due to its pro-inflammatory effects but also due to its involvement in T-cell apoptosis [23]. A pilot study was performed [24] to investigate safety and efficacy of a humanized anti-IL-6R monoclonal antibody in patients with CD. This target appeared to be promising in these studies with 80% of the patients treated for 12 weeks demonstrating clinical improvement as compared to 31% treated with placebo.

Interleukin-12

IL-12 is a heterodimeric molecule composed of IL-12 p40 and IL-12 p35 subunits. IL-12 is secreted by antigen-presenting cells such as monocytes, macrophages, and dendritic cells and to a lesser extent by NK cells. The most powerful inducers of IL-12 are bacteria, bacterial products, and parasites.

IL-12 is a pro-inflammatory cytokine that is important in the differentiation of naïve T cells into IFN-γ-producing pathogenic CD4+ Th1 cells [13, 25]. In peripheral lymphocytes of the Th1 T-helper cell type, IL-12 induces the synthesis of IFN-γ, IL-2, and TNF-α. TNF-α also appears to be involved in mediating the effects of IL-12 on natural killer cells since an antibody directed against TNF-α inhibits the effects of IL-12. IL-12 and TNF-α are costimulators for IFN-γ production with IL-12 maximizing the IFN-γ response; the production of IL-12, TNF-α, and IFN-γ is inhibited by

IL-10. In Th2 T-helper cells, IL-12 reduces the synthesis of IL-4, IL-5, and IL-10.

This cytokine is considered a driving force behind chronic intestinal inflammation. Evidence for this comes forth from murine models of colitis by demonstrating that disease development could be inhibited by treatment with anti-IL-12 p40 monoclonal antibodies [25]. In human studies, this master T-cell-differentiating cytokine has been shown to be produced in large amounts in the intestines of patients with CD [26]. In addition, this cytokine has been targeted in human CD using various anti-IL-12 p40 monoclonal antibodies and found to be effective in phase 2 and phase 3 multicenter trials [27, 28]. In the latter, significant clinical response and remission could be achieved in patients with moderate-to-severe active Crohn disease. Furthermore, the phase 3 UNITI trial also included a cohort of patients which failed TNF-α mAb, with significant response and remission rates demonstrated in this patient population. The long-lasting clinical effect observed may be due in part to the induction of apoptosis of the inflammatory effector cells. These studies suggest that in addition to IL-2, IL-12 is a necessary growth and survival factor for T cells [29]. It also brings forth the point that the mechanism of action of the various anti-biologic therapies lies not only in their capability to neutralize their respective cytokines but due to their ability to induce cell death of the inciting inflammatory effector cells. Interestingly, the p40 subunit is also found to be a portion of another significant pro-inflammatory master cytokine, IL-23. The positive effects observed of the anti-IL-12 p40 antibody may indeed be due to both the effect on IL-12 and IL-23 [26]. Further studies in models of colitis indicate that IL-23 is important in the inflammatory response in IBD in that it plays a significant role in the maintenance of Th-17 effective inflammatory cells [30].

Interleukin-17

The discovery of the Th17 cell lineage revolutionized our understanding of IBD pathogenesis. The Th17 type secretes IL-17 and IL-22. IL-17 has been associated with multiple immune regulatory functions. Most notably, IL-17 is involved in inducing and mediating pro-inflammatory responses. IL-17 induces the production of many other cytokines, such as IL-6, G-CSF, GM-CSF, IL-1β, TGF-β, and TNF-α; chemokines including IL-8, GRO-α, and MCP-1; and prostaglandins (e.g., PGE$_2$) from many cell types (fibroblasts, endothelial cells, epithelial cells, and macrophages). IL-17 expression is stimulated and/or maintained by IL-23 expression. These IL-17-expressing cells appear to be derived by a subset of CD4+ T Cells called T-helper-17 (Th17) cells, which are distinct from Th1 and Th2 cell lineage and need to be derived in the presence of IL-23; in addition IL-17 may be derived to a lesser degree from monocytes and neutrophils [31]. Increased expression of IL-17 has been reported in the intestinal mucosa of IBD patients [32]. Some reports suggest that IL-17 alone is capable of inducing autoimmune tissue reactivity, whereas other groups suggest that IL-17 and IFN-γ synergize to stimulate this autoimmune reactivity [33, 34]. In these studies it was indicated that T cells and monocytes in the intestinal mucosa produce IL-17. IL-17 binds to the IL-17 receptor on endothelial cells and epithelial cells to promote secretion of pro-inflammatory substances that recruit inflammatory cells to the site [35]. In studies where the gene for either IL-17A or IL-17F was deleted, mice continued to develop severe colitis, but when RORγτ (the transcription factor important for expression of all IL-17) genes were deleted, minimal inflammation occurred in colitis models which suggests that the different forms of IL-17 are redundant, but IL-17 together are important for the development of colitis. Unfortunately, as noted with other cytokines, it appears that IL-17 is not just simply an inflammatory cytokine. Recent murine studies in both chemically induced colitis and adoptive transfer colitis indicate that IL-17 plays a complex role in the inflammatory response. These studies showed that transfer of IL-17-deficient T cells into an immunodeficient mouse led to more rapid onset of colitis than transfer of cells from WT mice. One explanation of this could be that Th1 cells bear IL-17 receptors, and signaling through these receptors inhibits Th1 differentiation by suppressing the transcription factor Tbet. Thus, IL-17 may have pro- and anti-inflammatory properties.

As a result of these roles, the IL-17 family has been linked to many immune/autoimmune-related diseases including rheumatoid arthritis, asthma, and lupus. IL-17 expression is increased in patients with a variety of allergic and autoimmune diseases, such as RA, MS, inflammatory bowel disease (IBD), and asthma, suggesting the contribution of IL-17 to the induction and/or development of such diseases. It must be stated that IL-17 may not appear to be the main cytokine important for inflammation in IBD in that studies evaluating the effect of anti-IL-17A antibody secukinumab for the treatment of Crohn disease have been disappointing and do not appear to have a therapeutic effect. In a realm that is of interest in the development and progression of IBD, IL-17 has been identified as a key mediator of fibrosis in multiple organs including the intestine. As fibrosis is an important issue in IBD, this makes understanding of IL-17 even more critical. Recently, Biancheri et al. demonstrated that IL-17 is upregulated in strictured tissue and that myofibroblasts express receptors for IL-17A [36]. It remains the current hypothesis that while IL-17 plays a role in inflammation in Crohn disease, the role is complex, and it appears that Th1 cytokines such as IFN-γ may play a greater role.

Interleukin-23

IL-23 and IL-17 changed our view of the cytokines important in the development of IBD. Multiple murine colitis studies demonstrated that development of colitis appeared to be more dependent on IL-23 than on IL-12. IL-23 is a pro-inflammatory cytokine secreted by activated dendritic cells and macrophages that shares structural homology with IL-12; specifically it is composed of the p40 subunit and a unique p19 chain. Initial studies indicating an ameliorating effect of an anti-p40 antibody in murine models of inflammation were felt to be due to its effect on IL-12. However, this effect was reevaluated, and studies suggest that this ameliorating effect may be due to a decrease in IL-23 mediating effect. In these studies, mice deficient in the p19 subunit of IL-23 displayed attenuated inflammation in colitis models, whereas mice deficient in the p35 chain of IL-12 (therefore deficient in IL-12 but not IL-23) had no effect on colitis. These studies together suggest that the initial effects observed with anti-p40 in a variety of animal models may have been due to a decrease in IL-23. IL-23 promotes and stabilizes a novel subset of CD4+ T cells (Th17 cells) that is characterized by the production of IL-17, IL-6, and TNF-α and has been associated with autoimmune tissue inflammation [33]. Without IL-23, it has been noted that Th17 cells produce the anti-inflammatory cytokine IL-10. The exact mechanism by which IL-23 promotes the Th17 response has not been defined, but it appears TGF-β and IL-6 are important for the commitment into a Th17 cell, and IL-23 is important for the proliferation of this cell type [37, 38]. Furthermore, recent studies may indicate a separate role for IL-23 in the occurrence of IL-17-expressing cells [39], whereby IL-23 may have a direct effect on regulatory T-cell development. Thus, in these animal studies, mice that lack IL-23 fail to develop colitis; however, this may not be secondary to the inability to produce IL-17 but rather because of the development of a dominant regulatory T-cell response. Moreover, Sunjino et al. demonstrated a dominant role for T regulatory cells in the suppression of colitis by blocking differentiation of Th17 into alternative Th1 type cells, therefore establishing a significant role for this suppressive pathway [40].

IL-23 effect is not limited to Th17 cells but appears to have an effect of the innate immune system inducing monocytes and macrophages to produce pro-inflammatory cytokines such as IL-1, IL-6, and TNF-α as well. In murine colitis studies where either IL-23 or the IL-23 receptor was deleted, it was shown that IL-23 plays a major role in the development of colitis. These studies also have shown an increase in the number of anti-inflammatory Treg cells suggesting that IL-23 may play a role in suppressing this cell type.

In addition, in a genome-wide association study in adults [41] as well as in a pediatric population [42], the IL-23 receptor (IL-23R) gene on chromosome 1p31 has been shown to have a highly significant association with CD; specifically, an uncommon coding variant of the IL-23R gene was shown to confer protection. These data indicate that the IL-23 pathway may have a causal link to CD.

Interleukin-18

This cytokine initially identified as interferon-γ-inducing factor (IGIF) is similar to the IL-1 family in structure, processing, receptor, and pro-inflammatory properties. It is produced by intestinal epithelial cells and induces other pro-inflammatory cytokines and Th1 polarization. IL-12 and IL-18 have a synergistic relationship. Their production by activated macrophages appears to drive the development of Th1 CD4+ T-cell predominance in the intestinal mucosa. Recombinant IL-18 alone is able to induce a proliferative response in vitro in freshly isolated mucosal lymphocytes from patients with CD. The synergistic effect is likely due to the upregulation of the IL-18 receptor by IL-12.

Intestinal mucosa from patients with CD have been evaluated and found to have increased expression of IL-18 [43], and this was also noted in experimental murine colitis [44]. Tissues from CD patients have been shown in vitro to decrease suppressive cytokine IL-10 expression after treatment with IL-18 indicating one possible effector mechanism. IL-12 and IL-18 together appear to synergize to drive the lamina propria lymphocytes into a Th1-type response. IL-12 appears to induce increased IL-18 expression, thus the synergistic effect [45, 46]. Using models of colitis, multiple laboratories have tried to block IL-18, and the results indicate that IL-18 may have a role in the initiation of intestinal inflammation, while others have shown that IL-18 acts to reduce inflammation.

An additional source for IL-18 production is the inflammasome pathway. The role, however, of the inflammasome to induce secretion of cytokines such as IL-1β and IL-18 is complex. While IL-1β appears to function as a pro-inflammatory cytokine in murine models of colitis [47–50], the function of IL-18 remains a duality. Thus, whereas studies have demonstrated that IL-18 is necessary for the induction of DSS colitis [47, 51, 52], further studies have shown that a deficiency in IL-18 secretion affords mice more susceptibility rather than more resistance to DSS colitis [44, 53, 54]. This correlated to studies which show that a deficiency in NLRP3 inflammasome pathway leads to increased susceptibility to DSS colitis, which appears to be secondary to decreased IL-18 expression [44, 53]. Thus, although IL-18 may have pro-inflammatory properties, it also has an important role in epithelial cell restitution and repair after injury [54, 55].

In a separate but similar role IL-6, a cytokine that can also affect epithelial cells acts as a tumor promoter by affecting the carcinogenicity of these intestinal epithelial cells [56]. IL-18 can have effects on these cell types since IL-18$^{-/-}$ and IL-18R1$^{-/-}$ mice display increased susceptibility to DSS colitis-associated cancer [54]. This effect of IL-18 may be through the cytokine IL-22 and its IL-binding protein (22 bp), the latter a decoy protein that neutralizes IL-22. The interplay between these various cytokine pathways is shown by the fact that IL-22 and IL-22 bp can regulate epithelial cell growth/repair and control tumorigenesis, while these aforementioned factors can be regulated by IL-18 and the NLRP3 or NLRP6 inflammasomes [55].

Interleukin-13

IL-13 can have a dual functional role in that it can down-modulate macrophage activity, reducing the production of pro-inflammatory cytokines (IL-1, IL-6, IL-8, IL-10, IL-12) and chemokines (MIP-1, MCP) in response to IFN-γ or bacterial lipopolysaccharides. IL-13 can also enhance the production of the IL-1 receptor antagonist and decrease the production of nitric oxide by activated macrophages, leading to a decrease in parasiticidal activity. Yet, it appears that IL-13 is important in the development of Th2-type colitis such as the murine model of colitis oxazolone and its human component, UC [57]. In these studies, it was found that IL-13 produced by natural killer (NK) T cells, when neutralized, led to decreased inflammation in the oxazolone model of colitis. Furthermore and most importantly, in human studies, these IL-13-secreting NK T cells exhibited an increased cytolytic function against epithelial cell lines. Moreover, IL-13 itself has been shown to be directly toxic to epithelial cells as well as to cause increased permeability barrier functional defects [58]. Thus, in the oxazolone model of colitis and its human counterpart ulcerative colitis, it is believed that IL-13-secreting NK T cells play a role in the etiology of this disease entity. This is in contrast to the Th1/Th17 disease process discussed in the pathogenesis of CD. Although IL-13 can function as a pro-inflammatory molecule in UC, it may also play a role in innate tumor surveillance pathways. In studies by Schiechl et al., tumor formation was accompanied by the coappearance of F4/80+CD11bhigh Gr1low macrophages, cells that undergo differentiation and activation by IL-13 and subsequently produce a source of tumor-promoting factor such as IL-6 after such activation [59]. In a similar vein, F4/80+CD11bhigh Gr1intermediate macrophages after activation through IL-13 produced increased amounts of TGF-beta, a cytokine that inhibits tumor immunosurveillance.

Finally, clinical trials aimed at the IL-13 pathway have been performed. Although these trials did not meet their primary endpoints, they did reveal interesting findings concerning the IL-13 signaling pathway. In an initial trial, anrukinzumab, an agent that binds to the IL-4/IL-13Rα1 complex and blocks signaling of IL-13 via the IL-13Rα1 pathway, was utilized [60]. As noted by the authors, these complexes consist of study drug and IL-13, which may be subsequently cleared through another IL 13 receptor pathway, IL-13Rα2. More recent findings demonstrate that the latter IL-13 receptor pathway, IL-13Rα2, and not the IL-13Rα1 pathway appears to be involved in the activation and secretion of IL-13 in ulcerative colitis [61]. Thus, the decreased efficacy of this trap molecule antibody directed against the IL-13Rα1 pathway may be expected based upon the former findings. The dose-response curves demonstrate some efficacy at low doses but not that at higher levels. This might be explained by clearance of IL-13 initially but subsequently binding and activation of the aforementioned IL-13Rα2 pathway leading to decreased responses at higher doses. Finally, another monoclonal antibody, tralokinumab, directed at IL-13 itself had a significant remission rate as compared to placebo but did not achieve significance for response rate [62]. These results may demonstrate that a subgroup of patients may achieve a remission response; however, additional screening markers are necessary to evaluate these responder patients.

Interleukin-33

IL-33 is part of the IL-1 family and is expressed in various non-hematopoietic cells as well as in inflammatory cells (e.g., macrophages and dendritic cells) [63]. Similar to other IL-1 family members such as IL-1 and IL-18, IL-33 was originally thought to be synthesized as a 30-kDa precursor molecule then subsequently cleaved by caspase-1 upon inflammasome activation to its mature/bioactive 18-kDa form [64]. However, more recent studies have suggested that the full-length 30-kDa IL-33 (f-IL-33) is the bioactive form with decreased active forms (20–22 kDa) resulting from caspase cleavage [65, 66]. In addition, further reports indicate that the bioactive form may not depend upon any caspase cleavage [67]. Thus, IL-33 bioactive form can be regulated by cleavage through proteases, in particular neutrophil serine proteases cathepsin G or elastase c, both released from neutrophils. Therefore, the inflammatory milieu may play a role in the generation of highly active mature forms of IL-33.

The IL-1 receptor-related protein, ST2, is the IL-33 receptor and exists in two different splice variants. ST2L is a transmembrane receptor that confers IL-33's biological effects, and sST2 is a soluble molecule that serves as a decoy receptor [64]. Signaling through ST2 receptor can drive cytokine production in a host of cell populations, which include type 2 innate lymphoid cells (ILCs) (natural helper cells, nuocytes), T-helper lymphocytes, mast cells, basophils, eosinophils, and natural killer (NK) and invariant natural killer

T (iNK T) cells [68, 69]. Thus, the IL-33/ST2 axis appears to play an important role in several chronic inflammatory disorders through the induction of Th2 and/or Th17 cytokines responses such as IL-5, IL-13, and IL-17 [63, 64, 70, 71].

Increased IL-33 production has been noted in murine models of colitis (i.e., oxazolone colitis, SAMP1-yit) as well as in ulcerative colitis [72, 73]. Further studies of active UC patients reveal IL-33 production was localized to intestinal epithelial cells (IEC) and cells in colonic inflammatory infiltrates [70–73]. This increase appears to be regulated in part by TNF-α as the latter can upregulate both IL-33 and sST2 and treatment of patients with anti-TNF-α monoclonal antibody decreases circulating levels of these molecules [70].

Interleukin-9

IL-9 is another Th2-related cytokine that appears to be involved in IBD pathogenesis. Production of IL-9 is induced in naïve T cells by TGF-β and IL-4 in concert with additional cytokines (i.e., IL-1β and IL-25). This cytokine was initially identified as a Th2-type cytokine by its ability to induce Th2 inflammation in disease states such as parasitic infection, allergy, or autoimmune states [74–76]. Recent studies have elucidated the role of IL-9 in IBD, which demonstrated increased levels of this cytokine in UC (and to a lesser extent in CD) [77]. Studies of the murine colitis model, oxazolone colitis, revealed that mice lacking IL-9 develop no or reduced disease. However, mice deficient in IL-9 also manifest amelioration of several Th1/Th17 murine colitis models, including cell transfer colitis; thus, IL-9 contributes to inflammation in a variety of Th1/Th2/Th17 intestinal inflammatory conditions [78]. The mechanism by which IL-9 may have broad effects on intestinal inflammation is the ability to alter epithelial barrier function via effects on tight junction proteins.

Tumor Necrosis Factor-Like Ligand (TL1A)

TL1A is a cytokine that appears to contribute to intestinal inflammation; however, it does not appear to be uniquely associated with Th1/Th2 or Th17 cells and appears to be within the category of cytokines that can bridge the T-cell spectrum. This cytokine is secreted by T cells, antigen-presenting cells, and endothelial cells [79]. Studies involved in elucidating the exact function of TL1A indicate that TL1A enhances baseline T- and B-cell activation by T-cell receptor activation.

The significance of TL1A to intestinal inflammation is demonstrated in the studies where exogenous administration of TL1A to mice with dextran sodium sulfate (DSS) colitis increased both Th1 and Th17 responses. Furthermore, the administration of antibodies to TL1A led to the amelioration of colitis in the DSS and TNBS model of intestinal inflammation [80, 81]. While effects on Th1 and Th17 production have been associated with TL1A, in recent studies of mice carrying a transgene for TL1A, intestinal inflammation of the small intestine developed, which appeared dependent on IL-13 [81]. In separate studies, TL1A was found to inhibit the induction of new FoxP3⁺ regulatory cells and/or the expansion of existing subsets [82]. Thus, these studies suggest that TL1A is a cytokine that optimizes both Th1/Th2 and Th17 responses either through direct effects on these cell lineages or through effects on suppressor T regulatory cell pathway.

The costimulatory activities of TL1A induce cytokines associated with inflammation, such as IL-2, IFN-γ, IL-13, and IL-5 from T cells, while the latter (IL-5/IL-13) can also be generated from innate lymphoid cells (ILC type 2) [83–87]. TL1A can also costimulate additional intestinal innate lymphoid cell groups (ILC3), with divergent effects. In combination with the ILC stimulatory cytokine IL-23, TL1A can enhance the secretion of the regulatory cytokine IL-22 [87, 88]. IL-22, as noted above, can induce antimicrobial peptides, which can affect intestinal barrier homeostasis [86–88]. Therefore, TL1A can play a role in both pro-inflammatory and regulatory function through costimulation of ILC populations.

Turning to human studies, elevated TL1A has been noted in both CD and UC indicating again that TL1A is not associated with a unique T-cell differentiation cell lineage [79]. Furthermore, lamina propria CD14+ macrophages in CD patients produced increased amounts of TL1A, and the latter increased T-cell production of IFN-γ and IL-17 from alloantigen-stimulated T cells (but had no significant effect as a lone stimulus reiterating the mouse model data demonstrating a costimulatory effect of TL1A) [89]. Finally, polymorphisms in the TL1A gene have been observed in CD patients indicating a possible significant clinical function to this cytokine [90].

Anti-inflammatory Cytokines

As the host requires a pro-inflammatory response in the presence of a stimulating antigen, so too, the host requires a balancing anti-inflammatory response once the antigen has been dealt with or the offending infection has been cleared. Without the ability to turn off or downregulate the immune response, the inflammation becomes overwhelming and can be detrimental to the host. This issue is exemplified in patients with the disease known as IPEX (immunodysregulation, polyendocrinopathy enteropathy X-linked syndrome). This syndrome is characterized by the development of overwhelming systemic autoimmunity in the first year of life. It is associated with mutations identified in the *FOXP3* gene.

Foxp3 is a member of the forkhead/winged-helix family of transcriptional regulators known to be specific to regulatory T cells and important for their function. Without functional Treg cells, the activated immune system has little or no halt to the inflammatory process. Tolerance, in normal hosts, is mediated by these regulatory T cells, as well as B-lymphocytes, natural killer T cells, and dendritic cells that secrete transforming growth factor (TGF-β), interleukin (IL)-10, interferon (IFN)-α/β, and prostaglandin J2. Another mechanism for regulation is the secretion of anti-inflammatory cytokines. As these cytokines are defined, they are being evaluated for methods to increase their secretion or for systemic therapy with the cytokine itself to treat IBD.

Transforming Growth Factor Beta

TGF-β belongs to a family of multifunctional polypeptides produced by a wide variety of lymphoid and nonlymphoid cells. They exist in five different isoforms, three of which are expressed in mammals and designated as TGF-β1, TGF-β2, and TGF-β3 [1].

TGF-β can act in both autocrine and paracrine modes to control the differentiation, proliferation, and state of activation of immune cells. TGF-β can inhibit the production of and response to cytokines associated with CD4+ Th1 T cells and CD4+ Th2 T cells [91]. TGF-β inhibits the proliferation of T-lymphocytes by downregulating predominantly IL-2-mediated proliferative signals. It also inhibits the growth of natural killer cells in vivo and deactivates macrophages. Of significance, TGF-β has been shown to be important in stimulating the development of Foxp3⁺ T regulatory cells from naïve CD4+ T cells.

These activities have been verified by animal models of IBD [92]. These studies indicate that TGF-β production is relevant in the pathogenesis of experimental colitis. In two different models of Th1-mediated murine experimental colitis, it has been shown that protection from colitis development is strictly associated with the presence of increased numbers and/or upregulation of TGF-β1-producing cells. In these studies, T regulatory cells were first characterized by the surface marker CD25 and that transfer of CD4⁺ T cells depleted of CD4⁺CD25⁺ cells into recipient mice recovered their ability to induce intestinal inflammation in a murine cell transfer colitis model [93]. Recently, further studies reveal these CD25+ T cells are indeed the same T regulatory cells which bear the more familiar marker FoxP3. In addition, it has also been shown that TGF-β can be expressed on the surface of CD4⁺CD25⁺ T regulatory cells in association with latency-associated peptide (LAP), and it is LAP molecule, which mediates CD4⁺CD25⁺ T cell suppression in in vitro suppression assays and, furthermore, that CD4⁺LAP⁺, but not CD4⁺LAP⁻, T cells, can convey protection against the development of colitis in murine intestinal inflammatory models [94]. Recently, a novel therapy targeting TGF-β-expressing cells has been evaluated [95]. The target of this therapy is the expression of Smad7; Smad7 has been shown to inhibit the signaling of TGF-β in the setting of inflammation [96, 97]. The pharmaceutical mongersen (GED0301) has been developed as an antisense RNA to inhibit the expression of Smad7. By inhibiting the expression of Smad7, there is an increase in TGF-β expression and concurrent decrease in inflammation.

The Th17 T-cell pathway or specifically a major component of this pathway, IL-23, has been demonstrated to negatively influence regulatory T-cell development and/or responses. It has been demonstrated that IL-23 p19-deficient mice exhibit an increased number of T regulatory cells in the colon [98]. Furthermore, the numbers of Foxp3+ T regulatory cells in the colon of Rag-/- recipient mice (mice lacking T and B cells) reconstituted with IL-23 receptor-deficient T cells are increased [39]. Thus, these findings show that IL-23 skews the development of inflammation by mediating Th17 effector cell responses and by inhibiting Foxp3+ regulatory T-cell differentiation. Recent studies, however, have demonstrated that a cytokine constitutively expressed by epithelial cells, in the response to tissue damage, namely, IL-33, enhances regulatory T-cell stability and function in murine transfer cell colitis [67]; moreover, T regulatory cells, which lacked the IL-33 receptor (ST2), were shown to be unable to protect mice from development of colitis in the aforementioned transfer colitis model [99]. Of note, an important role for the transcription factor GATA-3 was found in regulatory T-cell function [100, 101] as ST2 expression in T regulatory cells was significantly dependent on GATA-3 [99]. Importantly, as noted above, IL-33 is found in inflamed tissues of IBD patients and may function to bring inflammation under control via T regulatory cell differentiation.

In humans, the data pertaining to regulatory cells remains sparse. In a single study, Maul et al. [102] have shown that there exists a decrease in Foxp3-expressing cells in the periphery of IBD patients. However, examination of mucosal tissue reveals that as compared to controls, IBD patients had a relative increase in these cells albeit this increase was less than that seen in other inflammatory disorders such as diverticulitis. The authors postulated that there is a relative lack of counter-regulation in IBD patients at the mucosal level and therefore an inability to increase the number of local resident regulatory cells in the face of inflammation. More recently, transcriptional gene network analysis revealed a close association of FoxP3 with EZH2 [103]. EZH2 is a gene that participates in DNA methylation and therefore transcriptional repression. Mutation or overexpression of EZH2 has been associated with many forms of cancer as EZH2 inhibits genes responsible for suppressing tumor development. In studies pertaining to regulatory cell generation and function,

potential coordinated functions between FoxP3 and EZH2 were identified. Genetic ablation of EZH2 resulted in T regulatory instability and conversion to Th1/Th17 effector cells in a murine model. Furthermore, these T regulatory cells failed to ameliorate DSS or T cell-mediated colitis. Thus, IBD may not be due to a failure in regulatory cells enumeration but suppressive function; however, this still requires further investigation.

Interleukin-4

IL-4 is produced mainly by a subpopulation of activated T cells (Th2), which are the biologically most active helper cells for B cells and which also secrete IL-5 and IL-6. Another subpopulation, Th1, also produces IL-4 albeit to a lesser extent. IL-4 is a stimulatory molecule for both B and T cells that has known immunosuppressive effects in the intestine; it promotes the proliferation and differentiation of activated B cells and the expression of MHC class 2 antigens.

IL-4 enhances expression of MHC class 2 antigens on B cells. It can promote their capacity to respond to other B-cell stimuli and to present antigens for T cells. While IL-4 is frequently described as an anti-inflammatory cytokine, recent studies have shown its capacity to perpetuate inflammatory diseases. Specifically, in a murine model of ileitis, a monoclonal antibody against IL-4 was shown to suppress disease severity [104]. Interestingly, IL-4-mediated disease in certain animal models appears to be most important in inflammation limited to the ileum and small intestine [105]. In the aforementioned oxazolone model of colitis, IL-4 is the predominant initial cytokine to appear in the mucosal lesions; however, this is subsequently superseded by an IL-13 response. This coincided with what one sees in the IBD disease entities as no significant measurable secreted levels of IL-4 have been found in either UC or CD patients to suggest a pathogenic role. Thus, IL-4, as with IL-13, displays both anti-inflammatory and inflammatory cytokine properties. Its targeting for therapy in animal studies has had some beneficial effects. Its targeting in human disease is not as clear.

Interleukin-10

IL-10 is a critical regulator of intestinal homeostasis and has been shown to inhibit pro-inflammatory cytokines and activate regulatory T-cell function and gene expression. IL-10 is produced by activated CD8+ peripheral blood T cells, by T-helper CD4+ T-cell clones after both antigen-specific and polyclonal activation. IL-10 is also produced by macrophages, dendritic cells, and B cells. IL-10 affects both innate and adaptive immune cells modulating multiple functions of pro-inflammatory cells. IL-10 inhibits the synthesis of a number of cytokines such as IFN-γ, IL-2, and TNF-α in Th1 T-helper subpopulations of T cells but not of Th2 T-helper cells. This activity is antagonized by IL-4. The inhibitory effect on IFN-γ production is indirect and appears to be the result of a suppression of IL-12 synthesis by accessory cells. In the human system, IL-10 is produced by, and downregulates the function of, Th1 and Th2 cells. In macrophages stimulated by bacterial lipopolysaccharides, it inhibits the synthesis of IL-1, IL-6, and TNF-α by promoting, among other things, the degradation of cytokine mRNA. It also leads to an inhibition of antigen presentation. The activation of macrophages can be prevented by IL-10. In human monocytes, IFN-γ and IL-10 antagonize each other's production and function. IL-10 has been shown also to be a physiologic antagonist of IL-12. In macrophages stimulated with bacterial lipopolysaccharides, IFN-gamma increases the synthesis of IL-6 by inhibiting the production of IL-10.

In B cells activated via their antigen receptors or via CD40, IL-10 induces the secretion of IgG, IgA, and IgM. This effect is synergized by IL-4, while the synthesis of immunoglobulins induced by IL-10 is antagonized by TGF-β. It has been shown that human IL-10 is a potent and specific chemoattractant for human T-lymphocytes. Finally, IL-10 also inhibits the chemotactic response of CD4(+) cells, but not of CD8(+) cells, toward IL-8.

In support of its role in IBD, mice deficient in IL-10 (IL-10-/-) gene spontaneously develop chronic colitis. In humans, patients with mutations in IL-10 or the IL-10 receptor (IL-10R) develop a severe form of IBD presenting in the first year of life demonstrating a critical anti-inflammatory pathway in IBD [106, 107]. With this information recombinant IL-10 has been used as therapy in patients with CD. While initial studies appeared positive, upon further evaluation in larger clinical trials, results were not noted to be significant. Due to the concern that IL-10 was not delivered in significant quantities to the local mucosal level, another approach was attempted using "Turbo Probiotics." This was done by engineering *Lactobacillus lactis* to secrete IL-10 specifically at the intestinal level. A similar construct has been tried in patients with IBD, but results are lacking. This novel approach has shown some promising results.

Interleukin 22

Interleukin-22 (IL-22) is a member of the IL-10 cytokine family [108]. IL-22 has been shown to induce proliferative, anti-apoptotic pathways as well as assist in tissue repair [109] and production of antimicrobial peptides [110]. IL-22 is secreted by both innate immune cells (NK cells and dendritic cell) and adaptive immune cells such as CD4+ and CD8+ cells. However, because its receptor is predominantly found on innate cell populations, it appears to regulate these cells and not adaptive immune cells [111]. IL-22 has been identified as an antimicrobial and proregenerative cytokine in IBD. This cytokine activates its function via the JAK/STAT pathways; specifically the STAT3 activation [112] appears to be quite strong similar to other IL-10 family members.

IL-22 is produced by a wide variety of cells, in innate lymphoid cells [113] in an IL-23-dependent manner, while it is produced by CD4+ T cells in an IL-6-dependent manner. Specifically, Th1 and Th17 cells [114] have been shown to secrete IL-22 after exposure to IL-6, and this secretion is somewhat inhibited by TGF-β. In addition, there is another Th cell type identified in human peripheral blood, which is defined by IL-22 secretion without IL-17 or IFN-γ secretion, now termed the Th22 cell [115], although their role is not well understood in the intestinal immune response.

Recent studies have identified a protective effect of IL-22 in IBD. In multiple models of colitis including epithelial cell disruption models as well as T-cell-mediated models of colitis, lack of IL-22 expression worsened the colitis or delayed recovery [116], and injection of IL-22 could ameliorate severe colitis. IL-22 also affects the production of antimicrobial proteins, which can protect against pathogenic bacteria and other infectious agents [117]. In humans, IL-22 has been associated by GWAS with multiple susceptibility genes including IL-23, IL-23R [118], as well as the IL-22 gene location within the ulcerative colitis risk locus at 12q15 [119]. No human studies to affect IL-22 expression or function are ongoing at this time in IBD, but studies in other diseases such as psoriasis are ongoing.

Summary

As evidenced above, there are a multitude of cytokines that are involved in the inflammatory response of the mucosa in inflammatory bowel disease. These cytokines can have pleiotropic effects including pro- and/or anti-inflammatory effects and are important in the pathogenesis of IBD as well as other autoimmune diseases. The above described cytokines are those that were deemed most significant to inflammatory bowel disease, but there are multiple other cytokines that are currently being evaluated or are as yet unknown that may in the future be targets for therapy of IBD.

References

1. Neurath MF et al. Experimental granulomatous colitis in mice is abrogated by induction of TGF-beta-mediated oral tolerance. J Exp Med. 1996;183(6):2605–16.
2. Reinecker HC et al. Enhanced secretion of tumour necrosis factor-alpha, IL-6, and IL-1 beta by isolated lamina propria mononuclear cells from patients with ulcerative colitis and Crohn's disease. Clin Exp Immunol. 1993;94(1):174–81.

3. Camoglio L et al. Altered expression of interferon-gamma and interleukin-4 in inflammatory bowel disease. Inflamm Bowel Dis. 1998;4(4):285–90.

4. Boirivant M et al. Oxazolone colitis: a murine model of T helper cell type 2 colitis treatable with antibodies to interleukin 4. J Exp Med. 1998;188(10):1929–39.

5. Shetty A, Forbes A. Pharmacogenomics of response to anti-tumor necrosis factor therapy in patients with Crohn's disease. Am J Pharmacogenomics. 2002;2(4):215–21.

6. Strober W et al. Reciprocal IFN-gamma and TGF-beta responses regulate the occurrence of mucosal inflammation. Immunol Today. 1997;18(2):61–4.

7. Neurath MF et al. Predominant pathogenic role of tumor necrosis factor in experimental colitis in mice. Eur J Immunol. 1997;27(7):1743–50.

8. Murch SH et al. Serum concentrations of tumour necrosis factor alpha in childhood chronic inflammatory bowel disease. Gut. 1991;32(8):913–7.

9. Reimund JM et al. Mucosal inflammatory cytokine production by intestinal biopsies in patients with ulcerative colitis and Crohn's disease. J Clin Immunol. 1996;16(3):144–50.

10. Targan SR et al. A short-term study of chimeric monoclonal antibody cA2 to tumor necrosis factor alpha for Crohn's disease. Crohn's Disease cA2 Study Group. N Engl J Med. 1997;337(15):1029–35.

11. Hanauer SB et al. Maintenance infliximab for Crohn's disease: the ACCENT I randomised trial. Lancet. 2002;359(9317):1541–9.

12. Colgan SP et al. Interferon-gamma induces a cell surface phenotype switch on T84 intestinal epithelial cells. Am J Physiol. 1994;267(2 Pt 1):C402–10.

13. Strober W, Fuss IJ, Blumberg RS. The immunology of mucosal models of inflammation. Annu Rev Immunol. 2002;20:495–549.

14. Reinisch W et al. A dose escalating, placebo controlled, double blind, single dose and multidose, safety and tolerability study of fontolizumab, a humanised anti-interferon gamma antibody, in patients with moderate to severe Crohn's disease. Gut. 2006;55(8):1138–44.

15. Hommes DW et al. Fontolizumab, a humanised anti-interferon gamma antibody, demonstrates safety and clinical activity in patients with moderate to severe Crohn's disease. Gut. 2006;55(8):1131–7.

16. Seo SU et al. Distinct commensals induce interleukin-1beta via NLRP3 inflammasome in inflammatory monocytes to promote intestinal inflammation in response to injury. Immunity. 2015;42(4):744–55.

17. Cominelli F, Pizarro TT. Interleukin-1 and interleukin-1 receptor antagonist in inflammatory bowel disease. Aliment Pharmacol Ther. 1996;10(Suppl 2):49–53; discussion 54.

18. Mahida YR, Wu K, Jewell DP. Enhanced production of interleukin 1-beta by mononuclear cells isolated from mucosa with active ulcerative colitis of Crohn's disease. Gut. 1989;30(6):835–8.

19. Andus T et al. Imbalance of the interleukin 1 system in colonic mucosa – association with intestinal inflammation and interleukin 1 receptor antagonist [corrected] genotype 2. Gut. 1997;41(5):651–7.

20. Van Assche G et al. A pilot study on the use of the humanized anti-interleukin-2 receptor antibody daclizumab in active ulcerative colitis. Am J Gastroenterol. 2003;98(2):369–76.

21. Van Assche G et al. Daclizumab, a humanised monoclonal antibody to the interleukin 2 receptor (CD25), for the treatment of moderately to severely active ulcerative colitis: a randomised, double blind, placebo controlled, dose ranging trial. Gut. 2006;55(11):1568–74.

22. Cantor MJ, Nickerson P, Bernstein CN. The role of cytokine gene polymorphisms in determining disease susceptibility and phenotype in inflammatory bowel disease. Am J Gastroenterol. 2005;100(5):1134–42.

23. Atreya R, Neurath MF. Involvement of IL-6 in the pathogenesis of inflammatory bowel disease and colon cancer. Clin Rev Allergy Immunol. 2005;28(3):187–96.

24. Ito H, et al. A pilot randomized trial of a human anti-interleukin-6 receptor monoclonal antibody in active Crohn's disease. Gastroenterology. 2004;126(4):989–96; discussion 947.

25. Bouma G, Strober W. The immunological and genetic basis of inflammatory bowel disease. Nat Rev Immunol. 2003;3(7):521–33.

26. Fuss IJ et al. Both IL-12p70 and IL-23 are synthesized during active Crohn's disease and are down-regulated by treatment with anti-IL-12 p40 monoclonal antibody. Inflamm Bowel Dis. 2006;12(1):9–15.

27. Mannon PJ et al. Anti-interleukin-12 antibody for active Crohn's disease. N Engl J Med. 2004;351(20):2069–79.

28. William Sandborn, Christopher Gasink, Marion Blank, Yinghua Lang, Jewel Johanns, Long-Long Gao, Bruce Sands, Stephen Hanauer, Brian Feagan, Stephan Targan, Subrata Ghosh, Wim de Villiers, Jean-Frédéric Colombel, Scott Lee, Pierre Desreumaux, Edward Loftus, Severine Vermeire, Paul Rutgeerts A Multicenter, Double-Blind, Placebo-Controlled Phase3 Study Of Ustekinumab, A Human Il-12/23P40 Mab, In Moderate-Service Crohn's Disease Refractory To Anti-Tfnα: Uniti- 1. Inflamm Bowel Dis 2016;22 Suppl 1:S1.

29. Fuss IJ et al. Anti-interleukin 12 treatment regulates apoptosis of Th1 T cells in experimental colitis in mice. Gastroenterology. 1999;117(5):1078–88.

30. Harrington LE et al. Interleukin 17-producing CD4+ effector T cells develop via a lineage distinct from the T helper type 1 and 2 lineages. Nat Immunol. 2005;6(11):1123–32.

31. Hue S et al. Interleukin-23 drives innate and T cell-mediated intestinal inflammation. J Exp Med. 2006;203(11):2473–83.

32. Fujino S et al. Increased expression of interleukin 17 in inflammatory bowel disease. Gut. 2003;52(1):65–70.

33. Langrish CL et al. IL-23 drives a pathogenic T cell population that induces autoimmune inflammation. J Exp Med. 2005;201(2):233–40.

34. Kullberg MC et al. IL-23 plays a key role in Helicobacter hepaticus-induced T cell-dependent colitis. J Exp Med. 2006;203(11):2485–94.

35. Kolls JK, Linden A. Interleukin-17 family members and inflammation. Immunity. 2004;21(4):467–76.

36. Biancheri P et al. The role of interleukin 17 in Crohn's disease-associated intestinal fibrosis. Fibrogenesis Tissue Repair. 2013;6(1):13.

37. Mangan PR et al. Transforming growth factor-beta induces development of the T(H)17 lineage. Nature. 2006;441(7090):231–4.

38. Bettelli E et al. Reciprocal developmental pathways for the generation of pathogenic effector TH17 and regulatory T cells. Nature. 2006;441(7090):235–8.

39. Ahern PP et al. Interleukin-23 drives intestinal inflammation through direct activity on T cells. Immunity. 2010;33(2):279–88.

40. Sujino T et al. Regulatory T cells suppress development of colitis, blocking differentiation of T-helper 17 into alternative T-helper 1 cells. Gastroenterology. 2011;141(3):1014–23.

41. Duerr RH et al. A genome-wide association study identifies IL23R as an inflammatory bowel disease gene. Science. 2006;314(5804):1461–3.

42. Wang K et al. Diverse genome-wide association studies associate the IL12/IL23 pathway with Crohn Disease. Am J Hum Genet. 2009;84(3):399–405.

43. Pizarro TT et al. IL-18, a novel immunoregulatory cytokine, is up-regulated in Crohn's disease: expression and localization in intestinal mucosal cells. J Immunol. 1999;162(11):6829–35.

44. Reuter BK, Pizarro TT. Commentary: the role of the IL-18 system and other members of the IL-1R/TLR superfamily in innate mucosal immunity and the pathogenesis of inflammatory bowel disease: friend or foe? Eur J Immunol. 2004;34(9):2347–55.

45. Okamura H et al. Regulation of interferon-gamma production by IL-12 and IL-18. Curr Opin Immunol. 1998;10(3):259–64.

46. Nakanishi K et al. Interleukin-18 is a unique cytokine that stimulates both Th1 and Th2 responses depending on its cytokine milieu. Cytokine Growth Factor Rev. 2001;12(1):53–72.

47. Siegmund B et al. IL-1 beta-converting enzyme (caspase-1) in intestinal inflammation. Proc Natl Acad Sci U S A. 2001;98(23): 13249–54.

48. Maeda S et al. Nod2 mutation in Crohn's disease potentiates NF-kappaB activity and IL-1beta processing. Science. 2005;307(5710):734–8.

49. Saitoh T et al. Loss of the autophagy protein Atg16L1 enhances endotoxin-induced IL-1beta production. Nature. 2008;456(7219): 264–8.

50. Bersudsky M et al. Non-redundant properties of IL-1alpha and IL-1beta during acute colon inflammation in mice. Gut. 2014;63(4):598–609.

51. Siegmund B, Fantuzzi G, Rieder F, Gamboni-Robertson F, Lehr HA, Hartmann G, Dinarello CA, Endres S, Eigler A. Neutralization of interleukin-18 reduces severity in murine colitis and intestinal IFN-gamma and TNF-alpha production. Am J Physiol Regul Integr Comp Physiol. 2001;281:R1264–73.

52. Sivakumar PV, Westrich GM, Kanaly S, Garka K, Born TL, Derry JM, Viney JL. Interleukin 18 is a primary mediator of the inflammation associated with dextran sulphate sodium induced colitis: blocking interleukin 18 attenuates intestinal damage. Gut. 2002;50:812–20.

53. Takagi H, Kanai T, Okazawa A, Kishi Y, Sato T, Takaishi H, Inoue N, Ogata H, Iwao Y, Hoshino K, Takeda K, Akira S, Watanabe M, Ishii H, Hibi T. Contrasting action of IL-12 and IL-18 in the development of dextran sodium sulphate colitis in mice. Scand J Gastroenterol. 2003;38:837–44.

54. Salcedo R, Worschech A, Cardone M, Jones Y, Gyulai Z, Dai RM, Wang E, Ma W, Haines D, O'HUigin C, Marincola FM, Trinchieri G. MyD88-mediated signaling prevents development of adenocarcinomas of the colon: role of interleukin 18. J Exp Med. 2010; 207:1625–36.

55. Huber S, Gagliani N, Zenewicz LA, Huber FJ, Bosurgi L, Hu B, Hedl M, Zhang W, O'Connor Jr W, Murphy AJ, Valenzuela DM, Yancopoulos GD, Booth CJ, Cho JH, Ouyang W, Abraham C, Flavell RA. IL-22BP is regulated by the inflammasome and modulates tumorigenesis in the intestine. Nature. 2012;491: 259–63.

56. Wang Y, Wang K, Han GC, Wang RX, Xiao H, Hou CM, Guo RF, Dou Y, Shen BF, Li Y, Chen GJ. Neutrophil infiltration favors colitis-associated tumorigenesis by activating the interleukin-1 (IL-1)/IL-6 axis. Mucosal Immunol. 2014;7:1106–15.

57. Fuss IJ et al. Nonclassical CD1d-restricted NK T cells that produce IL-13 characterize an atypical Th2 response in ulcerative colitis. J Clin Invest. 2004;113(10):1490–7.

58. Heller F et al. Interleukin-13 is the key effector Th2 cytokine in ulcerative colitis that affects epithelial tight junctions, apoptosis, and cell restitution. Gastroenterology. 2005;129(2): 550–64.

59. Schiechl G et al. Tumor development in murine ulcerative colitis depends on MyD88 signaling of colonic F4/80+CD11b(high) Gr1(low) macrophages. J Clin Invest. 2011;121(5):1692–708.

60. Reinisch W et al. Anrukinzumab, an anti-interleukin 13 monoclonal antibody, in active UC: efficacy and safety from a phase IIa randomised multicentre study. Gut. 2015;64(6):894–900.

61. Fuss I et al. IL-13Rα2-bearing, type II NKT cells reactive to sulfatide self-antigen populate the mucosa of ulcerative colitis. Gut. 2014;63(11):1728–36.

62. Danese S et al. Tralokinumab for moderate-to-severe UC: a randomised, double-blind, placebo-controlled, phase IIa study. Gut. 2015;64(2):243–9.

63. Guo L et al. IL-1 family members and STAT activators induce cytokine production by Th2, Th17, and Th1 cells. Proc Natl Acad Sci U S A. 2009;106:13463–8.

64. Schmitz J et al. IL-33, an interleukin-1-like cytokine that signals via the IL-1 receptor-related protein ST2 and induces T helper type 2-associated cytokines. Immunity. 2005;23:470–90.

65. Cayrol C, Girard JP. The IL-1-like cytokine IL-33 is inactivated after maturation by caspase-1. Proc Natl Acad Sci U S A. 2009;106:9021–6.

66. Lüthi AU et al. Suppression of interleukin-33 bioactivity through proteolysis by apoptotic caspases. Immunity. 2009;31:84–98.

67. Lefrancais E et al. IL-33 is processed into mature bioactive forms by neutrophil elastese and cathepsin G. Proc Natl Acad Sci U S A. 2012;109:1673–8.

68. Liew FY, Pitman NI, McInnes IB. Disease-associated functions of IL-33: the new kid in the IL-1 family. Nat Rev Immunol. 2010;10:103–10.

69. Smith DE. IL-33: a tissue derived cytokine pathway involved in allergic inflammation and asthma. Clin Exp Allergy. 2010;40:200–8.

70. Pastorelli L et al. Epithelial-derived IL-33 and its receptor ST2 are dysregulated in ulcerative colitis and in experimental Th1/Th2 driven enteritis. Proc Natl Acad Sci U S A. 2010;107: 8017–22.

71. Seidelin JB et al. IL-33 is upregulated in colonocytes of ulcerative colitis. Immunol Lett. 2010;128:80–5.

72. Rosen M et al. STAT6 deficiency ameliorates severity of oxazolone colitis by decreasing expression of claudin-2 and Th2-inducing cytokines. J Immunol. 2013;190(4):1849–58.

73. Kobori A, Yagi Y, Imaeda H, Ban H, Bamba S, Tsujikwa T, Saito Y, Fujiyama Y, Andoh A. Interleukin-33 expression is specifically enhanced in inflamed mucosa of ulcerative colitis. J Gastroenterol. 2010;45:999–1007.

74. Arendse B et al. IL-9 is a susceptibility factor in Leishmani major infection by promoting detrimental Th2/type 2 responses. J Immunol. 2005;174:2205–11.

75. Kim BS et al. Innate lymphoid cells and allergic inflammation. Curr Opin Immunol. 2013;25:738–44.

76. Kaplan MH. Th9 cells: differentiation and disease. Immunol Rev. 2013;252:104–15.

77. Gerlach K et al. TH9 cells that express the transcription factor PU.1 drive T cell-mediated colitis via IL-9 receptor signaling in intestinal epithelial cells. Nat Immunol. 2014;15(7):676–86.

78. Hundorfean G et al. Functional relevance of Th helper 17 (Th17) cells and the IL-17 cytokine family in inflammatory bowel disease. Inflamm Bowel Dis. 2012;18:180–6.

79. Prehn JL et al. The T cell costimulator TL1A is induced by FcgammaR signaling in human monocytes and dendritic cells. J Immunol. 2007;178(7):4033–8.

80. Takedatsu H et al. TL1A (TNFSF15) regulates the development of chronic colitis by modulating both T-helper 1 and T-helper 17 activation. Gastroenterology. 2008;135(2):552–67.

81. Meylan F et al. The TNF-family receptor DR3 is essential for diverse T cell-mediated inflammatory diseases. Immunity. 2008; 29(1):79–89.

82. Schreiber TH et al. Therapeutic Treg expansion in mice by TNFRSF25 prevents allergic lung inflammation. J Clin Invest. 2010;120(10):3629–40.

83. Meylan F et al. The TNF-family cytokine TL1A promotes allergic immunopathology through group 2 innate lymphoid cells. Mucosal Immunol. 2014;7:958–68.

84. Yu X et al. TNF superfamily member TL1A elicits type 2 innate lymphoid cells at mucosal barriers. Mucosal Immunol. 2014;7: 730–40.

85. Prehn JL et al. Potential role for TL1A, the new TNF-family member and potent costimulator of IFN-gamma, in mucosal inflammation. Clin Immunol. 2004;112:66–77.

86. Ahn YO et al. Human group3 innate lymphoid cells express DR3 and respond to TL1A with enhanced IL-22 production and IL-2-dependent proliferation. Eur J Immunol. 2015;45:2335–42.

87. Zheng Y et al. Interleukin 22 mediates early host defense against attaching and effacing bacterial pathogens. Nat Med. 2008;14:282–9.

88. Zenewicz LA et al. Innate and adaptive interleukin-22 protects mice from inflammatory bowel disease. Immunity. 2008;29:947–57.

89. Kamada N et al. TL1A produced by lamina propria macrophages induces Th1 and Th17 immune responses in cooperation with IL-23 in patients with Crohn's disease. Inflamm Bowel Dis. 2010;16(4):568–75.

90. Michelsen KS et al. IBD-associated TL1A gene (TNFSF15) haplotypes determine increased expression of TL1A protein. PLoS One. 2009;4(3):e4719.

91. McClane SJ, Rombeau JL. Cytokines and inflammatory bowel disease: a review. JPEN J Parenter Enteral Nutr. 1999;23(5 Suppl):S20–4.

92. Powrie F et al. A critical role for transforming growth factor-beta but not interleukin 4 in the suppression of T helper type 1-mediated colitis by CD45RB(low) CD4+ T cells. J Exp Med. 1996;183(6):2669–74.

93. Read S, Malmström V, et al. Cytotoxic T lymphocyte-associated antigen 4 plays an essential role in the function of CD25(+) CD4(+) regulatory cells that control intestinal inflammation. J Exp Med. 2000;192(2):295–302.

94. Nakamura K et al. TGF-beta 1 plays an important role in the mechanism of CD4+CD25+ regulatory T cell activity in both humans and mice. J Immunol. 2004;172(2):834–42.

95. Monteleone G et al. Mongersen, an oral SMAD7 antisense oligonucleotide, and Crohn's disease. N Engl J Med. 2015;372(12):1104–13.

96. Yan X, Liu Z, Chen Y. Regulation of TGF-beta signaling by Smad7. Acta Biochim Biophys Sin (Shanghai). 2009;41(4):263–72.

97. Boirivant M, Pallone F, Di Giacinto C. Inhibition of Smad7 with a specific antisense oligonucleotide facilitates TGF-beta1-mediated suppression of colitis. Gastroenterology. 2006;131(6):1786–98.

98. Izcue A et al. Interleukin-23 restrains regulatory T cell activity to drive T cell-dependent colitis. Immunity. 2008;28(4):559–70.

99. Schiering C et al. The alarmin IL-33 promotes regulatory T-cell function in the intestine. Nature. 2014;513(7519):564–8.

100. Wang Y et al. An essential role of the transcription factor GATA-3 for the function of regulatory T cells. Immunity. 2011;35(3):337–48.

101. Wohlfert EA et al. GATA3 controls Foxp3(+) regulatory T cell fate during inflammation in mice. J Clin Invest. 2011;121(11):4503–15.

102. Maul J et al. Peripheral and intestinal regulatory CD4+ CD25(high) T cells in inflammatory bowel disease. Gastroenterology. 2005;128(7):1868–78.

103. Sarmento O et al. Alterations in the FOXP3-EZH2 pathway associates with increased susceptibility to colitis in both mice and human. Inflamm Bowel Dis. 2016;22 suppl 1:S5–6.

104. Bamias G et al. Proinflammatory effects of TH2 cytokines in a murine model of chronic small intestinal inflammation. Gastroenterology. 2005;128(3):654–66.

105. Dohi T et al. T helper type-2 cells induce ileal villus atrophy, goblet cell metaplasia, and wasting disease in T cell-deficient mice. Gastroenterology. 2003;124(3):672–82.

106. Kotlarz D et al. Loss of interleukin-10 signaling and infantile inflammatory bowel disease: implications for diagnosis and therapy. Gastroenterology. 2012;143(2):347–55.

107. Moran CJ et al. IL-10R polymorphisms are associated with very-early-onset ulcerative colitis. Inflamm Bowel Dis. 2013;19(1):115–23.

108. Sonnenberg GF, Fouser LA, Artis D. Functional biology of the IL-22-IL-22R pathway in regulating immunity and inflammation at barrier surfaces. Adv Immunol. 2010;107:1–29.

109. Mizoguchi A. Healing of intestinal inflammation by IL-22. Inflamm Bowel Dis. 2012;18(9):1777–84.

110. Sonnenberg GF, Fouser LA, Artis D. Border patrol: regulation of immunity, inflammation and tissue homeostasis at barrier surfaces by IL-22. Nat Immunol. 2011;12(5):383–90.

111. Wolk K et al. Cutting edge: immune cells as sources and targets of the IL-10 family members? J Immunol. 2002;168(11):5397–402.

112. Pickert G et al. STAT3 links IL-22 signaling in intestinal epithelial cells to mucosal wound healing. J Exp Med. 2009;206(7):1465–72.

113. Longman RS et al. CX(3)CR1(+) mononuclear phagocytes support colitis-associated innate lymphoid cell production of IL-22. J Exp Med. 2014;211(8):1571–83.

114. Chung Y et al. Expression and regulation of IL-22 in the IL-17-producing CD4+ T lymphocytes. Cell Res. 2006;16(11):902–7.

115. Duhen T et al. Production of interleukin 22 but not interleukin 17 by a subset of human skin-homing memory T cells. Nat Immunol. 2009;10(8):857–63.

116. Sugimoto K et al. IL-22 ameliorates intestinal inflammation in a mouse model of ulcerative colitis. J Clin Invest. 2008;118(2):534–44.

117. Wilson MS et al. Redundant and pathogenic roles for IL-22 in mycobacterial, protozoan, and helminth infections. J Immunol. 2010;184(8):4378–90.

118. Zwiers A et al. Cutting edge: a variant of the IL-23R gene associated with inflammatory bowel disease induces loss of microRNA regulation and enhanced protein production. J Immunol. 2012;188(4):1573–7.

119. Silverberg MS et al. Ulcerative colitis-risk loci on chromosomes 1p36 and 12q15 found by genome-wide association study. Nat Genet. 2009;41(2):216–20.

The Gut Microbiota and Inflammatory Bowel Disease

4

Máire A. Conrad, Gary D. Wu, and Judith R. Kelsen

Abbreviations

AIEC	Adherent and invasive *E. coli*
AMP	Antimicrobial peptide
CD	Crohn disease
CDI	*C. difficile* infection
EN	Enteral nutrition therapy
FMT	Fecal microbiota transplantation
GWAS	Genome-wide array studies
IBD	Inflammatory bowel disease
ILC	Innate lymphoid cells
MAP	*Mycobacterium avium* subspecies *paratuberculosis*
NLR	Nucleotide-binding domain and leucine-rich repeat-containing receptor
NOD1	Nucleotide-binding oligomerization domain protein 1
PAMP	Pathogen-associated molecular pattern
PRR	Pattern recognition receptor
SCFA	Short-chain fatty acids
TLR	Toll-like receptor
TNF	Tumor necrosis factor
UC	Ulcerative colitis

Introduction

The inflammatory bowel diseases (IBDs), comprised of Crohn disease, ulcerative colitis, and indeterminate colitis, are chronic inflammatory diseases of the gastrointestinal tract. They are due to an aberrant immune response to

M.A. Conrad, MD (✉) • J.R. Kelsen, MD
Division of Gastroenterology, Hepatology and Nutrition, The Children's Hospital of Philadelphia, Perelman School of Medicine at the University of Pennsylvania, 3401 Civic Ctr. Blvd., Philadelphia, PA 19104, USA
e-mail: conradm@email.chop.edu

G.D. Wu, MD, PhD
Perelman School of Medicine at the University of Pennsylvania, Hospital of University of Pennsylvania, Philadelphia, PA, USA

environmental factors in a genetically susceptible host. The gut microbiota is thought to be a critical environmental factor in the development of IBD. Crohn disease (CD) can cause transmural inflammation throughout the GI tract and may be characterized histologically by granulomatous formation, as well as the presence of strictures and fistulae. Ulcerative colitis (UC) is typified by mucosal inflammation limited to the colon. A subset of patients are classified as "indeterminate colitis" based on having features of both CD and UC. However, within these classifications, there is significant heterogeneity in disease phenotype. This arises, in part, due to the host genomics, including multiple susceptibility genes, and possibly because of the variable composition of the gut microbiota [1].

There is significant evidence to support the role of gut microbes in the development of IBD. Animal studies of IBD have demonstrated that germ-free animals show little sign of inflammation [2]; however, inflammation develops with exposure to microbes [3]. Adaptive immune responses to bacterial antigens have been shown to lead to the spontaneous development of colitis through immune activation and/or the loss of immune tolerance in various models [4]. From a clinical standpoint, inflammation in CD and UC occurs predominantly in the terminal ileum (in CD) and colon (both UC and CD) where the greatest concentrations of bacteria are found. Antibiotics can have efficacy in the treatment of IBD [5–7], and recently, the therapy using a combination of antibiotics has been shown to be effective in patients with severe colonic disease [8]. Furthermore, the fecal flow exacerbates IBD and surgical diversion of the flow ameliorates the disease [9, 10]. From a more descriptive standpoint, studies have found that there are increased amounts of bacteria in the mucus layer in biopsy specimens of patients with IBD as compared to controls [11]. However, genetic studies have provided some of the strongest support for the role of the microbiota in the development of IBD. Genome-wide association studies (GWAS) have identified >200 genetic risk loci, with 28 shared between CD and UC [12, 13]. Many of

© Springer International Publishing AG 2017
P. Mamula et al. (eds.), *Pediatric Inflammatory Bowel Disease*, DOI 10.1007/978-3-319-49215-5_4

the genes and genetic loci identified involve pathways which are critical for the protection of the host against the gut microbiota, such as regulation of the epithelial barrier, microbial defense, and autophagy, as well as pathways involving regulation of the innate and adaptive immune systems [12]. Together, these aberrations support the notion that IBD is due to the inability of the host to protect against microbial invasion combined with an unrestrained immune activation.

Characteristics of the Gut Microbiome

The human gut microbiome is one of the most densely populated bacterial communities on Earth with up to 10^{11} organisms per gram of fecal weight composed of over 1000 species, most of which are obligate anaerobes [14, 15]. The bacterial concentration, as well as complexity, increases proximally from the stomach and duodenum, where there are approximately 10^2–10^3 aerobic organisms/gram luminal contents, to 10^{11}–10^{12} distally where anaerobic organisms predominate in the cecum and colon [4]. Throughout, the collective genome of the bacteria is 100-fold greater than that of its human host [16]. Indeed, humans should be viewed as a biologic "supraorganism" that is dynamic and carries out functions in parallel or cooperatively [17]. Roles of the microbiota include immune education and metabolism. Although there are over 50 bacterial phyla on Earth, the majority of the bacteria in the human adult gut largely belong to one of four phyla, *Actinobacteria*, *Firmicutes*, *Proteobacteria*, and *Bacteroidetes* [18, 19].

Most gut microbes are obligate anaerobes, many of which are fastidious and difficult to grow in vitro making traditional culture techniques of limited value in characterizing the composition of the gut microbiota. The development of culture-independent methods, mainly through the use of high-throughput DNA sequencing, has provided new means to evaluate the gut microbiome and its relationship to IBD. There are two primary methods that utilize deep-sequencing technologies to characterize the microbiome. The first approach uses small-subunit ribosomal RNA (16S rRNA gene sequences (for Archaea and Bacteria) or 18S rRNA gene sequences (for eukaryotes)) as stable phylogenetic markers to define the lineages present in a sample [20]. Another approach uses shotgun metagenomic sequencing. This sequences the total community DNA, thereby allowing for the microbial community structure and genomic representation of the community to be evaluated. The genomic community evaluation provides an understanding of the functions encoded by the genomes of the gut microbiota [16]. Metatranscriptomics and metaproteomics provide a deeper understanding of microbial function through direct evaluation of gene expression [21].

These advances in sequencing technologies have allowed investigators to characterize the bacterial composition of the gut throughout different stages of life, a critical step in the study of health and disease. Colonization of the gut begins at birth, and individual characteristics of the gut microbiome begin to arise during infancy and throughout the first year of life. This process is dependent on several factors including the mode of delivery and form of infant feeding. During the first year of life, the human gut microbiome becomes more stable and adult-like [22] concurrent with the introduction of solid foods into the diet [23]. Interindividual differences in the characteristics of the bacterial microbiota observed early in life, within months, persist at 1 year of life [22]. Indeed, interindividual differences in the gut microbiome are the largest source of variance among healthy individuals that appear to be relatively stable over time, at least in the short term [18].

The driving force behind interindividual variation remains to be determined; however, several studies provide indirect evidence that early environmental exposures may play a role. Palmer and colleagues studied the microbiome in 14 full-term healthy infants and discovered significant variability among the children, although marked similarity in bacterial communities in the one set of fraternal twins [22]. This suggests that interindividual characteristics of the gut microbiome may be shaped by environmental factors early in life. These characteristics may persist throughout the host's life and may be independent of genetic factors [18].

Diet and the Gut Microbiome

As the incidence of certain diseases has increased, there have been many environmental changes that have occurred over the last several decades. These changes in modern lifestyle have been implicated in the alteration of the gut microbiome, including improved sanitation, increase in antibiotic use, less crowded living conditions, decline in *H. pylori*, smaller family size, vaccinations, refrigeration, decline in parasite infections, sedentary lifestyle, cesarean section, food processing, and diet changes [24].

The development of agriculture and domestication of animals have been major factors in recent human evolution [25] with the resultant changes in diet perhaps altering the host-gut microbiome relationship [26]. Over time in industrialized nations, there has been a reduction in fiber consumption with an increase in simple sugars, fats, and proteins. It has been hypothesized that this change in diet may have altered the interaction of the host and the microbiota in a manner that has played a role in the increasing incidence of metabolic disorders [26]. Furthermore, fluctuations in diet may have consequences for the bacteria and the host, allowing for predisposition to invasion or inflammation [27].

There has been recent evidence demonstrating the relationship between the gut microbiota and diet. An analysis of fecal 16S rRNA sequences from 60 mammalian species indicated clustering according to host phylogeny as well as clustering according to diet (herbivore, carnivore, and omnivore) [28]. Cross-sectional studies using shotgun metagenomic sequencing have suggested that there has been a functional evolution of the gut microbiome in relation to diet [29]. Microbial genes encoding for enzymes involved in carbohydrate and amino acid metabolism are dissimilar between herbivores and carnivores [29].

A study by Wu et al. focusing on the effect of diet on the gut microbiome revealed differences in the impact of habitual long-term vs. short-term diet [30]. Long-term diet, similar to a "Westernized" diet (high in meats and fats, low in carbohydrates), was associated with high levels of *Bacteroides* and low levels of *Prevotella* genera. Diets high in carbohydrates but low in animal protein and fat had higher levels of the *Prevotella* and lower levels of *Bacteroides*. These results provide an explanation for previously described clustering of individuals into "enterotypes" dominated by *Bacteroides* and *Prevotella* based on the composition of the gut microbiota and not correlated to host properties such as age, gender, ethnicity, or body mass index [31]. These observations are also consistent with a study comparing the gut microbiome of children from a village in the West African country of Burkina Faso to those in Europe [32] where the inverse relationship between *Bacteroides* and *Prevotella* genera was also noted. These three studies suggest that long-term diet helps to distinguish a gut microbiota community or enterotype that is associated with a "Westernized" diet rich in *Bacteroides* from an enterotype associated with an agrarian diet where the bacteria of the *Prevotella* genus predominate. In addition, studies of monozygotic twins to assess host genotype influences on enterotypes showed most twin pairs had similar enterotypes longitudinally, although many of these subjects likely share similar diets and environments [33]. Enterotypes may function as a marker of disease; however, further studies are needed.

Gut Microbiota-Host Interactions at the Mucosal Interface

The alteration of the gut microbiota has had a direct effect on the host's immune system. Mammalian hosts have coevolved to exist with our gut microbiota in a mutualistic relationship where we provide a uniquely suited environment in return for physiological benefits provided to us by our gut microbiota [34]. Examples of the latter include the fermentation of

indigestible carbohydrates to produce short-chain fatty acids (SCFA) that are utilized by the host, biotransformation of conjugated bile acids, synthesis of certain vitamins, degradation of dietary oxalates, and education of the mucosal immune system [34]. Indeed, when viewed as a whole, the "supraorganism" of the gut can carry out enzymatic reactions distinct from those of the human genome and harvest energy that would otherwise be lost to the host. The consequences of these enzymatic reactions suggest that over the millennia, mammalian metabolism, physiology, and disease have shaped and have been shaped by the gut microbiota. Commensal bacteria may also directly inhibit the growth of specific pathogens, such as *Clostridium difficile*, by competitive inhibition thus preventing an adequate niche for expansion.

Relevant to pediatric IBD, the gut microbiota develops between birth and 3 years of life. In the case of very early-onset IBD, that is during the time period that the child presents with disease or develops symptoms, and each exposure to the infant results in a change in the microbial structure. There has been a drastic increase in the incidence of VEO-IBD, pointing to an environmental contribution to the disease despite the strong genetic drivers identified in this population. The relationship between host genetics and developing microbiome can be seen through germ-free (GF) murine models. GF mice have underdeveloped gut-associated lymphoid tissue. In an environment with specific defined flora, the gut microbiota elicits host-specific T-cell response and differentiation [35]. Concurrently, the aberrant T-cell development of GF mice shapes the gut microbiome, as seen by the different phylogenetic composition of the microbiota in Rag1-deficient mice [36]. Zebrafish models show similar findings, in which Rag1-deficient zebrafish had overgrowth of *Vibrio* species [37].

In general, the interaction between the gut microbiota and the mammalian host is complex but can be roughly divided into three major categories: the innate immune system, the adaptive immune system, and the intestinal epithelial interface.

The Innate Immune System

The innate immune response is the first line of defense against microbes and is a rapid response. It encompasses receptors that recognize the microbial patterns: pattern recognition receptors (PRRs) that serve as sensors of pathogen-associated molecular patterns (PAMPS) and reside in the lumen of the intestine [38]. The most studied PRRs are the Toll-like receptors (TLRs). PRRs are expressed on many cell types and activate an inflammatory response via NF-κβ activation, cytokine production, and recruitment of acute inflammatory cells [39]. TLR signaling in the intestine is important in homeostasis of the intestine through a variety of functions including epithelial cell proliferation [40], IgA production [41], antimicrobial cytokine production and peptide expression, and maintenance of tight junctions [42]. Nucleotide-binding domain and leucine-rich repeat-containing receptors (NLRs), another class of innate immune receptors, have the ability to respond to different stimuli with an inflammatory response. Examples of NLRs include nucleotide-binding oligomerization domain protein 1 (NOD1) and NOD2. NOD2 is highly expressed in monocytes and Paneth cells, and its ligand is common to both gram-positive and gram-negative bacteria. Relhman recently demonstrated via murine models that NOD2 is integral in the interaction between the host and the microbiota and for the development of the intestinal flora [43]. Disruptions in TLR and NLR expression have been associated with intestinal dysbiosis [44, 45].

The Adaptive Immune System

Innate immune signaling through the activation of PRRs or NLRs cannot distinguish between commensal and pathogenic bacteria. The adaptive immune system, involved in both humoral and cell-mediated immunity, has evolved to regulate immune responsiveness by selectively responding to or ignoring individual antigens based on previous encounters [46]. Failure to maintain the latter, known as immune tolerance, results in unrestrained immune activation and subsequent inflammation in the absence of a microbial pathogen, the hallmark of immune-mediated diseases such as IBD. Studies in germ-free mice demonstrate that the gut microbiota plays a critical role in helping to shape adaptive immune function through the production of IgA [47], development of Th17-producing lymphocytes [48], as well as T regulatory cells [49], which play a critical role in the maintenance of immune tolerance [50].

In addition, innate lymphoid cells (ILCs) are innate immune cells without antigen-specific responses. These are functionally associated with T cells with lymphoid lineage, of which there are three types, that also regulate effector T-cell response against commensal organisms. Group 3 ILCs are RORγt+ and produce IL-22 and/or IL-17 with stimulation by IL-23 and IL-1ß. ILCs are regulated by commensal organisms as the production of IL-22 is reduced in the absence of the microbiota [51]. Similar to the innate immune system, multiple gene variants associated with IBD involve components of the adaptive immune response including T- and B-cell regulation and the IL-23/Th17/T regulatory cell axis [12].

Intestinal Epithelium

The intestinal epithelium functions not only as a physical and chemical barrier to separate the luminal gut microbiota from the host, through mucus secretion, for example, but also produces antimicrobial peptides (AMPs) such as defensins, lysozyme, C-type lectins, and cathelicidin, some of which are produced by Paneth cells located at the base of small intestinal crypts [52]. Human genetic variants associated with IBD have been identified in a number of these pathways demonstrating that alterations in host innate immune protection from the gut microbiota play a role in the development of IBD. Among these include genes involved in epithelial barrier function, restitution, and solute transport as well as genes known to have an effect on the biology of Paneth cells [12, 53]. With respect to the latter, genetic polymorphisms in ATG16L1, associated with Crohn disease, lead to alterations in Paneth cells in both mice and humans that have functional consequences predisposing mice to the development of intestinal inflammation in response to bacteria and viruses [53, 54]. Paneth cell products, such as defensins, not only protect the host mucosal surface but can also help to shape the composition of the gut microbiome [55].

IBD and the Human Gut Microbiome

Epidemiological evidence provides strong evidence for the role of the environment in the pathogenesis of IBD. Over the last several decades, there has been an increase in the incidence of inflammatory bowel disease that is too rapid to be attributed solely to genetic factors. The association with residence in or immigration to industrialized nations [56], the consumption of a "Westernized" diet rich in fat and red meat [57], and the use of antibiotics at a young age [58] all implicate an alteration in the gut microbiota as a possible etiologic factor that may be playing a role in the increased incidence of IBD. Further support of this notion is the "hygiene hypothesis" suggesting that humans living in more industrialized societies are exposed to fewer microbes or less complex microbial communities at an early age leading to the development of an immune system less able to "tolerate" exposure to the microbial-laden environment in later life resulting in inappropriate immune activation [59].

Several theories have been suggested to explain the role of the gut microbiota in the pathogenesis of IBD: (1) specific microbial pathogens that induce intestinal inflammation, (2) host genetic defects in containing commensal microbiota in combination with defects in host mucosal immunoregulation, and (3) dysbiosis of commensal microbiota [4]. Multiple studies have been performed evaluating the role of specific bacteria in the development of IBD, such as *E. coli* and *Mycobacterium avium* subspecies *paratuberculosis* (MAP). In CD, there have been consistent findings of increased mucosa-associated *E. coli* in both the ileum and colon. The *E. coli* isolated in CD is often an adherent invasive *E. coli* (AIEC) phenotype, which is characterized by the invasion of epithelial cells and replication within macrophages [60] without causing cell death and induces the secretion of the tumor necrosis factor (TNF)-α [60, 61]. CD-associated AIEC strains are also capable of adhering to ileal enterocytes in patients with CD, however, not from control enterocytes [62].

MAP has also been implicated as a causal organism in the development of IBD. It is the known cause of Johne's disease in cattle which, similar to the histologic appearance of human CD, leads to chronic granulomatous enteritis. There have been multiple studies exploring the role of MAP in CD; however, controversy remains whether this organism indeed has a causal role. Some studies have shown remission in patients who have been treated with anti-MAP therapy; however, many argue that this has not proven causality. A large randomized controlled trial using combination antibiotics which have proven efficacy against MAP was performed by the Australian Antibiotic in Crohn's Disease Study Group [63]. This demonstrated an increase in steroid-induced remission; however, there was no significant effect on long-term maintenance of remission. Another criticism of this study was that patients were not assessed for the presence of MAP prior to initiation of therapy. As further studies are performed in MAP and IBD, perhaps a better understanding of this relationship will come to light [60].

Another consistent finding seen in multiple studies in patients with CD is that the phylum *Firmicutes* has been shown to be reduced [61, 64–68]. Specifically, *Faecalibacterium prausnitzii*, a *Firmicutes*, has been found to be decreased in IBD [69–71]. Furthermore, a decrease in *F. prausnitzii* was predictive of recurrence of disease in patients with CD undergoing ileal resection. There have also been studies that have shown a decrease in the presence of *Faecalibacterium prausnitzii* in fecal samples and biopsy specimens [69, 72]. In animal studies, *F. prausnitzii* can induce an anti-inflammatory response by increasing IL-10 as well as produce short-chain fatty acids, both of which may protect against the development of intestinal inflammation [61]. Concurrent with a reduction in *Firmicutes*, multiple studies have reported a concomitant increase in the abundance of *Proteobacteria* (including *E. coli*) [68, 73, 74] and *Enterobacteriaceae* [75, 76].

To control for the influence of genetics on the microbiome, there have been several studies performed comparing the microbiota of twin pairs. Dicksved and colleagues compared the intestinal microbiome of identical twins concordant or discordant for CD. Total bacterial diversity was decreased among patients with CD. Within twin sets, both healthy twins and twins concordant for CD had closely matched bacterial community profiles. In comparing the twin pairs discordant for CD, however, there was a difference between the fecal microbiome of those with CD and the healthy twin. This suggests that the structure of the bacterial communities is more closely associated with the disease activity rather than the genetics of the host [77]. In another study focusing on twins, Willing and colleagues characterized gut microbial communities in 40 twin pairs who were concordant or discordant for CD or UC. There were differences in the bacterial communities of patients with CD, and there were phenotypic differences as well among ileal and colonic disease as compared to the healthy subjects. There was a decrease in two genera of core commensals in patients with ileal CD, *Ruminococcaceae* family (including *Faecalibacterium*) and *Roseburia* (a member of the *Firmicutes* phylum) [78]. Consistent with prior studies, there was an increase in *Enterobacteriaceae*, including *E. coli* in some of the patients with ileal CD [79].

The alterations in the gut microbiome that are associated with IBD are often described as being "dysbiotic," implying that there is a functional imbalance between enteric bacteria with potentially pathogenic influences and bacteria who have a benign or beneficial effect on the host [80]. There is currently no clear evidence to confirm this notion in humans. An alternative explanation is that the observed alteration in the gut microbiome of patients with IBD is simply a consequence of the intestinal inflammatory response without consequence to the host. Additionally, in a human study of pediatric ulcerative colitis, evaluation of normal terminal ileum biopsies revealed a loss of goblet cells, depletion of the mucous layer, and loss of bacterial diversity despite a lack of inflammation in the sampled location, which may be due to a systemic effect to the gut epithelial lining independent of local inflammation [81].

There is, however, evidence for a functional effect of a "dysbiotic" intestinal microbiota in animal models. Investigators studying mice deficient in the immune regulatory transcription factor T-bet observed alterations in the intestinal microbiome that occurred simultaneously with the development of spontaneous colitis. Transfer of this bacterial community induced colitis in wild-type mice [82]. In a follow-up study, the investigators identified the presence of *Klebsiella pneumoniae* and *Proteus mirabilis* correlated with colitis in these mice [83]. Mice deficient in another immune regulator, the NLRP inflammasome, also develop spontaneous colitis, the susceptibility to which can also be transferred to wild-type mice [44]. Together, these studies suggest a causal role for the microbiota in IBD.

Diet, IBD, and the Gut Microbiome

Several investigators have examined the association of dietary patterns and the incidence of IBD [57, 84]. A systematic review of this subject found consistent results showing that high dietary intake of total fats, polyunsaturated fatty acids, omega-6 fatty acids, and meat was associated with an increased risk of CD and UC; high fiber and fruit intakes were associated with a decreased CD risk; and high vegetable intake was associated with a decreased UC risk [84]. These studies support a potential role for dietary patterns in the pathogenesis of IBD. Together with the recent data characterizing the impact of diet on the gut microbiome and its association with enterotypes [30], it is tempting to speculate that the alteration of gut microbiota community structure through the consumption of agrarian vs. a "Westernized" diet may play a role in either reducing or increasing, respectively, the risk for the development of IBD. This notion would be consistent with the increased incidence of IBD localized globally in more industrialized societies.

Enteral nutrition (EN) therapy, which has shown efficacy in the induction and maintenance of remission in patients with CD [85, 86], may ultimately provide additional support for the role of diet and the gut microbiota in the pathogenesis of IBD. As discussed in a separate chapter, EN is an attractive therapeutic option compared to pharmacological agents, as there are no serious associated side effects. While proven to be effective as therapy in CD, the mechanism of action of nutritional therapy has not been fully characterized. A recent study of pediatric CD patients on exclusive EN (90% of total caloric intake by dietary formula) compared to partial EN (53% by formula) was superior at improving symptoms and quality of life as well as inducing mucosal healing, suggesting that the elimination of solid table foods may be the key to why EN is therapeutic [87]. In addition, the alteration of the gut microbiota may be another possible mechanism of action. In the same study of pediatric CD patients, effective EN therapy changed the microbiota within 1 week and reduced the dysbiosis seen initially [88]. Leach and colleagues evaluated the fecal microbiome of patients with CD who were treated with EN and compared them to healthy control subjects on a regular diet [89]. Prior to initiation of EN, the two cohorts had similar diversity of bacteria present. At the 8-week follow-up, there was a significant decrease in diversity in the patients treated with EN that was sustained for several months following completion of therapy. Nutritional therapy highlights the importance of characterizing the interactions between diet, the gut microbiota, and the mucosal immune system.

The Gut Microbiota as a Therapeutic Strategy

Probiotics

One possible beneficial strategy for the treatment of IBD is probiotics. Probiotics are defined as living microorganisms that, when administered in adequate concentration, confer a health benefit on the host [90]. Probiotics have been shown to be effective in the treatment of pouchitis and possibly in UC [91–93]. Although evidence for the efficacy of probiotics in the treatment of IBD is currently equivocal, their beneficial effect in animal models is more consistent [94]. Possible mechanisms of action include the production of bacteriocins [95], the alteration of luminal pH of the intestine thereby altering the growth characteristics of some bacteria [96], and the enhancement of epithelial barrier function through the production of SCFA, a primary source of energy for colonocytes [97]. Numerous other proposed mechanisms of action have recently been reviewed [91, 97]. Prebiotics have also been investigated in the use of treatment of inflammatory bowel disease. Prebiotics are non-digestible food substances that stimulate the growth and/or activity of bacteria as well as the production of SCFA [97]. Prebiotics have been used with probiotics; this combination is called synbiotics. Several prebiotics that have been studied extensively and accepted in the European Union include fructooligosaccharides, galactooligosaccharides, and lactulose. The difficulty with these substances is ensuring the bacteria selectivity, i.e., only bacteria beneficial to the host will ferment the oligosaccharide and that the products of fermentation will promote the growth and activity of nonpathogenic organisms [98]. There have been several clinical trials using prebiotics as therapy [99–101], and some have shown promising results.

Bacterial Engineering

Another treatment in IBD utilizing the microbiome is bacterial engineering. In 2000, *Lactococcus lactis* was genetically engineered to secrete hIL-10 into the intestinal tissue in murine models. Colitis was prevented in IL-10 knockout mice, and there was a 50% reduction in inflammation in DSS-induced chronic colitis [102]. There have been clinical trials in humans that have shown promising results; however, further investigation is needed. Similarly, *Bacteroides ovatus* has been engineered to deliver TGF-β with good results in murine models [103]. There are ongoing trials in humans for the treatment of IBD.

Fecal Transplantation

Fecal microbiota transplantation (FMT) is another microbiota-based therapy that involves collecting stool from a healthy donor, preparing it in one of several ways, and transferring it to a patient with a disease or dysbiotic condition. The goal of FMT is to restore bacterial diversity through the microbiota of a healthy person. This healthy flora outcompetes *C. difficile* and produces secondary bile acids and antimicrobials that inhibit its growth. There remains no clear consensus regarding the mode of administration of fecal material. Possible delivery methods include upper endoscopy, nasogastric tube, nasointestinal tube, pill ingestion, colonoscopy to deliver to proximal colon, sigmoidoscopy, rectal tube, retention enema, or a combined approach. Patient comfort, safety, and cost-effectiveness should be considered when choosing how to deliver the material.

FMT was first safely described in humans in 1958 in the treatment of fulminant pseudomembranous enterocolitis [104]. Since then, there have been many published cases of *C. difficile* infection (CDI) and FMT, specifically for the treatment of recurrent or refractory CDI, which have been successful [105–107]. Multiple systemic reviews of fecal transplantation for CDI have demonstrated it to be safe, well tolerated, and effective with a mean cure rate of 87–90% and as high as 100% worldwide [108–110]. Moreover, the new healthy microbiota environment appears to be durable [107, 111]. In pediatric cases of recurrent CDI, there is limited data regarding safety and efficacy, but in all, a 92% cure rate has been reported without serious adverse events [112].

The effect seen in CDI may be possible in other dysbiotic conditions, particularly IBD. In 1989, Bennet and Brinkman published the first report of successfully treating UC with FMT, when Bennet successfully treated his own colitis [113]. In 2003, Borody and colleagues treated six patients with moderate to severe UC with FMT. All patients responded and remained in remission from 6 months to 13 years and had mucosal healing on endoscopy [114]. A review of several small studies of FMT as therapy for IBD showed mixed results; although the majority achieved clinical remission at least in the short term, none had serious adverse events, but there were several accounts of fever, chills, and gastrointestinal symptoms after, and one study reported worsening UC after FMT [115]. The largest studies of FMT for UC were randomized, placebo-controlled trials using FMT to induce remission in patients with mild to moderate UC which had mixed results regarding efficacy [116, 117].

A recent study showed that adult patients with IBD and parents of children with IBD were willing to consider fecal transplantation as therapy and felt that this was a safer option than many of the standard therapies [118]. In pediatric IBD,

the use of FMT has shown clinical benefit for a small cohort of 7/9 subjects with CD via nasogastric administration but not for UC subjects [119]. As with most pediatric therapies, the long-term consequences of FMT are unknown and should be better understood before implementing in conventional practice. There are currently no standard protocols, and further larger controlled studies are necessary; however, this therapy may hold promise for IBD as we learn more about the role of the gut microbiota and IBD pathogenesis.

Conclusions

Inflammatory bowel disease has been associated with both genetic and environmental factors. It has shown a dramatic increase in incidence over the past several decades. Effects of environmental changes in modern lifestyle, such as diet, sanitation, vaccinations, and antibiotics, have contributed to an alteration in the gut microbiome. While gut microbes very likely play a large role in the pathogenesis and propagation of the disease, their exact role requires further elucidation. The challenge remains to identify genetic, immunologic, environmental, and microbial triggers of disease development. As technologies such as DNA sequencing, metagenomics, transcriptomics, proteomics, and metabolomics continue to advance, along with the development of more sophisticated biocomputational tools, mechanisms by which the gut microbiota plays a role in the pathogenesis IBD will be better elucidated. In turn, this may provide novel insights into microbial-based methodologies that can be used to effectively prevent or treat IBD.

References

1. Bernstein CN, Shanahan F. Disorders of a modern lifestyle: reconciling the epidemiology of inflammatory bowel diseases. Gut. 2008;57(9):1185–91.
2. Sartor RB. Mechanisms of disease: pathogenesis of Crohn's disease and ulcerative colitis. Nat Clin Pract Gastroenterol Hepatol. 2006;3(7):390–407.
3. Rath HC, Herfarth HH, Ikeda JS, Grenther WB, Hamm Jr TE, Balish E, et al. Normal luminal bacteria, especially Bacteroides species, mediate chronic colitis, gastritis, and arthritis in HLA-B27/human beta2 microglobulin transgenic rats. J Clin Invest. 1996;98(4):945–53.
4. Sartor RB. Microbial influences in inflammatory bowel diseases. Gastroenterology. 2008;134(2):577–94.
5. Rutgeerts P, Hiele M, Geboes K, Peeters M, Penninckx F, Aerts R, et al. Controlled trial of metronidazole treatment for prevention of Crohn's recurrence after ileal resection. Gastroenterology. 1995;108(6):1617–21.
6. Rutgeerts P, Van Assche G, Vermeire S, D'Haens G, Baert F, Noman M, et al. Ornidazole for prophylaxis of postoperative Crohn's disease recurrence: a randomized, double-blind, placebo-controlled trial. Gastroenterology. 2005;128(4):856–61.

7. Sachar DB. Management of acute, severe ulcerative colitis. J Dig Dis. 2012;13(2):65–8.

8. Turner D, Levine A, Kolho KL, Shaoul R, Ledder O. Combination of oral antibiotics may be effective in severe pediatric ulcerative colitis: a preliminary report. J Crohns Colitis. 2014 Nov;8(11): 1464–70

9. Harper PH, Lee EC, Kettlewell MG, Bennett MK, Jewell DP. Role of the faecal stream in the maintenance of Crohn's colitis. Gut. 1985;26(3):279–84.

10. Rutgeerts P, Goboes K, Peeters M, Hiele M, Penninckx F, Aerts R, et al. Effect of faecal stream diversion on recurrence of Crohn's disease in the neoterminal ileum. Lancet. 1991;338(8770):771–4.

11. Swidsinski A, Loening-Baucke V, Theissig F, Engelhardt H, Bengmark S, Koch S, et al. Comparative study of the intestinal mucus barrier in normal and inflamed colon. Gut. 2007;56(3):343–50.

12. Khor B, Gardet A, Xavier RJ. Genetics and pathogenesis of inflammatory bowel disease. Nature. 2011;474(7351):307–17.

13. Liu JZ, van Sommeren S, Huang H, Ng SC, Alberts R, Takahashi A, et al. Association analyses identify 38 susceptibility loci for inflammatory bowel disease and highlight shared genetic risk across populations. Nat Genet. 2015;47(9):979–86.

14. Uhlig HH, Powrie F. Dendritic cells and the intestinal bacterial flora: a role for localized mucosal immune responses. J Clin Invest. 2003;112(5):648–51.

15. Lozupone CA, Knight R. Species divergence and the measurement of microbial diversity. FEMS Microbiol Rev. 2008;32(4):557–78.

16. Xu J, Gordon JI. Inaugural article: honor thy symbionts. Proc Natl Acad Sci U S A. 2003;100(18):10452–9.

17. Kelsen JR, Kim J, Latta D, Smathers S, McGowan KL, Zaoutis T, et al. Recurrence rate of clostridium difficile infection in hospitalized pediatric patients with inflammatory bowel disease. Inflamm Bowel Dis. 2011;17(1):50–5.

18. Costello EK, Lauber CL, Hamady M, Fierer N, Gordon JI, Knight R. Bacterial community variation in human body habitats across space and time. Science. 2009;326(5960):1694–7.

19. Reid G, Younes JA, Van der Mei HC, Gloor GB, Knight R, Busscher HJ. Microbiota restoration: natural and supplemented recovery of human microbial communities. Nat Rev Microbiol. 2011;9(1):27–38.

20. Marchesi JR. Prokaryotic and eukaryotic diversity of the human gut. Adv Appl Microbiol. 2010;72:43–62.

21. Hamady M, Knight R. Microbial community profiling for human microbiome projects: tools, techniques, and challenges. Genome Res. 2009;19(7):1141–52.

22. Palmer C, Bik EM, DiGiulio DB, Relman DA, Brown PO. Development of the human infant intestinal microbiota. PLoS Biol. 2007;5(7):e177.

23. Koenig JE, Spor A, Scalfone N, Fricker AD, Stombaugh J, Knight R, et al. Succession of microbial consortia in the developing infant gut microbiome. Proc Natl Acad Sci U S A. 2011;108(Suppl 1):4578–85.

24. Spor A, Koren O, Ley R. Unravelling the effects of the environment and host genotype on the gut microbiome. Nat Rev Microbiol. 2011;9(4):279–90.

25. Diamond J. Evolution, consequences and future of plant and animal domestication. Nature. 2002;418(6898):700–7.

26. Walter J, Ley R. The human gut microbiome: ecology and recent evolutionary changes. Annu Rev Microbiol. 2011;65:411–29.

27. Pflughoeft KJ, Versalovic J. Human microbiome in health and disease. Annu Rev Pathol. 2012;7:99–122.

28. Ley RE, Hamady M, Lozupone C, Turnbaugh PJ, Ramey RR, Bircher JS, et al. Evolution of mammals and their gut microbes. Science. 2008;320(5883):1647–51.

29. Muegge BD, Kuczynski J, Knights D, Clemente JC, Gonzalez A, Fontana L, et al. Diet drives convergence in gut microbiome functions across mammalian phylogeny and within humans. Science (New York, NY). 2011;332(6032):970–4.

30. Wu GD, Chen J, Hoffmann C, Bittinger K, Chen YY, Keilbaugh SA, et al. Linking long-term dietary patterns with gut microbial enterotypes. Science. 2011;334(6052):105–8.

31. Arumugam M, Raes J, Pelletier E, Le Paslier D, Yamada T, Mende DR, et al. Enterotypes of the human gut microbiome. Nature. 2011;473(7346):174–80.

32. De Filippo C, Cavalieri D, Di Paola M, Ramazzotti M, Poullet JB, Massart S, et al. Impact of diet in shaping gut microbiota revealed by a comparative study in children from Europe and rural Africa. Proc Natl Acad Sci U S A. 2010;107(33):14691–6.

33. Lim MY, Rho M, Song YM, Lee K, Sung J, Ko G. Stability of gut enterotypes in Korean monozygotic twins and their association with biomarkers and diet. Sci Rep. 2014;4:7348.

34. Hooper LV, Gordon JI. Commensal host-bacterial relationships in the gut. Science. 2001;292(5519):1115–8.

35. Round JL, Mazmanian SK. The gut microbiota shapes intestinal immune responses during health and disease. Nat Rev Immunol. 2009;9(5):313–23.

36. Zhang H, Sparks JB, Karyala SV, Settlage R, Luo XM. Host adaptive immunity alters gut microbiota. ISME J. 2015; 9(3):770–81.

37. Brugman S, Schneeberger K, Witte M, Klein MR, van den Bogert B, Boekhorst J, et al. T lymphocytes control microbial composition by regulating the abundance of Vibrio in the zebrafish gut. Gut Microbes. 2014;5(6):737–47.

38. Abraham C, Cho JH. Inflammatory bowel disease. N Engl J Med. 2009;361(21):2066–78.

39. Santaolalla R, Abreu MT. Innate immunity in the small intestine. Curr Opin Gastroenterol. 2012;28(2):124–9.

40. Fukata M, Chen A, Klepper A, Krishnareddy S, Vamadevan AS, Thomas LS, et al. Cox-2 is regulated by Toll-like receptor-4 (TLR4) signaling: role in proliferation and apoptosis in the intestine. Gastroenterology. 2006;131(3):862–77.

41. Shang L, Fukata M, Thirunarayanan N, Martin AP, Arnaboldi P, Maussang D, et al. Toll-like receptor signaling in small intestinal epithelium promotes B-cell recruitment and IgA production in lamina propria. Gastroenterology. 2008;135(2): 529–38.

42. Cario E, Gerken G, Podolsky DK. Toll-like receptor 2 enhances ZO-1-associated intestinal epithelial barrier integrity via protein kinase C. Gastroenterology. 2004;127(1):224–38.

43. Rehman A, Sina C, Gavrilova O, Hasler R, Ott S, Baines JF, et al. Nod2 is essential for temporal development of intestinal microbial communities. Gut. 2011;60(10):1354–62.

44. Elinav E, Strowig T, Kau AL, Henao-Mejia J, Thaiss CA, Booth CJ, et al. NLRP6 inflammasome regulates colonic microbial ecology and risk for colitis. Cell. 2011;145(5):745–57.

45. Vijay-Kumar M, Carvalho FA, Aitken JD, Fifadara NH, Gewirtz AT. TLR5 or NLRC4 is necessary and sufficient for promotion of humoral immunity by flagellin. Eur J Immunol. 2010;40(12):3528–34.

46. Neish AS. Microbes in gastrointestinal health and disease. Gastroenterology. 2009;136(1):65–80.

47. Peterson DA, McNulty NP, Guruge JL, Gordon JI. IgA response to symbiotic bacteria as a mediator of gut homeostasis. Cell Host Microbe. 2007;2(5):328–39.

48. Ivanov II, Atarashi K, Manel N, Brodie EL, Shima T, Karaoz U, et al. Induction of intestinal Th17 cells by segmented filamentous bacteria. Cell. 2009;139(3):485–98.

49. Surana NK, Kasper DL. The yin yang of bacterial polysaccharides: lessons learned from B. fragilis PSA. Immunol Rev. 2012;245(1):13–26.

50. Atarashi K, Tanoue T, Shima T, Imaoka A, Kuwahara T, Momose Y, et al. Induction of colonic regulatory T cells by indigenous Clostridium species. Science. 2011;331(6015):337–41.

51. Kamada N, Nunez G. Regulation of the immune system by the resident intestinal bacteria. Gastroenterology. 2014;146(6):1477–88.

52. Garrett WS, Gordon JI, Glimcher LH. Homeostasis and inflammation in the intestine. Cell. 2010;140(6):859–70.

53. Cadwell K, Liu JY, Brown SL, Miyoshi H, Loh J, Lennerz JK, et al. A key role for autophagy and the autophagy gene Atg16l1 in mouse and human intestinal Paneth cells. Nature. 2008;456(7219):259–63.

54. Cadwell K, Patel KK, Maloney NS, Liu TC, Ng AC, Storer CE, et al. Virus-plus-susceptibility gene interaction determines Crohn's disease gene Atg16L1 phenotypes in intestine. Cell. 2010;141(7):1135–45.

55. Salzman NH, Hung K, Haribhai D, Chu H, Karlsson-Sjoberg J, Amir E, et al. Enteric defensins are essential regulators of intestinal microbial ecology. Nat Immunol. 2010;11(1):76–83.

56. Molodecky NA, Soon IS, Rabi DM, Ghali WA, Ferris M, Chernoff G, et al. Increasing incidence and prevalence of the inflammatory bowel diseases with time, based on systematic review. Gastroenterology. 2012;142(1):46–54 e42. quiz e30

57. Chapman-Kiddell CA, Davies PS, Gillen L, Radford-Smith GL. Role of diet in the development of inflammatory bowel disease. Inflamm Bowel Dis. 2010;16(1):137–51.

58. Shaw SY, Blanchard JF, Bernstein CN. Association between the use of antibiotics and new diagnoses of Crohn's disease and ulcerative colitis. Am J Gastroenterol. 2011;106(12):2133–42.

59. Molodecky NA, Kaplan GG. Environmental risk factors for inflammatory bowel disease. Gastroenterol Hepatol (N Y). 2010;6(5):339–46.

60. Flanagan P, Campbell BJ, Rhodes JM. Bacteria in the pathogenesis of inflammatory bowel disease. Biochem Soc Trans. 2011;39(4):1067–72.

61. Vanderploeg R, Panaccione R, Ghosh S, Rioux K. Influences of intestinal bacteria in human inflammatory bowel disease. Infect Dis Clin North Am. 2010;24(4):977–93. ix

62. Barnich N, Carvalho FA, Glasser AL, Darcha C, Jantscheff P, Allez M, et al. CEACAM6 acts as a receptor for adherent-invasive E. coli, supporting ileal mucosa colonization in Crohn disease. J Clin Invest. 2007;117(6):1566–74.

63. Selby W, Pavli P, Crotty B, Florin T, Radford-Smith G, Gibson P, et al. Two-year combination antibiotic therapy with clarithromycin, rifabutin, and clofazimine for Crohn's disease. Gastroenterology. 2007;132(7):2313–9.

64. Van de Merwe JP, Schroder AM, Wensinck F, Hazenberg MP. The obligate anaerobic faecal flora of patients with Crohn's disease and their first-degree relatives. Scand J Gastroenterol. 1988;23(9):1125–31.

65. Walker AW, Sanderson JD, Churcher C, Parkes GC, Hudspith BN, Rayment N, et al. High-throughput clone library analysis of the mucosa-associated microbiota reveals dysbiosis and differences between inflamed and non-inflamed regions of the intestine in inflammatory bowel disease. BMC Microbiol. 2011;11:7.

66. Manichanh C, Rigottier-Gois L, Bonnaud E, Gloux K, Pelletier E, Frangeul L, et al. Reduced diversity of faecal microbiota in Crohn's disease revealed by a metagenomic approach. Gut. 2006;55(2):205–11.

67. Gophna U, Sommerfeld K, Gophna S, Doolittle WF, Veldhuyzen van Zanten SJ. Differences between tissue-associated intestinal microfloras of patients with Crohn's disease and ulcerative colitis. J Clin Microbiol. 2006;44(11):4136–41.

68. Frank DN, St Amand AL, Feldman RA, Boedeker EC, Harpaz N, Pace NR. Molecular-phylogenetic characterization of microbial community imbalances in human inflammatory bowel diseases. Proc Natl Acad Sci U S A. 2007;104(34):13780–5.

69. Martinez-Medina M, Aldeguer X, Gonzalez-Huix F, Acero D, Garcia-Gil LJ. Abnormal microbiota composition in the ileocolonic mucosa of Crohn's disease patients as revealed by polymerase chain reaction-denaturing gradient gel electrophoresis. Inflamm Bowel Dis. 2006;12(12):1136–45.

70. Prescott NJ, Fisher SA, Franke A, Hampe J, Onnie CM, Soars D, et al. A nonsynonymous SNP in ATG16L1 predisposes to ileal Crohn's disease and is independent of CARD15 and IBD5. Gastroenterology. 2007;132(5):1665–71.

71. Swidsinski A, Loening-Baucke V, Vaneechoutte M, Doerffel Y. Active Crohn's disease and ulcerative colitis can be specifically diagnosed and monitored based on the biostructure of the fecal flora. Inflamm Bowel Dis. 2008;14(2):147–61.

72. Sokol H, Pigneur B, Watterlot L, Lakhdari O, Bermudez-Humaran LG, Gratadoux JJ, et al. Faecalibacterium prausnitzii is an anti-inflammatory commensal bacterium identified by gut microbiota analysis of Crohn disease patients. Proc Natl Acad Sci U S A. 2008;105(43):16731–6.

73. Sartor RB. Therapeutic correction of bacterial dysbiosis discovered by molecular techniques. Proc Natl Acad Sci U S A. 2008;105(43):16413–4.

74. Mangin I, Bonnet R, Seksik P, Rigottier-Gois L, Sutren M, Bouhnik Y, et al. Molecular inventory of faecal microflora in patients with Crohn's disease. FEMS Microbiol Ecol. 2004;50(1):25–36.

75. Seksik P, Rigottier-Gois L, Gramet G, Sutren M, Pochart P, Marteau P, et al. Alterations of the dominant faecal bacterial groups in patients with Crohn's disease of the colon. Gut. 2003;52(2):237–42.

76. Baumgart M, Dogan B, Rishniw M, Weitzman G, Bosworth B, Yantiss R, et al. Culture independent analysis of ileal mucosa reveals a selective increase in invasive Escherichia coli of novel phylogeny relative to depletion of Clostridiales in Crohn's disease involving the ileum. ISME J. 2007;1(5):403–18.

77. Dicksved J, Halfvarson J, Rosenquist M, Jarnerot G, Tysk C, Apajalahti J, et al. Molecular analysis of the gut microbiota of identical twins with Crohn's disease. ISME J. 2008;2(7):716–27.

78. Sartor RB. Genetics and environmental interactions shape the intestinal microbiome to promote inflammatory bowel disease versus mucosal homeostasis. Gastroenterology. 2010;139(6):1816–9.

79. Willing BP, Dicksved J, Halfvarson J, Andersson AF, Lucio M, Zheng Z, et al. A pyrosequencing study in twins shows that gastrointestinal microbial profiles vary with inflammatory bowel disease phenotypes. Gastroenterology. 2010;139(6):1844–54 e1.

80. Tamboli CP, Neut C, Desreumaux P, Colombel JF. Dysbiosis in inflammatory bowel disease. Gut. 2004;53(1):1–4.

81. Alipour M, Zaidi D, Valcheva R, Jovel J, Martinez I, Sergi C, et al. Mucosal barrier depletion and loss of bacterial diversity are primary Abnormalities in paediatric ulcerative colitis. J Crohns Colitis. 2016;10(4):462–71.

82. Garrett WS, Lord GM, Punit S, Lugo-Villarino G, Mazmanian SK, Ito S, et al. Communicable ulcerative colitis induced by T-bet deficiency in the innate immune system. Cell. 2007;131(1):33–45.

83. Garrett WS, Gallini CA, Yatsunenko T, Michaud M, DuBois A, Delaney ML, et al. Enterobacteriaceae act in concert with the gut microbiota to induce spontaneous and maternally transmitted colitis. Cell Host Microbe. 2010;8(3):292–300.

84. Hou JK, Abraham B, El-Serag H. Dietary intake and risk of developing inflammatory bowel disease: a systematic review of the literature. Am J Gastroenterol. 2011;106(4):563–73.

85. Sandhu BK, Fell JM, Beattie RM, Mitton SG, Wilson DC, Jenkins H. Guidelines for the management of inflammatory bowel disease in children in the United Kingdom. J Pediatr Gastroenterol Nutr. 2010;50 Suppl 1:S1–13.

86. Caprilli R, Gassull MA, Escher JC, Moser G, Munkholm P, Forbes A, et al. European evidence based consensus on the diagnosis and management of Crohn's disease: special situations. Gut. 2006;55(Suppl 1):i36–58.

87. Lee D, Baldassano RN, Otley AR, Albenberg L, Griffiths AM, Compher C, et al. Comparative effectiveness of nutritional and biological therapy in North American children with active Crohn's disease. Inflamm Bowel Dis. 2015;21(8):1786–93.

88. Lewis JD, Chen EZ, Baldassano RN, Otley AR, Griffiths AM, Lee D, et al. Inflammation, antibiotics, and diet as environmental stressors of the gut microbiome in pediatric Crohn's disease. Cell Host Microbe. 2015;18(4):489–500.

89. Leach ST, Mitchell HM, Eng WR, Zhang L, Day AS. Sustained modulation of intestinal bacteria by exclusive enteral nutrition used to treat children with Crohn's disease. Aliment Pharmacol Ther. 2008;28(6):724–33.

90. Callaway TR, Edrington TS, Anderson RC, Harvey RB, Genovese KJ, Kennedy CN, et al. Probiotics, prebiotics and competitive exclusion for prophylaxis against bacterial disease. Anim Health Res Rev. 2008;9(2):217–25.

91. Haller D, Antoine JM, Bengmark S, Enck P, Rijkers GT, Lenoir-Wijnkoop I. Guidance for substantiating the evidence for beneficial effects of probiotics: probiotics in chronic inflammatory bowel disease and the functional disorder irritable bowel syndrome. J Nutr. 2010;140(3):690S–7S.

92. Bibiloni R, Fedorak RN, Tannock GW, Madsen KL, Gionchetti P, Campieri M, et al. VSL#3 probiotic-mixture induces remission in patients with active ulcerative colitis. Am J Gastroenterol. 2005;100(7):1539–46.

93. Tursi A, Brandimarte G, Giorgetti GM, Forti G, Modeo ME, Gigliobianco A. Low-dose balsalazide plus a high-potency probiotic preparation is more effective than balsalazide alone or mesalazine in the treatment of acute mild-to-moderate ulcerative colitis. Med Sci Monit. 2004;10(11):PI126–31.

94. Martin FP, Dumas ME, Wang Y, Legido-Quigley C, Yap IK, Tang H, et al. A top-down systems biology view of microbiome-mammalian metabolic interactions in a mouse model. Mol Syst Biol. 2007;3:112.

95. Spurbeck RR, Arvidson CG. Inhibition of Neisseria gonorrhoeae epithelial cell interactions by vaginal Lactobacillus species. Infect Immun. 2008;76(7):3124–30.

96. Medellin-Pena MJ, Wang H, Johnson R, Anand S, Griffiths MW. Probiotics affect virulence-related gene expression in *Escherichia coli* O157:H7. Appl Environ Microbiol. 2007;73(13):4259–67.

97. Sartor RB. Efficacy of probiotics for the management of inflammatory bowel disease. Gastroenterol Hepatol (N Y). 2011;7(9):606–8.

98. Kolida S, Gibson GR. Synbiotics in health and disease. Annu Rev Food Sci Technol. 2011;2:373–93.

99. Welters CF, Heineman E, Thunnissen FB, van den Bogaard AE, Soeters PB, Baeten CG. Effect of dietary inulin supplementation on inflammation of pouch mucosa in patients with an ileal pouch-anal anastomosis. Dis Colon Rectum. 2002;45(5):621–7.

100. Casellas F, Borruel N, Torrejon A, Varela E, Antolin M, Guarner F, et al. Oral oligofructose-enriched inulin supplementation in acute ulcerative colitis is well tolerated and associated with lowered faecal calprotectin. Aliment Pharmacol Ther. 2007;25(9):1061–7.

101. Lindsay JO, Whelan K, Stagg AJ, Gobin P, Al-Hassi HO, Rayment N, et al. Clinical, microbiological, and immunological effects of fructo-oligosaccharide in patients with Crohn's disease. Gut. 2006;55(3):348–55.

102. Steidler L, Hans W, Schotte L, Neirynck S, Obermeier F, Falk W, et al. Treatment of murine colitis by Lactococcus lactis secreting interleukin-10. Science (New York, NY). 2000;289(5483):1352–5.

103. Hamady ZZ, Scott N, Farrar MD, Wadhwa M, Dilger P, Whitehead TR, et al. Treatment of colitis with a commensal gut bacterium engineered to secrete human TGF-beta1 under the control of dietary xylan 1. Inflamm Bowel Dis. 2011;17(9):1925–35.

104. Eiseman B, Silen W, Bascom GS, Kauvar AJ. Fecal enema as an adjunct in the treatment of pseudomembranous enterocolitis. Surgery. 1958;44(5):854–9.

105. Garborg K, Waagsbo B, Stallemo A, Matre J, Sundoy A. Results of faecal donor instillation therapy for recurrent Clostridium difficile-associated diarrhoea. Scand J Infect Dis. 2010;42(11–12):857–61.

106. Rohlke F, Surawicz CM, Stollman N. Fecal flora reconstitution for recurrent Clostridium difficile infection: results and methodology. J Clin Gastroenterol. 2010;44(8):567–70.

107. Khoruts A, Dicksved J, Jansson JK, Sadowsky MJ. Changes in the composition of the human fecal microbiome after bacteriotherapy for recurrent Clostridium difficile-associated diarrhea. J Clin Gastroenterol. 2010;44(5):354–60.

108. Cammarota G, Ianiro G, Gasbarrini A. Fecal microbiota transplantation for the treatment of Clostridium difficile infection: a systematic review. J Clin Gastroenterol. 2014;48(8):693–702.

109. van Nood E, Dijkgraaf MG, Keller JJ. Duodenal infusion of feces for recurrent Clostridium difficile. N Engl J Med. 2013;368(22):2145.

110. Kassam Z, Lee CH, Yuan Y, Hunt RH. Navigating long-term safety in fecal microbiota transplantation. Am J Gastroenterol. 2013;108(9):1538.

111. Hamilton MJ, Weingarden AR, Unno T, Khoruts A, Sadowsky MJ. High-throughput DNA sequence analysis reveals stable engraftment of gut microbiota following transplantation of previously frozen fecal bacteria. Gut Microbes. 2013;4(2):125–35.

112. Kelly CR, Kahn S, Kashyap P, Laine L, Rubin D, Atreja A, et al. Update on fecal microbiota transplantation 2015: indications, methodologies, mechanisms, and outlook. Gastroenterology. 2015;149(1):223–37.

113. Bennet JD, Brinkman M. Treatment of ulcerative colitis by implantation of normal colonic flora. Lancet. 1989;1(8630):164.

114. Borody TJ, Warren EF, Leis S, Surace R, Ashman O. Treatment of ulcerative colitis using fecal bacteriotherapy. J Clin Gastroenterol. 2003;37(1):42–7.

115. Colman RJ, Rubin DT. Fecal microbiota transplantation as therapy for inflammatory bowel disease: a systematic review and meta-analysis. J Crohns Colitis. 2014;8(12):1569–81.

116. Moayyedi P, Surette MG, Kim PT, Libertucci J, Wolfe M, Onischi C, et al. Fecal microbiota transplantation induces remission in patients with active ulcerative colitis in a randomized controlled trial. Gastroenterology. 2015;149(1):102–9. e6

117. Rossen NG, Fuentes S, van der Spek MJ, Tijssen JG, Hartman JH, Duflou A, et al. Findings from a randomized controlled trial of fecal transplantation for patients with ulcerative colitis. Gastroenterology. 2015;149(1):110–8. e4

118. Kahn SA, Gorawara-Bhat R, Rubin DT. Fecal bacteriotherapy for ulcerative colitis: patients are ready, are we? Inflamm Bowel Dis. 2012;18(4):676–84.

119. Suskind DL, Brittnacher MJ, Wahbeh G, Shaffer ML, Hayden HS, Qin X, et al. Fecal microbial transplant effect on clinical outcomes and fecal microbiome in active Crohn's disease. Inflamm Bowel Dis. 2015;21(3):556–63.

Immune Dysregulation Associated with Very Early-Onset Inflammatory Bowel Disease

5

Judith Kelsen and Kathleen Sullivan

Introduction

An immunologic component to IBD has been recognized for many years. The strong association with specific MHC haplotypes underlies the presumption that T cells are involved in the pathogenesis [1, 2]. Additionally the serologic biomarkers also acknowledge that B cell responses are aberrant [2–4] Nevertheless, the exact pathogenesis of IBD remains elusive and even more so for VEO-IBD. Two lines of recent evidence support the hypothesis that immunologic dysfunction is fundamental to both the development and perpetuation of IBD. Genome-wide association studies have identified over 160 variants in teenage and adult cohorts, and the majority of those variants map to immunologically relevant genes [5–7]. These common variants are thought to synergistically interact with the microbiome to induce a state of susceptibility to IBD [8]. Some of these variants have independently been demonstrated to be associated with either impaired epithelial function or activation of immunologically competent cells [9, 10]. The effect size of each variant is rather small; however, it has been difficult to define the precise pathophysiologic contribution related to each independent variant. On the other side of the spectrum, monogenic disorders occur in which the penetrance of IBD is high. Understanding the mechanisms driving these rarer monogenic disorders has dramatically enhanced our understanding of IBD. A critical aspect of VEO-IBD is the hypothesis that genetic variants with a high penetrance for IBD dominate the susceptibility in young children, while adult-onset IBD is dominated by common variants with much lower relative risks for disease (Fig. 5.1).

J. Kelsen, MD (✉)
Division of Gastroenterology, Hepatology and Nutrition, The Children's Hospital of Philadelphia, Philadelphia, PA 19104, USA
e-mail: kelsen@email.chop.edu

K. Sullivan, MD, PhD
Division of Allergy and Immunology, The Children's Hospital of Philadelphia, Philadelphia, PA, USA

Genomics and VEO-IBD

Inflammatory bowel disease (IBD), comprised of Crohn disease, ulcerative colitis, and indeterminate colitis, is a multigenetic and environmentally triggered disease resulting in a dysregulated immune response to commensal or pathogenic microbes found in the gastrointestinal tract [6, 11–16]. Patients with IBD exhibit local and systemic immune reactivity to various microbes, have significant alterations in the composition of intestinal commensal bacteria, and can become colonized with pathogenic or opportunistic bacteria [17–24]. The multifactorial nature and environmental contribution to IBD is largely responsible for the increased incidence over the last several decades [25]. Despite this complex nature of the disease, it is becoming more apparent that host genetics may play a more prominent role in some subpopulations with the disease, particularly VEO-IBD [6, 26]. While this is a heterogeneous population, including some children with mild disease, patients with VEO-IBD can present with distinctive disease phenotypes, including extensive colonic involvement and more severe disease, than older children and adults [27, 28]. In addition, due to poor response to conventional therapies, severity of inflammation, and greater duration of disease, there are higher rates of morbidity in this population [27, 29, 30]. It is because of the aggressive disease phenotype, early age of onset, and strong family history of disease, that a portion of VEO-IBD is thought to be a monogenic disease, often involving genes associated with primary immunodeficiencies [31, 32]. The landmark discovery in 2009 was the first to demonstrate causal genetic defects, identifying several *IL10* [33], *IL10RA, and IL10RB* [30] gene mutations associated with a phenotype of severe perianal disease and colitis in infants with VEO-IBD. Additional underlying immunodeficiencies or genetic disorders may also present with an intestinal phenotype in patients with VEO-IBD [27, 32]. These include, but are not limited to, common variable immunodeficiency (CVID); Wiskott–Aldrich syndrome (WAS); immunodysregulation, polyendocrinopathy and enteropathy, X-linked (IPEX) syndrome;

© Springer International Publishing AG 2017
P. Mamula et al. (eds.), *Pediatric Inflammatory Bowel Disease*, DOI 10.1007/978-3-319-49215-5_5

Fig. 5.1 Inheritance and penetrance of variants related to IBD. VEO-IBD is thought to be enriched for monogenic disorders whereas adult-onset IBD has a polygenic inheritance with contributions from multiple variants, each of which may confer only a small increase in risk

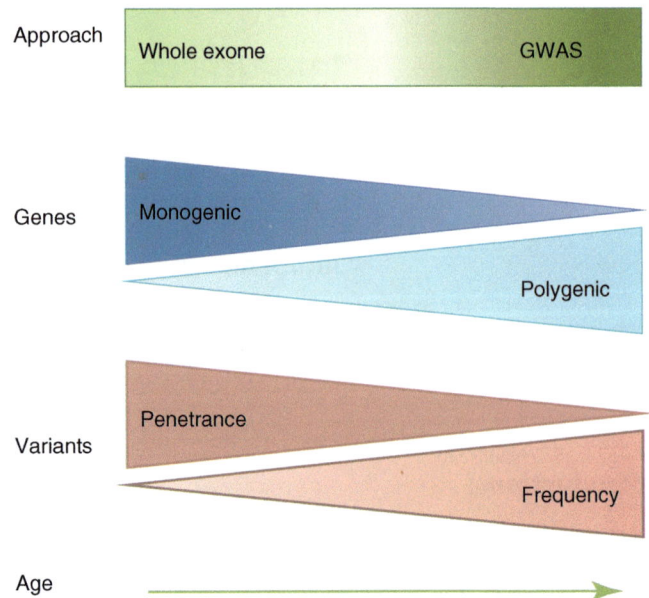

X-linked inhibitor of apoptosis (XIAP); and chronic granulomatous disease (CGD) [27, 29, 34].

Targeted genetic sequencing has been an extremely valuable approach to allow the identification and characterization of genetic variants associated with VEO-IBD. However, these approaches alone may not identify novel and rare gene variants. Recent advances in sequencing technology, such as whole exome sequencing (WES), have allowed an additional approach for an increased understanding of the pathogenesis of VEO-IBD and resulted in further discoveries of genes and pathways associated with the disease [34–38]. The genomic contribution of IBD has been extensively evaluated through genome-wide association studies (GWAS), and more than 200 IBD-associated risk loci [7] have been identified. Several genes located within the IBD-associated loci are critical in regulation of host defense, involving both the innate and adaptive immune response toward microbes [7]. However, GWAS were primarily performed in adult-onset IBD and children 10 years of age and greater, whose disease, as noted above, is most frequently a polygenic complex disease. Furthermore, GWAS often do not capture rare variants, specifically those with minor allele frequency (MAF) less than 5%. In contrast, as discussed above, a proportion of patients with VEO-IBD have a monogenic-driven disease or multigenic disease enriched with rare variants of the same or interacting immunologic pathways [30, 39]. Thus, as in the case of IL-10RA and IL10RB defects, the development of intestinal inflammation in VEO-IBD patients can be the direct result of defective immune responses [40]. While WES has revolutionized our ability to study rare variants and determine the genetic basis of disease, understanding the relevance of identified variants has remained challenging. The individual patient's phenotype may be shaped by mode of

inheritance, epigenetics, and gene–gene interaction. Environmental modifiers, such as the intestinal microbiota, antibiotic exposure, infection or diet, also significantly impact disease phenotype [26, 35]. Due to the clinical presentation, often of severe disease, together with the challenge of identifying the unique pathogenesis of the disease, there is currently no standard of care in the evaluation and treatment for VEO-IBD patients. Identifying the driving forces in patients with particularly severe early-onset disease may lead to group-specific therapeutic approaches.

Clinical Presentation of Very Early-Onset (VEO)-IBD

Pediatric IBD has increased in incidence and prevalence, and this phenomenon has included very young children [25, 40, 41]. Approximately 6–15% of the pediatric IBD population is less than 6 years old, and disease in the first year of life is rare [25, 41]. A subset of patients with VEO-IBD present with a phenotype that is distinct from older children and adults, including extensive colonic disease (pancolitis) that it is frequently difficult to differentiate ulcerative colitis (UC) from Crohn disease (CD), leading to a diagnosis of indeterminate colitis (Table 5.1) [27, 41]. At diagnosis, patients with VEO-IBD are more commonly diagnosed with UC (35–59%) as compared to older-onset IBD (older children >6 and adults) in which CD is more prevalent (55–60%). In contrast, approximately 30–35% of VEO-IBD patients are diagnosed with CD. Indeterminate colitis is also diagnosed more often in patients with VEO (11–22%) as compared to older onset IBD (4–10%) [42–45]. While formal guidelines or standards of care do not exist, disease evaluation of this

Table 5.1 Differences between VEO-IBD and older-onset IBD

VEO-IBD	Older-onset IBD

Disease presentation
  Predominately colonic
  Ileal involvement <20%
  Extensive at presentation
	Disease presentation
	  Ileocolonic
	  Less extensive at presentation

Disease classification
  CD: 30–35%
  UC: 35–39%
  IC: 11–22%
	Disease classification
	  CD: 55–60%
	  UC: 40–45%
	  IC: 4–10%

Histology
  Villous blunting
  Apoptosis
	Histology
	  Villous blunting/apoptosis
	  rarely seen

Positive family history
  40–50%
	Positive family history
	  10–20%

Therapeutic response to conventional therapy Decreased	

Surgical intervention
  70%
	Surgical intervention
	  55%

population includes laboratory, radiologic, and endoscopic evaluation (Table 5.2). Diagnosis at a very young age should trigger concern for a monogenic-driven disease, particularly in IBD diagnosed less than 2 years of age. Furthermore, extensive family history, including history of disease in male family members (such as in X-linked disease), history of infection, skin disease, or autoimmunity can help guide appropriate laboratory screening. One of the initial strategies to identify patients with primary immune deficiencies is to simply survey their immunologic function. The laboratory studies should include not only routine screening utilized for IBD diagnosis but also an immunological evaluation as well. This includes immunoglobulin profiles, vaccine titers, dihydrorhodamine (DHR) flow cytometry assay, analyses of B and T cell function, natural killer cell function, and, if necessary, more targeted phenotyping and functional profiling of the systemic and mucosal immune system.

While many of the defects may not have demonstrable effects on cells within the peripheral blood, many of the monogenic disorders will have an impact that can be appreciated through these simple screening studies. When those are not suggestive of a primary immune deficiency, in many cases WES will be pursued. This strategy is now sufficiently available, and the consequences of identification of a primary immune deficiency are sufficiently large, that it is appropriate to expand the energy and effort to obtain this type of sequencing.

Genetic Variants Associated with VEO-IBD and Their Immunologic Consequences

Immune defects that can present with the phenotype of intestinal inflammation include genes involved in intestinal epi-

thelial barrier function, phagocyte bacterial killing, hyper- or autoimmune inflammatory disorders and development and function of the adaptive immune system [39]. These defects can impact the developing gut microbiome and thus progression of intestinal inflammation. Therapeutic strategies for this unique cohort should be directed toward the underlying impaired pathway.

Genetic Variants Influencing Intestinal Epithelial Barrier Function

Defects in epithelial barrier function, lymphocyte signaling defects, regulatory T cell defects, innate responses to infection, and autoinflammatory disorders may seem to represent highly diverse types of defects leading to VEO-IBD. They come together at the epithelial surface where immune responses must be perfectly tuned to prevent inappropriate responses. Increased translocation of bacteria or translocation of inappropriate bacteria, as is the case in dysbiosis, drives an inflammatory loop. An important component of the integrity of the epithelial surface is the contribution of innate lymphoid cells. This cell type has not been previously discussed, and there are no known monogenic disorders that affect innate lymphoid cells; however, in murine models their role is now firmly established. These cells contribute to the maintenance of the epithelial layer as well as secretion of antimicrobial peptides and mucins. When this carefully constructed epithelial barrier is penetrated, cells of the innate immune system are activated and recruit additional cells to the inflammatory process. It may be that some of the signaling defects that have been described for conventional T cells also impact the function of innate lymphoid cells and contribute to the susceptibility of IBD through their roles in innate lymphoid cells more substantially than is currently appreciated. Within the lamina propria, T cells and innate lymphoid cells perform an intricate choreography mediated by the secretion of cytokines [46]. Many of the recognized cytokines are already being targeted through biologic therapies. From this framework, the high impact of the monogenic disorders may be appreciated.

Defects in the intestinal epithelial barrier function can present with inflammation in patients with VEO-IBD. These include loss-of-function mutations in *ADAM17* resulting in ADAM17 deficiency [47, 48], *IKBKG* (encoding NEMO) resulting in X-linked ectodermal dysplasia and immunodeficiency [49], *COL7A1* resulting in dystrophic epidermolysis bullosa [50], *FERMT1 resulting in* Kindler syndrome [51–53], and *TTC7A* [37] or gain-of-function mutations in *GUCY2* resulting in familial diarrhea [26, 54]. These defects have distinct deleterious effects on the integrity of the epithelial barrier: epithelial regeneration (*ADAM17*), [55], loss of signaling pathways involved in gene expression (*IKBKG*) [56, 57], altered cell adhesion, barrier formation and apoptosis (*COL7A1*, *FEMT1* and *TTC7A*) [37, 50–53], or impaired

Table 5.2 Primary immune deficiencies associated with IBD

Category	Gene name	Name of immune deficiency	Prevalence of IBD	Characteristics of IBD in this syndrome	Other features of the disorder	Other autoimmune manifestations
Central tolerance	AIRE	APECED	≈10%	Enteropathy with villous blunting	Candida, malabsorption	Autoimmune polyendocrinopathies
	RAG1/2	SCID, Leaky SCID	≈50%	Not reported	Low CD4/CD45RA cells, infections	Many types
Peripheral tolerance	FOXP3	IPEX	≈90%	Villous atrophy		Diabetes, autoimmune polyendocrinopathies
	STAT5b	STAT5b deficiency	Unknown	Villous atrophy	Post-natal growth retardation, lymphocytic interstitial pneumonitis, severe varicella	Arthritis, thyroiditis
	CD25	IL-2RA deficiency	≈90%	Villous atrophy	Viral infections	Various autoimmune
	CTLA4	CTLA4 haplosufficiency	≈80%	Villous blunting	Hypogammaglobulinemia, infections	Various autoimmune including granulomatous lung disease
	LRBA	LRBA deficiency	≈60%	Typical IBD and small bowel disease	Hypogammaglobulinemia, infections	
Apoptosis defects	FAS (TNFRSF6), FASLG (TNFSF6), somatic mutations of FAS in 30%	ALPS	≈1%	Not reported	Adenopathy, hepatosplenomegaly	Autoimmune cytopenias
	CYBA, CYBB, NCF1< NCF2, NCF4	CGD	≈10–50%	Villous blunting with acute inflammation common, pigmented macrophages in half, granulomas in half, eosinophils prominent in 25%	Fungal infections, abscesses	ITP rarely
	XIAP	XLP2	≈20%	Granulomas	HLH, hypogammaglobulinemia	None
Lymphocyte signaling defects	PLCG2	PLAID	≈5%	Not reported	Skin granulomas, cold urticaria, infections, hypogammaglobulinemia	Autoantibodies
	AID	AR Hyper-IgM syndrome	≈5–10%	Not reported	Adenopathy, high IgM, low IgG	Various autoimmune
	DOCK8	DOCK8 deficiency	≈5–10%	Not reported, may be secondary to infection	Severe infections	Vasculitis, autoimmune hemolytic anemia
	WAS	Wiskott–Aldrich syndrome	≈5–10%	Not reported	Small platelets with thrombocytopenia, infections, eczema	Various autoimmune
	NEMO (IKBKG), NFkB1A	Ectodermal dysplasia with immune deficiency	≈25%	Paucity of lymphocytes and relatively superficial neutrophil infiltrate	Infections are severe	Limited
	BTK	XLA	≈5–10%	Not reported	No B cells, hypogammaglobulinemia	Arthritis

Interferon hyper-production by lymphocytes	STAT1 GOF	STAT1 GOF	≈50%	Villous atrophy	Candida and other fungal infections	Diabetes common but other autoimmunity seen frequently
	STAT3 GOF	STAT3 GOF	60%	Villous atrophy	Short stature	Diabetes and other autoimmunity
	STAT3 LOF	Hyper-IgE syndrome	≈1–5%	Can be due to infection	Infections, eczema	Rare
Unknown mechanism		CVID	10–20%	Villous atrophy, collagenous colitis, typical IBD all seen	Usually adult onset, sinopulmonary infections	Autoimmune cytopenias, lymphoproliferation, granulomas
	DNMT3b, ZBTB24	ICF	50% have diarrhea	Not reported	Mild developmental delay, IgA deficiency	Rare

APECED autoimmune polyendocrinopathy, candidiasis, ectodermal dysplasia; *SCID* severe combined immune deficiency; *IPEX* immune dysregulation, polyendocrinopathy, X-linked syndrome; *ALPS* autoimmune lymphoproliferative syndrome; *CGD* chronic granulomatous disease; *XLP2* X-linked lymphoproliferative syndrome 2; *PLAID* phospholipase C-γ2–associated antibody deficiency and immune dysregulation; *XLA* X-linked agammaglobulinemia; *ICF* immunodeficiency, centromeric instability, facial anomalies syndrome

bacterial sensing and ion homeostasis (*GUCY2*), [26, 54]. The intestinal barrier is necessary to maintain a physical separation between commensal bacteria and the host immune system, and any break in this defense can lead to chronic intestinal inflammation [11, 13]. The intestinal barrier function is maintained through a number of physical and biochemical structures beyond the identified monogenic defects, including mucus production, intestinal epithelial cell tight junction proteins, immunoglobulin A (IgA), and antimicrobial peptides. Mouse models have illustrated the consequences of the disrupted epithelial barrier. Administration of dextran sodium sulfate (DSS) in the mice drinking water leads to disruption of the intestinal barrier and subsequent infiltration of commensal bacteria and activation of the innate immune system [58]. Chronic exposure to DSS can lead to activation of the adaptive immune response and the development pro-inflammatory, commensal bacteria-specific, B and T cell responses [17, 59], which are similar to that observed in IBD patients [17, 60]. Furthermore, murine models have shown the critical role of intestinal epithelial cells in regulation of intestinal immunologic homeostasis, through cell lineage-specific deletion of factors regulating the NFκB pathway, including NEMO and IKKβ, result in susceptibility to chronic intestinal inflammation [56, 57].

Patients with epithelial defects may have unique intestinal histology that can aid in diagnosis and therapy. Patients with *IKBKG* (NEMO) defects may have epithelial cell shedding or villous atrophy (as well as *TTC7A*) on pathology [61]. Histology in patients with *ADAM17* mutations may demonstrate hypoplastic crypts in small bowel secondary to a low rate of epithelial production, as *ADAM17* is necessary for TGF-α to be cleaved from the cell membrane [62, 63]. Although we know that loss of intestinal barrier function can directly cause intestinal inflammation, additional translational studies are needed to further define how these mutations in the above genes specifically lead to a break down in the barrier, and whether we can develop more targeted therapies to restore barrier integrity and limit chronic inflammation.

Genetic Variants Influencing Bacterial Recognition and Clearance

Chronic granulomatous disease (CGD) is a result of defective intestinal phagocytes, specifically the granulocytes responsible for bacterial killing and clearance [64]. The NADPH oxidase complex is responsible for killing of ingested microbes through its production of the respiratory burst. Mutations in any part of the complex molecules (CYBB, CYBA, NCF1, NCF2, NCF4) can result in intestinal inflammation as well as autoimmune disease [65, 66]. Intestinal inflammation can be observed in as high as 40% of patients with CGD [67–70]. Several variants have been associated with VEO-IBD, in particular defective NCF2 results in altered binding to RAC2 [71]. These patients can present

in the neonatal or first year of life with colitis, severe fistulizing perianal disease and structuring [69, 71]. Histology frequently demonstrates multiple granulomas that may not have associated inflammatory change [35, 71]. Critically, a recent study by Muise and colleagues identified that heterozygous loss of function mutations in components of the NADPH oxidase complex can determine susceptibility to VEO-IBD, without directly causing overt immunodeficiency [72]. Other neutrophil defects that are associated with VEO-IBD include leukocyte adhesion defect, due to mutation in ITGB2 [73, 74]. These patients can present with an IBD phenotype, history of bacterial infection and laboratory studies remarkable for increased peripheral granulocytes [75]. Glycogen storage disease type 1b, with the unique combination of neutropenia and neutrophil granulocyte dysfunction, can present with intestinal inflammation [76].

The reasons for why CGD and these other bacterial processing defects may manifest in intestinal inflammation is not fully clear; however, defective autophagy may play an important role. Furthermore, the therapies used to treat such patients need to be carefully considered. For example, anti-TNFα therapy is contraindicated in CGD. Though effective for intestinal disease, these agents can increase the risk of severe infections in these patients and can be fatal [77]. Other therapies include leukine, antibiotics, and allogenic hematopoietic stem cell transplantation, which have demonstrated some success [78]. IL-1R antagonists have been used in these patients with some positive results, by restoring autophagy and directly limiting inflammation [79].

Genetic Variants Impairing Development of the Adaptive Immune System

Several genetic variants can alter the development or function of adaptive immune cells in a cell-intrinsic or cell-extrinsic manner. Defects that affect development or function of B cells and T cells occur with loss-of-function mutations in recombination activating genes (*RAG1* or *RAG2*) or the IL-7R (*IL7R*) causing Omenn syndrome, or the *PTEN* gene causing PTEN syndrome. Defects in *RAG1*, *RAG2*, or *IL-7R* can cause cell-intrinsic defects in the development of both T cells and B cells, by blocking either early lymphocyte survival or recombination of the B cell receptor (BCR) or T cell receptor (TCR) [80–82]. Defects in B cell development lead to an absence of circulating mature B cells and antibody production, which have been linked to an IBD phenotype [83]. This includes agammaglobulinemia, which can also occur in X-linked agammaglobulinemia (XLA) [84] and common variable immune deficiency (CVID), a complex and heterogeneous disease, with the responsible mutations known for only a minority of cases [85]. Loss of function mutation in *LRBA*, resulting in multiple defects in immune cell populations, can result in a VEO-IBD phenotype [86]. In addition to CVID, antibody deficiency associated with IBD manifestations includes IgA deficiency and severe combined immunodeficiency (SCID). Multiple gene defects that impact the development or function of the adaptive immune system have been associated with SCID, including *RAG1, RAG2, JAK3, CD45, CD3G, ZAP70, ADA, DCLRE1C* and *DOCK8* [39, 83, 87]. Omenn syndrome, a recessive form of SCID, involves abnormal development of B cells and T cells, and can also be associated with intestinal disease as well as severe eczematous rash [87, 88]. Laboratory studies can show increased oligoclonal T cells and reduced B cells, and histology can show an intestinal graft versus host appearance [89, 90]. Aberrant function of immunoglobulins, such as in hyper-IgM and hyper-IgE syndromes, can also result in intestinal inflammation and an IBD phenotype [91]. While the exact mechanism leading to intestinal inflammation in these defects remains unclear, it may involve altered regulatory pathways, or chronic infections with pathogenic and opportunistic microbes. Additional studies are required to further interrogate the link of these mutations to intestinal inflammation.

Wiskott–Aldrich syndrome (WAS) results from a loss of function mutation in Wiskott–Aldrich syndrome protein (*WASP*), and patients can exhibit thrombocytopenia, eczema, immune deficiencies, and intestinal inflammation [92]. The clinical manifestation of patients with VEO-IBD with this genetic defect can be pancolitis in addition to other autoimmune processes. *WASP* is a critical cytoskeleton protein expressed in hematopoietic cells that is required for the normal development and function of multiple cell types [93, 94]. WASP is required for peripheral B cell development and function and subsequent response to antigens [95, 96]. Laboratory studies of these patients may show thrombocytopenia, low IgM levels, low marginal B cells, and lymphopenia [97]. Snapper and colleagues identified that intestinal inflammation in WASP-deficient mice was critically dependent upon inflammatory T cells [98], and may result from an impaired development of regulatory T cells (Tregs) in the thymus and periphery [99]. Surprisingly, absence of WASP in cells of the innate immune system directly contributed to the development of inflammatory T cell responses in mice, thus indicating that these defects are likely occurring in a cell extrinsic manner [100]. The causes of intestinal inflammation in other similar patient populations are less well understood, but defects in regulatory T cells, IgA, and abnormal selection of T cell and B cell specificities likely contribute. Additional translational and animal studies, such as those described above, are necessary to further define the causes of disease and potential therapeutic options in these patient populations.

Genetic Variants Impairing Regulatory T Cells

Defects in regulatory T cells can clinically present as colonic disease and well as an enteropathy. The prominence of villous atrophy is a clue to these disorders. Immunodysregulation, polyendocrinopathy, enteropathy X-linked syndrome (IPEX) is most often secondary to mutations of Forkhead box protein 3 (*FOXP3*) gene, a transcription factor that is essential for the development and immunosuppressive activity of CD4 Foxp3+ Tregs [88, 101–103]. There are over 20 mutations in *FOXP3* that have been identified in patients with IPEX [102], and patients frequently present with neonatal severe secretory diarrhea, failure to thrive, infection (due to defects in immunoregulation), skin rash, insulin-dependent diabetes, thyroiditis, cytopenias, and other autoimmune disorders [88]. Tregs are absent or dysfunctional in these patients, and in the intestine histologic analyses may reveal infiltration of inflammatory cells in the lamina propria and submucosa of the small bowel and colon as well as changes in the mucosa of the small bowel [104]. Other genetic defects have been found to cause IPEX-like disease, including loss of function mutations impacting IL-2–IL-2R interactions, STAT5b, and ITCH, or gain-of-function mutations in STAT1, all of which critically influence the development and function of Tregs [88]. Furthermore, Blumberg and colleagues identified a novel loss of function mutation in *CTLA4*, a surface molecule of regulatory T cells that directly suppresses effector T cell populations in VEO-IBD [105].

Murine models have helped characterize the mechanisms by which regulatory T cells limit intestinal inflammation. Regulatory T cells can develop in the thymus as "natural Tregs" and directly contribute to limiting pro-inflammatory T cells in the intestine [106]. The composition of commensal bacteria influences the repertoire of Tregs [106], and commensal bacteria-specific "induced Tregs" can also be generated in the periphery after interaction between commensal bacteria and dendritic cells in the intestine and migration to the mesenteric lymph node [11, 15, 103, 107]. Once generated, Tregs can then promote intestinal homeostasis through direct regulation of innate and adaptive immune cell responses to commensal bacteria, through cytokine production, direct cell–cell contact (in part through CTLA4), and sequestering of growth factors [11, 15, 103]. Consistent with a major role for regulatory T cells in limiting pro-inflammatory immune cell responses to commensal bacteria, mice deficient in IL-2 or FoxP3 develop significantly less intestinal inflammation when maintained in germ-free versus conventional housing conditions, but exhibit comparable levels of systemic autoimmunity [108, 109]. Murine models have also suggested the regulatory T cells function in the intestine, and ability to limit chronic inflammation is through balancing of tissue-specific IL-23 and IL-33 expression [110], although the role of these pathways in human VEO-IBD has not been extensively examined.

Genetic Variants in the IL-10-IL-10R Pathway and Related Cytokine Family Members

Homozygous loss of function mutations in *IL10* ligand and receptors *IL10RA* and *IL10RB* are associated with severe intestinal inflammation, particularly in neonatal or infantile

VEO-IBD, with a phenotype of severe enterocolitis and peri-anal disease [30, 33]. In addition, compound heterozygote loss of function mutations of *IL10RA* have been reported with neonatal Crohn disease and enterocolitis [111]. IL-10 is an anti-inflammatory cytokine secreted by a variety of cells, including dendritic cells, natural killer (NK) cells, eosino-phils, mast cells, macrophages, B cells, and CD4⁺ T cell sub-sets (including Th2 cells, Th1 cells, Th17 cells, and Treg) [112, 113]. IL-10 maintains homeostasis through suppres-sion of an excessive pro-inflammatory response and exerts its effect through binding to the IL-10 receptor, IL-10R, which is a tetrameric complex [114]. It is composed of two distinct chains, two molecules of IL-10R1 (α chain), and two molecules of IL-10R2 (β chain) [115]. IL-10 binding to IL-10R activates the JAK1/STAT3 cascade, which subse-quently limits pro-inflammatory gene expression [115]. In addition to intestinal inflammation, IL-10 defects are associ-ated with arthritis, folliculitis, and predisposition to lym-phoma [111, 116]. Hematopoietic stem cell transplantation has proven to be a successful treatment for this patients and potentially life-saving [117, 118].

An essential role for IL-10 in limiting intestinal inflam-mation was demonstrated by the spontaneous development of severe colitis in IL-10-deficient mice [119]. Furthermore, studies by Sartor and colleagues identified that the intestinal inflammation in IL-10-deficient mice was entirely dependent upon the presence of commensal bacteria [120]. Therefore, IL-10 plays a critical role in limiting dysregulated immune cell responses to intestinal commensal bacteria. Mouse stud-ies showing that permit conditional deletion of IL-10 and IL-10R have revealed an essential role of regulatory T cell-intrinsic IL-10 expression in preventing intestinal inflamma-tion in mice [121, 122]. Furthermore, IL-10R expression on myeloid cells in mice was shown to be critical in eliciting anti-inflammatory responses and limiting T cell-dependent intestinal inflammation [123, 124]. Patients with loss-of-function mutations in *IL10RA* or *IL10RB* also exhibited an impaired ability to differentiate anti-inflammatory myeloid cells in vitro, and exhibited increased pro-inflammatory properties, such as elevated expression of IL-6, IL-12, TNFα, MHCII, and co-stimulatory molecules [123].

IL-22 also plays a critical role in mediating intestinal homeostasis. It is a cytokine related to IL-10, shares the IL-10R2 chain with a unique IL-22R1, and signals through predominantly STAT3 [125]. However, IL-22 acts almost exclusively on intestinal epithelial cells to mediate innate immunity and intestinal barrier function and unlike IL-10, the complete IL-22R is restricted to non-hematopoietic cells [125]. IL-22 can be produced by Th17 cells and is predomi-nantly expressed by group 3 innate lymphoid cells (ILC3) [125, 126], a recently identified cell type of the innate immune system. This incredible finding has led to the identi-fication of other members of the innate lymphoid cell (ILC)

family, including group 1 ILCs (ILC1) that express T-bet and pro-inflammatory cytokines TNFα and IFNγ, and group 2 ILCs that express GATA3 and type 2 cytokines IL-4, IL-5, IL-9, and IL-13 [126, 127]. The ILC family is comparable to differentiated CD4 T cell subsets in its heterogeneity and plays a profound role in regulating intestinal health and dis-ease in mouse models [125–127]. Evidence suggests that ILC3 are a dominant source of IL-22 in the intestine of healthy humans, and that dysregulated ILC responses are observed in adult patients with IBD, a critical development in our understanding of the immunology of IBD [128–134]. ILC3 express MHCII and selective deletion of MHCII on ILC3 results in dysregulated CD4 T cell responses and spon-taneous intestinal inflammation, suggesting that these cells are essential for regulation of T cell-mediated inflammation in the gut [129]. MHCII⁺ ILC3 selectively induce cell death of pro-inflammatory, commensal bacteria-specific CD4 T cells in the intestine. MHCII was reduced on ILC3 from intestinal biopsies of pediatric IBD patients versus non-IBD controls and inversely correlated with levels of pro-inflam-matory Th17 cells [135]. Despite these advances, ILC and IL-22 responses have not yet been adequately explored in VEO-IBD, and given the importance of these pathways in mediating intestinal health and disease, it is likely the genetic variations associated with VEO-IBD may differentially influence ILC responses.

Autoimmune and Autoinflammatory Disorders

Autoimmune disease in general is strongly associated with variants related to immune deficiency. In a meta-analysis of rheumatoid arthritis, 377 candidate genes were identified as risk loci for rheumatoid arthritis. Among 98 genes with a relative risk greater than 2, 15 of those genes were related to primary immune deficiencies [136]. Therefore, it should come as no surprise that VEO-IBD is similarly enriched with gene defects related to primary immune deficiencies. The study of primary immune deficiencies and their association with VEO-IBD has illuminated the critical and delicate interaction of the immune system with the luminal contents of the gastrointestinal tract. Primary immune deficiencies no doubt increase the susceptibility to IBD through multiple mechanisms. Even a mild immune deficiency such as IgA deficiency has a significantly higher rate of IBD than the general population [137]. This may reflect changes to the microbiome due to the lack of selective pressure [138], increased microbial translocation, compromised signaling within the gastrointestinal tract, or stimulation of an aberrant response due to active infection. There are two compelling reasons to further understand defects in genes related to immunologic function in cohorts of patients with IBD. From a purely clinical perspective, identification of patients with monogenic disorders is critical to deliver optimal care. Whether it be through the use of targeted biologic therapy or

Fig. 5.2 Primary immune deficiencies have an increased frequency of autoimmune disease. The USIDNET registry was used to identify three types of autoimmune manifestations among different types of immune deficiencies. IBD occurs at a low frequency in many of the primary immune deficiencies. There is not a strong relationship between the three types of autoimmune disease, suggesting distinct mechanisms of disease

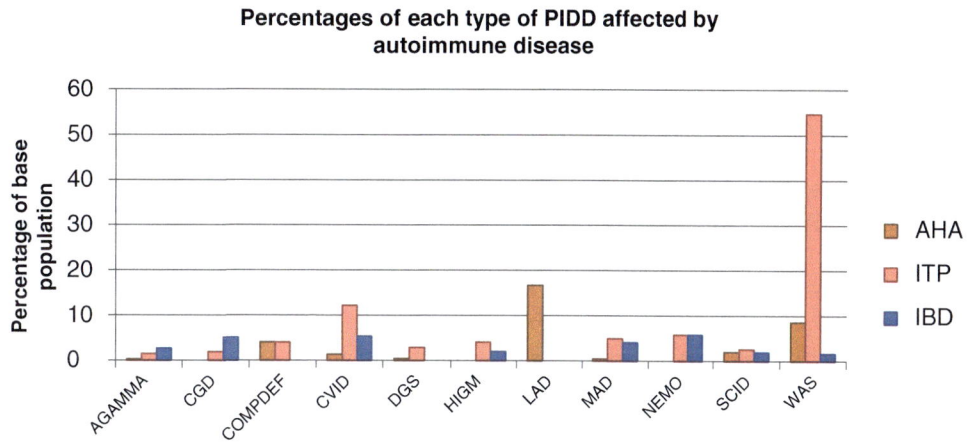

Percentages of each type of PIDD affected by autoimmune disease

hematopoietic stem cell transplantation, these patients clearly require a precise, targeted approach to their specific disease state. The second reason for the focus on monogenic disorders is the critical perspective that they provide for the population overall. As was shown above, many of the common variants as well as the monogenic disorders can be categorized according to pathologic pathways that drive the development of VEO-IBD. Even in those patients for which a monogenic cause is not found, these pathways contribute to greater insights and allow better selection of therapeutic approaches.

Several autoimmune/autoinflammatory diseases have been linked with intestinal inflammation in children with VEO-IBD. (Figure 5.2) These include mevalonate-kinase deficiency [139], familial Mediterranean fever (FMF) [140, 141], Hermansky-Pudlak syndrome [142], and X-linked lymphoproliferative syndrome (type 1 and 2), [34, 143, 144]. These diseases occur due to loss of function mutations in an enzyme critical for metabolism (mevalonate-kinase deficiency), cytoskeletal proteins (FMF), proteins involved in organelle fusion or biogenesis (Hermansky-Pudlak syndrome), or proteins involved in cell signaling or apoptosis (X-linked lymphoproliferative syndrome). While there are many additional clinical manifestations in these patients, 20% of patients with X-linked lymphoproliferative syndrome that have a loss of function defect in the gene X-linked inhibitor of apoptosis protein (*XIAP*) present with VEO-IBD [145]. *XIAP* is involved in NOD2-mediated NFkB signaling, and therefore these children may have an impaired ability to sense bacteria. In addition, as an inhibitor of apoptosis, it prevents apoptosis of activated T cells, thus allowing for expansion and survival of T cells in response to pathogens [146, 147]. Therefore, in XIAP deficiency, due to the inability to clear pathogens, there is a hyperinflammatory state, with increased production of cytokines resulting in an IBD phenotype [145, 147]. Children with these mutations can present with severe colonic and perianal fistualizing disease

[34, 148], and of great concern, EBV infection can result in fatal hemophagocytic lymphohistiocytosis [148].

TRIM22 has recently been identified as a causal single gene defect in patients with a phenotype of severe perianal disease and granulomatous colitis [149]. The authors demonstrated the fascinating TRIM22-NOD2 network and its role as an antiviral and mycobacterial regulator. TRIM22 is expressed in the intestine and macrophages, and involved in lymphocyte development [150, 151]. TRIM proteins are important components of both the innate and adaptive immune system, including cell proliferation, apoptosis, and autoimmunity [151, 152]. Defects in these proteins are involved in malignancies, autoimmune disease, and familial Mediterranean fever and Opitz syndrome type 1 [152]. Overexpression of TRIM22 can activate NF-kB and also critical for NOD2 function, partially through impairing NOD2-dependent NF-kB and interferon signaling [149]. Therefore, the authors demonstrate that mutations in TRIM22 not only result in VEO-IBD but can also play a role on older-onset disease as well.

While this is not an exhaustive description of the rare genomic drivers of VEO-IBD, it highlights the different components of the immune system, including innate and adaptive response, involved in this disease. Treatments guided toward the specific defect, such as IL-1 antagonists, colchicine, HSCT, or leukine, can be used if the defect is determined. Additionally, monitoring for potential complications associated with a genetic defect is essential, such as in XIAP, IL-10 gene variants, and CGD. In addition to these monogenic diseases, VEO-IBD has been shown to have a high degree of genetic heterogeneity. It is therefore likely that there are more pathways involved in VEO-IBD, and the outcome of therapeutic intervention can be improved through further study and identification of the associated variants. Utilizing next-generation sequencing (NGS) such as WES can improve detection of variants and diagnosis of disease. Furthermore, there is an urgent need to also directly translate genes-to-function and functionally profile the immunological significance of known genetic variations in intestinal inflammation.

Perspective and Future Directions in Genetic and Immunologic Analyses of VEO-IBD

In order to advance our understanding of VEO-IBD, new sequencing technology must be utilized to completely understand the genetic landscape of this disease, and immunologic studies spanning basic mouse models and translational patient-based approaches are required to determine the contribution of those genetic variations to human disease. Given that dysregulated interactions between the immune system and commensal bacteria underlie the pathogenesis of intestinal inflammation, it is also important to include analyses of composition and function of the microbiome. Given that these patient populations are studied worldwide, and sometimes in small numbers, an international registry containing the genetic, immunologic, and environmental results pertaining to VEO-IBD patients could provide significant benefit to a goal of better understanding the effects of different variants within known genes, and identifying new gene defects causing IBD through the study of mutations that arise in the same genes of multiple unrelated individuals. With increased understanding of the disease processes operating in VEO-IBD, we can begin to individualize therapies to the specific patient as well as employ unconventional therapies that are not routinely part of the IBD therapeutic arsenal. These approaches could provide a roadmap to establishing a standard of care for this disease and improving patient quality of life.

References

1. Goyette P, et al. High-density mapping of the MHC identifies a shared role for HLA-DRB1*01:03 in inflammatory bowel diseases and heterozygous advantage in ulcerative colitis. Nat Genet. 2015;47(2):172–9.
2. Stokkers PC, et al. HLA-DR and -DQ phenotypes in inflammatory bowel disease: a meta-analysis. Gut. 1999;45(3):395–401.
3. Sattler S, et al. IL-10-producing regulatory B cells induced by IL-33 (Breg(IL-33)) effectively attenuate mucosal inflammatory responses in the gut. J Autoimmun. 2014;50:107–22.
4. Saxon A, et al. A distinct subset of antineutrophil cytoplasmic antibodies is associated with inflammatory bowel disease. J Allergy Clin Immunol. 1990;86(2):202–10.
5. Cho JH, Brant SR. Recent insights into the genetics of inflammatory bowel disease. Gastroenterology. 2011;140(6):1704–12.
6. Khor B, Gardet A, Xavier RJ. Genetics and pathogenesis of inflammatory bowel disease. Nature. 2011;474(7351):307–17.
7. Jostins L, et al. Host-microbe interactions have shaped the genetic architecture of inflammatory bowel disease. Nature. 2012;491(7422):119–24.
8. Jacobs J, Braun J. Host genes and their effect on the intestinal microbiome garden. Genome Med. 2014;6(12):119.
9. D'Inca R, et al. Increased intestinal permeability and NOD2 variants in familial and sporadic Crohn's disease. Aliment Pharmacol Ther. 2006;23(10):1455–61.
10. Buhner S, et al. Genetic basis for increased intestinal permeability in families with Crohn's disease: role of CARD15 3020insC mutation? Gut. 2006;55(3):342–7.
11. Maloy KJ, Powrie F. Intestinal homeostasis and its breakdown in inflammatory bowel disease. Nature. 2011;474(7351):298–306.
12. Maynard CL, et al. Reciprocal interactions of the intestinal microbiota and immune system. Nature. 2012;489(7415):231–41.
13. Hooper LV, Macpherson AJ. Immune adaptations that maintain homeostasis with the intestinal microbiota. Nat Rev Immunol. 2010;10(3):159–69.
14. Hooper LV, Littman DR, Macpherson AJ. Interactions between the microbiota and the immune system. Science. 2012;336(6086):1268–73.
15. Belkaid Y, Hand TW. Role of the microbiota in immunity and inflammation. Cell. 2014;157(1):121–41.
16. Abraham C, Cho JH. Inflammatory bowel disease. N Engl J Med. 2009;361(21):2066–78.
17. Lodes MJ, et al. Bacterial flagellin is a dominant antigen in Crohn disease. J Clin Invest. 2004;113(9):1296–306.
18. Baumgart M, et al. Culture independent analysis of ileal mucosa reveals a selective increase in invasive Escherichia coli of novel phylogeny relative to depletion of Clostridiales in Crohn's disease involving the ileum. ISME J. 2007;1(5):403–18.
19. Darfeuille-Michaud A, et al. High prevalence of adherent-invasive Escherichia coli associated with ileal mucosa in Crohn's disease. Gastroenterology. 2004;127(2):412–21.
20. Dalwadi H, et al. The Crohn's disease-associated bacterial protein I2 is a novel enteric t cell superantigen. Immunity. 2001;15(1):149–58.
21. Walker AW, et al. High-throughput clone library analysis of the mucosa-associated microbiota reveals dysbiosis and differences between inflamed and non-inflamed regions of the intestine in inflammatory bowel disease. BMC Microbiol. 2011;11:7.
22. Willing B, et al. Twin studies reveal specific imbalances in the mucosa-associated microbiota of patients with ileal Crohn's disease. Inflamm Bowel Dis. 2009;15(5):653–60.
23. Willing BP, et al. A pyrosequencing study in twins shows that gastrointestinal microbial profiles vary with inflammatory bowel disease phenotypes. Gastroenterology. 2010;139(6):1844–1854 e1.
24. Martin HM, et al. Enhanced Escherichia coli adherence and invasion in Crohn's disease and colon cancer. Gastroenterology. 2004;127(1):80–93.
25. Benchimol EI, et al. Increasing incidence of paediatric inflammatory bowel disease in Ontario, Canada: evidence from health administrative data. Gut. 2009;58(11):1490–7.
26. Uhlig HH. Monogenic diseases associated with intestinal inflammation: implications for the understanding of inflammatory bowel disease. Gut. 2013;62(12):1795–805.
27. Glocker E, Grimbacher B. Inflammatory bowel disease: is it a primary immunodeficiency? Cell Mol Life Sci. 2012;69(1):41–8.
28. Ruemmele FM, et al. Characteristics of inflammatory bowel disease with onset during the first year of life. J Pediatr Gastroenterol Nutr. 2006;43(5):603–9.
29. Cannioto Z, et al. IBD and IBD mimicking enterocolitis in children younger than 2 years of age. Eur J Pediatr. 2009;168(2):149–55.
30. Glocker EO, et al. Inflammatory bowel disease and mutations affecting the interleukin-10 receptor. N Engl J Med. 2009;361(21):2033–45.

31. de Ridder L, et al. Genetic susceptibility has a more important role in pediatric-onset Crohn's disease than in adult-onset Crohn's disease. Inflamm Bowel Dis. 2007;13(9):1083–92.

32. Biank V, Broeckel U, Kugathasan S. Pediatric inflammatory bowel disease: clinical and molecular genetics. Inflamm Bowel Dis. 2007;13(11):1430–8.

33. Glocker EO, et al. Infant colitis – It's in the genes. Lancet. 2010;376(9748):1272.

34. Worthey EA, et al. Making a definitive diagnosis: successful clinical application of whole exome sequencing in a child with intractable inflammatory bowel disease. Genet Med. 2011;13(3):255–62.

35. Agarwal S, Mayer L. Diagnosis and treatment of gastrointestinal disorders in patients with primary immunodeficiency. Clin Gastroenterol Hepatol. 2013;11(9):1050–63.

36. Mao H, et al. Exome sequencing identifies novel compound heterozygous mutations of IL-10 receptor 1 in neonatal-onset Crohn's disease. Genes Immun. 2012;13(5):437–42.

37. Avitzur Y, et al. Mutations in tetratricopeptide repeat domain 7A result in a severe form of very early onset inflammatory bowel disease. Gastroenterology. 2014;146(4):1028–39.

38. Kammermeier J, et al. Targeted gene panel sequencing in children with very early onset inflammatory bowel disease-evaluation and prospective analysis. J Med Genet. 2014;51(11):748–55.

39. Durandy A, Kracker S, Fischer A. Primary antibody deficiencies. Nat Rev Immunol. 2013;13(7):519–33.

40. Muise AM, Snapper SB, Kugathasan S. The age of gene discovery in very early onset inflammatory bowel disease. Gastroenterology. 2012;143(2):285–8.

41. Uhlig HH, et al. The diagnostic approach to monogenic very early onset inflammatory bowel disease. Gastroenterology. 2014;147(5):990–1007 e3.

42. Heyman MB, et al. Children with early-onset inflammatory bowel disease (IBD): analysis of a pediatric IBD consortium registry. J Pediatr. 2005;146(1):35–40.

43. Mamula P, et al. Inflammatory bowel disease in children 5 years of age and younger. Am J Gastroenterol. 2002;97(8):2005–10.

44. Benchimol EI, et al. Incidence, outcomes, and health services burden of very early onset inflammatory bowel disease. Gastroenterol. 2014;147(4):803–13 e7; quiz e14–5.

45. Aloi M, et al. Phenotype and disease course of early-onset pediatric inflammatory bowel disease. Inflamm Bowel Dis. 2014;20(4):597–605.

46. Kelsen JR, et al. Maintaining intestinal health: the genetics and immunology of very early onset inflammatory bowel disease. Cell Mol Gastroenterol Hepatol. 2015;1(5):462–76.

47. Chalaris A, et al. ADAM17-mediated shedding of the IL6R induces cleavage of the membrane stub by gamma-secretase. Biochim Biophys Acta. 2010;1803(2):234–45.

48. Blaydon DC, et al. Inflammatory skin and bowel disease linked to ADAM17 deletion. N Engl J Med. 2011;365(16):1502–8.

49. Karamchandani-Patel G, et al. Congenital alterations of NEMO glutamic acid 223 result in hypohidrotic ectodermal dysplasia and immunodeficiency with normal serum IgG levels. Ann Allergy Asthma Immunol. 2011;107(1):50–6.

50. Zimmer KP, et al. Esophageal stenosis in childhood: dystrophic epidermolysis bullosa without skin blistering due to collagen VII mutations. Gastroenterology. 2002;122(1):220–5.

51. Sadler E, et al. Novel KIND1 gene mutation in Kindler syndrome with severe gastrointestinal tract involvement. Arch Dermatol. 2006;142(12):1619–24.

52. Ussar S, et al. Loss of Kindlin-1 causes skin atrophy and lethal neonatal intestinal epithelial dysfunction. PLoS Genet. 2008;4(12):e1000289.

53. Kern JS, et al. Chronic colitis due to an epithelial barrier defect: the role of kindlin-1 isoforms. J Pathol. 2007;213(4):462–70.

54. Fiskerstrand T, et al. Familial diarrhea syndrome caused by an activating GUCY2C mutation. N Engl J Med. 2012;366(17):1586–95.

55. Chalaris A, et al. Critical role of the disintegrin metalloprotease ADAM17 for intestinal inflammation and regeneration in mice. J Exp Med. 2010;207(8):1617–24.

56. Nenci A, et al. Epithelial NEMO links innate immunity to chronic intestinal inflammation. Nature. 2007;446(7135):557–61.

57. Zaph C, et al. Epithelial-cell-intrinsic IKK-beta expression regulates intestinal immune homeostasis. Nature. 2007;446(7135):552–6.

58. Strober W, Fuss IJ, Blumberg RS. The immunology of mucosal models of inflammation. Annu Rev Immunol. 2002;20:495–549.

59. Hand TW, et al. Acute gastrointestinal infection induces long-lived microbiota-specific T cell responses. Science. 2012;337(6101):1553–6.

60. Cong Y, et al. A dominant, coordinated T regulatory cell-IgA response to the intestinal microbiota. Proc Natl Acad Sci U S A. 2009;106(46):19256–61.

61. Cheng LE, et al. Persistent systemic inflammation and atypical enterocolitis in patients with NEMO syndrome. Clin Immunol. 2009;132(1):124–31.

62. Luetteke NC, et al. TGF alpha deficiency results in hair follicle and eye abnormalities in targeted and waved-1 mice. Cell. 1993;73(2):263–78.

63. Mann GB, et al. Mice with a null mutation of the TGF alpha gene have abnormal skin architecture, wavy hair, and curly whiskers and often develop corneal inflammation. Cell. 1993;73(2):249–61.

64. Kang EM, et al. Chronic granulomatous disease: overview and hematopoietic stem cell transplantation. J Allergy Clin Immunol. 2011;127(6):1319–26; quiz 1327–8.

65. Abo A, et al. Activation of the NADPH oxidase involves the small GTP-binding protein p21rac1. Nature. 1991;353(6345):668–70.

66. Matute JD, et al. A new genetic subgroup of chronic granulomatous disease with autosomal recessive mutations in p40 phox and selective defects in neutrophil NADPH oxidase activity. Blood. 2009;114(15):3309–15.

67. Marks DJ, et al. Inflammatory bowel disease in CGD reproduces the clinicopathological features of Crohn's disease. Am J Gastroenterol. 2009;104(1):117–24.

68. Jones LB, et al. Special article: chronic granulomatous disease in the United Kingdom and Ireland: a comprehensive national patient-based registry. Clin Exp Immunol. 2008;152(2):211–8.

69. Rosenzweig SD. Inflammatory manifestations in chronic granulomatous disease (CGD). J Clin Immunol. 2008;28(Suppl 1):S67–72.

70. Foster CB, et al. Host defense molecule polymorphisms influence the risk for immune-mediated complications in chronic granulomatous disease. J Clin Invest. 1998;102(12):2146–55.

71. Muise AM, et al. NADPH oxidase complex and IBD candidate gene studies: identification of a rare variant in NCF2 that results in reduced binding to RAC2. Gut. 2012;61(7):1028–35.

72. Dhillon SS, et al. Variants in nicotinamide adenine dinucleotide phosphate oxidase complex components determine susceptibility to very early onset inflammatory bowel disease. Gastroenterology. 2014;147(3):680–689 e2.

73. Roos D, Law SK. Hematologically important mutations: leukocyte adhesion deficiency. Blood Cells Mol Dis. 2001;27(6):1000–4.

74. van de Vijver E, et al. Hematologically important mutations: leukocyte adhesion deficiency (first update). Blood Cells Mol Dis. 2012;48(1):53–61.

75. Schmidt S, Moser M, Sperandio M. The molecular basis of leukocyte recruitment and its deficiencies. Mol Immunol. 2013;55(1):49–58.

76. Davis MK, et al. Adalimumab for the treatment of Crohn-like colitis and enteritis in glycogen storage disease type Ib. J Inherit Metab Dis. 2008;31 Suppl 3:505–9.

77. Uzel G, et al. Complications of tumor necrosis factor-alpha blockade in chronic granulomatous disease-related colitis. Clin Infect Dis. 2010;51(12):1429–34.

78. Kato K, et al. Successful allogeneic hematopoietic stem cell transplantation for chronic granulomatous disease with inflammatory complications and severe infection. Int J Hematol. 2011;94(5):479–82.

79. de Luca A, et al. IL-1 receptor blockade restores autophagy and reduces inflammation in chronic granulomatous disease in mice and in humans. Proc Natl Acad Sci U S A. 2014;111(9):3526–31.

80. Mombaerts P, et al. RAG-1-deficient mice have no mature B and T lymphocytes. Cell. 1992;68(5):869–77.

81. Shinkai Y, et al. RAG-2-deficient mice lack mature lymphocytes owing to inability to initiate V(D)J rearrangement. Cell. 1992;68(5):855–67.

82. Peschon JJ, et al. Early lymphocyte expansion is severely impaired in interleukin 7 receptor-deficient mice. J Exp Med. 1994;180(5):1955–60.

83. Pieper K, Grimbacher B, Eibel H. B-cell biology and development. J Allergy Clin Immunol. 2013;131(4):959–71.

84. Vetrie D, et al. The gene involved in X-linked agammaglobulinaemia is a member of the src family of protein-tyrosine kinases. Nature. 1993;361(6409):226–33.

85. Conley ME, Notarangelo LD, Etzioni A. Diagnostic criteria for primary immunodeficiencies. Representing PAGID (Pan-American Group for Immunodeficiency) and ESID (European Society for Immunodeficiencies). Clin Immunol. 1999;93(3):190–7.

86. Alangari A, et al. LPS-responsive beige-like anchor (LRBA) gene mutation in a family with inflammatory bowel disease and combined immunodeficiency. J Allergy Clin Immunol. 2012;130(2):481–8 e2.

87. Pai SY, Cowan MJ. Stem cell transplantation for primary immunodeficiency diseases: the North American experience. Curr Opin Allergy Clin Immunol. 2014;14(6):521–6.

88. Shearer WT, et al. Establishing diagnostic criteria for severe combined immunodeficiency disease (SCID), leaky SCID, and Omenn syndrome: the Primary Immune Deficiency Treatment Consortium experience. J Allergy Clin Immunol. 2014;133(4):1092–8.

89. Puel A, et al. Defective IL7R expression in T(−)B(+)NK(+) severe combined immunodeficiency. Nat Genet. 1998;20(4):394–7.

90. Dadi HK, Simon AJ, Roifman CM. Effect of CD3delta deficiency on maturation of alpha/beta and gamma/delta T-cell lineages in severe combined immunodeficiency. N Engl J Med. 2003;349(19):1821–8.

91. Nielsen C, et al. Immunodeficiency Associated with a Nonsense Mutation of IKBKB. J Clin Immunol. 2014;34(8):916–21.

92. Derry JM, Ochs HD, Francke U. Isolation of a novel gene mutated in Wiskott-Aldrich syndrome. Cell. 1994;79(5):following 922.

93. Watanabe Y, et al. T-cell receptor ligation causes Wiskott-Aldrich syndrome protein degradation and F-actin assembly downregulation. J Allergy Clin Immunol. 2013;132(3):648–655 e1.

94. Shimizu M, et al. Aberrant glycosylation of IgA in Wiskott-Aldrich syndrome and X-linked thrombocytopenia. J Allergy Clin Immunol. 2013;131(2):587–90 e1–3.

95. Westerberg LS, et al. Wiskott-Aldrich syndrome protein (WASP) and N-WASP are critical for peripheral B-cell development and function. Blood. 2012;119(17):3966–74.

96. Becker-Herman S, et al. WASp-deficient B cells play a critical, cell-intrinsic role in triggering autoimmunity. J Exp Med. 2011;208(10):2033–42.

97. Lanzi G, et al. A novel primary human immunodeficiency due to deficiency in the WASP-interacting protein WIP. J Exp Med. 2012;209(1):29–34.

98. Nguyen DD, et al. Lymphocyte-dependent and Th2 cytokine-associated colitis in mice deficient in Wiskott-Aldrich syndrome protein. Gastroenterology. 2007;133(4):1188–97.

99. Maillard MH, et al. The Wiskott-Aldrich syndrome protein is required for the function of CD4(+)CD25(+)Foxp3(+) regulatory T cells. J Exp Med. 2007;204(2):381–91.

100. Nguyen DD, et al. Wiskott-Aldrich syndrome protein deficiency in innate immune cells leads to mucosal immune dysregulation and colitis in mice. Gastroenterol. 2012;143(3):719–29 e1–2.

101. Chinen J, Notarangelo LD, Shearer WT. Advances in basic and clinical immunology in 2012. J Allergy Clin Immunol. 2013;131(3):675–82.

102. Barzaghi F, Passerini L, Bacchetta R. Immune dysregulation, polyendocrinopathy, enteropathy, x-linked syndrome: a paradigm of immunodeficiency with autoimmunity. Front Immunol. 2012;3:211.

103. Josefowicz SZ, Lu LF, Rudensky AY. Regulatory T cells: mechanisms of differentiation and function. Annu Rev Immunol. 2012;30:531–64.

104. van der Vliet HJ, Nieuwenhuis EE. IPEX as a result of mutations in FOXP3. Clin Dev Immunol. 2007;2007:89017.

105. Zeissig S, et al. Early-onset Crohn's disease and autoimmunity associated with a variant in CTLA-4. Gut. 2015;64(12):1889–97.

106. Cebula A, et al. Thymus-derived regulatory T cells contribute to tolerance to commensal microbiota. Nature. 2013;497(7448):258–62.

107. Lathrop SK, et al. Peripheral education of the immune system by colonic commensal microbiota. Nature. 2011;478(7368):250–4.

108. Chinen T, et al. A critical role for regulatory T cell-mediated control of inflammation in the absence of commensal microbiota. J Exp Med. 2010;207(11):2323–30.

109. Schultz M, et al. IL-2-deficient mice raised under germfree conditions develop delayed mild focal intestinal inflammation. Am J Phys. 1999;276(6 Pt 1):G1461–72.

110. Schiering C, et al. The alarmin IL-33 promotes regulatory T-cell function in the intestine. Nature. 2014;513(7519):564–8.

111. Shim JO, et al. Interleukin-10 receptor mutations in children with neonatal-onset Crohn's disease and intractable ulcerating enterocolitis. Eur J Gastroenterol Hepatol. 2013;25(10):1235–40.

112. Moore KW, et al. Interleukin-10 and the interleukin-10 receptor. Annu Rev Immunol. 2001;19:683–765.

113. Hutchins AP, Diez D, Miranda-Saavedra D. The IL-10/STAT3-mediated anti-inflammatory response: recent developments and future challenges. Brief Funct Genomics. 2013;12(6):489–98.

114. Engelhardt KR, Grimbacher B. IL-10 in humans: lessons from the gut, IL-10/IL-10 receptor deficiencies, and IL-10 polymorphisms. Curr Top Microbiol Immunol. 2014;380:1–18.

115. Murray PJ. The primary mechanism of the IL-10-regulated antiinflammatory response is to selectively inhibit transcription. Proc Natl Acad Sci U S A. 2005;102(24):8686–91.

116. Neven B, et al. A Mendelian predisposition to B-cell lymphoma caused by IL-10R deficiency. Blood. 2013;122(23):3713–22.

117. Engelhardt KR, et al. Clinical outcome in IL-10- and IL-10 receptor-deficient patients with or without hematopoietic stem cell transplantation. J Allergy Clin Immunol. 2013;131(3):825–30.

118. Murugan D, et al. Very early onset inflammatory bowel disease associated with aberrant trafficking of IL-10R1 and cure by T cell replete haploidentical bone marrow transplantation. J Clin Immunol. 2014;34(3):331–9.

119. Kuhn R, et al. Interleukin-10-deficient mice develop chronic enterocolitis. Cell. 1993;75(2):263–74.

120. Sellon RK, et al. Resident enteric bacteria are necessary for development of spontaneous colitis and immune system activation in interleukin-10-deficient mice. Infect Immun. 1998;66(11):5224–31.
121. Rubtsov YP, et al. Regulatory T cell-derived interleukin-10 limits inflammation at environmental interfaces. Immunity. 2008;28(4):546–58.
122. Roers A, et al. T cell-specific inactivation of the interleukin 10 gene in mice results in enhanced T cell responses but normal innate responses to lipopolysaccharide or skin irritation. J Exp Med. 2004;200(10):1289–97.
123. Shouval DS, et al. Interleukin-10 receptor signaling in innate immune cells regulates mucosal immune tolerance and anti-inflammatory macrophage function. Immunity. 2014;40(5):706–19.
124. Zigmond E, et al. Macrophage-restricted interleukin-10 receptor deficiency, but not IL-10 deficiency, causes severe spontaneous colitis. Immunity. 2014;40(5):720–33.
125. Sonnenberg GF, Fouser LA, Artis D. Border patrol: regulation of immunity, inflammation and tissue homeostasis at barrier surfaces by IL-22. Nat Immunol. 2011;12(5):383–90.
126. Sonnenberg GF, Artis D. Innate lymphoid cell interactions with microbiota: implications for intestinal health and disease. Immunity. 2012;37(4):601–10.
127. Spits H, et al. Innate lymphoid cells – A proposal for uniform nomenclature. Nat Rev Immunol. 2013;13(2):145–9.
128. Sonnenberg GF, et al. Innate lymphoid cells promote anatomical containment of lymphoid-resident commensal bacteria. Science. 2012;336(6086):1321–5.
129. Hepworth MR, et al. Innate lymphoid cells regulate CD4+ T-cell responses to intestinal commensal bacteria. Nature. 2013;498(7452):113–7.
130. Bernink JH, et al. Human type 1 innate lymphoid cells accumulate in inflamed mucosal tissues. Nat Immunol. 2013;14(3):221–9.
131. Geremia A, et al. IL-23-responsive innate lymphoid cells are increased in inflammatory bowel disease. J Exp Med. 2011;208(6):1127–33.
132. Takayama T, et al. Imbalance of NKp44(+)NKp46(−) and NKp44(−)NKp46(+) natural killer cells in the intestinal mucosa of patients with Crohn's disease. Gastroenterol. 2010;139(3):882–92, 892 e1–3.
133. Ciccia F, et al. Interleukin-22 and interleukin-22-producing NKp44+ natural killer cells in subclinical gut inflammation in ankylosing spondylitis. Arthritis Rheum. 2012;64(6):1869–78.
134. Fuchs A, et al. Intraepithelial type 1 innate lymphoid cells are a unique subset of IL-12- and IL-15-responsive IFN-gamma-producing cells. Immunity. 2013;38(4):769–81.
135. Hepworth MR, et al. Immune tolerance. Group 3 innate lymphoid cells mediate intestinal selection of commensal bacteria-specific CD4+ T cells. Science. 2015;348(6238):1031–5.
136. Okada Y, et al. Genetics of rheumatoid arthritis contributes to biology and drug discovery. Nature. 2014;506(7488):376–81.
137. Ludvigsson JF, Neovius M, Hammarstrom L. Association between IgA deficiency & other autoimmune conditions: a population-based matched cohort study. J Clin Immunol. 2014;34(4):444–51.
138. Palm NW, et al. Immunoglobulin A coating identifies colitogenic bacteria in inflammatory bowel disease. Cell. 2014;158(5):1000–10.
139. Bianco AM, et al. Mevalonate kinase deficiency and IBD: shared genetic background. Gut. 2014;63(8):1367–8.
140. Kuloglu Z, et al. An infant with severe refractory Crohn's disease and homozygous MEFV mutation who dramatically responded to colchicine. Rheumatol Int. 2012;32(3):783–5.
141. Beser OF, et al. Association of inflammatory bowel disease with familial Mediterranean fever in Turkish children. J Pediatr Gastroenterol Nutr. 2013;56(5):498–502.
142. Mora AJ, Wolfsohn DM. The management of gastrointestinal disease in Hermansky-Pudlak syndrome. J Clin Gastroenterol. 2011;45(8):700–2.
143. Almeida de Jesus A, Goldbach-Mansky R. Monogenic autoinflammatory diseases: concept and clinical manifestations. Clin Immunol. 2013;147(3):155–74.
144. Speckmann C, et al. X-linked inhibitor of apoptosis (XIAP) deficiency: the spectrum of presenting manifestations beyond hemophagocytic lymphohistiocytosis. Clin Immunol. 2013;149(1):133–41.
145. Latour S, Aguilar C. XIAP deficiency syndrome in humans. Semin Cell Dev Biol. 2015;39:115–23.
146. Pedersen J, et al. Inhibitors of apoptosis (IAPs) regulate intestinal immunity and inflammatory bowel disease (IBD) inflammation. Trends Mol Med. 2014;20(11):652–65.
147. Aguilar C, Latour S. X-linked inhibitor of apoptosis protein deficiency: more than an X-linked lymphoproliferative syndrome. J Clin Immunol. 2015;35(4):331–8.
148. Filipovich AH. The expanding spectrum of hemophagocytic lymphohistiocytosis. Curr Opin Allergy Clin Immunol. 2011;11(6):512–6.
149. Li Q, et al. Variants in TRIM22 that affect NOD2 signaling are associated with very-early-onset inflammatory bowel disease. Gastroenterology. 2016;150(5):1196–207.
150. Sawyer SL, Emerman M, Malik HS. Discordant evolution of the adjacent antiretroviral genes TRIM22 and TRIM5 in mammals. PLoS Pathog. 2007;3(12):e197.
151. Yu S, et al. Identification of tripartite motif-containing 22 (TRIM22) as a novel NF-kappaB activator. Biochem Biophys Res Commun. 2011;410(2):247–51.
152. Duan Z, et al. Identification of TRIM22 as a RING finger E3 ubiquitin ligase. Biochem Biophys Res Commun. 2008;374(3):502–6.

Epidemiology of Pediatric Inflammatory Bowel Disease

6

Shehzad A. Saeed and Subra Kugathasan

Introduction

Crohn disease (CD) and ulcerative colitis (UC), collectively known as inflammatory bowel diseases (IBD), are chronic inflammatory disorders of the gastrointestinal tract that occur commonly during the adolescent to young adult ages. Inflammatory bowel disease is characterized, respectively, by confluent inflammation of the colonic mucosa in UC and discontinuous transmural intestinal inflammation in CD. Approximately 25% of incident cases of IBD occur during childhood, and the rest occur throughout adulthood, peaking in the second and third decades of life [1].

Inflammation in IBD is thought to develop as a result of dysregulation of the immune response to "normal" gut flora in a genetically susceptible host. Emerging evidence over the last several years has better characterized these interactions, especially the interplay between genetic predispositions and their relationship with commensal bacteria. Serologic and immune markers have also been implicated in predicting the course of disease progression [2]. Some of the environmental triggers for IBD have been known and implicated as associated with either Crohn disease (e.g., smoking) or ulcerative colitis (e.g., appendectomy). Other triggers like breastfeeding, diet, drugs, stress, etc. have been associated with IBD, but the evidence seems to be conflicting and variable from study to study. Reactivity of commensal bacteria and the role of these in immune dysregulation as well as genetic predisposition are emerging as potential critical factors in the pathogenesis of IBD. The degree of reactivity of certain serological and immune markers may also indicate development of complicating disease characteristics and response to therapy [3]. A number of studies have identified newer risk polymorphisms for both CD and UC, most of them relating to commensal bacterial sensing, autophagy, and drug metabolism. These developments have enabled us to begin to think about individualized therapy selection, restricting aggressive and more potent therapies (e.g., biologics) for the patients who have a high risk profile and limiting the exposure of toxic medications.

The following observations underscore the importance of the environment on the development of IBD.

1. The concordance rate for CD in monozygotic twins is only 50% and even less for UC [4], suggesting that non-genetic factors may be at play leading to development of IBD.
2. The increasing incidence of IBD over the last 60 years, which is too fast to be explained by changes in our genetic makeup alone [5].
3. IBD is less common in developing countries, but as countries become more developed, the incidence of IBD also rises [6].
4. Second-generation immigrant children of those who immigrate from developing countries to Western countries exhibit an incidence of IBD similar to that of Western populations [7].

In this chapter, we will discuss the environmental triggers and descriptive epidemiology of childhood IBD, emerging and exciting areas of growth ("new epidemiology") including as-yet-unidentified environmental risk factors, clinical epidemiology (outcome of IBD) and also touch upon the emerging field of epigenetics, and risk prediction of complicating disease based on genetic and sero-immunologic profiles. Studies of epidemiology in children may therefore provide better clues as to the progression, predictors, and outcomes of IBD.

S.A. Saeed, MD
Division of Gastroenterology, Hepatology and Nutrition,
Cincinnati Children's Hospital Medical Center,
Cincinnati, OH, USA

S. Kugathasan, MD (✉)
Department of Pediatrics, Emory University School of Medicine
and Children's Healthcare of Atlanta, Atlanta, GA, USA

Emory University School of Medicine, Division of Pediatric
Gastroenterology, Emory Children's Center, 2015,
Uppergate Drive, Room 248, Atlanta, GA 30322, USA
e-mail: skugath@emory.edu

© Springer International Publishing AG 2017
P. Mamula et al. (eds.), *Pediatric Inflammatory Bowel Disease*, DOI 10.1007/978-3-319-49215-5_6

Descriptive Epidemiology

Descriptive epidemiology refers to the study of disease incidence, prevalence, temporal and geographical trends of disease, and demographic factors, such as age, gender, and race/ethnicity that may influence disease. Although emerging data from Asian-Pacific regions and South America suggest the incidence of IBD in children is increasing worldwide, most of the data regarding the descriptive epidemiology of IBD (including childhood onset) is derived from European and North American cohorts.

The US prevalence of CD and UC combined is estimated to be 400 cases per 100,000 persons, or 0.4%. Based on the current US population of 300 million, there are approximately 1.2 million Americans with IBD [6]. Accordingly, the age-specific incidence rates of IBD in North America for children aged 1–17 years old is approximately 2/100,000 for UC and 4.5/100,000 for CD [8]. About 30% of all patients with CD present before the age of 20 years. In addition, only 4% of pediatric IBD cases occur before the age of 5 years and 20% before the age of 10 years with a peak age of onset in the adolescent years [1]. Although there is no prevalence data of IBD among children available from North America, extrapolations of available data suggest that anywhere between 45,000 and 100,000 children and adolescents in North America are suffering from IBD and about 10,000 new cases are diagnosed annually [9]. In fact, IBD is one of the most common chronic gastrointestinal conditions being managed by gastroenterologists in the USA. The incidence and prevalence data from available pediatric studies from around the world is summarized in Table 6.1.

Time Trends in Pediatric IBD

Several studies from Europe have reported an increasing incidence of CD and UC. For instance, a Scottish cohort of hospitalized pediatric IBD patients noted a threefold increase in incidence of CD from 1968 to 1983, with essentially no change in incidence of UC [10]. A follow-up study in Scotland aimed at documenting the incidence of pediatric-onset IBD between 1981 and 1995 examined the temporal trends between 1968 and 1995 noting the increased incidence of pediatric-onset CD with rising prevalence by 30% since 1983 [11]. The authors further concluded that unlike the previous reports, the incidence of childhood-onset UC was also increasing. Whether this represents a real rise in incidence or merely the inclusion of milder cases remains uncertain. Additional evidence of the increasing incidence of CD comes from Sweden where the incidence of CD increased from 2.4/100,000 in 1990–1992 to 5.4/100,000 between 1996 and 1998. In contrast, the incidence of UC remained

stable over the same time period [12, 13] and from Southeastern Norway from 1990–1994 to 2005–2007 [14]. Data from Eastern Europe is similar with a Czech cohort [15] reporting an increased incidence from 0.25/100,000 to 1.25/100,000 in CD patients aged less than 15 years between 1990 and 2001. Although data from North America assessing time trends in pediatric IBD is sparse, similar increase in CD was reported from a community-based healthcare delivery system in Northern California, with annual incidence of CD increasing from 2.2 to 4.3/100,000 between 1996 and 2006 and from 1.8 to 4.9/100,000 for UC [16]. An extensive systematic review of published literature on pediatric onset IBD by Benchimol et al. has shown an overall increased incidence of pediatric IBD by 78% of the published studies dating back to 1950 till 2009 [17]. Sixty percent of the studies showed a statistically significant increase in CD incidence as opposed to only 20% for UC. The increasing incidence of IBD has been contradicted by other studies such as a cohort from Northern France, which documented no change in the incidence of CD over a 10-year period [18].

Geographical Trends of Pediatric IBD

Several studies have noted higher predisposition of IBD in northern latitudes as compared to southern regions [18, 19]. This gradient difference is even seen within countries. The study populations with the highest incidence and prevalence rates are reported from the northern latitudes. Although few pediatric studies have assessed this trend, a Scottish report noted a higher incidence of CD in Northern Scotland than in the southern regions of the country; this trend was not replicated for UC [20]. Again data are lacking from North America with no prospective multicenter assessment of this observation. A retrospective review of all hospitalized patients in the USA (including adults) over a 2-year period (1986–1987) noted higher frequencies of both CD and UC in northern regions and in urban areas [19].

Racial/Ethnicity Trends

Traditionally, IBD is thought to be less prevalent in non-Caucasian populations. This is most probably related to underrepresentations of non-Caucasians in the study populations/centers. An assessment of the epidemiology of these disorders in non-Caucasians is complicated by a wide range of factors including the absence of population-based registries in ethnically diverse regions, the use of retrospective data, and highly variable clinical presentations which may delay or obscure the diagnosis [21, 22]. In addition, two pediatric studies have also shown comparable incidence and disease characteristics in African-American compared with

Table 6.1 Available worldwide epidemiological data from pediatric studies

Authors and reference	Country	Year	IBD incidence (per 100,000)	IBD prevalence (per 100,00)	Other comments
Kugathasan et al. [8]	USA	2003	IBD 7.1 CD 4.5 UC 2.2	N/A	Prospective Population based

Malaty et al. [149]	USA	2010	IBD 1.1
			(1991–96)
			  2.44 (1997–02)
			CD 0.66
			(1991–96)
			  1.33 (1997–02)
			UC 0.34
			(1991–96)
			  0.45 (1997–02)
					Prospective

Benchimol et al. [158]	Canada	2008	IBD 9.5 (1994) 11.4 (2005)	IBD 42(1994) 56 (2005)	Health administrative data
Barton et al. [10]	UK	1989	IBD 3.9 CD 2.3 UC 1.6	N/A	Retrospective Population based
Cosgrove et al. [139]	UK	1996	IBD 3.81 CD 3.1 UC 0.71	CD-16.6 UC-3.4	Retrospective
Hassan et al. [146]	UK/Wales	2000	IBD 2.6 CD 1.36 UC 0.75	N/A	Prospective
Armitage et al. [11]	UK/Scotland	2001	IBD 3.8 CD 2.5 UC 1.3	N/A	Retrospective
Ahmed et al. [150]	UK/South Wales	2006	IBD 5.4 CD 3.6 UC 1.5	N/A	Prospective
Sawczenko et al. [151]	UK/Ireland	2001	IBD 5.2 CD 3.1 UC 1.4	N/A	Prospective
Askling et al. [12]	Sweden	1999	IBD 6.9 CD 3.8 UC 2.1 IC 1.1	N/A	Retrospective
Lindberg et al. [144]	Sweden	2000	IBD 4.5 CD1.3 UC3.2	N/A	Prospective
Hildebrand et al. [145]	Sweden	2003	IBD 7.4 CD 4.9 UC 2.2	N/A	Prospective

Jakobsen et al. [152]	Denmark	2008	IBD 4.3
			(1998–2000)
			  6.1 (2002–04)
			CD 2.3
			(1998–2000)
			  3.1 (2002–04)
			UC 1.8
			(1998–2000)
			  2.7 (2002–04)		

Størdal et al. [142]	Norway	2004	IBD 4.7 CD 2.7 UC 2.0	N/A	Prospective
Olafsdottir et al. [143]	Norway	1989	IBD 6.8 CD 2.5 UC 4.3	N/A	Prospective

Table 6.1 (continued)

Authors and reference	Country	Year	IBD incidence (per 100,000)	IBD prevalence (per 100,00)	Other comments
Pozler et al. [15]	Czech Republic	2006	CD 1.25	N/A	Partly retrospective and partly prospective
Kolek et al. [153]	Czech Republic	2004	IBD 2.24 CD 0.97 UC 1.12	N/A	Retrospective
Auvin et al. [18]	France	2005	IBD 3.1 CD 2.3 UC 0.8		Prospective
Bjornsson and Johannsson [140]	Iceland	2000	CD 8.5	N/A	Prospective Population based
Gottrand et al. [141]	France	1991	IBD 2.6 CD 2.1 UC 0.5	N/A	Published in French
Ott et al. [154]	Germany	2008	IBD 3.96 CD 2.44 UC 1.11	N/A	Prospective
Orel et al. [155]	Slovenia	2009	IBD 4.03 CD 2.42 UC 1.14	N/A	Retrospective
Arin Letamendia et al. [156]	Spain	2008	IBD 2.6 CD 1.74 UC 0.87	N/A	Prospective
Sood et al. [147]	India/Punjab	2003	UC 6.02	UC 44.3	Prospective
Phavichitr et al. [148]	Australia	2003	CD 2.0	N/A	Retrospective
Yap et al. [157]	New Zealand	2008	IBD 2.9 CD 1.9 UC 0.5	N/A	Prospective

N/A not applicable, *IBD* inflammatory bowel disease, *CD* Crohn's disease, *UC* ulcerative colitis, *IC* indeterminate colitis

Caucasian populations in two different geographical locations of the USA – Wisconsin [8] and Georgia [23]. These studies demonstrate differing proportions of African-Americans afflicted with IBD and therefore suggest IBD in African-Americans is not rare among pediatric populations. Another report of African-American patients from pediatric IBD consortium, comprising of six academic and community pediatric gastroenterology practices, has reported older age at diagnosis of CD in African-American patients versus non-African-American patients [24]. Differences in disease characteristics in Hispanic children have also been noted in a single-center study [25]. Hispanic children were noted to have the highest proportion of having UC and IBD unclassified than Caucasian or African-American children. They were also noted to be younger at diagnosis, despite having the same duration of disease, and were less likely to be treated with immunomodulators and biologics. Another interesting finding in this single-center study was the lack of familial history of IBD in Hispanic children.

Jewish ancestry is thought to confer increased susceptibility to IBD. One study showed lifetime risk of developing IBD in offspring of an affected non-Jewish parent to be 5% and 2% for CD and UC, respectively [26]. The risk increased to 8% and 5% if the affected parent happened to be Jewish. In addition, if both parents are affected, the lifetime risk of developing IBD increases to 33% by age 28.

Hygiene Hypothesis and Other Epidemiological Observations in IBD

A remarkable change in the types of diseases affecting humans has occurred in the developed world over the last century [27]. The most common illnesses responsible for the majority of morbidity and mortality have shifted from infectious diseases to chronic inflammatory diseases and cancer. This was initially noted in Northern Europe and North America, but since the end of World War II, this phenomenon has been observed in other parts of the world, such as, Japan, Eastern Europe, and some South American countries. The emergence of chronic autoimmune disorders and chronic inflammatory diseases (including IBD) throughout the world has been closely linked to social and economic progress. Keeping with this trend, the emergence of IBD has

Pre–World War II   **1950–1970**

1970–1990   **1990–present**

Legend:
☐ Light grey indicates low incidence of Inflammatory Bowel Disease
▨ Medium grey indicates moderate incidence of Inflammatory Bowel Disease
■ Black indicates high incidence of Inflammatory Bowel Disease

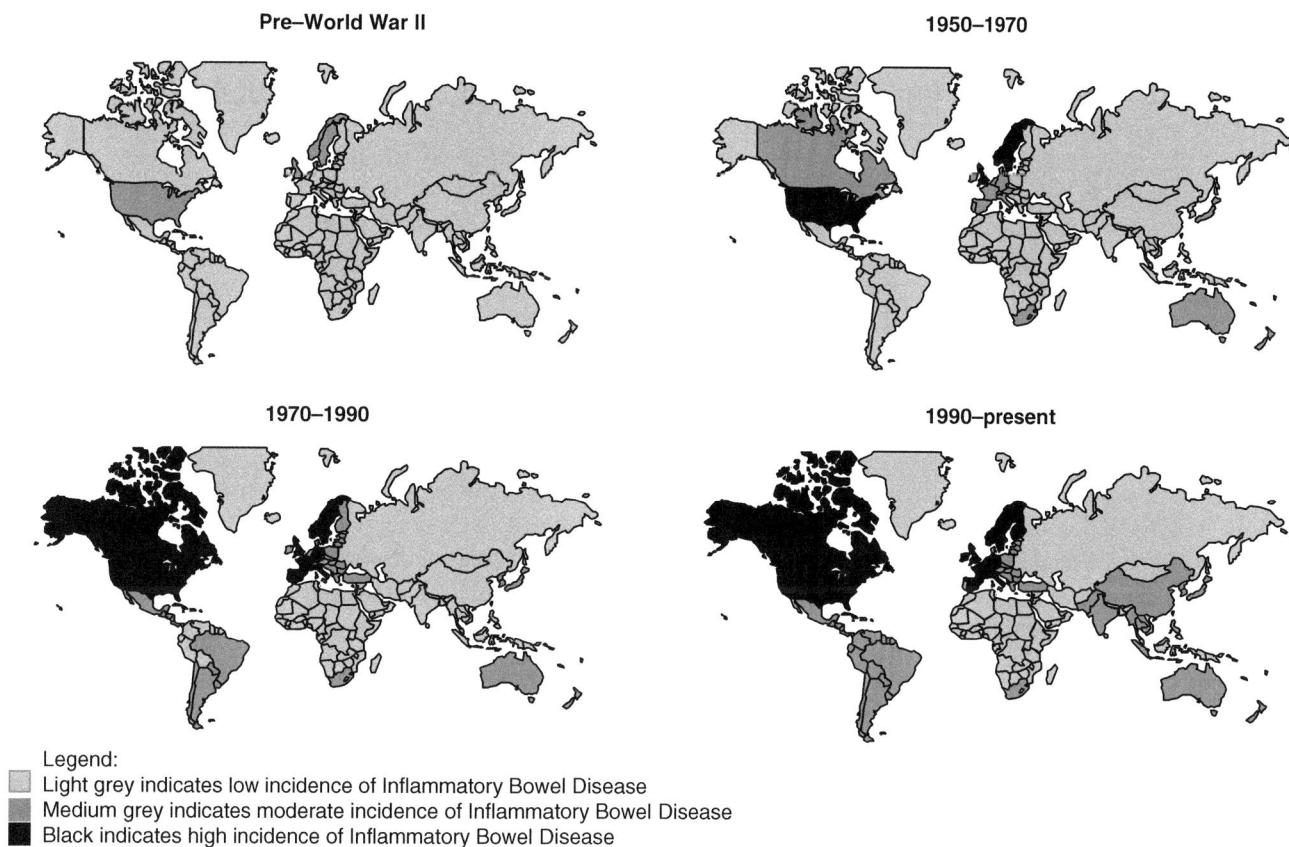

Fig. 6.1 Worldwide distribution of IBD since its description

most recently been observed in the Asian-Pacific region (Fig. 6.1) [28]. The "hygiene hypothesis" has been proposed as the probable underlying reason for the switch from infectious to chronic inflammatory diseases such as IBD and postulates that there has been a fundamental lifestyle change from one associated with high microbial exposure to one with low microbial exposure [29]. The lack of microbial antigens in infancy and childhood therefore leads to a less educated and weaker immune system poorly equipped to properly handle new challenges later on in life. This leads then to generating an ineffective immune response that is prolonged and inappropriate because it is powerless to eliminate the offending agent. Many environmental modifications have been ascribed to the hygiene hypothesis, including better and bigger housing, safe food and water, improved hygiene and sanitation, vaccines, widespread use of antibiotics leading to lack of parasites, fewer infections, and better nutrition [29, 30]. While contributing to the progressive decline of infectious diseases, these changes may have simultaneously contributed to a surge in allergic and immunologic diseases.

Environmental Risk Factors

Smoking

The most indisputable example of the influence of the environment on IBD is tobacco use, specifically, cigarette smoking. Smoking has a strikingly opposite effect on CD as compared to UC, supporting the notion that distinct mechanisms underlie the pathogenesis of each of these forms of IBD [30]. Notably, UC patients are frequently nonsmokers, and, furthermore, cessation of smoking increases the risk of developing UC. In fact, nicotine patches are currently being used to treat UC, supporting its protective role in this disease.

The role of passive smoking, particularly in children, as either a risk factor or protective factor for CD and/or UC is still a matter of controversy with none of the studies having quantitatively assessed passive smoke exposure. The mechanisms underlying the differential effect of smoking in CD or UC are also obscure. However, smoking has been demonstrated to affect both systemic and mucosal immunity, as well as alter a wide range of both innate and adaptive immune functions [31, 32]. For instance, smoking alters the ratio of T-helper to T-suppressor cells, reduces T-cell proliferation, modulates apoptosis, and significantly decreases serum and mucosal immunoglobulin levels. In animal models, smoking reduces mucosal cytokine production and promotes adhesion of leukocytes to endothelial cells. Furthermore, it enhances small bowel permeability and colonic mucus production. Interestingly, transdermal nicotine shows some beneficial effect in patients with mild to moderate UC. On the other hand, nicotine may be detrimental in CD by contributing to the hypercoagulability state present in this condition. A recent multicenter study from Europe reported a dose-dependent association between active smoking and extraintestinal manifestation in over 4000 CD and UC patients, with a rapid risk reduction in those patients who stopped smoking, down to never-smoked prevalence rates [33].

Taken together, these divergent effects of smoking in human IBD indicate a complex interaction between smoking and IBD [34]. In childhood IBD, a concerted effect should be made to study smoking exposure and the risks of IBD development, progression, as well as its interaction with an individual's genes in determining the eventual outcome.

Microbial Factors: Specific Infectious Agents

The search for specific infectious organisms as a cause of IBD has remained very attractive. The history of IBD is dotted by cyclic reports on the isolation of specific infectious agents thought to be responsible for CD or UC. Unfortunately, none of these initial reports have ever been reproducible. Several microorganisms have been proposed as having a potential etiologic role, such as *Listeria monocytogenes*, *Chlamydia trachomatis*, *Escherichia coli*, *Cytomegalovirus*, *Saccharomyces cerevisiae*, and others. Among those, the role of *Mycobacterium avium paratuberculosis* (MAP) in CD has been the center of major controversy. This bacterium is the causative agent of Johne's disease, a chronic granulomatous ileitis in ruminants that closely resembles CD. MAP was initially isolated from a few CD tissues [35], but follow-up studies that tried to culture *M. paratuberculosis* looked for specific DNA sequences in intestinal samples, or measured serum antibodies against *M. paratuberculosis* yielded conflicting or inconclusive results. In addition, controlled trials have repeatedly failed to show a therapeutic effect of antituberculous therapy in CD patients [36]. Recently, however, there has been a renewed interest in MAP as a cause of CD following the isolation of MAP by PCR in milk sold in supermarkets of California and Wisconsin [37].

In addition to bacteria, a few have proposed a viral etiology as the cause of IBD and specifically for CD. The finding of paramyxovirus-like particles in CD endothelial granulomas has led to the suggestion that CD is a chronic vasculitis caused by the persistence of the measles virus in the mucosa [38]. In support of this hypothesis, an association between perinatal measles and predisposition to CD was also advanced based on some epidemiological and serologic data [39]. Despite these preliminary findings, none were confirmed by later investigations [40].

Importantly, the progressive decline of measles virus infection in the last decades with the concomitant rise of CD during the same period of time speaks largely against an etiologic role of measles in CD. The hypothesis that measles vaccination, rather than measles infection, might be a risk factor for CD has also been raised, but again subsequent studies have failed to confirm any association [41]. A recent meta-analysis of eight case-control and three cohort studies again failed to show any association of risk of developing IBD with measles-containing vaccines, maybe putting to rest the argument of the putative role of vaccinations in the development of IBD [42].

Microbial Factors: Intestinal Commensal Flora

Over the past decade, there has been an exponential increase in interest about commensal bacteria as etiological agents of IBD. Based on fairly solid data, a substantial body of evidence has accumulated suggesting that the normal enteric flora plays a key role in the development of IBD [43]. In addition, the following clinical observations support this hypothesis:

1. That the beneficial effect of antibiotics in the treatment of CD, and now more recently with UC, has been appreciated for years.
2. Diversion of the fecal stream from inflamed bowel loops has been known to induce symptomatic improvement in CD patients, while relapse often occurs upon restoration of intestinal continuity.
3. Pouchitis, a chronic inflammation of a surgically constructed ileoanal pouch, develops in a considerable proportion of UC patients after proctocolectomy and is associated with a dysbiosis caused by the contact of the once near sterile small bowel mucosa with a rich colon-like flora repopulating the pouch after surgery [44]. Furthermore, the more recent demonstration that probiotics (primarily lactic acid bacteria), defined as live microbial feeds, beneficially affect the host by modulating gut microbial balance and improve both human IBD and experimental colitis and adds an important dimension to the role of gut flora in IBD. In addition, much larger numbers and concentrations of bacteria make up the biofilm covering the intestinal epithelium of IBD patients compared to the epithelium of healthy subjects [45], and loss

of immune tolerance against the autologous enteric aerobic and anaerobic flora has been reported [46]. Finally, and probably the most convincing is that in the majority of animal models of IBD, intestinal inflammation fail to develop when they are kept in a germfree environment [47]. A number of recent studies have noted decreased microbial diversity and the shift in intestinal microbiota from beneficial *Firmicutes* species to more pro-inflammatory *Proteobacteriacae* as compared to healthy subjects [48, 49]. *Faecalibacterium*, especially *F. prausnitzii*, which has been found to exhibit anti-inflammatory properties, is also noted to be in lower abundance in patients with CD [50]. Haberman et al. [51], combined host transcriptomic and microbial profiling to define core gene expression profiles and microbial communities in the ileum of patients with CD and noted a shift toward *Fusobacteria*, *Gemellaceae*, and *Proteobacteria* expansion. This pattern persisted in the ileum of patients with Crohn disease irrespective of the distribution of disease or the presence or severity of endoscopic and histologic ileal inflammation. Gene expression patterns differed between patients with CD, UC, and controls, but when patients with CD with an active ileitis were compared with those with a normal ileum but colonic CD, a similar pattern was observed. This suggests that gene expression profiles in CD are independent of clinical inflammation. They, as well as Kolho et al. [49], noted a differential microbial response to disease activity as well as anti-TNF therapy, with the former noting a reduction in abundance of *Firmicutes* and *Bacteroidetes* and an increase of *Proteobacteria* and the latter noting an abundance in *Eubacterium rectales* and *Bifidobacterium* spp. as predictors of response to anti-TNF medications.

Why there is an abnormal response to normal endogenous gut bacteria in IBD is not clear, but the discovery that CD is genetically associated with mutations of the NOD2 gene, whose products are bacteria-recognizing proteins, points to a link between gut inflammation and abnormal bacterial sensing [52]. Many other identified genes are also actively involved in regulating the interface between the intestinal epithelium and gut microorganisms. One model suggests a three-step scenario in which bacteria penetrate the epithelial barrier, provoking a weak inflammatory response with impaired clearance in certain persons, which in turn causes chronic inflammation, culminating in IBD [53].

Appendectomy

Protective effects of appendectomy upon UC have been well established in a number of adult and pediatric studies. A meta-analysis of 17 case-control studies showed a 69%

reduction in risk of subsequent development of UC in cases with appendectomy [54, 55]. This negative association is more pronounced in pediatric-onset UC. Duggan et al. [56] also noted a protective effect of appendectomy on development of UC, especially if performed during childhood. On the other hand, risk for CD is reported to be increased after appendectomy [57]. The reasons for these observed differences remain ill-defined with altered mucosal immunity in response to appendectomy as one of the proposed hypothesis.

Breastfeeding and Other Environmental Influences

Breastfeeding is thought to provide protection against infections and minimizes allergic triggers to a developing gut. It has also been suggested to provide long-term beneficial effects like improved cognitive functioning, prevention of chronic diseases like type I diabetes and celiac disease, lowering of blood pressure, and an improved cholesterol profile [58]. The role of breastfeeding (or lack thereof) has been reported to be associated with development of CD in a few pediatric studies. A meta-analysis by Klement et al. suggested protective effects of breastfeeding on later development of IBD [59]. This has been contradicted by a population-based case-control study which reported an increased risk of CD among breastfed infants [60]. They also reported increased risk of CD with eczema and BCG vaccines, but a protective effect of drinking tap water. Meanwhile, the risk of developing UC increased with family history of IBD, disease during pregnancy, and bedroom sharing, but appendectomy conferred a protective effect.

Dietary Factors

The gastrointestinal tract is constantly being exposed to dietary antigens, and hence, this exposure has generated a number of observations relating to the potential role of different dietary components in the pathogenesis of IBD. Given the location of IBD, this relationship between components of the diet and disease has been long considered, and immunologic mechanisms have been postulated to link food antigens and the development of intestinal inflammation. However, this logical and appealing explanation is far from proven. In addition, only a few unpersuasive studies provide only indirect evidence of a possible cause-and-effect relationship between specific dietary factors and IBD. Most of these case-control studies are limited by methodological problems including diet recall and role of pre-illness diet versus diet selection post diagnosis. Contrary to these case-control studies, a population-based study by Baron et al. [60] failed to identify any specific dietary factors as potential risk factors for development of IBD. However, a questionnaire-based, population case-control study from Manitoba, Canada, reported reduced ingestion of pork and unpasteurized milk as significantly associated with IBD compared to controls, while no difference was seen with beef or chicken meat ingestion, although the frequency of chicken intake was noted to be higher in patients with CD as compared to patients with UC [61]. Ingestion of refined sugars has also been reported to be associated with CD [61, 62]. Gilat et al. showed higher consumption of whole wheat bread and lower consumption of oatmeal cereals in CD patients [63]. Lastly, there is some evidence supporting the benefits of elemental and polymeric liquid diets as primary or adjuvant therapy for CD [64]. More detailed coverage of dietary therapy for treatment of IBD is covered in a later chapter.

Drugs

Oral contraceptives (OCPs) and nonsteroidal anti-inflammatory drugs (NSAIDs) are the two main classes of drugs that have been intensively studied for a possible epidemiological or causal relationship with IBD. Although there is no direct evidence for a causative relationship, the relative risk of CD in women taking oral contraceptives is about twice that of controls [65]. In contrast, prevalence of usage of OCPs in females in a case-control study from Canada [61] did not differ in patients with IBD compared with controls; however, CD patients were more likely to use OCPs than controls, and patients with IBD tended to start OCPs at an earlier age than the controls. Inverse causality has also been implicated in OCP use in patients with abdominal symptoms since they are routinely used to treat menstrual-associated complaints. The situation is less ambiguous in the case of NSAIDs, because their use is clearly associated with a higher risk of IBD. Primarily, IBD patients in clinical remission can relapse upon NSAIDs administration. In fact, IL-10 knockout mice spontaneously develop colitis when given NSAIDs and exhibit a far more rapid and severe form of colonic inflammation associated with blockade of protective prostaglandins and altered mucosal immune reactivity [66], suggesting a potential mechanism by which NSAIDs may worsen IBD. However, NSAIDs and OCPs are less likely to be an important contributing factor in childhood-onset IBD.

The role of antibiotics in causing or inducing IBD is also emerging. A meta-analysis of over 7,000 IBD patients reported the pooled odds ratio (OR) for IBD among patients exposed to any antibiotic was 1.57 (95% CI 1.27–1.94), with antibiotic exposure being significantly associated with CD (OR 1.74, 95% CI 1.35–2.23) versus UC (OR 1.08, 95% CI 0.91–1.27) [67]. Exposure to antibiotics most markedly increased the risk of CD in children (OR 2.75, 95% CI 1.72–

4.38) with all antibiotics (including metronidazole and fluoroquinolones) being associated with IBD, with the exception of penicillin. Another nested case-control study of over 2,000 patients in Canada found antibiotic dispensations to be associated with IBD with the association being nominally stronger in CD for ≥1 and ≥2 dispensations, as compared to UC where the association was found to be only stronger for ≥3 dispensations [68]. They also found a dose-dependent relationship between the number of antibiotic dispensations and the risk of IBD across all years investigated. These observations carry significant implications for an oft-repeated practice of treatment of IBD "flares" with antibiotics specially metronidazole and/or fluoroquinolones and guide us away from this practice. The role of antibiotics in treatment of IBD will be discussed later in another chapter.

Another medication that has been frequently associated with IBD is isotretinoin. The first case report of this association was reported in 1986 by Brodin [69]. Other cases then followed, leading to caution in using this medication as advertised by the drug manufacturer [70, 71]. However, a number of careful and systematic reviews have raised question about this association, and no evidence currently exists to convincingly support this [72, 73]. A recent meta-analysis showed no increased risk of developing IBD in patients exposed to isotretinoin compared with patients not exposed to isotretinoin [odds ratio (OR) 1.08, 95% confidence interval (CI) 0.82–1.42, $P = 0.59$] [74].

Furthermore, there was no increased risk of developing CD or UC in patients exposed to isotretinoin compared with those not exposed to the medication.

Risk Prediction of Disease Progression

The risk of surgery in CD patients has been studied in children and is reported to vary between 5% at 1 year after diagnosis and 36% at 5 years after diagnosis depending upon single-center or multicenter studies [75, 76]. The two multicenter studies [75, 77] have reported a 5-year risk of 17% and a 10-year risk of 28%. Clinical features that predict complicating disease (defined as stricturing or internal penetrating disease) in patients with CD include older age at onset, poor growth, small bowel disease, abscess, female gender, worsening disease activity as measured by physician global assessment (PGA), and presence of strictures and fistulae. Biochemical parameters predicting risk of surgery in children include leukocytosis and hypoalbuminemia. One caution that we have to exercise in these studies is the variability in defining the disease characteristics in that some of these studies have used descriptive disease location and are retrospective and others using Vienna classification [78]. Vernier-Massouille et al. [79] have also noted the shift of CD phenotype over time, with inflammatory CD tending to decrease, converging with the increasing prevalence of stric-turing. A newer, more consistent Paris classification [80] may help address some of these concerns and help in unify-ing these different phenotypes.

A number of serologic immune markers along with genetic polymorphisms have been associated with CD and UC. The sensitivity and specificity of these immune markers are variable and range from 65 to 80% for sensitivity and 92 to 94% for specificity [81–83]. These, therefore, are not use-ful as screening tests. Their utility, however, has been studied as markers for predicting disease complications. For exam-ple, it has been shown that ASCA is associated with small bowel disease location [84], risk of surgery [85], and compli-cated disease course [2]. High levels of pANCA and anti-CBir1 in UC patients are predictive of development of pouchitis after proctocolectomy [86]. However, these mark-ers are not specific for IBD and have been seen in non-IBD diseases like autoimmune hepatitis, primary sclerosing chol-angitis [87], ankylosing spondylitis, rheumatoid arthritis [88], diabetes [89], cystic fibrosis [90], and infections like tuberculosis [91].

So, how does these conflicting data help us in the man-agement and treatment of patients with IBD? The intrigu-ing emerging data has actually looked at the combination of the immune markers as predictive of complicating dis-ease behavior [3, 92, 93], showing that a combination of immune reactivity of these markers is predictive of com-plicating disease phenotype. In consort with these obser-vations in immune reactivity, a number of NOD2 genetic variants have also been associated with severe phenotypes of CD in both adults and pediatric patients, predicting stricturing and surgery and fistulizing disease [94–97]. Genome-wide association studies have identified 163 loci associated with IBD, with 110 conferring risks to both CD and UC, while 30 and 23 loci being unique to CD and UC, respectively [98]. These 163 loci account for only a mod-est proportion of disease variance – 13.6% for CD and 7.5% for UC. Some of these have been assessed for their relationship to CD phenotype and disease course. Weersma et al. [99] described association of genetic variants in NOD2/CARD15, *Drosophila* discs homolog 5 (DRG5), autophagy-related 16-like 1 gene (ATG16L1), and the interleukin-23 receptor gene (IL-23R) with an increase in the number of allelic variants or genotypes and an increased risk of developing CD and having a complicated disease course. These findings suggest that it is possible to assess a given patient's genetic profile to determine risk of com-plicated disease. NOD2/CARD15 variants seem to be more common in patients testing positive for multiple serologic markers, including those with high antibody lev-els (elevated quartile sum scores) [100, 101]. Ippoliti et al. [102] demonstrated that a combination of altered innate and adaptive immune responses synergistically increased

the likelihood of fibrostenosing CD, based on serologic quartile sum scores and presence or absence of NOD2/CARD15 variants. The odds ratios (ORs) were signifi-cantly greater among patients with the presence of NOD2 variants than those without. The ORs were also increased with higher quartile sum scores. Hence, it is theoretically possible to construct algorithms, based on these findings, to assign risk probability of severe disease. In fact, a new CD prognostic test has just been rolled out to actually achieve this same exact risk profile. This serogenetic panel comprises of seven assays for nine markers, including six serologic biomarkers, specifically ASCA-IgA, ASCA-IgG, anti-OmpC, anti-I2, anti-CBir1, and pANCA. In addition, the test recognizes three NOD2 gene variants. The prognostic panel calculates probability of complica-tions curve based on antibody quartile sum scores and NOD2/CARD15 mutation status. The results are then ana-lyzed by a logistic regression algorithm to quantify the likelihood that a patient will progress to a complicated CD phenotype. The test output is a probability score reflecting the likelihood of disease progression to complications [103].

Utility of Serologic and Genetic Markers in Predicting Drug Responsiveness

Patterns of serologic markers have also been studied to pre-dict drug responsiveness, raising the possibility of immuno-reactivity testing as predictor of drug responsiveness. One study showed an insignificant trend toward lower response rates to infliximab with the pANCA-positive/ASCA-negative combination in CD [104] and another associating the same combination with suboptimal early clinical response to inf-liximab in UC [105]. Other investigators have developed an algorithm to predict response to infliximab combining key clinical predictors (i.e., age <40 years, concurrent use of immunosuppressives, disease location, and CRP levels) and pharmacogenetic data of three apoptotic SNPs (Fas ligand-843 C/T, Fas-670 G/A, and Caspase9 93 C/T) [106]. The algorithm for inflammatory disease enabled prediction of response rates of 21–100% and remission rates of 16–86%, while the algorithm for fistulizing disease enabled prediction of response rates of 47–100% and remission rates of 20–58%. This has been replicated in children by Dubinsky et al. [107] indicating that a combination of a phenotype, serotype, and genotype is the best predictive model of nonresponse to anti-TNF-α agents in pediatric patients. Specifically, the most predictive model included the presence of three novel "phar-macogenetic" loci, the IBD-associated loci BRWD1, pANCA, and a UC diagnosis ($P < 0.05$ for all). The relative risk of nonresponse increased 15 times as the number of risk factors increased from 0–2 to ≥3.

New Epidemiology

We refer to "new epidemiology" as extensions and growth of descriptive epidemiology that advance our knowledge toward the pathogenesis of IBD. This will include genetic epidemiology, clinical epidemiology (outcome studies), some of the as-yet-identified environmental risk factors, studies of complex gene-environment interactions (epigenetics), as well as new approaches to analyze disease risk such as geocoding and small area geographical mapping of disease incidence.

Genetic Epidemiology and Its Impact on the Pathogenesis of IBD

Great advances have been made over the last decade to identify some of the candidate genes associated with IBD, and this topic will be discussed in greater depth in another chapter of this book. Although significant strides have occurred and candidate genes with biological significance have been discovered, it is very clear from twin studies that genetic determinants account for at most 50% of IBD susceptibility in CD and even significantly lower contributions in UC. This stresses the importance of environmental factors in the etiology of IBD. However, the best use of genetic knowledge in the context of epidemiology is likely to yield more useful information and breakthroughs in the pathogenesis of IBD [108]. Genome-wide association studies in early-onset pediatric IBD have identified and replicated previously unreported loci on chromosomes 20q13 and 21q22 located close to TNFRSF6B and PSMG1 genes [109]. Expanded GWAS, incorporating 3426 IBD cases from Canadian, Spanish, and US samples, identified five additional novel CD loci on chromosomes 16p11 near cytokine gene *IL27* and loci in 20q12, 10q22, 2q37, and 19q13.11 and for early-onset UC(<8 years of age) Toll-like receptor gene cluster [110]. These new loci highlight the dysregulated pathways implicated in the pathogenesis of IBD like Th17 effector cell physiology, autophagy, proteosomic degradation, and secondary immune responses. A number of recent studies have also identified homozygous, recessive loss-of-function mutations in the interleukin-10 receptor genes, IL-10RA and IL-10RB, as genetic defects in very early-onset IBD (VEO-IBD) [111]. Interestingly, a case report of a B-cell lymphoma in an adolescent patient with infantile IBD and IL-10 R deficiency has also been reported, highlighting the potential malignant potential of these genetic defects [112]. Other monogenic defects have also been reported, underscoring alternate inflammatory pathways as targets [113, 114]. Mature et al. [115] identified a case of early-onset CD with compound heterozygosity for frameshift mutation/missense R105Q in the PX domain of the NCF4 gene, associated with a defect in intracellular superoxide production during phagocytosis. Whole exome sequencing (WES) has emerged as a new way of surveying the whole genome for variants that may be at lower frequency and not well covered for detection by GWAS [116]. It was first described in a case of VEO-IBD associated with a rare mutation affecting the regulatory function of the X-linked inhibitor of apoptosis (XIAP) gene with subsequent identification of further rare functional variants in novel genes in VEO-IBD (FOXP3, IL-10RB) [117, 118].

Progress on The "Follow-Up GWAS"

The intestinal immune system modulates its response to maintain tolerance, as it is in constant flux with exposure to external stimuli like commensal microflora and pathogenic organisms. One important mediator of interactions between the environment and the genome is epigenetic factors. Epigenetics can be defined as mitotically heritable changes to phenotype (e.g., gene expression) without altering the DNA sequences [119]. These mechanisms operate at the interface between environmental stimuli and long-lasting molecular, cellular, and behavioral phenotypes, and these mechanisms are modulated by a process collectively termed as *epigenetics*. The main epigenetic modifications include DNA methylation, histone modifications, small and non-coding RNAs (microRNAs), and chromatin architecture, with DNA methylation implicated as the major mechanism in this gene-environment interaction [120–122]. Several studies have reported differential DNA methylation status between normal and inflamed tissues from CD and UC patients [123]. With the identification of differentially methylated genes in specific tissues and cells from, for example, discordant IBD twins [124], active versus inactive IBD [125], and Crohn disease versus ulcerative colitis [126], it is clear that the role of epigenetics in IBD pathogenesis is assuming increasing interest [127]. Another evidence of gene-environment interaction was provided by a largest-to-date study of 35,000 IBD patients undertaken by the International Inflammatory Bowel Disease Genetics Consortium (IIBDGC) [128]. Only very few significant genetic differences were observed: three loci (NOD2, major histocompatibility complex, and 3p21) were associated with IBD subphenotypes, primarily disease location. Essentially little to no genetic association with disease behavior remained after conditioning on disease location and age at onset. Predictive models based on the genetic risk score strongly distinguished colonic from ileal CD. A genetic risk score representing the 163 known IBD risk alleles showed that colonic Crohn disease was genetically intermediate between ileal Crohn disease and ulcerative colitis, suggesting that IBD be viewed as ileal CD, colonic CD, and UC instead of the current traditional distinction between CD and UC. Differential miRNA expression was also seen between ileal Crohn disease, colonic CD, and UC, supporting the likelihood that miRNAs influence differing inflammation-related gene expression in each IBD subtype [129]. This latter finding is also supported by the findings of Haberman et al. with distinctive genetic and microbial signature noted on newly diagnosed and treatment-naïve pediatric CD patients in the affected CD ilea that are preserved in the unaffected ilea of patients with colon-only CD but not present in those with UC or control individuals [51].

Together these findings suggested that disease location is a fundamental aspect of a patient's disease (such as age at diagnosis), and in part genetically determined, while disease behavior is more indicative of the stage of disease each patient has reached and more dependent on external influences such as treatment history and surgical interventions.

IBD Among New Populations

The most exciting and intriguing aspect of IBD is the apparent exponential increase in the incidence of IBD. IBD continues to become more common in formerly low-incidence areas such as Southern Europe, the Middle East, East Asia, the Indian subcontinent, Latin America, and Eastern Europe [130–135]. Although one can argue that improved methods of diagnosis and increased awareness among medical professionals are causes of this increase, the impact of IBD on the same "low-incidence" immigrant population living in the Western world is indisputable. It has been suggested, therefore, that studies of these "new populations" will likely yield more clues about the etiology of IBD than studying the stable IBD populations.

New Approaches

Geographical disease pattern analysis would be useful in epidemiological research of IBD to potentially identify locations of elevated disease incidence or "clusters." These areas could be later examined for associations with specific geographic variables, such as the type of water supply. It is essential to perform this type of analysis with close collaboration between IBD epidemiologists and geographic information systems experts. To date, however, studies of IBD clusters have remained outside the domain of medical geographers. Traditional disease-mapping strategies have used geopolitical boundaries such as countries, states or provinces, counties, or zip code areas to define incidence rates, but these arbitrary boundaries are unlikely to represent true distributions of disease. IBD cluster studies have been mostly limited to anecdotes of a few close individuals

who develop IBD, but these have been without demographic or geo-spatial context. A few reports of IBD clusters have been reported in small towns or villages [136], but these too have used political boundaries. Furthermore, these clusters were often identified prior to specific geographic boundary definition, having the effect of erroneously minimizing the at-risk denominator populations and thus increasing the apparent sizes of disease clusters. In many instances of cluster reporting, the terminology of cluster analysis has been applied loosely, with poor definitions of spatial boundaries. Modern geographic information systems (GIS) and spatial analytic technology offer a new, high-technology approach to disease cluster analysis [137] which could be applied to determining the pediatric IBD distribution within a defined location. Recently, Green et al. [138] reported another new approach to IBD epidemiology such as small area geographical mapping of disease incidence in the province of Manitoba, Canada, to look for etiological clues.

Summary and Conclusions

Inflammatory bowel disease is a complex disease with an unknown etiology. Strong environmental influences have been implicated as the reason for the observed exponential increased incidence of IBD over the last five decades since the genetic determinants do not change within this short period of time. However, most of the environmental risks and associations are reported from retrospective data collection or questionnaire-based adult studies and have not been systematically studied in a prospective and longitudinal format in a large population-based cohort. With the association and identification of potential genetic loci for IBD, complex interaction between the environmental and genetic influences may well be within our reach. Continued assessment of pediatric epidemiology is necessary as the clinical presentation, progression of disease, and risk factors for surgery and malignancy may drastically be altered in the next decade. It should be obvious to most people that if new discoveries are to be attained concerning the cause of IBD, the barriers to relaxing the assumptions of gene-environment interactions need immediate attention. The first design issue in studying a complex disorder like IBD is to identify and characterize the right population. Investigators should recognize this problem rather than simply work with convenient samples. For a variety of reasons, children with newly diagnosed IBD (incident cases) are ideally suited to carry out such investigations. It is imperative that pediatric-focused, multicenter consortia efforts be established and tasked to develop well-designed benchmarks for studying influences of environmental factors along with genetic determinants on early-onset IBD.

References

1. Baldassano RN, Piccoli DA. Inflammatory bowel disease in pediatric and adolescent patients. Gastroenterol Clin N Am. 1999;28:445–58.
2. Vasiliauskas EA, Kam LY, Karp LC, Gaiennie J, Yang H, Targan SR. Marker antibody expression stratifies Crohn's disease into immunologically homogeneous subgroups with distinct clinical characteristics. Gut. 2000;47(4):487–96.
3. Mow WS, Vasiliauskas EA, Lin YC, et al. Association of antibody responses to microbial antigens and complications of small bowel Crohn's disease. Gastroenterology. 2004;126(2):414–24.
4. Tysk C, Lindberg E, Järnerot G, Floderus-Myrhed B. Ulcerative colitis and Crohn's disease in an unselected population of monozygotic and dizygotic twins: a study of heritability and the influence of smoking. Gut. 1988;29(7):990–6.
5. Benchimol EI, Fortinsky KJ, Gozdyra P, Vanden Heuvel M, Van Limbergen J, Griffiths AM. Epidemiology of pediatric inflammatory bowel disease: a systematic review of international trends. Inflamm Bowel Dis. 2011;17(1):423–39.
6. Loftus EV. Clinical epidemiology of inflammatory bowel disease: incidence, prevalence, and environmental influences. Gastroenterology. 2004;126:1504–17.
7. Carr I, Mayberry JF. The effects of migration on ulcerative colitis: a three-year prospective study among Europeans and first- and second-generation South Asians in Leicester (1991-1994). Am J Gastroenterol. 1999;94(10):2918–22.
8. Kugathasan S, Judd RH, Hoffmann RG, et al. Epidemiologic and clinical characteristics of children with newly diagnosed inflammatory bowel disease in Wisconsin: a statewide population-based study. J Pediatr. 2003;143:525–31.
9. Markowitz JE, Mamula P, delRosario JF, Baldassano RN, Lewis JD, Jawad AF, Culton K, Strom BL. Patterns of complementary and alternative medicine use in a population of pediatric patients with inflammatory bowel disease. Inflamm Bowel Dis. 2004;10:599–605.
10. Barton JR, Gillon S, Ferguson A. Incidence of inflammatory bowel disease in Scottish children between 1968 and 1983; marginal fall in ulcerative colitis, three-fold rise in Crohn's disease. Gut. 1989;30:618–22.
11. Armitage E, Drummond HE, Wilson DC, Ghosh S. Increasing incidence of both juvenile-onset Crohn's disease and ulcerative colitis in Scotland. Eur J Gastroenterol Hepatol. 2001;13:1439–47.
12. Askling J, Grahnquist L, Ekbom A, Finkel Y. Incidence of paediatric Crohn's disease in Stockholm, Sweden. Lancet. 1999;354:1179. Furthermore, the incidence of pediatric IBD has almost doubled in Finland from 1987 to 2003, Turunen P, et al. Incidence of inflammatory bowel disease in Finnish children, 1987-2003. Inflamm Bowel Dis. 2006;12(8):677–83.
13. Turunen P, Kolho KL, Auvinen A, Iltanen S, Huhtala H, Ashorn M. Incidence of inflammatory bowel disease in Finnish children, 1987-2003. Inflamm Bowel Dis. 2006;12:677–83.
14. Perminow G, Brackmann S, Lyckander LG, et al. A characterization in childhood inflammatory bowel disease, a new population based inception cohort from South-Eastern Norway, 2005-07, showing increased incidence in Crohn's disease. Scand J Gastroenterol. 2009;44:446–56.
15. Pozler O, Maly J, Bonova O, et al. Incidence of Crohn disease in the Czech Republic in the years 1990 to 2001 and assessment of pediatric population with inflammatory bowel disease. J Pediatr Gastroenterol Nutr. 2006;42:186–9.
16. Abramson O, Durant M, Mow W, Finley A, et al. Incidence, prevalence, and time trends of pediatric inflammatory bowel disease in Northern California, 1996 to 2006. J Pediatr. 2010;157(2):233–9.
17. Benchimo EI, Fortinsky KJ, Gozdyra P, et al. Epidemiology of pediatric inflammatory bowel disease: a systematic review of international trends. Inflamm Bowel Dis. 2011;17:423–39.
18. Auvin S, Molinie F, Gower-Rousseau C, Brazier F, et al. Incidence, clinical presentation and location at diagnosis of pediatric inflammatory bowel disease: a prospective population-based study in northern France (1988-1999). J Pediatr Gastroenterol Nutr. 2005;41:49–55.
19. Sonnenberg A, McCarty DJ, Jacobsen SJ. Geographic variation of inflammatory bowel disease within the United States. Gastroenterology. 1991;100:143–9.
20. Armitage EL, Aldhous MC, Anderson N, Drummond HE, et al. Incidence of juvenile-onset Crohn's disease in Scotland: association with northern latitude and affluence. Gastroenterology. 2004;127:1051–7.
21. Reddy SI, Burakoff R. Inflammatory bowel disease in African Americans. Inflamm Bowel Dis. 2003;9:380–5.
22. Straus WL, Eisen GM, Sandler RS, Murray SC, Sessions JT. Crohn's disease: does race matter? The Mid-Atlantic Crohn's Disease Study Group. Am J Gastroenterol. 2000;95:479–83.
23. Ogunbi SO, Ransom JA, Sullivan K, Schoen BT, Gold BD. Inflammatory bowel disease in African-American children living in Georgia. J Pediatr. 1998;133:103–7.
24. White JM, O'Connor S, Winter HS, et al. Inflammatory bowel disease in African American children compared with other racial/ethnic groups in a multicenter study. Clin Gastroenterol Hepatol. 2008;6:1361–9.
25. Hattar LN, Abraham BP, Malaty HM, Smith EO, Ferry GD. Inflammatory bowel disease characteristics in Hispanic children in Texas. Inflamm Bowel Dis. 2012;18(3):546–54.
26. Fielding JF. The relative risk of inflammatory bowel disease among parents and siblings of Crohn's disease patients. J Clin Gastroenterol. 1986;8:655–7.
27. Cohen ML. Changing patterns of infectious disease. Nature. 2000;406:762–7.
28. Ouyang Q, Tandon R, Goh KL, Ooi CJ, Ogata H, Fiocchi C. The emergence of inflammatory bowel disease in the Asian Pacific region. Curr Opin Gastroenterol. 2005;21:408–13.
29. Bach JF. The effect of infections on susceptibility to autoimmune and allergic diseases. N Engl J Med. 2002;347:911–20.
30. Danese S, Fiocchi C. Etiopathogenesis of inflammatory bowel diseases. World J Gastroenterol. 2006;12:4807–12.
31. Thomas GA, Rhodes J, Green JT. Inflammatory bowel disease and smoking – a review. Am J Gastroenterol. 1998;93:144–9.
32. Rubin DT, Hanauer SB. Smoking and inflammatory bowel disease. Eur J Gastroenterol Hepatol. 2000;12:855–62.
33. Severs M, van Erp S, van der Valk ME, Mangen M, Fidder HH, et al. Smoking is associated with extra-intestinal manifestations in inflammatory bowel disease. Dutch Initiative on Crohn and Colitis. J Crohns Colitis. 2016;10(4):455–61. pii: jjv238.
34. Sopori ML, Kozak W, Savage SM, Geng Y, Kluger MJ. Nicotine-induced modulation of T Cell function. Implications for inflammation and infection. Adv Exp Med Biol. 1998;437:279–89.
35. Chiodini RJ, Van Kruiningen HJ, Thayer WR, Merkal RS, Coutu JA. Possible role of mycobacteria in inflammatory bowel disease. I. An unclassified Mycobacterium species isolated from patients with Crohn's disease. Dig Dis Sci. 1984;29:1073–9.
36. Thomas GA, Swift GL, Green JT, et al. Controlled trial of antituberculous chemotherapy in Crohn's disease: a five year follow up study. Gut. 1998;42:497–500.
37. Ellingson JL, Anderson JL, Koziczkowski JJ, et al. Detection of viable Mycobacterium avium subsp. paratuberculosis in retail

pasteurized whole milk by two culture methods and PCR. J Food Prot. 2005;68:966–72.

38. Wakefield AJ, Pittilo RM, Sim R, Cosby SL, et al. Evidence of persistent measles virus infection in Crohn's disease. J Med Virol. 1993;39:345–53.

39. Ekbom A, Daszak P, Kraaz W, Wakefield AJ. Crohn's disease after in-utero measles virus exposure. Lancet. 1996;348:515–7.

40. Fisher NC, Yee L, Nightingale P, McEwan R, Gibson JA. Measles virus serology in Crohn's disease. Gut. 1997;41:66–9.

41. Ghosh S, Armitage E, Wilson D, Minor PD, Afzal MA. Detection of persistent measles virus infection in Crohn's disease: current status of experimental work. Gut. 2001;48:748–52.

42. Pineton de Chambrun G, Dauchet L, Gower-Rousseau C, Cortot A, Colombel JF, Peyrin-Biroulet L. Vaccination and risk for developing inflammatory bowel disease: a meta-analysis of case-control and cohort studies. Clin Gastroenterol Hepatol. 2015;13(8):1405–15.

43. Guarner F, Malagelada JR. Gut flora in health and disease. Lancet. 2003;361:512–9.

44. Katz JA. Prevention is the best defense: probiotic prophylaxis of pouchitis. Gastroenterology. 2003;124:1535–8.

45. Swidsinski A, Ladhoff A, Pernthaler A, et al. Mucosal flora in inflammatory bowel disease. Gastroenterology. 2002;122:44–54.

46. Duchmann R, Kaiser I, Hermann E, Mayet W, et al. Tolerance exists towards resident intestinal flora but is broken in active inflammatory bowel disease (IBD). Clin Exp Immunol. 1995;102:448–55.

47. Taurog JD, Richardson JA, Croft JT, Simmons WA, et al. The germfree state prevents development of gut and joint inflammatory disease in HLA-B27 transgenic rats. J Exp Med. 1994;180:2359–64.

48. Daniel NF, Amand ALS, Feldman RA, Boedeker EC, Harpaz N, Pace NR. Molecular-phylogenetic characterization of microbial community imbalances in human inflammatory bowel diseases. Proc Natl Acad Sci. 2007;104:13780–5.

49. Kolho KL, Korpela K, Jaakkola T, Pichai MV, Zoetendal EG, Salonen A, de Vos WM. Fecal microbiota in pediatric inflammatory bowel disease and its relation to inflammation. Am J Gastroenterol. 2015;110(6):921–30.

50. Sokol H, Pigneur B, Watterlot L, et al. Faecalibacterium prausnitzii is an anti-inflammatory commensal bacterium identified by gut microbiota analysis of Crohn disease patients. Proc Natl Acad Sci U S A. 2008;105:16731–6.

51. Haberman Y, Tickle TL, Dexheimer PJ, Kim MO, Tang D, Karns R, et al. Pediatric Crohn disease patients exhibit specific ileal transcriptome and microbiome signature. J Clin Invest. 2014;124(8):3617–33. doi:10.1172/JCI75436. Epub 2014 Jul 8. Erratum in: J Clin Invest. 2015;125(3):1363.

52. Girardin SE, Hugot JP, Sansonctti PJ. Lessons from Nod2 studies: towards a link between Crohn's disease and bacterial sensing. Trends Immunol. 2003;24:652–8.

53. Sewell GW, Marks DJ, Segal AW. The immunopathogenesis of Crohn's disease: a three-stage model. Curr Opin Immunol. 2009;21:506–13.

54. Koutroubakis IE, Vlachonikolis IG, Kouroumalis EA. Role of appendicitis and appendectomy in the pathogenesis of ulcerative colitis: a critical review. Inflamm Bowel Dis. 2002;8:277–86.

55. Koutroubakis IE, Vlachonikolis IG. Appendectomy and the development of ulcerative colitis: results of a metaanalysis of published case-control studies. Am J Gastroenterol. 2000;95:171–6.

56. Duggan AE, Usmani I, Neal KR, Logan RF. Appendicectomy, childhood hygiene, Helicobacter pylori status, and risk of inflammatory bowel disease: a case control study. Gut. 1998;43:494–8.

57. Andersson RE, Olaison G, Tysk C, Ekbom A. Appendectomy is followed by increased risk of Crohn's disease. Gastroenterology. 2003;124:40–6.

58. Schack-Nielsen L, Michaelsen KF. Breast feeding and future health. Curr Opin Clin Nutr Metab Care. 2006;9:289–96.

59. Klement E, Cohen RV, Boxman J, Joseph A, Reif S. Breastfeeding and risk of inflammatory bowel disease: a systematic review with meta-analysis. Am J Clin Nutr. 2004;80:1342–52.

60. Baron S, Turck D, Leplat C, Merle V, et al. Environmental risk factors in paediatric inflammatory bowel diseases: a population based case control study. Gut. 2005;54:357–63.

61. Bernstein CN, Rawsthorne P, Cheang M, Blanchard JF. A population-based case control study of potential risk factors for IBD. Am J Gastroenterol. 2006;101:993–1002.

62. Martini GA, Brandes JW. Increased consumption of refined carbohydrates in patients with Crohn's disease. Klin Wochenschr. 1976;54:367–71.

63. Gilat T, Hacohen D, Lilos P, Langman MJ. Childhood factors in ulcerative colitis and Crohn's disease. An international cooperative study. Scand J Gastroenterol. 1987;22:1009–24.

64. Griffiths AM. Enteral nutrition in the management of Crohn's disease. JPEN J Parenter Enteral Nutr. 2005;29:S108–12; discussion S112–7, S184–8.

65. Godet PG, May GR, Sutherland LR. Meta-analysis of the role of oral contraceptive agents in inflammatory bowel disease. Gut. 1995;37:668–73.

66. Berg DJ, Zhang J, Weinstock JV, Ismail HF, et al. Rapid development of colitis in NSAID-treated IL-10-deficient mice. Gastroenterology. 2002;123:1527–42.

67. Ungaro R, Bernstein CN, Gearry R, Hviid A, Kolho KL, Kronman MP, Shaw S, Van Kruiningen H, Colombel JF, Atreja A. Antibiotics associated with increased risk of new-onset Crohn's disease but not ulcerative colitis: a meta-analysis. Am J Gastroenterol. 2014;109(11):1728–38.

68. Shaw S Y, Blanchard JF, Bernstein CN. Association between the use of antibiotics in the first year of life and pediatric inflammatory bowel disease. Am J Gastroenterol. 2010;105(12):2687–92.

69. Brodin MB. Inflammatory bowel disease and isotretinoin. J Am Acad Dermatol. 1986;14:843.

70. Reniers DE, Howard JM. Isotretinoin-induced inflammatory bowel disease in an adolescent. Ann Pharmacother. 2001;35:1214–6.

71. Reddy D, Siegel CA, Sands BE, et al. Possible association between isotretinoin and inflammatory bowel disease. Am J Gastroenterol. 2006;101:1569–73.

72. Bernstein CN, Nugent Z, Longobardi T, Blanchard JF. Isotretinoin is not associated with inflammatory bowel disease: a population-based case-control study. Am J Gastroenterol. 2009;104:2774–8.

73. Crockett SD, Gulati A, Sandler RS, MD K. A causal association between Accutane and IBD has yet to be established. Am J Gastroenterol. 2009;104(10):2387–93.

74. Lee SY, Jamal MM, Nguyen ET, Bechtold ML, Nguyen DL. Does exposure to isotretinoin increase the risk for the development of inflammatory bowel disease? A meta-analysis. Eur J Gastroenterol Hepatol. 2016;28(2):210–6.

75. Schaeffer ME, Machan JT, Kawatu D, Langton CR, et al. Factors that determine risk for surgery in pediatric patients with Crohn's disease. Clin Gastroenterol Hepatol. 2010;8:789–94.

76. Griffiths AM, Nguyen P, Smith C, MacMillan JH, Sherman PM. Growth and clinical course of children with Crohn's disease. Gut. 1993;34:939–43.

77. Gupta N, Cohen SA, Bostrom AG, Kirschner BS, Baldassano RN, et al. Risk factors for initial surgery in pediatric patients with Crohn's disease. Gastroenterology. 2006;130:1069–77.

78. Gasche C, Scholmerich J, Brynskov J, et al. A simple classification of Crohn's disease: report of the working party of the world congresses of gastroenterology, Vienna 1998. Inflamm Bowel Dis. 2000;6:8–15.

79. Vernier-Massouille G, Balde M, Salleron J, et al. Natural history of pediatric Crohn's disease: a population-based cohort study. Gastroenterology. 2008;135(4):1106–13.

80. Levine A, Griffiths A, Markowitz J, et al. Pediatric modification of the montreal classification of inflammatory bowel disease: the Paris classification. Inflamm Bowel Dis. 2011;17:1314–21.

81. Hoffenberg EJ, Fidanza S, Sauaia A. Serologic testing for inflammatory bowel disease. J Pediatr. 1999;134:447–52.

82. Khan K, Schwarzenberg SJ, Sharp H, Greenwood D, Weisdorf-Schindele S. Role of serology and routine laboratory tests in childhood inflammatory bowel disease. Inflamm Bowel Dis. 2002;8:325–9.

83. Zholudev A, Zurakowski D, Young W, Leichtner A, Bousvaros A. Serologic testing with ANCA, ASCA, and anti-OmpC in children and young adults with Crohn's disease and ulcerative colitis: diagnostic value and correlation with disease phenotype. Am J Gastroenterol. 2004;99:2235–41.

84. Klebl FH, Bataille F, Bertea CR, et al. Association of perinuclear anti-neutrophil cytoplasmic antibodies and anti-Saccharomyces cerevisiae antibodies with Vienna classification subtypes of Crohn's disease. Inflamm Bowel Dis. 2003;9(5):302–7.

85. Forcione DG, Rosen MJ, Kisiel JB, Sands BE. Anti-Saccharomyces cerevisiae antibody (ASCA) positivity is associated with increased risk for early surgery in Crohn's disease. Gut. 2004;53(8):1117–22.

86. Fleshner P, Ippoliti A, Dubinsky M, et al. Both preoperative perinuclear antineutrophil cytoplasmic antibody and anti-CBir1 expression in ulcerative colitis patients influence pouchitis development after ileal pouch-anal anastomosis. Clin Gastroenterol Hepatol. 2008;6(5):561–8.

87. Muratori P, Muratori L, Guidi M, et al. Anti-Saccharomyces cerevisiae antibodies (ASCA) and autoimmune liver diseases. Clin Exp Immunol. 2003;132(3):473–6.

88. Riente L, Chimenti D, Pratesi F, et al. Antibodies to tissue transglutaminase and Saccharomyces cerevisiae in ankylosing spondylitis and psoriatic arthritis. J Rheumatol. 2004;31(5):920–4.

89. Sakly W, Mankai A, Sakly N, et al. Anti-Saccharomyces cerevisiae antibodies are frequent in type 1 diabetes. Endocr Pathol. 2010;21(2):108–14.

90. Condino AA, Hoffenberg EJ, Accurso F, et al. Frequency of ASCA seropositivity in children with cystic fibrosis. J Pediatr Gastroenterol Nutr. 2005;41(1):23–6.

91. Makharia GK, Sachdev V, Gupta R, Lal S, Pandey RM. Anti-Saccharomyces cerevisiae antibody does not differentiate between Crohn's disease and intestinal tuberculosis. Dig Dis Sci. 2007;52(1):33–9.

92. Dubinsky MC, Lin YC, Dutridge D, et al. Serum immune responses predict rapid disease progression among children with Crohn's disease: immune responses predict disease progression. Am J Gastroenterol. 2006;101(2):360–7.

93. Dubinsky MC, Kugathasan S, Mei L, et al. Increased immune reactivity predicts aggressive complicating Crohn's disease in children. Clin Gastroenterol Hepatol. 2008;6(10):1105–11.

94. Abreu MT, Taylor KD, Lin YC, et al. Mutations in NOD2 are associated with fibrostenosing disease in patients with Crohn's disease. Gastroenterology. 2002;123(3):679–88.

95. Brant SR, Picco MF, Achkar JP, et al. Defining complex contributions of NOD2/CARD15 gene mutations, age at onset, and tobacco use on Crohn's disease phenotypes. Inflamm Bowel Dis. 2003;9(5):281–9.

96. Kugathasan S, Collins N, Maresso K, et al. Card15 gene mutations and risk for early surgery in pediatric onset Crohn's disease. Clin Gastroenterol Heaptol. 2004;2(11):1003–9.

97. Russell RK, Drummond HE, Nimmo EE, et al. Genotype-phenotype analysis in childhood-onset Crohn's disease: NOD2/CARD15 variants consistently predict phenotypic characteristics of severe disease. Inflamm Bowel Dis. 2005;11(11):955–64.

98. Jostins L, Ripke S, Weersma RK, Duerr RH, McGovern DP, Hui KY, Lee JC, Schumm LP, Sharma Y, Anderson CA, et al. Host-microbe interactions have shaped the genetic architecture of inflammatory bowel disease. Nature. 2012;491(7422):119–24.

99. Weersma RK, Stokkers PC, van Bodegraven AA, et al. Molecular prediction of disease risk and severity in a large Dutch Crohn's disease cohort. Gut. 2009;58(3):388–95.

100. Ippoliti AF, Devlin S, Yang H, et al. The relationship between abnormal innate and adaptive immune function and fibrostenosis in Crohn's disease patients [abstract 127]. Gastroenterology. 2006;130:A24–5.

101. Devlin SM, Yang H, Ippoliti A, et al. NOD2 variants and antibody response to microbial antigens in Crohn's disease patients and their unaffected relatives. Gastroenterology. 2007;132(2):576–86.

102. Ippoliti A, Devlin S, Mei L, et al. Combination of innate and adaptive immune alterations increased the likelihood of fibrostenosis in Crohn's disease. Inflamm Bowel Dis. 2010;16(8):1279–85.

103. Lichtenstein GR, Barken DM, Eggleston L, et al. A novel algorithm-based approach using clinical parameters, genetic and serological markers to effectively predict aggressive disease behavior in patients with Crohn's disease [abstract 207]. Presented at Digestive Disease Week, New Orleans, 1–6 May 2010.

104. Esters N, Vermeire S, Joossens S, et al. Serological markers for prediction of response to anti-tumor necrosis factor treatment in Crohn's disease. Am J Gastroenterol. 2002;97(6):1458–62.

105. Ferrante M, Vermeire S, Katsanos KH, et al. Predictors of early response to infliximab in patients with ulcerative colitis. Inflamm Bowel Dis. 2007;13(2):123–8.

106. Hlavaty T, Ferrante M, Henckaerts L, Pierik M, et al. Predictive model for the outcome of infliximab therapy in Crohn's disease based on apoptotic pharmacogenetic index and clinical predictors. Inflamm Bowel Dis. 2007;13(4):372–9.

107. Dubinsky MC, Mei L, Friedman M, et al. Genome wide association (GWA) predictors of anti-TNF alpha therapeutic responsiveness in pediatric inflammatory bowel disease. Inflamm Bowel Dis. 2009;16(8):1357–66.

108. Kugathasan S, Amre D. Inflammatory bowel disease – environmental modification and genetic determinants. Pediatr Clin N Am. 2006;53:727–49.

109. Kugathasan S, Baldassano RN, Bradfield JP, et al. Loci on 20q13 and 21q22 are associated with pediatric onset inflammatory bowel disease. Nat Genet. 2008;40(10):1211–5.

110. Imielinski M, Baldassano RN, Griffiths A, et al. Common variants at five new loci associated with early-onset inflammatory bowel disease. Nat Genet. 2009;41:1335–40.

111. Glocker EO, Kotlarz D, Boztug K, Gertz EM, et al. Inflammatory bowel disease and mutations affecting the interleukin-10 receptor. N Engl J Med. 2009;361:2033–45.

112. Shouval DS, Ebens CL, Murchie R, McCann K, Rabah R, Klein C, Muise A, Snapper SB. Large B-cell lymphoma in an adolescent patient with IL-10 receptor deficiency and history of infantile inflammatory bowel disease. J Pediatr Gastroenterol Nutr. 2016;63(1):e15–7.

113. Hayes P, Dhillon P, O'Neill K, Thoeni C et al. Defetcs in NADPH oxidase genes NOX1 and DUOX2 in very early onset inflmmatory bowel disease. Cell Mole Gastroenterol Hepatol 2015;1:489–502.

114. Uhlig HH. Monogenic diseases associated with intestinal inflammation: implications for the understanding of inflammatory bowel disease. Gut 2013;62:1795–805.

115. Mature JD, Arias AA, Wright NA, Wroble I et al. A new genetic subgroup of chronic granulamtous disease with autosomal recessive mutations in p40 phox and selective defects in neutrophil NADPH oxidase activity. Blood 2009;114:3309–15.

116. Worthey EA, Mayer AN, Syverson GD, Helbling D, Bonacci BB, Decker B, Serpe JM, et al. Making a definitive diagnosis: successful clinical application of whole exome sequencing in a child with intractable inflammatory bowel disease. Genet Med. 2011;13(3):255–62.

117. Okou DT, Mondal K, Faubion WA, Kobrynski LJ, Denson LA, Mulle JG, et al. Exome sequencing identifies a novel FOXP3 mutation in a 2-generation family with inflammatory bowel disease. J Pediatr Gastroenterol Nutr. 2014;58(5):561–8.

118. Moran CJ, Walters TD, Guo CH, Kugathasan S, Klein C, Turner D, Wolters VM, et al. IL-10R polymorphisms are associated with very-early-onset ulcerative colitis. Inflamm Bowel Dis. 2013;19(1):115–23.

119. Loddo I, Romano C. Inflammatory bowel disease: genetics, epigenetics and pathogenesis. Front Immunol. 2015;6:551.

120. Portela A, Esteller M. Epigenetic modifications and human disease. Nat Biotechnol. 2010;28:1057–68.

121. Wang Z, Zang C, Rosenfeld JA, et al. Combinatorial patterns of histone acetylations and methylations in the human genome. Nat Genet. 2008;40:897–903.

122. Bartel DP. MicroRNAs: genomics, biogenesis, mechanism, and function. Cell. 2004;116:281–97.

123. Karatzas PS, Gazouli M, Safioleas M, Mantzaris GJ. DNA methylation changes in inflammatory bowel disease. Ann Gastroenterol. 2014;27:125–32. 58.

124. Hasler R, Feng Z, Backdahl L, et al. A functional methylome map of ulcerative colitis. Genome Res. 2012;22:2130–7.

125. Cooke J, Zhang H, Greger L, et al. Mucosal genome-wide methylation changes in inflammatory bowel disease. Inflamm Bowel Dis. 2012;18:2128–37.

126. Karatzas PS, Mantzaris GJ, Safioleas M, Gazouli M. DNA methylation profile of genes involved in inflammation and autoimmunity in inflammatory bowel disease. Medicine. 2014;93:e309.

127. Ventham NT, Kennedy NA, Nimmo ER, Satsangi J. Beyond gene discovery in inflammatory bowel disease: the emerging role of epigenetics. Gastroenterology. 2013;145:293–308.

128. Cleynen I, Boucher G, Jostins L, Schumm LP, Zeissig S, Ahmad T, et al. Inherited determinants of Crohn's disease and ulcerative colitis phenotypes: a genetic association study. Lancet. 2016;387(10014):156–67. pii: S0140-6736(15)00465-1.

129. Wu F, Zhang S, Dassopoulos T, et al. Identification of microRNAs associated with ileal and colonic Crohn's disease. Inflamm Bowel Dis. 2010;16:1729–38.

130. Castro M, Papadatou B, Baldassare M, et al. Inflammatory bowel disease in children and adolescents in Italy: data from the pediatric national IBD register (1996-2003). Inflamm Bowel Dis. 2008;14(9):1246–52.

131. Tiemi J, Komati S, Sdepanian VL. Effectiveness of infliximab in Brazilian children and adolescents with Crohn disease and ulcerative colitis according to clinical manifestations, activity indices of inflammatory bowel disease, and corticosteroid use. J Pediatr Gastroenterol Nutr. 2010;50(6):628–33.

132. AL-Qabandi WA, Buhamrah EK, Hamdi KA, A-Osaimi SA, Al-Ruwayeh AA, Madda J. Inflammatory bowel disease in children, an evolving problem in Kuwait. Saudi J Gastroenetrol. 2011;17(5):323–7.

133. Kim BJ, Song SM, Kim KM, Lee YJ, Rhee KW, Jang JY, et al. Characteristics and trends in the incidence of inflammatory bowel disease in Korean children: a single-center experience. Dig Dis Sci. 2010;55(7):1989–95. Epub 2009 Sep 10.

134. Orel R, Kamhi T, Vidmar G, Mamula P. Epidemiology of pediatric chronic inflammatory bowel disease in central and western Slovenia, 1994-2005. J Pediatr Gastroenterol Nutr. 2009;48(5): 579–86.

135. Fallahi GH, Moazzami K, Tabatabaeiyan M, Zamani MM, Asgar-Shirazi M, et al. Clinical characteristics of Iranian pediatric patients with inflammatory bowel disease. Acta Gastroenterol Belg. 2009;72(2):230–4.

136. Van Kruiningen HJ, Freda BJ. A clustering of Crohn's disease in Mankato, Minnesota. Inflamm Bowel Dis. 2001;7:27–33.

137. Rushton G. Public health, GIS, and spatial analytic tools. Annu Rev Public Health. 2003;24:43–56.

138. Green C, Elliott L, Beaudoin C, Bernstein CN. A population-based ecologic study of inflammatory bowel disease: searching for etiologic clues. Am J Epidemiol. 2006;164:615–23; discussion 624–8.

139. Cosgrove M, Al-Atia RF, Jenkins HR. The epidemiology of paediatric inflammatory bowel disease. Arch Dis Child. 1996;74:460–1.

140. Bjornsson S, Johannsson JH. Inflammatory bowel disease in Iceland, 1990-1994: a prospective, nationwide, epidemiological study. Eur J Gastroenterol Hepatol. 2000;12:31–8.

141. Gottrand F, Colombel JF, Moreno L, Salomez JL, Farriaux JP, Cortot A. Incidence of inflammatory bowel diseases in children in the Nord-Pas-de-Calais region. Arch Fr Pediatr. 1991;48: 25–8.

142. Stordal K, Jahnsen J, Bentsen BS, Moum B. Pediatric inflammatory bowel disease in southeastern Norway: a five-year follow-up study. Digestion. 2004;70:226–30.

143. Olafsdottir EJ, Fluge G, Haug K. Chronic inflammatory bowel disease in children in western Norway. J Pediatr Gastroenterol Nutr. 1989;8:454–8.

144. Lindberg E, Lindquist B, Holmquist L, Hildebrand H. Inflammatory bowel disease in chilren and adolescents in Sweden, 1984-1995. J Pediatr Gastroenterol Nutr. 2000;30: 259–64.

145. Hildebrand H, Finkel Y, Grahnquist L, Lindholm J, Ekbom A, Askling J. Changing pattern of paediatric inflammatory bowel disease in northern Stockholm 1990-2001. Gut. 2003;52:1432–4.

146. Hassan K, Cowan FJ, Jenkins HR. The incidence of childhood inflammatory bowel disease in Wales. Eur J Pediatr. 2000;159:261–3.

147. Sood A, Midha V, Sood N, Bhatia AS, Avasthi G. Incidence and prevalence of ulcerative colitis in Punjab, North India. Gut. 2003;52:1587–90.

148. Phavichitr N, Cameron DJ, Catto-Smith AG. Increasing incidence of Crohn's disease in Vicorian children. J Gastroenterol Hepatol. 2003;18:329–32.

149. Malaty HM, Fan X, Opekun AR, et al. Rising incidence of inflammatory bowel disease among children: a 12 year study. J Pediatr Gastroenterol Nutr. 2010;50:27–31.

150. Ahmed M, Davies IH, Hood K, et al. Incidence of paediatric inflammatory bowel disease in South Wales. Arch Dis Child. 2006;91:344–5.

151. Sawczenko A, Sandhu BK, Logan RF, et al. Prospective survey of childhood inflammatory bowel disease in the British Isles. Lancet. 2001;357:1093–4.

152. Jakobsen C, Weaver V, Urne F, et al. Incidence of ulcerative colitis and Crohn's disease in Danish children: still rising or leveling out? J Crohn's Colitis. 2008;2:152–7.

153. Kolek A, Janout V, Tichy M, et al. The incidence of inflammatory bowel disease is increasing among children 15 years old and younger in the Czech Republic. J Pediatr Gastroenterol Nutr. 2004;38:362–3.

154. Ott C, Obermeier F, Thieler S, et al. The incidence of inflammatory bowel disease in a rural region of Southern Germany: a prospective population-based study. Eur J Gastroenetrol Hepatol. 2008;20:917–23.

155. Orel R, Kamhi T, Vidmar G, et al. Epidemiology of pediatric chronic inflammatory bowel disease in central and western Slovenia, 1994-2005. J Pediatr Gastroenterol Nutr. 2009;48:579–86.

156. Arin Letmendia A, Borda Celaya F, Burusco Paternain MJ, et al. High incidence rates of inflammatory bowel disease in Navarra (Spain). Results of a prospective, population-based study. Gastroenterol Hepatol. 2008;31:111–6.

157. Yap J, Wesley A, Mouat S, et al. Paediatric inflammatory bowel disease in New Zealand. N Z Med J. 2008;121:19–34.

158. Benchimol EI, Guttmann A, Griffiths AM, et al. Increasing incidence of paediatric inflammatory bowekl disease in Ontario, Canada: evidence from health administrative data. Gut. 2009;58:1490–7.

The Natural History of Crohn Disease in Children

7

Benjamin Sahn and James Markowitz

Abbreviations

Anti-TNF	Antitumor necrosis factor alpha
CD	Crohn disease
ECCDS	European Cooperative Crohn's Disease Study
HRQOL	Health-related quality of life
IBD	Inflammatory bowel disease
NCCDS	National Cooperative Crohn's Disease Study

Introduction

Determining the natural history of Crohn disease (CD) involves the consideration of a number of different factors: the disease activity over time, the frequency of complications, the need for surgery, and the risk of disease recurrence following both medically induced and surgically induced remission. In children, evaluation of the natural history also must include the effects of CD on growth and development and on quality of life.

The true natural history of CD remains largely unknown, however, primarily because there are virtually no data describing the long-term course of untreated children or adults with this illness. The data that do exist arise from early clinical experience treating patients with corticosteroids and 5-aminosalicylate medications and from a small number of placebo-controlled treatment trials. These data document that the natural history of CD is associated with significant

morbidity. As a consequence, one of the goals of current therapy includes improving the natural history of the disease. It is yet not clear, however, whether current therapy including the use of immunomodulatory or biologic medications, or the introduction of these agents earlier in the course of treatment, in fact, accomplishes this goal.

Disease Activity

Spontaneous remission in the absence of specific treatment can occur in Crohn disease. Two early adult trials, the National Cooperative Crohn's Disease Study (NCCDS) [1] and the European Cooperative Crohn's Disease Study (ECCDS) [2], included placebo treatment arms enrolling a total of less than 300 adult subjects. Among the 135 subjects with active disease at entry into the two trials, 26–42% achieved clinical remission after 3–4 months of placebo treatment, and 18% in both studies remained in clinical remission at 1 year [1, 2]. Prolonged spontaneous remission therefore appears to occur in only a small number of adults with CD. However, in the NCCDS, among the subgroup of 20 subjects with active disease who achieved clinical remission by 17 weeks, 75% remained in remission at 1 year, and 63% at 2 years [1]. Similarly, among the 153 subjects in the NCCDS and ECCDS who had inactive disease when randomized into the placebo arms of a maintenance study, 52–64% remained in remission at about 1 year and 35–40% at about 2 years [1, 2].

No comparable data from untreated or exclusively placebo treated children exist. However, in children with moderate-severe disease activity who achieve remission after a course of prednisone, the likelihood of prolonged remission without ongoing therapy appears lower than in adults. Newly diagnosed children randomized to the control arm of a multicenter trial received prednisone for induction of remission and were then maintained only on placebo [3]. One year following the course of corticosteroids, only 43% remained in remission. Similarly, 95% of a cohort of Italian

B. Sahn, MD MS (✉) • J. Markowitz, MD
Hofstra Northwell School of Medicine, Hempstead, NY, USA

Division of Pediatric Gastroenterology and Nutrition, Steven and Alexandra Cohen Children's Medical Center of NY, Northwell Health, 1991 Marcus Ave Suite M100, New Hyde Park, NY, 11042 USA
e-mail: bsahn@northwell.edu; Jmarkowi2@northwell.edu

© Springer International Publishing AG 2017
P. Mamula et al. (eds.), *Pediatric Inflammatory Bowel Disease*, DOI 10.1007/978-3-319-49215-5_7

children maintained on mesalamine following an 8-week course of corticosteroids relapsed by 1 year [4].

Whether specific genetic variants impact the likelihood of disease recurrence is only beginning to be investigated. In a study of 80 children with CD, the patients with homozygous ATG16L1 mutations had frequent relapses in the first year, while those with homozygous IRGM1 mutations had significantly fewer relapses in the first year [5].

Periods of active CD continue to be a problem beyond the first year after diagnosis. Disease activity over time has been described in a report derived from a large population-based inception cohort of patients with inflammatory bowel disease diagnosed and treated in Copenhagen County, Denmark, between 1962 and 1987 [6]. While useful, the data describing the course of pediatric CD in this study are based on observations of only 23 children. At diagnosis, 82.6% had disease activity characterized as moderate to severe. In each of the succeeding 9 years, only about 50% of the cohort was characterized as inactive during any given year, while roughly 20–35% had periods of high disease activity despite treatment [7] (Fig. 7.1).

Observations in the larger, primarily adult onset cohort from the same geographic area revealed that individual patients had different patterns of clinical activity over time: some experienced frequent relapses, some only occasional relapses, and others had prolonged periods of disease quiescence [7]. In this cohort, relapse in any given year after diagnosis increased the risk of relapse in the following year. Relapse rate in the first year after diagnosis also correlated with relapse rate in the next 5–7 years. A review of North American experience revealed similar patterns of disease, with most patients having a chronic intermittent disease course, but 13% of patients having an unremitting disease course and only 10% experiencing a prolonged remission [8].

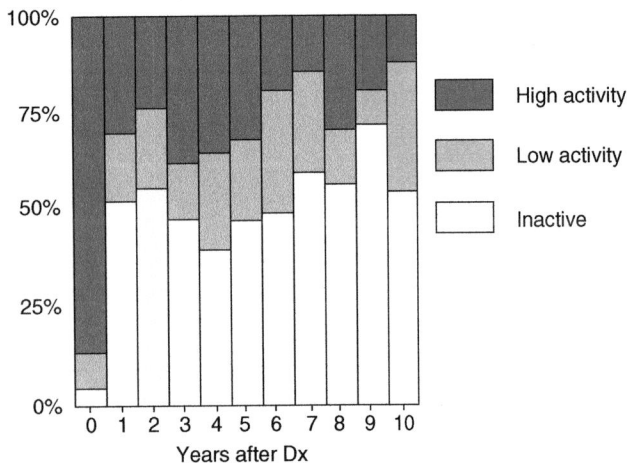

Fig. 7.1 Yearly Crohn disease activity over the first 10 years after diagnosis in a Danish population of children diagnosed prior to 15 years of age (Data from Langholz et al. [6])

Increased disease activity is often seen in those with earlier disease onset. In a study comparing the disease activity of 206 pediatric-onset patients with 412 adult-onset patients living in France between 1995–2007, a higher proportion of patient years was marked by active disease in those with pediatric-onset compared to those with adult-onset CD, 37% vs 31% of patient years ($p <0.001$), respectively [9]. In the study years 1999–2007, antitumor necrosis factor (anti-TNF) alpha therapy was required in 10.5% vs 3.5% patient years ($p <0.001$), respectively.

Evolution of Disease Phenotype

Disease location is highly variable at diagnosis and is not fixed over time. Data from a large multicenter European registry found the initial disease location of 582 children with Crohn disease to be widely distributed according to the Paris classification [10], with disease location L1 in 16%, L2 in 28%, L3 in 53%, and isolated L4a + L4b in 4% [11]. In a report from Scotland, at diagnosis extensive disease including the ileum, colon, and upper GI tract (disease location characterized as L3 + L4 by the Montreal classification [12]) was found in 31% of children [13]. However, among a subgroup of 149 children with less extensive disease at diagnosis who were followed at least 2 years after diagnosis, extension of CD was noted in 39% [13].

Disease behavior also evolves over time. At initial diagnosis, the vast majority of children have an inflammatory disease phenotype. However, as time goes on, an increasing proportion expresses a changing phenotype, characterized as either stricturing or penetrating. In a systematic review of the literature from years 1966 to 2010 evaluating 3505 pediatric-onset CD patients with at least 5 years of follow-up, development of stricture occurred in 24–43%, fistulae in 14–27%, and perianal disease in 25–30% of patients was found [14]. Similar disease behavior has also been documented clearly in data derived from the pooled observations from three multicenter North American pediatric IBD registries [15]. Among 796 children followed prospectively from diagnosis, 96 (12%) presented with a stricturing or penetrating CD phenotype. Among the 700 who had an inflammatory phenotype at presentation, 140 (20%) developed stricturing or penetrating disease after a mean of 32 months of follow-up [15], a finding strikingly similar to the 24% rate of complicated CD behavior described after 4 years in a pediatric study from Scotland [13]. Similar observations over extended periods of time have been reported in population-based studies in adults from both France [16] and New Zealand [17] (Fig. 7.2). In the latter study, a comparison of 630 subjects with adult-onset disease and 85 children diagnosed before age 17 years revealed no difference in the rate of progression

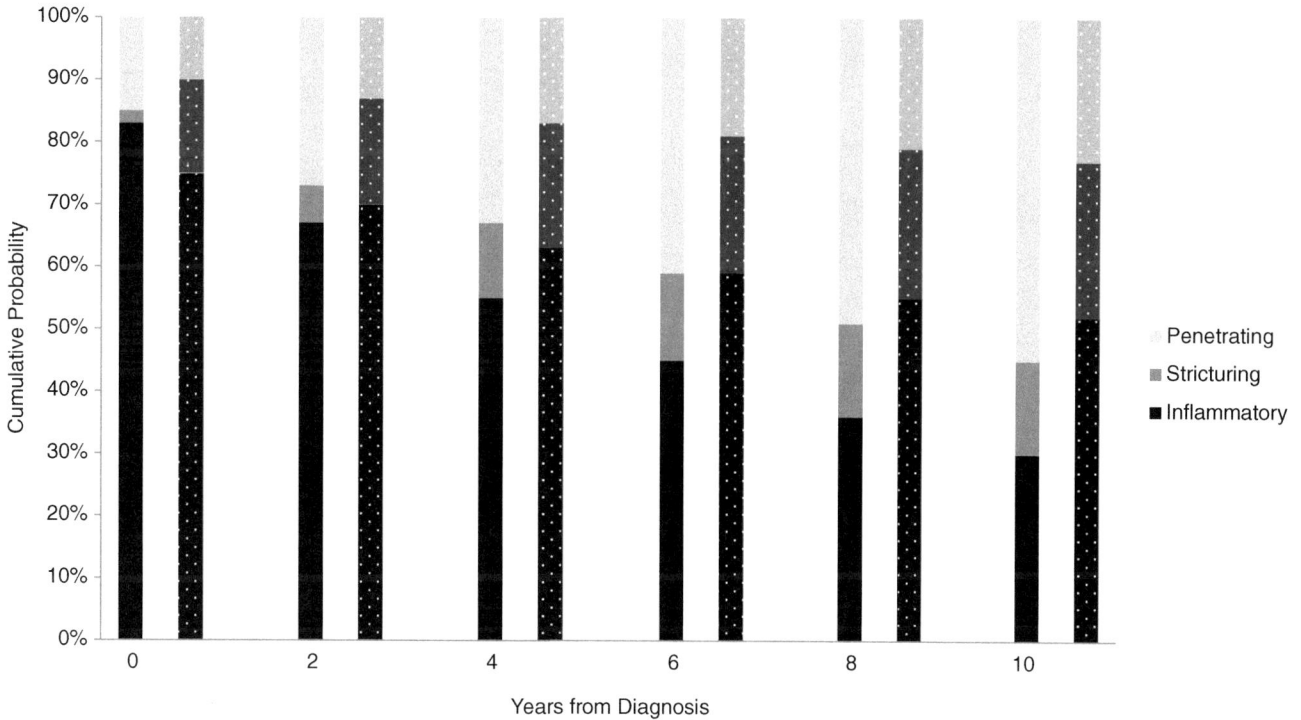

Fig. 7.2 Change in Crohn disease behavior over time (Adapted from Cosnes et al. [16] (*solid bars*) and Tarrant et al. [17] (*dotted bars*))

from inflammatory to either stricturing or penetrating disease phenotype [17].

Racial differences may affect the frequency of complicated CD, as a study from Baltimore has demonstrated more frequent stricturing and penetrating disease in black children compared to white children seen in the same university-based practice [18]. The risk for phenotypic change may also be associated with the presence of specific genetic allelic variants. Earlier reports suggested an increased risk of fibro-stenosis complications for patients with NOD2/CARD15 variants [19, 20], while those with abnormalities in the IBD5 gene may be more likely to develop perianal fistulae [21]. However, more recent studies only implicate NOD2/CARD15 mutation in risk of ileal disease location (which may be more likely to stricture compared to colonic disease) and not independently with increased risk of stricture [22, 23]. Crohn disease in children who are homozygous carriers of ATG16L1 mutation may have significantly increased stricturing behavior and have lower risk of perianal disease compared to wild-type patients [5]. In a small study of children and adults in Taiwan, homozygous mutation in the risk candidate gene SLCO3A1 was significantly associated with perforating disease compared to those with wild type who had more inflammatory disease [24]. Children at risk for stricturing or internal penetrating complications have also been shown to be more likely to have increased immune responses to microbial antigens, characterized by the presence of high-titer antibodies such as anti-ompC and anti-I2 [15, 25].

Growth

For a significant subgroup of children with CD, growth impairment is an important characteristic of the disease's natural history. While acute weight loss commonly is present in children with both ulcerative colitis and CD, impairment in linear growth is primarily a problem in the latter condition. At the time of initial diagnosis, about a third of children with CD have already dropped two or more major growth channels from their pre-illness growth percentiles [26, 27]. More dramatically, 88% have delayed height velocity at diagnosis [28]. Over time, periods of significantly impaired growth can be seen in about 60% of children and adolescents [27]. While catch-up growth is often possible, 7–35% of children diagnosed during the 1970s and 1980s had final adult heights that were significantly shorter than expected [27]. As a group, young adults who develop CD as children have adult heights skewed toward the lowest percentiles. In reports from both Chicago and New York, ~50% of young adults with childhood-onset CD have final adult heights less than the 10% for the general population, and ~25% have adult heights less than the 5% [26, 27]. While therapies including enteral nutrition [29], methotrexate [30], and infliximab [31, 32] have improved growth in the short to

Table 7.1 Surgical frequency in Crohn disease

Author	No. of children observed (period studied)	% Operated	% Permanent stomas
Farmer [37] (USA)	522 (1955–1974)	67	??
Ferguson [38] (UK)	50 (1968–1983)	78	30%
Griffiths [39] (Canada)	275 (1970–1987)	32	2%
Besnard [40] (France)	119 (1975–1994)	30	2%
Langholz [6] (Denmark)	23 (1962–1987)	43	??
Gupta [41] (USA)	989 (1987–2003)	13	10%

medium term, current therapies have not yet been demonstrated to provide a long-term reversal of growth impairment.

Corticosteroid Dependence

An important characteristic of Crohn disease in children as well as adults is the tendency to develop corticosteroid dependence. Population-based studies in adults from both Olmstead County, Minnesota [33], and Copenhagen County, Denmark [34], demonstrate similar findings; acute response to corticosteroid therapy in adults with CD is reasonably good (complete remission in 48–58%, partial remission in 26–32%, and no response in 12–20%). However, long-term response is less optimal, with rates of corticosteroid dependence of 28–36% at 1 year [33, 34].

A similar risk for corticosteroid dependence is evident in children. As in adults, acute response to a course of corticosteroids is good. In data derived from a multicenter North American observational registry, among 109 newly diagnosed children with moderate-severe CD activity treated with corticosteroids, 60% have a complete and 24% a partial clinical response by 3 months after initiation of treatment [35]. However, despite concomitant use of immunomodulators in many of these children, 31% are corticosteroid dependent at 1 year. In fact, without infliximab, only 46% of the children in this study maintained a corticosteroid-free remission to 1 year following an initial course of corticosteroids [35]. Similarly, in a French population-based study of 404 patients diagnosed before age 17 years, 24% were corticosteroid dependent, and 5% were corticosteroid resistant at 1 year from diagnosis [36]. In this cohort, corticosteroid use had a hazard ratio for intestinal surgery of 2.98 ($p < 0.01$).

Surgery

The need for surgery represents another important aspect of the natural history of Crohn disease in children. Table 7.1 summarizes published rates for surgery in children from a variety of different countries. Data from Denmark estimate a mean yearly operation rate of approximately 13%. The cumulative probability of surgery in this Danish cohort at 20 years was estimated to be 47% [6]. A multicenter pediatric experience from the USA estimates the cumulative incidence of surgery to be 6% at 1 year, 17% at 5 years, and 28% at 10 years after diagnosis [41]. Similarly, a pediatric study from Scotland noted resection rates of 20% at 5 years and 34% at 10 years [13]. The presence of variant NOD2/CARD15 [19, 20] and ATG16L1 [5] alleles appear to increase the risk for surgery, presumably due to the known association of these genetic polymorphisms with the development of fibrostenotic ileal disease. The presence of anti-Saccharomyces cerevisiae antibodies also appears to be associated with increased risk for surgery [15, 41].

The effect of immunomodulatory therapy on the need for surgery remains an open question. An analysis from France evaluated a series of successive 5-year adult CD cohorts [42]. Although there was a significant increase in the use of immunomodulatory therapy over time, there was no associated change in the rate of surgery [42]. By contrast, multivariate analysis from a similar series of 5-year adult CD cohorts from the UK identified the early use of thiopurines (within 3 months of diagnosis) to be associated with a marked reduction in the rate of surgery [43, 44].

The studies evaluating infliximab therapy in decreasing surgical rates are also mixed. In a Spanish retrospective assessment of infliximab therapy used in a "step-up" fashion, no significant decrease in surgical rates could be identified in patients receiving infliximab compared to those not receiving the treatment [45]. However, other studies reach the opposite conclusion. For instance, in a study utilizing data from a combined Danish and Czech collaboration, surgical rates in adults 40 months after starting infliximab were 20–23% in infliximab responders compared to 76% in non-responders [46]. In the ACCENT I [47] and ACCENT II [48] trials of adults with moderate to severe CD, and fistulizing CD, respectively, response to maintenance infliximab was associated with decreased surgery. Similar findings in children have been reported, with surgical rates 50 months after starting infliximab of 10% in patients maintained on the biologic compared to 70% in infliximab failures [49]. Further, in children with a favorable initial response, development of antibodies to infliximab led to loss of response and increased risk of surgical resections [50]. It remains to be determined if the recent trend toward early initiation of biological therapy ("top-down approach") will prove to result in decreased rates of surgery over time.

Postoperative Recurrence

Although there are little pediatric data published to document clinical experience, following surgery, the natural history of Crohn disease is to recur both endoscopically and symptomatically. The natural progression of CD following ileocolonic resection has been previously described by Rutgeerts and colleagues, with five levels of disease severity (i0–i4) found endoscopically. Postoperatively, disease appears to evolve from normal mucosa (i0) to the initial appearance of a few aphthous ulcers (i1–i2), followed by progressively more and/or deeper ulcerations until an area of confluent inflammation, large ulcers, or stricturing develop (i3–i4) [51]. CD recurrence is defined by an endoscopic score of i2, i3, or i4, while postoperative remission is defined by a score of i0 or i1.

In retrospective adult studies, symptomatic recurrence of CD following so-called curative resection (complete resection of all visibly evident disease) is reported to be 20–30% within the first year after surgery, with increasing likelihood in each subsequent year [52]. One or more additional surgeries are required in 15–45% of adults within 3 years, 26–65% in 10 years, and 33–82% in 15 years [34]. Controlled trials document severe endoscopic recurrence after placebo treatment in 43–79% of adult subjects by 1 year after surgery and in 42–85% of subjects after 2 years [53–58].

In children, the overall rate of clinical recurrence is estimated to be 50% at 5 years after initial resection [39]. However, the site and extent of preoperative CD can affect the recurrence-free interval such that it is estimated that 50% of children with extensive ileocolitis recur within 1 year, compared to a 50% recurrence rate after 5 years in children with ileocecal disease and a 50% recurrence rate after 6 years if preoperative disease is confined to the small bowel [39]. In a retrospective review of 30 children, multifocal preoperative disease, with perianal or upper gastrointestinal tract involvement, was a risk factor for postoperative recurrence after localized ileal or ileocecal resection [40]. Altering the natural history of postoperative CD and preventing recurrence have become an integral part of CD management. Use of mesalamine or thiopurines appears to have limited benefit [58, 59], while anti-TNF therapy may be highly effective [60, 61] in preventing CD recurrence.

Cancer Risk

Whether children with CD are at increased risk for malignancy over their lifetime is unknown. No data derived from a population with childhood-onset CD has been reported. In a recent retrospective multinational study from 2006 to 2011, including 20 European countries and Israel, 12 children with CD were identified with a malignancy prior to age 19 years [62]. Since the total number of children with CD during the study period could not be identified, the malignancy risk could not be reported. The majority of cancers were lymphoma or leukemia, and only three patients were not on immunomodulator therapy within 3 months of cancer diagnosis. The effect of CD independent of immunosuppression +/− Epstein-Barr virus infection in developing a malignancy could not be calculated, although the risk appeared to be small. Studies in adults, however, suggest that patients with CD do have an excess of malignancies compared to the general population. In a population-based cohort from the Uppsala region of Sweden, there was an increased relative risk of colorectal cancer of 2.5 (95% confidence interval (CI) 1.3–4.3) in patients with CD [63]. Duration of illness and gender did not affect risk, but those subjects with colonic disease had a greater risk of colorectal cancer than those with only small bowel involvement. Of note, however, among those subjects with any colonic involvement diagnosed with CD before the age of 30 years, the relative risk of colorectal cancer increased to 20.9 (95% CI 6.8–48.7) [63]. By contrast, a similar population-based study from Denmark identified a relative risk of colorectal cancer of only 1.1 (95% CI 0.6–1.9), and no risk differences were noted in different subgroups of patients [64]. A similar modest increase in colorectal cancer risk (1.9; 95% CI 0.7–4.1) was found in a population-based study from Olmstead County, Minnesota [65].

By contrast, the risk of small bowel cancer consistently appears increased in patients with CD. In part because the rate of small bowel cancer in the general population is very low (estimated to be 0.005% at 5 years and 0.03% at 25 years according to data cited in reference 62), there is a significantly elevated relative risk for small bowel cancers in patients with CD. In the Danish study cited above, the relative increased risk for small bowel cancer was 17.9 (95% CI 4.8–42) [64]. In Olmstead County, the relative risk was found to be 40.6 (95% CI 4.4–118) [65]. Duration of CD did not appear to influence risk of developing a small bowel cancer. Adenocarcinoma, carcinoid, leiomyosarcoma, and primary intestinal lymphoma have all been reported. The effect of age at CD onset on the risk of developing small bowel cancer has not been reported.

There may also be a slight increase in risk of developing lymphoma, although data is mixed and not always controlled for risk associated with therapeutic agents. In a single-center, retrospective study between 1979 and 2008 that included 791 children with CD followed in Boston, MA, one non-Hodgkin's lymphoma occurred in a patient receiving thiopurines; the overall cohort lymphoma risk did not meet statistical significance [66]. In a large population-based retrospective study of adults living in the UK between 1988 and 1997, seven patients with lymphoma were reported among 6605 patients with CD, and 0/7 were exposed to thiopurines. The risk of lymphoma in this cohort was not increased compared to the control population (relative risk 1.39; 95% CI 0.50–3.40) [67]. Among 454 adults living in Olmsted County who developed CD between 1950 and 1993, one developed a non-Hodgkin's lymphoma, resulting in a slight increase in relative risk (2.4; 95% CI 0.1–13), although not statistically significant compared to the general population [68]. In this report, however, the referral practice of the same group of investigators revealed that development of lymphoma was associated with treatment with immune modifiers in about 5% of cases [68].

A meta-analysis utilizing data from six studies estimates the risk of lymphoma in inflammatory bowel disease (IBD) patients treated with azathioprine or 6-mercaptopurine to be increased about fourfold (4.18; 95% CI 2.07–7.51) [69]. Infliximab in combination with thiopurine may add an additional element of risk, especially for children and young adults, in whom the development of hepatosplenic T-cell lymphoma has been described [70]. Whether these risks to children with CD are due to the nature of the illness in children, their frequent need for potent immune modifier and biological therapy, or both, is not known.

Quality of Life

In addition to imposing significant physical morbidity, CD in childhood imposes potentially dramatic psychosocial burdens as well. Health-related quality of life (HRQOL) scores, as measured by the IMPACT questionnaire (a validated, pediatric IBD health-related quality of life questionnaire) [71], correlate with physician's global assessment of disease severity, such that children with moderate-severe activity have the poorest HRQOL scores [72]. Over the first year after diagnosis, age also appears to be an independent factor affecting HRQOL scores, with older children reporting poorer IMPACT scores [72]. While treatment results in significant improvement in IMPACT scores in the first year after diagnosis, it is unknown whether further improvements in HRQOL occur over time. One by-product of increased disease severity is increased parental stress. The effect of parental stress was recently studied and found to partially contribute to lower HRQOL in children with active disease [73]. Children frequently report being bothered by having a chronic illness, having to undergo tests, and feeling tired. Over time, they also report feeling that their chronic illness is unfair and that they experience problems revolving around having to keep their illness a secret from others [72].

Other studies have noted that children with CD experience frequent absences from school, that they frequently require home tutoring, and that they commonly cannot participate fully at all in physical education classes [74, 75]. Children express fears concerning everyday childhood activities, schooling, and ability to get a job [76]. Fifty-seven percent of a cohort was reported to have had an absence from school of at least 2 months duration, and in this same cohort, 8% were involuntarily unemployed as young adults [77]. Similar impairments are described in adult CD populations, with 15% of a Danish population on disability by 15 years after diagnosis, 25% reporting some inability to work in any given year of follow-up, and 50% reporting one or more years during first decade of disease with at least some inability to work [7]. These latter studies [7, 74–77] report on patients treated in the prebiologic era, and the use of anti-TNF therapies appears to have significantly improved patient quality of life measures [78, 79].

References

1. Summers RW, Switz DM, Sessions Jr JT, et al. National Cooperative Crohn's Disease Study: results of drug treatment. Gastroenterology. 1979;77:847–69.
2. Malchow H, Ewe K, Brandes JW, et al. European Cooperative Crohn's Disease Study (ECCDS): results of drug treatment. Gastroenterology. 1984;86:249–66.

3. Markowitz J, Grancher K, Kohn N, et al. A multicenter trial of 6-mercaptopurine and prednisone in children with newly diagnosed Crohn's disease. Gastroenterology. 2000;119:895–902.
4. Romano C, Cucchiara S, Barabino A, et al. Usefulness of omega-3 fatty acid supplementation in addition to mesalazine in maintaining remission in pediatric Crohn's disease: a double-blind, randomized, placebo-controlled study. World J Gastroenterol. 2005;11:7118–21.
5. Strisciuglio C, Auricchio R, Martinelli M, et al. Autophagy genes variants and paediatric Crohn's disease phenotype: a single-centre experience. Dig Liver Dis. 2014;46:512–7.
6. Langholz E, Munkholm P, Krasilnikoff PA, Binder V. Inflammatory bowel diseases with onset in childhood. Clinical features, morbidity, and mortality in a regional cohort. Scand J Gastroenterol. 1997;32:139–47.
7. Munkholm P, Langholz E, Davidsen M, Binder V. Disease activity courses in a regional cohort of Crohn's disease patients. Scand J Gastroenterol. 1995;30:699–706.
8. Loftus Jr EV, Schoenfeld P, Sandborn WJ. The epidemiology and natural history of Crohn's disease in population-based patient cohorts from North America: a systematic review. Aliment Pharmacol Ther. 2002;16:51–60.
9. Pigneur B, Seksik P, Viola S, et al. Natural history of Crohn's disease: comparison between childhood- and adult-onset disease. Inflamm Bowel Dis. 2010;16:953–61.
10. Levine A, Griffiths A, Markowitz J, et al. Pediatric modification of the Montreal classification for inflammatory bowel disease: the Paris classification. Inflamm Bowel Dis. 2011;17:1314–21.
11. de Bie CI, Paerregaard A, Kolacek S, et al. Disease phenotype at diagnosis in pediatric Crohn's disease: 5-year analyses of the EUROKIDS Registry. Inflamm Bowel Dis. 2013;19:378–85.
12. Silverberg MS, Satsangi J, Ahmad T, et al. Toward an integrated clinical, molecular and serological classification of inflammatory bowel disease: report of a Working Party of the 2005 Montreal World Congress of Gastroenterology. Can J Gastroenterol 2005;19 Suppl A:5A–36A.
13. Van Limbergen J, Russell RK, Drummond HE, et al. Definition of phenotypic characteristics of childhood-onset inflammatory bowel disease. Gastroenterology. 2008;135:1114–22.
14. Abraham BP, Mehta S, El-Serag HB. Natural history of pediatric-onset inflammatory bowel disease: a systematic review. J Clin Gastroenterol. 2012;46:581–9.
15. Dubinsky MC, Kugathasan S, Mei L, et al. Increased immune reactivity predicts aggressive complicating Crohn's disease in children. Clin Gastroenterol Hepatol. 2008;6:1105–11.
16. Cosnes J, Cattan S, Blain A, et al. Long-term evolution of disease behavior of Crohn's disease. Inflamm Bowel Dis. 2002;8:244–50.
17. Tarrant KM, Barclay ML, Frampton CM, Gearry RB. Perianal disease predicts changes in Crohn's disease phenotype-results of a population-based study of inflammatory bowel disease phenotype. Am J Gastroenterol. 2008;103:3082–93.
18. Eidelwein AP, Thompson R, Fiorino K, et al. Disease presentation and clinical course in black and white children with inflammatory bowel disease. J Pediatr Gastroenterol Nutr. 2007;44:555–60.
19. Kugathasan S, Collins N, Maresso K, et al. CARD15 gene mutations and risk for early surgery in pediatric-onset Crohn's disease. Clin Gastroenterol Hepatol. 2004;2:1003–9.
20. Russell RK, Drummond HE, Nimmo EE, et al. Genotype-phenotype analysis in childhood-onset Crohn's disease: NOD2/CARD15 variants consistently predict phenotypic characteristics of severe disease. Inflamm Bowel Dis. 2005;11:955–64.
21. Vermeire S, Pierik M, Hlavaty T, et al. Association of organic cation transporter risk haplotype with perianal penetrating Crohn's disease but not with susceptibility to IBD. Gastroenterology. 2005;129:1845–53.
22. Cleynen I, Boucher G, Jostins L, et al. Inherited determinants of Crohn's disease and ulcerative colitis phenotypes: a genetic association study. Lancet. 2016;387:156–67.
23. Shaoul R, Karban A, Reif S, et al. Disease behavior in children with Crohn's disease: the effect of disease duration, ethnicity, genotype, and phenotype. Dig Dis Sci. 2009;54:142–50.
24. Wei SC, Tan YY, Weng MT, et al. SLCO3A1, A novel crohn's disease-associated gene, regulates nf-kappaB activity and associates with intestinal perforation. PLoS One. 2014;9:e100515.
25. Dubinsky MC, Lin YC, Dutridge D, et al. Serum immune responses predict rapid disease progression among children with Crohn's disease: immune responses predict disease progression. Am J Gastroenterol. 2006;101:360–7.
26. Kirschner BS. Growth and development in chronic inflammatory bowel disease. Acta Paediatr Scand Suppl. 1990;366:98–104.
27. Markowitz J, Grancher K, Rosa J, et al. Growth failure in pediatric inflammatory bowel disease. J Pediatr Gastroenterol Nutr. 1993;16:373–80.
28. Kanof ME, Lake AM, Bayless TM. Decreased height velocity in children and adolescents before the diagnosis of Crohn's disease. Gastroenterology. 1988;95:1523–7.
29. Sanderson IR, Udeen S, Davies PS, et al. Remission induced by an elemental diet in small bowel Crohn's disease. Arch Dis Child. 1987;62:123–7.
30. Turner D, Grossman AB, Rosh J, et al. Methotrexate following unsuccessful thiopurine therapy in pediatric Crohn's disease. Am J Gastroenterol. 2007;102:2804–12.
31. Hyams J, Crandall W, Kugathasan S, et al. Induction and maintenance infliximab therapy for the treatment of moderate-to-severe Crohn's disease in children. Gastroenterology. 2007;132:863–73.
32. Malik S, Wong SC, Bishop J, et al. Improvement in growth of children with Crohn disease following anti-TNF-alpha therapy can be independent of pubertal progress and glucocorticoid reduction. J Pediatr Gastroenterol Nutr. 2011;52:31–7.
33. Faubion Jr WA, Loftus Jr EV, Harmsen WS, Zinsmeis AR. The natural history of corticosteroid therapy for inflammatory bowel disease: a population-based study. Gastroenterology. 2001;121:255–60.
34. Munkholm P, Langholz E, Davidsen M, Binder V. Frequency of glucocorticoid resistance and dependency in Crohn's disease. Gut. 1994;35:360–2.
35. Markowitz J, Hyams J, Mack D, et al. Corticosteroid therapy in the age of infliximab: acute and 1-year outcomes in newly diagnosed children with Crohn's disease. Clin Gastroenterol Hepatol. 2006;4:1124–9.
36. Vernier-Massouille G, Balde M, Salleron J, et al. Natural history of pediatric Crohn's disease: a population-based cohort study. Gastroenterology. 2008;135:1106–13.
37. Farmer RG, Michener WM. Prognosis of Crohn's disease with onset in childhood or adolescence. Dig Dis Sci. 1979;24:752–7.
38. Ferguson A, Sedgwick DM. Juvenile-onset inflammatory bowel disease: predictors of morbidity and health status in early adult life. J R Coll Physicians Lond. 1994;28:220–7.
39. Griffiths AM. Factors that influence the postoperative recurrence of Crohn's disease in childhood. In: Hadziselimovic F, Herzog B, Burgin-Wolff A, editors. Inflammatory bowel disease and coeliac disease in children. Boston: Kluwer Academic Publishers; 1990. p. 131–6.
40. Besnard M, Jaby O, Mougenot JF, et al. Postoperative outcome of Crohn's disease in 30 children. Gut. 1998;43:634–8.
41. Gupta N, Cohen SA, Bostrom AG, et al. Risk factors for initial surgery in pediatric patients with Crohn's disease. Gastroenterology. 2006;130:1069–77.

42. Cosnes J, Nion-Larmurier I, Beaugerie L, Afchain P, et al. Impact of the increasing use of immunosuppressants in Crohn's disease on the need for intestinal surgery. Gut. 2005;54:237–41.

43. Ramadas AV, Gunesh S, Thomas GA, et al. Natural history of Crohn's disease in a population-based cohort from Cardiff (1986-2003): a study of changes in medical treatment and surgical resection rates. Gut. 2010;59:1200–6.

44. Picco MF, Zubiaurre I, Adluni M, et al. Immunomodulators are associated with a lower risk of first surgery among patients with non-penetrating non-stricturing Crohn's disease. Am J Gastroenterol. 2009;104:2754–9.

45. Domenech E, Zabana Y, Garcia-Planella E, et al. Clinical outcome of newly diagnosed Crohn's disease: a comparative, retrospective study before and after infliximab availability. Aliment Pharmacol Ther. 2010;31:233–9.

46. Pedersen N, Duricova D, Lenicek M, et al. Infliximab dependency is related to decreased surgical rates in adult Crohn's disease patients. Eur J Gastroenterol Hepatol. 2010;22:1196–203.

47. Rutgeerts P, Feagan BG, Lichtenstein GR, et al. Comparison of scheduled and episodic treatment strategies of infliximab in Crohn's disease. Gastroenterology. 2004;126:402–13.

48. Lichtenstein GR, Yan S, Bala M, et al. Infliximab maintenance treatment reduces hospitalizations, surgeries, and procedures in fistulizing Crohn's disease. Gastroenterology. 2005;128:862–9.

49. Duricova D, Pedersen N, Lenicek M, et al. Infliximab dependency in children with Crohn's disease. Aliment Pharmacol Ther. 2009;29:792–9.

50. Zitomersky NL, Atkinson BJ, Fournier K, et al. Antibodies to infliximab are associated with lower infliximab levels and increased likelihood of surgery in pediatric IBD. Inflamm Bowel Dis. 2015;21:307–14.

51. Rutgeerts P, Geboes K, Vantrappen G, et al. Predictability of the postoperative course of Crohn's disease. Gastroenterology. 1990;99:956–63.

52. Becker JM. Surgical therapy for ulcerative colitis and Crohn's disease. Gastroenterol Clin North Am. 1999;28:371–90. viii-ix

53. Chardavoyne R, Flint GW, Pollack S, Wise L. Factors affecting recurrence following resection for Crohn's disease. Dis Colon Rectum. 1986;29:495–502.

54. Brignola C, Cottone M, Pera A, et al. Mesalamine in the prevention of endoscopic recurrence after intestinal resection for Crohn's disease. Italian Cooperative Study Group. Gastroenterology. 1995;108:345–9.

55. Caprilli R, Andreoli A, Capurso L, et al. Oral mesalazine (5-aminosalicylic acid; Asacol) for the prevention of post-operative recurrence of Crohn's disease. Aliment Pharmacol Ther. 1994;8:35–43.

56. Rutgeerts P, Hiele M, Geboes K, et al. Controlled trial of metronidazole treatment for prevention of Crohn's recurrence after ileal resection. Gastroenterology. 1995;108:1617–21.

57. Rutgeerts P, Van Assche G, Vermeire S, et al. Ornidazole for prophylaxis of postoperative Crohn's disease recurrence: a randomized, double-blind, placebo-controlled trial. Gastroenterology. 2005;128:856–61.

58. Hanauer SB, Korelitz BI, Rutgeerts P, et al. Postoperative maintenance of Crohn's disease remission with 6-mercaptopurine, mesalamine, or placebo: a 2-year trial. Gastroenterology. 2004;127:723–9.

59. Ardizzone S, Maconi G, Sampietro GM, et al. Azathioprine and mesalamine for prevention of relapse after conservative surgery for Crohn's disease. Gastroenterology. 2004;127:730–40.

60. Regueiro M, Schraut W, Baidoo L, et al. Infliximab prevents Crohn's disease recurrence after ileal resection. Gastroenterology. 2009;136:441–50. e1

61. Carla-Moreau A, Paul S, Roblin X, et al. Prevention and treatment of postoperative Crohn's disease recurrence with anti-TNF therapy: a meta-analysis of controlled trials. Dig Liver Dis. 2015;47:191–6.

62. de Ridder L, Turner D, Wilson DC, et al. Malignancy and mortality in pediatric patients with inflammatory bowel disease: a multinational study from the porto pediatric IBD group. Inflamm Bowel Dis. 2014;20:291–300.

63. Ekbom A, Helmick C, Zack M, Adami HO. Increased risk of large-bowel cancer in Crohn's disease with colonic involvement. Lancet. 1990;336:357–9.

64. Mellemkjaer L, Johansen C, Gridley G, et al. Crohn's disease and cancer risk (Denmark). Cancer Causes Control. 2000;11:145–50.

65. Jess T, Loftus Jr EV, Velayos FS, et al. Risk of intestinal cancer in inflammatory bowel disease: a population-based study from olmsted county, Minnesota. Gastroenterology. 2006;130:1039–46.

66. Ashworth LA, Billett A, Mitchell P, et al. Lymphoma risk in children and young adults with inflammatory bowel disease: analysis of a large single-center cohort. Inflamm Bowel Dis. 2012;18:838–43.

67. Lewis JD, Bilker WB, Brensinger C, et al. Inflammatory bowel disease is not associated with an increased risk of lymphoma. Gastroenterology. 2001;121:1080–7.

68. Loftus Jr EV, Tremaine WJ, Habermann TM, et al. Risk of lymphoma in inflammatory bowel disease. Am J Gastroenterol. 2000;95:2308–12.

69. Kandiel A, Fraser AG, Korelitz BI, et al. Increased risk of lymphoma among inflammatory bowel disease patients treated with azathioprine and 6-mercaptopurine. Gut. 2005;54:1121–5.

70. Thayu M, Markowitz JE, Mamula P, et al. Hepatosplenic T-cell lymphoma in an adolescent patient after immunomodulator and biologic therapy for Crohn disease. J Pediatr Gastroenterol Nutr. 2005;40:220–2.

71. Otley A, Smith C, Nicholas D, et al. The IMPACT questionnaire: a valid measure of health-related quality of life in pediatric inflammatory bowel disease. J Pediatr Gastroenterol Nutr. 2002;35:557–63.

72. Otley AR, Griffiths AM, Hale S, et al. Health-related quality of life in the first year after a diagnosis of pediatric inflammatory bowel disease. Inflamm Bowel Dis. 2006;12:684–91.

73. Gray WN, Boyle SL, Graef DM, et al. Health-related quality of life in youth with Crohn disease: role of disease activity and parenting stress. J Pediatr Gastroenterol Nutr. 2015;60:749–53.

74. Rabbett H, Elbadri A, Thwaites R, et al. Quality of life in children with Crohn's disease. J Pediatr Gastroenterol Nutr. 1996;23:528–33.

75. Akobeng AK, Suresh-Babu MV, Firth D, Miller V, Mir P, Thomas AG. Quality of life in children with Crohn's disease: a pilot study. J Pediatr Gastroenterol Nutr. 1999;28:S37–9.

76. Moody G, Eaden JA, Mayberry JF. Social implications of childhood Crohn's disease. J Pediatr Gastroenterol Nutr. 1999;28:S43–5.

77. Ferguson A, Sedgwick DM, Drummond J. Morbidity of juvenile onset inflammatory bowel disease: effects on education and employment in early adult life. Gut. 1994;35:665–8.

78. Loftus EV, Feagan BG, Colombel JF, et al. Effects of adalimumab maintenance therapy on health-related quality of life of patients with Crohn's disease: patient-reported outcomes of the CHARM trial. Am J Gastroenterol. 2008;103:3132–41.

79. Louis E, Lofberg R, Reinisch W, et al. Adalimumab improves patient-reported outcomes and reduces indirect costs in patients with moderate to severe Crohn's disease: results from the CARE trial. J Crohns Colitis. 2013;7:34–43.

Natural History of Ulcerative Colitis in Children

Peter Townsend and Jeffrey S. Hyams

Introduction

Defining the natural history of a chronic disease is made difficult by the continuously changing landscape of available therapies, earlier recognition of disease by more sensitive diagnostic techniques, and changes in intrinsic biological behavior. The natural history of ulcerative colitis following therapy with aminosalicylates and corticosteroids from previous decades would be expected to differ from that following the current and increasingly widespread use of immunomodulators and biological therapy. The data presented in this chapter reflect what we know of natural history now and will likely be different than what we might describe 10 years from now. There are a number of aspects of ulcerative colitis whose natural history can be examined, including clinical indices, endoscopic measures, extraintestinal manifestations, and therapy changes. This chapter will focus on natural history elements pertaining to clinical remission, endoscopic remission, and colectomy. Discussion of drugs will mostly focus mainly on maintenance of remission. Lastly, possible methodology to predict response to therapy and alter natural history will be addressed.

Overview

Clinical reports from the 1970s describe a severe clinical course for children newly diagnosed with ulcerative colitis with chronic disease, recurrent hospitalizations, frequent

P. Townsend, MD • J.S. Hyams, MD (✉)
Division of Digestive Diseases, Hepatology, and Nutrition, Connecticut Children's Medical Center, Hartford, CT 06106, USA

University of Connecticut School of Medicine, Farmington, CT, USA
e-mail: jhyams@ccmckids.org

colectomy, and not rare deaths [1, 2]. Cohorts examined since the beginning of widespread use of immunomodulators have presented data with more encouraging outcomes. A report in 1996 of 171 subjects seen at two large pediatric inflammatory bowel disease centers in the Northeastern United States found that 43% of patients had mild disease and 57% moderate to severe disease at presentation [3]. Forty-three percent had pancolitis. Over 80% had resolution of symptoms within 6 months of diagnosis, and during subsequent yearly follow-up intervals, 55% were symptom free, 38% had chronic intermittent symptoms, and 7% had continuous symptoms. Corticosteroid therapy was used in 27% of those with initially mild disease and 70% of those with moderate/severe disease by 1 year. Eleven percent of those with moderate/severe disease received additional immunomodulatory therapy (azathioprine/6-mercaptopurine or cyclosporine) during the first year. By 1 year following diagnosis, 1% of those with initial mild disease and 8% of those with moderate/severe disease had required colectomy; at 5 years the risk of colectomy was 9% and 26% in the two groups, respectively. A report from Denmark in 1997 describing 80 children with ulcerative colitis demonstrated a cumulative colectomy rate of 6% and 23% at 1 and 5 years, respectively [4]. A report of a regional incident cohort from Northern France in 2009 on 113 pediatric patients showed evolution from initial extensive disease in 37% at diagnosis to 60% by last follow-up and a cumulative colectomy rate of 20% by 5 years [5]. In a population-based cohort in Texas, 25% of patients had proctitis, 40% had left-sided disease, and 35% had extensive colitis at presentation [6]. At a mean of 4.4 years, 20% of patients with proctitis initially progressed to left-sided disease, while 80% progressed to extensive disease; of those with left-sided colitis, 40% had progressed to extensive colitis. Colectomy rates in this cohort were 4.1% at 1 year and 16% at 10 years of follow-up.

A few recent cohorts from Europe and North America have encompassed populations that were all diagnosed in the era of biologic agents. In a Slovenian IBD cohort with 39 UC patients, only 5% of the patients had proctitis at diagnosis, while 69% had extensive colitis or pancolitis [7]. A portion of this cohort had colonoscopy >2 years from diagnosis; none of whom had proctitis, while 82% had extensive pancolitis. In this cohort, only one patient proceeded to colectomy. A prospective, population-based cohort in Wisconsin found 66% of patients with pancolitis versus 34% with left-sided disease [8]. While the authors deemed the data on progression insufficient for analysis, they did report a colectomy rate of 13% in a mean follow-up of 4 years. A prospective population-based cohort from Denmark found 8% of patients initially presenting with proctitis and 65% with extensive colitis [9]. Again, the study did not analyze disease progression, but found a 1-year colectomy rate of 2.4%. A colectomy rate of 9% for children diagnosed with ulcerative colitis was reported in a regional center in the United Kingdom [10]. All children underwent colectomy after failing maximal medical therapy. A review of the published literature on population-based natural history studies of pediatric ulcerative colitis suggested an overall colectomy rate of about 20% at 10 years follow-up [11].

As mentioned previously the natural history of ulcerative colitis is largely a function of the efficacy of medications used to treat it. Large-scale blinded, placebo-controlled trials are generally lacking in the pediatric population.

Aminosalicylates

Data supporting the use of 5-aminosalicylate (5-ASA) compounds for the induction and maintenance therapy in adult ulcerative colitis (UC) are strong [12, 13]. There are also data in adults suggesting that higher-dose 5-ASA may be more effective in inducing remission (4.8 g mesalamine vs. 2.4 g mesalamine), but this added efficacy seemed limited to patients with moderate disease and was not observed in those with mild disease [14].

In 1993, a small blinded pediatric study compared sulfasalazine (30 mg/kg/day) versus olsalazine (60 mg/kg/day [15]. Neither agent is in common use currently. A more recent study assessed the safety and efficacy of high- and low-dose oral delayed-release mesalamine in children with mild to moderately active ulcerative colitis [16]. Patients with a pediatric ulcerative colitis activity index (PUCAI) score of 10–55 received a weight-dependent low or high dose of delayed-release mesalamine. The primary outcome was achieving a PUCAI score of <10 at 6 weeks. No difference was found in the two dosing groups with each achieving a little over 50% remission. A limitation of this study was the wide range of dosing given even within each of the two dosing groups. Data on the use of aminosalicylates in a large, prospective North American observational cohort of 213 patients has been reported [17]. Children who received either

an aminosalicylate alone or aminosalicylate plus corticosteroid were followed; however, children who required additional therapy such as infliximab, calcineurin inhibitors, or surgery in the first 30 days were excluded from outcome analysis. The mean dose of 5-ASA used in the treated population was 52 mg/kg/day. The use of 5-ASA with or without CS in the first 30 days was associated with corticosteroid-free inactive disease at 1 year with no need for additional rescue therapy in approximately 40% of patients. Adherence was not monitored, and recent data show alarming rates of non-adherence into oral medications in children with IBD [18]. The effect of better adherence on long-term outcomes of children with newly diagnosed ulcerative colitis is an area currently being studied.

The use of rectal mesalamine therapy (suppositories, enemas) is often encouraged in those with largely limited distal disease or proctitis, but many children and adolescents prefer oral therapy instead.

Corticosteroids

Corticosteroids remain the mainstay of induction therapy for moderate to severe ulcerative colitis, and therefore understanding the course of disease following these medications is critical to understanding natural history. Traditional corticosteroid therapy has usually meant prednisone for moderate to severe disease though more recently budesonide MMX has been used for mild to moderate disease [19].

The outcome of corticosteroid therapy for adults with UC in a population-based study in Olmsted County, Minnesota, was published in 2001 [20]. In this study of 185 patients diagnosed with UC over a 23-year period, only 63 (34%) received corticosteroids. Fifty-four percent of subjects receiving corticosteroids had a complete clinical response by 30 days, 30% a partial response, and 16% no response. By 1 year, 49% had a prolonged response, 22% were termed corticosteroid-dependent, and 29% had undergone colectomy. Immunomodulators were used in very few of these patients. Corticosteroid use is more widespread in the treatment of pediatric ulcerative colitis compared with adults, with a rate of 79% reported in an observational registry [21]. This difference may be at least partially explained by the generally extensive and severe presentation of ulcerative colitis at diagnosis. In this registry report, 60% of children with ulcerative colitis treated with corticosteroids within 30 days of diagnosis were noted to have inactive disease activity at 3 months with mild disease in 27% and continued to moderate/severe activity in 11%. At 1 year, 31/62 (50%) of the corticosteroid-treated patients were considered corticosteroid-responsive and 28 (45%) corticosteroid-dependent. A total of four patients receiving corticosteroids (5%) required colectomy in the first year. Immunomodulators were used in 61% of all corticosteroid-treated patients. Optimal dosing regimens for corticosteroids have not been established though there appears to be little advantage to exceeding the equivalent of 40–60 mg/day in adults. The mechanisms underlying corticosteroid resistance are beyond the scope of this discussion and have been reviewed elsewhere [22]. In a study of 128 children hospitalized with ulcerative colitis and treated with intravenous corticosteroids, nonresponse to therapy was associated with overexpression of several genes involved in inflammatory pathways [23]. In vitro studies have identified expression of certain microRNAs as potential mediators of glucocorticoid resistance [24], but clinical studies have not been published that support this relationship.

Immunomodulators

The use of immunomodulators has become standard of care in corticosteroid-dependent ulcerative colitis in children and adults, though as discussed below, the emergence of newer biologic agents may be changing this paradigm. A review of seven blinded, controlled trials of azathioprine in ulcerative colitis highlighted the methodological issues with many early studies of adults which left unanswered the question of whether this drug was useful in maintaining remission [25]. A review of the 30-year experience with azathioprine in a large cohort of adult patients in Oxford, England, suggested significant utility of azathioprine in maintaining remission [26]. Almost two-thirds of patients maintained remission for up to 5 years and median time to relapse upon stopping the drug with 18 months. The addition of the 5-aminosalicylate olsalazine to azathioprine did not improve the maintenance of remission rate compared to azathioprine alone in steroid-dependent adults with ulcerative colitis. A recent meta-analysis supported the role of thiopurines in maintaining remission in adult ulcerative colitis [27].

Pediatric data are more limited. One report detailed their use in 133 children from an inception registry cohort in North America [28]. Of these, 65 (49%) had CS-free inactive UC without rescue therapy at 1 year from thiopurine start. CS-free inactive disease at 1 year after initiating thiopurine was not affected by starting thiopurine ≤3 months versus >3 months from diagnosis, gender, age, or concomitant treatment with 5-aminosalicylates. Kaplan-Meier analysis showed that the likelihood of remaining free of rescue therapy (surgery, calcineurin inhibitors, or biologic therapy) in the thiopurine-treated patients was 73% at 1 year. A French cohort reported a 54% success rate treating patients with azathioprine, with success defined as few to no symptoms and no corticosteroid rescue therapy, at a minimum of 2 years' follow-up [5]. A large population-based study from

Greece of children and young adults suggested that the use of thiopurines in ulcerative colitis therapy had not benefit in lowering the risk of colectomy [29].

The use of methotrexate as an immunomodulator for the treatment of ulcerative colitis remains controversial, and until recently little data were available. A recent randomized double-blind placebo-controlled study from Europe compared 25 mg of parenteral methotrexate weekly with placebo in adults with corticosteroid-dependent ulcerative colitis [30]. Steroid-free remission at week 16 was achieved by 19/60 patients given methotrexate (31.7%) and 10/51 patients given placebo (19.6%) – a difference of 12.1% (95% confidence interval [CI], −4.0% to 28.1%; P = .15). The proportions of patients in steroid-free clinical remission at week 16 were 41.7% in the methotrexate group and 23.5% in the placebo group, for a difference of 18.1% (95% CI, 1.1%–35.2%; P = .04). The proportions of patients with steroid-free endoscopic healing at week 16 were 35% in the methotrexate group and 25.5% in the placebo group-a difference of 9.5% (95% CI, −7.5% to 26.5%; P = .28). A Cochrane review meta-analysis of the literature prior to this report concluded there were insufficient data in the literature to support or refute a role for methotrexate in the management of ulcerative colitis in adults [31]. The use of methotrexate for the treatment of inflammatory bowel disease in general has recently been reviewed [32].

Though calcineurin inhibitors are widely accepted as effective therapy for inducing remission in severe ulcerative colitis [33–35], their use as maintenance therapy is uncommon. In children there are limited data on the use of these agents, and while short-term response averages about 80%, the majority of treated children still require colectomy within 2–3 years of their use [36, 37]. Additionally, because of their nephrotoxicity, increased susceptibility to infection, and other side effects, the use of calcineurin inhibitors is generally limited to several months as a bridge to other immunomodulators, infliximab, or surgery.

Biologics

There are ample data demonstrating the efficacy of anti-TNFα therapy in the treatment of adult [38] and pediatric ulcerative colitis [39]. In 2005, two randomized, double-blind, placebo-controlled studies, ACT 1 and ACT 2, were published in a single paper [38] evaluating the efficacy of infliximab for induction and maintenance in 728 adults with active ulcerative colitis (Mayo score 6–12). Clinical response at 8 weeks (decrease in Mayo score by 3 points) was observed in approximately 65% of subjects receiving a three-dose induction of infliximab (either 5 mg/kg/dose or 10 mg/kg/dose) compared to approximately 33% of placebo patients. Clinical remission at week 8 (Mayo score of 2 or lower, no item more than one) was observed in approximately 33% of infliximab-treated patients versus 10% in the placebo group. Mucosal healing at week 8 was seen in approximately 60% of infliximab-treated patients versus 30% of placebo treated patients. Week 54 data were available for 364 ACT 1 patients; 42% of infliximab-treated patients were in remission compared to 20% of those treated with placebo. Clinical remission without corticosteroids was seen in 9% of placebo-treated patients, 26% of those receiving 5 mg/kg maintenance doses of infliximab every 8 weeks, and 16% of those receiving 10 mg/kg doses. At the start of ACT 1 and ACT 2, approximately 30% of patients were felt to have corticosteroid refractory disease, 50–60% were taking corticosteroids at the time infliximab was initiated, 70% were receiving 5-aminosalicylate preparations, and 40–50% were taking immunomodulators. Average disease duration was approximately 6 years.

Subsequent observations since the ACT trials were published have greatly impacted the use of infliximab in the treatment of ulcerative colitis. It has been demonstrated that low serum trough levels of infliximab as well as the development of antibodies to infliximab negatively affect response and durability [40]. Rapid clearance of drug is noted in those patients with extensive disease and high C-reactive protein levels, likely through multiple mechanisms including the concept of a "large antigen sink" of TNF, hypoalbuminemia, and loss in the stool [40–43].

In a formal clinical trial of 60 children and adolescents with active ulcerative colitis despite treatment with corticosteroids, immunomodulators, and 5-aminosalicylates, a response as defined by a drop in Mayo score was seen at 8 weeks in 73% of patients following a three-dose induction of 5 mg/kg at 0, 2, and 6 weeks [39]. Clinical remission by Mayo score was seen in 40% at 8 weeks. At 54 weeks, in those patients treated with this induction regimen followed by maintenance therapy every 8 weeks, remission was noted in 38% of subjects. Similar to the experience in adults, a direct relationship was found between serum infliximab levels and a positive therapeutic response [44]. In a prospective observational registry, data on 51 children with ulcerative colitis treated with infliximab (65% corticosteroid refractory, 35% corticosteroid-dependent, 63% receiving immunomodulators) were available [45]. Inactive disease at 3 months following initiation of therapy was noted in 36% (26% also corticosteroid-free). At 12 months inactive disease was noted in 49% (38% corticosteroid-free).

There are no controlled pediatric data on the use of adalimumab to treat ulcerative colitis. In a controlled, randomized, placebo-controlled study of adult patients with moderate to severely active disease despite conventional therapy, adalimumab was associated with clinical remission in 16.5% of treated patients at 8 weeks compared to 9.3% treated with placebo; at 52 weeks the corresponding

remission rates were 17.3% and 8.5% [46]. Golimumab, another humanized IgG1 antibody to TNFα, has been shown to be more effective than placebo in inducing and maintaining remission [47, 48]. While direct comparison between infliximab, adalimumab, and golimumab is difficult because of differences in treatment design, a recent meta-analysis of data in adults suggested that infliximab was most likely of the three to prevent colectomy [49]. A lesson learned from all of these trials as well as real-world experience is the importance of achieving therapeutic drug levels no matter what agent is used [50].

Anti-integrin therapy has now shown efficacy in the treatment of adults with ulcerative colitis though there are no published data in children [51]. Response rates at week 6 were 47.1% and 25.5% among patients in the vedolizumab group and placebo group, respectively ($P < 0.001$). At week 52, 41.8% of patients who continued to receive vedolizumab every 8 weeks and 44.8% of patients who continued to receive vedolizumab every 4 weeks were in clinical remission, compared with 15.9% of patients who switched to placebo ($P < 0.001$). The frequency of adverse events was similar in the vedolizumab and placebo groups. Many patients in this study had previously been treated with anti-TNFα therapy.

It is quite likely that in the future both adult and pediatric patients with ulcerative colitis may cycle through several biologic agents, achieve clinical response or remission, have a good quality of life, and avoid colectomy.

Can We Predict the Course of Disease?

The wide range in phenotypic expression of pediatric ulcerative colitis and its response to therapy has heretofore made prediction of disease course difficult. Clinical factors examined have included features such as severity of disease (i.e., fulminant features requiring hospitalization), endoscopic appearance, laboratory markers, and early response to therapy [52–54]. Clinical severity, the need for hospitalization at diagnosis, and the need for rapid rescue with calcineurin inhibitors or anti-TNF agents remain the greatest risk factors for early colectomy. There are data in adults with ulcerative colitis suggesting that mucosal healing after a first course of corticosteroids for newly diagnosed ulcerative colitis is highly predictive of future course [55]. One hundred fifty-seven patients were followed for up to 5 years following their first course of corticosteroids. The group that displayed both clinical and endoscopic remission by 3 months had significantly lower rates of relapse, hospitalizations, and the need for immunosuppression than partial responders or non-responders. Moreover, the colectomy rate during follow-up was 3.3% in those with complete mucosal healing compared to 18% in partial responders and 17% in those without mucosal healing.

Attempts have also been made to try to correlate disease course with genetic profiles. An association between severe and extensive disease and the major histocompatibility complex (MHC) genes DRB1*0103 and DRB1*15 has been identified [56–58]. A structural polymorphism in the IKBL (inhibitor of κB-like) gene, located in the central region of the MHC locus, has also been associated with severe disease [59]. A genome-wide association study (GWAS) compared 324 adults with ulcerative colitis who required colectomy for refractory disease with 537 ulcerative colitis patients who did not [60]. A risk score determined from a combination of 46 single-nucleotide polymorphisms (SNPs) associated with the medically refractory group accounted for a little less than 50% of the variance for the colectomy risk. The sensitivity and specificity of the risk score were over 90%. Microarray of RNA isolated from colonic biopsy tissue has identified genes that may predict the response to infliximab in adults [61].

This panel of five genes (osteoprotegerin (OPG), stanniocalcin-1, prostaglandin-endoperoxide synthase 2 (COX2), interleukin 13 receptor alpha2, and interleukin 11) discriminated responders from non-responders with 95% sensitivity and 85% specificity. Another study of mucosal gene expression found a positive correlation between high IL-17 and IFN-γ expression and response to infliximab [62]. Variants of the IL-23R gene that increase susceptibility to UC seem to improve response to infliximab [63]. One study used a pharmacogenetics GWAS to evaluate infliximab non-response in a combined ulcerative colitis and Crohn disease group, finding BRWD1, TACR1, FAM19A4, and PHACTR3 to predict non-response [64].

In pediatric patients elevated fecal levels of OPG are associated with failure to respond to intravenous corticosteroids in children with severe ulcerative colitis [65]. Patients with colonic tissue that expresses high levels of the integrin αE gene (ITGAE) were shown to have improved response to a novel anti-integrin antibody, etrolizumab [66]. Emerging areas of research into biologic molecules (e.g., metabolomics, proteomics, epigenomics) have the potential to clarify disease phenotypes, behavior, and responsiveness to medications [67–69].

Summary

The optimal therapy for ulcerative colitis quickly induces and then effectively maintains remission with healing of the colonic mucosa and presents minimal toxicity to the patient. While 5-aminosalicylates are effective in inducing and maintaining remission in some patients, their efficacy in both aspects of therapy is limited for those with more severe disease. Nonetheless, 5-aminosalicylates should be the cornerstone of therapy if possible. Immunomodulators and anti-TNFα therapy are effective in many patients not maintained in remission on 5-aminosalicylates, but remission is noted in less than half of patients treated with these agents, and disease flares are still common. Evidence suggests that the short-term impact of biologic agents on disease course is positive, though it is not clear that disease course is altered for those who present with fulminant disease. This group continues to exhibit a greater degree of treatment unresponsiveness and has an unacceptably high rate of colectomy. Long-term observations will be required to better understand the changing natural history of ulcerative colitis in children with the emergence of new therapies. Current research holds the promise of development of risk assessment (e.g., gene expression, microbiome, genetics) promptly following diagnosis that will facilitate treatment design, decreasing the likelihood of treatment failure and complications of ineffective treatments.

References

1. Goel KM, Shanks RA. Long-term prognosis of children with ulcerative colitis. Arch Dis Child. 1973;48(5):337–42.
2. Michener WM, Farmer RG, Mortimer EA. Long-term prognosis of ulcerative colitis with onset in childhood or adolescence. J Clin Gastroenterol. 1979;1(4):301–5.
3. Hyams JS et al. Clinical outcome of ulcerative colitis in children. J Pediatr. 1996;129(1):81–8.
4. Langholz E et al. Inflammatory bowel diseases with onset in childhood. Clinical features, morbidity, and mortality in a regional cohort. Scand J Gastroenterol. 1997;32(2):139–47.
5. Gower-Rousseau C et al. The natural history of pediatric ulcerative colitis: a population-based cohort study. Am J Gastroenterol. 2009;104(8):2080–8.
6. Malaty HM et al. The natural history of ulcerative colitis in a pediatric population: a follow-up population-based cohort study. Clin Exp Gastroenterol. 2013;6:77–83.
7. Urlep D et al. Incidence and phenotypic characteristics of pediatric IBD in northeastern Slovenia, 2002-2010. J Pediatr Gastroenterol Nutr. 2014;58(3):325–32.
8. Adamiak T et al. Incidence, clinical characteristics, and natural history of pediatric IBD in Wisconsin: a population-based epidemiological study. Inflamm Bowel Dis. 2013;19(6):1218–23.
9. Jakobsen C et al. Pediatric inflammatory bowel disease: increasing incidence, decreasing surgery rate, and compromised nutritional status: a prospective population-based cohort study 2007-2009. Inflamm Bowel Dis. 2011;17(12):2541–50.
10. Ashton JJ et al. Colectomy in pediatric ulcerative colitis: a single center experience of indications, outcomes, and complications. J Pediatr Surg. 2016;51:277–81.
11. Fumery M et al. Review article: the natural history of paediatric-onset ulcerative colitis in population-based studies. Aliment Pharmacol Ther. 2016;3:346–55.
12. Sutherland L, Macdonald JK. Oral 5-aminosalicylic acid for induction of remission in ulcerative colitis. Cochrane Database Syst Rev. 2006;(2):CD000543.
13. Sutherland L, Macdonald JK. Oral 5-aminosalicylic acid for maintenance of remission in ulcerative colitis. Cochrane Database Syst Rev. 2006;(2):CD000544.
14. Hanauer SB et al. Delayed-release oral mesalamine at 4.8 g/day (800 mg tablet) for the treatment of moderately active ulcerative

colitis: the ASCEND II trial. Am J Gastroenterol. 2005;100(11):2478–85.

15. Ferry GD et al. Olsalazine versus sulfasalazine in mild to moderate childhood ulcerative colitis: results of the Pediatric Gastroenterology Collaborative Research Group Clinical Trial. J Pediatr Gastroenterol Nutr. 1993;17(1):32–8.

16. Winter HS et al. High- and low-dose oral delayed-release mesalamine in children with mild-to-moderately active ulcerative colitis. J Pediatr Gastroenterol Nutr. 2014;59(6):767–72.

17. Zeisler B et al. Outcome following aminosalicylate therapy in children newly diagnosed as having ulcerative colitis. J Pediatr Gastroenterol Nutr. 2013;56(1):12–8.

18. LeLeiko NS et al. Rates and predictors of oral medication adherence in pediatric patients with IBD. Inflamm Bowel Dis. 2013;19(4):832–9.

19. Lichtenstein GR. Budesonide multi-matrix for the treatment of patients with ulcerative colitis. Dig Dis Sci. 2016;61:358–7.

20. Faubion Jr WA et al. The natural history of corticosteroid therapy for inflammatory bowel disease: a population-based study. Gastroenterology. 2001;121(2):255–60.

21. Hyams J et al. The natural history of corticosteroid therapy for ulcerative colitis in children. Clin Gastroenterol Hepatol. 2006;4(9):1118–23.

22. De Iudicibus S et al. Molecular mechanism of glucocorticoid resistance in inflammatory bowel disease. World J Gastroenterol. 2011;17(9):1095–108.

23. Kabakchiev B, et al. Gene expression changes associated with resistance to intravenous corticosteroid therapy in children with severe ulcerative colitis. PLoS One. 2010;5(9):1–8.

24. De Iudicibus S et al. MicroRNAs as tools to predict glucocorticoid response in inflammatory bowel diseases. World J Gastroenterol. 2013;19(44):7947–54.

25. Sands BE. Immunosuppressive drugs in ulcerative colitis: twisting facts to suit theories? Gut. 2006;55(4):437–41.

26. Fraser AG, Orchard TR, Jewell DP. The efficacy of azathioprine for the treatment of inflammatory bowel disease: a 30 year review. Gut. 2002;50(4):485–9.

27. Khan KJ et al. Efficacy of immunosuppressive therapy for inflammatory bowel disease: a systematic review and meta-analysis. Am J Gastroenterol. 2011;106(4):630–42.

28. Hyams JS et al. Outcome following thiopurine use in children with ulcerative colitis: a prospective multicenter registry study. Am J Gastroenterol. 2011;106(5):981–7.

29. Chhaya V et al. The impact of timing and duration of thiopurine treatment on colectomy in ulcerative colitis: a national population-based study of incident cases between 1989–2009. Aliment Pharmacol Ther. 2015;41(1):87–98.

30. Carbonnel F et al. Methotrexate is not superior to placebo in inducing steroid-free remission, but induces steroid-free clinical remission in a larger proportion of patients with ulcerative colitis. Gastroenterology. 2016;150:380–8.

31. Wang Y, et al. Methotrexate for maintenance of remission in ulcerative colitis. Cochrane Database Syst Rev. 2015;8:CD007560.

32. Herfarth HH et al. Use of methotrexate in the treatment of inflammatory bowel diseases. Inflamm Bowel Dis. 2016;22(1):224–33.

33. Shibolet O, et al. Cyclosporine A for induction of remission in severe ulcerative colitis. Cochrane Database Syst Rev. 2005;(1):CD004277.

34. Navas-Lopez VM et al. Oral tacrolimus for pediatric steroid-resistant ulcerative colitis. J Crohns Colitis. 2014;8(1):64–9.

35. Kawakami K et al. Effects of oral tacrolimus as a rapid induction therapy in ulcerative colitis. World J Gastroenterol. 2015;21(6):1880–6.

36. Turner D et al. Consensus for managing acute severe ulcerative colitis in children: a systematic review and joint statement from ECCO, ESPGHAN, and the Porto IBD Working Group of ESPGHAN. Am J Gastroenterol. 2011;106(4):574–88.

37. Watson S et al. Outcomes and adverse events in children and young adults undergoing tacrolimus therapy for steroid-refractory colitis. Inflamm Bowel Dis. 2011;17(1):22–9.

38. Rutgeerts P et al. Infliximab for induction and maintenance therapy for ulcerative colitis. N Engl J Med. 2005;353(23):2462–76.

39. Hyams J et al. Induction and maintenance therapy with infliximab for children with moderate to severe ulcerative colitis. Clin Gastroenterol Hepatol. 2012;10(4):391–9. e1

40. Brandse JF et al. Pharmacokinetic features and presence of antidrug antibodies associate with response to infliximab induction therapy in patients with moderate to severe ulcerative colitis. Clin Gastroenterol Hepatol. 2016;14:251–8.

41. Hoekman DR et al. The association of infliximab trough levels with disease activity in pediatric inflammatory bowel disease. Scand J Gastroenterol. 2015;50(9):1110–7.

42. Brandse JF et al. Loss of infliximab into feces is associated with lack of response to therapy in patients with severe ulcerative colitis. Gastroenterology. 2015;149(2):350–5. e2

43. Ordas I, Feagan BG, Sandborn WJ. Therapeutic drug monitoring of tumor necrosis factor antagonists in inflammatory bowel disease. Clin Gastroenterol Hepatol. 2012;10(10):1079–87. ; quiz e85-6

44. Adedokun OJ et al. Pharmacokinetics of infliximab in children with moderate-to-severe ulcerative colitis: results from a randomized, multicenter, open-label, phase 3 study. Inflamm Bowel Dis. 2013;19(13):2753–62.

45. Hyams JS et al. Outcome following infliximab therapy in children with ulcerative colitis. Am J Gastroenterol. 2010;105(6):1430–6.

46. Sandborn WJ et al. Adalimumab induces and maintains clinical remission in patients with moderate-to-severe ulcerative colitis. Gastroenterology. 2012;142(2):257–65. e1-3

47. Sandborn WJ et al. Subcutaneous golimumab induces clinical response and remission in patients with moderate-to-severe ulcerative colitis. Gastroenterology. 2014;146(1):85–95. ; quiz e14-5

48. Sandborn WJ et al. Subcutaneous golimumab maintains clinical response in patients with moderate-to-severe ulcerative colitis. Gastroenterology. 2014;146(1):96–109. e1

49. Lopez A et al. Efficacy of tumour necrosis factor antagonists on remission, colectomy and hospitalisations in ulcerative colitis: meta-analysis of placebo-controlled trials. Dig Liver Dis. 2015;47(5):356–64.

50. Ungar B et al. Optimizing anti-TNFalpha therapy: serum levels of infliximab and adalimumab associate with mucosal healing in patients with inflammatory bowel diseases. Clin Gastroenterol Hepatol. 2015;14:550–7.

51. Feagan BG et al. Vedolizumab as induction and maintenance therapy for ulcerative colitis. N Engl J Med. 2013;369(8):699–710.

52. Turner D et al. Endoscopic and clinical variables that predict sustained remission in children with ulcerative colitis treated with infliximab. Clin Gastroenterol Hepatol. 2013;11(11):1460–5.

53. Schechter A et al. Early endoscopic, laboratory and clinical predictors of poor disease course in paediatric ulcerative colitis. Gut. 2015;64(4):580–8.

54. Kumar S et al. Severe ulcerative colitis: prospective study of parameters determining outcome. J Gastroenterol Hepatol. 2004;19(11):1247–52.

55. Ardizzone S et al. Mucosal healing predicts late outcomes after the first course of corticosteroids for newly diagnosed ulcerative colitis. Clin Gastroenterol Hepatol. 2011;9(6):483–9. e3

56. Bouma G et al. Genetic markers in clinically well defined patients with ulcerative colitis (UC). Clin Exp Immunol. 1999;115(2):294–300.

57. Trachtenberg EA et al. HLA class II haplotype associations with inflammatory bowel disease in Jewish (Ashkenazi) and non-Jewish caucasian populations. Hum Immunol. 2000;61(3):326–33.

58. Ahmad T et al. The contribution of human leucocyte antigen complex genes to disease phenotype in ulcerative colitis. Tissue Antigens. 2003;62(6):527–35.

59. de la Concha EG et al. Susceptibility to severe ulcerative colitis is associated with polymorphism in the central MHC gene IKBL. Gastroenterology. 2000;119(6):1491–5.

60. Haritunians T et al. Genetic predictors of medically refractory ulcerative colitis. Inflamm Bowel Dis. 2010;16(11):1830–40.

61. Arijs I et al. Mucosal gene signatures to predict response to infliximab in patients with ulcerative colitis. Gut. 2009;58(12): 1612–9.

62. Rismo R et al. Mucosal cytokine gene expression profiles as biomarkers of response to infliximab in ulcerative colitis. Scand J Gastroenterol. 2012;47(5):538–47.

63. Jurgens M et al. Disease activity, ANCA, and IL23R genotype status determine early response to infliximab in patients with ulcerative colitis. Am J Gastroenterol. 2010;105(8):1811–9.

64. Dubinsky MC et al. Genome wide association (GWA) predictors of anti-TNFalpha therapeutic responsiveness in pediatric inflammatory bowel disease. Inflamm Bowel Dis. 2010;16(8): 1357–66.

65. Sylvester FA et al. Fecal osteoprotegerin may guide the introduction of second-line therapy in hospitalized children with ulcerative colitis. Inflamm Bowel Dis. 2011;17(8):1726–30.

66. Tew GW et al. Association between response to etrolizumab and expression of integrin alphaE and granzyme A in colon biopsies of patients with ulcerative colitis. Gastroenterology. 2016;150: 477–87.

67. Fukuda K, Fujita Y. Determination of the discriminant score of intestinal microbiota as a biomarker of disease activity in patients with ulcerative colitis. BMC Gastroenterol. 2014;14:49.

68. Rantalainen M et al. Integrative transcriptomic and metabonomic molecular profiling of colonic mucosal biopsies indicates a unique molecular phenotype for ulcerative colitis. J Proteome Res. 2015;14(1):479–90.

69. Hasler R et al. A functional methylome map of ulcerative colitis. Genome Res. 2012;22(11):2130–7.

Natural History of Pediatric Indeterminate Colitis

9

Melissa A. Fernandes, Sofia Verstraete, and Melvin B. Heyman

Melissa A. Fernandes and Sofia Verstraete were supported in part by NIH Grant T32 DK007762.

Abbreviations

CD   Crohn's disease
IBD   Inflammatory bowel disease
IBD-U   Inflammatory bowel disease unclassified
IC   Indeterminate colitis
UC   Ulcerative colitis

Introduction

Indeterminate colitis (IC), as a classification of inflammatory bowel disease, was introduced by Kent in 1970 [1] and was intended to classify colectomy specimens that had histology findings suggestive of Crohn disease (CD), despite a patient's clinical history of ulcerative colitis (UC). Contemporarily, IC is used broadly for patients whose clinical, radiological, endoscopic, and histological findings provide a muddled picture. The 2014 Porto Criteria established a new terminology, inflammatory bowel disease unclassified (IBD-U), to reduce confusion among providers, researchers, and patients [2]. Additionally, the Paris Classification of Pediatric Inflammatory Bowel Disease strengthened the definitions of UC and CD in children to reduce misclassification [3]. However, random use of terms continues, with

M.A. Fernandes, MD • S. Verstraete, MD
Department of Pediatrics, University of California, San Francisco, San Francisco, CA, USA

M.B. Heyman, MD (✉)
Department of Pediatrics, University of California, San Francisco, San Francisco, CA, USA

Pediatric Gastroenterology/Nutrition, University of California, San Francisco, 550-16th Street, fifth floor, Mailstop 0136, San Francisco, CA 94143, USA
e-mail: mel.heyman@ucsf.edu

individuals using IC, IBD-U, uncertain colitis, and idiopathic chronic colitis interchangeably. Regardless, in adult patients, 10–15% of patients at diagnosis receive the classification of IBD-U [4], while in pediatrics this percentage is even greater, especially among those children who present with very early onset IBD [5]. In order to be consistent throughout this chapter, the diagnosis will be exclusively referred to as IBD-U, whether or not the original research classified patients as IC or IBD-U.

In this chapter, we review the clinical and histological criteria needed to establish the diagnosis of IBD-U, describe the factors that lead to the diagnosis of IBD-U, investigate occurrence of reclassification, and review the available literature about the natural history of this classification.

Definition and Diagnosis

In pediatrics, a subset of patients will be diagnosed with inflammatory bowel disease (IBD); however, they do not follow the classic definitions of CD or UC. These "in-between" patients challenge providers, as less is known about the natural history, prognosis, or efficacy of treatment of the disease. Both the 2014 Porto Criteria and European Crohn's and Colitis Organisation (ECCO) Guidelines established criteria for the diagnosis of IBD-U [2]. By providing specific criteria, a more homogenous group of patients will receive this diagnosis and potentially improve providers' ability to understand and manage the disease process.

To address the questions, inconsistencies, and controversies in the diagnosis and classification of pediatric inflammatory bowel disease, the North American Society for Pediatric Gastroenterology, Hepatology, and Nutrition and the Crohn's and Colitis Foundation of America jointly organized a working group of pediatric gastroenterologists and GI pathologists in 2003 and 2007. The goals of this working group were to establish an agreed-upon set of definitions and phenotypes and to develop an algorithm that would improve interobserver agreement in the diagnosis and classification of CD, UC, and IBD-U.

Although the working group was unable to find enough data in the literature to state a definition of IBD-U, they posited several general recommendations: (1) Clinicians should try to avoid overuse of the diagnosis of IBD-U. The recommendations specifically state that the following criteria do not preclude a diagnosis of UC in children with colitis: backwash ileitis, rectal sparing, histological patchiness, periappendiceal inflammation, and gastritis. (2) For patients diagnosed with IBD-U based on findings highly atypical for UC, such as ileal aphthae, backwash ileitis in a patient with left-sided colitis, profound growth failure, large oral aphthae, or absolute rectal sparing, clinicians should precisely specify the reason(s) for the diagnosis of IBD-U rather than UC or CD. (3) Patients given a provisional diagnosis of IBD-U should undergo additional endoscopic and radiographic evaluations after 1 year or during the next disease exacerbation to try to establish a definitive diagnosis, while acknowledging that partially treated disease may have a patchy distribution [6].

The 2014 Porto Guidelines and the Paris Classification provided pediatric specific definitions of CD and UC, decreasing confusion about proper classification. According to the Porto Criteria, IBD-U is a term that applies to patients who have definite IBD with inflammatory changes limited to the colon, but certain features render the differentiation between UC and CD difficult despite complete evaluation [2]. IBD remains a clinical diagnosis dependent on comprehensive evaluation – physical examination, radiological images, and macroscopic and microscopic endoscopic findings of both the upper and lower gastrointestinal tract. While accepted criteria can establish the diagnosis of UC and CD, several macroscopic and microscopic histological findings can make it difficult to distinguish between UC and CD in the pediatric population. We will first discuss atypical presentations of UC, obscured findings in fulminant colitis, and lack of specific findings in CD, each of which can lead to the IBD-U classification.

Pediatric UC patients provide a unique challenge, because they often deviate from classic definitions. Patients may have discontinuous disease at diagnosis, challenging accepted definitions of UC that may delay a patient's diagnosis and leading them to have a temporary diagnosis of IBD-U. In a study of the EUROKIDS registry, 5% of pediatric UC patients had rectal sparing defined as macroscopic normal disease with abnormal microscopic findings [7]. These children tended to be younger and have more extensive disease. In the same study, "backwash ileitis," or abnormal macroscopic findings in the ileum in the setting of pancolitis involving the cecum, was found in 10% of children with UC [7]. The existence of inflammation in the

cecum and ascending colon in a patient with left-sided UC has been well described, often termed the "cecal patch" [8]. Newer pediatric IBD guidelines, such as the Paris Classification, encourage practitioners to label a patient with UC rather than a temporary IBD-U diagnosis in these specific instances.

Resected colectomy specimens from patients with fulminant colitis can have nonspecific histological findings [9]. Macroscopic features of IBD-U include extensive ulceration, more severe involvement of the transverse and right colon, >50% of mucosal surface involvement, diffuse disease with possible rectal sparing, and toxic dilation [10]. Microscopic findings consist of extensive v-shaped ulcerations with sharp transitions to normal adjacent mucosa, transmural lymphoid inflammation with an absence of lymphoid aggregates, absence of well-defined epithelioid granulomas distant from crypts (or histiocytic collections adjacent to injured crypts), and knife-like deep penetrating fissures [10].

Finally, patients with a clinical presentation strongly suggestive of CD might receive a diagnosis of IBD-U if no pathognomonic findings such as granulomas are seen on histology. Ideally, initial histological evaluation is completed prior to initiation of treatment; however, even in this instance, sampling error is a problem with CD, given the patchy nature of the disease [11]. Endoscopic biopsies are confined to superficial and interspersed findings, thus not providing sufficient tissue sample to evaluate for transmural inflammatory changes and sometimes identification of granulomas [12]. In one study, only 20.5% of initial colonic biopsies of untreated pediatric patients later found to have CD had granulomas. The inclusion of upper gastrointestinal tract and terminal ileal biopsies increased identification of granulomas to 61% [13]. Comprehensive evaluation should include endoscopic and radiological examination of the upper gastrointestinal tract and intubation of the ileum.

Epidemiology

Disagreement concerning the definition of IBD-U has led to varying estimates of the incidence and prevalence of this disorder. In 2009, all children and adults newly diagnosed with UC, IBD-U, or CD in specific regions of southeastern Norway were enrolled into a prospective study in order to evaluate change in IBD diagnosis. At enrollment, 843 cases of IBD were identified: 518 patients with UC, 221 patients with CD, 40 patients with IBD-U, and 64 patients with possible IBD. At 5-year follow-up, 36 (35%) patients from the IBD-U and possible IBD group ($n = 104$) were diagnosed with UC and 8 (8%) with CD. It should be noted that the average age of onset was 42.6 years, indicating that the study population was predominantly adult [14]. A study by Bardhan et al. created a database of IBD patients across the United Kingdom. The study collected information on 11,432 patients with IBD, with 474 (4%) of participants classified as having IBD-U, with an average age of onset of 41 years [15].

Incidence data for IBD-U is even more varied in pediatric studies. In a Wisconsin-based pediatric study, 10 out of 199 incident IBD cases (5%) were classified as IBD-U, with an overall incidence of 0.35 per 100,000. A similar pediatric study in Poland enrolled 491 IBD patients, with 144 classified as IBD-U, with an overall incidence of all types of IBD of 2.7 cases per 100,000 and incidence of IC of 0.8 per 100,000 (29.3% of all IBD cases) [16]. Additional reports from the pediatric literature estimate the proportion of newly diagnosed IBD cases categorized as IBD-U to be anywhere between 3.3 and 30%, depending in part on the age of the population [17–22].

A meta-analysis published in 2008 by Prenzel and Uhlig, including 6262 pediatric patients and 15,776 adults with IBD, found a statistically different frequency of IBD-U (12.7% in children and 6.0% in adults, $p < 0.0001$). Also, that same study suggested a correlation between the age of a patient and the frequency of IBD-U, with younger patients more likely to be diagnosed with IBD-U. In children 0–2 years old, 34% of the 133 identified patients were diagnosed with IBD-U, compared with 21% of patients 0–5 years old [5].

It is postulated that differences in the proportion of incident IBD cases categorized as IBD-U, despite relatively similar overall IBD incidence rates, represent extremes in diagnosis and categorization rather than actual "biological" differences. This variation underscores not only the heterogeneity of conditions labeled as IBD-U, but also the inadequacy of the current classification system, especially with regard to the pediatric population. Newby in 2008 suggested that for pediatric patients in particular, the training of the medical provider may also play a role in the initial diagnosis, with a "specialist pediatric unit" being less likely to diagnose IBD-U, compared with nonpediatric providers [23].

The prevalence of IBD-U is affected not only by the number of new cases, but also by the number of cases exiting the prevalent pool. Because of the chronic nature of this illness, patients leave the pediatric prevalence pool only under a limited number of circumstances: (1) becoming adults, (2) death (uncommon), and (3) having their diagnosis changed to CD or UC. Therefore, estimates of prevalence are limited not only by the diagnostic concerns addressed above, but also by the natural history and disease evolution.

Noninvasive Diagnostic Tools

Serology

While IBD remains a clinical diagnosis, a number of serum antibodies have been identified that can help differentiate CD from UC. For example, particular patterns of anti-*Saccharomyces cerevisiae* antibodies (ASCA), perinuclear

antineutrophil cytoplasmic antibody (pANCA), and anti-outer membrane porin C antibody (anti-OmpC) have been noted in CD and UC. Recent studies have also attempted to determine if a unifying pattern exists for patients diagnosed with IBD-U or if antibody serology can provide an appropriate classification. Sura et al. found that the presence of pANCA was associated with an ultimate diagnosis of UC in patients diagnosed with IBD-U, who had a high clinical suspicion of UC [4, 24]. To date, no genetic or immunological markers have been shown to reliably differentiate between CD, UC, and IBD-U.

Capsule Endoscopy

Capsule endoscopy is another noninvasive modality that has been suggested to evaluate patients with IBD-U. In 2003, the FDA approved capsule endoscopy in pediatrics. In recent studies, capsule endoscopy has provided additional information, either confirming a diagnosis of CD or leading to reclassification of CD from UC or IBD-U [25–27]. Larger studies of the pediatric IBD-U population are needed to validate these findings.

Microbiome

Ongoing investigation and understanding about the fecal microbiome, virome, and fungal communities might also yield information on differentiating subtypes of pediatric IBD. Current research has suggested a bacterial dysbiosis exists in patients with IBD, and recent studies report unique phage patterns in patients with UC and CD [28, 29]. However, at this time, no unique fecal pattern has been identified that can distinguish IBD-U from CD or UC. Ongoing developments in this expanding area of research may allow identification of disease classification from a fecal sample.

Electron Microscopy

Application of electron microscopy has been proposed to gain more information from endoscopically obtained mucosal biopsies. Evaluation of endoscopic biopsy results using electron microscopy may facilitate detection of unique proteomic patterns that could help define a patient's IBD classification [30].

Medical Management

With uncertainty around the diagnosis of IBD-U, patients are often excluded from randomized clinical trials or grouped with UC patients. Results of large studies, retrospective reviews, and observational studies may also be limited by inadvertent inclusion of IBD-U patients. From published studies and anecdotal experience, patients with IBD-U are exposed to and respond to the same classes of medications as children with UC or CD, that is, corticosteroids, aminosalicylates, immunosuppressants, and biological agents. However, no algorithms or guidelines exist for medical management of IBD-U.

Papadakis et al. [31] investigated the use of infliximab in steroid-refractory IBD-U. Of the 20 patients treated with infliximab, 14 had a complete response, 2 had a partial response, and 4 had no response. Interestingly, 10 of the 20 patients (50%) ultimately received a diagnosis of CD [31]. A retrospective study by Willot et al. [32] investigated tolerance and safety of methotrexate in children with IBD. In the study, 11 of the 79 patients had IBD-U [32]. As in many studies, the IBD-U patients were grouped together with the UC patients; however, IBD-U patients (n = 11) outnumbered the UC patients (n = 5). IBD-U patients had similar outcomes to Crohn's patients at final follow-up in terms of efficacy, tolerance, and safety of methotrexate [33]. Ultimately, few studies focus on investigating the medical management of children with IBD-U.

Surgical Outcomes

Surgeons are typically reluctant to offer surgical options to IBD-U patients, given the uncertainty of the diagnosis. However, numerous studies have investigated outcomes for ileal pouch anal anastomosis (IPAA) and have shown equivalent functional outcomes as patients with UC [34–36], although increased complications such as anal fistula formation and development of CD have been reported. Most striking though, Delany et al. reported that 93% of all subjects themselves would opt to undergo the surgery again, regardless of the outcome [34].

Summary

Children classified as having IBD-U are a heterogeneous group of patients. Variability in the application of this term among clinicians has resulted in general misconceptions, including widespread differences in the reported prevalence and confusion regarding the natural history of IBD-U. Patients with IBD-U are often excluded from clinical trials, thus interfering with our ability to gain knowledge regarding the clinical course and the efficacy of treatment regimens in these patients. While efforts have been made to standardize diagnostic criteria of IBD-U, disagreement and confusion persist. Additionally, the often-transient nature of this diagnosis makes prospectively observational and randomized studies a

challenge. Pediatric patients with IBD-U are typically reclassified as UC or CD, with children under 6 years of age having a greater predisposition for eventual diagnosis of CD. Emerging understanding of noninvasive diagnostic tools such as serological and fecal markers should improve initial diagnostic classification of pediatric IBD and thus decrease the number of patients classified as IBD-U. We suspect that patients who, despite new technologies, maintain a diagnosis of IBD-U will be a more homogenous group of patients, potentially with a distinct disease entity.

Given current knowledge of IBD-U, we suggest utilization of medical management with agents that are effective in both CD and UC (i.e. steroids, salicylates, immunomodulators, and infliximab); specific therapies should be chosen based on disease location, severity, estimation of risk for recurrence, and potentially yet to be defined biomarkers. Although IBD-U patients who undergo surgical therapy such as colectomy and IPAA may be at higher risk of postoperative complications, these patients appear to have similar functional outcomes. Therefore, surgical therapy should not be withheld from IBD-U patients with refractory disease, once an attempt has been made to reclassify their disease status.

References

1. Kent TH, Ammon RK, DenBesten L. Differentiation of ulcerative colitis and regional enteritis of colon. Arch Pathol. 1970;89(1):20–9.
2. Levine A, Koletzko S, Turner D, Escher JC, Cucchiara S, de Ridder L, et al. ESPGHAN revised porto criteria for the diagnosis of inflammatory bowel disease in children and adolescents. J Pediatr Gastroenterol Nutr. 2014;58(6):795–806.
3. Levine A, Griffiths A, Markowitz J, Wilson DC, Turner D, Russell RK, et al. Pediatric modification of the Montreal classification for inflammatory bowel disease: the Paris classification. Inflamm Bowel Dis. 2011;17(6):1314–21.
4. Sura SP, Ahmed A, Cheifetz AS, Moss AC. Characteristics of inflammatory bowel disease serology in patients with indeterminate colitis. J Clin Gastroenterol. 2014;48(4):351–5.
5. Prenzel F, Uhlig HH. Frequency of indeterminate colitis in children and adults with IBD – a metaanalysis. J Crohns Colitis. 2009;3(4):277–81.
6. North American Society for Pediatric Gastroenterology, Hepatology, and Nutrition, Colitis Foundation of America, Bousvaros A, Antonioli DA, Colletti RB, Dubinsky MC, et al. Differentiating ulcerative colitis from Crohn disease in children and young adults: report of a working group of the North American Society for Pediatric Gastroenterology, Hepatology, and Nutrition and the Crohn's and Colitis Foundation of America. J Pediatr Gastroenterol Nutr. 2007;44(5):653–74.
7. Levine A, de Bie CI, Turner D, Cucchiara S, Sladek M, Murphy MS, et al. Atypical disease phenotypes in pediatric ulcerative colitis: 5-year analyses of the EUROKIDS Registry. Inflamm Bowel Dis. 2013;19(2):370–7.
8. Mutinga ML, Odze RD, Wang HH, Hornick JL, Farraye FA. The clinical significance of right-sided colonic inflammation in patients with left-sided chronic ulcerative colitis. Inflamm Bowel Dis. 2004;10(3):215–9.

9. Odze RD. A contemporary and critical appraisal of 'indeterminate colitis'. Mod Pathol. 2015;28(Suppl 1):S30–46.

10. Martland GT, Shepherd NA. Indeterminate colitis: definition, diagnosis, implications and a plea for nosological sanity. Histopathology. 2007;50(1):83–96.

11. Langner C, Magro F, Driessen A, Ensari A, Mantzaris GJ, Villanacci V, et al. The histopathological approach to inflammatory bowel disease: a practice guide. Virchows Arch. 2014;464(5):511–27.

12. DeRoche TC, Xiao SY, Liu X. Histological evaluation in ulcerative colitis. Gastroenterol Rep (Oxf). 2014;2(3):178–92.

13. De Matos V, Russo PA, Cohen AB, Mamula P, Baldassano RN, Piccoli DA. Frequency and clinical correlations of granulomas in children with Crohn disease. J Pediatr Gastroenterol Nutr. 2008;46(4):392–8.

14. Henriksen M, Jahnsen J, Lygren I, Sauar J, Schulz T, Stray N, et al. Change of diagnosis during the first five years after onset of inflammatory bowel disease: results of a prospective follow-up study (the IBSEN Study). Scand J Gastroenterol. 2006;41(9):1037–43.

15. Bardhan KD, Simmonds N, Royston C, Dhar A, Edwards CM, Rotherham IBD Database Users Group. A United Kingdom inflammatory bowel disease database: making the effort worthwhile. J Crohns Colitis. 2010;4(4):405–12.

16. Karolewska-Bochenek K, Lazowska-Przeorek I, Albrecht P, Grzybowska K, Ryzko J, Szamotulska K, et al. Epidemiology of inflammatory bowel disease among children in Poland. A prospective, population-based, 2-year study, 2002-2004. Digestion. 2009;79(2):121–9.

17. Heyman MB, Kirschner BS, Gold BD, Ferry G, Baldassano R, Cohen SA, et al. Children with early-onset inflammatory bowel disease (IBD): analysis of a pediatric IBD consortium registry. J Pediatr. 2005;146(1):35–40.

18. Hildebrand H, Finkel Y, Grahnquist L, Lindholm J, Ekbom A, Askling J. Changing pattern of paediatric inflammatory bowel disease in northern Stockholm 1990-2001. Gut. 2003;52(10):1432–4.

19. van der Zaag-Loonen HJ, Casparie M, Taminiau JA, Escher JC, Pereira RR, Derkx HH. The incidence of pediatric inflammatory bowel disease in the Netherlands: 1999-2001. J Pediatr Gastroenterol Nutr. 2004;38(3):302–7.

20. Carvalho RS, Abadom V, Dilworth HP, Thompson R, Oliva-Hemker M, Cuffari C. Indeterminate colitis: a significant subgroup of pediatric IBD. Inflamm Bowel Dis. 2006;12(4):258–62.

21. Malaty HM, Fan X, Opekun AR, Thibodeaux C, Ferry GD. Rising incidence of inflammatory bowel disease among children: a 12-year study. J Pediatr Gastroenterol Nutr. 2010;50(1):27–31.

22. Castro M, Papadatou B, Baldassare M, Balli F, Barabino A, Barbera C, et al. Inflammatory bowel disease in children and adolescents in Italy: data from the pediatric national IBD register (1996-2003). Inflamm Bowel Dis. 2008;14(9):1246–52.

23. Newby EA, Croft NM, Green M, Hassan K, Heuschkel RB, Jenkins H, et al. Natural history of paediatric inflammatory bowel diseases over a 5-year follow-up: a retrospective review of data from the register of paediatric inflammatory bowel diseases. J Pediatr Gastroenterol Nutr. 2008;46(5):539–45.

24. Joossens S, Reinisch W, Vermeire S, Sendid B, Poulain D, Peeters M, et al. The value of serologic markers in indeterminate colitis: a prospective follow-up study. Gastroenterology. 2002;122(5):1242–7.

25. Long MD, Barnes E, Isaacs K, Morgan D, Herfarth HH. Impact of capsule endoscopy on management of inflammatory bowel disease: a single tertiary care center experience. Inflamm Bowel Dis. 2011;17(9):1855–62.

26. Cohen SA, Gralnek IM, Ephrath H, Saripkin L, Meyers W, Sherrod O, et al. Capsule endoscopy may reclassify pediatric inflammatory bowel disease: a historical analysis. J Pediatr Gastroenterol Nutr. 2008;47(1):31–6.

27. Gralnek IM, Cohen SA, Ephrath H, Napier A, Gobin T, Sherrod O, et al. Small bowel capsule endoscopy impacts diagnosis and management of pediatric inflammatory bowel disease: a prospective study. Dig Dis Sci. 2012;57(2):465–71.

28. Norman JM, Handley SA, Baldridge MT, Droit L, Liu CY, Keller BC, et al. Disease-specific alterations in the enteric virome in inflammatory bowel disease. Cell. 2015;160(3):447–60.

29. Sheehan D, Moran C, Shanahan F. The microbiota in inflammatory bowel disease. J Gastroenterol. 2015;50(5):495–507.

30. Ballard BR, M'Koma AE. Gastrointestinal endoscopy biopsy derived proteomic patterns predict indeterminate colitis into ulcerative colitis and Crohn's colitis. World J Gastrointest Endosc. 2015;7(7):670–4.

31. Papadakis KA, Treyzon L, Abreu MT, Fleshner PR, Targan SR, Vasiliauskas EA. Infliximab in the treatment of medically refractory indeterminate colitis. Aliment Pharmacol Ther. 2003;18(7):741–7.

32. Willot S, Noble A, Deslandres C. Methotrexate in the treatment of inflammatory bowel disease: an 8-year retrospective study in a Canadian pediatric IBD center. Inflamm Bowel Dis. 2011;17(12):2521–6.

33. Assa A, Hartman C, Weiss B, Broide E, Rosenbach Y, Zevit N, et al. Long-term outcome of tumor necrosis factor alpha antagonist's treatment in pediatric Crohn's disease. J Crohns Colitis. 2013;7(5):369–76.

34. Delaney CP, Remzi FH, Gramlich T, Dadvand B, Fazio VW. Equivalent function, quality of life and pouch survival rates after ileal pouch-anal anastomosis for indeterminate and ulcerative colitis. Ann Surg. 2002;236(1):43–8.

35. Yu CS, Pemberton JH, Larson D. Ileal pouch-anal anastomosis in patients with indeterminate colitis: long-term results. Dis Colon Rectum. 2000;43(11):1487–96.

36. Turina M, Remzi FH. The J-pouch for patients with Crohn's disease and indeterminate colitis: (when) is it an option? J Gastrointest Surg. 2014;18(7):1343–4.

Shervin Rabizadeh and Maria Oliva-Hemker

Introduction

Inflammatory bowel disease (IBD) is not just a disorder of one organ system, but rather a multisystem disease. In addition to the more typical gastrointestinal involvement, which can present with symptoms such as abdominal pain, chronic diarrhea, or bloody stools, several other organs can be involved as well, including the eyes, skin, joints, kidneys, and liver. In fact, these extraintestinal manifestations may be the presenting symptoms and become the predominant source of morbidity for a given patient. These manifestations have been classified in various ways such as their relationship with the degree of inflammation of the underlying bowel disease or by the location of the bowel disease, for example, colonic versus small intestinal [1]. They can also be divided by whether or not they are a consequence of the IBD itself. Extraintestinal manifestations affecting the joints, skin, hepatobiliary system, and eye can be differentiated from those that are complications of the disease such as malabsorption leading to osteoporosis, growth issues, kidney stones, etc.

The pathogenesis of the extraintestinal manifestations, like the etiology of IBD, is unknown. However, possible hypotheses include abnormal immune self-recognition, antibody production against specific extraintestinal organs that cross-react with gastrointestinal antigens, and/or genetic susceptibility. It is postulated that the inflammatory response in patients with IBD leads to the inability of the intestine to act as a selective barrier. Hence, the uptake of bacterial products or dietary antigens can induce circulating immune complexes or a systemic inflammatory response [2]. Another theory involves the cross-reaction with a bacterial epitope leading to autoimmunity directed against an antigen shared among the intestine, skin, synovium, eye, and biliary system [3]. An autoimmune reaction to an isoform of tropomyosin, which is expressed in the eye (non-pigmented ciliary epithelium), skin (keratinocytes), joints (chondrocytes), biliary epithelium, and the gut, is speculated as the focal point for this theory [4]. Similarly, extraintestinal manifestations may share a common pathway with the bowel disease in that recruitment of mucosal memory and/or effector T cells to various tissues via the expression of endothelial adhesion molecules that are usually restricted to the gut may lead to destruction from the influx of inflammatory cells [5]. One mechanism does not explain all of the different extraintestinal symptoms described in IBD patients. This is supported by the lack of uniform response to treatment. For example, one-half of patients with Crohn disease had complete resolution of their extraintestinal manifestations with adalimumab treatment. There was a significant reduction in arthralgias, arthritis, oral aphthous ulcers, and erythema nodosum, but not ankylosing spondylitis, iritis, or uveitis [6].

There is a strong genetic influence on extraintestinal manifestations, with reports of 70% concordance between parent–child pairs and 83% concordance between siblings [7, 8]. The human leukocyte antigen (HLA) system is postulated as a link between IBD and certain extraintestinal manifestations, especially ocular and articular manifestations [7]. HLA-A2, -DR1, and -DQw5 are more commonly associated with extraintestinal comorbidities in Crohn disease. On the other hand, genotypes HLA-DRB1, -B27, and -B58 are linked with extraintestinal manifestations of ulcerative colitis. Primary sclerosing cholangitis as well as other autoimmune disorders (e.g. celiac disease, autoimmune hepatitis, myasthenia gravis) have been associated with IBD patients with haplotype HLA-B8/DR3, while HLA-B27 is reported in 50–80% of IBD patients with ankylosing spondylitis [4].

S. Rabizadeh, MD, MBA (✉)
Pediatric Inflammatory Bowel Disease Program, Department of Pediatrics, Cedars-Sinai Medical Center, 8635 W 3rd Street; Suite 1165W, Los Angeles, CA 90077, USA
e-mail: Shervin.Rabizadeh@cshs.org

M. Oliva-Hemker, MD
Division of Pediatric Gastroenterology and Nutrition, The Johns Hopkins University School of Medicine, 600 N Wolfe St., CMSC 2-116, Baltimore, MD 21287-2631, USA
e-mail: moliva@jhmi.edu

Table 10.1 Common extraintestinal manifestations of IBD in children and their relative prevalence

Extraintestinal manifestation	Prevalence
Growth failure	++++
Sacroiliitis	++++
Osteoporosis/osteopenia	+++
Peripheral joint inflammation	+++
Aphthous ulcers	+++
Primary sclerosing cholangitis	++
Granulomatous skin lesion	++
Erythema nodosum	++
Pyoderma gangrenosum	+
Uveitis/episcleritis	+
Ankylosing spondylitis	+

The incidence of developing any extraintestinal manifestation in IBD is estimated to be as high as 40% in predominately adult studies, and it can be the presenting symptom in one out of four patients with IBD [9, 10]. Two pediatric studies have shown similar rates. In a retrospective study of over 1,600 pediatric IBD patients, the incidence of extraintestinal manifestations was 29% at 15 years post diagnosis [11]. These complications were more common in older patients, and 6% of the patients had extraintestinal symptoms prior to diagnosis. In another prospective study of over 1,000 pediatric IBD patients, the incidence of extraintestinal manifestations was 28%, with the majority (87%) occurring in the first year after diagnosis [12]. Interestingly, patients with more severe disease had a higher likelihood of having an extraintestinal manifestation. Further, the presence of one extraintestinal manifestation confers a risk to develop other manifestations [10].

Over 130 extraintestinal manifestations have been reported in the literature associated with IBD, but fortunately, most of these are rare [13]. Several excellent comprehensive reviews are available on the extraintestinal manifestations of IBD [8, 13, 14, 15, 16, 17, 18, 19]. This chapter will focus on the more common extraintestinal manifestations found in the pediatric population and present them by the affected system and descending order of prevalence (Table 10.1).

Growth Failure

Extraintestinal manifestations of pediatric IBD patients cannot be discussed without first mentioning growth failure, which is estimated to occur in 30% of children with Crohn disease and in 5–10% of those with ulcerative colitis [9]. Children can present with an obvious lack of growth, such as a height below the 5th percentile for age, or growth changes can be more subtle with a gradual flattening of the child's height velocity which is only evident upon plotting multiple height measurements on a growth chart and comparison to midparental height. Some children can have delays in bone maturation and pubertal development. It is important to not merely assume that growth failure is a consequence of gastrointestinal manifestations, as decreases in weight and height velocities can precede any clinical evidence of bowel disease [20]. Thus, the concept of viewing growth failure as an independent manifestation of IBD will help health care providers develop a higher index of suspicion for the diagnosis of IBD in children presenting in this manner, even if they do not have gastrointestinal complaints.

IBD-associated growth failure could be secondary to deficient nutrient intake, poor digestion and absorption, as well as increased metabolic demands; however, the most likely etiology remains chronic caloric insufficiency [21]. Unfortunately, certain treatments for IBD, such as chronic corticosteroids, can have deleterious effects on overall growth, and these need to be weighed against the detrimental effects of the inflammatory process on growth. In addition to the consideration of immunomodulator (such as 6-mercaptopurine/azathioprine or methotrexate) and tumor necrosis factor alpha (TNFα) antagonists earlier in the disease course of pediatric patients, administration of oral or enteral formula feedings should be considered to rehabilitate the growth-stunted patient. A more extensive review can be found in the chapter devoted to growth issues in pediatric IBD.

Joint Manifestations

Joint inflammation is a commonly seen extraintestinal manifestation of IBD in both adults and children, with arthritis or joint pain occurring in 16–33% of children with IBD [9, 22, 23]. Similar to most other extraintestinal manifestations, symptoms of joint inflammation may occur before or after the development of bowel disease. Besides joint inflammation, one in five pediatric patients report enthesitis, inflammation at the bony insertion sites of ligaments, tendons, and fascia [24]. Joint manifestations can be divided into an axial form (involvement of the axial spine and sacroiliac joints) and a peripheral form (involvement of larger joints such as the knees, ankles, hips, wrists, and elbows).

The axial form of joint involvement includes ankylosing spondylitis and sacroiliitis. Ankylosing spondylitis, which is associated with the HLA-B27 antigen, is more commonly associated with ulcerative colitis and occurs in less than 2% of IBD patients. Symptoms include back stiffness, pain, and eventually stooped posture as well as peripheral joint complaints. Almost all of these patients will have involvement in their sacroiliac joints. On the other hand, asymptomatic sacroiliitis is more common with an estimated incidence of 10–52% [7]. Sacroiliitis is rarely diagnosed, especially in the early stages, unless sought after with bone scans or noted on computed tomography enterography [25]. Isolated sacroiliitis seems not to be associated with HLA-B27 [4]. Asymptomatic HLA-B27 negative patients with normal spinal mobility do not require specific treatment. Though ankylosing spondylitis has been shown to respond to sulfasalazine in multiple double-blind studies, none of the studies addressed ankylosing spondylitis in IBD patients [26]. Small studies have demonstrated a role of TNFα antagonist therapy in patients with IBD and ankylosing spondylitis [23]. Physical therapy and an exercise program to stop the progression of any disability and deformity remain a mainstay of treatment as well.

Peripheral joint inflammation is most frequently reported with Crohn disease and is most typically associated with colonic inflammation, although it can also be associated with small bowel disease [7]. The patient usually presents with erythema, swelling, and decreased range of motion in an asymmetric pauciarticular pattern. Fortunately, joint deformity is uncommon. The arthritis tends to worsen during times of increasing bowel disease, and there is an association with other extraintestinal manifestations such as those of the skin, mouth, and ocular systems. In fact, patients with involvement of these systems can share serological markers such as elevations in antibody levels against exocrine pancreas compared to other IBD and non-IBD patients [27].

Primary treatment of the bowel inflammation with 5-aminosalicylate medications, corticosteroids, immunomodulating agents, or TNFα antagonists is the first course of action for peripheral joint inflammation [9]. Resolution is commonly achieved with this approach in <8 weeks [22]. Studies have shown that infliximab is efficacious in the treatment of spondyloarthropathies, such as the articular and musculoskeletal findings in IBD [7]. Treatments with non-steroidal anti-inflammatory agents and cyclooxygenase-2-inhibitors have the potential for gastrointestinal mucosal injury and should be avoided if possible. In refractory cases, consideration is given to methotrexate and intraarticular corticosteroid injections.

Bone Disease

There has been increasing interest in identifying osteopenia and osteoporosis in patients with IBD, especially given that IBD commonly presents during adolescence and young adulthood when bone mass is being rapidly attained. In adult populations, the overall prevalence of osteoporosis in IBD is estimated between 4 and 40%, with increasing prevalence in older patients [4]. A large population-based adult study reported an osteoporosis prevalence of 15% and relative risk of 1.4 for fractures in IBD patients compared to the general population [28]. Prevalence of osteopenia and osteoporosis in the pediatric population is estimated between 8 and 30%, based on several smaller studies [11, 29]. The increased risk of eventually developing osteoporosis in IBD patients, especially those with Crohn disease, is secondary to multiple factors, including inadequate intake or malabsorption of calcium and vitamin D, corticosteroid use, low estrogen states in females, and negative effects of circulating proinflammatory cytokines [30]. This osteoporosis can make the patients prone to bone fracture, bone deformities, and chronic pain.

Diagnosis of osteopenia/osteoporosis is made with dual-energy x-ray absorptiometry (DEXA), which measures bone mineral density in the spine, femoral neck, or other bones rapidly and with low amounts of radiation. Treatment with calcium and vitamin D may prevent further deterioration of bone, but not necessarily help in the recovery of lost bone density, though some pediatric studies have suggested bone recovery in children with IBD on treatments [31]. Prevention has not been well studied in IBD patients, but it would be prudent to ensure intake of at least the recommended daily requirement for age of calcium and vitamin D, proper exercise, and minimization of corticosteroid usage to maximize the pediatric patient's potential in achieving an appropriate peak bone mass. The role of bone-protecting agents in IBD, especially pediatrics, is unknown so far.

Other bone complications in IBD patients include osteonecrosis of the femoral head, hypertrophic osteoarthropathy, and chronic recurrent multifocal osteomyelitis (CRMO). Osteonecrosis of the femoral head is usually associated with patients who have received chronic steroids and have complaints of hip or knee pain. Clubbing or hypertrophic osteoarthropathy is another bone manifestation associated with IBD, especially with small intestinal Crohn disease. The etiology, though unknown, is postulated to involve increased blood flow to the fingers, and hence increased connective tissue growth secondary to circulating cytokine production [7].

Chronic recurrent multifocal osteomyelitis (CRMO), rarely described in children with IBD, is an aseptic inflammatory bone disease that typically affects the long bones and clavicles [32].

Oral Lesions

Oral lesions can arise at anytime in patients with IBD and at any age, but they occur more commonly in children and are often independent of the intestinal disease severity [33]. Though the incidence can vary, the highest report rate was 48% in a pediatric age group study [34]. Recurrent aphthous lesions are the most common oral lesions associated with IBD, with a reported incidence of approximately 8–14% in pediatric IBD patients with higher rates in Crohn disease compared to ulcerative colitis [11–13]. Aphthous lesions tend to parallel intestinal disease, though they often can predate intestinal symptoms. Other oral lesions can consist of lip swelling, fissures, and gingivitis, which can demonstrate granulomas on histology [35]. Orofacial granulomatosis is a rare syndrome with chronic swelling of the lips and lower half of the face combined with oral ulcerations, and hyperplastic gingivitis that has been reported in three dozen Crohn cases [36]. Orofacial granulomatosis can be seen in other disorders such as foreign body reaction, tuberculosis, sarcoidosis, and idiopathic causes which share similar histopathological features [33]. Another rare disorder seen in association with ulcerative colitis patients is pyostomatitis vegetans which can present with oral and cutaneous findings in the axillae, genital areas, and scalp. The oral lesions consist of multiple neutrophil-filled and eosinophil-filled pustules on erythematous bases which can erode and fuse to form shallow ulcers that have been described as being "snail track" configuration [37]. Oral lesions in IBD patients could also be a result of nutritional deficiencies, specifically low levels of zinc, folic acid, niacin, and vitamin B-12 [33].

Treatment of oral lesions is usually reserved for those causing significant discomfort, and may involve topical, intralesional or systemic corticosteroids, dapsone, or preparations directed at the bowel disease including immunomodulators, TNFα antagonists, and thalidomide [33, 38].

Skin Lesions

Cutaneous manifestations of IBD can be classified into three principal groups: granulomatous, reactive, and secondary to nutritional deficiency. Granulomatous skin manifestations have the same histological features as the bowel disease and can include perianal and peristomal ulcers and fistulas, oral granulomatous ulcers, epidermolysis bullosa acquisita, and

metastatic Crohn disease. The latter is a rare complication that manifests as subcutaneous nodules or ulcers mainly in the lower extremities, and occasionally can occur in the genital areas. It appears unrelated to bowel activity and can be treated successfully with corticosteroids, antibiotics, azathioprine, methotrexate, and infliximab [7].

Of all the skin manifestations associated with IBD, erythema nodosum (Fig. 10.1) and pyoderma gangrenosum (Fig. 10.2) are the most common. In the pediatric patient, erythema nodosum, which is more commonly associated with Crohn disease than with ulcerative colitis, is encountered more frequently [9, 11]. Erythema nodosum presents as tender, subcutaneous, erythematous nodules, usually on the extremities, especially the lower legs, and the majority of patients with this skin manifestation will have associated joint pain or develop arthritis. Children may appear systemically ill with fever. Over days to weeks, the nodules will flatten, turn brown or gray, and can be mistaken for bruises. Histologically, erythema nodosum is a septal panniculitis consisting of a lymphohistiocytic infiltrate. The prevalence in all IBD patients, adult and pediatric, is estimated between 3% and 15% [28]. Exacerbations of erythema nodosum correlate most often with increased intestinal inflammation; hence, treatment toward the bowels is considered a primary

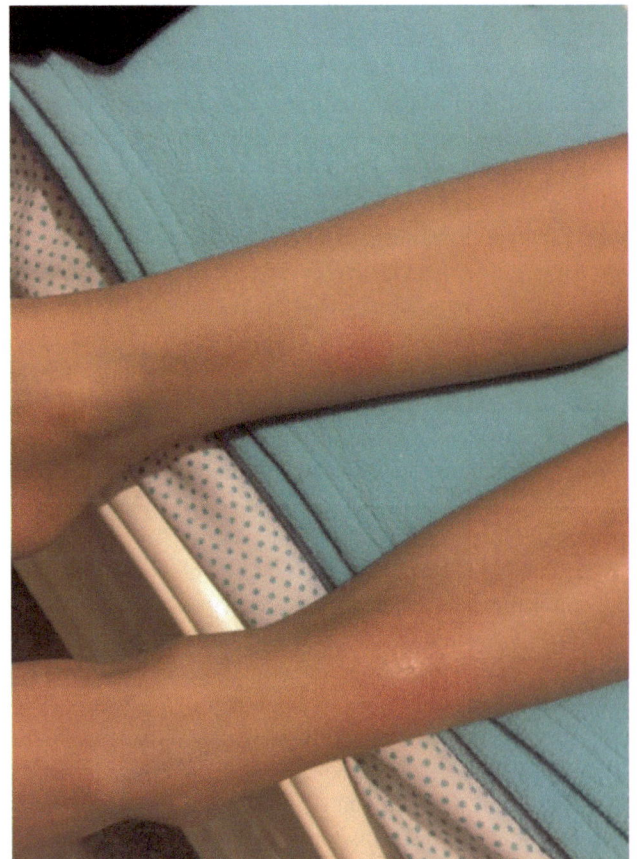

Fig. 10.1 Erythema nodosum (Courtesy of Dr. Susan M. Rabizadeh)

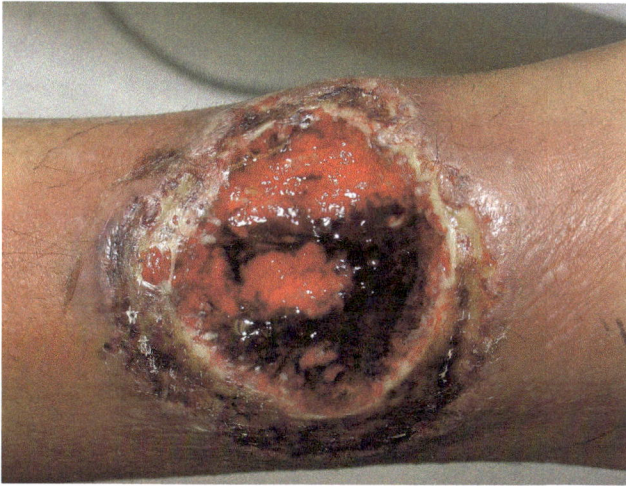

Fig. 10.2 Pyoderma gangrenosum (Courtesy of Dr. Rachel Nussbaum, Johns Hopkins University)

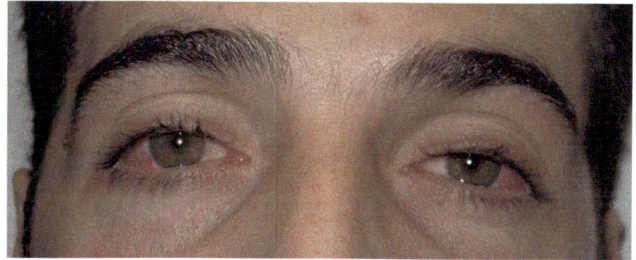

Fig. 10.3 Episcleritis (Courtesy of Dr. Rachel Nussbaum, Johns Hopkins University)

Vulvar lesions have also been associated with IBD in patients presenting with vulvar ulcers, labial swelling, exophytic lesions, condylomatous lesions, and abnormalities on pap smear. Most often, the histopathology demonstrates noncaseating vulvar granulomas, but dysplasia and carcinoma have also been reported [42].

form of management. Recent reports in children have shown good response to infliximab [39].

Pyoderma gangrenosum is an ulcerating lesion often correlating with exacerbations of the bowel disease. However, it can persist for long periods, while the intestinal inflammation is clinically quiescent. Fortunately, it is relatively rare with a reported incidence of 2% in UC patients and a smaller number in Crohn patients [39]. The lesions are often painful and located on the lower extremities. Histopathology reveals endothelial injury with fibrinoid necrosis of blood vessels and marked neutrophilic and lymphocytic infiltrates. Treatment is difficult, and patients may require large doses of systemic corticosteroids or immunomodulators as well as topical ulcer care. Infliximab has shown to be effective in refractory cases; however, some extreme cases might require grafting [7, 39].

Sweet's syndrome is another very rare reactive cutaneous disorder associated with IBD. It is a neutrophilic dermatosis presenting with painful erythematous plaques or nodules often associated with fever and leukocytosis. Usually, there is good response to corticosteroids, and a study has demonstrated benefit of cyclophosphamide in steroid refractory patients [40].

Psoriasis is seen commonly in patients with IBD [41]. In addition, therapy-related psoriasiform skin lesions have been reported in patients undergoing TNFα antagonist therapy. Anti-IL-12/IL-23 therapy may have a role in the treatment of these patients from an intestinal and skin standpoint [41].

Nutritional issues, such as trace mineral and vitamin deficiencies, occur in children with IBD, especially Crohn disease; however, skin disorders secondary to these are unusual. There are rare reported cases of acrodermatitis enteropathica, pellagra, and scurvy, secondary to zinc, niacin, and vitamin C deficiency, respectively.

Eye Lesions

The most common eye manifestations of IBD are episcleritis and uveitis [9]. These are often associated with other extraintestinal manifestations, especially arthritis and erythema nodosum. Episcleritis (Fig. 10.3), inflammation of the blood-rich episclera, tends to parallel bowel activity and is often confused with conjunctivitis as the patients present with eye redness and burning. Episcleritis does not impair vision and usually responds clinically to topical corticosteroids. If visual impairment is present, the possibility of scleritis, which can occur with protracted intestinal disease, needs to be considered, and an emergent evaluation by an ophthalmologist is required to evaluate for retinal detachment or optic nerve swelling.

Uveitis, unlike episcleritis, is usually independent of the bowel activity and inflammation. Anterior uveitis involves inflammation of the iris and the ciliary body. Symptoms can include acute or subacute eye pain, headache, photophobia, and blurred vision, or occasionally decreased vision; however, many patients may be asymptomatic. Complications of uveitis can be serious and include iris atrophy, synechiae, pigment deposits, glaucoma, cataracts, and permanent visual deficits. Attention must be paid for early signs of uveitis, which can include a cellular or proteinaceous exudate of inflammatory cells in the anterior chamber of the eye. An evaluation of 147 children with IBD who had no ophthalmological complaints revealed a prevalence of uveitis of 6.1% in patients with Crohn disease [43]. Like scleritis, acute anterior uveitis is an ophthalmological emergency. Treatment involves covering the eye to reduce pain and photophobia, pupillary dilatation, and the use of topical or systemic corticosteroids.

Liver Disease

Liver pathology, including hepatitis, fatty liver, cholelithiasis, amyloidosis, and primary sclerosing cholangitis, is found in <5–10% of patients with IBD [9, 11]. Screening with periodic checks of serum aminotransferases, alkaline phosphatase, gamma glutamyltransferase, and bilirubin is necessary, as many of the children with liver disease are asymptomatic. A more extensive review of this extraintestinal manifestation can be found in another chapter devoted to liver disease in pediatric IBD.

Hematological Abnormalities

Anemia, thrombocytosis, and leukocytosis are common hematological abnormalities in IBD patients and can be seen in up to half the patients with active disease [9]. Usually, the anemia is secondary to iron, vitamin B12, and folic acid deficiency, as well as anemia of chronic disease. The thrombocytosis is postulated to result from circulating inflammatory cytokines that stimulate platelet production. Similarly, leukocytosis can occur as a result of generalized inflammation. On the other hand, patients should be monitored for leukopenia with certain therapies such as use of thiopurine immunomodulators (e.g. 6-mercatopurine or azathioprine) or methotrexate. Further information can be found in the laboratory evaluation in pediatric IBD chapter.

Other Extraintestinal Manifestations

Many other systems, listed below, have had reported involvement in IBD, but they have been reported to occur in <1% of pediatric IBD patients [9].

Vascular

Patients with IBD have been reported to have a threefold increased risk of venous thrombosis compared to matched controls [44]. Interestingly, this increased risk is specific for IBD, as it is not seen with other inflammatory conditions such as rheumatoid arthritis or other bowel disorders such as celiac disease. Deep venous thrombosis and pulmonary embolism are the most common complications resulting from an overall increased coagulation.

Coagulation factors may be elevated as part of an acute phase response. Factor V Leiden, a genetic disorder characterized by an impaired anticoagulant response to protein C leading to a prothrombotic state, may be increased in Crohn disease patients [44]. Furthermore, IBD patients might have higher levels of homocysteine, which can be a potential cause of thrombosis [44]. Another vascular complication, arteritis of small or large vessels, has been reported in children with IBD [45].

Pancreatitis

The incidence of pancreatic involvement in IBD varies but is estimated to be 0.7–1.6% in children [46]. The most likely etiologies are medications, anatomical, immunological, or gallstones secondary to ileal disease. Although patients with IBD appear to have a small increased risk for idiopathic pancreatitis, the most common cause of pancreatitis in IBD appears to be associated with medications such as 5-aminosalicylate preparations or 6-mercaptopurine. As this is presumed to be an idiosyncratic reaction, discontinuation of the medication is indicated. Although pancreatic autoantibodies have been found in up to 40% of Crohn disease patients, their significance remains unclear. In one series, patients with Crohn disease who were pancreatic antibody-positive had a higher rate of pancreatic exocrine insufficiency than those who were antibody-negative [4]. Furthermore, chronic pancreatitis has also been reported in a series of six adult IBD patients, five of whom had changes on pancreatic pathology samples [47].

Renal

IBD patients, especially those with extensive ileal disease or ileal resection with significant fat malabsorption or fluid losses, are at risk for developing calcium oxalate and uric acid stones. Glomerulonephritis with immune complex deposition can also be seen which can progress to severe renal disease. Other renal diseases, described in children with IBD, include renal artery stenosis, amyloidosis leading to renal failure, ureteral compression, and perinephritic abscesses secondary to abscesses, or inflammation surrounding the terminal ileum [48].

Pulmonary

Pulmonary manifestations associated with IBD are reported less frequently in children than adults, though the scope of disorders is similar. Reactive airway disease, bronchitis, bronchiectasis, tracheal obstruction, granulomatous lung disease, interstitial or hypersensitivity pneumonitis, and bronchiolitis obliterans are being reported at an increasing frequency [4, 9, 49–51]. However, the latter two have been associated with 5-aminosalicylate products and methotrexate treatment [4, 51]. Similar to other extraintestinal manifestations, pulmonary disease can predate the bowel disease by months or years. Most pulmonary manifestations respond to corticosteroids via an inhaled, oral, or intravenous route.

Neurological

Peripheral nerve disorders, cardiovascular disorders, myopathy, multiple sclerosis, optic neuritis, and epilepsy have been described in IBD patients [52]. Peripheral neuropathies are the most common neurological disorders reported, while cardiovascular disorders with neurological morbidities have been documented in up to 4% of patients [53]. A retrospective cross-sectional study of adult patients with IBD reported an odds ratio of 1.67 for developing multiple sclerosis, optic neuritis, or a demyelinating disorder [4]. An interesting future focus will center around the role of medication treatments for IBD and neurological adverse events especially given the risk of progressive multifocal leukoencephalopathy related to the anti-alpha 4 integrin antibody natalizumab.

Cardiac

Rarely, children with IBD can develop myopericarditis and pleuropericarditis with symptoms of chest pain and dyspnea. Cardiac manifestations are not necessarily associated with active bowel disease and respond to corticosteroids and non-steroidal anti-inflammatory agents, which need to be used with caution in IBD patients. An active area of research is the risk of cardiovascular events in patients with IBD. A recent study showed an increased incidence in coronary artery disease in adults with IBD [54]. Interestingly, the IBD patients had significantly lower rates of traditional coronary artery disease risk factors such as hypertension, diabetes, obesity, and dyslipidemia. Further work will help determine the affect of various treatments on decreasing risk of cardiac disease.

Summary

Given that Crohn disease and ulcerative colitis are associated with numerous extraintestinal manifestations, it is clearly evident that IBD is a multisystem disease that stretches beyond the gastrointestinal tract. Knowledge about extraintestinal manifestations is critical, as patients can present with these instead of more classic bowel symptoms. Furthermore, the extraintestinal manifestations of IBD can be a cause of major morbidity in patients and need to be considered and addressed at all points of care.

References

1. Lichtman SN, Sartor RB. Extraintestinal manifestations of inflammatory bowel disease: clinical aspects and natural history. In: Targan S, Shanahan F, editors. Inflammatory bowel disease: from bench to bedside. Baltimore: Williams & Wilkins; 1994.
2. Levine JB, Lukawski-Trubish D. Extraintestinal considerations in inflammatory bowel disease. Gastroenterol Clin North Am. 1995;24:633.
3. Bhagat S, Das KM. A shared and unique peptide in the human colon, eye, and joint detected by a monoclonal antibody. Gastroenterology. 1994;107:103.
4. Rothfuss KS, Stange EF, Herrlinger KR. Extraintestinal manifestations and complications in inflammatory bowel disease. World J Gastroenterol. 2006;12:4819.
5. Adams DH, Eksteen B. Aberrant homing of mucosal T cells and extra-intestinal manifestations of inflammatory bowel disease. Nat Rev Immunol. 2006;6:244.
6. Lofberg R, Louis EV, Reinish W, Robinson AM, Kron M, Camez A, Pollack PF. Adalimumab produces clinical remission and reduces extraintestinal manifestations in Crohn disease: results from CARE. Inflamm Bowel Dis. 2012;18:1–9.
7. Danese S, Semeraro S, Papa A, Roberto I, Scaldaferri F, Fedeli G, Gasbarrini G, Gasbarrini A. Extraintestinal manifestations in inflammatory bowel disease. World J Gastroenterol. 2005;11:7227.
8. Vavricka S, Schoepfer A, Scharl M, Lakatos PL, Navarini A, Rogler G. Extraintestinal manifestations of inflammatory bowel disease. Inflamm Bowel Dis. 2015;21:1982–92.
9. Oliva-Hemker M. More than a gut reaction: extraintestinal complications of IBD. Contemp Pediatr. 1999;16:45.
10. Vavricka SR, Brun L, Ballabeni P, Pittet V, Vavricka BMP, Zeitz J, Rogler G, Schoepfer AM, Swiss IBD Cohort Study Group. Frequency and risk factors for extraintestinal manifestations in the Swiss inflammatory bowel disease cohort. Am J Gastroenterol. 2011;106:110–9.
11. Jose FA, Garnett EA, Vittinghoff E, Ferry GD, Winter HS, Baldassano RN, Kirschner BS, Cohen SA, Gold BD, Abramson O, Heyman MB. Development of extraintestinal manifestations in pediatric patients with inflammatory bowel disease. Inflamm Bowel Dis. 2009;15:63–8.
12. Dotson JL, Hyams JS, Markowitz J, LeLeiko NS, Mack DR, Evans JS, Pfefferkorn MD, Griffiths AM, Otley AR, Bousvaros A, Kugathasan S, Rosh JR, Keljo D, Carvalho RS, Tomer G, Mamula P, Kay MH, Kerzner B, Oliva-Hemker M, Langton CR, Crandall W. Extraintestinal manifestations of pediatric inflammatory bowel disease and their relation to disease type and severity. JPGN. 2010;51:140–5.
13. Hyams JS. Extraintestinal manifestations of inflammatory bowel disease in children. J Pediatr Gastroenterol Nutr. 1994;19:7.
14. Kethu SR. Extraintestinal manifestations of inflammatory bowel disease. J Clin Gastroenterol. 2006;40:467.
15. Urlep D, Mamula P, Baldassano R. Extraintestinal manifestations of inflammatory bowel disease. Minerva Gastroenterol Dietol. 2005;51:147.

16. Loftus EV. Management of extraintestinal manifestations and other complications of inflammatory bowel disease. Curr Gastroenterol Rep. 2004;6:506.

17. Hoffmann RM, Kruis W. Rare extraintestinal manifestations of inflammatory bowel disease. Inflamm Bowel Dis. 2004;10:140.

18. Su CG, Judge TA, Lichtenstein GR. Extraintestinal manifestations of inflammatory bowel disease. Gastroenterol Clin North Am. 2002;31:307.

19. Jose FA, Heyman MB. Extraintestinal manifestations of inflammatory bowel disease. JPGN. 2008;46:124–33.

20. Kanof ME, Lake AM, Bayles TM. Decreased height velocity in children and adolescents before the diagnosis of Crohn disease. Gastroenterology. 1988;95:1523.

21. Conklin LS, Oliva-Hemker M. Nutritional considerations in pediatric inflammatory bowel disease. Expert Rev Gastroenterol Hepatol. 2010;4:305–17.

22. Passo MH, Fitzgerald JF, Brandt KD. Arthritis associated with inflammatory bowel disease in children—relationship of joint disease to activity and severity of bowel lesion. Dig Dis Sci. 1986;31:492.

23. Cardile S, Romana C. Current issues in pediatric inflammatory bowel disease-associated arthropathies. World J Gastroenterol. 2014;20(1):45–52.

24. Horton DB, Sherry DD, Baldassano RN, Weiss PF. Enthesitis is an extraintestinal manifestation of pediatric inflammatory bowel disease. Ann Paediatr Rheumatol. 2012;1(4):214–21.

25. Paparo F, Bacigalupo L, Garello I, Biscaldi E, Cimmino MA, Marinaro E, Rollandi GA. Crohn disease: prevalence of intestinal and extraintestinal manifestations detected by computed tomography enterography with water enema. Abdom Imaging. 2012;37(3):326–37.

26. Juillerat P, Mottet C, Froehlich F, Felley C, Vader J, Burnand B, Gonvers J, Michetti P. Extraintestinal manifestations of Crohn disease. Digestion. 2005;71:31–6.

27. Lakatos PL, Altorjay I, Szamosi T, Palatka K, Vitalis Z, Tumpek J, Sipka S, Udvardy M, Dinya T, Lakatos L, Kovacs A, Molnar T, Tulassay Z, Miheller P, Barta Z, Stocker W, Papp J, Veres G, Papp M, Hungarian IBD Study Group. Pancreatic autoantibodies are associated with reactivity to microbial antibodies, penetrating disease behavior, perianal disease, and extraintestinal manifestations, but not with NOD2/CARD15 or TLR4 genotype in a Hungarian IBD cohort. Inflamm Bowel Dis. 2009;15:365–74.

28. Bernstein CN. Osteoporosis and other complications of inflammatory bowel disease. Curr Opin Gastroenterol. 2002;18:428.

29. Gokhale R, Favus MJ, Karrison T, et al. Bone mineral density assessment in children with inflammatory bowel disease. Gastroenterology. 1998;114:902.

30. Hyams JS, Wyzga N, Kreutzer DL, et al. Alterations in bone metabolism in children with inflammatory bowel disease: an in vitro study. J Pediatr Gastroenterol Nutr. 1997;24:289.

31. Gasparetto M, Guariso G. Crohn's disease and growth deficiency in children and adolescents. World J Gastroenterol. 2014;20(37):13219–33.

32. Bousvaros A, Marcon M, Treem W, Waters P, Issenman R, Couper R, Burnell R, Rosenberg A, Rabinovish E, Kirschner B. Chronic recurrent multifocal osteomyelitis associated with chronic inflammatory bowel disease in children. Dig Dis Sci. 1999;44:2500–7.

33. Fatahzadeh M, Schwartz RA, Kapila R, Rochford C. Orofacial Crohn disease: an oral enigma. Acta Dermatoveneral Croat. 2009;17:289–300.

34. Lankarani KB, Sivandzadeh GR, Hassanpour S. Oral manifestation in inflammatory bowel disease: a review. World J Gastroenterol. 2013;19(46):8571–9.

35. Plauth M, Jenss H, Meyle J. Oral manifestations of Crohn disease. J Clin Gastroenterol. 1991;13:29.

36. Grilich C, Bogenrieder T, Palitzsch KD, Scholmerich J, Lock G. Orofacial granulomatosis as initial manifestation of Crohn disease: a report of two cases. Eur J Gastroenterol Hepatol. 2002;13:873–6.

37. Storwick GS, Prihoda MB, Fulton RJ, et al. Pyodermatitis-pyostomatitis vegetans: a specific marker for inflammatory bowel disease. J Am Acad Dermatol. 1994;31:336.

38. Lynde CB, Brue AJ, Rogers RS. Successful treatment of complex aphthous with colchicine and dapsone. Arch Dermatol. 2009;145:273–6.

39. Kugathasan S, Miranda A, Nocton J, Drolet BA, Raasch C, Binion DG. Dermatologic manifestations of Crohn disease in children: response to infliximab. J Pediatr Gastroenterol Nutr. 2003;37:150–4.

40. Meinhardt C, Buning J, Fellermann K, Lehnert H, Schmidt KJ. Cyclophosphamide therapy in Sweet's syndrome complicating refractory Crohn disease – efficacy and mechanism of action. J Crohns Colitis. 2011;6:633–7.

41. Hagen JW, Swoger JM, Grandinetti LM. Cutaneous manifestations of Crohn disease. Dermatol Clin. 2015;33:417–31.

42. Foo WC, Papalas JA, Robboy SJ, Selim MA. Vulvar manifestations of Crohn disease. Am J Dermatopathol. 2011;33:588–93.

43. Hofley P, Roarty J, McGinnity G, et al. Asymptomatic uveitis in children with chronic inflammatory bowel disease. J Pediatr Gastroenterol Nutr. 1993;17:397.

44. Purnak T, Yuksel O. Overview of venous thrombosis in inflammatory bowel disease. Inflamm Bowel Dis. 2015;21:1195–203.

45. Mader R, Segol O, Adawi M, Trougoboff P, Nussinson E. Arthritis or vasculitis as presenting symptoms of Crohn disease. Rheumatol Int. 2005;25:401–5.

46. Cardile S, Randazzo A, Valenti S, Romano C. Pancreatic involvement in pediatric inflammatory bowel diseases. World J Pediatr. 2015;11(3):207–11.

47. Barthet M, Hastier P, Bernard JP, et al. Chronic pancreatitis and inflammatory bowel disease: true or coincidental association? Am J Gastroenterol. 1999;94:2141–8.

48. Kuzmic AC, Kolacek S, Brkljacic B, Juzjak N. Renal artery stenosis associated with Crohn disease. Pediatr Nephrol. 2001;16:371–3.

49. Camus P, Piard F, Ashcroft T, et al. The lung in inflammatory bowel disease. Medicine. 1993;72:151.

50. Al-Binali AM, Scott B, Al-Garni A, Montgomery M, Robertson M. Granulomatous pulmonary disease in a child: an unusual presentation of Crohn disease. Pediatr Pulmonol. 2003;36:76–80.

51. Haralambou G, Teirstein AS, Gil J, Present D. Bronchiolitis obliterans in a patient with ulcerative colitis receiving mesalamine. Mt Sinai J Med. 2001;68:384–8.

52. Lossos A, River Y, Eliakim A, et al. Neurologic aspects of inflammatory bowel disease. Neurology. 1995;45:416.

53. Zois CD, Katsanos KH, Kosmidou M, Tsianos EV. Neurologic manifestations in inflammatory bowel disease: current knowledge and novel insights. J Crohns Colitis. 2010;4:115–24.

54. Yarur AJ, Deshpande AR, Pechman DM, Tamariz L, Abreu MT. Inflammatory bowel disease is associated with an increased incidence of cardiovascular events. Am J Gastroenterol. 2011;106:741–7.

Liver Disease in Pediatric Inflammatory Bowel Disease

Amanda Ricciuto and Binita M. Kamath

Introduction

Diseases involving the hepatobiliary system are among the most common extraintestinal manifestations of inflammatory bowel disease (IBD). They can be classified into a few broad categories: (1) liver diseases that may share a common pathogenic mechanism with IBD, such as primary sclerosing cholangitis (PSC), autoimmune hepatitis (AIH), and PSC/AIH overlap, also known as autoimmune sclerosing cholangitis (ASC); (2) liver diseases that reflect the pathophysiology of IBD, such as cholelithiasis and portal vein thrombosis; and (3) liver diseases that result from the adverse effects of IBD therapy, such as drug-induced hepatitis [1]. In addition, an association has been noted between a number of other less common hepatobiliary diseases and IBD, including IgG4-associated cholangitis (IAC). Some of the conditions listed above are observed more frequently in Crohn disease (CD) or ulcerative colitis (UC), while others occur at similar rates in both types of IBD (Table 11.1). Liver enzyme abnormalities are common in IBD and, while often transient and inconsequential, deranged hepatic biochemistry may herald serious underlying liver disease, such as PSC. The challenge lies in determining which patients merit further work-up versus observation. No standardized algorithm exists to guide clinicians in this decision-making process, particularly in children, in whom there is a relative paucity of data. This chapter strives to facilitate this task by providing an overview of liver disease occurring in association with pediatric IBD.

A. Ricciuto, MDCM, FRCP(C) • B.M. Kamath, MBBChir, MRCP, MTR (✉)
Division of Gastroenterology, Hepatology and Nutrition, The Hospital for Sick Children, Toronto, Canada

University of Toronto, Toronto, Canada
e-mail: binita.kamath@sickkids.ca

Abnormal Liver Chemistry

Abnormal liver chemistry is common in IBD. Liver enzyme abnormalities (any value exceeding the upper limit of normal (ULN)) have been reported in 15–40% of adults with IBD over 1–5 years of follow-up [2–4], with more marked elevations (>2× the ULN) occurring in 5% [2]. Abnormal liver biochemistry appears to be similarly frequent in pediatric IBD. Nemeth described "pathological liver function tests" in 52% of his 46-patient cohort in 1990 [5], and similar findings have since been reproduced by two large retrospective pediatric studies, in which at least one liver enzyme elevation was observed in 40–60% of children with IBD over 3 years [6, 7], even after excluding patients with PSC/ASC. No differences were observed between patients with CD and UC. Liver enzyme elevations >2× the ULN occur in a smaller proportion of children, roughly 15–30% [7, 8]. The pattern of biochemical injury is typically hepatocellular, but can be mixed or, less commonly, cholestatic [4, 6]. ALT is the most frequently abnormal test [7], with the caveat that ALT also tends to be measured more often than other tests, like GGT. The majority of these biochemical abnormalities are mild, transient, and benign in nature [4, 6–8,]. The degree of transaminase elevation appears to correlate with the likelihood of identifying underlying liver disease; in one study, 95% of children with peak ALT <2× ULN were found to have no specific liver disease [6], and conversely, in another, 93% of children with PSC or ASC had liver enzymes 2× the ULN or greater, sustained for 30–90 days [7]. In this latter study, GGT was found to be particularly useful for identifying PSC/ASC, with a value of 252 U/L, having a sensitivity of 99% and specificity of 77% for PSC or ASC [7].

Well-defined chronic liver disease (PSC/ASC and AIH) accounts for only 1.4–6% of elevated liver enzymes in pediatric IBD, whereas the majority of cases remain idiopathic [6, 7, 9]. The most common etiology, when one is identified, is drug toxicity [2, 6, 8]. In children, steroids,

Table 11.1 Hepatobiliary diseases associated with pediatric IBD

Hepatobiliary disease	Ulcerative colitis	Crohn disease
Primary sclerosing cholangitis (PSC)	++	+
Autoimmune hepatitis (AIH)	++	++
Autoimmune sclerosing cholangitis (ASC)	++	+
IgG4-associated cholangitis (IAC)	++	+
Cholelithiasis	−	++
Portal vein thrombosis and hepatic abscess	+	++
Drug-induced hepatitis	++	++
Hepatitis B reactivation (infliximab)	++	++
Hepatosplenic T-cell lymphoma	+/−	+
Fatty liver	++	++
Hepatic amyloidosis	−	++
Granulomatous hepatitis	−	++
Primary biliary cholangitis (PBC)	++	−

antibiotics, methotrexate, adalimumab, as well as exclusive enteral nutrition, have been positively associated with liver enzyme abnormalities [7]. Conversely, liver enzyme abnormalities appear to be less frequent in children taking 5-ASA and sulfasalazine, although these agents may simply be surrogates for milder IBD [3, 7]. Other less common causes of deranged hepatic biochemistry in pediatric IBD include infection (particularly CMV and EBV), nonalcoholic fatty liver disease (NAFLD), cholelithiasis, and vascular abnormalities [6]. Active IBD has also been proposed as a cause of abnormal liver enzymes, but the evidence is conflicting; several studies lend support to this hypothesis [4, 8, 10], while others refute it. One such study in adults actually found a higher prevalence of liver enzyme abnormalities in patients in remission compared to those with active IBD [3]. In children, biochemical abnormalities do not appear to be associated with IBD duration or extent [5, 6, 9]. With regard to prognosis, death was found to be 4.8 times higher in adults with abnormal liver biochemistry, even after excluding those with any diagnosis of liver disease [3]. No equivalent pediatric data exist.

In summary, abnormal liver biochemistry is common in children with IBD. Most cases are mild and resolve spontaneously, and such cases tend to be associated with undefined etiologies. However, a small subset of patients with more severe, prolonged derangements has serious disease or medication adverse effects. Given this, it seems reasonable to adopt a period of watchful waiting in patients with mild elevations (<2× the ULN) unless there are overt signs of underlying liver disease. More marked or persistent (>1 month) abnormalities may warrant further investigation. We suggest obtaining a liver biochemical panel, including ALT and GGT, in all newly diagnosed IBD patients and repeating this at least every 6–12 months for surveillance.

Primary Sclerosing Cholangitis

Epidemiology and Pathogenesis

Primary sclerosing cholangitis (PSC) is a chronic, progressive, cholestatic liver disease characterized by inflammation and obliterative fibrosis of the intrahepatic and/or extrahepatic biliary tree, resulting in multifocal strictures and dilatation. It is a rare disease, with an incidence and prevalence of 0.1–0.2 and 1.5 per 100,000 children, respectively, which is substantially lower than in adults [11–13]. Pediatric PSC typically presents early in the second decade of life and has a modest male predominance, as in adults [12, 14–16]. The link between PSC and IBD has been known for greater than five decades [17]. As many as 60–80% of adults with PSC in North America and Northern Europe have IBD, primarily ulcerative colitis (UC) [18, 19]. The prevalence of IBD in children with PSC is also very high, >50% in most series and up to 97% in a recent population study [12, 14–16, 20]. Conversely, only a minority of children with colitis, <10% in most series, have or develop concurrent PSC [7, 12, 21, 22]. However, these reports may underestimate the true prevalence of PSC in IBD as neither adult nor pediatric IBD patients are systematically investigated with liver biopsy and cholangiography to screen for liver disease. Most patients are found to have PSC within a year of their IBD diagnosis [12], but the two can occur years apart, and PSC can manifest first, in which case a full colonoscopy is recommended to screen for IBD [23].

The pathogenesis of PSC remains incompletely understood. Genomewide association studies have identified a number of HLA and non-HLA risk loci [24, 25], some of which are shared with IBD, and a hallmark paper in 2004 reported an accumulation of gut-homing CCR9-positive T cells in explanted human livers of patients with PSC [26], findings that point to both a genetic and immunological basis for PSC. In addition, there is growing evidence for the role of the "gut-liver" axis in the pathogenesis of PSC. Several animal models and human tissue-based translational studies support that enteric microbial molecules/dysbiosis can lead to PSC-like hepatobiliary inflammation [27].

Primary Sclerosing Cholangitis and IBD

The intestinal inflammation in individuals with PSC and colitis may represent a distinct IBD phenotype, termed PSC-IBD. This has been well characterized in adults as extensive colonic involvement, often worse on the right, and relatively frequent "backwash ileitis," rectal sparing, and pouchitis post colectomy [28]. Crohn disease (CD) is uncommon in the setting of PSC, but, when it does occur, it too tends to have an extensive colonic distribution; isolated small bowel, perianal, and fistulizing disease are uncommon [29]. Despite the extensive nature of the colonic inflammation, PSC-IBD tends to have a relatively mild clinical course with a paucity of overt clinical symptoms [30, 31]. There are significantly less data pertaining to the phenotype of pediatric PSC-IBD, but findings analogous to those in adults have been reported in two small studies [32, 33]. In addition, a recent study specifically aimed at investigating the phenotype of pediatric PSC-IBD compared 37 children with IBD and PSC or ASC to 137 non-PSC matched IBD controls. In keeping with the above, the authors found a higher proportion of pancolitis in the PSC-IBD group, although this was only marginally statistically significant. In contrast to some of the adult evidence, both groups were similar in terms of the proportion of patients with rectal sparing (defined histologically) and disease activity, as reflected by physician's global assessment, Mayo endoscopic scores, admission rates, and colonic surgery rates [34].

The interplay between IBD and PSC remains to be elucidated. Adults with severe PSC requiring liver transplant (LT) have been found to have milder UC than patients with less severe liver disease, suggesting that PSC may have a "protective" effect on colonic disease [35]. Furthermore, while it has long been maintained that PSC and IBD progress independently, as supported by older studies indicating that the natural history of PSC is unaffected by colectomy [36], more recent findings suggest that colectomy may reduce the risk of PSC recurrence post LT [37]. The interaction between PSC and IBD, including the effect of ongoing colonic inflammation on PSC progression, if any, requires further clarification.

Diagnosis

The diagnosis of PSC in a child is based on a compatible clinical presentation and biochemistry, with characteristic changes on cholangiography and/or liver biopsy, after excluding secondary causes of sclerosing cholangitis. The most common presenting symptoms and signs are hepatomegaly and abdominal pain, followed by diarrhea, splenomegaly, fatigue, pruritus, weight loss, impaired growth, and jaundice [15]. The presenting features may also, uncommonly, be those of advanced liver disease, such as gastrointestinal bleeding and cholangitis, or those of associated colitis, especially bloody diarrhea. About 20% of children with PSC are asymptomatic at presentation and come to medical attention solely due to deranged liver biochemistry. Transaminases are often modestly elevated, with a predominantly cholestatic pattern [15]. GGT is more reliable in children as ALP elevations may reflect bone growth. The odds of PSC are 660-fold greater in children with ALT and GGT elevations >50 U/L within 3 months of their IBD diagnosis compared to children whose values remain <50 U/L [9]. INR, albumin, and conjugated bilirubin, which reflect synthetic function, are generally normal at presentation. Elevated conjugated bilirubin may signal a stricture, cholangitis, or a mass, and warrants further work-up. Serum immunoglobulin G (IgG) levels may be elevated, and a variety of autoantibodies may be present, the most common of which is anti-neutrophil cytoplasmic antibody (ANCA), usually with an atypical perinuclear ("p") pattern, which is found in up to 80% of patients. None of these are specific to PSC, however [12, 23]. Serum IgG4 should be measured at least once in children with PSC. An elevated IgG4 may denote IgG4-associated cholangitis (IAC), which has important implications, given its favorable response to corticosteroids [38]. Ultrasound is a reasonable initial imaging modality; it may reveal bile duct wall thickening, focal bile duct dilatations, and/or gallbladder changes, including wall thickening, enlargement, cholecystitis, and mass lesions. It is also useful for ruling out alternate etiologies. However, none of these findings are diagnostic, and ultrasound may be normal in the setting of PSC [23]. Cholangiography, preferably by magnetic resonance cholangiopancreatography (MRCP), which has supplanted endoscopic retrograde cholangiopancreatography (ERCP) as the first-line diagnostic imaging modality due its less invasive nature and lower cost, is a vital component of the PSC diagnostic work-up [39]. Characteristic cholangiographic findings include multifocal, short strictures alternating with normal or dilated segments, producing a "beaded" appearance (Fig. 11.1) [23]. The gallbladder, cystic duct, and pancreatic duct may also be abnormal [40]. Contrary to adult guidelines, a liver biopsy is almost always performed in a child with suspected PSC. Histopathological assessment is necessary to distinguish PSC from autoimmune sclerosing cholangitis (ASC), which occurs frequently in children and mandates different treatment. A liver biopsy is also useful to diagnose small-duct PSC, a label applied to cases with compatible histological changes but without cholangiographic abnormalities, and to stage the degree of fibrosis. Periductular concentric fibrosis, or "onion-skinning" (Fig. 11.2), is pathognomonic for PSC, but not always observed. Other, nonspecific findings may include ductular proliferation or periductular inflammation, with variable types of portal inflammation and fibrosis. The diagnostic work-up for suspected PSC in children is illustrated in Fig. 11.3.

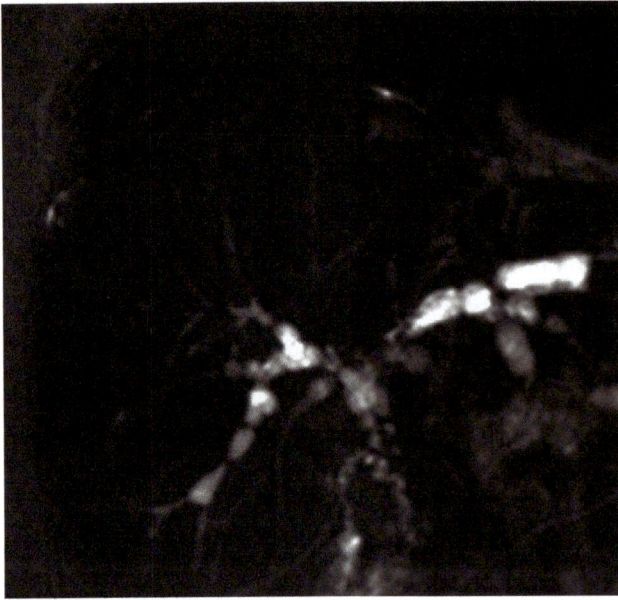

Fig. 11.1 Cholangiographic appearance of PSC with typical "beading"

Outcomes

PSC is one of the most important sources of morbidity and mortality in IBD, but few studies have examined its natural history in children. Based on limited data, the probability of developing complicated liver disease, defined as clinical portal hypertension, obstructive cholangitis, cholangiocarcinoma, liver transplant, or death, over 5 years in children with PSC, is 37% [12]. About 20% of children with PSC ultimately require a liver transplant (LT), a figure that has remained fairly constant over the past 20 years. The median time from diagnosis to LT is 7–12 years [14–16, 41]. Survival is significantly shorter in children with PSC compared to age-matched and gender-matched American children. Lower platelet count, splenomegaly, and older age are associated with shorter survival [14]. Adults with UC and PSC have an almost five times greater risk of colorectal neoplasia compared to adults with UC alone [42]. Surveillance colonoscopies every 1–2 years from the time of diagnosis are recommended in adults [23]. No equivalent pediatric guidelines exist, but it seems reasonable for similar screening practices to be applied to older children and teenagers. There is a markedly increased risk of cholangiocarcinoma in adults with PSC [43], but this malignancy is exceedingly rare in children. Nevertheless, a handful of cases has been reported in older teenagers [12]. While adult guidelines suggest consideration be given to screening for cholangiocarcinoma with regular cross-sectional imaging and CA 19-9, this is not routinely recommended in children [23, 39]. However, based on clinical experience and expert opinion, the authors suggest an ultrasound yearly, an MRI every 2 years, and CA 19-9 levels yearly in children with PSC to screen for cholangiocarcinoma.

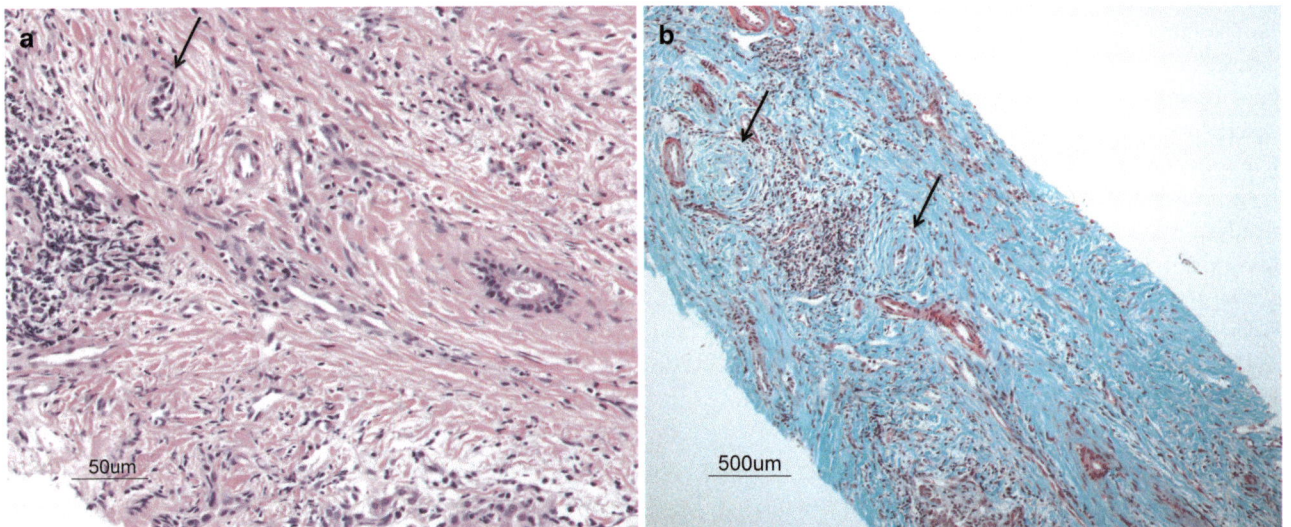

Fig. 11.2 Liver biopsy showing typical histological changes of PSC, including periductular concentric fibrosis denoted by the arrows with (**a**) H&E and (**b**) trichrome staining

```
┌─────────────────────────────────────────────────┐
│ PSC suspected based on symptoms, signs and        │
│ biochemistry (particularly elevated GGT)          │
└─────────────────────────────────────────────────┘
                        │
                        ▼
┌─────────────────────────────────────────────────┐
│ Obtain full liver panel if not already performed  │
│ (ALT, AST, ALP, GGT, INR, bilirubin, albumin) and │
│ additional labs (ANA, anti-SMA, anti-LKM1, ANCA,  │
│ IgG, IgG4)                                         │
└─────────────────────────────────────────────────┘
                        │
                        ▼
┌─────────────────────────────────────────────────┐
│ Obtain abdominal ultrasound (look for supporting  │
│ features and rule out alternate etiologies)       │
└─────────────────────────────────────────────────┘
                        │
                        ▼
┌─────────────────────────────────────────────────┐
│ Obtain MRCP (look for supporting features)        │
└─────────────────────────────────────────────────┘
                        │
                        ▼
┌─────────────────────────────────────────────────┐
│ Obtain liver biopsy (look for supporting features,│
│ evidence of autoimmune hepatitis overlap, small   │
│ duct PSC if imaging normal, degree of fibrosis)   │
└─────────────────────────────────────────────────┘
```

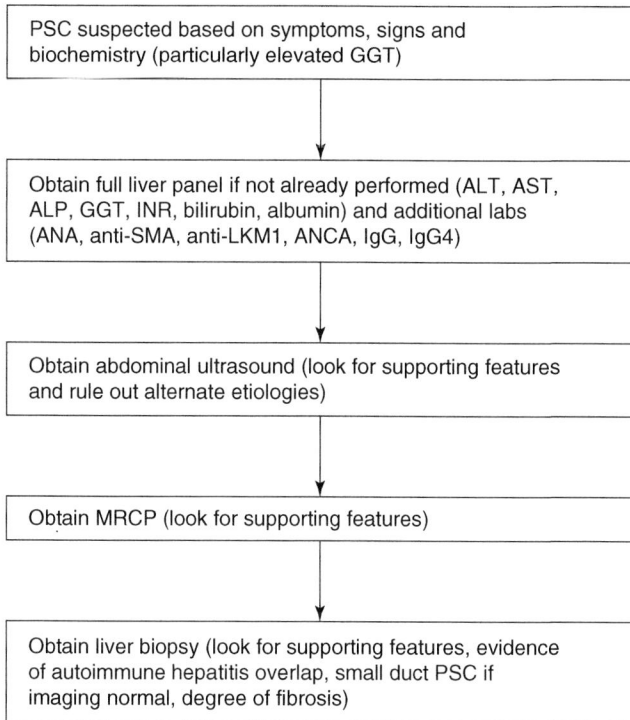

Fig. 11.3 Diagnostic work-up for suspected pediatric PSC. *ANA* antinuclear antibody, *ANCA* antineutrophil cytoplasmic antibody, *LKM1* liver kidney microsomal type 1, *MRCP* magnetic resonance cholangiopancreatography, *PSC* primary sclerosing cholangitis, *SMA* smooth muscle antibody

Small-duct PSC may have a more favorable prognosis than classic PSC. It has been associated with a longer transplant-free survival in adults, and there have been no reports of cholangiocarcinoma occurring with small-duct PSC. However, small-duct PSC can progress to classic PSC with cholangiographic abnormalities over time, and it can recur post transplant [44]. It is unclear whether small-duct PSC represents an early stage of classic PSC or a distinct entity.

Treatment

Data pertaining to the medical management of PSC in children are scarce, and current practices largely derive from adult studies. No medical therapy currently exists to reverse or halt the progression of PSC liver disease. As such, treatment is mainly supportive. Although numerous aspects of PSC invoke an autoimmune basis for the disease, thus far, no single immunosuppressive or immune-modulating agent has been found to be efficacious [45].

Ursodeoxycholic acid (UDCA) is widely used in adults and children with cholestatic liver disease, including PSC. Although biochemical improvement has been demonstrated in children, a beneficial effect on the natural history of PSC, as reflected by a decrease in mortality and/or LT rates, has never been shown [14, 15, 46]. Similarly, adult studies have documented improvements in biochemistry, but not in hard outcomes [47]. Furthermore, the use of high-dose UDCA >28 mg/kg has been associated with a twofold increased risk of death/transplant and a fourfold increased risk of colorectal cancer in adults [48]. There is no consensus regarding the use of UDCA in adults with PSC, with one expert group advising against its use entirely [23] and another merely recommending against the use of high doses [39]. In light of this, it appears prudent to avoid high-dose UDCA in children with PSC, but continued use of low-to-moderate doses, not exceeding 20 mg/kg/day, is reasonable.

Limited anecdotal evidence supports the use of oral vancomycin for treating pediatric PSC [49–51]. Oral vancomycin's therapeutic effect may occur through immunomodulation, by increasing transforming growth factor-β (TGF-β) and peripheral levels of regulatory T cells [52]. Data from prospective pediatric trials are pending. Metronidazole and minocycline, but not rifaximin, have also been associated with improved liver biochemistry in adults with PSC [53–55]. At the current time, the use of oral antibiotics for pediatric PSC remains experimental, as a benefit beyond biochemical has yet to be demonstrated.

Dominant strictures are less common in children than adults, but should, when identified in association with symptoms or signs such as cholangitis, jaundice, pruritus, right upper quadrant pain, or worsening biochemistry, be managed with ERCP and balloon dilatation, often with sphincterotomy, with or without stent placement [23]. This may prolong symptom-free intervals prior to LT [56]. Although cholangiocarcinoma is rare in pediatrics, brush cytology in the setting of a dominant stricture remains important. ERCP should be performed by a physician who is adequately trained in and experienced with the procedure, which often requires collaboration with an adult gastroenterologist.

Liver transplant remains the only definitive treatment for PSC and should be considered for children with decompensated cirrhosis, recurrent or chronic cholangitis refractory to ERCP, hilar cholangiocarcinoma, and intractable pruritus [23, 57]. PSC accounts for 2.6% of pediatric transplants [58]. The mean age at transplant is 12.6 years. Patient and graft survival after LT for PSC is comparable to that for non-PSC pediatric indications, with 1-year and 5-year patient and graft survival rates of 99% and 97%, and 93% and 76%, respectively. However, a diagnosis of IBD prior to LT is associated with an increased risk of death post LT. Intrahepatic biliary strictures and cholangitis are more common in the first 6 months post LT in children with PSC compared to other liver diseases [59]. Furthermore, PSC recurs in about 10% of children post LT [14, 59, 60]. A diagnosis of IBD and younger age have been linked with an increased risk of PSC recurrence [59, 60]. As mentioned above, colectomy prior to or during LT may decrease the risk of PSC recurrence [37].

Other Autoimmune Liver Diseases

Autoimmune Hepatitis

Epidemiology and Pathogenesis
Autoimmune hepatitis (AIH) is an idiopathic, progressive, inflammatory liver disease characterized by elevated transaminases, interface hepatitis on biopsy, hypergammaglobulinemia, and autoantibody positivity. It is the most common pediatric autoimmune liver disease, with an incidence and prevalence of 0.23–0.4 and 3 per 100,000 children, respectively [12, 61]. The prevalence of IBD in children with AIH, which approaches 20% [61–63], exceeds that in the general pediatric population, but the magnitude of the association between AIH and IBD is less than that between PSC and IBD. Only 0.3–0.6% of children with IBD develop AIH and, unlike in PSC, this proportion does not differ substantially between children with UC and CD [12]. Two main types of AIH are recognized: AIH type 1 (AIH-1), which accounts for the majority (60–87%) of cases, is characterized by positive antinuclear (ANA) and/or anti-smooth muscle (SMA) autoantibodies, whereas AIH-2 is distinguished by positive antiliver kidney microsomal type 1 (LKM-1) and/or antiliver cytosol type 1 (LC-1) autoantibodies. Of note, lower antibody titers are considered significant in children, namely, 1:20 for ANA and SMA, and 1:10 for LKM1 and LC-1, compared to a threshold of 1:40 in adults [64]. Both types of AIH have a female predominance [61], although it is not clear whether this is also true of cases associated with IBD [61, 62, 65]. The pathogenesis of AIH is unknown, but is likely multifactorial, involving genetic susceptibility and immune dysregulation, modified by environmental factors. An aberrant immune response targeting liver autoantigens has been implicated [66].

Diagnosis
Pediatric AIH can present in a highly variable manner, ranging from nonspecific insidious symptoms to fulminant liver failure. The most common presenting symptoms are fatigue, jaundice, and abdominal pain, which occur in about half of patients. Hepatomegaly and splenomegaly are the most frequently observed abnormalities on physical exam [61]. In the context of IBD, however, AIH typically comes to light as a result of elevated transaminases, which can fluctuate over time. The pattern of injury is predominantly hepatocellular, with AST and ALT values typically in the several hundred range. Conjugated bilirubin is generally normal, but GGT can be modestly elevated. Serum IgG is elevated in 80% of

cases, but a normal result does not rule out AIH. Although none of the autoantibodies listed above are entirely specific to AIH, the presence of high-titer autoantibodies, in combination with compatible clinical features and histological findings, strongly supports a diagnosis of AIH. A liver biopsy is typically performed to confirm a diagnosis of AIH and to establish the severity of liver damage. Characteristic findings include interface hepatitis, lymphoplasmacytic infiltrates, and rosetting of hepatocytes. Biliary changes, such as ductular proliferation, can be seen, as well as fibrosis. Cirrhosis is observed in 20–80% of children at presentation and is more common in AIH-1 [61, 67, 68]. Of note, the distinction between AIH and drug-induced liver injury, which is particularly relevant in children with IBD, can be very challenging. In addition to the AIH work-up presented above, it is recommended that all children with presumed AIH undergo cholangiography to investigate for ASC or PSC.

Outcomes and Treatment
Although a significant fraction of children with AIH present with cirrhosis and AIH has an aggressive natural history in children, when treatment is instituted promptly, outcomes are usually favorable. Conventional treatment is with prednisone 2 mg/kg/day (maximum 60 mg/day) to induce remission, decreased over 4–8 weeks, and then continued at a lower dose (0.1–0.2 mg/kg/day, or 2.5–5 mg/day) as maintenance, often with azathioprine. Azathioprine is generally started at a dose of 0.5–1 mg/kg/day and increased to a maximum of 2–2.5 mg/kg/day until remission is achieved [69, 70]. Thiopurine methyltransferase (TMPT) activity may be verified prior to initiating azathioprine to identify patients at heightened risk of myleosuppression, but this is not routinely recommended [66]. This treatment regimen is associated with biochemical remission (normalization of liver enzymes and IgG) rates >80% in children with AIH, although this can take several months, and relapses requiring temporary increases in immunosuppression are common [61, 65]. The optimal duration of treatment is not known. In patients who have had sustained biochemical remission for 2–3 years, a liver biopsy may be performed and, if resolution of histological inflammation has occurred, treatment withdrawal may be attempted [70].

Children with AIH have an approximately 15% probability of developing complicated liver disease, as defined above, over 5 years [12]. Transplant rates for AIH are variable, but range from 5 to 10% in recent studies [12, 61]. AIH can recur post transplant with recurrence rates varying between 12 and 46% [71]. It is therefore recommended that steroid-based immunosuppression be maintained at a higher dose than that used for non-AIH transplants [72]. At the current time, it is unclear whether the disease course of AIH occurring in association with IBD differs from that in children without IBD.

Autoimmune Sclerosing Cholangitis

Epidemiology and Pathogenesis

Autoimmune sclerosing cholangitis (ASC) is an overlap condition between AIH and PSC, characterized by the combination of autoimmune features, namely, positive autoantibodies (especially ANA and SMA), hypergammaglobulinemia and interface hepatitis on liver biopsy, and cholangiopathy, as demonstrated by an abnormal cholangiogram or histological evidence of ductal involvement [63]. However, there are no clear diagnostic criteria for ASC. The International Autoimmune Hepatitis Group (IAIHG) suggests that conditions with overlapping features between autoimmune liver diseases not be considered separate diagnostic entities [73]. Rather, ASC may exist along a continuum of pathological changes between AIH and PSC. This concept of a spectrum of autoimmune liver disease is supported by the observation of a child progressing from AIH to ASC after 8 years in a prospective study [62]. Given the lack of established diagnostic criteria, the epidemiology of ASC is difficult to ascertain. However, a recent population study reported an incidence and prevalence of 0.1 and 0.6 per 100,000 children, respectively [12]. ASC appears to occur predominantly in children and young adults: a quarter to a third of children with sclerosing cholangitis have autoimmune overlap features [14–16], compared to only 1.4–17% of adults [23]. Conversely, almost half of 55 children with features of autoimmune liver disease were found to have cholangiographic abnormalities compatible with ASC in a prospective study in the United Kingdom [62]. Similar to PSC, ASC is typically diagnosed in the first half of the second decade of life, but, unlike PSC, it tends to affect both sexes fairly equally [12, 15, 62]. A definite association exists between ASC and IBD, the magnitude of which appears to be intermediate between that of PSC and AIH. Up to 75% of children with ASC have IBD. Conversely, 1.5–1.7% of children with IBD, mostly UC, have ASC [7, 12]. Given this, all children with ASC should undergo an evaluation for IBD, even if asymptomatic.

Diagnosis

The clinical presentation of ASC in children is similar to that described above. Biochemistry can provide some guidance in distinguishing ASC from AIH and PSC. Compared to AIH, ASC is typically associated with a higher ALP to AST ratio (around 4), and p-ANCA positivity is more common (74% compared to 36% of cases). Anti-LKM1, on the other hand, is more specific to AIH [63]. Clues of a possible diagnosis of ASC rather than PSC include higher transaminases, elevated serum IgG, and high-titer ANA and SMA autoantibodies. However, none of these biochemical parameters is sufficiently specific to make a diagnosis of ASC. The ability to firmly diagnose ASC and to differentiate it from AIH and PSC requires both cholangiography and liver biopsy. This is particularly relevant in children with IBD given the known association between ASC and IBD.

Outcomes and Treatment

An accurate diagnosis of ASC is essential as it has important prognostic and therapeutic implications. ASC may respond to the immunosuppressive regimen outlined above for AIH and, as such, may have a more favorable prognosis than PSC. A trial of corticosteroids with or without azathioprine is generally warranted [74]. However, the biliary disease in ASC progresses in 50% of children despite treatment [62]. UDCA is often used at doses of 15–20 mg/kg/day to address the biliary component of the disease, but, as with PSC, there is no evidence that biochemical improvement translates into a positive effect on natural history [75]. Twenty-five percent of children with ASC develop complicated liver disease, as defined above, within 5 years of diagnosis, a rate that is intermediate between that for PSC and AIH [12]. Given the lack of well-defined diagnostic criteria, it is difficult to comment on precise LT and mortality outcomes in children with ASC and studies to date have yielded conflicting results. An older series reported a 65% 10-year survival with native liver, distinctly worse than the 100% survival in children with AIH [62], whereas a more recent study found a 90% 5-year survival with native liver, comparable to the rate observed in children with AIH. Overall, it is believed that transplant rates in ASC are similar to those in PSC, around 20% [63]. As with PSC and AIH, ASC can recur post LT, a phenomenon that has been observed in up to 70% of cases [71]. Uncontrolled intestinal inflammation in patients with IBD is thought to be a risk factor for ASC recurrence, but direct evidence to this effect is lacking [63].

IgG4-Associated Cholangitis

IgG4-associated cholangitis (IAC) is a rare inflammatory disorder of the biliary tree, characterized by elevated serum IgG4 levels and infiltration of IgG4+ plasma cells in the bile duct walls, causing thickening and stenoses. IAC is often associated with type 1 autoimmune pancreatitis (AIP), the pancreatic manifestation of IgG4-related disease (IgG4-RD), a systemic multiorgan disorder only defined during the last decade [76]. The typical IAC/IgG4-RD patient profile is that of an elderly man with obstructive jaundice, weight loss, and abdominal discomfort. However, IAC occurring in association with UC has been reported, including in children [77]. The clinical and cholangiographic presentation of IAC is often indistinguishable from that of PSC. Furthermore, 9–36% of patients with PSC have elevated serum IgG4 levels (although usually lower than in IAC) [78, 79], and IgG4+ plasma cells have been documented on liver biopsy in PSC patients [80], further blurring the relationship between the two. However, PSC and IAC appear to be distinct entities, as evidenced by their very different response to corticosteroids; in contrast to PSC, IAC typically shows excellent response to immunosuppressive treatment, including resolution of strictures. However, relapse is common after tapering immunosuppression; long-term low-dose therapy with corticosteroids/azathioprine is often needed, analogous to the management of autoimmune hepatitis [81]. Diagnostic criteria have been proposed for IAC; these combine biochemical, radiographic, and histopathological characteristics with multiorgan involvement of IgG4-RD and responsiveness to immunosuppressive treatment [82].

Figure 11.4 graphically depicts the relationship between autoimmune liver diseases and IBD.

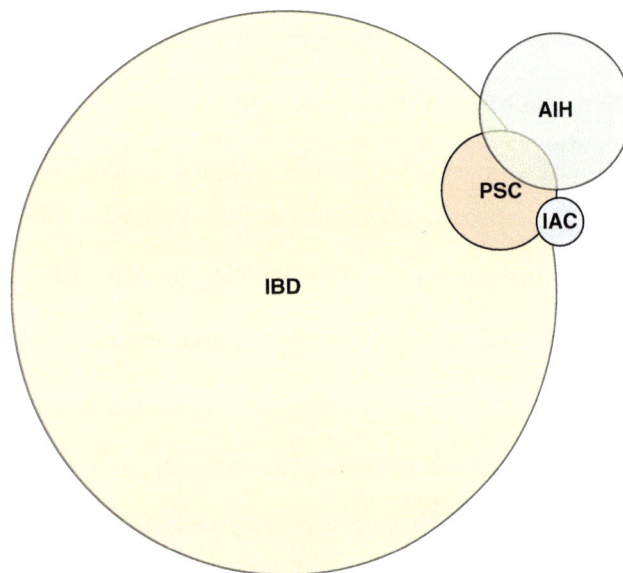

Fig. 11.4 The relationship between autoimmune liver disease and IBD. *AIH* autoimmune hepatitis, *IAC* IgG4-associated cholangitis, *IBD* inflammatory bowel disease, *PSC* primary sclerosing cholangitis

Drug Hepatotoxicity (Table 11.2)

Methotrexate

A recent systematic review and meta-analysis examining 32 randomized controlled trials, including a total of 13,177 adults primarily with rheumatological indications for treatment, demonstrated an increased risk of liver enzyme abnormalities in patients treated with methotrexate compared to a comparator agent, but no difference in the risk of liver failure, cirrhosis, or death [83]. The results of two adult IBD studies, in which fairly large numbers of liver biopsies were performed, also found very low rates of hepatic fibrosis in patients receiving methotrexate [84, 85], indicating that hepatic fibrosis is not as commonly observed in methotrexate users as suggested by older studies.

Pediatric IBD studies have found varying rates of biochemical liver abnormalities in children treated with methotrexate, ranging from 10% in a recent systematic review to 39% in a multicenter retrospective comparison of oral and subcutaneous methotrexate. Most resolved spontaneously or with dosage adjustment; medication discontinuation was required in only a minority (<5%) [86–88]. These studies are limited, however, by their retrospective nature, the inability to correlate biochemistry with histopathology, and the inability to definitively ascribe the biochemical abnormalities to methotrexate given the absence of documented normal laboratories prior to medication initiation in most cases. Conflicting data exist regarding whether higher methotrexate doses and parenteral versus oral administration are associated with a greater risk of hepatotoxicity [84, 87, 89]. The risk of hepatotoxicity may be higher in the immediate period after starting methotrexate [90]. Importantly, abnormal liver biochemistry does not reliably identify methotrexate-associated fibrosis.

Based on the available evidence, when initiating methotrexate in children with IBD, the authors recommend obtaining liver biochemistry at baseline, weekly for the first month and

Table 11.2 Differential diagnosis of clinical syndromes associated with IBD drugs causing liver injury

Syndrome	Drug
Acute hypersensitivity reaction	Sulfasalazine, mesalamine, thiopurines
Acute granulomatous hepatitis	Sulfasalazine, mesalamine
Autoimmune hepatitis-like	Anti-TNF
Noncirrhotic portal hypertension	Thiopurines
Fibrosis/cirrhosis	Methotrexate
Cholestatic jaundice	Sulfasalazine, mesalamine, thiopurines, anti-TNF
Sinusoidal obstruction syndrome	Thiopurines
Hepatic rupture	Thiopurines (peliosis)
Hepatic mass on imaging	Thiopurines (peliosis), anti-TNF/thiopurines (HSTCL)
Hepatitis B reactivation	Anti-TNF

HSTCL hepatosplenic T-cell lymphoma

every 2–3 months thereafter. In cases of persistent moderate enzyme elevations (up to 2–3× ULN), the dose of methotrexate can be adjusted, preferably in consultation with a pediatric hepatologist, whereas, when faced with more marked elevations (>5× ULN), methotrexate should be entirely held, at least temporarily. A liver biopsy should be performed in cases in which liver enzymes remain abnormal despite medication cessation, or when methotrexate discontinuation would be deleterious to IBD management. The use of methotrexate in patients with underlying liver disease, such as PSC, should generally be avoided, if possible.

Thiopurines

Azathioprine (AZA) is a prodrug for 6-mercaptopurine (6-MP), which is, in turn, converted to 6-thioguanine (6-TG), the final effector metabolite. The enzyme thiopurine methyltransferase (TPMT) catalyzes the formation of 6-methylmercaptopurine (6-MMP) and 6-methylmercaptopurine ribonucleotides (6-MMPR) [91]. A systematic review, including 34 mostly adult IBD studies, found a mean overall prevalence of AZA/6-MP-induced "liver disorder" of 3.4% and a mean annual rate of abnormal liver tests (up to 2× ULN) per patient-year of 1.4%, suggesting that thiopurine-associated hepatotoxicity is relatively uncommon. However, most studies did not provide definitions for "liver disorder" and were retrospective in design [92]. Two large pediatric studies examining the use of thiopurines in IBD also found fairly low rates of hepatotoxicity, namely, 4.6% and <3%, respectively [93, 94].

Thiopurine-induced hepatotoxicity can be grouped into three syndromes: (1) hypersensitivity reactions; (2) idiosyncratic cholestatic reactions; and (3) presumed endothelial cell injury. Hypersensitivity reactions usually have their onset within 2–3 weeks. Non-allergic cholestatic injuries are characterized by increased serum bilirubin and ALP, with or without moderate aminotransferase elevations, and typically occur within 2–5 months of therapy initiation. Variable parenchymal cell necrosis is typically seen on liver biopsy. Jaundice regression is not universal upon medication cessation [92]. Nodular regenerative hyperplasia (NRH), peliosis hepatis, sinusoidal dilatation, and sinusoidal obstruction syndrome (SOS, or veno-occlusive disease) fall into the latter category and are felt to be dose-dependent. The inciting injury in this group of vascular pathology is at the level of the endothelial cells lining the sinusoids and terminal hepatic venules and tends to occur between 3 months and 3 years of treatment [95]. More specifically, NRH is thought to result from areas of hepatocyte hypoperfusion and atrophy alternating with adaptive hepatocyte hyperplasia. IBD patients treated with AZA have a cumulative incidence of NRH of approximately 0.6 and 1.3% at 5

and 10 years, respectively [96]. Patients with NRH may be asymptomatic with normal or only mild elevations in liver function tests or isolated thrombocytopenia, or may present with clinically evident portal hypertension (PHT). NRH can be detected on liver biopsy, which demonstrates diffuse transformation of normal hepatic parenchyma into small, regenerative nodules with little or no fibrosis [97], and on MRI, which shows multiple fine, nonenhancing nodules [98]. The course is usually indolent, but, rarely, NRH may progress to end-stage liver disease requiring LT [99]. NRH has also been postulated to be a preneoplastic condition, which may predispose some individuals to developing hepatocellular carcinoma [100]. Thiopurine cessation in patients with NRH is generally followed by biochemical normalization, but patients with PHT have a variable course, with resolution of PHT in some, but persistence in others. Peliosis hepatis results in multiple cystic blood-filled spaces in the liver, spleen, lymph nodes, and other organs, which can lead to hepatic hematomas and, rarely, hepatic rupture [101]. SOS typically presents with a Budd-Chiari like picture, with the triad of rapid-onset ascites, painful hepatomegaly, and jaundice.

A reasonable monitoring strategy when initiating thiopurine therapy might include liver biochemistry at baseline, weekly for the first month, biweekly for the second and third months, and monthly thereafter. 6-MMP levels >5700 pmol/8 × 10^8 red blood cells have been linked with liver toxicity in children [102], but this finding has not been consistent across all studies [103]. If available, metabolite levels may be used to complement liver enzyme monitoring, and TPMT genotype or activity may be determined prior to initiating therapy, but this remains controversial. Mild liver enzyme abnormalities in children on thiopurine therapy may be observed with repeat blood work, but the authors suggest that the dose of thiopurine be reduced by about 50% in patients with more marked derangements. If this does not result in biochemical normalization after several weeks to months, therapy should be withdrawn entirely. Immediate thiopurine discontinuation should be the approach in any patient with clinically overt jaundice. Liver biopsy should be considered if liver tests fail to normalize after medication withdrawal or if there is any suggestion of PHT, even in patients with normal laboratory parameters.

Antitumor Necrosis Factor α (Anti-TNFα)

Based on postmarketing surveillance, the Food and Drug Administration (FDA) has issued warnings about the potential risk of serious liver injury with the use of anti-TNFα antibodies [104]. TNFα plays an important role in many aspects of immune response regulation. The association between anti-TNFα use and the development of autoantibodies is well known, although the pathological role of these antibodies remains unclear [105]. Anti-TNFα related hepatotoxicity does not appear to be dose-dependent, but instead is thought to occur in genetically susceptible individuals who generate an idiosyncratic immune response after inhibition of the TNFα pathway. The release and presentation of hepatic auto-antigens by immune cells may be involved [106].

Infliximab (IFX) and adalimumab (ADA) have been implicated in drug-induced liver injury (DILI) in both rheumatology and IBD populations. The median latency period is 13–18 weeks, but is hugely variable; DILI may have its onset after a single infusion/injection, but 20% occur more than 6 months into therapy [107, 108]. DILI seems to occur more frequently with IFX than ADA; the rate of DILI has been found to be 1/120 IFX-treated patients compared to 1/270 ADA-treated patients [109]. This is in keeping with the findings of a large retrospective review of adult IBD patients, in which IFX accounted for a disproportionate fraction of the 2.7% of patients who developed significant liver enzyme elevations felt to be secondary to anti-TNFα therapy [108]. The most common presentation is an autoimmune phenotype with primarily hepatocellular injury, high rates of autoantibody (especially ANA) positivity, and histological findings compatible with autoimmune hepatitis. However, mixed nonautoimmune and predominantly cholestatic patterns also occur. Cases with autoimmune features may have a longer latency and higher peak ALT [107]. Autoantibody positivity prior to anti-TNFα initiation does not appear to predict the risk of DILI [109]. Cases of DILI with AIH features should be managed with anti-TNFα discontinuation, in which case the prognosis is favorable. Some patients benefit from treatment with corticosteroids [107]. Anti-TNFα associated DILI does not seem to be a class effect, and switching to a different anti-TNFα, with close observation, appears safe. Milder cases of hepatotoxicity without overt autoimmune features often resolve spontaneously without anti-TNFα discontinuation [108]. No data currently exist regarding anti-TNFα associated liver injury in pediatric IBD.

Another concern with anti-TNFα agents is the risk of viral reactivation, in patients with chronic hepatitis B (HBV) infection, particularly those who are HBsAg-positive. Approximately one-third of HBsAg-positive IBD patients were observed to develop liver dysfunction while receiving immunosuppressive therapy, including anti-TNFα [110]. Treatment with anti-TNFα in IBD patients with hepatitis C (HCV) appears to be less of a concern and is generally well tolerated, with most patients displaying either unchanged or even improved biochemistry while receiving anti-TNF therapy [111]. Notably, no pediatric data exist regarding the outcomes of children with IBD and HBV or HCV receiving anti-TNFα. Strong consideration should be given to treating chronic HBV infection in children who are to commence anti-TNF therapy, whereas this may not be necessary in chil-

dren with HCV. Regardless, routine surveillance with liver enzymes and viral loads should be performed regularly in such children.

A child's immunization history should be carefully reviewed at the time of IBD diagnosis, and laboratory investigations, including HBsAb, HBsAg, anti-HBc, and anti-HCV, should be obtained. Although it is preferable to vaccinate for hepatitis A (HAV) prior to anti-TNFα initiation, seroconversion is still likely once on therapy and should be attempted regardless [112]. Patients with IBD who have nonimmune HBsAb levels (<10 mIU/mL) should be revaccinated with the routine three-dose regimen.

Sulfasalazine and Mesalamine

Sulfasalazine causes two main forms of hepatic injury. First, acute hepatocellular damage may develop as part of a generalized hypersensitivity reaction. This reaction, sometimes referred to as DRESS (drug rash with eosinophilia and systemic symptoms), is characterized by fever, rash, hepatomegaly, lymphadenopathy, atypical lymphocytosis, and eosinophilia, and is thought to be due to the sulfapyridine moiety [113]. The injury typically manifests within 2 months of starting therapy, with a shorter latency upon re-exposure [114]. This reaction is uncommon with data from the UK suggesting an incidence of 0.4% [115]. Prompt sulfasalazine discontinuation is critical, and corticosteroids may be helpful. However, progression to acute liver failure and death has been reported [115, 116]. Second, acute granulomatous hepatitis, characterized by fever, malaise, right upper quadrant pain, variable transaminases, and ALP and noncaseating granulomas on biopsy, may also occur [117]. In addition, cholestatic injury has been described with sulfasalazine use [118]. Mesalamine-induced hepatotoxicity is rare. A UK audit reported an incidence of 3.2 cases per million prescriptions, which was not statistically different from the six cases per million for sulfasalazine [119]. Cholestatic injury, with or without granulomatous hepatitis, resolving upon mesalamine discontinuation has been reported [120–122]. An apparent cross-reactive hypersensitivity reaction with mesalamine after a reaction to sulfasalazine [123] and a case of chronic hepatitis with autoimmune features have also been described [124].

Glucocorticoids

It is postulated that glucocorticoid-related alterations in hepatic lipid metabolism may lead to hepatic steatosis. Steroid use has been identified as an independent risk factor for nonalcoholic fatty liver disease (NAFLD) identified by abdominal imaging in IBD patients [125].

Hepatosplenic T-Cell Lymphoma

Hepatosplenic T-cell lymphoma (HSTCL) is a rare, aggressive, and almost uniformly fatal extranodal lymphoma. The usual presentation includes fever, fatigue, abnormal liver tests, hepatosplenomegaly, and pancytopenia. Between 1996 and 2011, 36 cases of HSTCL were reported in IBD patients, the majority of whom were young (<35 years) male patients with Crohn disease. Sixteen had received thiopurine monotherapy, and 20 had received a combination of anti-TNF and thiopurine (all had been exposed to IFX) [126]. The absolute risk of HSTCL in all patients receiving thiopurines has been estimated to be 1:45,000 compared to 1:7404 in men <35 years old, whereas the absolute risk for all patients receiving concomitant thiopurine and anti-TNF has been estimated to be slightly less than 1:22,000 compared to approximately 1:3534 in men <35 years [127]. In keeping with this, in a case-control study, anti-TNF combined with thiopurine therapy was associated with a higher risk of HSTCL compared to infliximab alone. At the current time, the role of anti-TNF agents, if any, in the development of HSTCL is uncertain, but the risk appears to be greater with combination therapy [128]. A high degree of suspicion must be maintained for this diagnosis, especially in young males.

Other Liver Diseases and IBD

Cholelithiasis

CD patients have an increased risk of gallstone disease, particularly in the setting of ileal disease and postileal resection. The incidence and prevalence of cholelithiasis in CD patients is 14.35 per 1000 person-years and 11–34%, respectively, compared to 7.75 per 1000 person-years and 5.5–15%, respectively, in controls [129, 130]. Overall, the odds of gallstones are 2.1-fold higher in CD patients compared to the general population. In contrast, definite evidence of an association between UC and cholelithiasis is lacking [129]. Although gallstones are relatively unusual in pediatric populations, 2.3% of children with IBD in an American consortium developed cholelithiasis [22], which significantly exceeds the population prevalence of 0.88–0.99% in individuals <30 years [131]. Bile in patients with CD postileal resection contains higher concentrations of bilirubin, suggesting an increased risk of developing pigment stones. Findings regarding the cholesterol component have been contradictory, with some studies reporting higher, and others lower, cholesterol saturation. The bile composition in patients with UC has not been consistently shown to differ from controls. Previous intestinal resection is the strongest risk factor for gallstone disease in patients with CD, with an ileal resection >30 cm increasing the odds of cholelithiasis

sevenfold. Other risk factors include disease location and duration, age, number of clinical recurrences and hospitalizations, total parenteral nutrition, prolonged hospitalization, and female sex. Impaired gallbladder emptying may also be a contributing factor [129]. Symptomatic cholelithiasis should prompt a referral to a pediatric surgeon. Children may also present with cholecystitis, which should be managed with broad-spectrum antibiotics and a general surgery consultation to guide eventual cholecystectomy.

Liver Abscess

Liver abscess is a rare complication of IBD. The precise incidence and prevalence are unknown, but it is more common in CD and in males and tends to occur in the setting of active disease. There is a tendency to develop multiple abscesses, which almost invariably involve the right lobe. The presentation is similar to that in non-IBD patients, but the diagnosis can be challenging and is often overlooked. Investigations, when suspected, should include an ultrasound and blood cultures, which are positive in 50% of cases. Compared to hepatic abscesses in the general population, which are usually polymicrobial, a single pathogen, often *Streptococcus milleri*, is frequently isolated in patients with IBD. Treatment is with prolonged parenteral antibiotics (commonly 4–8 weeks) with or without drainage, preferably percutaneously. An intra-abdominal source should be ruled out. Risk factors for liver abscess in IBD include intra-abdominal abscesses, fistulizing disease, intestinal perforation, abdominal surgery, and malnutrition [129, 132].

Portal Vein Thrombosis and Budd-Chiari Syndrome

Adult and pediatric patients with CD and UC are at increased risk of thromboembolism (TE). In a Danish cohort study using administrative data, the odds of thrombotic events were 1.5–1.8 times higher in IBD patients ≤20 years compared to controls [133]. The relative risk of TE was found to be slightly higher than this in hospitalized children with IBD, namely, 2.36, with an incidence of 118 per 10,000 [134]. Although the incidence of TE is lower in pediatric than adult IBD patients, the relative risk is higher in young patients with IBD [133]. To date, the mechanism behind this prothrombotic state is not fully understood, but it is likely multifactorial and related to the inflammatory state. The potential etiologies for increased thrombosis in IBD include thrombocytosis/platelet activation, hyperhomocysteinemia, increased fibrinogen, impaired fibrinolysis, increased procoagulation factors, decreased anticoagulation factors, and procoagulation mutations. The extent of IBD has also been shown to correlate with the risk of TE, but TE can occur in patients with UC even after proctocolectomy [134].

Portal vein thrombosis (PVT) appears to occur at higher rates in the IBD population, particularly postoperatively. Most studies suggest it is a rare complication, with a prevalence of 0.1–1% in IBD [135]. The incidence specifically in pediatric IBD patients has been reported to be 9 per 10,000 hospitalizations, with sixfold increased odds compared to non-IBD controls [134]. Overall, the precise epidemiology of the condition is difficult to ascertain as most patients are asymptomatic. The diagnosis may be made at the chronic stage, at which time cavernomatous transformation of the portal vein may be evident on imaging. A variety of imaging modalities can be used to make the diagnosis, including ultrasound with Doppler, contrast-enhanced CT, and MR angiography. Treatment is generally with anticoagulation, although the duration is not well established. While older studies suggested high mortality rates with this complication, more recent publications indicate a more benign natural history [135].

Budd-Chiari syndrome is a rare complication of UC, mostly in adults, but has been reported in a small number of children as well, with an incidence of 2.1 per 10,000 hospitalized pediatric IBD patients [134, 136–138]. It typically presents with hepatomegaly, right upper quadrant pain, and rapid-onset ascites with abnormal liver tests, but 25% can be asymptomatic. Diagnosis is supported by imaging and/or liver biopsy. Therapy may include thrombolysis, anticoagulation, angioplasty, or vascular stents. More definitive treatment, such as porto-/mesocaval shunts, or even liver transplant, may be required in medically refractory cases. Symptomatic treatment of ascites is with diuretics and paracentesis. While outcomes have often been poor in adults, the pediatric cases reported to date have had a favorable evolution with resolution, with anticoagulation or even spontaneously.

Nonalcoholic Fatty Liver Disease

The prevalence of nonalcoholic fatty liver disease (NAFLD) in IBD has varied widely across different studies, ranging from 13 to 100% [1], depending on the diagnostic modality employed and the indication for screening/testing. According to a systematic review, the mean prevalence of fatty liver disease in adults is 23% in UC and 1.5–39.5% in CD, in comparison to 20% in the general population [129]. The prevalence of NAFLD in pediatric IBD patients has never been specifically examined. Overall, it would appear that fatty liver is common in the IBD population, but definitive evidence that the prevalence of NALFD in IBD exceeds that in the general population is lacking. Patients with metabolic risk factors, such as obesity and hypertension, are at

increased risk, but these risk factors are not universally present in IBD patients with NAFLD. Coupled with the asymptomatic nature of NAFLD, a high degree of suspicion must to be maintained, particularly in the setting of raised liver enzymes. Diagnostic confirmation requires histopathological assessment, but screening can be performed with transaminases, GGT, and triglycerides. Management includes attaining adequate IBD control and working toward a healthy BMI in patients who are overweight, in conjunction with a pediatric dietitian.

Granulomatous Hepatitis

Granulomatous hepatitis is estimated to occur in <1% of IBD patients, primarily those with CD. It tends to present with a cholestatic picture, especially elevated ALP. The diagnosis is confirmed by visualizing granulomas on liver biopsy. The most common cause in the setting of IBD is medications, especially sulfasalazine, but granulomatous hepatitis can also be an extraintestinal manifestation of IBD, and can be associated with malignancy or infections. Corticosteroids and immunosuppressive agents have been used as treatment [1].

Hepatic Amyloidosis

Amyloidosis is a rare but serious complication of IBD, especially CD. It has a prevalence of 0.5% in IBD, more specifically 0.9–3% in CD, and 0–0.07% in UC [139–141]. The pathogenesis remains unclear. Patients are usually male with extensive, long-standing disease, although amyloidosis may be present at the time of, or even prior to, the diagnosis of IBD. Fistulae and/or abscesses, as well as other extraintestinal manifestations, are common. Amyloidosis is predominantly a disease of the kidneys, but hepatic involvement has been described in a small subset of patients, including in children [141]. Signs and symptoms of hepatic amyloidosis are few, and liver tests are generally normal. The diagnosis is established by biopsy, and, often, only comes to light at the time of autopsy. Mortality is intricately tied to the renal disease, but hepatic involvement is associated with a reduced likelihood of survival [142].

Primary Biliary Cholangitis (Previously Termed Primary Biliary Cirrhosis)

Primary biliary cholangitis (PBC) is characterized by chronic inflammatory destruction of the intrahepatic bile ducts and infiltration by lymphocytes and plasma cells into the portal tract. To date, there have been approximately 20 reports of PBC occurring in association with UC, none of which have involved children [143, 144]. PBC associated with UC has less of a female predominance, and affects younger patients than PBC in the general population. In addition, the colitis tends to be mild, often limited to the rectum. The typical features of PBC include pruritus, cholestasis, and increased IgM, but these can be seen in other hepatobiliary disorders associated with UC, such as PSC. Serum antimitochondrial antibody (AMA), which is almost always positive in PBC, but generally negative in PSC, is very helpful for distinguishing the two. Liver biopsy can also provide additional useful information; it typically shows granulomatous inflammation of the periportal area in PBC.

A Clinical Approach to Children with IBD and Liver Abnormalities

Children with IBD who develop abnormal liver biochemistry or physical stigmata of liver disease may have a wide range of potential underlying diagnoses, as reviewed in this chapter. Based on the available but limited evidence presented, the authors suggest the following approach to liver disease in pediatric IBD (Fig. 11.5). All children with IBD should have routine liver biochemistry with ALT, AST, GGT, ALP, fractionated bilirubin, and albumin measured every 6–12 months when the child is well. The frequency of blood work can be increased if the child is unwell or receiving medications with known potential hepatotoxicity, as

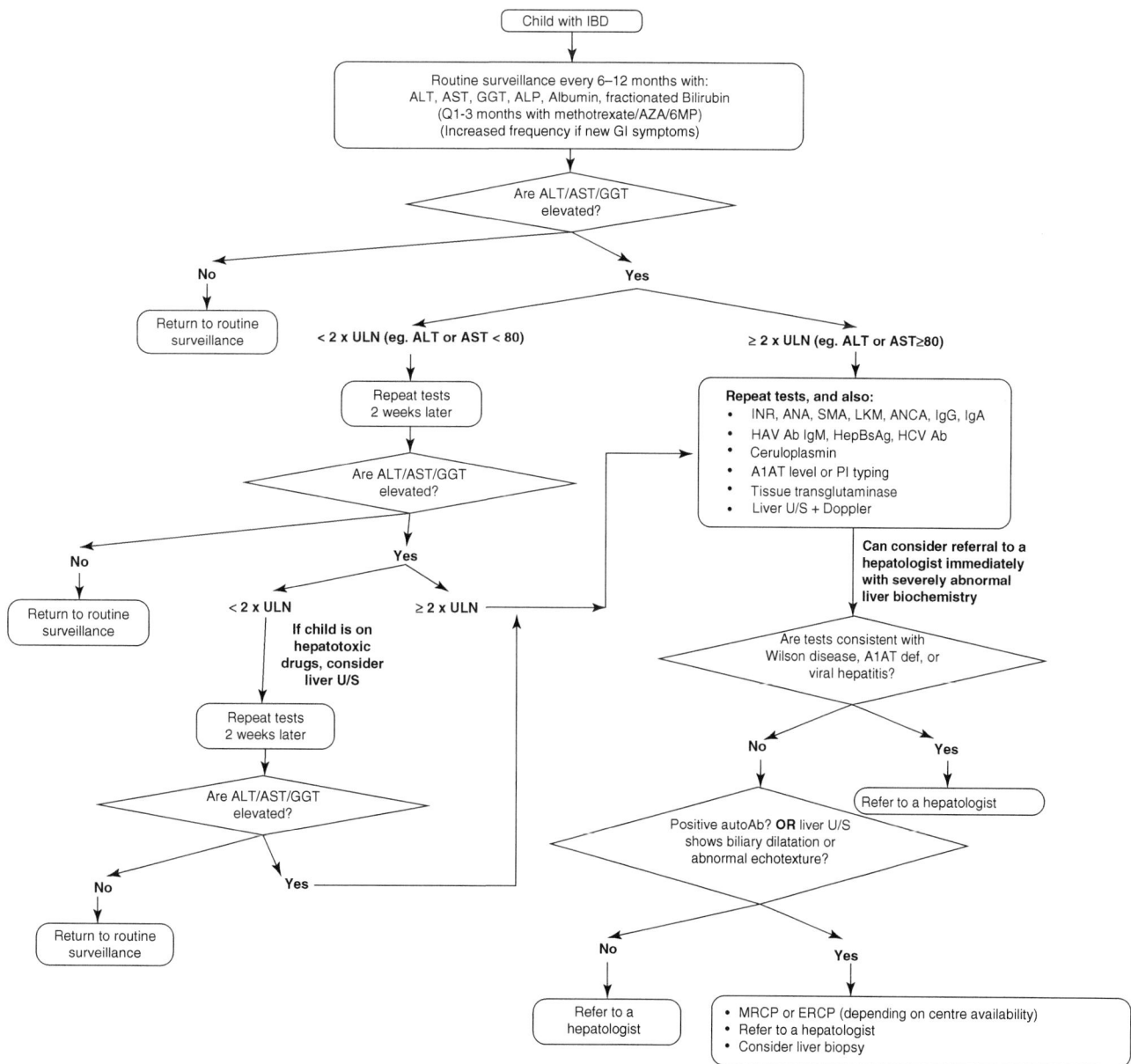

Fig. 11.5 Suggested approach to liver disease in pediatric IBD

detailed above. If low-grade abnormalities are detected, liver tests should be repeated in 1–2 weeks to ensure they are not rising acutely and subsequently followed for the first few months. With more marked elevations, or clinically overt evidence of liver disease, such as hepatosplenomegaly or jaundice, further investigations should be considered, including autoantibodies (ANA, SMA, LKM1, ANCA), serum IgG, viral hepatitis serologies, celiac serology, ceruloplasmin, and alpha-1 antitrypsin level, along with abdominal ultrasound. Depending on the clinical context, MRCP and/or liver biopsy may also be indicated. If medications are felt to be a potential contributor, a trial of reducing the dose or holding the medication entirely (if this is not felt to be detrimental to the child's IBD care) should be performed. The distinction between "low" and "high-grade" elevations is controversial. The authors propose that elevations >2–3× ULN are significant and require further investigation. Additional studies in pediatric IBD populations are required to construct truly evidence-based algorithms to guide the work-up and management of abnormal liver biochemistry and liver disease in children with IBD.

References

1. Navaneethan U, Shen B. Hepatopancreatobiliary manifestations and complications associated with inflammatory bowel disease. Inflamm Bowel Dis. 2010;16:1598–619. doi:10.1002/ibd.21219.
2. Gisbert JP, Luna M, Gonzalez-Lama Y, Pousa ID, Velasco M, Moreno-Otero R, Mate J. Liver injury in inflammatory bowel disease: long-term follow-up study of 786 patients. Inflamm Bowel Dis. 2007;13:1106–14. doi:10.1002/ibd.20160.
3. Mendes FD, Levy C, Enders FB, Loftus Jr EV, Angulo P, Lindor KD. Abnormal hepatic biochemistries in patients with inflammatory bowel disease. Am J Gastroenterol. 2007;102:344–50. doi:10.1111/j.1572-0241.2006.00947.x.
4. Yamamoto-Furusho JK, Sanchez-Osorio M, Uribe M. Prevalence and factors associated with the presence of abnormal function liver tests in patients with ulcerative colitis. Ann Hepatol. 2010;9:397–401.
5. Nemeth A, Ejderhamn J, Glaumann H, Strandvik B. Liver damage in juvenile inflammatory bowel disease. Liver. 1990;10:239–48.
6. Pusateri AJ, Kim SC, Dotson JL, Balint JP, Potter CJ, Boyle BM, Crandall WV. Incidence, pattern, and etiology of elevated liver enzymes in pediatric inflammatory bowel disease. J Pediatr Gastroenterol Nutr. 2015;60:592–7. doi:10.1097/MPG.0000000000000672.
7. Valentino PL, Feldman BM, Walters TD, Griffiths AM, Ling SC, Pullenayegum EM, Kamath BM. Abnormal liver biochemistry is common in pediatric inflammatory bowel disease: prevalence and associations. Inflamm Bowel Dis. 2015; doi:10.1097/MIB.0000000000000558.
8. Hyams J, Markowitz J, Treem W, Davis P, Grancher K, Daum F. Characterization of hepatic abnormalities in children with inflammatory bowel disease. Inflamm Bowel Dis. 1995;1:27–33.
9. Goyal A, Hyams JS, Lerer T, et al. Liver enzyme elevations within 3 months of diagnosis of inflammatory bowel disease and likelihood of liver disease. J Pediatr Gastroenterol Nutr. 2014;59:321–3. doi:10.1097/mpg.0000000000000409.
10. Riegler G, D'Inca R, Sturniolo GC, et al. Hepatobiliary alterations in patients with inflammatory bowel disease: a multicenter study. Caprilli & Gruppo Italiano Studio Colon-Retto. Scand J Gastroenterol. 1998;33:93–8.
11. Card TR, Solaymani-Dodaran M, West J. Incidence and mortality of primary sclerosing cholangitis in the UK: a population-based cohort study. J Hepatol. 2008;48:939–44. doi:10.1016/j.jhep.2008.02.017.
12. Deneau M, Jensen MK, Holmen J, Williams MS, Book LS, Guthery SL. Primary sclerosing cholangitis, autoimmune hepatitis, and overlap in Utah children: epidemiology and natural history. Hepatology. 2013;58:1392–400. doi:10.1002/hep.26454.
13. Kaplan GG, Laupland KB, Butzner D, Urbanski SJ, Lee SS. The burden of large and small duct primary sclerosing cholangitis in adults and children: a population-based analysis. Am J Gastroenterol. 2007;102:1042–9. doi:10.1111/j.1572-0241.2007.01103.x.
14. Feldstein AE, Perrault J, El-Youssif M, Lindor KD, Freese DK, Angulo P. Primary sclerosing cholangitis in children: a long-term follow-up study. Hepatology. 2003;38:210–7. doi:10.1053/jhep.2003.50289.
15. Miloh T, Arnon R, Shneider B, Suchy F, Kerkar N. A retrospective single-center review of primary sclerosing cholangitis in children. Clin Gastroenterol Hepatol. 2009;7:239–45. doi:10.1016/j.cgh.2008.10.019.
16. Wilschanski M, Chait P, Wade JA, et al. Primary sclerosing cholangitis in 32 children: clinical, laboratory, and radiographic features, with survival analysis. Hepatology. 1995;22:1415–22.
17. Warren KW, Athanassiades S, Monge JI. Primary sclerosing cholangitis. A study of forty-two cases. Am J Surg. 1966;111:23–38.
18. Boonstra K, Beuers U, Ponsioen CY. Epidemiology of primary sclerosing cholangitis and primary biliary cirrhosis: a systematic review. J Hepatol. 2012;56:1181–8. doi:10.1016/j.jhep.2011.10.025.
19. Schrumpf E, Boberg KM. Epidemiology of primary sclerosing cholangitis. Best Pract Res Clin Gastroenterol. 2001;15:553–62. doi:10.1053/bega.2001.0204.
20. Batres LA, Russo P, Mathews M, Piccoli DA, Chuang E, Ruchelli E. Primary sclerosing cholangitis in children: a histologic follow-up study. Pediatr Dev Pathol. 2005;8:568–76. doi:10.1007/s10024-005-0020-0.
21. Dotson JL, Hyams JS, Markowitz J, et al. Extraintestinal manifestations of pediatric inflammatory bowel disease and their relation to disease type and severity. J Pediatr Gastroenterol Nutr. 2010;51:140–5. doi:10.1097/MPG.0b013e3181ca4db4.
22. Jose FA, Garnett EA, Vittinghoff E, et al. Development of extraintestinal manifestations in pediatric patients with inflammatory bowel disease. Inflamm Bowel Dis. 2009;15:63–8. doi:10.1002/ibd.20604.
23. Chapman R, Fevery J, Kalloo A, Nagorney DM, Boberg KM, Shneider B, Gores GJ. Diagnosis and management of primary sclerosing cholangitis. Hepatology. 2010;51:660–78. doi:10.1002/hep.23294.
24. Mells GF, Kaser A, Karlsen TH. Novel insights into autoimmune liver diseases provided by genome-wide association studies. J Autoimmun. 2013;46:41–54. doi:10.1016/j.jaut.2013.07.004.
25. Williamson KD, Chapman RW. Primary sclerosing cholangitis: a clinical update. Br Med Bull. 2015;114:53–64. doi:10.1093/bmb/ldv019.
26. Eksteen B, Grant AJ, Miles A, et al. Hepatic endothelial CCL25 mediates the recruitment of CCR9+ gut-homing lymphocytes to the liver in primary sclerosing cholangitis. J Exp Med. 2004;200:1511–7. doi:10.1084/jem.20041035.
27. Tabibian JH, O'Hara SP, Lindor KD. Primary sclerosing cholangitis and the microbiota: current knowledge and perspectives on

etiopathogenesis and emerging therapies. Scand J Gastroenterol. 2014;49:901–8. doi:10.3109/00365521.2014.913189.

28. Loftus Jr EV, Harewood GC, Loftus CG, et al. PSC-IBD: a unique form of inflammatory bowel disease associated with primary sclerosing cholangitis. Gut. 2005;54:91–6. doi:10.1136/gut.2004.046615.

29. Halliday JS, Djordjevic J, Lust M, Culver EL, Braden B, Travis SP, Chapman RW. A unique clinical phenotype of primary sclerosing cholangitis associated with Crohn disease. J Crohn Colitis. 2012;6:174–81. doi: http://dx.doi.org/10.1016/j.crohns.2011.07.015.

30. Lundqvist K, Broome U. Differences in colonic disease activity in patients with ulcerative colitis with and without primary sclerosing cholangitis: a case control study. Dis Colon Rectum. 1997;40:451–6.

31. Schaeffer DF, Win LL, Hafezi-Bakhtiari S, Cino M, Hirschfield GM, El-Zimaity H. The phenotypic expression of inflammatory bowel disease in patients with primary sclerosing cholangitis differs in the distribution of colitis. Dig Dis Sci. 2013;58:2608–14. doi:10.1007/s10620-013-2697-7.

32. Faubion Jr WA, Loftus EV, Sandborn WJ, Freese DK, Perrault J. Pediatric "PSC-IBD": a descriptive report of associated inflammatory bowel disease among pediatric patients with psc. J Pediatr Gastroenterol Nutr. 2001;33:296–300.

33. Ordonez F, Lacaille F, Canioni D, et al. Pediatric ulcerative colitis associated with autoimmune diseases: a distinct form of inflammatory bowel disease? Inflamm Bowel Dis. 2012;18:1809–17. doi:10.1002/ibd.22864.

34. Lascurain L, Jensen MK, Guthery SL, Holmen J, Deneau M. Inflammatory bowel disease phenotype in pediatric primary sclerosing cholangitis. Inflamm Bowel Dis. 2016;22:146–50. doi:10.1097/MIB.0000000000000586.

35. Marelli L, Xirouchakis E, Kalambokis G, Cholongitas E, Hamilton MI, Burroughs AK. Does the severity of primary sclerosing cholangitis influence the clinical course of associated ulcerative colitis? Gut. 2011;60:1224–8. doi:10.1136/gut.2010.235408.

36. Cangemi JR, Wiesner RH, Beaver SJ, et al. Effect of proctocolectomy for chronic ulcerative colitis on the natural history of primary sclerosing cholangitis. Gastroenterology. 1989;96:790–4.

37. Cholongitas E, Shusang V, Papatheodoridis GV, et al. Risk factors for recurrence of primary sclerosing cholangitis after liver transplantation. Liver Transpl. 2008;14:138–43. doi:10.1002/lt.21260.

38. Bjornsson E, Chari S, Silveira M, Gossard A, Takahashi N, Smyrk T, Lindor K. Primary sclerosing cholangitis associated with elevated immunoglobulin G4: clinical characteristics and response to therapy. Am J Ther. 2011;18:198–205. doi:10.1097/MJT.0b013e3181c9dac6.

39. Lindor KD, Kowdley KV, Harrison ME. ACG Clinical Guideline: primary sclerosing cholangitis. Am J Gastroenterol. 2015;110:646–59. quiz 660 doi:10.1038/ajg.2015.112.

40. MacCarty RL, LaRusso NF, Wiesner RH, Ludwig J. Primary sclerosing cholangitis: findings on cholangiography and pancreatography. Radiology. 1983;149:39–44. doi:10.1148/radiology.149.1.6412283.

41. Deneau M, Adler DG, Schwartz JJ, et al. Cholangiocarcinoma in a 17-year-old boy with primary sclerosing cholangitis and inflammatory bowel disease. J Pediatr Gastroenterol Nutr. 2011;52:617–20. doi:10.1097/MPG.0b013e3181f9a5d2.

42. Soetikno RM, Lin OS, Heidenreich PA, Young HS, Blackstone MO. Increased risk of colorectal neoplasia in patients with primary sclerosing cholangitis and ulcerative colitis: a meta-analysis. Gastrointest Endosc. 2002;56:48–54.

43. Ponsioen CY, Vrouenraets SM, Prawirodirdjo W, et al. Natural history of primary sclerosing cholangitis and prognostic value of cholangiography in a Dutch population. Gut. 2002;51:562–6.

44. Bjornsson E, Olsson R, Bergquist A, et al. The natural history of small-duct primary sclerosing cholangitis. Gastroenterology. 2008;134:975–80. doi:10.1053/j.gastro.2008.01.042.

45. Tabibian JH, Lindor KD. Primary sclerosing cholangitis: a review and update on therapeutic developments. Expert Rev Gastroenterol Hepatol. 2013;7:103–14. doi:10.1586/egh.12.80.

46. Gilger MA, Gann ME, Opekun AR, Gleason Jr WA. Efficacy of ursodeoxycholic acid in the treatment of primary sclerosing cholangitis in children. J Pediatr Gastroenterol Nutr. 2000;31:136–41.

47. Triantos CK, Koukias NM, Nikolopoulou VN, Burroughs AK. Meta-analysis: ursodeoxycholic acid for primary sclerosing cholangitis. Aliment Pharmacol Ther. 2011;34:901–10. doi:10.1111/j.1365-2036.2011.04822.x.

48. Lindor KD, Kowdley KV, Luketic VA, et al. High-dose ursodeoxycholic acid for the treatment of primary sclerosing cholangitis. Hepatology. 2009;50:808–14. doi:10.1002/hep.23082.

49. Cox KL, Cox KM. Oral vancomycin: treatment of primary sclerosing cholangitis in children with inflammatory bowel disease. J Pediatr Gastroenterol Nutr. 1998;27:580–3.

50. Davies YK, Cox KM, Abdullah BA, Safta A, Terry AB, Cox KL. Long-term treatment of primary sclerosing cholangitis in children with oral vancomycin: an immunomodulating antibiotic. J Pediatr Gastroenterol Nutr. 2008;47:61–7. doi:10.1097/MPG.0b013e31816fee95.

51. Tabibian JH, Weeding E, Jorgensen RA, Petz JL, Keach JC, Talwalkar JA, Lindor KD. Randomised clinical trial: vancomycin or metronidazole in patients with primary sclerosing cholangitis – a pilot study. Aliment Pharmacol Ther. 2013;37:604–12. doi:10.1111/apt.12232.

52. Abarbanel DN, Seki SM, Davies Y, et al. Immunomodulatory effect of vancomycin on Treg in pediatric inflammatory bowel disease and primary sclerosing cholangitis. J Clin Immunol. 2013;33:397–406. doi:10.1007/s10875-012-9801-1.

53. Farkkila M, Karvonen AL, Nurmi H, Nuutinen H, Taavitsainen M, Pikkarainen P, Karkkainen P. Metronidazole and ursodeoxycholic acid for primary sclerosing cholangitis: a randomized placebo-controlled trial. Hepatology. 2004;40:1379–86. doi:10.1002/hep.20457.

54. Silveira MG, Torok NJ, Gossard AA, Keach JC, Jorgensen RA, Petz JL, Lindor KD. Minocycline in the treatment of patients with primary sclerosing cholangitis: results of a pilot study. Am J Gastroenterol. 2009;104:83–8. doi:10.1038/ajg.2008.14.

55. Tabibian JH, Gossard A, El-Youssef M, et al. Prospective clinical trial of rifaximin therapy for patients with primary sclerosing cholangitis. Am J Ther. 2014;doi:10.1097/mjt.0000000000000102.

56. Johnson GK, Saeian K, Geenen JE. Primary sclerosing cholangitis treated by endoscopic biliary dilation: review and long-term follow-up evaluation. Curr Gastroenterol Rep. 2006;8:147–55.

57. Venkat VL, Ranganathan S, Sindhi R. The challenges of liver transplantation in children with primary sclerosing cholangitis. Expert Rev Gastroenterol Hepatol. 2015;9:289–94. doi:10.1586/17474124.2015.1002085.

58. Squires RH, Ng V, Romero R, Ekong U, Hardikar W, Emre S, Mazariegos GV. Evaluation of the pediatric patient for liver transplantation: 2014 practice guideline by the American Association for the Study of Liver Diseases, American Society of Transplantation and the North American Society for Pediatric Gastroenterology, Hepatology, and Nutrition. J Pediatr Gastroenterol Nutr. 2014;59:112–31. doi:10.1097/mpg.0000000000000431.

59. Miloh T, Anand R, Yin W, Vos M, Kerkar N, Alonso E, Studies of Pediatric Liver Transplantation Research Group. Pediatric liver transplantation for primary sclerosing cholangitis. Liver Transpl. 2011;17:925–33. doi:10.1002/lt.22320.

60. Venkat VL, Ranganathan S, Mazariegos GV, Sun Q, Sindhi R. Recurrence of primary sclerosing cholangitis in pediatric liver

transplant recipients. Liver Transpl. 2014;20:679–86. doi:10.1002/lt.23868.

61. Jimenez-Rivera C, Ling SC, Ahmed N, et al. Incidence and characteristics of autoimmune hepatitis. Pediatrics. 2015; doi:10.1542/peds.2015-0578.

62. Gregorio GV, Portmann B, Karani J, Harrison P, Donaldson PT, Vergani D, Mieli-Vergani G. Autoimmune hepatitis/sclerosing cholangitis overlap syndrome in childhood: a 16-year prospective study. Hepatology. 2001;33:544–53. doi:10.1053/jhep.2001.22131.

63. Mieli-Vergani G, Vergani D. Paediatric autoimmune liver disease. Arch Dis Child. 2013;98:1012–7. doi:10.1136/archdischild-2013-303848.

64. Mieli-Vergani G, Vergani D. Autoimmune hepatitis in children: what is different from adult AIH? Semin Liver Dis. 2009;29:297–306. doi:10.1055/s-0029-1233529.

65. Gregorio GV, Portmann B, Reid F, et al. Autoimmune hepatitis in childhood: a 20-year experience. Hepatology. 1997;25:541–7. doi:10.1002/hep.510250308.

66. Manns MP, Lohse AW, Vergani D. Autoimmune hepatitis–update 2015. J Hepatol. 2015;62:S100–11. doi:10.1016/j.jhep.2015.03.005.

67. Mieli-Vergani G, Vergani D. Autoimmune hepatitis. Nat Rev Gastroenterol Hepatol. 2011;8:320–9. doi:10.1038/nrgastro.2011.69.

68. Radhakrishnan KR, Alkhouri N, Worley S, et al. Autoimmune hepatitis in children–impact of cirrhosis at presentation on natural history and long-term outcome. Dig Liver Dis. 2010;42:724–8. doi:10.1016/j.dld.2010.01.002.

69. Floreani A, Liberal R, Vergani D, Mieli-Vergani G. Autoimmune hepatitis: contrasts and comparisons in children and adults – a comprehensive review. J Autoimmun. 2013;46:7–16. doi:10.1016/j.jaut.2013.08.004.

70. Manns MP, Woynarowski M, Kreisel W, et al. Budesonide induces remission more effectively than prednisone in a controlled trial of patients with autoimmune hepatitis. Gastroenterology. 2010;139:1198–206. doi:10.1053/j.gastro.2010.06.046.

71. Liberal R, Longhi MS, Grant CR, Mieli-Vergani G, Vergani D. Autoimmune hepatitis after liver transplantation. Clin Gastroenterol Hepatol. 2012;10:346–53. doi:10.1016/j.cgh.2011.10.028.

72. Liberal R, Zen Y, Mieli-Vergani G, Vergani D. Liver transplantation and autoimmune liver diseases. Liver Transpl. 2013;19:1065–77. doi:10.1002/lt.23704.

73. Boberg KM, Chapman RW, Hirschfield GM, Lohse AW, Manns MP, Schrumpf E. Overlap syndromes: the International Autoimmune Hepatitis Group (IAIHG) position statement on a controversial issue. J Hepatol. 2011;54:374–85. doi:10.1016/j.jhep.2010.09.002.

74. Manns MP, Czaja AJ, Gorham JD, et al. Diagnosis and management of autoimmune hepatitis. Hepatology. 2010;51:2193–213. doi:10.1002/hep.23584.

75. European Association for the Study of the Liver. EASL Clinical Practice Guidelines: management of cholestatic liver diseases. J Hepatol. 2009;51:237–67. doi:10.1016/j.jhep.2009.04.009.

76. Beuers U, Hubers LM, Doorenspleet M, et al. IgG4-associated cholangitis – a mimic of PSC. Dig Dis. 2015;33(Suppl 2):176–80. doi:10.1159/000440830.

77. Dastis SN, Latinne D, Sempoux C, Geubel AP. Ulcerative colitis associated with IgG4 cholangitis: similar features in two HLA identical siblings. J Hepatol. 2009;51:601–5. doi:10.1016/j.jhep.2009.05.032.

78. Hirano K, Kawabe T, Yamamoto N, et al. Serum IgG4 concentrations in pancreatic and biliary diseases. Clin Chim Acta. 2006;367:181–4. doi:10.1016/j.cca.2005.11.031.

79. Mendes FD, Jorgensen R, Keach J, et al. Elevated serum IgG4 concentration in patients with primary sclerosing cholangitis. Am J Gastroenterol. 2006;101:2070–5. doi:10.1111/j.1572-0241.2006.00772.x.

80. Zhang L, Lewis JT, Abraham SC, et al. IgG4+ plasma cell infiltrates in liver explants with primary sclerosing cholangitis. Am J Surg Pathol. 2010;34:88–94. doi:10.1097/PAS.0b013e3181c6c09a.

81. Ghazale A, Chari ST, Zhang L, et al. Immunoglobulin G4-associated cholangitis: clinical profile and response to therapy. Gastroenterology. 2008;134:706–15. doi:10.1053/j.gastro.2007.12.009.

82. Ohara H, Okazaki K, Tsubouchi H, et al. Clinical diagnostic criteria of IgG4-related sclerosing cholangitis 2012. J Hepatobiliary Pancreat Sci. 2012;19:536–42. doi:10.1007/s00534-012-0521-y.

83. Conway R, Low C, Coughlan RJ, O'Donnell MJ, Carey JJ. Risk of liver injury among methotrexate users: a meta-analysis of randomised controlled trials. Semin Arthritis Rheum. 2015;45:156–62. doi:10.1016/j.semarthrit.2015.05.003.

84. Fournier MR, Klein J, Minuk GY, Bernstein CN. Changes in liver biochemistry during methotrexate use for inflammatory bowel disease. Am J Gastroenterol. 2010;105:1620–6. doi:10.1038/ajg.2010.21.

85. Te HS, Schiano TD, Kuan SF, Hanauer SB, Conjeevaram HS, Baker AL. Hepatic effects of long-term methotrexate use in the treatment of inflammatory bowel disease. Am J Gastroenterol. 2000;95:3150–6. doi:10.1111/j.1572-0241.2000.03287.x.

86. Sunseri W, Hyams JS, Lerer T, et al. Retrospective cohort study of methotrexate use in the treatment of pediatric Crohn disease. Inflamm Bowel Dis. 2014;20:1341–5. doi:10.1097/mib.0000000000000102.

87. Turner D, Doveh E, Cohen A, et al. Efficacy of oral methotrexate in paediatric Crohn disease: a multicentre propensity score study. Gut. 2015;64(12):1898–904. doi:10.1136/gutjnl-2014-307964. Epub 2014 Nov 21.

88. Valentino PL, Church PC, Shah PS, Beyene J, Griffiths AM, Feldman BM, Kamath BM. Hepatotoxicity caused by methotrexate therapy in children with inflammatory bowel disease: a systematic review and meta-analysis. Inflamm Bowel Dis. 2014;20:47–59. doi:10.1097/01.MIB.0000436953.88522.3e.

89. Khan N, Abbas AM, Whang N, Balart LA, Bazzano LA, Kelly TN. Incidence of liver toxicity in inflammatory bowel disease patients treated with methotrexate: a meta-analysis of clinical trials. Inflamm Bowel Dis. 2012;18:359–67. doi:10.1002/ibd.21820.

90. Kalb RE, Strober B, Weinstein G, Lebwohl M. Methotrexate and psoriasis: 2009 National Psoriasis Foundation Consensus Conference. J Am Acad Dermatol. 2009;60:824–37. doi:10.1016/j.jaad.2008.11.906.

91. Bousvaros A. Use of immunomodulators and biologic therapies in children with inflammatory bowel disease. Expert Rev Clin Immunol. 2010;6:659–66. doi:10.1586/eci.10.46.

92. Gisbert JP, Gonzalez-Lama Y, Mate J. Thiopurine-induced liver injury in patients with inflammatory bowel disease: a systematic review. Am J Gastroenterol. 2007;102:1518–27. doi:10.1111/j.1572-0241.2007.01187.x.

93. Lee MN, Kang B, Choi SY, et al. Relationship between azathioprine dosage, 6-thioguanine nucleotide levels, and therapeutic response in pediatric patients with IBD treated with azathioprine. Inflamm Bowel Dis. 2015;21:1054–62. doi:10.1097/MIB.0000000000000347.

94. Riello L, Talbotec C, Garnier-Lengline H, et al. Tolerance and efficacy of azathioprine in pediatric Crohn disease. Inflamm Bowel Dis. 2011;17:2138–43. doi:10.1002/ibd.21612.

95. Haboubi NY, Ali HH, Whitwell HL, Ackrill P. Role of endothelial cell injury in the spectrum of azathioprine-induced liver disease after renal transplant: light microscopy and ultrastructural observations. Am J Gastroenterol. 1988;83:256–61.

96. Dubinsky MC, Vasiliauskas EA, Singh H, et al. 6-thioguanine can cause serious liver injury in inflammatory bowel disease patients. Gastroenterology. 2003;125:298–303. doi:10.1016/s0016-5085(03)00938-7.

97. Calabrese E, Hanauer SB. Assessment of non-cirrhotic portal hypertension associated with thiopurine therapy in inflammatory bowel disease. J Crohns Colitis. 2011;5:48–53. doi:10.1016/j.crohns.2010.08.007.
98. Seiderer J, Zech CJ, Reinisch W, et al. A multicenter assessment of liver toxicity by MRI and biopsy in IBD patients on 6-thioguanine. J Hepatol. 2005;43:303–9. doi:10.1016/j.jhep.2005.02.051.
99. Musumba CO. Review article: the association between nodular regenerative hyperplasia, inflammatory bowel disease and thiopurine therapy. Aliment Pharmacol Ther. 2013;38:1025–37. doi:10.1111/apt.12490.
100. Russmann S, Zimmermann A, Krähenbühl S, Kern B, Reichen J. Veno-occlusive disease, nodular regenerative hyperplasia and hepatocellular carcinoma after azathioprine treatment in a patient with ulcerative colitis. Eur J Gastroenterol Hepatol. 2001;13:287–90.
101. Khokhar OS, Lewis JH. Hepatotoxicity of agents used in the management of inflammatory bowel disease. Dig Dis. 2010;28:508–18. doi:10.1159/000320410.
102. Dubinsky MC, Lamothe S, Yang HY, Targan SR, Sinnett D, Theoret Y, Seidman EG. Pharmacogenomics and metabolite measurement for 6-mercaptopurine therapy in inflammatory bowel disease. Gastroenterology. 2000;118:705–13.
103. Konidari A, Anagnostopoulos A, Bonnett LJ, Pirmohamed M, El-Matary W. Thiopurine monitoring in children with inflammatory bowel disease: a systematic review. Br J Clin Pharmacol. 2014;78:467–76. doi:10.1111/bcp.12365.
104. Connor V. Anti-TNF therapies: a comprehensive analysis of adverse effects associated with immunosuppression. Rheumatol Int. 2011;31:327–37. doi:10.1007/s00296-009-1292-x.
105. Vaz JL, Fernandes V, Nogueira F, Arnobio A, Levy RA. Infliximab-induced autoantibodies: a multicenter study. Clin Rheumatol. 2015; doi:10.1007/s10067-015-3140-6.
106. Weiler-Normann C, Schramm C, Quaas A, et al. Infliximab as a rescue treatment in difficult-to-treat autoimmune hepatitis. J Hepatol. 2013;58:529–34. doi:10.1016/j.jhep.2012.11.010.
107. Ghabril M, Bonkovsky HL, Kum C, et al. Liver injury from tumor necrosis factor-alpha antagonists: analysis of thirty-four cases. Clin Gastroenterol Hepatol. 2013;11:558–564.e553. doi:10.1016/j.cgh.2012.12.025.
108. Shelton E, Chaudrey K, Sauk J, et al. New onset idiosyncratic liver enzyme elevations with biological therapy in inflammatory bowel disease. Aliment Pharmacol Ther. 2015;41:972–9. doi:10.1111/apt.13159.
109. Bjornsson ES, Gunnarsson BI, Grondal G, et al. Risk of drug-induced liver injury from tumor necrosis factor antagonists. Clin Gastroenterol Hepatol. 2015;13:602–8. doi:10.1016/j.cgh.2014.07.062.
110. Loras C, Gisbert JP, Minguez M, et al. Liver dysfunction related to hepatitis B and C in patients with inflammatory bowel disease treated with immunosuppressive therapy. Gut. 2010;59:1340–6. doi:10.1136/gut.2010.208413.
111. Lin MV, Blonski W, Buchner AM, Reddy KR, Lichtenstein GR. The influence of anti-TNF therapy on the course of chronic hepatitis C virus infection in patients with inflammatory bowel disease. Dig Dis Sci. 2013;58:1149–56.
112. Park SH, Yang SK, Park SK, et al. Efficacy of hepatitis A vaccination and factors impacting on seroconversion in patients with inflammatory bowel disease. Inflamm Bowel Dis. 2014;20:69–74. doi:10.1097/01.MIB.0000437736.91712.a1.
113. Boyer DL, Li BU, Fyda JN, Friedman RA. Sulfasalazine-induced hepatotoxicity in children with inflammatory bowel disease. J Pediatr Gastroenterol Nutr. 1989;8:528–32.
114. Bashir RM, Lewis JH. Hepatotoxicity of drugs used in the treatment of gastrointestinal disorders. Gastroenterol Clin North Am. 1995;24:937–67.
115. Jobanputra P, Amarasena R, Maggs F, et al. Hepatotoxicity associated with sulfasalazine in inflammatory arthritis: a case series
from a local surveillance of serious adverse events. BMC Musculoskelet Disord. 2008;9:48. doi:10.1186/1471-2474-9-48.
116. Ribe J, Benkov KJ, Thung SN, Shen SC, LeLeiko NS. Fatal massive hepatic necrosis: a probable hypersensitivity reaction to sulfasalazine. Am J Gastroenterol. 1986;81:205–8.
117. Namias A, Bhalotra R, Donowitz M. Reversible sulfasalazine induced granulomatous hepatitis. J Clin Gastroenterol. 1981;3:193–8.
118. Quallich LG, Greenson J, Haftel HM, Fontana RJ. Is it Crohn disease? A severe systemic granulomatous reaction to sulfasalazine in patient with rheumatoid arthritis. BMC Gastroenterol. 2001;1:8.
119. Ransford RA, Langman MJ. Sulphasalazine and mesalazine: serious adverse reactions re-evaluated on the basis of suspected adverse reaction reports to the Committee on Safety of Medicines. Gut. 2002;51:536–9.
120. Braun M, Fraser GM, Kunin M, Salamon F, Tur-Kaspa R. Mesalamine-induced granulomatous hepatitis. Am J Gastroenterol. 1999;94:1973–4. doi:10.1111/j.1572-0241.1999.01245.x.
121. Stelzer T, Kohler S, Marques Maggio E, Heuss LT. An unusual cause of febrile hepatitis. BMJ Case Rep. 2015; 2015. doi:10.1136/bcr-2014-205857.
122. Stoschus B, Meybehm M, Spengler U, Scheurlen C, Sauerbruch T. Cholestasis associated with mesalazine therapy in a patient with Crohn disease. J Hepatol. 1997;26:425–8.
123. Hautekeete ML, Bourgeois N, Potvin P, et al. Hypersensitivity with hepatotoxicity to mesalazine after hypersensitivity to sulfasalazine. Gastroenterology. 1992;103:1925–7.
124. Deltenre P, Berson A, Marcellin P, Degott C, Biour M, Pessayre D. Mesalazine (5-aminosalicylic acid) induced chronic hepatitis. Gut. 1999;44:886–8.
125. Sourianarayanane A, Garg G, Smith TH, Butt MI, McCullough AJ, Shen B. Risk factors of non-alcoholic fatty liver disease in patients with inflammatory bowel disease. J Crohns Colitis. 2013;7:e279–85. doi:10.1016/j.crohns.2012.10.015.
126. Kotlyar DS, Osterman MT, Diamond RH, et al. A systematic review of factors that contribute to hepatosplenic T-cell lymphoma in patients with inflammatory bowel disease. Clin Gastroenterol Hepatol. 2011;9:36–41 e31. doi:10.1016/j.cgh.2010.09.016.
127. Mason M, Siegel CA. Do inflammatory bowel disease therapies cause cancer? Inflamm Bowel Dis. 2013;19:1306–21. doi:10.1097/MIB.0b013e3182807618.
128. Deepak P, Sifuentes H, Sherid M, Stobaugh D, Sadozai Y, Ehrenpreis ED. T-cell non-Hodgkin's lymphomas reported to the FDA AERS with tumor necrosis factor-alpha (TNF-alpha) inhibitors: results of the REFURBISH study. Am J Gastroenterol. 2013;108:99–105. doi:10.1038/ajg.2012.334.
129. Gizard E, Ford AC, Bronowicki JP, Peyrin-Biroulet L. Systematic review: the epidemiology of the hepatobiliary manifestations in patients with inflammatory bowel disease. Aliment Pharmacol Ther. 2014;40:3–15. doi:10.1111/apt.12794.
130. Parente F, Pastore L, Bargiggia S, et al. Incidence and risk factors for gallstones in patients with inflammatory bowel disease: a large case-control study. Hepatology. 2007;45:1267–74. doi:10.1002/hep.21537.
131. Ehlin AG, Montgomery SM, Ekbom A, Pounder RE, Wakefield AJ. Prevalence of gastrointestinal diseases in two British national birth cohorts. Gut. 2003;52:1117–21.
132. Margalit M, Elinav H, Ilan Y, Shalit M. Liver abscess in inflammatory bowel disease: report of two cases and review of the literature. J Gastroenterol Hepatol. 2004;19:1338–42. doi:10.1111/j.1440-1746.2004.03368.x.
133. Kappelman MD, Horvath-Puho E, Sandler RS, et al. Thromboembolic risk among Danish children and adults with inflammatory bowel diseases: a population-based nationwide study. Gut. 2011;60:937–43. doi:10.1136/gut.2010.228585.
134. Nylund CM, Goudie A, Garza JM, Crouch G, Denson LA. Venous thrombotic events in hospitalized children and adolescents with inflammatory bowel disease. J Pediatr Gastroenterol Nutr. 2013;56:485–91. doi:10.1097/MPG.0b013e3182801e43.

135. Maconi G, Bolzacchini E, Dell'Era A, Russo U, Ardizzone S, de Franchis R. Portal vein thrombosis in inflammatory bowel diseases: a single-center case series. J Crohns Colitis. 2012;6:362–7. doi:10.1016/j.crohns.2011.10.003.

136. Kraut J, Berman JH, Gunasekaran TS, Allen R, McFadden J, Messersmith R, Pellettiere E. Hepatic vein thrombosis (Budd-Chiari syndrome) in an adolescent with ulcerative colitis. J Pediatr Gastroenterol Nutr. 1997;25:417–20.

137. Rahhal RM, Pashankar DS, Bishop WP. Ulcerative colitis complicated by ischemic colitis and Budd Chiari syndrome. J Pediatr Gastroenterol Nutr. 2005;40:94–7.

138. Socha P, Ryzko J, Janczyk W, Dzik E, Iwanczak B, Krzesiek E. Hepatic vein thrombosis as a complication of ulcerative colitis in a 12-year-old patient. Dig Dis Sci. 2007;52:1293–8. doi:10.1007/s10620-006-9503-8.

139. Greenstein AJ, Sachar DB, Panday AK, et al. Amyloidosis and inflammatory bowel disease. A 50-year experience with 25 patients. Medicine (Baltimore). 1992;71:261–70.

140. Serra I, Oller B, Manosa M, Naves JE, Zabana Y, Cabre E, Domenech E. Systemic amyloidosis in inflammatory bowel disease: retrospective study on its prevalence, clinical presentation, and outcome. J Crohns Colitis. 2010;4:269–74. doi:10.1016/j.crohns.2009.11.009.

141. Wester AL, Vatn MH, Fausa O. Secondary amyloidosis in inflammatory bowel disease: a study of 18 patients admitted to Rikshospitalet University Hospital, Oslo, from 1962 to 1998. Inflamm Bowel Dis. 2001;7:295–300.

142. Sattianayagam PT, Gillmore JD, Pinney JH, et al. Inflammatory bowel disease and systemic AA amyloidosis. Dig Dis Sci. 2013;58:1689–97. doi:10.1007/s10620-012-2549-x.

143. Tada F, Abe M, Nunoi H, et al. Ulcerative colitis complicated with primary biliary cirrhosis. Intern Med. 2011;50:2323–7. doi:10.2169/internalmedicine.50.5919.

144. Xiao WB, Liu YL. Primary biliary cirrhosis and ulcerative colitis: a case report and review of literature. World J Gastroenterol. 2003;9:878–80.

Growth Impairment in Pediatric Inflammatory Bowel Disease

Thomas D. Walters and Anne M. Griffiths

Introduction

The clinical course and severity of inflammatory bowel disease (IBD) vary widely in children and in adults [1, 2]. Unique to pediatric patient populations, however, is the potential for linear growth impairment as a complication of chronic intestinal inflammation. The challenge in treating each child or adolescent is to employ pharmacological, nutritional, and where appropriate, surgical interventions, to not only decrease mucosal inflammation and thereby alleviate symptoms, but also to optimize growth and normalize associated pubertal and social development. Indeed, normal growth is a marker of therapeutic success. This chapter reviews the prevalence of growth impairment in pediatric IBD, discusses its pathophysiology, and outlines strategies for its prevention and management.

Normal Growth and Pubertal Development

"Normal" children grow at very different rates. Patterns of growth and pubertal progression in young patients with IBD can only be accurately recognized as pathological, if the variations in normal development of healthy children and adolescents are first appreciated. A child's growth is the result of both genes and environment; it appears principally mediated by hormones and nutrition [3]. Linear growth can be represented by stature (attained height) or by the rate of growth (height velocity). A child's attained height represents the culmination of

growth in all preceding years; height velocity reflects growth status at a particular point in time.

Normal Growth Patterns

Growth can be conceptualized as the product of three overlapping biological phases: infancy, childhood, and puberty. Final height represents the sum of each of the individual components.

Linear growth velocity decreases from birth onwards, punctuated by a short period of growth acceleration (the "adolescent growth spurt") just prior to completion of growth. As the rapid growth of infancy tails off, the steady growth of childhood predominates. Healthy children grow at a consistent rate in the range of 4–6 cm annually from 6 years of age until the onset of puberty [4].

At puberty, there is a rapid alteration in body size, shape, and composition; for a year or more, height velocity approximately doubles. Puberty depends on a healthy hypothalamic-pituitary-gonadal (HPG) axis and is marked by the return of gonadotropin-releasing hormone (GnRH) secretion. GnRH stimulates the secretion of luteinizing and follicle-stimulating hormones, which then stimulate gonadal maturation and sex steroid production [5]. Although much is known about the components of the HPG axis, the factors that trigger pubertal onset remain elusive [5]. The age of onset of puberty, and hence of the pubertal growth spurt, varies among normal individuals and between ethnic populations. Puberty begins earlier in girls than in boys; moreover, the pubertal growth spurt occurs in midpuberty (prior to menarche) in girls but in late puberty (after Tanner stage 4) in boys [4]. There is hence quite consistently a 2-year difference in the timing of peak height velocity (PHV) in girls compared to boys [4]. In North American females, PHV occurs at a mean age of 11.5 years, but in males not until 13.5 years (2SD = 1.8 years) [4]. The occurrence of menarche is an indication that linear growth is nearing completion; usually girls gain only 5–8 cm more in height within the 2 subsequent years [4].

T.D. Walters, MBBS, MSc, FRACP (✉)
A.M. Griffiths, MD, FRAP(C)
Division of Gastroenterology, Hepatology and Nutrition, The Hospital for Sick Children, University of Toronto, 555 University Avenue, Toronto, ON M5G 1X8, Canada
e-mail: thomas.walters@sickkids.ca

© Springer International Publishing AG 2017
P. Mamula et al. (eds.), *Pediatric Inflammatory Bowel Disease*, DOI 10.1007/978-3-319-49215-5_12

Normal Growth Physiology

To understand the mechanisms by which growth is inhibited in children with IBD, and to thoughtfully consider solutions by which it might be corrected, it is necessary to understand the normal physiology and regulation of growth. The growth hormone/insulin-like growth factor-1 (GH/IGF-1) axis plays a pivotal role in normal postnatal growth. Thyroxine, cortisol, and the sex steroids are also implicated in the maintenance of normal linear growth.

The GH/IGF-1 Axis

The Somatomedin Hypothesis
In 1956, Daughaday and Salmon proposed that an intermediate hormone they termed "somatomedin C" mediated all the growth-promoting effects of growth hormone (GH). This hormone was subsequently purified and named "insulin-like growth factor-1" (IGF-1) [6–8] and found to act in both an "endocrine" fashion, via its hepatic generation and subsequent release into the circulation, as well as in an "autocrine/paracrine" fashion, through its local generation within target organs [9, 10]. More recent work has determined that, by acting on different cell types, both hormones (GH and IGF-1) can directly stimulate longitudinal growth: GH induces differentiation of epiphyseal growth plate precursor cells toward chondrocytes, which in turn become responsive to IGF-1, while IGF-1 stimulates the clonal expansion of differentiated chondrocytes [10, 11] (Fig. 12.1).

Growth Hormone and IGF-1
The precise mechanism by which GH is released and subsequently stimulates the release of IGF-1 is now well established [12–16] (Fig. 12.2). In humans, the majority of circulating IGF-1 is synthesized in the liver, although a low level of GH-dependent and GH-independent IGF-1 expression does occur in extrahepatic tissues.

Gender Differences in the GH/IGF-1 Pathway
GH is released in a pulsatile pattern that is gender-specific, with males experiencing higher peaks and deeper troughs compared to females [18]. Interestingly, STAT5 exists in two genetically distinct, although highly homologous, forms (STAT5A and STAT5B) [19], which are known to differ somewhat in their tissue distribution [20]. Of note, while STAT5A and STAT5B are both required for normal GH-dependent growth, STAT5B is responsive to pulsatile GH, whereas STAT5A is not. Indeed, STAT5B-deficient male mice have pronounced growth impairment, and tend to grow at a rate similar to normal females. Thus, the complex regulation of sexually dimorphic growth appears to be mediated, at least in part, by STAT5B "interpreting" the differing GH pulsatile secretion patterns of males versus

females [19]. Given this, it seems plausible that any interference within the GH/STAT5B/IGF-1 pathway is likely to have a more pronounced effect on growth patterns in males than females.

Insulin-like Growth Factor Binding Proteins (IGFBPs)
The bioavailability of IGF-1 depends on its unbound or "free" fraction. Six specific high-affinity IGF-1 binding proteins (IGFBP-1 to IGFBP-6) are present within the circulation and can each bind IGF-1 with an affinity at least equal to the binding of IGF-1 to the IGF receptor [21]. The IGFBPs are each regulated by specific proteases that dramatically reduce their IGF-1 binding affinity. The specific function and structure of the six IGFBPs differ significantly [22]. IGFBP-1,-2,-4, and -6 primarily inhibit IGF-1 by tightly binding to it and preventing it from binding to its receptor [21, 23, 24]. Conversely, IGFBP-3 potentiates the action of IGF-1 by "loosely" binding to it, thus prolonging the time it is available within the circulation to interact with its receptor. About 75% of IGF-1 circulates as a 150 kDa ternary complex composed of IGF-1, acid-labile subunit (ALS), and IGFBP-3 [21]. This large complex, which cannot cross the endothelial barrier [25], significantly increases the half-life of IGF-1 from <10 min to >16 h [21]. Caloric and protein restriction can cause a reduction in the levels of IGFBP-3 [26, 27].

Growth Plate Proliferation, Senescence, and Fusion
The normal age-dependent decline in growth rate is due primarily to a senescent decline in the rate of growth plate chondrocyte proliferation [28, 29] referred to as "growth plate senescence" [30–32]. The proliferative capacity of the "stem-like" cells within the resting zone of the growth plate is finite. Thus, "senescence" is not a function of time per se, but of proliferative cycle number. Given this, it becomes apparent that interventions that slow the proliferation rate of growth plate chondrocytes, such as glucocorticoid exposure, will also slow the rate of growth plate senescence [31, 33]. That is to say, following transient growth inhibition, growth plates are "less senescent," retaining a greater proliferative capacity than expected for age. Thus, in the "postinhibitory period," the growth plate will show a greater growth rate than expected for age, resulting in "catch-up growth," the apparently "accelerated" linear growth that occurs after resolution of a growth-inhibiting condition [32, 34].

The pubertal growth spurt is primarily induced by estrogen, which acts to increase the activity of the GH/IGF-1 axis [35, 36]. In addition, the sex steroids, especially the androgens, appear to stimulate growth by a direct effect on growth plate chondrocytes [37–39]. Estrogen is also known to be the key hormone that promotes epiphyseal fusion [30].

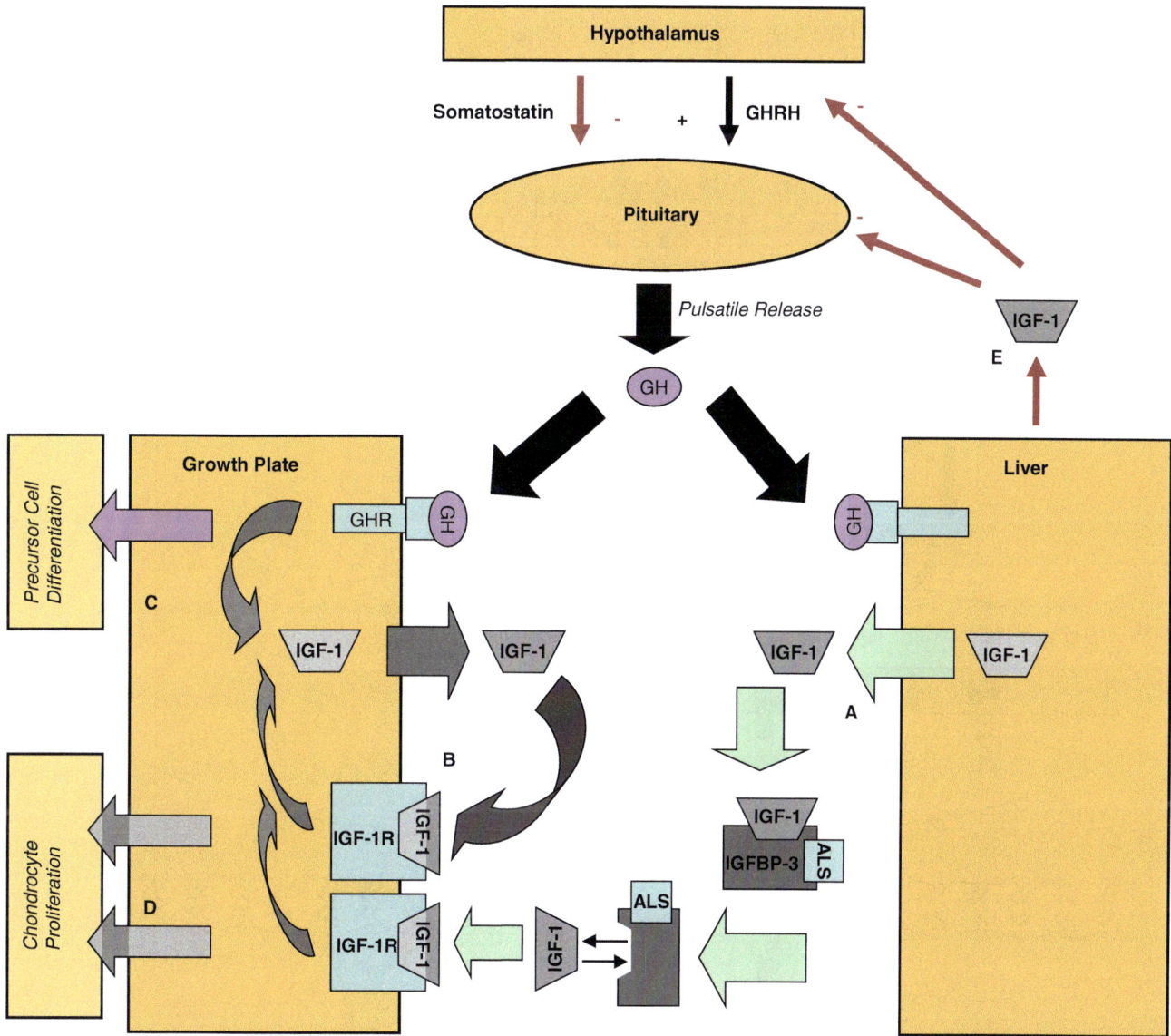

Fig. 12.1 The GH/IGF-1 axis and its role in linear growth. The hypothalamic release of growth hormone releasing hormone (*GHRH*) stimulates the pulsatile release of growth hormone (*GH*) from the pituitary. The GH cell surface receptor (*GHR*) is widely expressed throughout the body. GH binds to the extracellular domain of GHR, inducing the upregulation of various anabolic target genes including insulin-like growth factor 1 (*IGF-1*). The majority of circulating IGF-1 forms a ternary complex with acid-labile subunit (*ALS*) and insulin-like growth factor binding protein-3 (*IGFBP-3*). IGF-1 acts in both an "endocrine fashion" (process *A*) and "autocrine/paracrine" fashion (process *B*). In addition to upregulating IGF-1 production, GH contributes directly to linear growth by inducing differentiation of the precursor cells within the growth plate toward chondrocytes [*C*]. IGF-1 stimulates mitosis of epiphyseal chondrocytes [*D*] and also mediates the negative feedback of GH [*E*]

Monitoring and Assessment of Growth

Standardized charts are available for graphically recording height, weight, and height velocity, such that an individual child's growth can be compared to normative values [40–42]. Wherever possible, reference data most appropriate to the child being monitored should be utilized. An individual child's growth measurement can be represented as a percentile or as a standard deviation score, a quantitative expression of distance from the reference population mean (50th percentile) for the same age and gender [43]. Healthy children grow steadily along the same height percentile and hence maintain the same standard deviation score for height from early childhood through until adulthood. Combined parental heights can be used to estimate a child's potential height [43]. Some temporary deviation from the usual growth channel may occur if the pubertal growth spurt occurs particularly early (temporary increase in height velocity and height centiles) or late (temporary decrease in height velocity and height centiles).

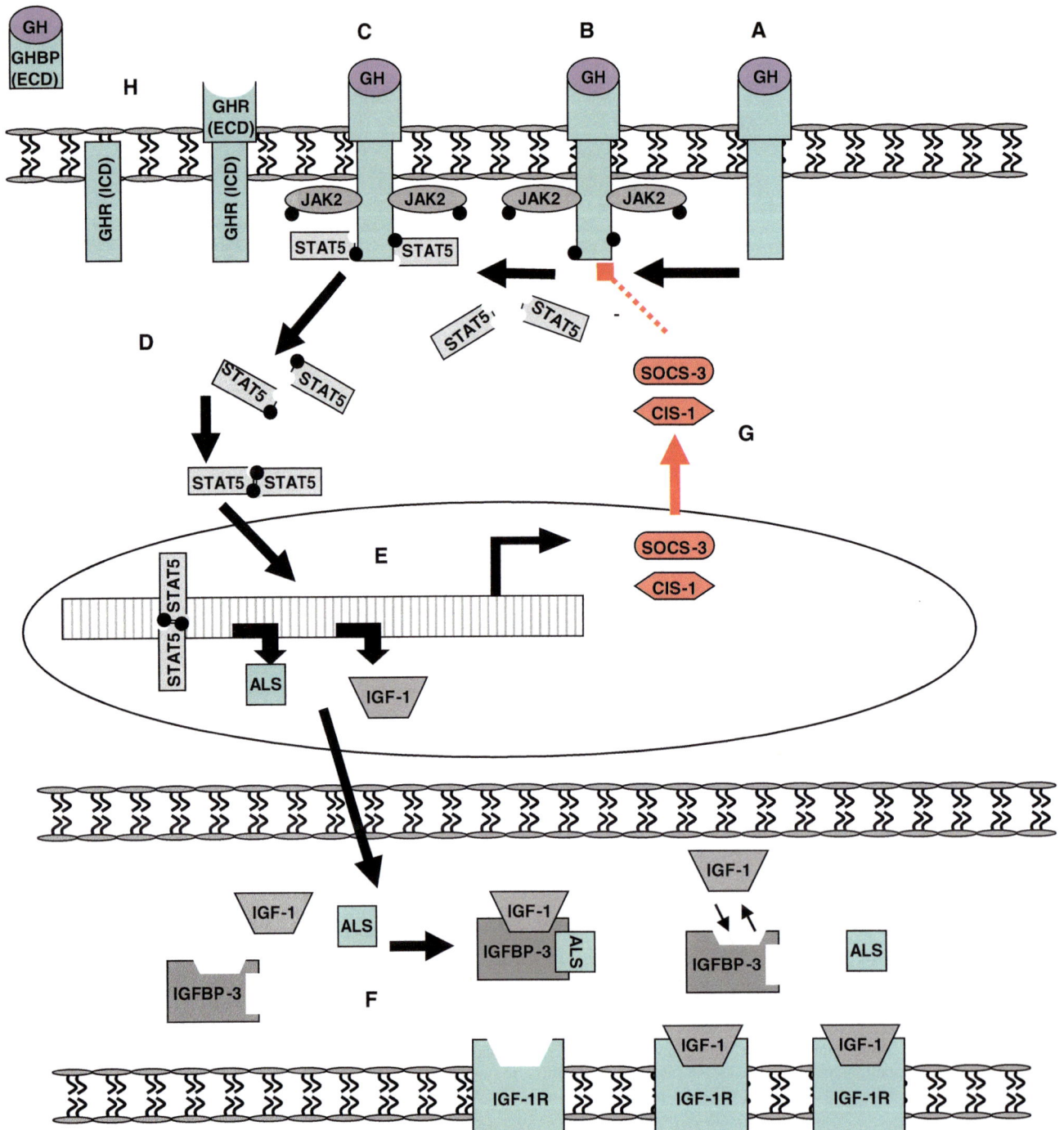

Fig. 12.2 The growth hormone receptor and JAK2/STAT5 signaling pathway. [A] Within its various target tissues, GH binds to the extracellular domain of the growth hormone receptor (*GHR*), [B] inducing the intracellular autophosphorylation of Janus kinase 2 (JAK2). [C] In turn, phosphorylated JAK2, in association with activated GHR, leads to the phosphorylation of signal transducer and activator of transcription protein 5 (*STAT5*). [D] Activated STAT5 dimerizes and then [E] translocates to the nucleus, resulting in the upregulation of various anabolic target genes including IGF-1 and acid-labile subunit (*ALS*) [13–15]. [F] IGF-1 and ALS pass to the circulation and form ternary complexes with insulin-like growth factor binding protein (*IGFBP*), about 75% as a 150 kDa complex with IGFBP-3. [G]

Suppressors of cytokine signaling (*SOCS*) proteins are postreceptor inhibitors of cell signaling that mediate their effect via the JAK/STAT pathway [16]. GH rapidly and prominently induces expression of SOCS-3 and cytokine-inducible SH2-containing protein-1 (*CIS-1*) within the liver as part of a negative feedback loop that functions by blocking the phosphorylation of STAT5. SOCS-3 inhibits JAK2 by a mechanism requiring GHR. [H] The GHR has both an intracellular and extracellular domain (*ICD* and *ECD*). Growth hormone receptor binding protein (*GHBP*), present within the circulation, is produced by the inducible metalloproteolytic cleavage of the GHR's extracellular domain. Serum concentrations of this protein are thought to reflect GHR density [17]

Definitions of Impaired Growth

Within a large patient group, skewing of standard deviation scores (SDS) for height below population reference values is evidence of disease-associated growth impairment. Mean height SDS of a population characterized by normal growth approximates zero. Growth disturbance in an individual child is indicated by an abnormal growth rate [43]. A definition in terms of static height measurement, although sometimes used, may be misleading, since it is so influenced by parental heights. An individual child may be normally short; conversely, a previously tall child may not have increased his height in 2 years, but still be of average stature. A shift from higher to lower centiles on a growth chart of height attained more sensibly signifies growth faltering. Height velocity, expressed either as a centile or as a standard deviation score for age and gender, is the most sensitive parameter by which to recognize impaired growth.

Growth in Pediatric IBD

Prevalence of Growth Impairment in IBD

Inflammatory disease occurring during early adolescence is likely to have a major impact on nutritional status and growth because of the very rapid accumulation of lean body mass that normally occurs at this time. Further, boys are more vulnerable to disturbances in growth than girls, because their growth spurt comes later and is ultimately longer and greater [4, 44].

Crohn Disease

Several studies have characterized the growth of children with Crohn disease as treated in the 1980s and into the 1990s [1, 45–50]. These studies are important as a benchmark of outcomes with traditional therapy. It is to be hoped that the now better understanding of the pathogenesis of growth impairment, together with the greater efficacy of current therapeutic regimens in healing intestinal inflammation, may lead to enhanced growth of young patients diagnosed now.

As summarized in Table 12.1,

The estimated percentage of patients with Crohn disease, whose growth is affected, varies with the time of assessment, the definition of growth impairment, and with the nature of the population under study (tertiary referral center versus population-based) [1, 45–55]. It has nevertheless been consistently observed that impairment of linear growth is common prior to recognition of Crohn disease as well as during the subsequent years, and that height at maturity has often been compromised [1, 45–52, 54–57]. More recent

Table 12.1 Prevalence of linear growth impairment in pediatric Crohn disease

Study details (Ref.)	Time of assessment	Patients studied	n	Definition of linear growth impairment	Percentage with growth impairment (%)
Baltimore, USA 1961–1985 [46]	At diagnosis	Prepubertal (Tanner 1 or 2)	50	Decrease in height velocity prior to diagnosis	88
Toronto, Canada 1980–1988 [1]	During follow-up	Prepubertal (Tanner 1 or 2)	100	Height velocity ≤2 SD for age ≥2 years	49
Sweden 1983–1987 [47]	During follow-up	Population-based cohort <16 years at Dx	46	Height velocity ≤ 2 SD for age 1 year	65
New York, USA 1979–1989 [48]	At maturity	Children in tertiary care	38	Failure to reach predicted adult height	37
Toronto, Canada 1990–1999 [50]	During follow-up	Prepubertal (Tanner 1 or 2)	161	Height velocity ≤ 2 SD for age ≥ 2 years	54
United Kingdom 1998–1999 [51]	At diagnosis	Population-based cohort <16 years at Dx	338	Height SDS <−1.96	13
Israel 1991–2003 [52]	At diagnosis	Children in tertiary care	93	Height SDS <−2.0	20
France 1988–2004 [53]	At diagnosis	Population-based cohort <17 years at Dx	261	Height SDS <−2.0	9.5

Varying definitions and times of assessment (at the time of diagnosis and during follow-up) are applied

data from the UK and the USA suggest that the degree of deficit at maturity may be slowly reducing [57, 58]. It is also apparent that these problems are, and remain, more frequent among males than females, independent of the disease location or severity [1, 53, 56, 59–62]. The basis of this observed gender difference is yet to be fully elucidated. Interestingly, as the incidence of CD increases in geographical regions where it was previously rare, reports demonstrate that similar patterns of impaired growth are being observed [63, 64].

At the time of diagnosis, mean standard deviation score (SDS) for height is reduced among children with Crohn's disease as a group compared to reference populations (Table 12.2),

an indication of the growth retardation occurring prior to recognition and treatment of intestinal inflammation [1, 46, 47, 50–52]. During the decade 1990–1999, in Toronto, mean SDS for height at the time of diagnosis among 161 Tanner stage 1 or 2 children was -0.74 ± 1.2 [50], indicating overall lesser growth delay in comparison to the earlier decade [1]. Nevertheless, the percentage of children with height less than the 5th centile (SDS score <-1.8), based on the Center for Disease Control 2000 data, was still 22% [50]. Mean

SDS for height among 333 patients aged <16 years was -0.54 (95% CI -0.67 to -0.41) in a 1998–1999 population-based surveillance study of incident IBD in the United Kingdom [51]. Thirteen percent were below the third centile (SDS <-1.96) for height based on data from Child Growth Foundation, London [51]. In Israel, SDS for height at diagnosis among a cohort of 93 patients aged <18 years was -0.56 ± 1.16, but 20% had SDS score <-2.0 [52]. Taken together, these data confirm that growth delay prior to diagnosis remains a challenge [50–52].

Delay in epiphyseal closure allows growth to continue longer than normal. Hence, mean SDS for height may improve over the course of treatment, when the chronic inflammation can be controlled [1, 47, 50]. No population-based cohort studies have compared pre-illness height centiles with final adult stature in order to determine how often catch-up growth is complete. In spite of gains, past and current reports suggest that the mean adult height of patients with prepubertal onset of disease remains reduced compared to population reference data [1, 47, 50, 54–58]. Studies suggesting otherwise have included patients with postpubertal onset of disease, and therefore not at risk for growth impairment [65].

Table 12.2 Mean height standard deviation scores for height in children diagnosed with Crohn disease prior to or in early puberty (Tanner stage 1 or 2)

Study (Ref.)	Patients studied	n	Mean height SDS (SD)	
			at diagnosis	at maturity
Baltimore, USA 1961–1985 [46]	Prepubertal (Tanner 1 or 2)	50	−0.48	Not assessed
Toronto, Canada 1980–1988 [1]	Prepubertal (Tanner 1 or 2)	100	−1.1 (1.3)	−0.82 (1.1)
Sweden 1983–1987 [47]	Population-based cohort <16 years at Dx	46	−0.5 (1.4)	−0.4 (1.1)
Toronto, Canada 1990–1999 [50]	Prepubertal (Tanner 1 or 2)	161	−0.74 (1.2)	−0.70 (1.2)
United Kingdom 1998–1999 [51]	Population-based cohort <16 years at Dx	338	−0.54	Not assessed
Israel 1991–2003 [52]	Children in tertiary care	93	−0.56 (1.16)	Not assessed
Leiden, The Netherlands Reported in 2002 [55]	Children in tertiary care	64	Not reported	−0.9 (1.2)
London, UK 1996–2002 [54]	Prepubertal children in tertiary care	20	Not reported	−0.57 (0.3)
Finland 1987–2003 [56]	Population-based cohort <17 years at Dx	128	Not reported	Male: −0.56 Female: −0.24

Ulcerative Colitis

Cohort data are sparse in comparison to Crohn disease, but in general, at diagnosis, no significant reduction is observed in height-for-age standard deviation scores among young patients with ulcerative colitis compared to the reference population [47, 49, 51]. As an example, SDS for height was not reduced (mean −0.12, 95% CI −0.30 to 0.05) in 143 children and adolescents with incident UC in the British pediatric surveillance study [51].

In follow-up, growth impairment remains a less frequent complication, although relatively few studies have carefully described linear growth in ulcerative colitis as compared to the abundance of studies in Crohn disease. Hildebrand et al. observed that 11 (24%) of 45 children had a height velocity <−2.0 SD during at least 1 year [47]. Final attained mean height was comparable to reference population data in this study [47].

Why linear growth impairment is less common in ulcerative colitis than in Crohn disease is not entirely clear. Certainly, the interval between symptom onset and diagnosis correlates with the degree of growth impairment [51, 58, 66]. The usual colitic symptom of bloody diarrhea in ulcerative colitis is more promptly investigated than the often subtle presenting symptoms of Crohn disease, particularly the nonspecific abdominal pain and anorexia associated with small bowel Crohn disease, and this may account at least in part for the lesser effect on growth prior to diagnosis. Disease-related differences in cytokine production are likely also important. Notably, pubertal delay can contribute to growth impairment, and Crohn disease is more frequently associated with delayed puberty [44, 67, 68].

Sex Differences in Linear Growth Impairment

As mentioned, growth impairment is both more frequent and more severe in boys compared to girls with Crohn disease [1, 62]. These differences persist post diagnosis [56].

Pathophysiology of Growth Impairment in IBD

As summarized in Table 12.3, several interrelated factors contribute to linear growth impairment in children with IBD.

The fundamental mechanisms have recently been comprehensively reviewed [69].

Chronic Caloric Insufficiency

Growth requires energy. Chronic undernutrition has long been implicated and remains an important and remediable cause of growth retardation [70]. Multiple factors contribute to malnutrition [71]. However, reduced intake, rather than excessive loss or increased need, is generally the major cause of the caloric insufficiency [72, 73]. Kirschner et al. reported

Table 12.3 Factors contributing to growth impairment in children with Crohn disease

Factor	Explanation
Proinflammatory cytokines	Direct interference with IGF-1 mediation of linear growth
Decreased food intake	Cytokine-mediated anorexia, fear of worsening gastrointestinal symptoms
Stool losses	Mucosal damage leading to protein-losing enteropathy; diffuse small intestinal disease or resection leading to steatorrhea
Increased nutritional needs	Fever; required catch-up growth
Corticosteroid treatment	Interference with growth hormone and insulin-like growth factor-1

caloric intakes of growth-impaired patients to average 54% of that recommended for children of similar height age [74]. Food restriction may be deliberate, to avoid symptoms. More importantly, cytokine-mediated disease-related anorexia may be profound. Work in a rat model of colitis suggests that tumor necrosis factor alpha (TNFα) and interleukin-1 interact with hypothalamic appetite pathways via serotonin receptors [75, 76]. Human studies have demonstrated an association between inflammatory cytokines and alterations in gut hormones related to appetite such as ghrelin [77] and polypeptide YY [78]. While clinical studies have demonstrated that significant intestinal fat malabsorption is uncommon [79], leakage of protein is frequent [80]. However, neither have been shown to be common causes of undernutrition in Crohn disease. In general, resting energy expenditure (REE) does not differ from normal in patients with inactive disease, but can exceed predicted rates in the presence of fever and sepsis [81]. Moreover, malnourished adolescents with CD fail to reduce their REE as efficiently as comparably malnourished patients with anorexia nervosa [81]. Reduction in REE is a normal biological response to conserve energy. This relative failure of a compensatory mechanism has, again, been attributed to the effects of proinflammatory cytokines.

Direct Cytokine Effects

A simple nutritional hypothesis, where adequate caloric delivery would remediate any growth impairment, fails to explain all the observations related to growth patterns among children with IBD. To date, a variety of cytokines have been implicated in the pathogenesis of IBD including tumor necrosis factor alpha (TNFα), interferon-gamma (IFN-gamma), and multiple interleukins (including IL-6, IL-12, IL-17, and IL-23). The direct growth-inhibiting effects of proinflammatory cytokines released from the inflamed intestine have been increasingly recognized [82–85].

Disruption of the GH/IGF-1 Axis

As described above, IGF-1, produced by the liver in response to GH stimulation, is the key mediator of GH effects at the growth plate of bones. An association between impaired growth in children with Crohn disease and low IGF-1 levels is well recognized [86]. However, GH production in this setting has been shown to be normal [87]. The molecular mechanisms by which cytokines induce this state of "GH resistance" have not yet been completely elucidated. Conceptually, they could involve downregulation of the GH receptor (GHR), upregulation of postreceptor inhibitory proteins, reduced protein synthesis, and/or increased protein degradation. Information from both animal models and/or human studies supports each of these potential mechanisms [15, 16, 82, 84, 88–101] (Fig. 12.3).

IGF-1 Independent Mechanisms

Inflammatory cytokines inhibit linear growth through pathways other than IGF-1 production. Animal experiments have shown that TNFα and interleukin-1 (IL-1) increase chondro-

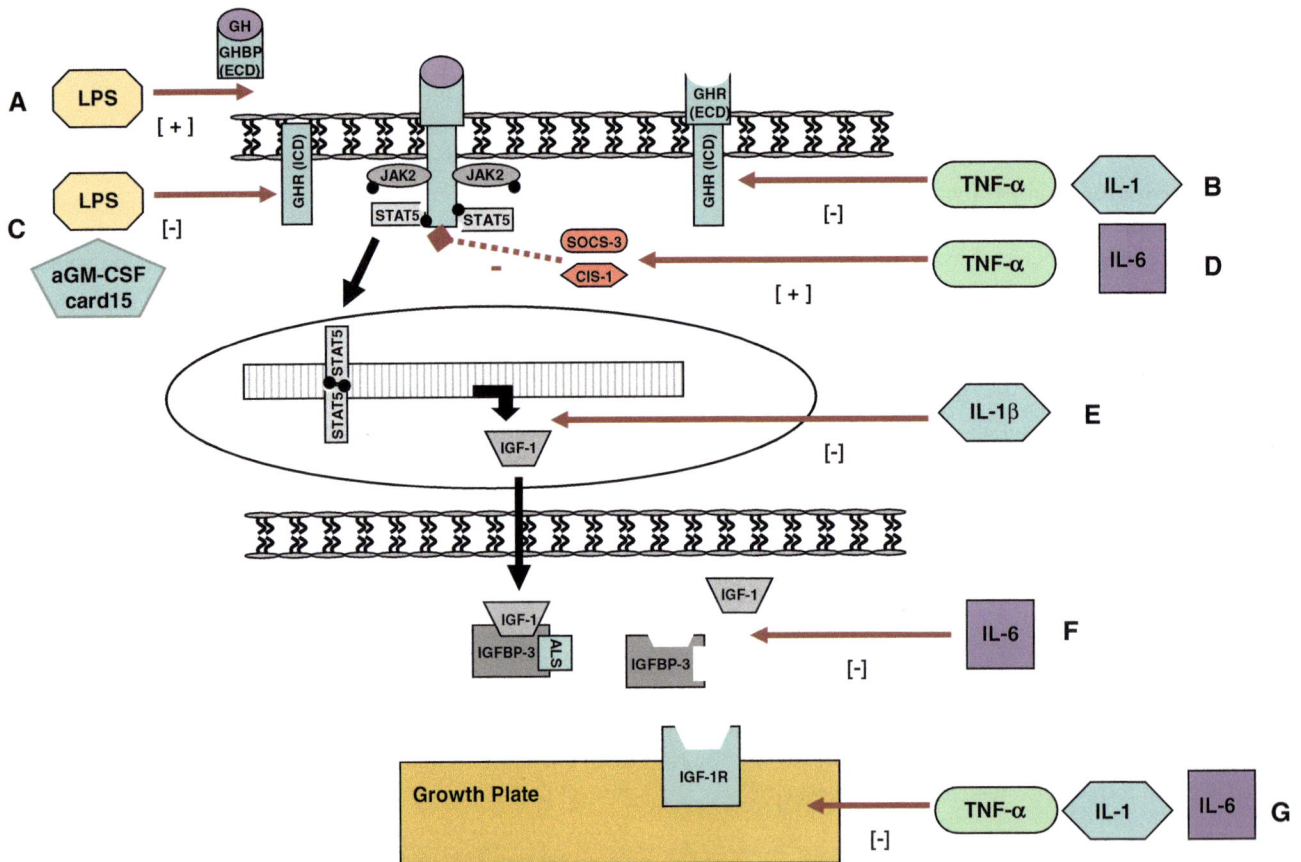

Fig. 12.3 Confirmed and potential molecular mechanisms that underpin the development of GH resistance in Crohn disease: *At the growth hormone receptor*: [A] Endotoxin exposure, specifically lipopolysaccharide (*LPS*), reduces GHR density by inducing GHR proteolysis and increasing the shedding of GHBP [88] (mechanism not yet ascertained). [B] TNFα has been demonstrated to downregulate GHR formation via inhibition of Sp1/Sp3's ability to transactivate the *GHR* gene [89]. IL-1 suppresses GHR promoter activity [89]. [C] LPS can directly inhibit GHR gene expression via a cytokine-independent mechanism through the TLR-4/MD2 signaling pathway that results in a cytokine response, significant reduction in GHR promoter activity. Importantly, the addition of anti-TNFα antibody failed to abrogate this effect [90]. Innate immune pathways associated with granulocyte-macrophage colony-stimulating factor autoantibodies and card15 deficiency can also reduce GHR expression [101]. *Via postreceptor inhibitory proteins*: [D] IL-6 and TNFα can upregulate the expression of SOCS-3 and cytokine-inducible SH2-containing protein (*CIS*)1 [15, 91]. Both of these proteins have, in turn, been shown to inhibit GH signaling by blocking the phosphorylation of STAT5 [16, 92, 93]. *Via reduced protein synthesis*: [E] IL-1β has been shown to reduce IGF-1 mRNA levels. The mechanism is yet to be elucidated, but does not appear to be via upregulation of SOCS nor by impairment of JAK2/STAT5 signaling [94]. *Via increased protein clearance*: [F] IL-6 has been implicated in a reduction in IGFBP-3 levels due to either reduced production and/or increased proteolysis [95]. Previously, low levels of IGFBP-3 have been associated with accelerated clearance, and hence lower levels, of IGF-1 [95]. *Via IGF-1 independent mechanisms*: [G] Animal experiments have shown that TNFα and interleukin-1 (IL-1) increase chondrocyte death and thus may have a deleterious effect on growth [84]. Cytokines appear to impair end-organ responsiveness to circulating testosterone [96]. IL-6 exposure promotes osteoclast maturation and activation, affects osteoblasts, is associated with osteoclast/osteoblast uncoupling, and results in thinning of the growth plates [82, 97–100]. Although the mechanism is yet to be determined, laboratory evidence suggests that it is independent of IGF-1 [97]

cyte death, and thus may have a deleterious effect on growth [84]. In an organ culture model of fetal rat parietal bone, marked impairment in osteoblast function and bone growth was observed with the addition of serum from children with CD, but not from children with ulcerative colitis, nor from healthy controls [85]. Finally, cytokines appear to impair end-organ responsiveness to circulating testosterone, thereby compounding the effects of undernutrition in delaying progression through puberty [96].

The Role of IL-6 in Growth Impairment

As with a number of chronic inflammatory conditions, IL-6 is known to be elevated in the serum of pediatric patients with active CD and predictive of clinical relapse [102]. IL-6 activates STAT3 via the glycoprotein 130 signaling receptor (gp130), a process that is negatively regulated by SOCS-3 [103–105]. SOCS-3 is also a negative regulator of GH signaling. Very recently, it was confirmed that IL-6:STAT3 activation correlates with mucosal inflammation in active pediatric-onset CD [106, 107].

Transgenic mice with defective growth have been found to overexpress interleukin-6 (IL-6). Antibody to IL-6 partially corrected the growth defect, whereas administration of IL-6 led to a decrease in IGF-1 before food intake was affected [82]. Similar to CD, children with juvenile idiopathic arthritis (JIA) also present with linear growth failure [108, 109]. Of note, IGF-1 levels are negatively correlated with IL-6 among this patient group [82]. The exact mechanism underpinning this observation, however, is not completely clear. While these, and other data [110], suggest an IL-6 mediated decrease in IGF-1 *production* [82] work by DeBenedetti et al. suggests that the primary mechanism is a reduction in IGFBP-3 levels due to reduced production and/or increased proteolysis of this binding protein [95]. Previously, low levels of IGFBP-3 have been associated with accelerated clearance, and hence, low levels of IGF-1 [95].

Recent studies in both these pediatric patient groups have demonstrated a significant "uncoupling" of osteoblast and osteoclast activities [97, 111–113]. Concurrent mouse and human studies have shown that chronic IL-6 exposure promotes osteoclast maturation and activation, affects osteoblasts, and is associated with osteoclast/osteoblast uncoupling, and results in thinning of the growth plates [82, 97–100]. Again, while the mechanism is yet to be determined, laboratory evidence suggests that it is independent of IGF-1 [97].

Taken together, these data suggest that increased IL-6 may represent a major generalized mechanism by which chronic inflammation affects the developing skeleton. This would imply that anti-IL6 therapeutic approaches, which have shown promising anti-inflammatory efficacy in CD, rheumatoid arthritis, and systemic JIA [114–117], may also specifically address the problem of growth impairment.

Notably, in a rat model with TNBS-induced colitis and poor growth, treatment with an anti-IL6 antibody enhanced IGF-1 expression and growth without reducing intestinal inflammation [110].

The Interplay Between Nutrition and Cytokines

Thus, inflammation may have a direct effect on linear growth, via the mechanisms described above, as well as an indirect effect via its effect on the appetite centers of the brain and subsequent reduction in caloric intake. The relative contributions of malnutrition and inflammation to linear growth delay were explored by Ballinger et al. using a rat model of TNBS colitis [83]. Two control groups were used: healthy controls with free access to food, and a pair-fed group comprised of healthy animals with daily food intake restricted to match that of colitic rats [83]. In the colitic rats, IGF-1 levels were reduced to 35% of control values. Comparison with the healthy but undernourished pair-fed rats suggested that malnutrition accounted for 53% of the total depression of IGF-1 in colitic rats, with the remaining 47% directly attributable to inflammation [83].

Disruption of the GH/IGF-1 Axis by Cytokine-Independent Molecular Pathways

Impaired intestinal barrier function is a recognized feature in some patients with CD, and may predispose them to chronic, subclinical, endotoxin exposure, specifically lipopolysaccharide (LPS) [118]. Various groups are currently investigating whether LPS directly interferes with the GH/IGF-1 axis via cytokine-independent mechanisms. To date, in vivo data from a mouse model have demonstrated that LPS exposure reduces GHR density by inducing GHR proteolysis, probably via the metalloprotease cleavage site, resulting in the increased shedding of GHBP [88]. More recent in vitro data demonstrate that LPS can directly inhibit GHR promoter activity and subsequent expression through an effect on the TLR-4 signaling pathway [90]. Both mechanisms are seemingly independent of the inflammatory cytokine cascade, and the addition of anti-TNFα antibody failed to abrogate the effect [90]. Although intriguing, the clinical significance of these findings and their relative importance in the setting of growth impairment and CD are yet to be determined.

Corticosteroid Suppression of Linear Growth

The growth-suppressive effects of glucocorticoids are multifactorial, and can occur at virtually any point along the growth axis (Table 12.4)

A [119]. In general, exogenous corticosteroids are considered to create a state of functional GH deficiency [67]. Dose, preparation, and timing of glucocorticoids all influence the degree of growth suppression observed. It appears that concentrations of glucocorticoids required to exert direct suppression on the growth plate may be lower than those

Table 12.4 Effects of exogenous glucocorticoid therapy related to linear growth [119]

GH/IGF-1 axis
Inhibit endogenous GH secretion
Reduce pulsatile release of GH
Increase somatostatin
Interference with the GHR
Reduce GHR expression
Reduce GHR binding
Uncouple GHR from signal transduction components
Reduce IGF-1 activity levels
Reduced activation of STAT5b
Increased levels of IGFBP-3
Skeletal system
Growth plate
Inhibit chondrocyte mitosis
Inhibit IGF-1-induced chondrocyte proliferation
Inhibit epiphyseal maturation
Skeletal matrix
Diminish activity of enzymes required for posttranslational procollagen chain modification
Inhibit collagen synthesis
Increase collagen degradation
Inhibit osteoblast function
Peripheral tissues
Calcium balance
Decrease intestinal calcium absorption
Increase urinary calcium excretion
Body composition
Increase protein catabolism
Decrease lipid oxidation
Inhibit secretion of adrenal sex steroids
Reduce direct growth stimulatory effect of sex steroids
Reduce usual augmentation of GH release

Adapted from Allen [119]

required to suppress GH secretion. Growth, particularly in prepubertal children, can be impaired by relatively modest daily doses of prednisone (3–5 mg/m²) [119]. This effect may be reduced, but is not necessarily eliminated, by alternate-day therapy. Selectively eliminating evening administration may avoid blunting of both nocturnal GH secretion and/or ACTH-induced adrenal androgen production [119]. Catch-up growth, following the cessation of glucocorticoid therapy, does not always fully compensate for growth deficits, particularly when treatment occurs during puberty. Although chronic daily dosing and frequent induction courses of steroids have been shown to lead to bone demineralization, at present, there is *no* good evidence that short-term use of steroids for the induction of remission in CD is detrimental to long-term growth.

The Pathogenesis of Pubertal Delay and Its Influence on Growth Impairment

Puberty is frequently delayed in young patients with CD [67]. It not only results in linear growth impairment, but

decreases bone mineralization and can significantly impact a patient's quality of life and psychological health [68]. In girls with Crohn disease, a delay in menarche is closely related to delays in skeletal maturity [120]. Pubertal delay is defined as the absence of testicular enlargement in boys or breast development in girls at an age that is 2–2.5 standard deviations later than the population mean [5]. Traditionally, the mean age has been 14 years in boys and 13 years in girls; however, with recent downward trends in pubertal timing in many countries, some observers are advocating for younger age cutoffs [5, 121, 122].

As alluded to earlier, the factors that trigger normal pubertal onset remain elusive [5], thus impeding our comprehension and complete understanding of the mechanisms that underlie pubertal delay in CD. Similar to linear growth impairment, although undernutrition has been frequently considered the main reason for delayed puberty in children with CD, there is a group of patients with persistently active disease who do not enter puberty despite the provision of adequate energy [123]. Experimental colitis models demonstrate that inflammatory mediators potentiate the puberty-delaying effects of undernutrition [67, 124–126] via alterations in gonadotropin-releasing hormone (GnRH) secretion patterns, although which specific inflammatory cytokines impact on puberty are yet to be determined. However, both human and experimental data suggest that there is also an element of gonadotropin resistance in pubertal delay, and in vitro studies implicate TNFα in the downregulation of androgen gene expression [127]. Although Cushing's disease has been associated with pubertal delay [128, 129], it is not known whether the doses of corticosteroid used in the management of CD are sufficient to delay either the onset or progression of puberty [67].

Influence of Genetic Factors

A number of genetic polymorphisms have been implicated in CD susceptibility and pathogenesis, the most prominent of which are within the *NOD2* gene. While some investigators [130, 131] have suggested that CD-associated NOD2 polymorphisms may be determinants of growth impairment, neither analysis controlled for disease location. A subsequent careful analysis of growth prior to and following diagnosis found no such association [52]. Scottish pediatric data suggest an association between polymorphisms in the IBD5 susceptibility locus and low anthropometric centiles at diagnosis [132]. Similarly, data from Boston, examining 14 different CD susceptibility genes, highlight a potential association with the CD susceptibility allele within ATG16L1 [133].

It is feasible that common genetic polymorphisms which alter cytokine expression may contribute to growth impairment but not influence overall susceptibility to CD. A recent study of Israeli patients suggests that relatively common variations in the promoter region for TNFα may have an independent effect on linear growth outcomes [134].

Similarly, data from Sawczenko et al. demonstrate a potential causal relationship between variation in the promoter region for IL-6, subsequent IL-6 expression, and a differential in linear growth impairment during active inflammation [110]. Confirmation of these and similar findings is awaited, and may help better elucidate the complex molecular interactions pertinent to the pathophysiology of growth impairment.

Facilitation of Normal Growth in IBD

The Importance of Prompt Recognition of IBD

The clinical presentation of childhood Crohn's disease may be subtle and varied. Impairment of linear growth and concomitant delay in sexual maturation may precede the development of intestinal symptoms and dominate the presentation. Prompt diagnosis is important in avoiding a long period of growth retardation. The greater the height deficit at diagnosis, the greater is the demand for catch-up growth.

The Importance of Monitoring Growth

In caring for children with IBD, it is important to obtain pre-illness and parental heights [57], so that the impact of the chronic intestinal inflammation can be fully appreciated. Following diagnosis and institution of treatment, regular measurement and charting of height, together with calculation of height velocity, are central to management. A properly calibrated wall-mounted stadiometer is required for accurate and reproducible serial measurements.

Part of the assessment of response to therapy in children with IBD is a regular analysis of whether rate of growth is normal for age and pubertal stage and whether catch-up growth to pre-illness centiles is being achieved. Height velocity should be appraised in the context of current pubertal stage, because of the variation in normal rates of growth before puberty, during puberty, and near the end of puberty. If growth and puberty appear either delayed or very advanced, radiological determination of bone age can be used to indicate the remaining growth potential. Delayed radiological bone age suggests greater potential for catch-up growth than may be anticipated for the subject's chronological age. Conversely, in the subject with growth failure and a normal bone age, the potential window to achieve any growth catch-up may be very small.

One of the difficulties in evaluating growth in response to a therapy is the relatively long interval of time required for valid assessment. Published normal standards for height velocity throughout childhood are based on height increments during 12-month periods [135]. When growth velocity is calculated over short time periods, small errors in

Table 12.5 Techniques to assess and monitor linear growth in children with CD

Initial evaluation
Accurate measurement of the patient's height and weight by trained staff using reliable equipment
Accurate pubertal assessment
Accurate measurement of the biological parents' heights, and calculation of midparental height (MPH) *Formula to estimate a subject's potential adult height* Male: MPH plus 6.5 cm; Female: MPH minus 6.5 cm
Obtain pre-illness anthropological (height, weight) data on the patient
Radiological bone age estimation
Dietetic assessment of caloric, Ca, Vitamin D, and micronutrient intake
Ongoing monitoring
Accurate height and weight measurements by trained staff using reliable equipment
Calculate height velocity
Calculate z-score for height, weight, and height velocity data and/or plot sequentially on gender-specific, ethnically appropriate reference curve
Accurate pubertal assessment
Consider repeat bone age estimation
Endeavor to follow until adult height achieved (Tanner stage 5 and <0.5 cm linear growth annually)

individual measurements are significantly magnified, and the normal seasonal variation in growth is overlooked. The consensus from pediatric endocrinologists is that height velocity should be calculated over intervals no shorter than 6 months [135]. On a research basis, efforts to reflect growth changes over intervals shorter than 6 months have focused on measuring changes in lower leg length by knemometry and on determination of circulating levels of markers of bone and collagen metabolism [135–137]. The clinical utility of routine serial assessment of the GH/IGF-1 axis is yet to be ascertained [138]. A valid indicator of contemporaneous linear growth would allow for a more timely change in therapy. A summary of techniques that should be employed to clinically assess and monitor linear growth through to adulthood, based on the management guidelines by Heuschkel and colleagues, is presented [139] in Table 12.5.

Psychosocial Impact of Impaired Growth

Growth impairment and accompanying pubertal delay have a significant psychosocial impact on adolescents, as the physical differences between them and healthy peers become progressively more obvious. In the development process of a disease-specific health-related quality-of-life instrument for pediatric IBD, body image issues including height and weight were among the concerns most frequently cited by adolescents with Crohn's disease [140].

General Principles of Management

Prior to recognition of the direct influences of proinflammatory cytokines on linear growth, management of growth-impaired children focused on nutritional restitution [70, 74]. Improved growth following supplementary enteral or parenteral nutrition is well documented [141–143]. Decreases in inflammatory parameters and increases in IGF-1 occur very early during exclusive enteral nutrition and precede changes in nutritional parameters [144], highlighting that nutrition and inflammation constitute a bidirectional pathway [145]. Nevertheless, a subset of patients fails to grow despite nutritional repletion, presumably because intestinal inflammation remains chronically active. Hence, in the management or prevention of growth impairment, attention needs to focus on providing adequate nutritional support, as well as treating inflammatory disease using the most appropriate pharmacological, nutritional, or surgical interventions available [139, 146] (Table 12.6).

A comprehensive management guideline is available for children with IBD-related growth failure [139].

Anti-inflammatory Treatments and Effects on Growth

Few interventions have been tested in the randomized controlled trial setting in children, and hence the effects of therapies on growth have seldom been rigorously assessed. The one exception is enteral nutrition as the primary therapy for pediatric Crohn disease. For most other therapies, until recently, growth outcomes have been reported only in observational/retrospective studies. However, given the importance of persistent inflammation in the pathogenesis of growth impairment, it is intuitive that therapies which achieve mucosal healing are more likely to facilitate normal growth. When assessing the available evidence of any treatment's impact on linear growth, two important questions need to be considered: Were the population of patients being studied growth-impaired prior to commencing therapy (recognizing that linear growth impairment is not a universal feature of all young patients with active CD)? Did the population being studied still have enough remaining "growth potential" for any therapeutic impact to be measureable? Below, treatments of pediatric IBD will be briefly discussed with respect to their potential effects on growth. A detailed Cochrane review by Newby and colleagues is available [147] for reference.

Enteral Nutrition

Prior to the availability of biological therapies, acute treatment options for moderate-to-severe active Crohn disease were limited. "Exclusive enteral nutrition" (EEN) refers to

Table 12.6 Strategies for managing growth failure in children with CD

Initial evaluation
Detailed assessment of disease activity and distribution
Ensure optimal nutrition (supplement energy and/or substrates as required)
Induction of remission
Aim for the rapid induction of a complete remission
Endeavor to avoid/minimize steroid usage (enteral therapy)
Consider surgical resection, especially in cases of limited localized ileal/ileocecal disease
Use biological therapies when other medical options have failed and surgery is not appropriate
Monitor closely and ensure remission is achieved in a timely fashion
Maintenance of remission
Aim for a prolonged, ongoing continuous remission
Consider the early introduction of immunomodulator therapy
Ensure optimal nutrition (supplement energy and/or substrates as required)
Monitor closely to ensure the persistence of remission and the timely reinduction of remission in the event of disease relapse.
Persistent growth failure in the setting of clinically quiescent CD
Ensure optimal nutrition (supplement energy and/or substrates as required)
Detailed reassessment of disease activity and distribution
Consider alternative causes of poor growth (including endocrinological and psychosocial)

the administration of formulated food as sole source nutrition. It has been shown to decrease mucosal cytokine production and induce endoscopic healing [148]. The appeal of EEN among pediatric patients primarily relates to avoidance of steroid therapy [146]. Amino acid based and peptide-based formulae are administered by nocturnal nasogastric infusion, but more palatable polymeric formulae can be consumed orally and appear comparably efficacious [149]. Some have argued that active Crohn disease occurring in children is more responsive to enteral nutrition than that occurring in adults, where corticosteroid therapy more often induces clinical remission [150, 151]. It seems likely, however, that other factors, such as small bowel localization and recent onset of Crohn disease, rather than young age per se, influence responsiveness of intestinal inflammation to exclusive enteral nutrition [152, 153]. Nevertheless, enteral nutrition does seem to be more feasible in pediatric patients. Children quickly become adept at swallowing the silastic catheter required for nasogastric feeding regimens, and can remove it each morning before school.

If enteral nutrition is to facilitate growth, remission must be maintained. One of the limitations of liquid diet therapy has been the observed tendency for symptoms to recur promptly following its cessation [154]. Chronic intermittent bowel rest with nocturnal infusion of an elemental diet 1 month out of four has been reported as a means of sustaining remission and facilitating growth [142]. Another nutritional strategy, continuation of nocturnal nasogastric feeding four to five times weekly as a supplement to an unrestricted ad lib daytime diet, was also associated with prolonged disease quiescence and improved growth in a historical cohort study [143]. Maintenance of EEN, however, is not always well tolerated by patients.

Corticosteroids

Conventional corticosteroids are still the most commonly used drugs to treat acute disease exacerbations of pediatric Crohn disease and ulcerative colitis. Resolution of inflammation, if sustained following a short course of steroids, will be associated with normal linear growth. Chronic daily administration of corticosteroids to control intestinal inflammation is clearly contraindicated in pediatric IBD because of the interference with linear growth in addition to the other unwanted long-term adverse effects common to children and adults. Children with moderate symptoms of active Crohn disease localized to the ileum and/or right colon may respond to short-term treatment with controlled ileal release budesonide. Similarly, extended release budesonide utilizing MMX technology can be used in patients with colonic disease. Cosmetic effects of steroids are spared in this context, even if efficacy is overall less than that with conventional corticosteroids [155, 156]. Studies in adults demonstrate little benefit in comparison to placebo in maintaining remission. Limited clinical experience with maintenance budesonide in children raised concern that linear growth was impaired during therapy in spite of good weight gain [157].

Immunomodulatory Drugs

The steroid-sparing roles of immunomodulatory drugs, azathioprine, 6-mercaptopurine, and methotrexate, are well documented [158, 159]. In a multicenter trial, newly diagnosed children with moderately severe Crohn disease treated with an initial course of prednisone were randomized to receive either concomitant 6-mercaptopurine or placebo [158]. A beneficial effect on linear growth was not clearly apparent in this study in spite of the steroid-sparing effect and improved control of intestinal inflammation, perhaps a function of sample size and difficulties inherent in comparing growth rates among patients of varying ages and pubertal stages [135]. Retrospective data have shown enhancement of linear growth, when methotrexate was given to young CD patients intolerant of or refractory to thiopurine therapy [159], a finding replicated in a recent prospective observational cohort [160].

Antitumor Necrosis Factor Alpha (Anti-TNFα)

The development of anticytokine therapies, such as infliximab and adalimumab, with the potential to achieve mucosal healing, even in otherwise treatment-refractory patients constitutes a tremendous advance. The efficacy of anti-TNF agents in pediatric as well as adult patients is well established [161]. Considering the role cytokines, including TNFα, play in growth impairment, and the ability of anti-TNFα antibodies to achieve mucosal healing, it is of little surprise that both observational [160, 162–171] and clinical trial [172–174] data demonstrate a beneficial effect on linear growth, if treatment is undertaken early enough prior to or during puberty. Complementary data have demonstrated a restoration of hepatic GH signaling and improved anabolic metabolism in the setting of TNFα blockade [175]. Furthermore, and consistent with our evolving mechanistic understanding of IBD-related growth impairment, improvement in height velocity with the use of TNFα therapy has been correlated with increases in IGF-1 and IGFBP-3 levels, with no accompanying change in serum GH levels [176]. These observations are cause for optimism that the medical therapy for Crohn disease available in the present decade will reduce the prevalence of sustained growth impairment in pediatric patients.

Surgery

Optimal management of young patients with IBD includes appropriate and timely referral for intestinal resection. Sustained steroid-dependency and associated impairment of linear growth should not be tolerated in children with ulcerative colitis, where colectomy cures the disease and restores growth [177]. For some children with Crohn disease, notably those with localized internal penetrating or stricturing disease, timely surgical intervention is a very attractive therapeutic option. Despite the almost inevitable endoscopic and subsequent clinical recurrence of CD, the significant period of postoperative remission that can be anticipated in many patients allows important catch-up growth in patients undergoing operation prior to or during early puberty [178–180].

Hormonal Interventions

The potential therapeutic role of GH and IGF-1 in pediatric IBD patients with persistent growth impairment is an alluring prospect. There have been increasing pediatric data exploring this over the last several decades [181–184] culminating in three small randomized trials [185–187]. These data have been recently reviewed by Vortia and colleagues [188]. The rationale for pursuing GH therapy (GHT) in growth-impaired IBD patients is strengthened by the improved growth that has been recently observed following GHT in children with juvenile idiopathic arthritis [189] and cystic fibrosis [190] To date, while demonstrating that GHT can improve short-term linear growth in select CD patients, it should be emphasized that there are no data yet available to suggest that GHT will alter the final adult height of children with IBD-associated growth disturbance. There is a small experience with the supplemental use of GH during ongoing steroid therapy in a number of pediatric conditions [96] including steroid-dependent CD [191], again without evidence that final adult height is impacted.

Beyond its "antiglucocorticoid" effects, it is possible that GHT has a direct anti-inflammatory effect in IBD. A randomized controlled clinical trial by Slonim in 2000 demonstrated a possible positive effect of GHT on disease activity in adults with Crohn disease [192]. Recent experimental data support this finding, wherein GHT was demonstrated to reduce mucosal inflammation in an experimental colitis via an IGF-1 independent mechanism that downregulated IL-6/STAT3 [193] but did not reverse local inflammatory resistance to the GH upregulation of IGF-1 [193]. However, clinical data in pediatrics are scant, and the observations conflicting [186, 187]. Despite the possible benefits, GHT may also introduce a variety of risks and complications. Described adverse systemic effects of GHT include altered carbohydrate metabolism with glucose intolerance, a transient increase in total body fluid, hypertension, cardiac disease, stimulation of autoimmune disease, and increased malignancy risk. Given the variety of potential risks and complications, GHT, as either an adjunct to support linear growth or as a form of anti-inflammatory therapy, should be considered experimental in the setting of IBD, and is still best limited to formal investigative study settings.

Studies on the utility of recombinant IGF-1 on growth in CD have not been described to date. This is likely due to the theoretical risk of colon cancer with high circulating levels of IGF-1. A model has recently been formulated that allows for the calculation of a dose in children with active CD that would maintain IGF-1 levels within normal limits [194]. It remains to be seen whether future studies determine this to be any more effective than GH therapy.

Although there are no controlled clinical studies, 3–6 months of testosterone therapy, carefully supervised by pediatric endocrinologists, has been used in boys with extreme delay of puberty and has been associated with a significant growth spurt [67, 195].

It must be emphasized, however, that children requiring consideration of these adjunctive hormonal therapies should be encountered increasingly less commonly. Treatment of intestinal inflammation and assurance of adequate nutrition are of much greater importance. However, targeted therapies based on our current understanding of the GH-IGF-1 axis may be important for patients with significant linear growth impairment, whose inflammation remains refractory to best current anti-inflammatory therapies.

Summary

Increased understanding of the mechanisms of linear growth impairment associated with chronic inflammatory disease points the way toward better management. Early recognition of Crohn disease remains an important challenge. Following diagnosis of IBD, restoration and maintenance of a child's pre-illness growth pattern indicate success of therapy. Current treatment regimens limit the use of corticosteroids, via optimization of immunomodulatory drugs, use of enteral nutrition in Crohn disease, and, if necessary, surgery for ulcerative colitis and for intestinal complications of localized Crohn disease. Biological agents with the potential for mucosal healing hold promise of growth enhancement even among patients with otherwise refractory disease, whose growth was previously compromised. For all interventions, there is a window of opportunity, which must be taken advantage of before puberty is too advanced.

References

1. Griffiths AM, Nguyen P, Smith C, MacMillan JH, Sherman PM. Growth and clinical course of children with Crohn's disease. Gut. 1993;34:939–43.
2. Hyams JS, Davis P, Grancher K, Lerer T, Justinich CJ, Markowitz J. Clinical outcome of ulcerative colitis in children. J Pediatr. 1996;129:81–8.
3. Karlberg J, Jalil F, Lam B, Low L, Yeung CY. Linear growth retardation in relation to the three phases of growth. Eur J Clin Nutr 1994;48 Suppl 1:S25–43; discussion S-4.
4. Rogol AD, Roemmich JN, Clark PA. Growth at puberty. J Adolesc Health. 2002;31:192–200.
5. Palmert MR, Dunkel L. Clinical practice. Delayed puberty. N Engl J Med. 2012;366:443–53.
6. Salmon Jr WD, Daughaday WH. A hormonally controlled serum factor which stimulates sulfate incorporation by cartilage in vitro. 1956. J Lab Clin Med. 1990;116:408–19.
7. Daughaday WH. A personal history of the origin of the somatomedin hypothesis and recent challenges to its validity. Perspect Biol Med. 1989;32:194–211.
8. Rinderknecht E, Humbel RE. The amino acid sequence of human insulin-like growth factor I and its structural homology with proinsulin. J Biol Chem. 1978;253:2769–76.
9. Isaksson OG, Jansson JO, Gause IA. Growth hormone stimulates longitudinal bone growth directly. Science. 1982;216:1237–9.
10. Isaksson OG, Lindahl A, Nilsson A, Isgaard J. Mechanism of the stimulatory effect of growth hormone on longitudinal bone growth. Endocr Rev. 1987;8:426–38.
11. Green H, Morikawa M, Nixon T. A dual effector theory of growth-hormone action. Differentiation. 1985;29:195–8.
12. Frank SJ, Messina JL, Baumann G, Black RA, Bertics PJ. Insights into modulation of (and by) growth hormone signaling. J Lab Clin Med. 2000;136:14–20.
13. Teglund S, McKay C, Schuetz E, et al. Stat5a and Stat5b proteins have essential and nonessential, or redundant, roles in cytokine responses. Cell. 1998;93:841–50.
14. Bergad PL, Schwarzenberg SJ, Humbert JT, et al. Inhibition of growth hormone action in models of inflammation. Am J Physiol Cell Physiol. 2000;279:C1906–17.

15. Denson LA, Held MA, Menon RK, Frank SJ, Parlow AF, Arnold DL. Interleukin-6 inhibits hepatic growth hormone signaling via upregulation of Cis and Socs-3. Am J Physiol Gastrointest Liver Physiol. 2003;284:G646–54.

16. Ram PA, Waxman DJ. SOCS/CIS protein inhibition of growth hormone stimulated STAT5 signaling by multiple mechanisms. J Biol Chem. 1999;274:35553–61.

17. Leung DW, Spencer SA, Cachianes G, et al. Growth hormone receptor and serum binding protein: purification, cloning and expression. Nature. 1987;330:537–43.

18. Asplin CM, Faria AC, Carlsen EC, et al. Alterations in the pulsatile mode of growth hormone release in men and women with insulin-dependent diabetes mellitus. J Clin Endocrinol Metab. 1989;69:239–45.

19. Herrington J, Smit LS, Schwartz J, Carter-Su C. The role of STAT proteins in growth hormone signaling. Oncogene. 2000;19:2585–97.

20. Liu X, Robinson GW, Gouilleux F, Groner B, Hennighausen L. Cloning and expression of Stat5 and an additional homologue (Stat5b) involved in prolactin signal transduction in mouse mammary tissue. Proc Natl Acad Sci U S A. 1995;92:8831–5.

21. Jones JI, Clemmons DR. Insulin-like growth factors and their binding proteins: biological actions. Endocr Rev. 1995;16:3–34.

22. Govoni KE, Baylink DJ, Mohan S. The multi-functional role of insulin-like growth factor binding proteins in bone. Pediatr Nephrol. 2005;20:261–8.

23. Rechler MM. Insulin-like growth factor binding proteins. Vitam Horm. 1993;47:1–114.

24. Miyakoshi N, Richman C, Qin X, Baylink DJ, Mohan S. Effects of recombinant insulin-like growth factor-binding protein-4 on bone formation parameters in mice. Endocrinology. 1999;140:5719–28.

25. Rajaram S, Baylink DJ, Mohan S. Insulin-like growth factor-binding proteins in serum and other biological fluids: regulation and functions. Endocr Rev. 1997;18:801–31.

26. Thissen JP, Davenport ML, Pucilowska JB, Miles MV, Underwood LE. Increased serum clearance and degradation of 125I-labeled IGF-I in protein-restricted rats. Am J Phys. 1992;262:E406–11.

27. Underwood LE, Thissen JP, Lemozy S, Ketelslegers JM, Clemmons DR. Hormonal and nutritional regulation of IGF-I and its binding proteins. Horm Res. 1994;42:145–51.

28. Nilsson O, Baron J. Impact of growth plate senescence on catch-up growth and epiphyseal fusion. Pediatr Nephrol. 2005;20:319–22.

29. Walker KV, Kember NF. Cell kinetics of growth cartilage in the rat tibia. II. Measurements during ageing. Cell Tissue Kinet. 1972;5:409–19.

30. Weise M, De-Levi S, Barnes KM, Gafni RI, Abad V, Baron J. Effects of estrogen on growth plate senescence and epiphyseal fusion. Proc Natl Acad Sci U S A. 2001;98:6871–6.

31. Gafni RI, Weise M, Robrecht DT, et al. Catch-up growth is associated with delayed senescence of the growth plate in rabbits. Pediatr Res. 2001;50:618–23.

32. Baron J, Klein KO, Colli MJ, et al. Catch-up growth after glucocorticoid excess: a mechanism intrinsic to the growth plate. Endocrinology. 1994;135:1367–71.

33. Wei W, Sedivy JM. Differentiation between senescence (M1) and crisis (M2) in human fibroblast cultures. Exp Cell Res. 1999;253:519–22.

34. Prader A, Tanner JM, von Harnack G. Catch-up growth following illness or starvation. An example of developmental canalization in man. J Pediatr. 1963;62:646–59.

35. Cutler Jr GB. The role of estrogen in bone growth and maturation during childhood and adolescence. J Steroid Biochem Mol Biol. 1997;61:141–4.

36. Veldhuis JD, Bowers CY. Three-peptide control of pulsatile and entropic feedback-sensitive modes of growth hormone secretion: modulation by estrogen and aromatizable androgen. J Pediatr Endocrinol Metab. 2003;16(Suppl 3):587–605.

37. Keenan BS, Richards GE, Ponder SW, Dallas JS, Nagamani M, Smith ER. Androgen-stimulated pubertal growth: the effects of testosterone and dihydrotestosterone on growth hormone and insulin-like growth factor-I in the treatment of short stature and delayed puberty. J Clin Endocrinol Metab. 1993;76:996–1001.

38. Nilsson KO, Albertsson-Wikland K, Alm J, et al. Improved final height in girls with Turner's syndrome treated with growth hormone and oxandrolone. J Clin Endocrinol Metab. 1996;81:635–40.

39. Stanhope R, Buchanan CR, Fenn GC, Preece MA. Double blind placebo controlled trial of low dose oxandrolone in the treatment of boys with constitutional delay of growth and puberty. Arch Dis Child. 1988;63:501–5.

40. Tanner JM, Whitehouse RH. Clinical longitudinal standards for height, weight, height velocity, weight velocity, and stages of puberty. Arch Dis Child. 1976;51:170–9.

41. Centers for Disease Control and Prevention NCfHS. CDC growth charts: United States, http://www.cdc.gov/growthcharts/.30-5-2000.

42. Freeman JV, Cole TJ, Chinn S, Jones PR, White EM, Preece MA. Cross sectional stature and weight reference curves for the UK, 1990. Arch Dis Child. 1995;73:17–24.

43. Zeferino AM, Barros Filho AA, Bettiol H, Barbieri MA. Monitoring growth. J Pediatr (Rio J). 2003;79 Suppl 1:S23–32.

44. Mason A, Malik S, Russell RK, Bishop J, McGrogan P, Ahmed SF. Impact of inflammatory bowel disease on pubertal growth. Horm Res Paediatr. 2011;76:293–9.

45. Kirschner BS. Growth and development in chronic inflammatory bowel disease. Acta Paediatr Scand Suppl 1990;366:98–104; discussion 105.

46. Kanof ME, Lake AM, Bayless TM. Decreased height velocity in children and adolescents before the diagnosis of Crohn's disease. Gastroenterology. 1988;95:1523–7.

47. Hildebrand H, Karlberg J, Kristiansson B. Longitudinal growth in children and adolescents with inflammatory bowel disease. J Pediatr Gastroenterol Nutr. 1994;18:165–73.

48. Markowitz J, Grancher K, Rosa J, Aiges H, Daum F. Growth failure in pediatric inflammatory bowel disease. J Pediatr Gastroenterol Nutr. 1993;16:373–80.

49. Motil KJ, Grand RJ, Davis-Kraft L, Ferlic LL, Smith EO. Growth failure in children with inflammatory bowel disease: a prospective study. Gastroenterology. 1993;105:681–91.

50. Kundhal P, Critch J, Hack C, Griffiths A. Clinical course and growth of children with Crohn's disease. Can J Gastroenterol. 2002;V16(Suppl):77S.

51. Sawczenko A, Sandhu BK. Presenting features of inflammatory bowel disease in Great Britain and Ireland. Arch Dis Child. 2003;88:995–1000.

52. Wine E, Reif SS, Leshinsky-Silver E, et al. Pediatric Crohn's disease and growth retardation: the role of genotype, phenotype, and disease severity. Pediatrics. 2004;114:1281–6.

53. Vasseur F, Gower-Rousseau C, Vernier-Massouille G, et al. Nutritional status and growth in pediatric Crohn's disease: a population-based study. Am J Gastroenterol. 2010;105:1893–900.

54. Sawczenko A, Ballinger AB, Croft NM, Sanderson IR, Savage MO. Adult height in patients with early onset of Crohn's disease. Gut. 2003;52:454–5; author reply 5.

55. Alemzadeh N, Rekers-Mombarg LT, Mearin ML, Wit JM, Lamers CB, van Hogezand RA. Adult height in patients with early onset of Crohn's disease. Gut. 2002;51:26–9.

56. Turunen P, Ashorn M, Auvinen A, Iltanen S, Huhtala H, Kolho KL. Long-term health outcomes in pediatric inflammatory bowel disease: a population-based study. Inflamm Bowel Dis. 2009; 15:56–62.

57. Lee JJ, Escher JC, Shuman MJ, et al. Final adult height of children with inflammatory bowel disease is predicted by parental height and patient minimum height Z-score. Inflamm Bowel Dis. 2010;16:1669–77.

58. Sawczenko A, Ballinger AB, Savage MO, Sanderson IR. Clinical features affecting final adult height in patients with pediatric-onset Crohn's disease. Pediatrics. 2006;118:124–9.

59. Gupta N, Lustig RH, Kohn MA, McCracken M, Vittinghoff E. Sex differences in statural growth impairment in Crohn's disease: role of IGF-1. Inflamm Bowel Dis. 2011;17:2318–25.

60. Sentongo TA, Semeao EJ, Piccoli DA, Stallings VA, Zemel BS. Growth, body composition, and nutritional status in children and adolescents with Crohn's disease. J Pediatr Gastroenterol Nutr. 2000;31:33–40.

61. Pigneur B, Seksik P, Viola S, et al. Natural history of Crohn's disease: comparison between childhood- and adult-onset disease. Inflamm Bowel Dis. 2010;16:953–61.

62. Gupta N, Bostrom AG, Kirschner BS, et al. Gender differences in presentation and course of disease in pediatric patients with Crohn disease. Pediatrics. 2007;120:e1418–25.

63. Shono T, Kato M, Aoyagi Y, et al. Assessment of growth disturbance in Japanese children with IBD. Int J Pediatr. 2010; 2010:958915.

64. Kim BJ, Song SM, Kim KM, et al. Characteristics and trends in the incidence of inflammatory bowel disease in Korean children: a single-center experience. Dig Dis Sci. 2010;55:1989–95.

65. Ferguson A, Sedgwick DM. Juvenile onset inflammatory bowel disease: height and body mass index in adult life. BMJ. 1994;308:1259–63.

66. Timmer A, Behrens R, Buderus S, et al. Childhood onset inflammatory bowel disease: predictors of delayed diagnosis from the CEDATA German-language pediatric inflammatory bowel disease registry. J Pediatr. 2011;158:467–73. e2

67. Ballinger AB, Savage MO, Sanderson IR. Delayed puberty associated with inflammatory bowel disease. Pediatr Res. 2003;53:205–10.

68. DeBoer MD, Denson LA. Delays in puberty, growth, and accrual of bone mineral density in pediatric Crohn's disease: despite temporal changes in disease severity, the need for monitoring remains. J Pediatr. 2013;163:17–22.

69. Walters TD, Griffiths AM. Mechanisms of growth impairment in pediatric Crohn's disease. Nat Rev Gastroenterol Hepatol. 2009; 6:513–23.

70. Kelts DG, Grand RJ, Shen G, Watkins JB, Werlin SL, Boehme C. Nutritional basis of growth failure in children and adolescents with Crohn's disease. Gastroenterology. 1979;76:720–7.

71. Hill RJ, Lewindon PJ, Withers GD, et al. Ability of commonly used prediction equations to predict resting energy expenditure in children with inflammatory bowel disease. Inflamm Bowel Dis. 2011;17:1587–93.

72. Gerasimidis K, McGrogan P, Edwards CA. The aetiology and impact of malnutrition in paediatric inflammatory bowel disease. J Hum Nutr Diet. 2011;24:313–26.

73. Pons R, Whitten KE, Woodhead H, Leach ST, Lemberg DA, Day AS. Dietary intakes of children with Crohn's disease. Br J Nutr. 2009;102:1052–7.

74. Kirschner BS, Klich JR, Kalman SS, deFavaro MV, Rosenberg IH. Reversal of growth retardation in Crohn's disease with therapy emphasizing oral nutritional restitution. Gastroenterology. 1981; 80:10–5.

75. Ballinger A, El-Haj T, Perrett D, et al. The role of medial hypothalamic serotonin in the suppression of feeding in a rat model of colitis. Gastroenterology. 2000;118:544–53.

76. El-Haj T, Poole S, Farthing MJ, Ballinger AB. Anorexia in a rat model of colitis: interaction of interleukin-1 and hypothalamic serotonin. Brain Res. 2002;927:1–7.

77. Ates Y, Degertekin B, Erdil A, Yaman H, Dagalp K. Serum ghrelin levels in inflammatory bowel disease with relation to disease activity and nutritional status. Dig Dis Sci. 2008;53:2215–21.

78. Moran GW, Leslie FC, McLaughlin JT. Crohn's disease affecting the small bowel is associated with reduced appetite and elevated levels of circulating gut peptides. Clin Nutr. 2013;32:404–11.

79. Filipsson S, Hulten L, Lindstedt G. Malabsorption of fat and vitamin B12 before and after intestinal resection for Crohn's disease. Scand J Gastroenterol. 1978;13:529–36.

80. Griffiths AM, Drobnies A, Soldin SJ, Hamilton JR. Enteric protein loss measured by fecal alpha 1-antitrypsin clearance in the assessment of Crohn's disease activity: a study of children and adolescents. J Pediatr Gastroenterol Nutr. 1986;5:907–11.

81. Azcue M, Rashid M, Griffiths A, Pencharz PB. Energy expenditure and body composition in children with Crohn's disease: effect of enteral nutrition and treatment with prednisolone. Gut. 1997;41:203–8.

82. De Benedetti F, Alonzi T, Moretta A, et al. Interleukin 6 causes growth impairment in transgenic mice through a decrease in insulin-like growth factor-I. A model for stunted growth in children with chronic inflammation. J Clin Invest. 1997;99:643–50.

83. Ballinger AB, Azooz O, El-Haj T, Poole S, Farthing MJ. Growth failure occurs through a decrease in insulin-like growth factor 1 which is independent of undernutrition in a rat model of colitis. Gut. 2000;46:694–700.

84. Martensson K, Chrysis D, Savendahl L. Interleukin-1beta and TNF-alpha act in synergy to inhibit longitudinal growth in fetal rat metatarsal bones. J Bone Miner Res. 2004;19:1805–12.

85. Varghese S, Wyzga N, Griffiths AM, Sylvester FA. Effects of serum from children with newly diagnosed Crohn disease on primary cultures of rat osteoblasts. J Pediatr Gastroenterol Nutr. 2002;35:641–8.

86. Kirschner BS, Sutton MM. Somatomedin-C levels in growth-impaired children and adolescents with chronic inflammatory bowel disease. Gastroenterology. 1986;91:830–6.

87. Tenore A, Berman WF, Parks JS, Bongiovanni AM. Basal and stimulated serum growth hormone concentrations in inflammatory bowel disease. J Clin Endocrinol Metab. 1977;44:622–8.

88. Wang X, Jiang J, Warram J, et al. Endotoxin-induced proteolytic reduction in hepatic growth hormone (GH) receptor: a novel mechanism for GH insensitivity. Mol Endocrinol. 2008;22: 1427–37.

89. Denson LA, Menon RK, Shaufl A, Bajwa HS, Williams CR, Karpen SJ. TNF-alpha downregulates murine hepatic growth hormone receptor expression by inhibiting Sp1 and Sp3 binding. J Clin Invest. 2001;107:1451–8.

90. Dejkhamron P, Thimmarayappa J, Kotlyarevska K, et al. Lipopolysaccharide (LPS) directly suppresses growth hormone receptor (GHR) expression through MyD88-dependent and -independent Toll-like receptor-4/MD2 complex signaling pathways. Mol Cell Endocrinol. 2007;274:35–42.

91. Colson A, Le Cam A, Maiter D, Edery M, Thissen JP. Potentiation of growth hormone-induced liver suppressors of cytokine signaling messenger ribonucleic acid by cytokines. Endocrinology. 2000;141:3687–95.

92. Cohney SJ, Sanden D, Cacalano NA, et al. SOCS-3 is tyrosine phosphorylated in response to interleukin-2 and suppresses STAT5 phosphorylation and lymphocyte proliferation. Mol Cell Biol. 1999;19:4980–8.

93. Ram PA, Waxman DJ. Role of the cytokine-inducible SH2 protein CIS in desensitization of STAT5b signaling by continuous growth hormone. J Biol Chem. 2000;275:39487–96.

94. Shumate ML, Yumet G, Ahmed TA, Cooney RN. Interleukin-1 inhibits the induction of insulin-like growth factor-I by growth

hormone in CWSV-1 hepatocytes. Am J Physiol Gastrointest Liver Physiol. 2005;289:G227–39.

95. De Benedetti F, Meazza C, Oliveri M, et al. Effect of IL-6 on IGF binding protein-3: a study in IL-6 transgenic mice and in patients with systemic juvenile idiopathic arthritis. Endocrinology. 2001;142:4818–26.

96. Mauras N. Growth hormone therapy in the glucocorticosteroid-dependent child: metabolic and linear growth effects. Horm Res. 2001;56(Suppl 1):13–8.

97. De Benedetti F, Rucci N, Del Fattore A, et al. Impaired skeletal development in interleukin-6-transgenic mice: a model for the impact of chronic inflammation on the growing skeletal system. Arthritis Rheum. 2006;54:3551–63.

98. Kamimura D, Ishihara K, Hirano T. IL-6 signal transduction and its physiological roles: the signal orchestration model. Rev Physiol Biochem Pharmacol. 2003;149:1–38.

99. Tamura T, Udagawa N, Takahashi N, et al. Soluble interleukin-6 receptor triggers osteoclast formation by interleukin 6. Proc Natl Acad Sci U S A. 1993;90:11924–8.

100. Franchimont N, Wertz S, Malaise M. Interleukin-6: An osteotropic factor influencing bone formation? Bone. 2005;37:601–6.

101. D'Mello S, Trauernicht A, Ryan A, et al. Innate dysfunction promotes linear growth failure in pediatric Crohn's disease and growth hormone resistance in murine ileitis. Inflamm Bowel Dis. 2012;18:236–45.

102. Bross DA, Leichtner AM, Zurakowski D, Law T, Bousvaros A. Elevation of serum interleukin-6 but not serum-soluble interleukin-2 receptor in children with Crohn's disease. J Pediatr Gastroenterol Nutr. 1996;23:164–71.

103. Suzuki A, Hanada T, Mitsuyama K, et al. CIS3/SOCS3/SSI3 plays a negative regulatory role in STAT3 activation and intestinal inflammation. J Exp Med. 2001;193:471–81.

104. Tebbutt NC, Giraud AS, Inglese M, et al. Reciprocal regulation of gastrointestinal homeostasis by SHP2 and STAT-mediated trefoil gene activation in gp130 mutant mice. Nat Med. 2002;8:1089–97.

105. Nicholson SE, De Souza D, Fabri LJ, et al. Suppressor of cytokine signaling-3 preferentially binds to the SHP-2-binding site on the shared cytokine receptor subunit gp130. Proc Natl Acad Sci U S A. 2000;97:6493–8.

106. Carey R, Jurickova I, Ballard E, et al. Activation of an IL-6:STAT3-dependent transcriptome in pediatric-onset inflammatory bowel disease. Inflamm Bowel Dis. 2008;14:446–57.

107. Mudter J, Weigmann B, Bartsch B, et al. Activation pattern of signal transducers and activators of transcription (STAT) factors in inflammatory bowel diseases. Am J Gastroenterol. 2005;100:64–72.

108. Cassidy JT, Hillman LS. Abnormalities in skeletal growth in children with juvenile rheumatoid arthritis. Rheum Dis Clin N Am. 1997;23:499–522.

109. MacRae VE, Farquharson C, Ahmed SF. The pathophysiology of the growth plate in juvenile idiopathic arthritis. Rheumatology (Oxford). 2006;45:11–9.

110. Sawczenko A, Azooz O, Paraszczuk J, et al. Intestinal inflammation-induced growth retardation acts through IL-6 in rats and depends on the −174 IL-6 G/C polymorphism in children. Proc Natl Acad Sci U S A. 2005;102:13260–5.

111. Cezard JP, Touati G, Alberti C, Hugot JP, Brinon C, Czernichow P. Growth in paediatric Crohn's disease. Horm Res. 2002;58 (Suppl 1):11–5.

112. Bernstein CN, Leslie WD. The pathophysiology of bone disease in gastrointestinal disease. Eur J Gastroenterol Hepatol. 2003;15:857–64.

113. Lien G, Selvaag AM, Flato B, et al. A two-year prospective controlled study of bone mass and bone turnover in children with early juvenile idiopathic arthritis. Arthritis Rheum. 2005;52:833–40.

114. Ito H, Takazoe M, Fukuda Y, et al. A pilot randomized trial of a human anti-interleukin-6 receptor monoclonal antibody in active Crohn's disease. Gastroenterology. 2004;126:989–96. discussion 47

115. Nishimoto N, Kishimoto T. Inhibition of IL-6 for the treatment of inflammatory diseases. Curr Opin Pharmacol. 2004;4:386–91.

116. Nishimoto N, Yoshizaki K, Miyasaka N, et al. Treatment of rheumatoid arthritis with humanized anti-interleukin-6 receptor antibody: a multicenter, double-blind, placebo-controlled trial. Arthritis Rheum. 2004;50:1761–9.

117. Yokota S, Miyamae T, Imagawa T, et al. Therapeutic efficacy of humanized recombinant anti-interleukin-6 receptor antibody in children with systemic-onset juvenile idiopathic arthritis. Arthritis Rheum. 2005;52:818–25.

118. Wolk K, Witte E, Hoffmann U, et al. IL-22 induces lipopolysaccharide-binding protein in hepatocytes: a potential systemic role of IL-22 in Crohn's disease. J Immunol. 2007;178:5973–81.

119. Allen DB. Influence of inhaled corticosteroids on growth: a pediatric endocrinologist's perspective. Acta Paediatr. 1998;87:123–9.

120. Gupta N, Lustig RH, Kohn MA, Vittinghoff E. Menarche in pediatric patients with Crohn's disease. Dig Dis Sci. 2012;57:2975–81.

121. Wu T, Mendola P, Buck GM. Ethnic differences in the presence of secondary sex characteristics and menarche among US girls: the Third National Health and Nutrition Examination Survey, 1988-1994. Pediatrics. 2002;110:752–7.

122. Susman EJ, Houts RM, Steinberg L, et al. Longitudinal development of secondary sexual characteristics in girls and boys between ages 91/2 and 151/2 years. Arch Pediatr Adolesc Med. 2010;164:166–73.

123. Brain CE, Savage MO. Growth and puberty in chronic inflammatory bowel disease. Baillieres Clin Gastroenterol. 1994;8:83–100.

124. Azooz OG, Farthing MJ, Savage MO, Ballinger AB. Delayed puberty and response to testosterone in a rat model of colitis. Am J Physiol Regul Integr Comp Physiol. 2001;281:R1483–91.

125. DeBoer MD, Li Y, Cohn S. Colitis causes delay in puberty in female mice out of proportion to changes in leptin and corticosterone. J Gastroenterol. 2010;45:277–84.

126. Deboer MD, Li Y. Puberty is delayed in male mice with dextran sodium sulfate colitis out of proportion to changes in food intake, body weight, and serum levels of leptin. Pediatr Res. 2011;69:34–9.

127. Mizokami A, Gotoh A, Yamada H, Keller ET, Matsumoto T. Tumor necrosis factor-alpha represses androgen sensitivity in the LNCaP prostate cancer cell line. J Urol. 2000;164:800–5.

128. Zadik Z, Cooper M, Chen M, Stern N. Cushing's disease presenting as pubertal arrest. J Pediatr Endocrinol. 1993;6:201–4.

129. Deboer MD, Steinman J, Li Y. Partial normalization of pubertal timing in female mice with DSS colitis treated with anti-TNF-alpha antibody. J Gastroenterol. 2012;47:647–54.

130. Russell RK, Drummond HE, Nimmo EE, et al. Genotype-phenotype analysis in childhood-onset Crohn's disease: NOD2/CARD15 variants consistently predict phenotypic characteristics of severe disease. Inflamm Bowel Dis. 2005;11:955–64.

131. Tomer G, Ceballos C, Concepcion E, Benkov KJ. NOD2/CARD15 variants are associated with lower weight at diagnosis in children with Crohn's disease. Am J Gastroenterol. 2003;98:2479–84.

132. Russell RK, Drummond HE, Nimmo ER, et al. Analysis of the influence of OCTN1/2 variants within the IBD5 locus on disease susceptibility and growth indices in early onset inflammatory bowel disease. Gut. 2006;55:1114–23.

133. Lee JJ, Essers JB, Kugathasan S, et al. Association of linear growth impairment in pediatric Crohn's disease and a known height locus: a pilot study. Ann Hum Genet. 2010;74:489–97.

134. Levine A, Shamir R, Wine E, et al. TNF promoter polymorphisms and modulation of growth retardation and disease severity in pediatric Crohn's disease. Am J Gastroenterol. 2005;100:1598–604.

135. Griffiths AM, Otley AR, Hyams J, et al. A review of activity indices and end points for clinical trials in children with Crohn's disease. Inflamm Bowel Dis. 2005;11:185–96.

136. Tuchman S, Thayu M, Shults J, Zemel BS, Burnham JM, Leonard MB. Interpretation of biomarkers of bone metabolism in children: impact of growth velocity and body size in healthy children and chronic disease. J Pediatr. 2008;153:484–90.

137. Thayu M, Leonard MB, Hyams JS, et al. Improvement in biomarkers of bone formation during infliximab therapy in pediatric Crohn's disease: results of the REACH study. Clin Gastroenterol Hepatol. 2008;6:1378–84.

138. Wong SC, Smyth A, McNeill E, et al. The growth hormone insulin-like growth factor 1 axis in children and adolescents with inflammatory bowel disease and growth retardation. Clin Endocrinol (Oxf). 2010;73:220–8.

139. Heuschkel R, Salvestrini C, Beattie RM, Hildebrand H, Walters T, Griffiths A. Guidelines for the management of growth failure in childhood inflammatory bowel disease. Inflamm Bowel Dis. 2008;14:839–49.

140. Griffiths AM, Nicholas D, Smith C, et al. Development of a quality-of-life index for pediatric inflammatory bowel disease: dealing with differences related to age and IBD type. J Pediatr Gastroenterol Nutr. 1999;28:S46–52.

141. Aiges H, Markowitz J, Rosa J, Daum F. Home nocturnal supplemental nasogastric feedings in growth-retarded adolescents with Crohn's disease. Gastroenterology. 1989;97:905–10.

142. Belli DC, Seidman E, Bouthillier L, et al. Chronic intermittent elemental diet improves growth failure in children with Crohn's disease. Gastroenterology. 1988;94:603–10.

143. Wilschanski M, Sherman P, Pencharz P, Davis L, Corey M, Griffiths A. Supplementary enteral nutrition maintains remission in paediatric Crohn's disease. Gut. 1996;38:543–8.

144. Bannerjee K, Camacho-Hubner C, Babinska K, et al. Anti-inflammatory and growth-stimulating effects precede nutritional restitution during enteral feeding in Crohn disease. J Pediatr Gastroenterol Nutr. 2004;38:270–5.

145. Gassull MA, Stange EF. Nutrition and diet in inflammatory bowel disease. In: Satsangi J, Sutherland LR, editors. Inflammatory bowel diseases. London: Elsevier; 2003. p. 461–74.

146. Walker-Smith JA. Management of growth failure in Crohn's disease. Arch Dis Child. 1996;75:351–4.

147. Newby E, Sawczenko A, Thomas A, Wilson D. Interventions for growth failure in childhood Crohn's disease. Cochrane Database Syst Rev. 2005;(3):CD003873.

148. Fell JM, Paintin M, Arnaud-Battandier F, et al. Mucosal healing and a fall in mucosal pro-inflammatory cytokine mRNA induced by a specific oral polymeric diet in paediatric Crohn's disease. Aliment Pharmacol Ther. 2000;14:281–9.

149. Zachos M, Tondeur M, AM G. Enteral nutritional therapy for inducing remission of Crohn's disease. Cochrane Database Syst Rev. 2001;(1):CD000542.

150. Heuschkel RB, Menache CC, Megerian JT, Baird AE. Enteral nutrition and corticosteroids in the treatment of acute Crohn's disease in children. J Pediatr Gastroenterol Nutr. 2000;31:8–15.

151. Griffiths AM, Ohlsson A, Sherman PM, Sutherland LR. Meta-analysis of enteral nutrition as a primary treatment of active Crohn's disease. Gastroenterology. 1995;108:1056–67.

152. Seidman E, Griffiths AM, Jones A. Semi-elemntal diet versus prednisone in the treatment of acute Crohn's disease in children and adolescents. Gastroenterology. 1993;104:A778.

153. Griffiths AM. Enteral nutrition: the neglected primary therapy of active Crohn's disease. J Pediatr Gastroenterol Nutr. 2000;31:3–5.

154. Rigaud D, Cosnes J, Le Quintrec Y, Rene E, Gendre JP, Mignon M. Controlled trial comparing two types of enteral nutrition in treatment of active Crohn's disease: elemental versus polymeric diet. Gut. 1991;32:1492–7.

155. Escher JC. Budesonide versus prednisolone for the treatment of active Crohn's disease in children: a randomized, double-blind, controlled, multicentre trial. Eur J Gastroenterol Hepatol. 2004;16:47–54.

156. Papi C, Luchetti R, Gili L, Montanti S, Koch M, Capurso L. Budesonide in the treatment of Crohn's disease: a meta-analysis. Aliment Pharmacol Ther. 2000;14:1419–28.

157. Kundhal P, Zachos M, Holmes JL, Griffiths AM. Controlled ileal release budesonide in pediatric Crohn disease: efficacy and effect on growth. J Pediatr Gastroenterol Nutr. 2001;33:75–80.

158. Markowitz J, Grancher K, Kohn N, Lesser M, Daum F. A multicenter trial of 6-mercaptopurine and prednisone in children with newly diagnosed Crohn's disease. Gastroenterology. 2000;119: 895–902.

159. Turner D, Grossman AB, Rosh J, et al. Methotrexate following unsuccessful thiopurine therapy in pediatric Crohn's disease. Am J Gastroenterol 2007;102:2804–12; quiz 2803, 2813.

160. Thayu M, Denson LA, Shults J, et al. Determinants of changes in linear growth and body composition in incident pediatric Crohn's disease. Gastroenterology. 2010;139:430–8.

161. Hyams J, Crandall W, Kugathasan S, et al. Induction and maintenance infliximab therapy for the treatment of moderate-to-severe Crohn's disease in children. Gastroenterology 2007;132:863–73; quiz 1165–6.

162. Walters TD, Gilman AR, Griffiths A. Infliximab Therapy Restores Normal Growth in Children with Chronically Active Severe Crohn Disease Refractory to Immunomodulatory Therapy. Gastroenterology. 2005;128 Suppl 2:A27.

163. de Ridder L, Escher JC, Bouquet J, et al. Infliximab therapy in 30 patients with refractory pediatric crohn disease with and without fistulas in The Netherlands. J Pediatr Gastroenterol Nutr. 2004;39:46–52.

164. Borrelli O, Bascietto C, Viola F, et al. Infliximab heals intestinal inflammatory lesions and restores growth in children with Crohn's disease. Dig Liver Dis. 2004;36:342–7.

165. Cezard JP, Nouaili N, Talbotec C, et al. A prospective study of the efficacy and tolerance of a chimeric antibody to tumor necrosis factors (remicade) in severe pediatric crohn disease. J Pediatr Gastroenterol Nutr. 2003;36:632–6.

166. Wanty C, Stephenne X, Sokal E, Smets F. Long-term outcome of infliximab therapy in pediatric Crohn disease. Arch Pediatr. 2011;18:863–9.

167. Malik S, Wong SC, Bishop J, et al. Improvement in growth of children with Crohn disease following anti-TNF-alpha therapy can be independent of pubertal progress and glucocorticoid reduction. J Pediatr Gastroenterol Nutr. 2011;52:31–7.

168. Malik S, Ahmed SF, Wilson ML, et al. The effects of anti-TNF-alpha treatment with adalimumab on growth in children with Crohn's disease (CD). J Crohns Colitis. 2012;6:337–44.

169. Church PC, Guan J, Walters TD, et al. Infliximab maintains durable response and facilitates catch-up growth in luminal pediatric Crohn's disease. Inflamm Bowel Dis. 2014;20:1177–86.

170. Walters TD, Hyams JS. Can early anti-TNF-alpha treatment be an effective therapeutic strategy in children with Crohn's disease? Immunotherapy. 2014;6:799–802.

171. Crombe V, Salleron J, Savoye G, et al. Long-term outcome of treatment with infliximab in pediatric-onset Crohn's disease: a population-based study. Inflamm Bowel Dis. 2011;17: 2144–52.

172. Griffiths AM, Hyams JS, Crandall W. Height of children with Active Crohn's Disease Improves During Treatment with Infliximab. Gastroenterology. 2006;130 Suppl 2:59.

173. Hyams J, Walters TD, Crandall W, et al. Safety and efficacy of maintenance infliximab therapy for moderate-to-severe Crohn's disease in children: REACH open-label extension. Curr Med Res Opin. 2011;27:651–62.

174. Hyams JS, Griffiths A, Markowitz J, et al. Safety and efficacy of adalimumab for moderate to severe Crohn's disease in children. Gastroenterology. 2012;143:365–74.e2.
175. DiFedele LM, He J, Bonkowski EL, et al. Tumor necrosis factor alpha blockade restores growth hormone signaling in murine colitis. Gastroenterology. 2005;128:1278–91.
176. Vespasiani Gentilucci U, Caviglia R, Picardi A, et al. Infliximab reverses growth hormone resistance associated with inflammatory bowel disease. Aliment Pharmacol Ther. 2005;21:1063–71.
177. Nicholls S, Vieira MC, Majrowski WH, Shand WS, Savage MO, Walker-Smith JA. Linear growth after colectomy for ulcerative colitis in childhood. J Pediatr Gastroenterol Nutr. 1995;21:82–6.
178. Griffiths AM, Wesson DE, Shandling B, Corey M, Sherman PM. Factors influencing postoperative recurrence of Crohn's disease in childhood. Gut. 1991;32:491–5.
179. Davies G, Evans CM, Shand WS, Walker-Smith JA. Surgery for Crohn's disease in childhood: influence of site of disease and operative procedure on outcome. Br J Surg. 1990;77:891–4.
180. Baldassano RN, Han PD, Jeshion WC, et al. Pediatric Crohn's disease: risk factors for postoperative recurrence. Am J Gastroenterol. 2001;96:2169–76.
181. McCaffery Jr TD, Nasr K, Lawrence AM, Kirsner JB. Effect of administered human growth hormone on growth retardation in inflammatory bowel disease. Am J Dig Dis. 1974;19:411–6.
182. Henker J. Therapy with recombinant growth hormone in children with Crohn disease and growth failure. Eur J Pediatr. 1996;155:1066–7.
183. Henker J. Effect of growth hormone therapy in patients with Crohn disease. J Pediatr Gastroenterol Nutr. 2002;34:424–5.
184. Heyman MB, Garnett EA, Wojcicki J, et al. Growth hormone treatment for growth failure in pediatric patients with Crohn's disease. J Pediatr 2008;153:651–8, 658.e1–3
185. Calenda KA, Schornagel IL, Sadeghi-Nejad A, Grand RJ. Effect of recombinant growth hormone treatment on children with Crohn's disease and short stature: a pilot study. Inflamm Bowel Dis. 2005;11:435–41.
186. Denson LA, Kim MO, Bezold R, et al. A randomized controlled trial of growth hormone in active pediatric Crohn disease. J Pediatr Gastroenterol Nutr. 2010;51:130–9.
187. Wong SC, Kumar P, Galloway PJ, et al. A preliminary trial of the effect of recombinant human growth hormone on short-term linear growth and glucose homeostasis in children with Crohn's disease. Clin Endocrinol (Oxf). 2011;74:599–607.
188. Vortia E, Kay M, Wyllie R. The role of growth hormone and insulin-like growth factor-1 in Crohn's disease: implications for therapeutic use of human growth hormone in pediatric patients. Curr Opin Pediatr. 2011;23:545–51.
189. Bechtold S, Ripperger P, Dalla Pozza R, et al. Dynamics of body composition and bone in patients with juvenile idiopathic arthritis treated with growth hormone. J Clin Endocrinol Metab. 2010;95:178–85.
190. Phung OJ, Coleman CI, Baker EL, et al. Recombinant human growth hormone in the treatment of patients with cystic fibrosis. Pediatrics. 2010;126:e1211–26.
191. Mauras N, George D, Evans J, et al. Growth hormone has anabolic effects in glucocorticosteroid-dependent children with inflammatory bowel disease: a pilot study. Metabolism. 2002;51:127–35.
192. Slonim AE, Bulone L, Damore MB, Goldberg T, Wingertzahn MA, McKinley MJ. A preliminary study of growth hormone therapy for Crohn's disease. N Engl J Med. 2000;342:1633–7.
193. Han X, Sosnowska D, Bonkowski EL, Denson LA. Growth hormone inhibits signal transducer and activator of transcription 3 activation and reduces disease activity in murine colitis. Gastroenterology. 2005;129:185–203.
194. Rao A, Standing JF, Naik S, Savage MO, Sanderson IR. Mathematical modelling to restore circulating IGF-1 concentrations in children with Crohn's disease-induced growth failure: a pharmacokinetic study. BMJ Open. 2013;3:e002737.
195. Mason A, Wong SC, McGrogan P, Ahmed SF. Effect of testosterone therapy for delayed growth and puberty in boys with inflammatory bowel disease. Horm Res Paediatr. 2011;75:8–13.

Inflammatory Bowel Diseases and Skeletal Health

Francisco Sylvester

Introduction

The skeleton is a scaffold for soft tissue but is also the largest calcium reservoir in the body, and it harbors and interacts with the hematopoietic bone marrow. In addition, bone tissue is metabolically active and susceptible to regulation by local and systemic signals, including those generated during active intestinal inflammation. Moreover, mechanical strain exerted by skeletal muscle is anabolic to bone, and muscle mass is frequently decreased in inflammatory bowel disease (IBD). In addition, children with IBD can have deficiencies in macro- and micronutrients that impact the availability of protein to synthesize bone matrix and calcium and phosphate to mineralize it. Consequently, the integrity of the skeleton is vulnerable to the effects of IBD on bone cell function and muscle mass. In addition, IBD may influence bone indirectly, by inhibiting key endocrine axes, such as insulin-like growth factor 1 (IGF-1) and sex steroids, which are critical for bone formation and maintenance of skeletal mass. Childhood is characterized by active bone metabolism and growth in size and width due to the combined activities of bone cells and the growth plate. *Bone modeling*, which is the main process responsible for bone tissue expansion in childhood until skeletal maturity is reached, involves both bone-forming osteoblasts, bone-resorbing osteoclasts, and osteocytes, with all cell types being active at the same time on different bone surfaces, with net gain in bone mass (Fig. 13.1) [1]. Osteoblasts, osteoclasts, osteocytes, and chondrocytes may be sensitive to disease and treatment effects in children with IBD, impairing both bone formation and linear growth [2]. *Bone remodeling*, which occurs in both adults and children, is on the other hand a slower process that aims to repair and maintain existing bone mass and architecture. It involves the sequential activities of osteoclasts and osteoblasts under the direction of osteocytes on the same bone surface. Osteoclasts first dissolve stressed or microfractured bone, which is then followed by bone matrix formation by osteoblasts to fill the gap. This process is orchestrated by osteocytes embedded in the bone matrix [3]. In children with active IBD, both bone metabolic activity and linear growth are impaired [4]. Both modeling and remodeling may be affected by multiple influences, including malnutrition, inflammation, inactivity, hypogonadism, and medications such as corticosteroids [2]. In this chapter, we will review current clinical and experimental evidence of the effects of IBD on the pediatric skeleton.

Growth and Bone Modeling and Remodeling

Childhood is a time of active skeletal growth and maturation. After rapid growth in the third trimester of gestation and in the early neonatal period, bone growth rates fall sharply until puberty. Sexual maturation during puberty is associated with a dramatic acceleration in longitudinal bone growth until it ceases when growth plates become fused. The structure of bone changes during growth, with expansion of the medullary cavity and thickening of the cortical shell and of existing bone trabeculae. Consequently, the mechanical properties of bone evolve rapidly during adolescence. Bone mineralization lags behind linear growth, resulting in a relative structural weakness that increases fracture risk during adolescence [5–7]. Peak bone mass is achieved after a period of consolidation at the end of the second decade of life in females and at the beginning of the third decade of life in males [8, 9]. Consequently, gains in skeletal mass may occur after epiphyseal closure and cessation of linear growth. After a period of stability that lasts for about two decades, bone loss occurs after menopause in women and in elderly men. In adults, loss of mineral mass is accompanied by deterioration of bone microarchitecture and increased propensity to fractures with age, leading to osteoporosis [10]. Bone deterioration may be

F. Sylvester, MD
The University of North Carolina at Chapel Hill,
333 South Columbia Street 247 MacNider Hall, Chapel Hill,
NC, USA
e-mail: fsylvester@unc.edu

© Springer International Publishing AG 2017
P. Mamula et al. (eds.), *Pediatric Inflammatory Bowel Disease*, DOI 10.1007/978-3-319-49215-5_13

Fig. 13.1 Bone modeling and remodeling. (**a**) Bone remodeling takes place in both adults and children. It can occur in either trabecular or cortical bone as a consequence of microfractures, mechanical stress, or triggered to replace old bone. Small amounts of bone are dissolved by osteoclasts, which are followed by a wave of bone-forming osteoblasts. The protein matrix secreted by osteoblasts then becomes calcified, restoring the original bone mass. (**b**) Bone modeling occurs uniquely in children and results from the combined activities of osteoblasts, osteoclasts, osteocytes, and growth plate cells. As a result, bone grows in length and width and is reshaped. Compared to remodeling, bone modeling is a fast process in which all bone surfaces are active and osteoblasts and osteoclasts work at the same time

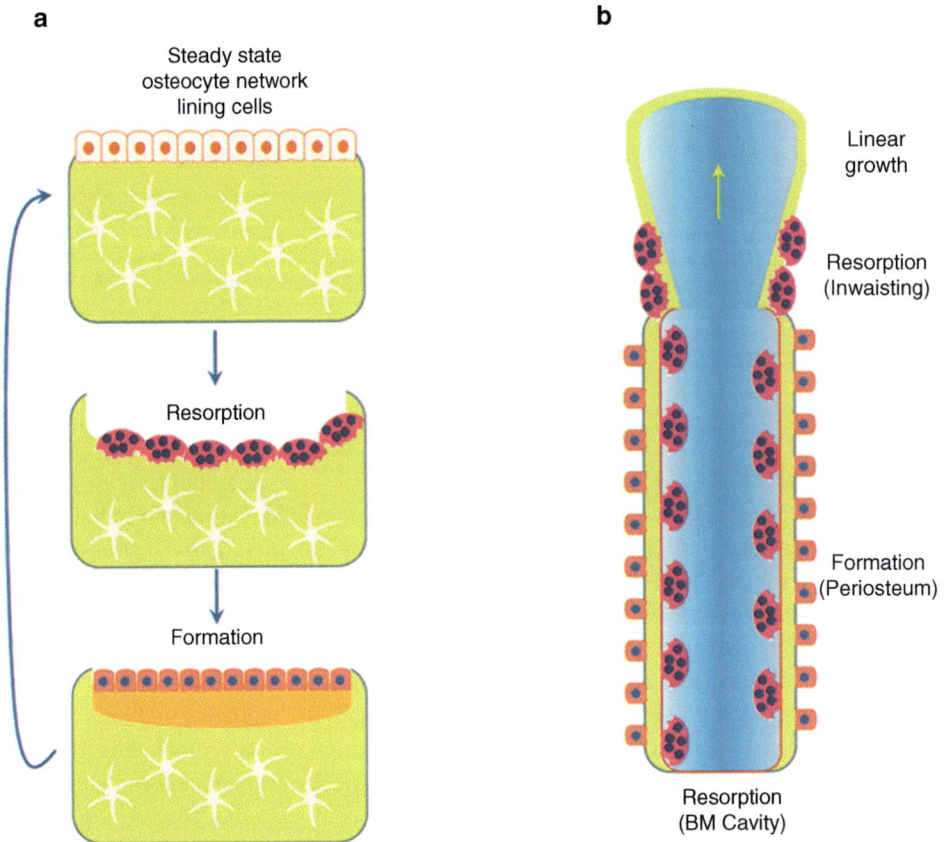

enhanced by IBD in adults, but the effects of the disease in children are probably different due to the unique features of skeletal biology in individuals that are still growing compared to adults.

Bone mass is maintained by bone remodeling, characterized by the formation of a functional unit that consists of osteoclasts and osteoblasts, under the direction of osteocytes (the bone-remodeling unit) (Fig. 13.1) [3]. In response to damage or mechanical strain, osteoclasts resorb bone and form resorption pits. This is followed by a decrease in sclerostin from osteocytes [11], which removes a break for bone formation. There is consequent recruitment of osteoblasts that fill the bone divots with a specialized protein matrix (osteoid, composed primarily of type I collagen). Osteoid later becomes mineralized by deposition of hydroxyapatite, a calcium and phosphate crystal [12]. Some osteoblasts undergo apoptosis, while others become embedded in the newly formed bone matrix and become osteocytes. Osteocytes become interconnected by dendrites, sense mechanical strain, and direct the cells of the bone-remodeling unit with mediators such as sclerostin [3]. The process of remodeling typically takes several months and generates small amounts of bone. In bone remodeling, the activities of osteoblasts and osteoclasts are sequentially coordinated, so formation normally follows resorption. Only about 20% of bone surfaces in the

body are actively engaged in this process at any given time. Bone remodeling occurs both in adults and children and takes place in both cortical and trabecular bone [13]. Importantly, bone cells involved in remodeling cross talk with bone marrow cells [14]. The bone marrow harbors T cells that may be generated in the inflamed intestine. Colitogenic CD4+ T central memory cells and T effector memory cells have been reported in the bone marrow of mouse models of colitis [15, 16]. Interleukin-7 (IL-7) produced by bone marrow stromal cells is required to maintain these cells [17]. In the IL-2$^{-/-}$ model of inflammation, activated T cells accumulate in the bone marrow and produce receptor activator of nuclear factor κB ligand (RANKL) [18]. T regulatory cells also exist in the bone marrow [19, 20]. Therefore, it is possible that T cells that migrated from the inflamed gut to the bone marrow influence bone remodeling.

Gains in bone mass in childhood are largely due a combination of the action of the growth plate and a distinct process called bone modeling, which is normally exclusive to children (Fig. 13.1). Bone modeling can be compared to the process of erecting a skyscraper, which requires a large amount of new material and connecting diverse structure elements. Bone remodeling on the other hand is akin to maintaining the building's structural integrity over time by scheduled and unscheduled repairs (prompted by damage).

In children, accumulation of bone mass is largely a consequence of linear growth and bone modeling [1]. Longitudinal growth is triggered by hormonal signals and involves the production of a cartilaginous scaffold by the growth plate that is calcified, remodeled by osteoclasts, and turned into trabecular bone. Trabeculae act as struts, plates, and joists to distribute mechanical load from the epiphysis to the compact bone shaft, which carries the majority of the load. Linear growth and bone modeling occur simultaneously, with osteoblasts laying down new bone matrix in the periosteal surface, while osteoclasts reshape the bone by resorbing endosteal and metaphyseal bone (resulting in the expansion of the medullary cavity and metaphyseal inwaisting, respectively). Bone modeling occurs in 100% of bone surfaces, with both osteoclasts and osteoblasts being active at the same time, and is faster than bone remodeling [21].

These significant physiological differences between pediatric and adult bone have important implications for children with IBD. Disease and treatment factors influence both modeling and remodeling, but the major impact in children is likely to be on growth plate cells and bone modeling, the two most active processes in bone during growth. Moreover, IBD in children is associated with significant deficits in muscle mass, leading to a decrease in mechanical strain on bone and a consequent reduction in bone modeling, and weight loss associated with IBD decreases gravitational forces on the skeleton that are anabolic.

The measurement of true volumetric bone density with peripheral computed tomography is not routinely available clinically. Instead, dual X-ray absorptiometry (DXA), a precise and accurate method commonly used to assess bone mass, measures bone mineral content, which is divided by bone area (e.g., DXA "density" is expressed as g/cm^2, or "areal" bone density, not a true material density). DXA produces a two-dimensional projection of the three-dimensional skeleton, so larger bones with equal material density than smaller bones will be measured as "denser" by DXA. Therefore, diseases like IBD that can affect linear growth and bone size may affect DXA measurements by underestimating bone mass in smaller children. This requires correction of DXA readings for patient's size, sex, and sexual maturation [22] (please see Chap. 24 "Bone Health Assessment in Pediatric Inflammatory Bowel Disease" for more information).

Bone Cells and Inflammation

Osteoclasts and the RANKL/OPG System

Both bone remodeling and modeling involve the activity of osteoclasts and osteoblasts. Osteoclasts secrete enzymes

(e.g., cathepsin K) and acid that dissolve the bone mineral and degrade the bone matrix. This releases collagen split products and growth factors (such as transforming growth factor-β) embedded in the bone matrix that stimulate osteoblast recruitment to the resorption site. Osteoclasts are cells from the macrophage/monocyte (myeloid) lineage, which secrete and are regulated by cytokines [23]. Osteoclasts are formed primarily by stimulation of hematopoietic precursors with RANKL in the presence of macrophage stimulating factor (M-CSF) (Fig. 13.2). RANKL, a member of the tumor necrosis factor receptor superfamily, is produced by osteoblasts, stromal cells, fibroblasts, and activated T cells [24, 25] and stimulates osteoclast differentiation, activation, and survival. A complex network of cytokines and immune receptors regulate osteoclast formation and activity either directly or indirectly via RANKL [26–31]. RANKL-deficient mice have hyperdense bones secondary to lack of osteoclasts [25]. RANKL has been implicated as a key factor in the pathogenesis of bone loss associated with increased resorption, including postmenopausal osteoporosis and rheumatoid arthritis. A monoclonal antibody to RANKL, denosumab, is used to treat postmenopausal osteoporosis and bone loss associated with rheumatoid arthritis [32, 33].

Osteoprotegerin (OPG) is a soluble decoy receptor for RANKL produced by osteoblasts and stromal cells [34]. OPG is a potent inhibitor of osteoclast development. OPG transgenic mice have hyperdense bones, a phenotype that can be replicated by systemic administration of OPG to normal mice. OPG-null mice on the other hand are profoundly osteopenic due to unopposed osteoclast activity [35, 36]. Besides OPG, another control switch in osteoclast development is interferon (IFN)-β, which is induced by RANKL binding to its receptor RANK on osteoclast precursors [37]. IFN-β interferes with the activity of c-fos, a transcription factor that is essential for osteoclast formation. Other factors, such as transforming growth factor-β (TGF-β) and Wnt, inhibit osteoclastogenesis by upregulating the production of OPG by osteoblasts [38]. Wnt also directly represses RANKL expression via the Wnt canonical pathway [39, 40], while Wnt5a, a typical non-canonical Wnt ligand, enhances the expression of RANK in osteoclast precursors [41]. In addition, several cytokines relevant to the pathogenesis of IBD inhibit osteoclast differentiation, including interferon-γ (IFN-γ) [42], IL-10 [43, 44], IL-12 [45, 46], and IL-17 [47, 48]. Moreover, osteoclast differentiation involves transcription factors such as NFκB, AP-1, and NFATc1, as well as co-stimulation via immunoglobulin-like receptors and activation of the phosphatase calcineurin, which can be regulated by inflammation [47, 49–52]. Therefore, osteoclast formation is subject to multiple regulatory controls by cytokines, transcription factors, and enzymes that play key roles in

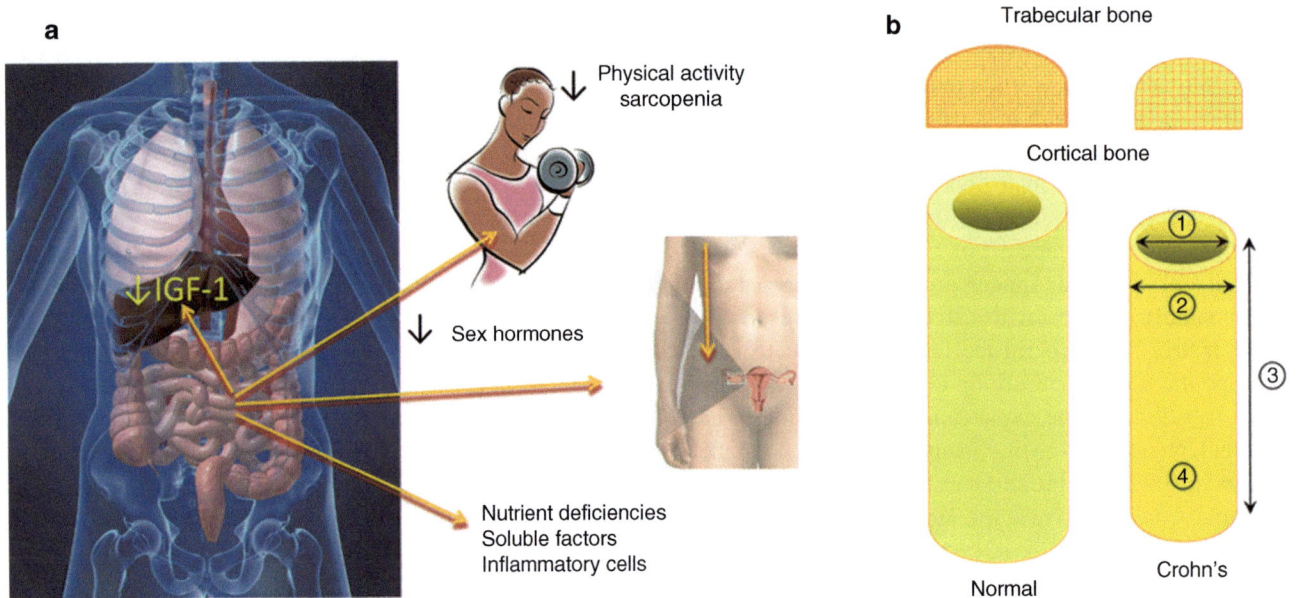

Fig. 13.2 Effects of IBD on the muscle-bone unit. (**a**) Active inflammation in IBD can affect the skeleton by multiple mechanisms, including blocking the formation of IGF-1 in the liver, delaying puberty, and affecting bone cell function via immune cells and cytokines. A decrease in muscle mass (sarcopenia) can impair bone development. Active IBD can also cause fatigue and decreased weight-bearing activity. Corticosteroids to treat IBD can primarily impair bone formation and secondarily increase bone resorption. Malnutrition can affect the availability of protein, calcium, and vitamin D; they are essential for normal bone formation. Therefore, IBD constitutes a multipronged attack on the integrity of the muscle-bone unit and puts at risk the acquisition of genetically programmed peak bone mass. (**b**) At diagnosis, children with Crohn disease have significant bone mass deficits and alterations in bone geometry. In cortical bone, these include ① increased endosteal surface probably due to increased bone resorption, ② decreased periosteal circumference secondary to decreased bone formation, ③ reduced bone length due to growth plate inactivity, and ④ increased cortical bone density, likely a result of reduced bone remodeling. Trabecular bone is less dense ⑤. Some of these abnormalities can be partially reversible with anti-inflammatory therapy (resulting in reduction in endosteal surface, improved bone length, increased trabecular bone density, and decreased cortical bone density), but periosteal circumference can remain lower than normal

IBD. In addition, osteoclasts interact closely with the hematopoietic stem cells niche [53, 54]. These pathways are an example of the close physiological ties between the immune system and bone cells. However, it is not yet known whether these mechanisms are engaged in regulating bone mass in children with IBD.

The RANKL/OPG system also plays important roles outside of bone. This is evidenced by the lack of peripheral lymph nodes and impaired development of lactating mammary glands in RANKL or RANK-null mice [55]. In addition, RANKL/OPG may be involved in the formation of calcified atherosclerotic plaques, and serum OPG is emerging as a marker of cardiovascular mortality [56, 57]. The balance between RANKL and OPG may affect the severity of bone metastases of several cancers [58]. RANKL contributes to normal dendritic cell function and survival and the early development of B and T cells [25, 59, 60]. In addition, RANKL/RANK may play a role in intestinal mucosal tolerance [60]. OPG also has a role in the regulation of the immune response. Both B cells and dendritic cells secrete OPG, and this secretion is regulated by the CD40 receptor [61]. Also, dendritic cells isolated from OPG$^{-/-}$ mice more efficiently present antigen in vitro and secrete more inflammatory cytokines when stimulated with bacterial products or soluble RANKL in vitro [62]. Collectively, this evidence suggests that RANKL/RANK/OPG plays an important role in the regulation of the immune response and in pathways involving the mobilization of calcium [63].

A role for the RANKL/OPG system is emerging in IBD. Circulating OPG levels are elevated in patients with IBD [64, 65], and expression of OPG and RANKL is increased in colonic macrophages, dendritic cells, and epithelial cells [66, 67]. High fecal OPG (which probably comes from the inflamed colonic epithelium) predicts resistance to corticosteroids and to infliximab in patients with IBD [68, 69]. In addition, fecal OPG decreases in children with IBD in remission [65]. Currently it is not clear whether circulating OPG in patients with IBD represents spillover from intestinal inflammatory activity or it comes from bone or other tissues (e.g., the endothelium or the liver) or from lipopolysaccharide that permeates into the systemic circulation from the inflamed gut. The function of RANKL/OPG in the pathogenesis of intestinal inflammation deserves further study.

Osteoblasts

Osteoblasts are cells from mesenchymal origin that lay down bone matrix that is rich in type 1 collagen. Several factors and hormones regulate osteoblast formation, both systemic and in the bone microenvironment [70]. Insulin-like growth factor-1 (IGF-1) is secreted by the liver in response to stimulation by growth hormone and enhances the expression of the mature osteoblast phenotype [71]. Serum IGF-1 is frequently reduced in children with active IBD due to growth hormone insensitivity in the liver and malnutrition [72]. Consequently, relative IGF-1 deficiency in children with IBD may negatively affect osteoblast differentiation and function. Tumor necrosis factor-α (TNF-α), an important cytokine in the pathogenesis of IBD, inhibits osteoblast development by inducing the degradation of Runx2 [73], a critical transcription factor in osteoblast development [73] and suppression of osteogenic factor signaling including Wnt [29] and bone morphogenetic protein-2 [74, 75]. TNF-α also regulates a number of inflammatory chemokines and cytokines, inflammatory genes, transcriptional regulators, bone-remodeling genes, signal transducers, cytoskeletal genes, and genes involved in apoptosis in pre-osteoblasts [76]. TNF-α and colitis decrease the expression of *Phex* in osteoblasts, which affects their mineralization function [77, 78]. TNF-α induces cAMP response element-binding protein H (CREBH), which blocks the anabolic effects of bone morphogenetic protein-2 on osteoblast precursors by inducing the Smurf1-mediated degradation of Smad1 [79]. In children, TNF-α blockade leads to a brisk increase in biomarkers of bone formation and significant linear growth, suggesting an activation of bone modeling [80, 81]. However, the effects of infliximab may be a product of improved disease control and not specific effects of this drug on bone metabolism in these patients. Besides their bone-forming activity, osteoblasts also interact with hematopoietic cells in the bone marrow [82].

T Cells and Bone Loss

T cells are emerging as important regulators of bone cell function [83]. Activated T cells can regulate osteoclast formation and activity by several mechanisms, both RANKL dependent and independent. Activated T cells secrete RANKL and consequently can promote osteoclast differentiation and survival. Both soluble and membrane-bound RANKL are produced by activated CD4+ and CD8+ T cells [24]. T cell-induced bone resorption has been implicated in tissue injury in animal models of arthritis and periodontal disease [84]. CD4+ Th17 T cells may be the most

pro-resorptive T cell in the bone marrow [47] probably due to their ability to secrete cytokines that stimulate osteoclast formation and activity [85], upregulation of RANK in osteoclast precursors [86], and increased expression of RANKL in osteocytes [87]. This is significant given the importance of Th17 cells in the pathogenesis of IBD [88]. T cells may also play an important role in bone loss associated with estrogen deficiency, where osteoclast activity is upregulated. This is suggested by experiments performed in ovariectomized mice, where absence of T cells prevents bone loss [89]. In this model, the expansion of a TNF-α-producing T-cell pool appears to be essential and may occur as a result of upregulation of antigen presentation. The nature of the activating antigen(s) is not yet known, but it is possible that both self and foreign epitopes (including intestinal bacterial products) may play a role [90]. The concept that T cells activated by bacterial antigens may regulate bone cell function is intriguing in the setting of IBD, due to the defects in microbial recognition and processing that have been identified in this condition [91]. In IBD, it is possible that activated T cells may serve as "inflammatory shuttles" between the intestine and bone, since circulating T cells produce cytokines that can regulate both osteoblasts and osteoclasts. Ciucci et al. have shown that bone marrow IL-17/TNF-α-producing CD4+ T cells from IL-10$^{-/-}$ mice with colitis (but not from IL-10$^{-/-}$ without colitis or wild-type mice) induce osteoclast formation in vitro without addition of RANKL/M-CSF. These cells express membrane-bound RANKL and secrete M-CSF [16]. In addition, it is possible that circulating antigens may trigger immune responses via T-cell memory cells in the bone marrow that affect bone cell function. The activation state of T cells may also be important in their interaction with osteoclasts, since resting T cells inhibit osteoclastogenesis [92]. T regulatory cells (Treg) are present in the bone marrow and are potent inhibitors of bone resorption [93] probably due to their secretion of IL-4, IL-10, and TGF-β. In addition, T cells may also regulate bone formation by osteoblasts. For example, bone marrow CD8+ T cells stimulated by intermittent parathyroid hormone administration activate anabolic canonical Wnt signaling in pre-osteoblasts by CD8+ T cells [94]. Moreover, bone cells can influence T-cell differentiation and activity. Osteoclasts affect the differentiation and activity of $\gamma\delta$ T cells from peripheral blood in vitro via soluble factors and cell-to-cell contact [95]. Osteoclasts can function as antigen-presenting cells and direct the formation of effector CD4+ and CD8+ cells [96] and induce FoxP3 expression in CD8+ cells [97]. Osteoclasts can also induce the formation of anti-resorptive CD8+ Treg [98], in a process that involves permissive levels of RANKL [99]. Examining these complex mechanisms in the context of IBD awaits additional research.

Novel Pathogenic Pathways in IBD: Bone Connections

Genome-wide association studies have identified a number of unsuspected pathogenic pathways in IBD. Among them are endoplasmic reticulum (ER) stress, the unfolded protein response (UPR), and autophagy [100]. These pathways regulate the function of highly secretory cells such as Paneth cells and goblet cells in the intestinal lining and innate immune cells in the intestinal lamina propria [101]. When there is an overabundance of unfolded and misfolded proteins in the ER, the ER becomes stressed. The UPR is triggered, involving the activation of inositol-requiring kinase 1 α (IRE1α), pancreatic ER eIF2α kinase (PERK), and activating transcription factor 6 α (ATF6α) [102]. Each pathway leads to separate transcriptional events. The UPR aims to restore homeostasis to the ER by decreasing transcription and protein synthesis, degradation of proteins inside the ER, and shuttling of proteins away from the ER with chaperones. When ER stress is chronic and homeostasis cannot be achieved by the UPR, the cell goes into apoptosis. Osteoblasts secrete large amounts of collagen (osteoid, the bone matrix) and other factors and might be affected by defects in ER stress and the UPR found in IBD [103]. Bone morphogenetic protein-2 (BMP-2, a stimulator of osteoblast development and activity) induces the expression of ER stress transducers, such as old astrocyte specifically induced substance [104] and ATF [105]. The inositol-requiring protein 1α (IRE1α) and its target transcription factor X-box binding protein 1 (XBP1) are essential for BMP-2 -induced osteoblast differentiation [106]. The BMP-2 signaling pathway also activates the UPR during osteogenesis [105, 106], which induces the synthesis of RANKL and osteoclastogenesis [107]. To date, it is not known whether defects in the UPR that occur in IBD affect osteoblast function. Mature osteoclasts actively secrete acid and proteolytic enzymes such as cathepsin K to degrade the bone matrix and are also sensitive to ER stress. The IRE1α/XBP1-mediated branch is important in osteoclast development [108] and is involved in parathyroid hormone-induced osteoclast formation [107]. Therefore, defects in the UPR and ER stress present in IBD may affect the development and activity of both osteoblasts and osteoclasts.

Autophagy is a process by which cells recycle old proteins, damaged organelles, and other cellular debris. These elements are encircled by double-membrane vesicles called the autophagosomes, which fuse with lysosomes to become autolysosomes. Their content is recycled and returned back to the cell. Autophagy also plays a role in bacterial digestion after phagocytosis. The mammalian target of rapamycin (mTOR) is an important regulator of autophagy. In addition to controlling cell growth and metabolism, mTOR negatively regulates autophagy when nutrients and growth factors are abundant [109]. In IBD autophagy can be deficient, leading to persistence of bacteria inside of cells. It is possible that defects in autophagy in IBD may affect bone cell function.

For example, induction of autophagy in osteoclasts decreases bone resorption [110]. On the other hand, autophagy induces osteoclast formation during hypoxia [111] and microgravity [112]. Autophagy is important for osteoblast differentiation [113, 114] and bone mineralization [115]. Therefore, it is possible that altered autophagy in IBD impairs normal osteoid mineralization by osteoblasts. Moreover, GWAS suggests that genes involved in autophagy regulate bone mineral density in humans [116]. In summary, pathogenic pathways involved in IBD may establish novel osteoimmune connections, an area that deserves additional study.

Cytokines produced by the inflamed intestine can regulate bone cell activity. IL-6, IL-17, and TNF-α induce osteoclast formation in vitro [16, 117, 118]. However, indirect effects of cytokines mediated through osteoblasts may affect their ultimate influence on osteoclasts. For example, IL-17 stimulates osteoblasts to secrete GM-CSF in the presence of vitamin D, resulting in inhibition of osteoclast formation in vitro [119]. IL-17 can also induce mesenchymal stromal cells and osteoblasts to secrete RANKL, which would stimulate osteoclastogenesis and bone resorption [47, 120]. In a mouse model of colitis, Th17 cells in the bone marrow that produce TNF-α and RANKL increase osteoclast formation; this effect can be blocked by an anti-IL-17 antibody, suggesting that IL-17 is an important pathogenic factor that reduces bone mass in this model [16]. Oncostatin M (OSM), a cytokine of the IL-6 family, is a major coupling factor produced by activated circulating CD14+ or bone marrow CD11b+ monocytes/macrophages upon activation of toll-like receptors (TLRs) by lipopolysaccharide or endogenous ligands that induce osteoblast differentiation and matrix mineralization from human mesenchymal stem cells [121].

Innate immune responses can be activated by toll-like receptors (TLRs). The mechanism of pathogen-induced bone disease includes activation of TLRs in immune cells by pathogen-derived molecules [122]. This activation results in synthesis and release of inflammatory cytokines that are capable of stimulating osteoclastic bone resorption, thus causing bone loss. Osteoclasts express functional TLRs. TLR ligands (CpG-ODN, LPS, Poly(I:C)) exert dual effect on osteoclast precursors. They inhibit the activity of the physiological osteoclast differentiation factor, RANKL, in early precursors, but strongly increase osteoclastogenesis in RANKL-pretreated osteoclast precursors [123–126].

The gut microbiome probably plays an important role in the pathogenesis of IBD. The study of the effects of the intestinal microbiota on bone development is in its early stages however. A report by Sjogren et al. suggests that gut bacteria are essential for normal postnatal bone remodeling [127]. Britton et al. showed that a strain of *Lactobacillus reuteri* can reverse osteoporosis caused by ovariectomy in mice [128]. The same group has treated bone loss associated by experimental type 1 diabetes in mice [129]. Collectively this evidence offers proof of principle that enteric organisms have the potential to regulate bone cell activity. More research is needed in this important area that is very relevant to human IBD.

Effects of Intestinal Inflammation on Bone

Animal Models

IBD is a complex clinical entity, where multiple disease and treatment factors contribute to affect bone cell biology and ultimately skeletal health. In an effort to study mechanistic questions, animal models of intestinal inflammation have been used by several groups. A brief description of their observations follows.

Studies in both rat and mouse models suggest that intestinal inflammation can decrease bone mass by impairing bone formation. Lin et al. induced colitis in rats by rectal instillation of TNBS [130] to study its effects on bone mass, assessed by quantitative histomorphometry. After 3 weeks, rats with colitis had a 33% loss of trabecular bone loss in the tibia compared with age-matched, pair-fed control animals. This was associated with a marked suppression of the trabecular bone formation rate. As the colitis healed, bone formation became more active and bone mass normalized after 12 weeks. In IL-10$^{-/-}$ mice with colitis, Dresner-Pollak et al. performed bone densitometry, ash weight, histomorphometry analysis, and mechanical fragility testing [131]. They observed that bone mass decreased secondary to decreased bone formation in 8- and 12-week-old mice; bone resorption was not increased in mice with colitis compared to wild-type controls. Long bones were more fragile in IL-10$^{-/-}$ with colitis, and ash weight was reduced. However, since these studies did not include IL-10$^{-/-}$ mice without colitis, it was not clear if at least some of the observations in the skeleton of IL-10$^{-/-}$ mice were due to the IL-10 deficiency. More recently, Ciucci et al. addressed this gap and reported significant decreases in trabecular thickness, trabecular number, trabecular bone surface density, and trabecular bone volume per tissue volume in IL-10$^{-/-}$ mice with colitis, but not in IL-10$^{-/-}$ mice without colitis [16], suggesting that in this model bone effects are due to colitis and not IL-10 deficiency. IL-10$^{-/-}$ mice with colitis harbor in their bone marrow IL-17/TNF-α-producing CD4$^+$ T cells that attract osteoclast precursors. In addition, bone marrow mesenchymal stromal cells produce chemokines that may attract additional osteoclast precursors in this model [16]. Harris et al. have demonstrated that the inhibition of bone formation and bone modeling is reversible with healing of colitis in mice [132].

Three reports using adoptive transfer models of colitis suggest that bone mass decreases secondary to increased bone resorption. In the first paper, Ashcroft et al. studied IL-2$^{-/-}$ mice with colitis at 4, 7, and 9 weeks of age and compared X-ray and histomorphometry with IL-2$^{-/+}$ and wild-type mice. IL-2$^{-/-}$ mice develop colitis and also have splenomegaly, anemia, and other signs of systemic inflammation [18]. They observed a decrease in trabecular bone volume in IL-2$^{-/-}$ with colitis compared with the other two groups of mice at 7 and 9 weeks of age. C57BL/6-Rag1$^{-/-}$ mice transplanted with CD3$^+$ cells from IL-2$^{-/-}$ had significantly lower femoral BMD and % trabecular volume 6–8 weeks post-grafting. Serum OPG and osteoclast number were significantly higher in mice engrafted with T cells from IL-2$^{-/-}$ mice compared to IL-2$^{+/+}$. In this model, treatment with OPG was associated with both improved bone mass and decreased intestinal inflammation. These results point to a possible role of T cells in bone loss in the context of intestinal inflammation and suggest a possible anti-inflammatory role for OPG. In the second study, Byrne et al. transferred CD4$^+$CD45RB^{Hi} or CD4$^+$CD45RB^{Lo} from CB6F1 mice to C.B.17 scid/scid mice [133]. CD4$^+$CD45RB^{Hi}, but not CD4$^+$CD45RB^{Lo}, caused colitis in recipient mice, and mice with colitis had lower bone mineral density in the femur/tibia. To treat bone loss, mice received Fc-OPG 3.4–5 mg/kg SC three times weekly for 34 days. OPG had no effect on the severity of colitis but significantly improved BMD. In the third study, Ciucci et al. reported CD4$^+$T cells in the bone marrow of mice with colitis that produce IL-17 and TNF-α, capable of stimulating osteoclastogenesis in vitro [16].

Collectively, these observations suggest that intestinal inflammation can directly affect bone mass in rodents. Mechanisms may include decreased bone formation or increased bone resorption, depending on the model. It appears that intestinal inflammation present at an early age is associated with decreased bone formation. Administration of exogenous OPG increases bone mass in older mice with certain forms of colitis. However, this may be a nonspecific effect of OPG on normally active osteoclasts and by itself does not establish that increased bone resorption is responsible for bone loss in rodent models of colitis. In addition, in adoptive transfer models of colitis, it is not possible to distinguish whether intestinal inflammation in the recipient animals caused bone loss or if colitogenic T cells directly migrated into the bone marrow, influencing bone cell function. However, it is interesting that in the CD4$^+$CD45RB^{Hi} model there is an inflammatory infiltrate in the bone marrow containing TNF-α-producing cells [133]. This provides proof of principle that intestinal inflammation is associated with the presence of activated T cells in the bone marrow that secrete pro-inflammatory cytokines which may influence the function of bone cells. The presence of these cells awaits studies in other animal models of intestinal inflammation and in humans.

Human Studies

Several studies have measured bone mineral density in children with IBD, both in incident and in prevalent cohorts (Table 13.1). The studies, which have been either longitudinal

Table 13.1 Studies on bone density in children with IBD

	Cohort	n	Age (years)	M/F	Normative data	Z-score	Risk factors	Ref
CD	Iᵃ	17	Mean 13.9 ± 2.1	17	Healthy controls	Lower bone mineral content/bone width	N/A	[134]
CD UC	I Pᵇ	123	(Mean ± SD) Crohn 11.8 ± 2.9 (M), 11.9 ± 2.4 (F), UC10.1 ± 2.8 (M), 11.7 ± 2.6 (F)	Crohn 43/39, UC 22/19	Hologic database Healthy controls	Crohn, spine Z-score −1.44 ± 0.97 (M), −1.37 ± 1.22 (F)ᶜ. UC, spine Z-score −0.93 ± 1.10 (M), Z-score −0.56 ± 0.89 (F)	Male Relatively young at diagnosis No immunomodulator	[135]
CD	I	18	Mean (range)12.9 (5.5–16.8)	11/7	GE Lunar Database	Body −0.24 ± 0.79 Spine −0.99 ± 1.1**	Low BMI, low weight, height, and lean body mass Delayed puberty Decreased physical activity	[136]
CD	I	23	Mean ± SD 12.58 ± 2.37	15/8	Healthy controls; Van der Sluis [137]	Body 0.36 ± 1.99 Spine −0.14 ± 1.04	Low BMI	[64]
CD UC	I	58 CD 18 UC 49 Control			GE Lunar Database	Body CD −0.78 ± 1.02ˣ UC −0.46 ± 1.14 Control −0.17 ± 0.95	Low BMI High IL-6	[4]
CD UC	P	47 CD 26 UC		46/27	GE Lunar Database	ᵈCD −2.0 (−3.8, −0.3) UC 1.2 (−3.2, 0.8)	Short stature Low BMI	[138]
CD	P	29	Median (range)15.18 (13.85–17.18)	20/9	GE Lunar Database	ᵉBody −1.20 Spine −2.10	Corticosteroids	[139]
CD UC	P	28 CD 10 UC	Median (range)13 (5–18)	N/A	Faulkner [92]	18/28 CD 8/10 UC had "low Z-scores"	N/A	[140]
CD	P	119		72/47		38/119 <−2.0 81/119 <−1.0	Low weight and height Z-scores, male sex	[141]
CD	I	78	12 (5–18)	44/34	CHOP	pQCT of the tibia Decreased trabecular BMD Increased cortical BMD Increased endocortical circumference Decreased periosteal circumference	Low serum albumin, anemia	[142]
CD UC	P	22 CD 33 UC	4–18	34/21		Body SDS −0.95 Spine SDS −0.75	Corticosteroids, low BMI SDS, Crohn disease	[143]
CD	P Treated with anti-TNF-α for 12 months	74	11.8 (5–17.6)	47/27	CHOP	Significant increase in bone metabolic activity and height. pQCT showed significant increases in trabecular BMD and cortical area Z-scores.	Gains in trabecular BMD correlated with linear growth	[81]

Table 13.1 (continued)

	Cohort	n	Age (years)	M/F	Normative data	Z-score	Risk factors	Ref
CD	I	65	12.7 ± 2.5	54/11	CHOP	Comparison of pQCT measures of trabecular BMD and three different DXA measures of spine BMD	Gains in BMD correlated with increases in height Z-score at 12 months	[144]
CD UC	P	45 CD 83 UC	14.2 (6–19)	93/51	GE Lunar Database	DXA: lower BMD mean Z-score for the lumbar spine	Gains in BMD correlated with increases in height Z-score at 12 months. Disease duration and male sex positive correlated with BMD	[145]
CD UC	I	82 CD 20 UC	14.1 (6.9–20.1)	67/35	Neu [146]	pQCT (adjusted for height) Decreased trabecular BMD Decreased cortical cross-sectional area Reduced muscle cross-sectional area Lower grip strength	Persistent deficits in trabecular bone BMD and muscle cross-sectional area	[147]

I incident cohort, *P* prevalent cohort, *CD* Crohn disease, *UC* ulcerative colitis, N/A not available

[a]Single photon densitometry was used to measure bone mineral mass at the one third distal radius. Longitudinal 2-year study

[b]Mean follow-up approximately 4 years

[c]Spine BMD Z-score significantly lower in children with Crohn than in those with UC

[d]BMD expressed as median standard deviation score (90th percentile, 10th percentile), CD significantly different than UC ($P < 0.05$)

[e]Results expressed as median

[&]$p < 0.01$

[**]$P = 0.002$

or cross-sectional and have used primarily DXA or pQCT to image bone, suggest that decreased bone mineral density is common in children with Crohn disease at the time of diagnosis, especially in patients with delays in growth and sexual maturation, active disease, and those with decreased lean tissue mass [4, 142, 148, 149]. Studies performed in incident cohorts of treatment-naïve patients suggest that disease factors can affect bone mass in children with IBD prior to the initiation of treatment. Collectively, this work suggests that children with Crohn disease are at greater risk for decreased bone mass than children with ulcerative colitis, probably because Crohn disease is more likely to affect linear growth. Patients with low body mass index, low serum albumin, and active severe IBD appear to be at particular risk for decreased BMD. The role of corticosteroids on BMD in pediatric Crohn disease, however, is not clear. The attainment of peak bone mass in Crohn disease is at risk, which may affect fracture risk later in life [150].

According to recent guidelines by the International Society for Clinical Densitometry, children with IBD should have DXA scanning if in the clinician's judgment the measurement may influence the patients' management [22]. In addition to measuring bone mass, body composition data provided by DXA may be helpful in guiding the nutritional rehabilitation of these patients. It is important to DXA BMD measurements to patient size, gender, and sexual maturation, because in any given patient with IBD, the challenge is to distinguish between small, normally mineralized bones and abnormally thin and weak bones [151]. Taken together, these studies indicate that the observed reduction of BMD in children with IBD can be attributed in part to decreased bone size due to growth delay. However, it is important to note that smaller bones may be weaker, and their physical properties may not be normal. It is not yet known whether smaller bone size leads to increased fracture risk in children with IBD. Conversely, increases in height track with significant improvements in BMD, especially in trabecular bone (Table 13.1).

Indirect markers of bone cell function, including osteocalcin and bone alkaline phosphatase for osteoblasts and products of type I collagen degradation for osteoclasts, can be used to infer bone-remodeling activity in adults. In children, however, bone biomarkers cannot distinguish between bone modeling, bone remodeling, and bone growth. Nonetheless, significant reductions in the concentration of bone metabolic activity markers suggest that children with Crohn disease have decreased bone turnover at diagnosis [4]. This indicates that the observed reduction in BMD in children with IBD is probably secondary to a combination of decreased net bone formation and linear growth. A study reported the results of histomorphometry in transiliac bone biopsies of 20 children with newly diagnosed Crohn disease and confirmed that bone formation and resorption is reduced at diagnosis; in addition, there was cortical thinning, but trabecular thickness and number was unaffected [152]. Longitudinal studies of incident cohorts of children with Crohn disease have revealed significant alterations in bone geometry of long bones, including decreased periosteal circumference (due to reduced bone formation), expanded endosteal surface (due to increased bone resorption), and increases in cortical bone density (probably due to decreased cortical bone remodeling) [142, 153]. Treatment with anti-TNF-α antibodies for 12 months was associated with improved bone length, reduction of the endosteal surface, and decreased cortical bone density (likely due to increased bone cell activity and rapid growth, respectively), but not a significant increase in periosteal circumference compared to normal controls [81]. Periosteal circumference may be responsive to gains in muscle mass that occur as a result of sustained disease remission.

Laboratory observations suggest that systemic factors impair bone formation in IBD. For example, serum from newly diagnosed children demonstrates decreased markers of osteoblastic activity in bone explants [154] and in osteoblasts [155], while indicators of bone resorption are not increased. IL-6, a pro-inflammatory cytokine, appears to play an important role in these effects, in cooperation with other factors present in intact bone [156]. In consequence, IBD may have systemic effects on linear growth and direct effects on bone cells in children, thereby decreasing bone mass. Although globally both bone formation and bone resorption appear lower in children with IBD at diagnosis, it is possible that in some regions of the skeleton bone resorption may be increased, resulting in thinner bone cortices and mechanical fragility.

While systemic and local humoral factors can directly influence bone cell function in IBD, other influences, albeit indirect, may also be significant. For example, an important stimulus for bone formation is mechanical loading by the expanding muscle forces during puberty [157]. Muscle volume (lean body mass) normally expands during sexual maturation, and its expansion precedes gains in bone mass. Children with IBD often present with malnutrition, with significant losses in both the fat and lean tissue compartments and decreased body mass index. With treatment and clinical improvement, children gain weight but deficits in lean body

mass persist [149, 158, 159]. This may result in decreased mechanical loading on bone and be a reason for decreased bone formation in children. In addition, children with IBD may be less active than their peers when they don't feel well, which may also affect gains in muscle and bone mass over time.

Nutritional factors can also negatively impact bone mass. For example, vitamin D is essential for normal calcium absorption and may have immunoregulatory effects in the gut [160, 161]. Vitamin D deficiency may be common in children with IBD, especially in high latitudes [162] and in African-American children [163]. These patients may spend more time indoors during disease exacerbations, affecting their exposure to sunlight and cutaneous synthesis of vitamin D. Their intake of dairy products fortified with vitamin D may be limited due to secondary lactase deficiency. Vitamin K deficiency is prevalent in children with IBD [164] and may compromise the normal γ-carboxylation of osteocalcin, a mineralization factor [165].

It is not clear whether children with IBD are at increased risk of fractures. Population-based studies in adults with IBD suggest that the risk of clinically apparent fractures appears to be modestly increased [166] or not elevated [167]. Two pediatric studies examining the prevalence of long bone fractures, one by a questionnaire and the other an analysis of an administrative database, found no increase in the frequency of fractures in children with IBD [168, 169]. One should consider that long bone fractures are very common in active children. Consequently, demonstrating an effect of IBD on long bone fracture risk in children may be very difficult because of the number of children in the study to show a significant effect size of the disease. Risk factors for fractures for adults and children with IBD may be different, and the risk of fracture for a given decrease in bone mass may vary depending on age.

However, a study of vertebral fracture assessment in adults with Crohn disease indicated high prevalence of asymptomatic vertebral fractures, even in patients with normal bone density by DXA [170]. Vertebral fractures have been reported in children as well [171]. Children who report back pain, have pain upon palpation of the spinal processes, or have a reduction in height should have spine films to screen for vertebral fractures.

Treatment

In children with IBD who have a significant decrease in BMD (Z-score adjust for height Z-score < − 2 in the total body and/or lumbar spine), disease and treatment factors that can impair the acquisition of bone mineral should be identified and corrected. These include active inflammation, malnutrition, specific nutrient deficiencies (calcium, vitamin D and vitamin K), and corticosteroid use [172]. High doses of vitamin D may be required to replenish vitamin D stores [173]. Weight-bearing physical activity should be encouraged. Treatment modalities such as exclusive enteral nutrition and anti-TNF-α antibodies have positive effects on linear growth and BMD [81, 174] and should be considered in children with IBD with very low BMD.

In children with "clinically significant fractures" (vertebral fractures, fractures of lower extremity bones with low trauma) with or without low BMD, it is important to evaluate for primary bone disease in addition to establishing measures to optimize nutrition, reduce inflammation with corticosteroid-spearing strategies, and improve physical activity. A partnership with an endocrinologist knowledgeable in pediatric bone disorders is important, especially if bone-active agents are being considered (bisphosphonates) for therapy [175].

Conclusions

Inflammatory bowel disease can negatively affect bone development in children through multiple mechanisms. Due to differences in bone metabolism in children and adults, IBD impacts bone metabolism differently in these two age groups. In children, decreased BMD is probably the result of impaired growth, a primary decrease in osteoblast function, and reduced mechanical strain on bone. Current therapies, including corticosteroids and immunomodulators, may not be optimal for promoting normal body composition and skeletal health in children with IBD. Preliminary data indicate that TNF-α blockade may be more effective in this regard. In children, careful attention to disease control, nutrition (including calcium and vitamin D), and activity level is probably appropriate to improve skeletal mass. Anti-resorptive agents such as bisphosphonates may be helpful in selected children (e.g., those with fragility fractures, especially if they have growth potential) [88] but should not be started in children without input from experts in pediatric metabolic bone diseases.

References

1. Seeman E. Bone modeling and remodeling. Crit Rev Eukaryot Gene Expr. 2009;19(3):219–33.
2. Sylvester FA, Gordon CM, Thayu M, Burnham JM, Denson LA, Essers J, et al. Report of the CCFA pediatric bone, growth and muscle health workshop, New York City, November 11-12, 2011, with updates. Inflamm Bowel Dis. 2013;19(13):2919–26.
3. Bellido T. Osteocyte-driven bone remodeling. Calcif Tissue Int. 2014;94(1):25–34.
4. Sylvester FA, Wyzga N, Hyams JS, Davis PM, Lerer T, Vance K, et al. Natural history of bone metabolism and bone mineral density in children with inflammatory bowel disease. Inflamm Bowel Dis. 2007;13(1):42–50.
5. Wang Q, Seeman E. Skeletal growth and peak bone strength. Best Pract Res Clin Endocrinol Metab. 2008;22(5):687–700.
6. Wang Q, Wang XF, Iuliano-Burns S, Ghasem-Zadeh A, Zebaze R, Seeman E. Rapid growth produces transient cortical weakness: a risk factor for metaphyseal fractures during puberty. J Bone Miner Res. 2010;25(7):1521–6.
7. Wang Q, Ghasem-Zadeh A, Wang XF, Iuliano-Burns S, Seeman E. Trabecular bone of growth plate origin influences both trabecular and cortical morphology in adulthood. J Bone Miner Res. 2011;26(7):1577–83.
8. Ohlsson C, Darelid A, Nilsson M, Melin J, Mellstrom D, Lorentzon M. Cortical consolidation due to increased mineralization and endosteal contraction in young adult men: a five-year longitudinal study. J Clin Endocrinol Metab. 2011;96(7):2262–9.
9. Walsh JS, Paggiosi MA, Eastell R. Cortical consolidation of the radius and tibia in young men and women. J Clin Endocrinol Metab. 2012;97(9):3342–8.
10. Black DM, Rosen CJ. Clinical practice. Postmenopausal osteoporosis. N Engl J Med. 2016;374(3):254–62.
11. Winkler DG, Sutherland MK, Geoghegan JC, Yu C, Hayes T, Skonier JE, et al. Osteocyte control of bone formation via sclerostin, a novel BMP antagonist. EMBO J. 2003;22(23):6267–76.
12. Bala Y, Seeman E. Bone's material constituents and their contribution to bone strength in health, disease, and treatment. Calcif Tissue Int. 2015;97(3):308–26.
13. Parfitt AM, Travers R, Rauch F, Glorieux FH. Structural and cellular changes during bone growth in healthy children. Bone. 2000;27(4):487–94.
14. Mendelson A, Frenette PS. Hematopoietic stem cell niche maintenance during homeostasis and regeneration. Nat Med. 2014;20(8):833–46.
15. Nemoto Y, Kanai T, Makita S, Okamoto R, Totsuka T, Takeda K, et al. Bone marrow retaining colitogenic CD4+ T cells may be a pathogenic reservoir for chronic colitis. Gastroenterology. 2007;132(1):176–89.
16. Ciucci T, Ibanez L, Boucoiran A, Birgy-Barelli E, Pene J, Abou-Ezzi G, et al. Bone marrow Th17 TNFalpha cells induce osteoclast differentiation, and link bone destruction to IBD. Gut. 2015;64(7):1072–81.
17. Nemoto Y, Kanai T, Takahara M, Oshima S, Nakamura T, Okamoto R, et al. Bone marrow-mesenchymal stem cells are a major source of interleukin-7 and sustain colitis by forming the niche for colitogenic CD4 memory T cells. Gut. 2013;62(8):1142–52.
18. Ashcroft AJ, Cruickshank SM, Croucher PI, Perry MJ, Rollinson S, Lippitt JM, et al. Colonic dendritic cells, intestinal inflammation, and T cell-mediated bone destruction are modulated by recombinant osteoprotegerin. Immunity. 2003;19(6):849–61.
19. Zou L, Barnett B, Safah H, Larussa VF, Evdemon-Hogan M, Mottram P, et al. Bone marrow is a reservoir for CD4+CD25+ regulatory T cells that traffic through CXCL12/CXCR4 signals. Cancer Res. 2004;64(22):8451–5.
20. Tokoyoda K, Zehentmeier S, Hegazy AN, Albrecht I, Grun JR, Lohning M, et al. Professional memory CD4+ T lymphocytes preferentially reside and rest in the bone marrow. Immunity. 2009;30(5):721–30.
21. Rauch F. The dynamics of bone structure development during pubertal growth. J Musculoskelet Neuronal Interact. 2012;12(1):1–6.
22. Bianchi ML, Baim S, Bishop NJ, Gordon CM, Hans DB, Langman CB, et al. Official positions of the International Society for Clinical Densitometry (ISCD) on DXA evaluation in children and adolescents. Pediatr Nephrol. 2010;25(1):37–47.
23. Ikeda K, Takeshita S. The role of osteoclast differentiation and function in skeletal homeostasis. J Biochem. 2016;159(1):1–8.

24. Kong YY, Feige U, Sarosi I, Bolon B, Tafuri A, Morony S, et al. Activated T cells regulate bone loss and joint destruction in adjuvant arthritis through osteoprotegerin ligand. Nature. 1999;402(6759):304–9.

25. Kong YY, Yoshida H, Sarosi I, Tan HL, Timms E, Capparelli C, et al. OPGL is a key regulator of osteoclastogenesis, lymphocyte development and lymph-node organogenesis. Nature. 1999;397(6717):315–23.

26. Watanabe Y, Namba A, Aida Y, Honda K, Tanaka H, Suzuki N, et al. IL-1beta suppresses the formation of osteoclasts by increasing OPG production via an autocrine mechanism involving celecoxib-related prostaglandins in chondrocytes. Mediators Inflamm. 2009;2009:308596.

27. Hoshino A, Iimura T, Ueha S, Hanada S, Maruoka Y, Mayahara M, et al. Deficiency of chemokine receptor CCR1 causes osteopenia due to impaired functions of osteoclasts and osteoblasts. J Biol Chem. 2010;285(37):28826–37.

28. Mun SH, Ko NY, Kim HS, Kim JW, Kim DK, Kim AR, et al. Interleukin-33 stimulates formation of functional osteoclasts from human CD14(+) monocytes. Cell Mol Life Sci. 2010;67:3883–92.

29. Gilbert LC, Chen H, Lu X, Nanes MS. Chronic low dose tumor necrosis factor-alpha (TNF) suppresses early bone accrual in young mice by inhibiting osteoblasts without affecting osteoclasts. Bone. 2013;56(1):174–83.

30. Ota K, Quint P, Weivoda MM, Ruan M, Pederson L, Westendorf JJ, et al. Transforming growth factor beta 1 induces CXCL16 and leukemia inhibitory factor expression in osteoclasts to modulate migration of osteoblast progenitors. Bone. 2013;57:68–75.

31. Humphrey MB, Nakamura MC. A comprehensive review of immunoreceptor regulation of osteoclasts. Clin Rev Allergy Immunol. 2016;51:48–58.

32. McClung MR, Lewiecki EM, Cohen SB, Bolognese MA, Woodson GC, Moffett AH, et al. Denosumab in postmenopausal women with low bone mineral density. N Engl J Med. 2006;354(8):821–31.

33. Dore RK, Cohen SB, Lane NE, Palmer W, Shergy W, Zhou L, et al. Effects of denosumab on bone mineral density and bone turnover in patients with rheumatoid arthritis receiving concurrent glucocorticoids or bisphosphonates. Ann Rheum Dis. 2010;69(5):872–5.

34. Simonet WS, Lacey DL, Dunstan CR, Kelley M, Chang MS, Luthy R, et al. Osteoprotegerin: a novel secreted protein involved in the regulation of bone density. Cell. 1997;89(2):309–19.

35. Bucay N, Sarosi I, Dunstan CR, Morony S, Tarpley J, Capparelli C, et al. osteoprotegerin-deficient mice develop early onset osteoporosis and arterial calcification. Genes Dev. 1998;12(9):1260–8.

36. Mizuno A, Amizuka N, Irie K, Murakami A, Fujise N, Kanno T, et al. Severe osteoporosis in mice lacking osteoclastogenesis inhibitory factor/osteoprotegerin. Biochem Biophys Res Commun. 1998;247(3):610–5.

37. Takayanagi H, Kim S, Matsuo K, Suzuki H, Suzuki T, Sato K, et al. RANKL maintains bone homeostasis through c-Fos-dependent induction of interferon-beta. Nature. 2002;416(6882):744–9.

38. Quinn JM, Itoh K, Udagawa N, Hausler K, Yasuda H, Shima N, et al. Transforming growth factor beta affects osteoclast differentiation via direct and indirect actions. J Bone Miner Res. 2001;16(10):1787–94.

39. Spencer GJ, Utting JC, Etheridge SL, Arnett TR, Genever PG. Wnt signalling in osteoblasts regulates expression of the receptor activator of NFkappaB ligand and inhibits osteoclastogenesis in vitro. J Cell Sci. 2006;119(Pt 7):1283–96.

40. Moverare-Skrtic S, Henning P, Liu X, Nagano K, Saito H, Borjesson AE, et al. Osteoblast-derived WNT16 represses osteoclastogenesis and prevents cortical bone fragility fractures. Nat Med. 2014;20(11):1279–88.

41. Maeda K, Kobayashi Y, Udagawa N, Uehara S, Ishihara A, Mizoguchi T, et al. Wnt5a-Ror2 signaling between osteoblast-lineage cells and osteoclast precursors enhances osteoclastogenesis. Nat Med. 2012;18(3):405–12.

42. Takayanagi H, Ogasawara K, Hida S, Chiba T, Murata S, Sato K, et al. T-cell-mediated regulation of osteoclastogenesis by signalling cross-talk between RANKL and IFN-gamma. Nature. 2000;408(6812):600–5.

43. Sasaki H, Hou L, Belani A, Wang CY, Uchiyama T, Muller R, et al. IL-10, but not IL-4, suppresses infection-stimulated bone resorption in vivo. J Immunol. 2000;165(7):3626–30.

44. Park-Min KH, Ji JD, Antoniv T, Reid AC, Silver RB, Humphrey MB, et al. IL-10 suppresses calcium-mediated costimulation of receptor activator NF-kappa B signaling during human osteoclast differentiation by inhibiting TREM-2 expression. J Immunol. 2009;183(4):2444–55.

45. Yoshimatsu M, Kitaura H, Fujimura Y, Eguchi T, Kohara H, Morita Y, et al. IL-12 inhibits TNF-alpha induced osteoclastogenesis via a T cell-independent mechanism in vivo. Bone. 2009;45(5):1010–6.

46. Kitaura H, Fujimura Y, Yoshimatsu M, Kohara H, Morita Y, Aonuma T, et al. IL-12- and IL-18-mediated, nitric oxide-induced apoptosis in TNF-alpha-mediated osteoclastogenesis of bone marrow cells. Calcif Tissue Int. 2011;89(1):65–73.

47. Sato K, Suematsu A, Okamoto K, Yamaguchi A, Morishita Y, Kadono Y, et al. Th17 functions as an osteoclastogenic helper T cell subset that links T cell activation and bone destruction. J Exp Med. 2006;203(12):2673–82.

48. Tyagi AM, Mansoori MN, Srivastava K, Khan MP, Kureel J, Dixit M, et al. Enhanced immunoprotective effects by anti-IL-17 antibody translates to improved skeletal parameters under estrogen deficiency compared with anti-RANKL and anti-TNF-alpha antibodies. J Bone Miner Res. 2014;29(9):1981–92.

49. Shinohara M, Koga T, Okamoto K, Sakaguchi S, Arai K, Yasuda H, et al. Tyrosine kinases Btk and Tec regulate osteoclast differentiation by linking RANK and ITAM signals. Cell. 2008;132(5):794–806.

50. Kim HS, Kim DK, Kim AR, Mun SH, Lee SK, Kim JH, et al. Fyn positively regulates the activation of DAP12 and FcRgamma-mediated costimulatory signals by RANKL during osteoclastogenesis. Cell Signal. 2012;24(6):1306–14.

51. Kim H, Kim T, Jeong BC, Cho IT, Han D, Takegahara N, et al. Tmem64 modulates calcium signaling during RANKL-mediated osteoclast differentiation. Cell Metab. 2013;17(2):249–60.

52. Decker CE, Yang Z, Rimer R, Park-Min KH, Macaubas C, Mellins ED, et al. Tmem178 acts in a novel negative feedback loop targeting NFATc1 to regulate bone mass. Proc Natl Acad Sci U S A. 2015;112(51):15654–9.

53. Kollet O, Dar A, Shivtiel S, Kalinkovich A, Lapid K, Sztainberg Y, et al. Osteoclasts degrade endosteal components and promote mobilization of hematopoietic progenitor cells. Nat Med. 2006;12(6):657–64.

54. Mansour A, Abou-Ezzi G, Sitnicka E, Jacobsen SE, Wakkach A, Blin-Wakkach C. Osteoclasts promote the formation of hematopoietic stem cell niches in the bone marrow. J Exp Med. 2012;209(3):537–49.

55. Fata JE, Kong YY, Li J, Sasaki T, Irie-Sasaki J, Moorehead RA, et al. The osteoclast differentiation factor osteoprotegerin-ligand is essential for mammary gland development. Cell. 2000;103(1):41–50.

56. Roysland R, Masson S, Omland T, Milani V, Bjerre M, Flyvbjerg A, et al. Prognostic value of osteoprotegerin in chronic heart failure: the GISSI-HF trial. Am Heart J. 2010;160(2):286–93.

57. Montagnana M, Lippi G, Danese E, Guidi GC. The role of osteoprotegerin in cardiovascular disease. Ann Med. 2013;45(3):254–64.
58. Walsh MC, Choi Y. Biology of the RANKL-RANK-OPG system in immunity, bone, and beyond. Front Immunol. 2014;5:511.
59. Anderson DM, Maraskovsky E, Billingsley WL, Dougall WC, Tometsko ME, Roux ER, et al. A homologue of the TNF receptor and its ligand enhance T-cell growth and dendritic-cell function. Nature. 1997;390(6656):175–9.
60. Summers deLuca L, Gommerman JL. Fine-tuning of dendritic cell biology by the TNF superfamily. Nat Rev Immunol. 2012;12(5):339–51.
61. Yun TJ, Chaudhary PM, Shu GL, Frazer JK, Ewings MK, Schwartz SM, et al. OPG/FDCR-1, a TNF receptor family member, is expressed in lymphoid cells and is up-regulated by ligating CD40. J Immunol. 1998;161(11):6113–21.
62. Chino T, Draves KE, Clark EA. Regulation of dendritic cell survival and cytokine production by osteoprotegerin. J Leukoc Biol. 2009;86(4):933–40.
63. Jones D, Glimcher LH, Aliprantis AO. Osteoimmunology at the nexus of arthritis, osteoporosis, cancer, and infection. J Clin Invest. 2011;121(7):2534–42.
64. Sylvester FA, Davis PM, Wyzga N, Hyams JS, Lerer T. Are activated T cells regulators of bone metabolism in children with Crohn disease? J Pediatr. 2006;148(4):461–6.
65. Nahidi L, Leach ST, Sidler MA, Levin A, Lemberg DA, Day AS. Osteoprotegerin in pediatric Crohn's disease and the effects of exclusive enteral nutrition. Inflamm Bowel Dis. 2011;17(2):516–23.
66. Franchimont N, Reenaers C, Lambert C, Belaiche J, Bours V, Malaise M, et al. Increased expression of receptor activator of NF-kappaB ligand (RANKL), its receptor RANK and its decoy receptor osteoprotegerin in the colon of Crohn's disease patients. Clin Exp Immunol. 2004;138(3):491–8.
67. Moschen AR, Kaser A, Enrich B, Ludwiczek O, Gabriel M, Obrist P, et al. The RANKL/OPG system is activated in inflammatory bowel disease and relates to the state of bone loss. Gut. 2005;54(4):479–87.
68. Arijs I, Li K, Toedter G, Quintens R, Van Lommel L, Van Steen K, et al. Mucosal gene signatures to predict response to infliximab in patients with ulcerative colitis. Gut. 2009;58:1612–9.
69. Sylvester FA, Turner D, Draghi 2nd A, Uuosoe K, McLernon R, Koproske K, et al. Fecal osteoprotegerin may guide the introduction of second-line therapy in hospitalized children with ulcerative colitis. Inflamm Bowel Dis. 2011;17(8):1726–30.
70. Abdallah BM, Jafari A, Zaher W, Qiu W, Kassem M. Skeletal (stromal) stem cells: an update on intracellular signaling pathways controlling osteoblast differentiation. Bone. 2015;70:28–36.
71. Zhao G, Monier-Faugere MC, Langub MC, Geng Z, Nakayama T, Pike JW, et al. Targeted overexpression of insulin-like growth factor I to osteoblasts of transgenic mice: increased trabecular bone volume without increased osteoblast proliferation. Endocrinology. 2000;141(7):2674–82.
72. Difedele LM, He J, Bonkowski EL, Han X, Held MA, Bohan A, et al. Tumor necrosis factor-a blockade restores growth hormone signaling in murine colitis. Gastroenterology. 2005;128(5):1278–91.
73. Kaneki H, Guo R, Chen D, Yao Z, Schwarz EM, Zhang YE, et al. Tumor necrosis factor promotes Runx2 degradation through up-regulation of Smurf1 and Smurf2 in osteoblasts. J Biol Chem. 2006;281(7):4326–33.
74. Yamazaki M, Fukushima H, Shin M, Katagiri T, Doi T, Takahashi T, et al. Tumor necrosis factor alpha represses bone morphogenetic protein (BMP) signaling by interfering with the DNA binding of Smads through the activation of NF-kappaB. J Biol Chem. 2009;284(51):35987–95.
75. Lee HL, Yi T, Woo KM, Ryoo HM, Kim GS, Baek JH. Msx2 mediates the inhibitory action of TNF-alpha on osteoblast differentiation. Exp Mol Med. 2010;42(6):437–45.
76. Shen F, Ruddy MJ, Plamondon P, Gaffen SL. Cytokines link osteoblasts and inflammation: microarray analysis of interleukin-17- and TNF-a-induced genes in bone cells. J Leukoc Biol. 2005;77(3):388–99.
77. Uno JK, Kolek OI, Hines ER, Xu H, Timmermann BN, Kiela PR, et al. The role of tumor necrosis factor-a in down-regulation of osteoblast Phex gene expression in experimental murine colitis. Gastroenterology. 2006;131(2):497–509.
78. Majewski PM, Thurston RD, Ramalingam R, Kiela PR, Ghishan FK. Cooperative role of NF-{kappa}B and poly(ADP-ribose) polymerase 1 (PARP-1) in the TNF-induced inhibition of PHEX expression in osteoblasts. J Biol Chem. 2010;285(45):34828–38.
79. Jang WG, Jeong BC, Kim EJ, Choi H, Oh SH, Kim DK, et al. Cyclic AMP Response Element-binding Protein H (CREBH) mediates the inhibitory actions of tumor necrosis factor alpha in osteoblast differentiation by stimulating Smad1 degradation. J Biol Chem. 2015;290(21):13556–66.
80. Thayu M, Leonard MB, Hyams JS, Crandall WV, Kugathasan S, Otley AR, et al. Improvement in biomarkers of bone formation during infliximab therapy in pediatric Crohn's disease: results of the REACH study. Clin Gastroenterol Hepatol. 2008;6(12):1378–84.
81. Griffin LM, Thayu M, Baldassano RN, DeBoer MD, Zemel BS, Denburg MR, et al. Improvements in bone density and structure during anti-TNF-alpha therapy in pediatric Crohn's disease. J Clin Endocrinol Metab. 2015;100(7):2630–9.
82. Calvi LM. Osteolineage cells and regulation of the hematopoietic stem cell. Best Pract Res Clin Haematol. 2013;26(3):249–52.
83. Pacifici R. T cells, osteoblasts, and osteocytes: interacting lineages key for the bone anabolic and catabolic activities of parathyroid hormone. Ann N Y Acad Sci. 2016;1364:11–24.
84. Takayanagi H. Osteoimmunology in 2014: two-faced immunology-from osteogenesis to bone resorption. Nat Rev Rheumatol. 2015;11(2):74–6.
85. Jovanovic DV, Di Battista JA, Martel-Pelletier J, Jolicoeur FC, He Y, Zhang M, et al. IL-17 stimulates the production and expression of proinflammatory cytokines, IL-beta and TNF-alpha, by human macrophages. J Immunol. 1998;160(7):3513–21.
86. Adamopoulos IE, Chao CC, Geissler R, Laface D, Blumenschein W, Iwakura Y, et al. Interleukin-17A upregulates receptor activator of NF-kappaB on osteoclast precursors. Arthritis Res Ther. 2010;12(1):R29.
87. Li JY, D'Amelio P, Robinson J, Walker LD, Vaccaro C, Luo T, et al. IL-17A is increased in humans with primary hyperparathyroidism and mediates PTH-induced bone loss in mice. Cell Metab. 2015;22(5):799–810.
88. Harbour SN, Maynard CL, Zindl CL, Schoeb TR, Weaver CT. Th17 cells give rise to Th1 cells that are required for the pathogenesis of colitis. Proc Natl Acad Sci U S A. 2015;112(22):7061–6.
89. Cenci S, Weitzmann MN, Roggia C, Namba N, Novack D, Woodring J, et al. Estrogen deficiency induces bone loss by enhancing T-cell production of TNF-alpha. J Clin Invest. 2000;106(10):1229–37.
90. Pacifici R. Role of T cells in ovariectomy induced bone loss–revisited. J Bone Miner Res. 2012;27(2):231–9.
91. Cleynen I, Boucher G, Jostins L, Schumm LP, Zeissig S, Ahmad T, et al. Inherited determinants of Crohn's disease and ulcerative colitis phenotypes: a genetic association study. Lancet. 2016;387:156–67.
92. Li Y, Toraldo G, Li A, Yang X, Zhang H, Qian WP, et al. B cells and T cells are critical for the preservation of bone homeostasis

and attainment of peak bone mass in vivo. Blood. 2007;109(9):3839–48.

93. Kelchtermans H, Geboes L, Mitera T, Huskens D, Leclercq G, Matthys P. Activated CD4+CD25+ regulatory T cells inhibit osteoclastogenesis and collagen-induced arthritis. Ann Rheum Dis. 2009;68(5):744–50.

94. Terauchi M, Li JY, Bedi B, Baek KH, Tawfeek H, Galley S, et al. T lymphocytes amplify the anabolic activity of parathyroid hormone through Wnt10b signaling. Cell Metab. 2009;10(3):229–40.

95. Pappalardo A, Thompson K. Novel immunostimulatory effects of osteoclasts and macrophages on human gammadelta T cells. Bone. 2015;71:180–8.

96. Li H, Hong S, Qian J, Zheng Y, Yang J, Yi Q. Cross talk between the bone and immune systems: osteoclasts function as antigen-presenting cells and activate CD4+ and CD8+ T cells. Blood. 2010;116(2):210–7.

97. Kiesel JR, Buchwald ZS, Aurora R. Cross-presentation by osteoclasts induces FoxP3 in CD8+ T cells. J Immunol. 2009;182(9):5477–87.

98. Buchwald ZS, Kiesel JR, DiPaolo R, Pagadala MS, Aurora R. Osteoclast activated FoxP3+ CD8+ T-cells suppress bone resorption in vitro. PLoS One. 2012;7(6):e38199.

99. Buchwald ZS, Yang C, Nellore S, Shashkova EV, Davis JL, Cline A, et al. A bone anabolic effect of RANKL in a murine model of osteoporosis mediated through FoxP3+ CD8 T cells. J Bone Miner Res. 2015;30(8):1508–22.

100. Jostins L, Ripke S, Weersma RK, Duerr RH, McGovern DP, Hui KY, et al. Host-microbe interactions have shaped the genetic architecture of inflammatory bowel disease. Nature. 2012;491(7422):119–24.

101. Adolph TE, Tomczak MF, Niederreiter L, Ko HJ, Bock J, Martinez-Naves E, et al. Paneth cells as a site of origin for intestinal inflammation. Nature. 2013;503(7475):272–6.

102. Cao SS. Endoplasmic reticulum stress and unfolded protein response in inflammatory bowel disease. Inflamm Bowel Dis. 2015;21:636–44.

103. Wu Y, Yang M, Fan J, Peng Y, Deng L, Ding Y, et al. Deficiency of osteoblastic Arl6ip5 impaired osteoblast differentiation and enhanced osteoclastogenesis via disturbance of ER calcium homeostasis and induction of ER stress-mediated apoptosis. Cell Death Dis. 2014;5:e1464.

104. Murakami T, Saito A, Hino S, Kondo S, Kanemoto S, Chihara K, et al. Signalling mediated by the endoplasmic reticulum stress transducer OASIS is involved in bone formation. Nat Cell Biol. 2009;11(10):1205–11.

105. Saito A, Ochiai K, Kondo S, Tsumagari K, Murakami T, Cavener DR, et al. Endoplasmic reticulum stress response mediated by the PERK-eIF2(alpha)-ATF4 pathway is involved in osteoblast differentiation induced by BMP2. J Biol Chem. 2011;286(6):4809–18.

106. Tohmonda T, Miyauchi Y, Ghosh R, Yoda M, Uchikawa S, Takito J, et al. The IRE1alpha-XBP1 pathway is essential for osteoblast differentiation through promoting transcription of Osterix. EMBO Rep. 2011;12(5):451–7.

107. Tohmonda T, Yoda M, Mizuochi H, Morioka H, Matsumoto M, Urano F, et al. The IRE1alpha-XBP1 pathway positively regulates parathyroid hormone (PTH)/PTH-related peptide receptor expression and is involved in pth-induced osteoclastogenesis. J Biol Chem. 2013;288(3):1691–5.

108. Tohmonda T, Yoda M, Iwawaki T, Matsumoto M, Nakamura M, Mikoshiba K, et al. IRE1alpha/XBP1-mediated branch of the unfolded protein response regulates osteoclastogenesis. J Clin Invest. 2015;125(8):3269–79.

109. Cao SS, Luo KL, Shi L. Endoplasmic reticulum stress interacts with inflammation in human diseases. J Cell Physiol. 2016;231(2):288–94.

110. Kneissel M, Luong-Nguyen NH, Baptist M, Cortesi R, Zumstein-Mecker S, Kossida S, et al. Everolimus suppresses cancellous bone loss, bone resorption, and cathepsin K expression by osteoclasts. Bone. 2004;35(5):1144–56.

111. Zhao Y, Chen G, Zhang W, Xu N, Zhu JY, Jia J, et al. Autophagy regulates hypoxia-induced osteoclastogenesis through the HIF-1alpha/BNIP3 signaling pathway. J Cell Physiol. 2012;227(2):639–48.

112. Sambandam Y, Townsend MT, Pierce JJ, Lipman CM, Haque A, Bateman TA, et al. Microgravity control of autophagy modulates osteoclastogenesis. Bone. 2014;61:125–31.

113. Liu F, Fang F, Yuan H, Yang D, Chen Y, Williams L, et al. Suppression of autophagy by FIP200 deletion leads to osteopenia in mice through the inhibition of osteoblast terminal differentiation. J Bone Miner Res. 2013;28(11):2414–30.

114. Pantovic A, Krstic A, Janjetovic K, Kocic J, Harhaji-Trajkovic L, Bugarski D, et al. Coordinated time-dependent modulation of AMPK/Akt/mTOR signaling and autophagy controls osteogenic differentiation of human mesenchymal stem cells. Bone. 2013;52(1):524–31.

115. Nollet M, Santucci-Darmanin S, Breuil V, Al-Sahlanee R, Cros C, Topi M, et al. Autophagy in osteoblasts is involved in mineralization and bone homeostasis. Autophagy. 2014;10(11):1965–77.

116. Zhang L, Guo YF, Liu YZ, Liu YJ, Xiong DH, Liu XG, et al. Pathway-based genome-wide association analysis identified the importance of regulation-of-autophagy pathway for ultradistal radius BMD. J Bone Miner Res. 2010;25(7):1572–80.

117. Van bezooijen RL, Farih-Sips HC, Papapoulos SE, Lowik CW. Interleukin-17: a new bone acting cytokine in vitro. J Bone Miner Res. 1999;14(9):1513–21.

118. Yago T, Nanke Y, Ichikawa N, Kobashigawa T, Mogi M, Kamatani N, et al. IL-17 induces osteoclastogenesis from human monocytes alone in the absence of osteoblasts, which is potently inhibited by anti-TNF-alpha antibody: a novel mechanism of osteoclastogenesis by IL-17. J Cell Biochem. 2009;108(4):947–55.

119. Balani D, Aeberli D, Hofstetter W, Seitz M. Interleukin-17A stimulates granulocyte-macrophage colony-stimulating factor release by murine osteoblasts in the presence of 1,25-dihydroxyvitamin D(3) and inhibits murine osteoclast development in vitro. Arthritis Rheum. 2013;65(2):436–46.

120. Kotake S, Udagawa N, Takahashi N, Matsuzaki K, Itoh K, Ishiyama S, et al. IL-17 in synovial fluids from patients with rheumatoid arthritis is a potent stimulator of osteoclastogenesis. J Clin Invest. 1999;103(9):1345–52.

121. Guihard P, Danger Y, Brounais B, David E, Brion R, Delecrin J, et al. Induction of osteogenesis in mesenchymal stem cells by activated monocytes/macrophages depends on oncostatin M signaling. Stem Cells. 2012;30(4):762–72.

122. Jimenez-Dalmaroni MJ, Gershwin ME, Adamopoulos IE. The critical role of toll-like receptors–From microbial recognition to autoimmunity: a comprehensive review. Autoimmun Rev. 2016;15(1):1–8.

123. Takami M, Kim N, Rho J, Choi Y. Stimulation by toll-like receptors inhibits osteoclast differentiation. J Immunol. 2002;169(3):1516–23.

124. Zou W, Bar-Shavit Z. Dual modulation of osteoclast differentiation by lipopolysaccharide. J Bone Miner Res. 2002;17(7):1211–8.

125. Zou W, Schwartz H, Endres S, Hartmann G, Bar-Shavit Z. CpG oligonucleotides: novel regulators of osteoclast differentiation. FASEB J. 2002;16(3):274–82.

126. Krisher T, Bar-Shavit Z. Regulation of osteoclastogenesis by integrated signals from toll-like receptors. J Cell Biochem. 2014;115(12):2146–54.

127. Sjogren K, Engdahl C, Henning P, Lerner UH, Tremaroli V, Lagerquist MK, et al. The gut microbiota regulates bone mass in

mice. J Bone Miner Res Off J Am Soc Bone Miner Res. 2012;27(6):1357–67.

128. Britton RA, Irwin R, Quach D, Schaefer L, Zhang J, Lee T, et al. Probiotic L. reuteri treatment prevents bone loss in a menopausal ovariectomized mouse model. J Cell Physiol. 2014;229:1822–30.

129. Zhang J, Motyl KJ, Irwin R, MacDougald OA, Britton RA, McCabe LR. Loss of Bone and Wnt10b Expression in Male Type 1 Diabetic Mice Is Blocked by the Probiotic Lactobacillus reuteri. Endocrinology. 2015;156(9):3169–82.

130. Lin CL, Moniz C, Chambers TJ, Chow JW. Colitis causes bone loss in rats through suppression of bone formation. Gastroenterology. 1996;111(5):1263–71.

131. Dresner-Pollak R, Gelb N, Rachmilewitz D, Karmeli F, Weinreb M. Interleukin 10-deficient mice develop osteopenia, decreased bone formation, and mechanical fragility of long bones. Gastroenterology. 2004;127(3):792–801.

132. Harris L, Senagore P, Young VB, McCabe LR. Inflammatory bowel disease causes reversible suppression of osteoblast and chondrocyte function in mice. Am J Physiol Gastrointest Liver Physiol. 2009;296(5):G1020–9.

133. Byrne FR, Morony S, Warmington K, Geng Z, Brown HL, Flores SA, et al. CD4+CD45RBHi T cell transfer induced colitis in mice is accompanied by osteopenia which is treatable with recombinant human osteoprotegerin. Gut. 2005;54(1):78–86.

134. Issenman RM, Atkinson SA, Radoja C, Fraher L. Longitudinal assessment of growth, mineral metabolism, and bone mass in pediatric Crohn's disease. J Pediatr Gastroenterol Nutr. 1993;17(4):401–6.

135. Gupta A, Paski S, Issenman R, Webber C. Lumbar spine bone mineral density at diagnosis and during follow-up in children with IBD. J Clin Densitom. 2004;7(3):290–5.

136. Harpavat M, Greenspan SL, O'Brien C, Chang CC, Bowen A, Keljo DJ. Altered bone mass in children at diagnosis of Crohn disease: a pilot study. J Pediatr Gastroenterol Nutr. 2005;40(3):295–300.

137. van der Sluis IM, de Ridder MA, Boot AM, Krenning EP, de Muinck Keizer-Schrama SM. Reference data for bone density and body composition measured with dual energy x ray absorptiometry in white children and young adults. Arch Dis Child. 2002;87(4):341–7; discussion 341–7.

138. Ahmed SF, Horrocks IA, Patterson T, Zaidi S, Ling SC, McGrogan P, et al. Bone mineral assessment by dual energy X-ray absorptiometry in children with inflammatory bowel disease: evaluation by age or bone area. J Pediatr Gastroenterol Nutr. 2004;38(3):276–80.

139. Bourges O, Dorgeret S, Alberti C, Hugot JP, Sebag G, Cezard JP. Low bone mineral density in children with Crohn's disease. Arch Pediatr. 2004;11(7):800–6.

140. Scheer K, Kratzsch J, Deutscher J, Gelbrich G, Borte G, Kiess W. Bone metabolism in 53 children and adolescents with chronic inflammatory bowel disease. Klin Padiatr. 2004;216(2):62–6.

141. Semeao EJ, Jawad AF, Zemel BS, Neiswender KM, Piccoli DA, Stallings VA. Bone mineral density in children and young adults with Crohn's disease. Inflamm Bowel Dis. 1999;5(3):161–6.

142. Dubner SE, Shults J, Baldassano RN, Zemel BS, Thayu M, Burnham JM, et al. Longitudinal assessment of bone density and structure in an incident cohort of children with Crohn's disease. Gastroenterology. 2009;136(1):123–30.

143. Boot AM, Bouquet J, Krenning EP, de Muinck Keizer-Schrama SM. Bone mineral density and nutritional status in children with chronic inflammatory bowel disease. Gut. 1998;42(2):188–94.

144. Tsampalieros A, Berkenstock MK, Zemel BS, Griffin L, Shults J, Burnham JM, et al. Changes in trabecular bone density in incident pediatric Crohn's disease: a comparison of imaging methods. Osteoporos Int. 2014;25(7):1875–83.

145. Schmidt S, Mellstrom D, Norjavaara E, Sundh V, Saalman R. Longitudinal assessment of bone mineral density in children

and adolescents with inflammatory bowel disease. J Pediatr Gastroenterol Nutr. 2012;55(5):511–8.

146. Neu CM, Manz F, Rauch F, Merkel A, Schoenau E. Bone densities and bone size at the distal radius in healthy children and adolescents: a study using peripheral quantitative computed tomography. Bone. 2001;28(2):227–32.

147. Werkstetter KJ, Pozza SB, Filipiak-Pittroff B, Schatz SB, Prell C, Bufler P, et al. Long-term development of bone geometry and muscle in pediatric inflammatory bowel disease. Am J Gastroenterol. 2011;106(5):988–98.

148. Thayu M, Shults J, Burnham JM, Zemel BS, Baldassano RN, Leonard MB. Gender differences in body composition deficits at diagnosis in children and adolescents with Crohn's disease. Inflamm Bowel Dis. 2007;13(9):1121–8.

149. Sylvester FA, Leopold S, Lincoln M, Hyams JS, Griffiths AM, Lerer T. A two-year longitudinal study of persistent lean tissue deficits in children with Crohn's disease. Clin Gastroenterol Hepatol. 2009;7(4):452–5.

150. Laakso S, Valta H, Verkasalo M, Toiviainen-Salo S, Makitie O. Compromised peak bone mass in patients with inflammatory bowel disease – a prospective study. J Pediatr. 2014;164(6):1436–43.e1.

151. Pappa H, Thayu M, Sylvester F, Leonard M, Zemel B, Gordon C. Skeletal health of children and adolescents with inflammatory bowel disease. J Pediatr Gastroenterol Nutr. 2011;53(1):11–25.

152. Ward LM, Rauch F, Matzinger MA, Benchimol EI, Boland M, Mack DR. Iliac bone histomorphometry in children with newly diagnosed inflammatory bowel disease. Osteoporos Int. 2010;21:331–7.

153. Bechtold S, Alberer M, Arenz T, Putzker S, Filipiak-Pittroff B, Schwarz HP, et al. Reduced muscle mass and bone size in pediatric patients with inflammatory bowel disease. Inflamm Bowel Dis. 2010;16(2):216–25.

154. Hyams JS, Wyzga N, Kreutzer DL, Justinich CJ, Gronowicz GA. Alterations in bone metabolism in children with inflammatory bowel disease: an in vitro study. J Pediatr Gastroenterol Nutr. 1997;24(3):289–95.

155. Varghese S, Wyzga N, Griffiths AM, Sylvester FA. Effects of serum from children with newly diagnosed Crohn disease on primary cultures of rat osteoblasts. J Pediatr Gastroenterol Nutr. 2002;35(5):641–8.

156. Sylvester FA, Wyzga N, Hyams JS, Gronowicz GA. Effect of Crohn's disease on bone metabolism in vitro: a role for interleukin-6. J Bone Miner Res. 2002;17(4):695–702.

157. Laurent MR, Dubois V, Claessens F, Verschueren SM, Vanderschueren D, Gielen E, et al. Muscle-bone interactions: from experimental models to the clinic? A critical update. Mol Cell Endocrinol. 2016;432:14–36.

158. Thayu M, Denson LA, Shults J, Zemel BS, Burnham JM, Baldassano RN, et al. Determinants of changes in linear growth and body composition in incident pediatric Crohn's disease. Gastroenterology. 2010;139:430–8.

159. Werkstetter KJ, Ullrich J, Schatz SB, Prell C, Koletzko B, Koletzko S. Lean body mass, physical activity and quality of life in paediatric patients with inflammatory bowel disease and in healthy controls. J Crohns Colitis. 2012;6:665–73.

160. Reich KM, Fedorak RN, Madsen K, Kroeker KI. Vitamin D improves inflammatory bowel disease outcomes: Basic science and clinical review. World J Gastroenterol WJG. 2014;20(17):4934–47.

161. Meeker S, Seamons A, Maggio-Price L, Paik J. Protective links between vitamin D, inflammatory bowel disease and colon cancer. World J Gastroenterol. 2016;22(3):933–48.

162. Prosnitz AR, Leonard MB, Shults J, Zemel BS, Hollis BW, Denson LA, et al. Changes in vitamin D and parathyroid hormone metabolism in incident pediatric Crohn's disease. Inflamm Bowel Dis. 2013;19(1):45–53.

163. Middleton JP, Bhagavathula AP, Gaye B, Alvarez JA, Huang CS, Sauer CG, et al. Vitamin D status and bone mineral density in African American children with Crohn disease. J Pediatr Gastroenterol Nutr. 2013;57(5):587–93.

164. Nowak JK, Grzybowska-Chlebowczyk U, Landowski P, Szaflarska-Poplawska A, Klincewicz B, Adamczak D, et al. Prevalence and correlates of vitamin K deficiency in children with inflammatory bowel disease. Sci Rep. 2014;4:4768.

165. Nakajima S, Iijima H, Egawa S, Shinzaki S, Kondo J, Inoue T, et al. Association of vitamin K deficiency with bone metabolism and clinical disease activity in inflammatory bowel disease. Nutrition. 2011;27(10):1023–8.

166. Bernstein CN, Blanchard JF, Leslie W, Wajda A, Yu BN. The incidence of fracture among patients with inflammatory bowel disease. A population-based cohort study. Ann Intern Med. 2000;133(10):795–9.

167. Loftus EJ, Crowson CS, Sandborn WJ, Tremaine WJ, O'Fallon WM, Melton 3rd LJ. Long-term fracture risk in patients with Crohn's disease: a population-based study in Olmsted County, Minnesota. Gastroenterology. 2002;123(2):468–75.

168. Persad R, Jaffer I, Issenman RM. The prevalence of long bone fractures in pediatric inflammatory bowel disease. J Pediatr Gastroenterol Nutr. 2006;43(5):597–602.

169. Kappelman MD, Galanko JA, Porter CQ, Sandler RS. Risk of diagnosed fractures in children with inflammatory bowel diseases. Inflamm Bowel Dis. 2011;17:1125–30.

170. Siffledeen JS, Siminoski K, Jen H, Fedorak RN. Vertebral fractures and role of low bone mineral density in Crohn's disease. Clin Gastroenterol Hepatol. 2007;5(6):721–8.

171. Semeao EJ, Stallings VA, Peck SN, Piccoli DA. Vertebral compression fractures in pediatric patients with Crohn's disease. Gastroenterology. 1997;112(5):1710–3.

172. Tsampalieros A, Lam CK, Spencer JC, Thayu M, Shults J, Zemel BS, et al. Long-term inflammation and glucocorticoid therapy impair skeletal modeling during growth in childhood Crohn disease. J Clin Endocrinol Metab. 2013;98(8):3438–45.

173. Al-Shaar L, Mneimneh R, Nabulsi M, Maalouf J, Fuleihan GH. Vitamin D3 dose requirement to raise 25-hydroxyvitamin D to desirable levels in adolescents: results from a randomized controlled trial. J Bone Miner Res. 2014;29(4):944–51.

174. Werkstetter KJ, Schatz SB, Alberer M, Filipiak-Pittroff B, Koletzko S. Influence of exclusive enteral nutrition therapy on bone density and geometry in newly diagnosed pediatric Crohn's disease patients. Ann Nutr Metab. 2013;63(1–2):10–6.

175. Bernstein CN, Targownik LE, Leslie WD. What is the role for bisphosphonates in IBD? Gut. 2014;63(9):1369–70.

Puberty and Pediatric-Onset Inflammatory Bowel Disease

14

Dianne Deplewski, Neera Gupta, and Barbara S. Kirschner

The Pubertal Process in Healthy Children and Adolescents

Puberty is defined as the developmental stage during which sequential biological processes occur that ultimately lead to reproductive capacity [1]. The onset of puberty is initiated following increased synthesis and secretion of gonadotropin releasing hormone (GnRH) in the hypothalamus and its transport to gonadotrophs within the anterior pituitary. In response to pulsatile GnRH, the gonadotrophs secrete luteinizing hormone (LH) and follicle stimulating hormone (FSH), which in turn regulate ovarian and testicular functions. Pituitary sensitivity to GnRH varies throughout life, but increases prior to the onset of puberty. At this time, LH is secreted in a pulsatile manner, primarily during sleep, but subsequently changes to a pulsatile pattern throughout the day as puberty progresses [2]. In females, LH stimulates theca cells in the ovary to produce androgens, which diffuse to granulosa cells for conversion into estrogens. FSH causes growth of granulosa cells in the ovarian follicle and estrogen production (estrone or E1 and estradiol or E2). The estrogen elaborated in large amounts by the ovaries leads to feminization in girls. In males, LH stimulates testosterone production by Leydig cells in the testis. Testosterone subsequently undergoes 5α-reduction to dihydrotestosterone, which induces secondary sex characteristics. FSH acts on Sertoli cells in the seminiferous tubules of the testes to stimulate sperm production and testicular enlargement.

Adrenarche involves maturation of the adrenal gland with increased secretion of 17-ketosteroid and androgen production in response to ACTH. Adrenarche most often occurs between 6 and 9 years of age with elevation of circulating dehydroepiandrosterone sulfate (DHEAS) [3]. This results in the growth of pubic and axillary hair. Adrenarche is typically temporally related to pubertal maturation of the hypothalamic–pituitary–gonadal (HPG) axis, but is not causally related to maturation of this axis. While adrenal androgen production is a minor component of the midpubertal male testosterone level, the adrenal gland contributes about half the total testosterone produced in the female. Since adrenal androgen production is ACTH- dependent, this synthesis is subject to suppression with exogenous glucocorticoid therapy. In normal maturation, DHEAS is the most abundant circulating adrenal steroid after the onset of adrenarche and often reflects endogenous glucocorticoid secretory capacity. Adrenal androgen production has also been shown to be affected by other hormones, such as insulin, growth hormone (GH), and insulin-like growth factor 1 (IGF-1), and indirectly to nutritional status [4].

Since in early puberty increased gonadotropin pulse amplitude increases first during sleep, gonadal steroid secretion at this point of development is maximal in the very early morning hours and may wane to low, prepubertal levels by 0900. Thus, it is important to assay gonadotropin and sex steroid levels in the early morning. In addition, it is important to perform these assays in a specialty laboratory with sensitive pediatric assays to detect the normally low prepubertal and early pubertal levels. The adrenal steroid DHEAS does not follow this pattern because of its long plasma half-life, and a meaningful level may be determined throughout the day. A summary of normal hormone levels in puberty is seen in Table 14.1.

Although puberty typically occurs between the ages of 9–12 in girls and 10–13 in boys, the factors in the brain that trigger the onset of the pulsatile GnRH secretion at the time

D. Deplewski, MD (✉)
Section of Adult and Pediatric Endocrinology, Diabetes and Metabolism, University of Chicago, Chicago, IL, USA
e-mail: ddeplcws@peds.bsd.uchicago.edu

N. Gupta, MD, MAS
Pediatric Gastroenterology and Nutrition, Weill Cornell Medicine, New York, NY, USA
e-mail: neg9020@med.cornell.edu

B.S. Kirschner, MD
Section of Gastroenerology, Hepatology and Nutrition, University of Chicago, Chicago, IL, USA
e-mail: bkirschn@peds.bsd.uchicago.edu

© Springer International Publishing AG 2017
P. Mamula et al. (eds.), *Pediatric Inflammatory Bowel Disease*, DOI 10.1007/978-3-319-49215-5_14

Table 14.1 Hormone levels in puberty

Hormone	Stage/age	Male	Female
Dehydroepiandrosterone	Tanner I	<89	<46
Sulfate (DHAS) (mcg/dl)	Tanner II	<81	15–113
	Tanner III	22–126	42–162
	Tanner IV	33–117	42–241
	Tanner V	110–510	45–320
Luteinizing hormone	3–7 years	<0.26	<0.26
(LH)	8–9 years	<0.46	<0.69
Pediatric – IU/L	10–11 years	<3.31	<4.38
	12–14 years	0.23–4.41	0.04–10.8
	15–17 years	0.29–4.77	0.97–14.7
Follicle stimulating	5–9 years	0.21–4.33	0.72–5.33
hormone (FSH)	10–13 years	0.53–4.92	0.87–9.16
Pediatric (IU/L)	14–17 years	0.85–8.74	0.64–10.98
Estradiol (E2)	Prepubertal	<4	<16
Pediatric (pg/ml)	10–11 years	<12	<65
	12–14 years	<24	<142
	15–17 years	<31	<283
Estrone (E1) (pg/ml)	Prepubertal	<10	<34
	10–11 years	<12	<72
	12–14 years	<28	<75
	15–17 years	<64	<188
Testosterone (Te)	Tanner I	<5	<8
(ng/dl)	Tanner II	<167	<24
	Tanner III	21–719	<28
	Tanner IV	25–912	<31
	Tanner V	110–975	<33
IGF-1 (ng/ml)	Tanner I	96–341	105–359
	Tanner II	101–478	99–451
	Tanner III	101–478	197–642
	Tanner IV	318–765	330–776
	Tanner V	318–765	330–776

Modified from Nakamoto and Mason [82], and Quest Diagnostics Reference Ranges, Quest Diagnostics Inc., San Juan Capistrano CA Caution is suggested in differentiating puberty from prepuberty, especially with regard to LH, FSH, E2, and Te. The assays must be sufficiently specific as well as sensitive for the normally low prepubertal and early pubertal levels. In addition, these hormones are secreted episodically with short half-lives in the blood. Early morning testing is recommended

of puberty are still not completely understood. Leptin is a peptide hormone expressed predominantly in adipocytes that regulates food intake and energy expenditure at the hypothalamic level [5]. Serum leptin levels have been shown to correlate closely with body fat content. Leptin is thought to be an important link between nutrition and the attainment and maintenance of reproductive function, as patients with leptin deficiency have been shown to not only be obese, but to also have gonadotropin deficiency [6]. However, while leptin levels normally rise throughout childhood and puberty, a rise in leptin is not required to trigger puberty. Thus, leptin likely functions as a permissive factor rather than a trigger in the

onset of human puberty. In late 2003, loss of function mutations of GPR54 (a G-protein coupled receptor) were described in patients with hypogonadotropic hypogonadism [7]. This discovery led to the finding that GPR54 and its ligand (kisspeptin) act as a signal for pubertal GnRH release. Further research suggests that kisspeptin influences the timing of puberty and the integration of nutritional and energy status, likely indirectly through leptin expression. However, what controls the regulation of kisspeptin expression at the time of puberty is not completely known.

Neuropeptide Y (NPY), a potent appetite-stimulating agent found in the hypothalamus, may also mediate the effects of leptin on puberty. Based on studies in prepubertal rats, Pralong et al. suggested that NPY may inhibit GnRH secretion and delay sexual maturation [8]. In a limited study, girls with constitutional delay in puberty were found to have higher levels of NPY than those with a normal course of puberty [9].

The onset of puberty is associated with Tanner stage II for breast development in girls and testicular volume of 4 ml or length of 2.6 cm in boys [10, 11]. The current best estimates for the mean age of onset of puberty in healthy children in the United States are 10.2 years for girls and 11.5 years for boys [10]. The mean age of menarche is 12.6 years in Caucasian girls, 12.3 years in Mexican-American girls, and 12.1 years in African-American girls of normal weight [12]. The mean age for spermarche in boys is between 13.5 and 14.5 years [13]. The average duration of puberty in girls is 4 years (range 1.5–8 years) and for boys 3 years (range 2–5 years) [13]. This is important as it reflects the wide range in maturation of normal, healthy individuals as well as the variation in duration to completion [14–16].

The standard deviation for all pubertal milestones is about 1 year [17, 18]. Thus, girls older than 13 years and boys older than 14 years without evidence of Tanner II development are considered to have delayed puberty. The most common cause of delayed puberty in otherwise healthy children is an extreme variant of normal known as constitutional delay of growth and puberty (CDGP). This occurs due to an unexplained delayed activation of the hypothalamic–pituitary–gonadal axis. A family history of delayed puberty can usually be elicited. In a large case series, CDGP was found to be the cause of delayed puberty in 53% of the subjects (approximately 63% of boys and 30% of girls) [19]. The second most common cause of delayed puberty in the case series was functional gonadotropin deficiency, which affected 19% of subjects. Functional gonadotropin deficiency can be seen in chronic illness, especially in conditions that are also associated with decreased body fat. Other less common causes of delayed puberty include primary gonadal failure and gonadotropin deficiency.

For distinguishing different phases of pubertal development, most reports in the pediatric gastroenterology literature have used Tanner stages which rely on visual observation of the progression of pubic hair character and distribution, breast size and contour, and testicular size [20]. Schall et al. studied the validity of self-assessment of sexual maturity in 100 patients, age 8–18 years, with Crohn's disease [21]. The instrument included drawings and written description of Tanner stages. Patients' self-assessments were compared with those of a designated pediatrician. Agreement varied between 74% and 85%, depending on the sex and sexual maturity status with younger children and overweight boys tending to overestimate their sexual maturity status (SMS). Rapkin et al. also noted that self-staging of Tanner stage was as accurate as circulating estradiol and FSH measurements in 124 healthy girls, aged 8–18 years [22]. However, one needs to be cautious with Tanner staging of breasts in overweight girls by self-report, as adipose tissue in the chest can be mistaken for early breasts. This emphasizes the necessity of palpation to identify true breast bud tissue in girls.

Thus, puberty involves a change in the balance of inhibitory and stimulatory signals that impact the GnRH neuron. Genetic factors, ethnicity, nutrition, and environmental chemicals are important in the pubertal process. However, the mechanisms by which neuroendocrine and genetic factors control pubertal development are yet to be fully elucidated.

The Influence of Inflammatory Bowel Disease on Puberty

Delayed puberty and poor growth often complicate the clinical course of children diagnosed with IBD, especially children diagnosed with Crohn disease (CD). As progression through puberty and increased growth velocity are intricately linked, most studies that look at the effects of IBD on puberty examine both growth and pubertal progress. Normal prepubertal growth velocity after 3 years of age averages about 5–6.5 cm/year. The pubertal growth spurt provides an additional 15–25 cm of growth [9, 12–14]. Delayed puberty is often associated with lower peak height velocity. Midparental target heights can be calculated with the following formulas: for boys, add 13 cm to the mother's height and average it with the father's height; for girls, subtract 13 cm from the father's height and average it with the mother's height. Most children will fall within ±8.5 cm of this prediction.

From the viewpoint of the authors, one of the most interesting studies which assessed the effect of IBD on puberty is that of Hildebrand et al. [23]. This study obtained height and weight data collected from birth through final adult height in 46 patients with childhood-onset Crohn disease (CD) and 60 patients with childhood-onset ulcerative colitis (UC) from a defined area in Sweden. In this study, the age at peak height velocity (PHV) was stated to represent the middle of puberty.

Individual values for height were converted into standard deviation scores (SDS) using the infancy–childhood–puberty growth standard of Karlberg et al. [24]. The PHV for healthy children in Sweden was reported to be 12.05 ± 0.88 years for girls and 14.15 ± 0.98 for boys. Delayed puberty was defined as a delayed age at PHV of >2.0 SDS. No significant delay was noted in children with UC with age at PHV 11.9 ± 1.1 years for girls and 14.0 ± 1.2 years for boys. However, mean age at PHV was later in patients with CD: 12.7 ± 1.4 years for girls and 14.9 ± 1.2 years for boys, and 23% of these children with CD had a delayed age of PHV of >2.0 SDS.

Brain et al. also observed several alterations in the pattern of puberty among pediatric patients with IBD [11]. The mean age of onset of puberty was delayed for both female and male patients when compared to healthy controls: 12.6 years versus 11.1 years in girls and 13.2 years versus 12.4 years in boys. In addition, the duration of puberty was prolonged, especially in adolescents with frequent relapses during puberty [11]. Some patients with IBD took up to 4 years to progress from Tanner stage II to stage IV. Peak height velocities during puberty reached rates >12 cm/year in patients who remained in remission in contrast to as little as 1–2 cm/year in those with relapsing disease. When surgical resection was performed in 11 prepubertal children with CD, puberty started within 1 year of resection. The authors postulated that if the onset of puberty was delayed beyond 14 years, then the final height may be "irreparably compromised." Our data would confirm that statement, as we observed that there was a strong correlation between age at menarche and height gain [25]. When menarche occurred at <13 years of age, the mean increment in height was 10 cm compared with only 3.0 cm in those aged >15 years. Homer et al. also noted that catch-up growth, even in prepubertal patients, occurred only in those with sustained clinical remission [26].

Ferguson and Sedgwick described delayed puberty in IBD based on a retrospective survey of adults with a history of pediatric-onset UC and CD [27]. Their results were different from other published reports in several ways. Adult stature achieved by 67 of 70 patients was similar to normal adults, and no difference was seen whether the patients had CD or UC. Delayed puberty was based on patients' recall many years later. Pubertal delay was reported as follows: Crohn disease, 11/28 (39%) of men and 13/22 (59%) of women compared with 2/9 (22%) of men and 3/11 (27%) of women with UC. These numbers were not statistically different. Age at menarche was reported to be >16 years in 8 of 11 (73%) women whose menarche occurred after the diagnosis of CD.

More recently, Gupta et al. compared the age at menarche in 34 patients with CD with that for 545 controls, using data from the National Health and Nutrition Examination Survey (NHANES) [28]. They found that the median chronological age at menarche (13.9 years) in CD was older than that in the NHANES sample (12.0 years). In CD patients, the cumulative incidence of menarche was 10% at chronological age 12 years, 51% at chronological age 14 years, and 100% at chronological age 16 years. Sixty-eight percent reached menarche by bone age 13.5 years and 100% by bone age >14 years. Menarche occurred earliest in South Asians, followed by East Asians, and then Caucasians. They suggested if menarche has not occurred by bone age >14 years, endocrinology referral should be considered.

Other studies also show that onset of IBD during the prepubertal period is frequently associated with subnormal growth. In the Hildebrand et al. study, growth velocity in children diagnosed with IBD during the prepubertal period was −2.0 SDS in 24% of children with UC and 40% of children with CD [23]. Kanoff et al. and Kirschner also reported impaired growth in 68–88% of prepubertal children with CD [29, 30]. In addition, within a group of prepubertal patients, Saha et al. noted the poorest growth in those with severe CD when compared with UC [31]. In this study, no difference was seen between patients with and without corticosteroid treatment. In contrast, Motil et al. and Sentongo et al. reported that the prevalence of growth failure was equal regardless of the stage of pubertal development [32, 33]. Sawczenko et al. studied the effect of CD on final height in 123 patients who were designated "prepubertal" based on age at onset of symptoms: <13 years for boys and <11 years for girls [34]. Nineteen percent had a final height 8.0 cm or more below the targeted or midparental height. Those children who received steroid therapy were not found to be significantly shorter than other children at final height, suggesting that the judicious use of systemic steroids should not lead to significant long-term growth delay. However, of the shorter children in their study, boys were overrepresented with an OR of 3.70.

Several additional studies have suggested that boys with CD are more likely to have abnormalities of growth, especially while their disease is active. In an earlier report, Griffiths et al. had also observed less catch-up growth in boys than girls [35]. More recently, Gupta et al. reported that serum IGF-1 levels were reduced in males with IBD for both chronological and skeletal age when compared with female patients with IBD, and this may explain, at least in part, why male children with CD achieve less catch-up growth and have lower ultimate height Z-scores than females [36]. Gupta et al. subsequently reported that mean bone age Z-scores were lower in females, perhaps providing an opportunity for greater catch-up growth for females, once they are in remission [37]. To determine if some of the newer therapies in use for CD lead to improvements in growth and normal advancement in puberty, Pfefferkorn et al. analyzed growth outcomes in children with newly diagnosed CD [38]. They found that despite improvements in disease activity, mean height SDS

scores did not change significantly, and pubertal progression remained slow. Children diagnosed with CD prior to 9 years of age had a higher mean growth velocity 2 years after diagnosis, as compared to children diagnosed after 9 years of age. Children who required prolonged corticosteroid therapy (longer than 6 months) had poorer growth outcomes. These data suggest that despite advances in nutritional and anti-inflammatory therapies for CD, growth and pubertal delays continue to persist in these children with CD.

In contrast, a study by Malik et al. suggested that children who had a clinical response to infliximab therapy had improvement in their linear growth that was independent of their pubertal progression [39]. In addition, children who had not been exposed to exogenous glucocorticoids also exhibited better growth with infliximab therapy, suggesting that the effect on growth was not simply related to a decrease in glucocorticoid use. In a more recent study, Mason et al. followed 63 adolescents with IBD (CD, n = 45 [23 males] and UC, n = 18 [12 males]), median age 13.4 years (range 10–16.6 years) over 12 months [40]. Interestingly, they reported no significant delay in puberty in their subjects. However, attenuation of the pubertal growth spurt was evident in these subjects. In the adolescents with IBD, the median IGF-1 SDS score was lower and IGFBP-3 higher than the control group, suggesting an abnormality of IGF-1 bioavailability.

Pubertal Arrest

Pubertal delay in IBD can have many etiologies, and poor nutritional status is often thought to be the major cause, as optimal nutrition is necessary for the initiation and maintenance of reproductive function. GnRH secretion is blunted in the malnourished state which leads to pubertal arrest, and secretion of GnRH normalizes with weight gain [41]. However, the delay of puberty in IBD presents a more complex issue, with weight not the sole independent variable. Stress and inflammation likely also have important roles. In addition to delays in the onset of puberty, slowing or cessation of sexual maturation may occur in patients with IBD. For example, secondary amenorrhea is a well-recognized complication of weight loss.

Potential Causes of Pubertal Delay in Patients with IBD

The complex interactions between severity of disease, fluctuations in inflammatory cytokines, and their effect on nutritional status and hormonal profile make it difficult to determine how individual factors influence the onset and progression of puberty in pediatric patients with IBD. As a consequence, while nutritional deficits are well described in patients, other aspects such as the potential role of inflammatory cytokines on puberty are often extrapolated from animal models [42].

Nutritional Causes of Pubertal Delay

In otherwise healthy children, undernutrition may cause a delay in sexual maturation and menarche. Important studies done by Frisch and colleagues demonstrated that the age of pubertal growth and menarche in girls correlated more closely to weight than to chronological age [43–45]. During the adolescent growth spurt prior to menarche, girls had a continuous decline in the percent body water and increase in body fat, resulting in a change in the ratio of lean body weight from 5:1 to 3:1 and a mean percent body fat at menarche of 22% [43–45]. The investigators noted that the mean weight at menarche in girls in the United States was 47.8 ± 0.5 kg [43–45]. A possible relationship between body fat and menarche was suggested by adipose tissue being a significant extragonadal site of estrogen production through conversion of androgen into estrogen. She postulated that the decrease in age at menarche (approximately 3–4 months each decade over the past 100 years) is due to girls reaching the "critical" weight earlier, secondary to improved nutrition. In girls with primary amenorrhea due to undernutrition, a minimal equivalent of 17% body fat may be necessary for menarche to occur [43–45]. For girls experiencing secondary amenorrhea, resumption of menses usually occurred when weight gain was 10% higher than the weight at menarche.

Dreizen et al. compared the age at menarche of 30 girls with "chronic undernutrition" with 30 "well-nourished" girls living in north central Alabama [46]. The average age at menarche was 14.5 years in the former group and 12.4 years in the latter group. Interestingly, standing heights that had differed by 9.2 cm at 12.5 years decreased to a difference of only 3.5 cm at 14.5 years and were not significantly different (1.1 cm) at 17 years. Similarly, skeletal age was delayed in the undernourished group, but at the time of menarche, the bone age in the undernourished girls was only 3.8 months more advanced than the well-nourished group. Complete fusion of the epiphyses was delayed in the malnourished group to 17.6 years versus 15.9 years for healthy controls. Therefore, although the timing of the adolescent growth spurt was delayed by undernutrition, final height (in the absence of underlying disease) was not significantly reduced. An earlier study by the same authors in undernourished boys also showed delayed epiphyseal fusion to 18.7 years versus 17.0 years and a mean difference in height between the groups of 2.68 inches at 16 years [47]. Unfortunately, final adult heights were not reported.

Similar delays in menarche (with onset averaging 15.1 ± 0.5 years) are seen in ballet dancers, swimmers, and runners whose training and low calorie intakes begin prior to menarche [44, 45]. Frisch postulated that these females have a raised lean/fat ratio. Both increased nutrition and reduction in the intensity of training may restore menses. Athletic amenorrhea is a hypothalamic reversion to a more immature pattern in GnRH response. Normalization may occur with reduction in exercise and/or other stress without the weight change estimated by Frisch.

Reduction in calorie intake has been documented in many studies of pediatric-onset IBD, especially CD [48–50]. Thus, undernutrition is likely to be one of the contributing factors leading to delay in the onset and progression of puberty. Similarly, secondary amenorrhea seen in female patients with IBD may be caused by weight loss, a frequent complication of IBD in adolescents.

Sentongo et al. used dual energy x-ray absorptiometry (DEXA) and anthropometric measures to compare fat mass (FM) and fat-free mass (FFM) in 132 pediatric patients with IBD and 66 healthy controls [33]. They found that patients had normal fat stores but reduced FFM, consistent with "inflammatory cachexia" [33]. They cited data suggesting that proinflammatory muscle-active cytokines may impair accretion of lean tissue.

Burnham et al. compared 104 North American patients with CD to 233 healthy control subjects and documented delayed sexual maturation in the CD group [51]. Patients within Tanner stages II–IV averaged 1.4–1.5 years older than control subjects at the same pubertal stages. Lean mass was reduced by 8% in the patient CD group. It is the opinion of the authors that the role of undernutrition in both growth failure and sexual maturation may be underestimated if these complications are compared only with documented weight loss. Failure to gain weight (without a history of weight loss) may also adversely affect the timing of menarche and the progression of puberty.

Advancement in puberty may also be related to excess weight gain [12, 52]. Early adrenarche appears to be related to excess weight gain and may be accompanied by skeletal advancement and possibly earlier true puberty. This may be related to peripheral aromatization of adrenal androgens to estrogens in fat.

Endocrine Aspects of Pubertal Delay

Most studies of endocrine function in children and adolescents with IBD have been performed to investigate the causes of growth failure rather than the onset and progression of puberty [48–50, 53–57]. An intact growth hormone/insulin-like growth factor I (IGF-I) axis is necessary for normal postnatal growth. Thyroid hormone and cortisol are also important, as are the sex steroids at the time of puberty. IGF-I is produced in the liver under the stimulation of GH, and is thought to be the key mediator of the growth-promoting effects of GH. Reports in growth-impaired patients with IBD have generally demonstrated normal GH secretion, thyroid function, cortisol response to hypoglycemia, and gonadotropin response to GnRH. What changes were observed such as reduced amplitude of the GH pulse or increase in reverse triiodothyronine (rT3) were not associated with reduced growth velocity [55]. We observed that weight loss could be associated with prepubertal levels of circulating sex hormones despite previous physical signs of pubertal progression [56]. IGF-1 levels have been shown to be reduced in children and adolescents with IBD [42, 56, 58, 59]. This usually occurs despite the presence of adequate circulating levels of GH and is known as "growth hormone resistance." Since IGF-1 is modulated by both GH and nutritional status, it is not clear whether the reduction of IGF-1 seen in this population is secondary to active disease or to the decrease in calorie intake (or both) [42, 56]. An increase in IGF-1 occurs following nutritional restitution in children with IBD. Some have suggested that the IGF-1 rise following enteral nutrition or surgical resection in children with active IBD precedes improvement in nutritional status (based on anthropometric measures); however, more rapid indices of nutritional restitution such as prealbumin were not measured in those studies. Corkins et al. noted the major binding protein for IGF-1 (IGFBP-3) was also reduced at diagnosis in children with IBD which would result in a reduced half-life for circulating IGF-1 [58]. Evidence using a knockout mouse lacking only liver-derived IGF-1 demonstrated normal growth and development, suggesting an important role for paracrine or autocrine production of IGF-1 by nonhepatic tissues [60]. The use of IGF-1 as a potential therapeutic agent to enhance growth in childhood IBD is hampered by concerns regarding a potential increased risk for colon cancer and other malignancies in this population [61].

In a trinitrobenzene sulfonate (TNBS) model of experimental colitis in rats, Azooz et al. noted that puberty was delayed but plasma concentrations of gonadotropins were similar to healthy controls [62]. Interestingly, delayed puberty and reduced levels of plasma testosterone and 17β-estriol levels were present in both colitic and noncolitic pair-fed rats, compared to healthy controls, emphasizing the importance of caloric sufficiency. However, the frequency of delayed puberty was less in the food-restricted rats (28%) versus the colitis rats (57%), suggesting an independent role for inflammation in this process. The authors demonstrated that the administration of testosterone subcutaneously on a daily basis to the colitis rats normalized the onset of puberty. Similar results were recently reported by DeBoer and colleagues comparing pubertal progression in dextran sodium sulfate (DSS) induced colitis, food-restricted mice, and free-feeding control mice.

Pubertal progression in male mice was measured by separation of the prepuce from the glans penis and in female mice by the timing of the vaginal opening. For both sexes, puberty was more delayed in the colitis model than the food-restricted animals, despite similar leptin levels [63, 64].

Proinflammatory Cytokines–Endocrine Interactions

Several in vitro studies have elucidated ways in which proinflammatory cytokines (such as tumor necrosis factor-α (TNF-α), interleukin-6 (IL-6), and interleukin-1β (IL-1 β)), elevated in patients with IBD, affect endocrine function. Elevations of these cytokines have been shown to lead to altered gonadal function and reduced sex steroid synthesis [65]. Several of these findings may be applicable to explaining pubertal delay in patients with chronic inflammatory bowel disease.

TNF-α has inhibitory effects on GH and sex hormone function. Transgenic mice overexpressing TNF-α (or IL-6) are growth-impaired and have low IGF-1 levels despite normal GH because of inhibition of GH signaling within hepatocytes [66]. Denson et al. showed that TNF-α suppressed GH receptor expression by inhibiting Sp1/Sp3 transactivators [67]. IL-6 inhibits hepatic GH signaling by inducing a suppressor of cytokine-inducible signaling (SOCS-3) and reduces the half-life of IGF-1 by increasing the catabolism of its binding protein, IGFBP-3. TNF-α and IL-6 also reduce IGF-1 action by inhibiting insulin receptor substrate 1 which influences IGF-1 binding to its receptors and interleukin-1β (IL-1 β). TNF-α and IL-1β have also been shown to induce anorexia. It has been suggested that GH therapy may overcome hepatic GH resistance induced by IL-6 [68].

TNF-α has also been shown to decrease androgen receptor protein as well as dihydrotestosterone activation. TNF-α, IL-6, and IL-1 β reduce testosterone synthesis in Leydig cells and steroidogenesis in cells in the ovary. DeBoer et al. recently reported partial normalization of puberty in female mice with dextran sodium sulfate (DSS) colitis treated with anti-TNF-α, when compared to a placebo-treated group. The authors utilized the day of life of the vaginal opening as the validated measure of puberty in female mice: day 30 in controls, day 31 in DSS colitis with anti-TNF-α, and day 33 or later in DSS and placebo. The DSS colitis mice controls and those treated with anti-TNF-α maintained similar weights throughout the study, but the DSS–placebo mice had higher IL-6 levels [69].

Psychosocial Issues and Puberty

There is extensive literature describing dynamic changes in the psychosocial interests and concerns of adolescents. Shafer and Irwin addressed these issues and emphasized how they develop and are different among adolescents during early adolescence (ages 10–13 years), middle adolescence (ages 14–16 years), and late adolescence (ages 17–21 years) [13]. Nottelmann et al. studied the relationship between adolescent psychosocial adjustment and chronological age, pubertal status, and serum hormone levels [70]. In boys, adjustment problems were associated with low sex hormones or lower pubertal stage in conjunction with higher chronological age. These included sadness/anxiety and problems with body and self-image. In girls, adjustment problems in social relationships were also associated with lower pubertal stage and higher age. Both groups had elevated levels of androstenedione, an adrenal hormone responsive to stress, which the authors suggested may be due to self-comparison with same-age peers. They speculated that boys may be more sensitive to hormonal influences and girls to environmental influences.

Delayed sexual maturation may have significant adverse effects on self-esteem and socialization, as the child with delayed puberty looks younger than their chronological age, and often are treated as such [71]. Thus, an adolescent with IBD must cope not only with the impact of having a chronic disease, but also with the psychological issues of delayed puberty.

In addition to the psychological response to pubertal delay, stress itself may interfere with the functioning of the brain–pituitary–gonadal axis. Evidence suggests that this may be mediated by elevated cortisol levels over a protracted period of time. Consten et al. noted that cortisol administration to male carp caused delayed testicular development, reduced testosterone levels, and impaired maturation of pituitary gonadotrophs [72].

Therapeutic Approach to Addressing Pubertal Issues in IBD

The observations and studies described above suggest that prolonged control of active inflammation and providing adequate nutrient intake are both essential in promoting normal puberty. Alperstein et al. reported that it took 2.5–10 years for five of nine children with growth delay who were in Tanner stage I to attain their pre-illness height percentile following surgery [73]. Thus, optimal control of IBD and optimization of nutritional status are paramount in adolescents with IBD and delayed puberty.

Although experience with GH treatment in pediatric patients with IBD is limited, improvement of growth velocity may be observed when there is reasonable disease control with reduced corticosteroid exposure. Furthermore, steroid-related growth effects may be in part ameliorated with GH treatment [74–76]. In one recent study, a trend was observed that improved growth velocity was greater in Tanner stage I

and II patients who received GH as compared to those who were in the later stages of puberty [76].

Often, final height preservation is at odds with the child's desire to proceed through puberty. Artificial induction of puberty with estrogen or testosterone runs the risk of skeletal advancement without commensurate growth. An anabolic steroid such as oxandrolone (Anavar®), which does not advance bone maturation as much as testosterone in modest dose, might be of some small value. Mason et al. described a retrospective study of eight boys with IBD (seven of whom were prepubertal at 13.6–15.6 years of age) who received testosterone therapy for pubertal induction [77]. Testosterone dose and route of administration were either monthly injections of testosterone enanthate 50 mg (five patients) or transdermal testosterone patch 2.5 mg daily (two patients) or 5.0 mg daily (one patient). Following 6 months of treatment, seven out of eight boys progressed in puberty to Tanner stage II–IV, and the median height velocity increased from 1.6 to 6.9 cm/year. There was a significant correlation between C-reactive protein levels and height velocity.

Ballinger et al. describe their approach to "young patients with IBD" as including a 3 to 6 month course of 100–125 mg/month of intramuscular testosterone ester (enanthate or cypionate) in boys and ethynyl estradiol 4–6 mcg/day orally for the same length of time in girls [78]. Our current therapy for pubertal induction in selected male patients with delayed puberty consists of a 6-month course of 50 mg/m^2 intramuscular testosterone ester. For girls with either functional gonadotropin deficiency or constitutional delay of puberty, it is reasonable to offer a 6-month course of either a low dose of IM depot estradiol (0.2–0.4 mg monthly), or a low dose estrogen patch (applying a 25 mcg patch twice weekly for 1 week out of the month) for pubertal induction. As opposed to boys, there are few studies that report the outcome of a brief exposure to sex steroid therapy for girls with delayed puberty. The response to this approach in pediatric patients with IBD has not been studied.

The relationship between puberty and its effects on bone density in children with IBD has not been addressed in this chapter as the topic is discussed in depth elsewhere in this text. Although pubertal delay has been associated with reduced BMD in adult men, its impact on peak bone mass in pediatric patients with IBD has not been determined [79, 80]. Bernstein et al. compared BMD T scores of the lumbar spine, femoral neck, total hip, and total body in a series of 70 adult women with IBD, who were <45 years of age. They observed no significant differences between 12 patients with disease onset before puberty compared with 58 whose disease was diagnosed after puberty [81]. More long-range data is needed on the relationship between pubertal delay and bone mineralization in adulthood.

For the reasons stated above, assessment of pubertal staging should be an integral part of the monitoring of pediatric patients with inflammatory bowel disease. Referral to a pediatric endocrinologist should be considered in boys who have reached 14 years and girls who have reached 13 years without evidence of any physical changes of puberty. Patients who are delayed in puberty, but showing evidence of pubertal progression on physical examination, need not be referred, unless the puberty appears to stall.

References

1. Bordini B, Rosenfield RL. Normal pubertal development: part I: the endocrine basis of puberty. Pediatr Rev. 2011;32(6):223–9.
2. Boyar R, Finkelstein J, Roffwarg H, Kapen S, Weitzman E, Hellman L. Synchronization of augmented luteinizing hormone secretion with sleep during puberty. N Engl J Med. 1972;287(12):582–6.
3. Reiter EO, Fuldauer VG, Root AW. Secretion of the adrenal androgen, dehydroepiandrosterone sulfate, during normal infancy, childhood, and adolescence, in sick infants, and in children with endocrinologic abnormalities. J Pediatr. 1977;90(5):766–70.
4. Guercio G, Rivarola MA, Chaler E, Maceiras M, Belgorosky A. Relationship between the growth hormone/insulin-like growth factor-I axis, insulin sensitivity, and adrenal androgens in normal prepubertal and pubertal girls. J Clin Endocrinol Metab. 2003;88(3):1389–93.
5. Friedman JM. The function of leptin in nutrition, weight, and physiology. Nutr Rev. 2002;60(10 Pt 2):S1–14; discussion S68–84, 85–7.
6. Farooqi IS. Leptin and the onset of puberty: insights from rodent and human genetics. Semin Reprod Med. 2002;20(2):139–44.
7. Seminara SB, Messager S, Chatzidaki EE, Thresher RR, Acierno Jr JS, Shagoury JK, et al. The GPR54 gene as a regulator of puberty. N Engl J Med. 2003;349(17):1614–27.
8. Pralong FP, Voirol M, Giacomini M, et al. Acceleration of pubertal development following central blockade of the Y1 subtype of neuropeptide Y receptors. Regul Pept. 2000;95(1–3):47–52.
9. Blogowska A, Rzepka-Gorska I, Krzyzanowska-Swiniarska B. Is neuropeptide Y responsible for constitutional delay of puberty in girls? A preliminary report. Gynecol Endocrinol. 2004;19(1): 22–5.
10. Bordini B, Rosenfield RL. Normal pubertal development: part II: clinical aspects of puberty. Pediatr Rev. 2011;32(7):281–92.
11. Brain CE, Savage MO. Growth and puberty in chronic inflammatory bowel disease. Baillieres Clin Gastroenterol. 1994;8(1): 83–100.
12. Rosenfield RL, Lipton RB, Drum ML. Thelarche, pubarche, and menarche attainment in children with normal and elevated body mass index. Pediatrics. 2009;123(1):84–8.
13. Irwin Jr CE, Shafer M. Adolescent health problems. Harrison's principals of internal medicine. 14th ed. New York: McGraw Hill; 1998. p. 30–3.
14. Marshall WA, Tanner JM. Variations in pattern of pubertal changes in girls. Arch Dis Child. 1969;44(235):291–303.
15. Marshall WA, Tanner JM. Variations in the pattern of pubertal changes in boys. Arch Dis Child. 1970;45(239):13–23.
16. Tanner JM, Whitehouse RH. Clinical longitudinal standards for height, weight, height velocity, weight velocity, and stages of puberty. Arch Dis Child. 1976;51(3):170–9.
17. MacMahon B. Age at Menarche: United States, 1960-1970. Vital Health Stat 11. 1973;133:1–36.
18. Tanner JM, Davies PS. Clinical longitudinal standards for height and height velocity for North American children. J Pediatr. 1985;107(3):317–29.
19. Sedlmeyer IL, Palmert MR. Delayed puberty: analysis of a large case series from an academic center. J Clin Endocrinol Metab. 2002;87(4):1613–20.
20. Tanner JM. Growth at adolescence. 2nd ed. Oxford: Blackwell Scientific Publications; 1962.
21. Schall JI, Semeao EJ, Stallings VA, et al. Self-assessment of sexual maturity status in children with Crohn's disease. J Pediatr. 2002;141(2):223–9.
22. Rapkin AJ, Tsao JC, Turk N, et al. Relationships among self-rated tanner staging, hormones, and psychosocial factors in healthy female adolescents. J Pediatr Adolesc Gynecol. 2006;19(3):181–7.
23. Hildebrand H, Karlberg J, Kristiansson B. Longitudinal growth in children and adolescents with inflammatory bowel disease. J Pediatr Gastroenterol Nutr. 1994;18(2):165–73.
24. Karlberg J, Fryer JG, Engstrom I, et al. Analysis of linear growth using a mathematical model. II. From 3 to 21 years of age. Acta Paediatr Scand Suppl. 1987;337:12–29.
25. Kirschner BS, Uebler N, Sutton MM. Growth after menarche in pediatric patients with chronic inflammatory bowel disease. Gastroenterology. 1993;104:A629.
26. Homer DR, Grand RJ, Colodny AH. Growth, course, and prognosis after surgery for Crohn's disease in children and adolescents. Pediatrics. 1977;59(5):717–25.
27. Ferguson A, Sedgwick DM. Juvenile onset inflammatory bowel disease: height and body mass index in adult life. BMJ. 1994;308(6939):1259–63.
28. Gupta N, Lustig RH, Kohn MA, Vittinghoff E. Menarche in pediatric patients with Crohn's disease. Dig Dis Sci. 2012;57(11): 2975–81.
29. Kanof ME, Lake AM, Bayless TM. Decreased height velocity in children and adolescents before the diagnosis of Crohn's disease. Gastroenterology. 1988;95(6):1523–7.
30. Kirschner BS. Growth and development in chronic inflammatory bowel disease. Acta Paediatr Scand Suppl. 1990;366:98–104. discussion 5
31. Saha MT, Ruuska T, Laippala P, et al. Growth of prepubertal children with inflammatory bowel disease. J Pediatr Gastroenterol Nutr. 1998;26(3):310–4.
32. Motil KJ, Grand RJ, Davis-Kraft L, et al. Growth failure in children with inflammatory bowel disease: a prospective study. Gastroenterology. 1993;105(3):681–91.
33. Sentongo TA, Semeao EJ, Piccoli DA, et al. Growth, body composition, and nutritional status in children and adolescents with Crohn's disease. J Pediatr Gastroenterol Nutr. 2000;31(1):33–40.
34. Sawczenko A, Ballinger AB, Savage MO, et al. Clinical features affecting final adult height in patients with pediatric-onset Crohn's disease. Pediatrics. 2006;118(1):124–9.
35. Griffiths AM, Nguyen P, Smith C, et al. Growth and clinical course of children with Crohn's disease. Gut. 1993;34(7):939–43.
36. Gupta N, Lustig RH, Kohn MA, McCracken M, Vittinghoff E. Sex differences in statural growth impairment in Crohn's disease: role of IGF-1. Inflamm Bowel Dis. 2011;17(11):2318–25.
37. Gupta N, Lustig RH, Kohn MA, Vittinghoff E. Determination of bone age in pediatric patients with Crohn's disease should become part of routine care. Inflamm Bowel Dis. 2013;19(1):61–5.
38. Pfefferkorn M, Burke G, Griffiths A, Markowitz J, Rosh J, Mack D, et al. Growth abnormalities persist in newly diagnosed children with Crohn disease despite current treatment paradigms. J Pediatr Gastroenterol Nutr. 2009;48(2):168–74.
39. Malik S, Wong SC, Bishop J, Hassan K, McGrogan P, Ahmed SF, et al. Improvement in growth of children with Crohn disease following anti-TNF-alpha therapy can be independent of pubertal progress and glucocorticoid reduction. J Pediatr Gastroenterol Nutr. 2011;52(1):31–7.
40. Mason A, Malik S, McMillan M, McNeilly JD, Bishop J, McGrogan P, et al. A prospective longitudinal study of growth and pubertal

progress in adolescents with inflammatory bowel disease. Horm Res Paediatr. 2015;83(1):45–54.

41. Beumont PJ, George GC, Pimstone BL, Vinik AI. Body weight and the pituitary response to hypothalamic releasing hormones in patients with anorexia nervosa. J Clin Endocrinol Metab. 1976;43(3):487–96.

42. Ballinger AB, Camacho-Hubner C, Croft NM. Growth failure and intestinal inflammation. QJM. 2001;94(3):121–5.

43. Frisch RE. Fatness, menarche, and female fertility. Perspect Biol Med. 1985;28(4):611–33.

44. Frisch RE, Gotz-Welbergen AV, McArthur JW, Albright T, Witschi J, Bullen B, et al. Delayed menarche and amenorrhea of college athletes in relation to age of onset of training. JAMA. 1981;246(14):1559–63.

45. Frisch RE, Wyshak G, Vincent L. Delayed menarche and amenorrhea in ballet dancers. N Engl J Med. 1980;303(1):17–9.

46. Dreizen S, Spirakis CN, Stone RE. A comparison of skeletal growth and maturation in undernourished and well-nourished girls before and after menarche. J Pediatr. 1967;70(2):256–63.

47. Dreizen S, Stone R. Human nutritive and growth failure. Postgrad Med; 1962;32(4):381–6.

48. Kelts DG, Grand RJ, Shen G, et al. Nutritional basis of growth failure in children and adolescents with Crohn's disease. Gastroenterology. 1979;76(4):720–7.

49. Kirschner BS, Voinchet O, Rosenberg IH. Growth retardation in inflammatory bowel disease. Gastroenterology. 1978;75(3):504–11.

50. Thomas AG, Taylor F, Miller V. Dietary intake and nutritional treatment in childhood Crohn's disease. J Pediatr Gastroenterol Nutr. 1993;17(1):75–81.

51. Burnham JM, Shults J, Semeao E, Foster B, Zemel BS, Stallings VA, et al. Whole body BMC in pediatric Crohn disease: independent effects of altered growth, maturation, and body composition. J Bone Miner Res. 2004;19(12):1961–8.

52. Kaplowitz P. Clinical characteristics of 104 children referred for evaluation of precocious puberty. J Clin Endocrinol Metab. 2004;89(8):3644–50.

53. Chong SK, Grossman A, Walker-Smith JA, et al. Endocrine dysfunction in children with Crohn's disease. J Pediatr Gastroenterol Nutr. 1984;3(4):529–34.

54. Farthing MJ, Campbell CA, Walker-Smith J, et al. Nocturnal growth hormone and gonadotrophin secretion in growth retarded children with Crohn's disease. Gut. 1981;22(11):933–8.

55. Gotlin RW, Dubois RS. Nyctohemeral growth hormone levels in children with growth retardation and inflammatory bowel disease. Gut. 1973;14(3):191–5.

56. Kirschner BS, Sutton MM. Somatomedin-C levels in growth-impaired children and adolescents with chronic inflammatory bowel disease. Gastroenterology. 1986;91(4):830–6.

57. Tenore A, Berman WF, Parks JS, et al. Basal and stimulated serum growth hormone concentrations in inflammatory bowel disease. J Clin Endocrinol Metab. 1977;44(4):622–8.

58. Corkins MR, Gohil AD, Fitzgerald JF. The insulin-like growth factor axis in children with inflammatory bowel disease. J Pediatr Gastroenterol Nutr. 2003;36(2):228–34.

59. Thomas AG, Holly JM, Taylor F, et al. Insulin like growth factor-I, insulin like growth factor binding protein-1, and insulin in childhood Crohn's disease. Gut. 1993;34(7):944–7.

60. Yakar S, Liu JL, Stannard B, Butler A, Accili D, Sauer B, et al. Normal growth and development in the absence of hepatic insulin-like growth factor I. Proc Natl Acad Sci U S A. 1999;96(13):7324–9.

61. Giovannucci E. Insulin, insulin-like growth factors and colon cancer: a review of the evidence. J Nutr. 2001;131(11 Suppl):3109S–20S.

62. Azooz OG, Farthing MJ, Savage MO, et al. Delayed puberty and response to testosterone in a rat model of colitis. Am J Physiol Regul Integr Comp Physiol. 2001;281(5):R1483–91.

63. DeBoer MD, Li Y. Puberty is delayed in male mice with dextran sodium sulfate colitis out of proportion to changes in food intake, body weight, and serum levels of leptin. Pediatr Res. 2011;69(1):34–9.

64. DeBoer MD, Li Y, Cohn S. Colitis causes delay in puberty in female mice out of proportion to changes in leptin and corticosterone. J Gastroenterol. 2010;45(3):277–84.

65. Wong SC, Macrae VE, McGrogan P, Ahmed SF. The role of pro-inflammatory cytokines in inflammatory bowel disease growth retardation. J Pediatr Gastroenterol Nutr. 2006;43(2):144–55.

66. Wang P, Li N, Li JS, Li WQ. The role of endotoxin, TNF-alpha, and IL-6 in inducing the state of growth hormone insensitivity. World J Gastroenterol. 2002;8(3):531–6.

67. Denson LA, Menon RK, Shaufl A, et al. TNF-alpha downregulates murine hepatic growth hormone receptor expression by inhibiting Sp1 and Sp3 binding. J Clin Invest. 2001;107(11):1451–8.

68. Theiss AL, Fruchtman S, Lund PK. Growth factors in inflammatory bowel disease: the actions and interactions of growth hormone and insulin-like growth factor-I. Inflamm Bowel Dis. 2004;10(6):871–80.

69. DeBoer MD, Steinman J, Li Y. Partial normalization of pubertal timing in female mice with DSS colitis treated with anti-TNF-alpha antibody. J Gastroenterol. 2012;47(6):647–54.

70. Nottelmann ED, Susman EJ, Inoff-Germain G, et al. Developmental processes in early adolescence: relationships between adolescent adjustment problems and chronologic age, pubertal stage, and puberty-related serum hormone levels. J Pediatr. 1987;110(3):473–80.

71. Mamula P, Markowitz JE, Baldassano RN. Inflammatory bowel disease in early childhood and adolescence: special considerations. Gastroenterol Clin N Am. 2003;32(3):967–995, viii.

72. Consten D, Bogerd J, Komen J, et al. Long-term cortisol treatment inhibits pubertal development in male common carp, Cyprinus carpio L. Biol Reprod. 2001;64(4):1063–71.

73. Alperstein G, Daum F, Fisher SE, Aiges H, Markowitz J, Becker J, et al. Linear growth following surgery in children and adolescents with Crohn's disease: relationship to pubertal status. J Pediatr Surg. 1985;20(2):129–33.

74. Allen DB, Julius JR, Breen TJ, Attie KM. Treatment of glucocorticoid-induced growth suppression with growth hormone. National Cooperative Growth Study. J Clin Endocrinol Metab. 1998;83(8):2824–9.

75. Heyman MB, Garnett EA, Wojcicki J, Gupta N, Davis C, Cohen SA, et al. Growth hormone treatment for growth failure in pediatric patients with Crohn's disease. J Pediatr. 2008;153(5):651–8, 658. e1–3.

76. Denson LA, Kim MO, Bezold R, Carey R, Osuntokun B, Nylund C, et al. A randomized controlled trial of growth hormone in active pediatric Crohn disease. J Pediatr Gastroenterol Nutr. 2010;51(2):130–9.

77. Mason A, Wong SC, McGrogan P, Ahmed SF. Effect of testosterone therapy for delayed growth and puberty in boys with inflammatory bowel disease. Horm Res Paediatr. 2011;75(1):8–13.

78. Ballinger AB, Savage MO, Sanderson IR. Delayed puberty associated with inflammatory bowel disease. Pediatr Res. 2003;53(2):205–10.

79. Finkelstein JS, Klibanski A, Neer RM. A longitudinal evaluation of bone mineral density in adult men with histories of delayed puberty. J Clin Endocrinol Metab. 1996;81(3):1152–5.

80. Pappa H, Thayu M, Sylvester F, Leonard M, Zemel B, Gordon C. Skeletal health of children and adolescents with inflammatory bowel disease. J Pediatr Gastroenterol Nutr. 2011;53(1):11–25.

81. Bernstein CN, Leslie WD, Taback SP. Bone density in a population-based cohort of premenopausal adult women with early onset inflammatory bowel disease. Am J Gastroenterol. 2003;98(5):1094–100.

82. Nakamoto JM, Mason PW, editors. Endocrinology: quest diagnostics manual. 5th ed. San Juan Capistrano: Quest Diagnostics Inc.; 2012.

Classification of Inflammatory Bowel Disease in Children

Mary E. Sherlock and Eric I. Benchimol

Introduction

Inflammatory bowel disease (IBD) comprises a group of disorders characterized by chronic inflammation of the gastrointestinal tract. In approximately 25% of patients, symptoms begin during childhood or adolescence [1]. Although the labels ulcerative colitis (UC) and Crohn's disease (CD) are applied to differentiate the two major phenotypic forms, it is recognized that both, and particularly CD, comprise a spectrum of chronic intestinal inflammation, with tremendous variation in phenotypic characteristics such as disease location and extent, behavior (inflammatory, stricturing, or penetrating), severity, responsiveness to therapies, and associations with extraintestinal manifestations [1, 2]. Between 5% and 10% of patients have colitis, but the clinical or histological features make it difficult to assign a diagnosis of either CD or UC, and a diagnosis of inflammatory bowel disease type unclassified (IBDU) is assigned [3, 4]. Rates of IBDU may be higher in very young children with one study describing this phenotype at diagnosis in 12 of 54 (22%) children presenting prior to 6 years of age [5]. Over time, the true type of IBD may become more evident, and the patient can be categorized as having either CD or UC. In the EUROKIDS registry, which prospectively collects data on newly diagnosed pediatric patients with IBD in Europe and Israel, the rate of IBDU decreased from 7.7% (265/3461) at diagnosis to 5.6% over the course of follow-up when diagnostic workup was complete [4].

The first question for the physician is whether or not the patient has inflammatory bowel disease or if the presentation represents an acute, self-limiting colitis, possibly secondary to infection, ischemia, or other pathology. Increasingly we are recognizing a primary immune dysfunction or deficiency as a cause for the "IBD" phenotype in very young children presenting with IBD-like symptoms, and physicians need to be aware of this patient group, as immunosuppressive medication may be harmful in this setting.

The next step, once a diagnosis of IBD has been confirmed using a combination of clinical, endoscopic, and radiologic assessments, is to apply a diagnostic label of CD, UC, or IBDU. Where possible, the physician should strive to assign a diagnosis of either CD or UC as this may have therapeutic implications, but is particularly important if surgical intervention is considered. In addition, assigning a diagnosis of IBDU could render a patient ineligible to participate in a research study, depending on inclusion criteria [2]. Deciding on the type of IBD can be challenging unless features which are diagnostic of CD are present, such as stenosing or penetrating disease behavior, macroscopic skip lesions or small intestinal disease, perianal disease, and granulomata on histology. In addition, there are a number of features such as relative or absolute rectal sparing, peri-appendiceal inflammation (the "cecal patch"), backwash ileitis, and the presence of upper GI tract findings that can make determining the type of IBD challenging. These features are discussed in more detail later in this chapter.

Within each diagnostic category, of either CD or UC, phenotypic classification systems aim to delineate disease location and behavior in CD and disease extent in UC. While classification systems were initially developed with adult patients in mind, more recently, a pediatric IBD classification system (the Paris modification of the Montreal classification, hereafter referred to as the Paris classification) was developed and is now in widespread use in both the clinical and research setting [6].

M.E. Sherlock, MB BCh BAO, PhD, FRCPC (✉)
Division of Gastroenterology and Nutrition, Hamilton Health Sciences, McMaster Children's Hospital,
Hamilton, ON L8S 4K1, Canada
e-mail: sherlom@mcmaster.ca

E.I. Benchimol
Division of Gastroenterology, Hepatology and Nutrition, Children's Hospital of Eastern Ontario, Department of Pediatrics and School of Epidemiology, Public Health and Preventive Medicine, University of Ottawa, 401 Smyth Road,
Ottawa, ON K1H 8L1, Canada
e-mail: ebenchimol@cheo.on.ca

© Springer International Publishing AG 2017
P. Mamula et al. (eds.), *Pediatric Inflammatory Bowel Disease*, DOI 10.1007/978-3-319-49215-5_15

In 2007, the North American Society for Pediatric Gastroenterology, Hepatology and Nutrition, led by Dr. Athos Bousvaros (author of the previous edition of this chapter), developed a detailed document that provided recommendations for assisting pediatric gastroenterologists in distinguishing CD from UC and provided detailed evidence-based directions in the grey areas. The authors of this chapter would like to direct readers to this publication as well as the Paris classification and the revised Porto criteria, all of which contributed to the drafting of this chapter [2, 6, 7].

The first part of the chapter will review various guideline documents, which aim to assist physicians when applying a phenotypic classification to pediatric patients with IBD. The second part of this chapter will describe the development and refinement of IBD phenotypic classifications.

Guideline Documents for Making the Diagnosis of Type of IBD in Pediatric Patients

A working group comprising pediatric gastroenterologists and pathologists, commissioned by the North American Society for Pediatric Gastroenterology, Hepatology and Nutrition (NASPGHAN) and the Crohn's and Colitis Foundation of America, following critical literature review, produced detailed guidelines for diagnosing and distinguishing CD from UC in pediatric patients [2]. The paper focused on areas of potential controversy when assigning a definitive diagnosis of UC, CD, or IBDU. Findings that can make it difficult to categorize the type of IBD include the presence of peri-appendiceal inflammation ("cecal patch"), backwash ileitis, rectal sparing, and upper GI tract inflammation.

Cecal Patch

A cecal patch, also known as peri-appendiceal inflammation, seen in association with left-sided ulcerative colitis, was identified in the 1950s [8]. The frequency of this finding is variable. Park, Loftus, and Yang reviewed the literature extensively on this topic and summarized reports published before 2012 [9]. The prevalence of the peri-appendiceal inflammation in colectomy specimens was found to be anywhere between 5% and 88%, but many of the specimens included in these retrospective studies had pan-colonic inflammation and therefore don't meet our current understanding of a cecal patch (inflammation around the peri-appendiceal orifice in association with UC which does not involve the entire colon and thus has normal intervening mucosa). Studies looking at endoscopic assessments describe this finding in 8–75%. However, the majority of studies reported peri-appendiceal inflammation to be present in

under 25% of cases [9]. A large prospective study of 279 adult patients described the presence of peri-appendiceal inflammation in 54 (19.4%) patients, 33 of whom had left-sided disease or proctitis [10]. The largest retrospective review of 379 colonoscopies described peri-appendiceal inflammation in 29 (7.9%) patients [11]. Based on available evidence, disease severity and progression do not appear to be influenced by the presence or absence of a cecal patch [12, 13]. The prevalence of a cecal patch in pediatric patients with UC is much lower than rates reported for adult patients. The EUROKIDS Registry assessed 643 pediatric patients with UC and found that only 2% met criteria for a cecal patch [14]. This likely reflects the fact that most pediatric patients with UC have pancolitis at presentation [3, 14, 15].

Backwash Ileitis

This is a nonspecific ileitis which can be seen in the setting of pancolitis. There are no deep ulcerations, cobblestones, or strictures, which may be seen in Crohn's ileitis. Inflammation is typically limited to the distal 10 cm of terminal ileum, and the macroscopic appearance may demonstrate erythema or granularity, or the inflammation may only be evident on histology [2]. The largest study in adult patients by Heuschen et al. [16] found that backwash ileitis was present in 107 of 476 (22%) patients undergoing colectomy for pancolitis in contrast to 0 of 114 patients with disease limited to the left side of the colon. The NASPGHAN working group recommended that the label of "histologic backwash ileitis" be assigned to those patients with a normal macroscopic appearance of the terminal ileum but with histologic features of inflammation and the term "endoscopic and histologic backwash ileitis" be assigned to those patients with macroscopic evidence of inflammation (erythema and granularity) in addition to the microscopic findings [2].

Haskell et al. [17] examined colectomy specimens from 200 patients with UC who underwent a colectomy. Ileal inflammation was noted in 34 (17%) of patients. The most common histologic finding (present in 62% of the patients) was neutrophilic cryptitis and/or crypt abscess formation without surface ulceration. Twelve percent of the patients showed surface ulceration. None of the patients with surface ulceration were subsequently diagnosed with CD after a mean follow-up of 48 months (range 26–102 months). Other features included regenerative crypt changes and villous atrophy in some patients. In the absence of cecal inflammation, a diagnosis of backwash ileitis should not be made, and a diagnosis of CD should be considered. In the Haskell study [17], the presence of backwash ileitis was not associated with an increase in complications, dysplasia, or carcinoma. Alexander et al. [18] reviewed outcomes of 151 young UC patients (mean age 18 years) undergoing ileoanal pouch anastomosis and found that 15% (16 of 109) of patients with a 5-year follow-up had evidence of backwash ileitis. This finding was not associated with increased pouch complications or with the subsequent development of Crohn's disease. In the EUROKIDS registry, endoscopic evaluation of the terminal ileum was available in 296 of 397 (75%) patients with UC. Macroscopic abnormalities in the terminal ileum were described in 10% of these patients [14].

Rectal Sparing

Absolute rectal sparing refers to normal macroscopic and microscopic findings in the rectum, while relative rectal sparing is said to be present when inflammation in the rectum is less severe than the remainder of the colon [2]. In the majority of patients, the presence of absolute rectal sparing will point a physician toward a diagnosis of CD or at least IBDU. However, there are a minority of UC patients who have relative rectal sparing. Glickman [19] compared mucosal biopsies from 73 pediatric and 38 adult patients newly diagnosed with UC. Among the pediatric group, relative rectal sparing was present in 23% of patients and absolute rectal sparing in 3% of patients, features which were not seen in the adult group [19]. Washington et al. [20] also examined rectal biopsy specimens from adult and pediatric patients with UC and found that children more frequently lacked classic histologic features and felt this may have been the result of shorter duration of inflammation in the pediatric group prior to diagnosis. In a small series of 30 pediatric patients with newly diagnosed UC, Rajwal et al. [21] found that 7% had macroscopic rectal sparing. The EUROKIDS registry described macroscopic rectal sparing in 28 of 553 (5%) UC patients. Rectal sparing was more common in younger patients (mean age of 9.9 years versus 11.8 years at diagnosis). The finding was also more prevalent in those with extensive (E3) or pancolitis (E4) than those with left-sided disease (6% versus 1%, $P = 0.04$). Rectal sparing was also more likely to be present in patients diagnosed earlier in their disease course [14].

Upper GI Tract Inflammation

Histologic inflammation of upper GI tract sites is very commonly found in both CD and UC [22]. The reported prevalence of upper GI tract disease in pediatric IBD patients is variable and may be related to the definitions used, with some centers reporting upper GI tract disease only when macroscopic disease is present, whereas other investigators consider upper GI tract disease to be present even when findings are only histologic. The EUROKIDS registry found that 18% of newly diagnosed pediatric CD patients had macroscopic evidence of gastric inflammation. Findings included

ulcers, erosions, aphthous lesions, and cobblestone mucosa [23]. Nonspecific macroscopic upper GI tract inflammation is present in up to 30–64% of CD patients [24, 25] and up to 50% of patients with UC [22, 26]. While deep ulceration and granulomas in the esophagus, stomach, or duodenum are suggestive of CD, the presence of nonspecific or microscopic inflammation in the upper GI tract should not preclude a diagnosis of UC if other features best fit this diagnosis.

The Porto Criteria and the Revised Porto Criteria

In 2005, the European Society for Pediatric Gastroenterology, Hepatology and Nutrition (ESPGHAN) working group, consisting of 23 pediatric gastroenterologists from 12 European countries, published the Porto criteria which outlined criteria for diagnosing IBD and made recommendations for diagnostic workup [27]. The group recommended that symptoms should be present for a minimum of 4 weeks or that episodes have occurred at least twice within a 6-month period. Typical presenting symptoms of IBD, which are discussed in greater detail in another chapter of this book, include abdominal pain, diarrhea, weight loss, extraintestinal manifestations, and growth failure, the latter being more prominent in Crohn's disease [25]. Other symptoms such as malaise, vague abdominal pain, unexplained anemia (in the absence of gastrointestinal symptoms), and delayed puberty may also be manifestations of IBD, and physicians should maintain an index of suspicion when investigating patients with these symptoms.

Upper endoscopy is always required in the diagnostic workup as up to 30% of children will have isolated upper gastrointestinal tract Crohn's disease [28–30]. While the original Porto criteria recommend small bowel imaging in the setting where the diagnosis of UC is not definite, we would suggest imaging of the small bowel in all cases. Imaging may consist of magnetic resonance enterography, computed tomography enterography, video capsule endoscopy (in the confirmed absence of strictures or narrowing of the small intestine), small bowel ultrasound, or small bowel follow-through x-ray with barium. Young children with IBD often present with extensive colitis, without skip areas, making it difficult to distinguish those with CD from those with UC [31, 32]. Therefore, the presence of macroscopic inflammation or ulceration of the esophagus or small bowel would support a diagnosis of CD, and not UC.

The Porto criteria were revised in 2014, using an extensive evidence-based and iterative approach to develop recommendations and an algorithm for the evaluation of a pediatric patient with suspected IBD [7]. The new criteria consist of 12 recommendations, incorporating the Paris modification of the Montreal classification (see below), the original Porto criteria, and consideration of fecal and serum biomarkers [7]. In addition, the group advocated for upper endoscopy for all patients with suspected IBD and the use of small bowel imaging unless the diagnosis favors typical UC. Typical UC consists of continuous inflammation extending proximally from the rectum, without small intestinal inflammation with the exception of backwash ileitis.

The revised Porto criteria [7] introduced the idea of typical and atypical UC as a new category for "type of IBD." Figure 15.1, from the Porto Group, provides an algorithm for assigning type of IBD, which considers atypical variants of UC. Five different "atypical UC" variants are presented:

1. The presence of macroscopic rectal sparing. The Paris classification [6] specifies that there must be at least microscopic inflammation in order to still consider a diagnosis of UC.
2. Disease may be patchy (histologically), early in the disease course when the duration of symptoms is short. Macroscopically the inflammation is continuous, but may

have relative rectal sparing. In addition, features of chronicity may be absent.
3. Cecal patch – features of left-sided UC and isolated inflammation in the cecum, usually peri-appendiceal, with normal intervening mucosa [9, 33, 34].
4. Involvement of the upper GI tract – up to half of all UC patients will have evidence of upper GI tract inflammation on histology [22]. The EUROKIDS registry described gastric erosions or small ulcers in 4.2% of pediatric UC patients [14]. The presence of focal active gastritis alone can be present in both UC and CD [35].
5. Transmural inflammation with or without deep ulcers may be present in acute severe UC. The ulcers may be fissuring or V-shaped and lymphoid aggregates may be absent. In reality, these patients would likely be given the diagnostic label "IBDU," but the disease may declare itself as UC over time.

The typical features of classic CD are described elsewhere in this book, but there would be no dispute on diagnostic

JPGN • Volume 58, Number 6, June 2014   *ESPGHAN Revised Porto Criteria for Diagnosis of IBD*

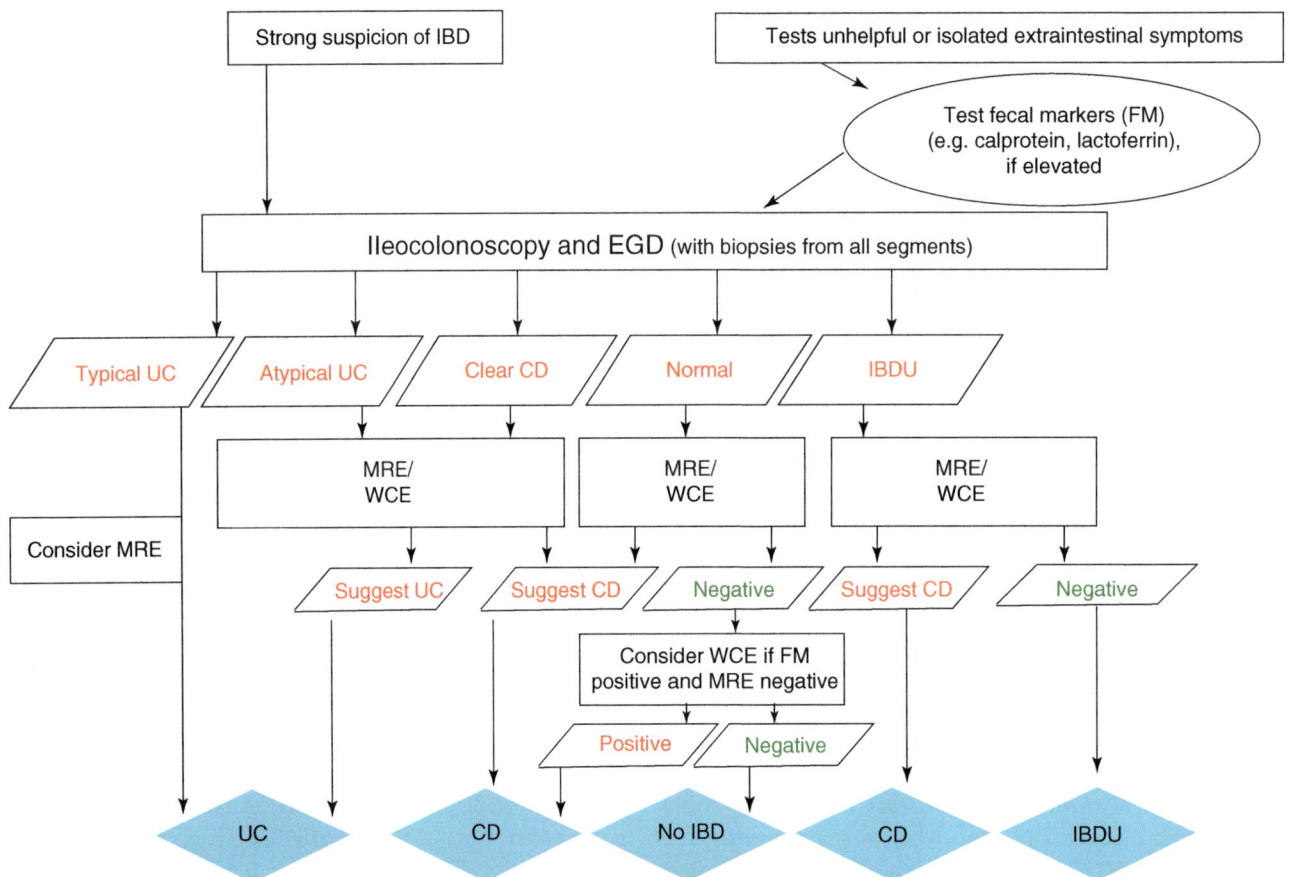

Fig. 15.1 Evaluation of child with suspected IBD. Atypical UC is a new IBD category consisting of 5 phenotypes and reflects a phenotype that should be treated as UC. IBD-U may be entertained as a tentative diagnosis after endoscopy and can be used as a final diagnosis after imaging and a full endoscopic workup. UC is divided into UC and atypical UC. *CD* Crohn's disease, *EGD* esophagogastroduodenoscopy, *FM* fecal marker, *IBD* inflammatory bowel disease, *MRE* magnetic resonance enterography, *UC* ulcerative colitis, *WCE* wireless capsule endoscopy (Reprinted from Levine et al. [7], Fig. 1, page 797, with permission)

classification for patients with cobblestoning of the small bowel mucosa, skip lesions, perianal disease (fistulae, abscesses, or large inflamed skin tags), and the presence of complicated disease behaviors such as stricturing or penetrating disease. Involvement of the small intestine with reliable interpretation of imaging would also point to a diagnosis of CD. However, particularly in young children, colonic involvement in CD may be continuous, making it difficult to distinguish from UC, and consideration for the diagnosis of IBDU should be applied. Figure 15.2, from the ESPGHAN revised Porto criteria, provides criteria to assist the treating physician when assigning the label of CD, UC, or IBDU.

Phenotypic Classification of IBD: A Historical Perspective

For decades, CD was considered a relatively homogeneous condition, without attempts to further subclassify the phenotype. In 1975, Farmer et al. [36] were among the first to recognize that CD is not a homogeneous entity, hypothesizing that sites of inflammation influenced outcomes and disease behavior. The group categorized CD into (1) ileocolonic, (2) small intestinal, (3) isolated colonic, and (4) isolated anorectal disease. The authors attempted to correlate clinical symptoms at presentation with disease location in their clinical cohort and described the evolution of disease over time including the development of rectal and internal intestinal fistulae, growth impairment, intestinal obstruction, and need for surgery. By using categories of disease location, the authors provide some of the earliest data on the potential relationship between phenotype and clinical outcomes and recognized that such correlations might facilitate therapeutic decisions for these patients.

Further consideration toward a phenotypic classification of CD came from Greenstein et al. [37] who described two disease behavior patterns, perforating and non-perforating, using a cohort of 770 patients undergoing surgery. Site of inflammation (categorized as ileitis, colitis, or ileocolitis) was associated with type of surgery with patients with ileal

---

JPGN • Volume 58, Number 6, June 2014   *ESPGHAN Revised Porto Criteria for Diagnosis of IBD*

TABLE 3. Diagnostic features in a child with untreated colitis phenotype at diagnosis

Likelihood of occurring in UC	Feature	Diagnostic approach
Class 1: Nonexistent	Well-formed granulomas anywhere in the GI tract, remote from ruptured crypt	Diagnose as CD
	Deep serpentine ulcerations, cobblestoning or stenosis anywhere in the SB or UGI tract	
	Fistulizing disease (internal or perianal)	
	Any ileal inflammation in the presence of normal cecum (ie, incompatible with backwash ileitis)	
	Thickened jejunal or ileal bowel loops or other evidence of significant SB inflammation (more than a few scattered erosions) not compatible with backwash ileitis*	
	Macroscopically and microscopically normal appearing skip lesions in untreated IBD (except with macroscopic rectal sparing and cecal patch)	
	Large inflamed perianal skin tags	
Class 2: Rare with UC (<5%)	Combined (macroscopic and microscopic) rectal sparing, all other features are consistent with UC	Diagnose as IBD-U, if at least 1 class 2 feature exists**
	Significant growth delay (height velocity <2 SDS), not explained by other causes	
	Transmural inflammation in the absence of severe colitis, all other features are consistent with UC	
	Duodenal or esophageal ulcers, not explained by other causes (eg, *Helicobacter pylori*, NSAIDs and celiac disease)	
	Multiple aphthous ulcerations in the stomach, not explained by other causes (eg, *H pylori* and NSAIDs)	
	Positive ASCA in the presence of negative pANCA	
Class 3: Uncommon (~5%–10%)	Reverse gradient of mucosal inflammation (proximal >distal (except rectal sparing))	Diagnose as IBD-U, if at least 2–3 feature exists
	Severe scalloping of the stomach or duodenum, not explained by other causes (eg, celiac disease and *H pylori*)	
	Focal chronic duodenitis on multiple biopsies or marked scalloping of the duodenum, not explained by other causes (eg, celiac disease and *H pylori*)	
	Focal active colitis on histology in more than 1 biopsy from macroscopically inflamed site	
	Non-bloody diarrhea	
	Aphthous ulceratons in the colon or UGI tract	

ASCA = anti-*Saccharomyces cerevisiae* antibody; GI = gastrointestinal; IBD = inflammatory bowel disease; NSAID = nonsteroidal anti-inflammatory drug; pANCA = perinuclear antineutrophil cytoplasmic antibody; SB = small bowel; SDS = standard deviation score; UC = ulcerative colitis.
* After full diagnostic workup including SB imaging.
** The likelihood of CD increases with increasing number of class 2 features.

Fig. 15.2 Diagnostic characteristics associated with different types of IBD (Reprinted from Levine et al. [7], Table 3, page 799, with permission)

disease more likely to require surgery for obstructive symptoms in comparison with ileocolonic disease where fistulizing disease was the main surgical indication.

These observations that disease location and behavior influence outcomes became the basis of the more rigorously developed Vienna, Montreal and Paris classifications for IBD [6, 38, 39].

The Vienna Classification

Between 1996 and 1998, an international working group was established to develop and validate a phenotypic classification for CD [38]. The final included categories were age at diagnosis (<40 or ≥40 years), disease location (terminal ileum, colonic, ileocolonic, or involvement of the upper GI tract), and disease behavior (non-stricturing non-penetrating, stricturing, or penetrating). While great efforts were made to develop a reproducible and validated phenotypic classification, there were some limitations. The Vienna classification cannot distinguish disease location when disease is present in both the upper GI tract and other intestinal regions or when it occurs in isolation. Likewise, perianal disease is not considered a separate category; rather it is categorized as "perforating" disease behavior making it impossible to distinguish whether a patient has perianal disease, internal intestinal fistulizing disease, or both.

The Montreal Classification

The Montreal classification was developed to provide a uniform system of designating subgroups of patients with IBD, with the aim of facilitating multicenter genotype-phenotype correlation studies. It is the most commonly used classification for adult patients. Unlike the Vienna classification and its predecessors, which focused on CD classification, the Montreal classification includes a phenotypic classification for UC and makes recommendations for assigning the diagnostic label of "inflammatory bowel disease-type unclassified" (IBDU) [39].

For CD, modifications to the Vienna classification included (1) an additional category to classify children diagnosed at ≤16 years of age, (2) allow for upper GI tract disease to be classified independently of ileocolonic and colonic involvement, and (3) classify perianal disease as a category independent of the "penetrating disease behavior" category.

The group proposed that the maximal disease extent prior to first resection in those undergoing surgery be used when considering the variable "disease location." Given the propensity for disease behavior to evolve over time [40], the recommendation of the working group is to wait a minimum of 5 years before definitively assigning a disease behavior for the non-stricturing, non-penetrating category, particularly when data are used as part of research studies.

For UC, the group proposed that patients be classified according to maximal extent of inflammation at any time during follow-up. Maximal disease extent is E3, which denotes any disease extending proximal to the splenic flexure.

When a principal diagnosis of UC or CD cannot be established, the group recommends that the term colonic "IBD-type unclassified (IBDU)" be assigned and the term "indeterminate colitis" be reserved for use only after colectomy has been performed, when features of both CD and UC coexist.

The Paris Modification of the Montreal Classification for Pediatric IBD

In 2009 an international group of pediatric IBD experts took on the task of modifying the Montreal classification, to capture aspects of disease phenotype that are pertinent to pediatric patients. Following an extensive review of the literature, with attention focused on pediatric data, where available, and including recommendations from expert opinion and narrative review, the Paris classification of pediatric inflammatory bowel disease was published in 2011 [6]. The committee also reviewed, and was in agreement with, the 2007 paper put forward by NASPGHAN and the Crohn's and Colitis Foundation of America (CCFA), which provided recommendations for differentiating UC from CD [2].

Novel Features of the Paris Classification

1. A new age category, allowing differentiation between patients presenting prior to or after their 10th birthday, was introduced. The new classification proposed that children presenting prior to 10 years of age are designated to the age category A1a and those presenting from 10 to 17 years of age be assigned to the category A1b. Disease location in CD at diagnosis appears to be different in these two age categories with the younger group being more likely to have isolated colonic disease rather than ileal involvement. Ileal disease (whether isolated or in conjunction with disease in other locations) is more common in the older age group [5, 15, 41, 42]. For ulcerative colitis, the Pediatric Inflammatory Bowel Disease Collaborative Research Registry found the youngest patients, diagnosed aged 1–5 had greater use of mesalamine and thiopurines [43]. A Canadian population-based study found lower colectomy rates in children diagnosed under 10 years of age [44].

2. The Paris group recognized that the Montreal classification did not optimally describe disease location, particularly regarding the upper GI tract category (L4), which is

unable to distinguish between disease of the small intestine and disease proximal to the ligament of Treitz. The Paris classification recommends that the presence of upper GI tract disease only be assigned in the presence of macroscopic disease as there is no literature to suggest that histologic involvement alone influences disease progression or phenotypic classification over time. The presence of mucosal erythema or granularity is not sufficient to be considered as macroscopic disease. The Paris group subdivided the L4 Montreal category for upper GI tract disease into L4a (denoting disease proximal to the ligament of Treitz) and L4b (denoting disease distal to the ligament of Treitz).

3. Disease behavior is inflammatory (B1) at diagnosis for the majority of patients, but may evolve into a more complicated phenotype, stricturing (B2), or penetrating (B3) over time. Some patients have a complicated disease phenotype at presentation. The Paris classification also allows capture of patients who have both concomitant stricturing and penetrating behavior (B2B3 category).

4. Since the majority of pediatric patients with UC have extensive disease at presentation (in comparison to adult patients, many of whom have less extensive disease), the Paris classification includes an additional category for disease extension proximal to the hepatic flexure (E4) [14, 15, 42, 45].

5. Regarding UC disease behavior, the Pediatric Ulcerative Colitis Activity Index (PUCAI) [46] is used to determine whether or not a patient has ever had severe disease (PUCAI ≥ 65) as studies have found that colectomy rates are higher in patients who have had severe disease [47].

6. Pertinent to pediatric patients is the ability to capture growth impairment when classifying disease [48, 49]. A growth category was introduced which allows normal growth at diagnosis and over the course of follow-up (G0) or impaired linear growth, using height velocity Z-scores (G1) at any time point, to be captured. Z-scores should be adjusted for age (or bone age when delayed) and sex.

The Paris group described a list of clinical features, which when present do not support a diagnosis of UC:

1. Perianal disease
2. Microscopic skip lesions
3. Stenosis, cobblestoned mucosa, and linear ileal ulcers (even in the setting of pancolitis)
4. Macroscopic inflammation of the ileum in the absence of cecal inflammation
5. Presence of a well-formed granuloma at a site that is not adjacent to a ruptured crypt
6. Absolute rectal sparing (no macroscopic or histologic features of inflammation)

The group advised that the finding of a few small ulcers in the small intestine during capsule endoscopy should not preclude the diagnosis of UC (if other features point to this diagnosis) since these may be nonspecific and are sometimes seen in healthy people.

Evolution of Disease Phenotype

Disease phenotype in both adult and pediatric patents is not static [15, 40, 50, 51]. This represents a challenge when phenotyping both adult and pediatric patients. When the Montreal classification was proposed, the authors recommended waiting for 5 years, or until the time of surgery (whichever was sooner), before assigning a disease behavior. However, in reality, increasingly pediatric patients are being entered into prospective registries requiring a phenotypic classification at diagnosis be assigned. It is important that such registries have the ability to capture the evolution of disease phenotype such as disease extension in UC as well as CD, in addition to change in behavior to a more complicated phenotype (stricturing and/or penetrating) in CD. It is important to remember that IBD phenotype may evolve over time particularly in children [15, 42, 52, 53]. A population-based study determined that the diagnosis (CD, UC, or IBDU) of children <6 years changed in 16.2% of cases, compared with 18.1% of children diagnosed 6–10 years, and 13.8% of children diagnosed ≥10 years ($P = 0.007$) [44]. In addition, adult CD studies have demonstrated a change from non-stricturing to stricturing disease in 27% and penetrating disease in 28% [40]. In UC, other population-based studies demonstrated that more than half of the patients with initial proctosigmoiditis eventually extended more proximally, but 75% of extensive cases regressed [54].

A summary of the Paris classification of pediatric IBD is represented in Fig. 15.3.

Future Directions

Classification of IBD has progressed well beyond the classic categories of CD, UC, or indeterminate colitis. The advent of the Montreal classification and the subsequent Paris modification for pediatric IBD have allowed for granularity in the description of IBD phenotype for both clinical and research purposes. While these classification systems have been extremely valuable, disease location and severity do not tell the full story of IBD. Some have suggested adding histology to the macroscopic description of the Paris modification to improve granularity and descriptive capability [55]. In addition, with advances in characterization of the role of gene, environment, and microbiome interactions and their effect on disease phenotype, we anticipate that future classification

Crohn's disease

Age at Diagnosis	Location
A1a < 10 years	L1 distal 1/3 ileum ± limited cecal disease
A1b 10 - <17 years	L2 colonic
A2 17 - 40 years	L3 ileocolonic
A3 > 40 years	L4a* upper GI disease proximal to Ligament of Treitz
	L4b* upper GI disease distal to Ligament of Treitz but
	proximal to distal 1/3 ileum
Behaviour	**Growth**
B1 Non-stricturing, non-penetrating	G0: No evidence of growth delay at diagnosis and subsequently
B2 Stricturing	G1: Growth delay at any time (at diagnosis or over the course of follow-up)
B3 Penetrating	
B2B3 Stricturing **and** penetrating	
p perianal disease modifier	

Footnotes
* L4a and L4b can coexist with L1, L2 or L3 or can occur in isolation
§ perianal disease can coexist with any behaviour, B1, B2, B3, B2B3
Perianal disease is present if there are fistulae, abscesses or anal canal ulcers. Skin tags do not form
part of the definition of perianal disease

Ulcerative Colitis

Disease Extent	Definition
E1 Ulcerative Proctitis	Disease limited to the rectum
E2 Left-sided Disease	Disease distal to the splenic flexure
E3 Extensive disease	Disease proximal to the splenic flexure but not extending proximal to the hepatic flexure
E4 Pancolitis	Disease extends proximal to the hepatic flexure
Severity	**Definition**
S0	Never severe (PUCAI score never ≥ 65)
S1	Ever Severe (PUCAI score ≥ 65 at least once during course of follow-up)

Fig. 15.3 Paris classification of inflammatory bowel disease (Adapted from Levine et al. [6])

systems will incorporate new disease location categories, histology findings, protein expression characteristics, and other factors. In the era of personalized medicine, treatment choice will depend on many more factors than those described in current classification systems. We anticipate that definition of the inflammatory bowel diseases will consist of a continuum of categories resulting in even more power to describe the disease characteristics of a child with IBD.

Acknowledgments We are grateful to Dr. Athos Bousvaros who authored the first edition of this chapter and allowed its use as the basis for this new edition. Eric Benchimol is supported by a New Investigator Award from the Canadian Institutes of Health Research, Crohn's and Colitis Canada, and the Canadian Association of Gastroenterology.

References

1. Griffiths AM. Specificities of inflammatory bowel disease in childhood. Best Pract Res Clin Gastroenterol. 2004;18:509–23. doi:10.1016/j.bpg.2004.01.002.

2. North American Society for Pediatric Gastroenterology, Hepatology, and Nutrition; Colitis Foundation of America, Bousvaros A, Antonioli DA, Colletti RB, Dubinsky MC, Glickman JN, Gold BD, Griffiths AM, Jevon GP, Higuchi LM, Hyams JS, Kirschner BS, Kugathasan S, Baldassano RN, Russo PA. Differentiating ulcerative colitis from Crohn disease in children and young adults: report of a working group of the North American Society for Pediatric Gastroenterology, Hepatology, and Nutrition and the Crohn's and Colitis Foundation of America. J Pediatr Gastroenterol Nutr. 2007;44:653–74. doi:10.1097/MPG.0b013e31805563f3.

3. Muller KE, Lakatos PL, Arato A, Kovacs JB, Varkonyi A, Szucs D, Szakos E, Solyom E, Kovacs M, Polgar M, Nemes E, Guthy I, Tokodi I, Toth G, Horvath A, Tarnok A, Csoszanszki N, Balogh M, Vass N, Bodi P, Dezsofi A, Gardos L, Micskey E, Papp M, Cseh A, Szabo D, Voros P, Veres G, Hungarian IBDRG. Incidence, Paris classification, and follow-up in a nationwide incident cohort of pediatric patients with inflammatory bowel disease. J Pediatr Gastroenterol Nutr. 2013;57:576–82. doi:10.1097/MPG.0b013e31829f7d8c.

4. Winter DA, Karolewska-Bochenek K, Lazowska-Przeorek I, Lionetti P, Mearin ML, Chong SK, Roma-Giannikou E, Maly J, Kolho KL, Shaoul R, Staiano A, Damen GM, de Meij T, Hendriks D, George EK, Turner D, Escher JC. Pediatric IBD-unclassified is less common than previously reported; results of an 8-year audit of the EUROKIDS registry. Inflamm Bowel Dis. 2015;21:2145–53. doi:10.1097/MIB.0000000000000483.

5. Aloi M, Lionetti P, Barabino A, Guariso G, Costa S, Fontana M, Romano C, Lombardi G, Miele E, Alvisi P, Diaferia P, Baldi M, Romagnoli V, Gasparetto M, Di Paola M, Muraca M, Pellegrino S, Cucchiara S, Martelossi S, SIGENP IBD Group. Phenotype and disease course of early-onset pediatric inflammatory bowel disease. Inflamm Bowel Dis. 2014;20:597–605. doi:10.1097/01.MIB.0000442921.77945.09.

6. Levine A, Griffiths A, Markowitz J, Wilson DC, Turner D, Russell RK, Fell J, Ruemmele FM, Walters T, Sherlock M, Dubinsky M, Hyams JS. Pediatric modification of the Montreal classification for inflammatory bowel disease: the Paris classification. Inflamm Bowel Dis. 2011;17(6):1314–21. doi:10.1002/ibd.21493.

7. Levine A, Koletzko S, Turner D, Escher JC, Cucchiara S, de Ridder L, Kolho KL, Veres G, Russell RK, Paerregaard A, Buderus S, Greer ML, Dias JA, Veereman-Wauters G, Lionetti P, Sladek M, Martin de Carpi J, Staiano A, Ruemmele FM, Wilson

DC, European Society of Pediatric Gastroenterology, Hepatology, and Nutrition. ESPGHAN revised porto criteria for the diagnosis of inflammatory bowel disease in children and adolescents. J Pediatr Gastroenterol Nutr. 2014;58(6):795–806. doi:10.1097/MPG.0000000000000239.

8. Lumb G, Protheroe RH. Ulcerative colitis; a pathologic study of 152 surgical specimens. Gastroenterology. 1958;34:381–407.

9. Park SH, Loftus Jr EV, Yang SK. Appendiceal skip inflammation and ulcerative colitis. Dig Dis Sci. 2014;59:2050–7. doi:10.1007/s10620-014-3129-z.

10. Yamagishi N, Iizuka B, Nakamura T, Suzuki S, Hayashi N. Clinical and colonoscopic investigation of skipped periappendiceal lesions in ulcerative colitis. Scand J Gastroenterol. 2002;37:177–82.

11. Rubin DT, Rothe JA. The peri-appendiceal red patch in ulcerative colitis: review of the University of Chicago experience. Dig Dis Sci. 2010;55:3495–501. doi:10.1007/s10620-010-1424-x.

12. Byeon JS, Yang SK, Myung SJ, Pyo SI, Park HJ, Kim YM, Lee YJ, Hong SS, Kim KJ, Lee GH, Jung HY, Hong WS, Kim JH, Min YI. Clinical course of distal ulcerative colitis in relation to appendiceal orifice inflammation status. Inflamm Bowel Dis. 2005;11:366–71.

13. Naves JE, Lorenzo-Zuniga V, Marin L, Manosa M, Oller B, Moreno V, Zabana Y, Boix J, Cabre E, Domenech E. Long-term outcome of patients with distal ulcerative colitis and inflammation of the appendiceal orifice. J Gastrointestin Liver Dis. 2011;20:355–8.

14. Levine A, de Bie CI, Turner D, Cucchiara S, Sladek M, Murphy MS, Escher JC, EUROKIDS Porto IBD Working Group of ESPGHAN. Atypical disease phenotypes in pediatric ulcerative colitis: 5-year analyses of the EUROKIDS Registry. Inflamm Bowel Dis. 2013;19:370–7. doi:10.1002/ibd.23013.

15. Van Limbergen J, Russell RK, Drummond HE, Aldhous MC, Round NK, Nimmo ER, Smith L, Gillett PM, McGrogan P, Weaver LT, Bisset WM, Mahdi G, Arnott ID, Satsangi J, Wilson DC. Definition of phenotypic characteristics of childhood-onset inflammatory bowel disease. Gastroenterology. 2008;135:1114–22. doi:10.1053/j.gastro.2008.06.081.

16. Heuschen UA, Hinz U, Allemeyer EH, Stern J, Lucas M, Autschbach F, Herfarth C, Heuschen G. Backwash ileitis is strongly associated with colorectal carcinoma in ulcerative colitis. Gastroenterology. 2001;120:841–7.

17. Haskell H, Andrews Jr CW, Reddy SI, Dendrinos K, Farraye FA, Stucchi AF, Becker JM, Odze RD. Pathologic features and clinical significance of "backwash" ileitis in ulcerative colitis. Am J Surg Pathol. 2005;29:1472–81.

18. Alexander F, Sarigol S, DiFiore J, Stallion A, Cotman K, Clark H, Lydzinski B, Fazio V. Fate of the pouch in 151 pediatric patients after ileal pouch anal anastomosis. J Pediatr Surg. 2003;38:78–82. doi:10.1053/jpsu.2003.50015.

19. Glickman JN, Bousvaros A, Farraye FA, Zholudev A, Friedman S, Wang HH, Leichtner AM, Odze RD. Pediatric patients with untreated ulcerative colitis may present initially with unusual morphologic findings. Am J Surg Pathol. 2004;28:190–7.

20. Washington K, Greenson JK, Montgomery E, Shyr Y, Crissinger KD, Polk DB, Barnard J, Lauwers GY. Histopathology of ulcerative colitis in initial rectal biopsy in children. Am J Surg Pathol. 2002;26:1441–9.

21. Rajwal SR, Puntis JW, McClean P, Davison SM, Newell SJ, Sugarman I, Stringer MD. Endoscopic rectal sparing in children with untreated ulcerative colitis. J Pediatr Gastroenterol Nutr. 2004;38:66–9.

22. Tobin JM, Sinha B, Ramani P, Saleh AR, Murphy MS. Upper gastrointestinal mucosal disease in pediatric Crohn disease and ulcerative colitis: a blinded, controlled study. J Pediatr Gastroenterol Nutr. 2001;32:443–8.

23. de Bie CI, Paerregaard A, Kolacek S, Ruemmele FM, Koletzko S, Fell JM, Escher JC, EUROKIDS Porto IBD Working Group of ESPGHAN. Disease phenotype at diagnosis in pediatric Crohn's

disease: 5-year analyses of the EUROKIDS Registry. Inflamm Bowel Dis. 2013;19:378–85. doi:10.1002/ibd.23008.

24. Lenaerts C, Roy CC, Vaillancourt M, Weber AM, Morin CL, Seidman E. High incidence of upper gastrointestinal tract involvement in children with Crohn disease. Pediatrics. 1989;83:777–81.

25. Sawczenko A, Sandhu BK. Presenting features of inflammatory bowel disease in Great Britain and Ireland. Arch Dis Child. 2003;88:995–1000.

26. Ruuska T, Vaajalahti P, Arajarvi P, Maki M. Prospective evaluation of upper gastrointestinal mucosal lesions in children with ulcerative colitis and Crohn's disease. J Pediatr Gastroenterol Nutr. 1994;19:181–6.

27. Inflammatory bowel disease in children and adolescents: recommendations for diagnosis–the Portocriteria. IBD Working Group of the European Society for Paediatric Gastroenterology, Hepatology and Nutrition. J Pediatr Gastroenterol Nutr. 2005;41(1):1–7.

28. Abdullah BA, Gupta SK, Croffie JM, Pfefferkorn MD, Molleston JP, Corkins MR, Fitzgerald JF. The role of esophagogastroduodenoscopy in the initial evaluation of childhood inflammatory bowel disease: a 7-year study. J Pediatr Gastroenterol Nutr. 2002;35:636–40.

29. Kovacs M, Muller KE, Arato A, Lakatos PL, Kovacs JB, Varkonyi A, Solyom E, Polgar M, Nemes E, Guthy I, Tokodi I, Toth G, Horvath A, Tarnok A, Tomsits E, Csoszanszky N, Balogh M, Vass N, Bodi P, Dezsofi A, Gardos L, Micskey E, Papp M, Szucs D, Cseh A, Molnar K, Szabo D, Veres G, Hungarian IBDRG. Diagnostic yield of upper endoscopy in paediatric patients with Crohn's disease and ulcerative colitis. Subanalysis of the HUPIR registry. J Crohns Colitis. 2012;6:86–94. doi:10.1016/j.crohns.2011.07.008.

30. Turner D, Griffiths AM. Esophageal, gastric, and duodenal manifestations of IBD and the role of upper endoscopy in IBD diagnosis. Curr Gastroenterol Rep. 2009;11:234–7.

31. Prenzel F, Uhlig HH. Frequency of indeterminate colitis in children and adults with IBD - a metaanalysis. J Crohns Colitis. 2009;3:277–81. doi:10.1016/j.crohns.2009.07.001.

32. Uhlig HH, Schwerd T, Koletzko S, Shah N, Kammermeier J, Elkadri A, Ouahed J, Wilson DC, Travis SP, Turner D, Klein C, Snapper SB, Muise AM, COLORS in IBD Study Group and NEOPICS. The diagnostic approach to monogenic very early onset inflammatory bowel disease. Gastroenterology. 2014;147:990–1007.e3. doi:10.1053/j.gastro.2014.07.023.

33. Dendrinos K, Cerda S, Farraye FA (2008) The "cecal patch" in patients with ulcerative colitis. Gastrointest Endosc 68: 1006–7; discussion 1007. doi: 10.1016/j.gie.2008.04.003

34. Paine ER. Colonoscopic evaluation in ulcerative colitis. Gastroenterol Rep (Oxf). 2014;2:161–8. doi:10.1093/gastro/gou028.

35. Xin W, Greenson JK. The clinical significance of focally enhanced gastritis. Am J Surg Pathol. 2004;28:1347–51.

36. Farmer RG, Hawk WA, Turnbull Jr RB. Clinical patterns in Crohn's disease: a statistical study of 615 cases. Gastroenterology. 1975;68:627–35.

37. Greenstein AJ, Lachman P, Sachar DB, Springhorn J, Heimann T, Janowitz HD, Aufses Jr AH. Perforating and non-perforating indications for repeated operations in Crohn's disease: evidence for two clinical forms. Gut. 1988;29:588–92.

38. Gasche C, Scholmerich J, Brynskov J, D'Haens G, Hanauer SB, Irvine EJ, Jewell DP, Rachmilewitz D, Sachar DB, Sandborn WJ, Sutherland LR. A simple classification of Crohn's disease: report of the Working Party for the World Congresses of Gastroenterology, Vienna 1998. Inflamm Bowel Dis. 2000;6:8–15.

39. Silverberg MS, Satsangi J, Ahmad T, Arnott ID, Bernstein CN, Brant SR, Caprilli R, Colombel JF, Gasche C, Geboes K, Jewell DP, Karban A, Loftus Jr EV, Pena AS, Riddell RH, Sachar DB,

Schreiber S, Steinhart AH, Targan SR, Vermeire S, Warren BF. Toward an integrated clinical, molecular and serological classification of inflammatory bowel disease: Report of a Working Party of the 2005 Montreal World Congress of Gastroenterology. Can J Gastroenterol. 2005;19 Suppl A:5–36.

40. Louis E, Collard A, Oger AF, Degroote E, Aboul Nasr El Yafi FA, Belaiche J. Behaviour of Crohn's disease according to the Vienna classification: changing pattern over the course of the disease. Gut. 2001;49:777–82.

41. Levine A, Kugathasan S, Annese V, Biank V, Leshinsky-Silver E, Davidovich O, Kimmel G, Shamir R, Palmieri O, Karban A, Broeckel U, Cucchiara S. Pediatric onset Crohn's colitis is characterized by genotype-dependent age-related susceptibility. Inflamm Bowel Dis. 2007;13:1509–15. doi:10.1002/ibd.20244.

42. Vernier-Massouille G, Balde M, Salleron J, Turck D, Dupas JL, Mouterde O, Merle V, Salomez JL, Branche J, Marti R, Lerebours E, Cortot A, Gower-Rousseau C, Colombel JF. Natural history of pediatric Crohn's disease: a population-based cohort study. Gastroenterology. 2008;135:1106–13. doi:10.1053/j.gastro.2008.06.079.

43. Oliva-Hemker M, Hutfless S, Al Kazzi ES, Lerer T, Mack D, LeLeiko N, Griffiths A, Cabrera J, Otley A, Rick J, Bousvaros A, Rosh J, Grossman A, Saeed S, Kay M, Carvalho R, Keljo D, Pfefferkorn M, Faubion W Jr, Kappelman M, Sudel B, Schaefer ME, Markowitz J, Hyams JS. Clinical Presentation and Five-Year Therapeutic Management of Very Early-Onset Inflammatory Bowel Disease in a Large North American Cohort. J Pediatr. 2015;167(3):527–32.e1–3. doi:10.1016/j.jpeds.2015.04.045. Epub 2015 May 15.

44. Benchimol EI, Mack DR, Nguyen GC, Snapper SB, Li W, Mojaverian N, Quach P, Muise AM (2014) Incidence, outcomes, and health services burden of very early onset inflammatory bowel disease. Gastroenterology 147: 803–813.e7; quiz e14–5. doi: 10.1053/j.gastro.2014.06.023

45. Romberg-Camps MJ, Dagnelie PC, Kester AD, Hesselink-van de Kruijs MA, Cilissen M, Engels LG, Van Deursen C, Hameeteman WH, Wolters FL, Russel MG, Stockbrugger RW. Influence of phenotype at diagnosis and of other potential prognostic factors on the course of inflammatory bowel disease. Am J Gastroenterol. 2009;104:371–83. doi:10.1038/ajg.2008.38.

46. Turner D, Otley AR, Mack D, Hyams J, de Bruijne J, Uusoue K, Walters TD, Zachos M, Mamula P, Beaton DE, Steinhart AH, Griffiths AM. Development, validation, and evaluation of a pediatric ulcerative colitis activity index: a prospective multicenter study. Gastroenterology. 2007;133:423–32. doi:10.1053/j.gastro.2007.05.029.

47. Turner D, Mack D, Leleiko N, Walters TD, Uusoue K, Leach ST, Day AS, Crandall W, Silverberg MS, Markowitz J, Otley AR, Keljo D, Mamula P, Kugathasan S, Hyams J, Griffiths AM (2010) Severe pediatric ulcerative colitis: a prospective multicenter study of outcomes and predictors of response. Gastroenterology 138: 2282–2291. doi: S0016–5085(10)00313–6 [pii]. 10.1053/j.gastro.2010.02.047 [doi]

48. Pfefferkorn M, Burke G, Griffiths A, Markowitz J, Rosh J, Mack D, Otley A, Kugathasan S, Evans J, Bousvaros A, Moyer MS, Wyllie R, Oliva-Hemker M, Carvalho R, Crandall W, Keljo D, Walters TD, LeLeiko N, Hyams J. Growth abnormalities persist in newly diagnosed children with crohn disease despite current treatment paradigms. J Pediatr Gastroenterol Nutr. 2009;48:168–74. doi:10.1097/MPG.0b013e318175ca7f.

49. Walters TD, Griffiths AM. Mechanisms of growth impairment in pediatric Crohn's disease. Nat Rev Gastroenterol Hepatol. 2009;6:513–23. doi:10.1038/nrgastro.2009.124.

50. Cosnes J, Cattan S, Blain A, Beaugerie L, Carbonnel F, Parc R, Gendre JP. Long-term evolution of disease behavior of Crohn's disease. Inflamm Bowel Dis. 2002;8:244–50.

51. Papi C, Festa V, Fagnani C, Stazi A, Antonelli G, Moretti A, Koch M, Capurso L. Evolution of clinical behaviour in Crohn's disease: predictive factors of penetrating complications. Dig Liver Dis. 2005;37:247–53. doi:10.1016/j.dld.2004.10.012.

52. Gupta N, Bostrom AG, Kirschner BS, Cohen SA, Abramson O, Ferry GD, Gold BD, Winter HS, Baldassano RN, Smith T, Heyman MB (2008) Presentation and disease course in early- compared to later-onset pediatric Crohn's disease. Am J Gastroenterol 103: 2092–2098. doi: AJG2000 [pii]. 10.1111/j.1572-0241.2008.02000.x [doi]

53. Pigneur B, Seksik P, Viola S, Viala J, Beaugerie L, Girardet JP, Ruemmele FM, Cosnes J. Natural history of Crohn's disease: comparison between childhood- and adult-onset disease. Inflamm Bowel Dis. 2010;16:953–61. doi:10.1002/ibd.21152.

54. Langholz E, Munkholm P, Davidsen M, Nielsen OH, Binder V. Changes in extent of ulcerative colitis: a study on the course and prognostic factors. Scand J Gastroenterol. 1996; 31:260–6.

55. Fernandes MA, Verstraete SG, Garnett EA, Heyman MB. Addition of histology to the Paris classification of pediatric Crohn disease Alters classification of disease location. J Pediatr Gastroenterol Nutr. 2016;62:242–5. doi:10.1097/mpg.0000000000000967.

The History and Physical Exam

Alka Goyal

Introduction

The history and physical exam form the foundation for medical evaluation. Physicians learn that a good history and physical exam can point to a diagnosis, even before other investigations have been undertaken. This is particularly true for the diagnosis of inflammatory bowel disease (IBD).

There are some challenges in obtaining a good history, which are more frequent in pediatric patients. Children are often too young or shy to provide the pertinent information. Parents and caregivers are frequently relied upon to provide the necessary details, and their skills as observers and reporters can vary widely. Many gastrointestinal disorders, such as functional abdominal pain, irritable bowel syndrome, infectious gastroenteritis or eosinophilic enteritis, may mimic the signs and symptoms of IBD. The index of suspicion for diagnosis of IBD is considerably lower in children, which can significantly delay the diagnosis. Within the spectrum of IBD, Crohn disease (CD) and ulcerative colitis (UC) may have overlapping clinical presentations as well as similar extraintestinal manifestations. A proper history and physical exam will help narrow the differential diagnosis that can lead to a correct diagnosis and proper treatment.

History

Consensus-based criteria for establishing the diagnosis of IBD were developed by the European Society of Pediatric Gastroenterology Hepatology and Nutrition (ESPGHAN). These criteria were based on a review of a prospective registry of children with IBD [1]. The group suggested that there should be a clinical suspicion of IBD in any child with persistent (≥4 weeks) or recurrent (≥2 episodes in 6 months) symptoms of abdominal pain, diarrhea, hematochezia, and weight loss [1]. Other supporting symptoms and signs were poor growth, lethargy, and anorexia.

While abdominal pain, weight loss, rectal bleeding, and diarrhea are the symptoms most frequently associated with IBD, only 25% of patients diagnosed with CD had a typical presentation. The symptoms could differ between Crohn disease and ulcerative colitis. Weight loss, malaise, and abdominal pain are the most common presenting symptoms with Crohn disease, while diarrhea and rectal bleeding are more likely in ulcerative colitis. Children with IBD may also present with sole findings of perirectal abscess, anemia, growth failure, delayed puberty, arthritis, recurrent fever, vomiting, amenorrhea, weight loss, lip swelling, or other extraintestinal symptoms. Table 16.1 summarizes the frequency of symptoms in studies from Wisconsin, United States, and the United Kingdom [2, 3].

Careful attention to pain patterns can yield important information. Patients with esophageal ulcerations may complain of odynophagia or dysphagia while eating, or heartburn after eating. Gastritis or duodenitis may result in early satiety or vomiting. Distal ileal stenosis or strictures can be associated with pain and nausea beginning within an hour or more after a meal and may also be associated with weight loss, bloating and vomiting. Small bowel inflammation is frequently associated with a sensation of nausea, bloating and generalized malaise. Nocturnal awakening due to pain is unlikely to be functional in nature. Crampy lower abdominal pain reflecting colonic inflammation and rectal inflammation will additionally be marked by urgency of stooling, or tenesmus, and more commonly by hematochezia. It is important to note that young children are frequently stoic and may underreport pain. They will also be less able than older children to describe or localize their pain.

Questions regarding patient's bowel movements are sometimes difficult to address but are necessary. Parents do not generally witness their child's stools once toilet training has been completed, and many adolescents never look at

A. Goyal, MD
Department of Gastroenterology, Hepatology and Nutrition,
Children's Mercy Hospital, 2401 Gillham Road,
Kansas City, MO 64108, USA
e-mail: agoyal@cmh.edu

© Springer International Publishing AG 2017
P. Mamula et al. (eds.), *Pediatric Inflammatory Bowel Disease*, DOI 10.1007/978-3-319-49215-5_16

Table 16.1 Frequency of symptoms in newly diagnosed patients with inflammatory bowel disease in Wisconsin, United States, and United Kingdom

	Wisconsin *N* = 199		Great Britain *N* = 739		
	UC (%)	CD (%)	UC *n* = 172 (%)	IC *n* = 72 (%)	CD *n* = 379 (%)
Abdominal pain	43	67	72	75	72
Diarrhea	98	30	74	78	56
Rectal bleeding	83	43	84	68	22
Weight loss	38	55	31	35	58
Fatigue	2	13	12	14	27
Aphthous lesions	13	5			
Anorexia			6	13	25
Arthritis		1	6	4	7.5
Nausea/vomiting			0.5	1	6
Constipation/soiling					1
Anal fistula					4.5
Growth failure and delayed puberty				1	4
Anal abscess, ulcer					2
Erythema nodosum, rash		1.5	0.5		1.5
Liver disease		2	3	3	
Toxic megacolon			0.5		

UC ulcerative colitis, *CD* Crohn disease, *IC* indeterminate colitis

their stools let alone talk about them. It is required not only to ask about the frequency of stooling but also to ask about the quality of the stool. Individuals have different definitions of diarrhea; so, it is important to ask a patient or caregiver to describe the bowel movement in some detail. "Does it fall apart when it hits the water?" is a question which is useful to distinguish between formed and loose stools. Nocturnal bowel movements are never normal, often reflect inflammation in the colon, and are highly suspicious for IBD. School-aged children may be afraid to report blood in the stools, and adolescents may not look at their stools, so it is necessary to ask the patient if they even look at their stools when asking about presence of bloody stools. Quantity of blood (Is it mostly blood or mostly stool?) and frequency of stooling can help to assess the severity of colitis. Urgency, increased stooling frequency, and tenesmus are symptoms indicative of rectal inflammation and may be seen in either CD or UC.

Children with IBD often present with weight loss or poor weight gain, growth failure, and pubertal delay. Growth failure is a unique characteristic of pediatric IBD, as opposed to adult IBD, and occurs in 10–40% of patients at the time of presentation [1]. While it can be seen both in CD and UC, it is more common in CD. When loss of appetite, early satiety, or weight loss is the only symptom, IBD could be misdiagnosed as anorexia nervosa.

IBD patients may present with nonspecific symptoms or solely with the extraintestinal manifestations of IBD. Fever of unknown origin (FUO) is defined as documented daily temperatures >101 °F persisting for >3 weeks without a cause despite an extensive workup. It has been estimated that 5% of children with FUO will ultimately be diagnosed with

inflammatory bowel disease and that roughly 2% of patients diagnosed with IBD will present with fever alone [4].

Approximately 5% of patients with IBD will present with a predominant symptom of arthritis. The arthritis of IBD is typically pauciarticular and involves large joints. Arthritis pain tends to be worse in the morning. Distinction from infectious arthritis is obviously important [5].

Patients with Crohn disease may present first to the surgeon with recurrent perianal abscess, small bowel obstruction, or an appendicitis-like picture. Free perforations are occasionally seen. Patients with IBD can develop fistulas, or communications between bowel and bowel, bowel and skin, or bowel and urinary tract. Unless specifically asked, patients may not mention air or feces in the urine.

Patients may be seen first by the dermatologists, with painful and nonspecific rashes, especially on the lower extremities. A large fraction of patients with erythema nodosum (Fig. 16.1) or pyoderma gangrenosum (Fig. 16.2) will be found to have IBD. Some patients will have swelling of the lips as the only external manifestation of IBD.

Along with the history of present illness, the family history is important, especially in children. Somewhere between 11% and 29% of newly diagnosed IBD patients will have a first or second degree relative with a history of IBD [2, 6]. Many parents with IBD worry about IBD in their children when they have any GI complaint. Symptoms in subsequent siblings tend to be more rapidly recognized than symptoms in probands. Social history and review of systems including a detailed allergy history should be routinely obtained.

There is an increasing incidence of IBD in very young children, who often present with colitis or perianal disease. It is

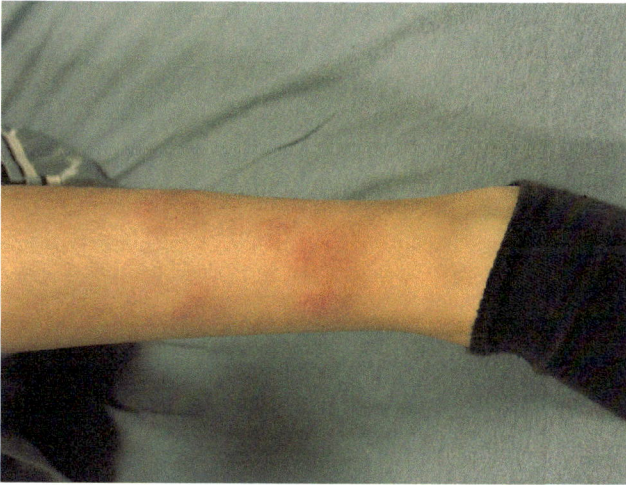

Fig. 16.1 A 10-year-old boy with Crohn disease and erythema nodosum lesions on his lower leg

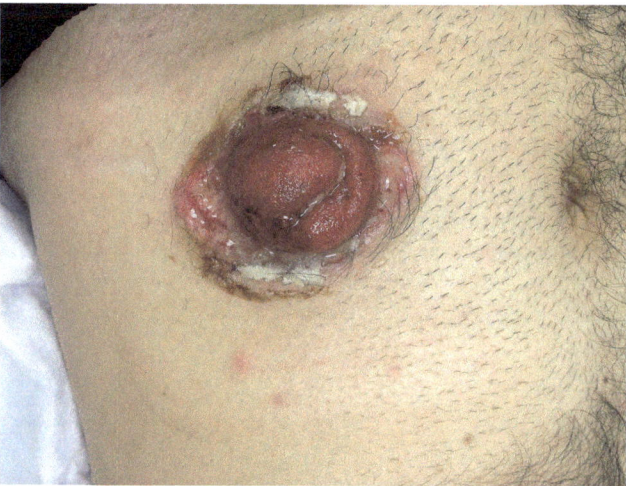

Fig. 16.2 A 18-year-old male with peristomal pyoderma gangrenosum

therefore important to keep IBD in the differential diagnosis even in infants and toddlers having suspicious symptoms like bloody diarrhea, perianal deep fissures, fistulae, abscess or tags, poor growth, or other extraintestinal symptoms [6, 7].

Physical Exam

The physical exam often confirms your suspicion after taking a thorough and complete history. The patient's general appearance may reflect illness. Affect and energy are often lacking in ill patients. Significant anemia can manifest as pallor. Children with growth and pubertal delay may look much younger than their stated age. While the eye is a sensitive tool for nutritional assessment, careful measurement of height and weight is as important as obtaining historical

growth data. These must be plotted on growth and on height velocity charts. Decreased growth velocity is an important indicator of disease activity. With the recent increase in obesity incidence, normal nutritional status or even obesity does not exclude the possibility of IBD. Important changes may be seen in vital signs. Fever can be a presenting sign of IBD and should be noted on exam. Tachycardia can indicate fever, anemia, hypoproteinemia, or dehydration.

Ocular findings of IBD include uveitis and episcleritis. A patient with newly diagnosed IBD should be referred to an ophthalmologist for a complete eye examination to evaluate for these extraintestinal manifestations of IBD and for baseline assessment for cataracts and glaucoma, which can follow steroid therapy. Because these can be clinically silent, patients should follow up with their ophthalmologist yearly.

The oropharynx needs to be thoroughly examined looking for evidence of gingival hypertrophy or apthous lesions. Orofacial granulomatosis is an uncommon presentation of Crohn disease and appears as nonspecific lip swelling and oral ulcers [8].

It is important to assess cardiopulmonary status in any patient. Patients with IBD will rarely develop interstitial pneumonitis which may have minimal findings on exam or pericardial effusions manifested by friction rubs, muffled heart sounds, or paradoxical changes in the blood pressure with respiration.

The abdominal exam may be deceiving, because the exam may be normal or exhibit only nonspecific tenderness. Abdominal distension may be seen with obstruction, ileus, perforation, or toxic megacolon. The pitch of bowel sounds may be increased with distension of bowel loops. Bowel sounds may be diminished in frequency or absent with severe inflammation, peritonitis, or ileus caused by medication or electrolyte imbalance. A "fullness" felt in the right lower quadrant may indicate thickened bowel in the area of the terminal ileum, an area often inflamed in patients with Crohn disease. A tender inflammatory mass may be clearly palpable in patients with CD, which may indicate active inflammation or an abscess. Tenderness over an inflamed colon, while frequent in patients with Crohn colitis, is seen only with severe disease in patients with ulcerative colitis.

A visual perianal exam and digital rectal exam, while unpleasant for the patient, are critical parts of the examination of patients with the potential diagnosis of IBD. Hemorrhoids are uncommon in children, are usually present only when straining, and have the bluish discoloration reflecting venous distention. Small (<0.5 cm) skin tags may be present most commonly at 12 o'clock in patients with chronic constipation. Larger skin tags or skin tags in other locations are suggestive of Crohn disease. Deep perianal fissures are suggestive, and anal fistulae almost pathognomonic, of Crohn disease. Occasionally, perianal Crohn disease may not be painful, and a patient may be unaware of the extent of their perianal disease. Perianal abscesses are generally marked by erythema, induration, fluctuance, and severe tenderness. With significant perianal disease, it may be impossible to perform a rectal exam in a conscious patient. When it can be performed reasonably comfortably, it may reveal important information regarding the presence or absence of blood in the stool, and presence or absence of anal stenosis. If the anal canal is stenotic and the small finger will pass through the anal canal, the stenosis is usually not limiting of stool passage. During a digital rectal exam, the palpation of a tender mass or collection in the pelvis may suggest the possibility of a ruptured appendix rather than IBD as a cause of tenesmus. It is also important to examine secondary sexual development and assess Tanner staging, which may often be delayed in a teenager with long-standing disease.

Examination of the skin, nails, and joints may reveal important information. Finger clubbing may be present. Rashes, such as erythema nodosum and pyoderma gangrenosum, are found in patients with IBD and are relatively easily distinguishable from other, more common rashes. Joint effusions may be subtle.

Conclusion

A careful history and physical examination may reveal important information regarding the diagnosis of IBD, distinguish between Crohn disease and ulcerative colitis, and even indicate location of disease. Accurate assessment of disease activity and detection of complications can be facilitated by careful serial assessments of history and physical examination.

References

1. IBD Working Group of the European Society for Paediatric Gastroenterology Hepatology and Nutrition. Inflammatory bowel disease in children and adolescents: recommendations for diagnosis – the Porto criteria. J Pediatr Gastroenterol Nutr. 2005;41(1):1–7.
2. Kugathasan S, Judd RH, Hoffmann RG, et al. Epidemiologic and clinical characteristics of children with newly diagnosed inflammatory bowel disease in Wisconsin: a statewide population-based study. J Pediatr. 2003;143(4):525–31.
3. Sawczenko A, Sandhu BK. Presenting features of inflammatory bowel disease in Great Britain and Ireland. Arch Dis Child. 2003;88(11):995–1000.
4. Miller LC, Sisson BA, Tucker LB, et al. Prolonged fevers of unknown origin in children: patterns of presentation and outcome. J Pediatr. 1996;129(3):419–23.
5. Paraskevi V. Voulgari. Rheumatological manifestations in inflammatory bowel disease. Annals of Gastroenterology. 2011;24:173–80.
6. Heyman MB, Kirschner BS, Gold BD, et al. Children with early-onset inflammatory bowel disease (IBD): analysis of a pediatric IBD consortium registry. J Pediatr. 2005;146(1):35–40.
7. Uhlig HH. Monogenic diseases associated with intestinal inflammation: implications for the understanding of inflammatory bowel disease. Gut. 2013;62:1795–805.
8. Khouri JM, Bohane TD, Day AS. Is orofacial granulomatosis in children a feature of Crohn's disease? Acta Paediatr. 2005;94(4):501–4.

Differential Diagnosis of Inflammatory Bowel Disease

17

Thierry Lamireau and Raphael Enaud

A diagnosis of inflammatory bowel disease (IBD) is usually suspected in patients with chronic digestive symptoms, especially diarrhea (with or without blood in the stools), abdominal pain, and poor weight gain. Numerous other diseases can have similar symptoms. For some of them, laboratory investigations, endoscopic, and even histological features may be difficult to distinguish from those of ulcerative colitis (UC) or Crohn's disease (CD).

In the short term, the most important challenge is to rule out an infectious disease. In the long term, the differential diagnosis with other chronic diseases, such as eosinophilic gastroenteropathy, vasculitis, lymphoma, or immunodeficiency syndromes, may cause some difficulties.

In some cases, the possibility of IBD, mostly CD, is considered in a child presenting with abdominal mass, isolated esophagogastroduodenal, or perineal involvement.

Acute Onset Diarrhea

In 10–20% of adults with IBD, patients present with apparently transient diarrhea, abdominal cramps, and low-grade fever [1]. In this acute-onset disease, the diagnoses to be considered are mostly intestinal infection, food allergy, and acute appendicitis.

Intestinal Infection

In the case of acute diarrhea, patients are thought to have *viral gastroenteritis*, particularly if they appear to recover promptly. However, prolonged diarrhea, right lower quadrant tenderness, or a slow recovery should alert the physician to

the possibility of early IBD (although in this setting a *bacterial or parasitic infection* of the intestine is more likely to be responsible for prolonged symptoms). Stool sample should therefore be collected for culture and toxin assays that can identify one of the numerous pathogens responsible for intestinal infection (Table 17.1). According to the age of the patient, the severity of symptoms, and the type of bacteria, an appropriate antibiotic treatment may then be initiated. When no pathogen is present in the stools, imaging such as an abdominal ultrasound is usually performed. It can show enlarged mesenteric lymph nodes and thickening of the colonic and/or ileal wall, but these findings can be seen in infectious diseases as well as in IBD. In this setting, colonoscopy is useful, enabling the visualization of colonic lesions and collection of biopsy samples for histology and culture. The endoscopist should describe the lesions precisely without directly stating a final diagnosis of IBD. Besides *Clostridium difficile,* which is responsible for the typical pseudomembranous colitis, infection with numerous bacteria or parasites may lead to colonic lesions that can be very similar to those of UC or CD [2] (Table 17.2). Moreover, intestinal infection is part of initial manifestations in 10–20% cases of IBD. When symptoms are severe, it may be justified to propose a short-course empiric treatment with broad-spectrum antibiotics, with activity against enteric pathogens (e.g., ceftriaxone, ciprofloxacin – usually after 15 years of age, and metronidazole).

If laboratory tests and evolution of symptoms do not confirm the hypothesis of infection, the diagnosis can be changed to IBD based on histological findings. Acute inflammatory changes of cryptitis, and crypt abscesses with neutrophilic infiltration, are not specific and are seen in both entities. The more discriminatory findings in favor of a first manifestation of IBD are the presence of glandular bifurcations and distortions, an infiltration of the mucosa with plasmocytes, and the presence of granulomata [3, 4]. However, these findings are rarely seen when endoscopy is performed at an early stage, and, in adults, most acute episodes of colitis remain initially unclassified. Half of these patients will relapse in the follow-

T. Lamireau, MD, PhD (✉) • R. Enaud
Unit of Pediatric Gastroenterology and Nutrition,
Children's Hospital, Amelie Raba Leon 33076 Bordeaux, France
e-mail: thierry.lamireau@chu-bordeaux.fr;
raphael.enaud@chu-bordeaux.fr

© Springer International Publishing AG 2017
P. Mamula et al. (eds.), *Pediatric Inflammatory Bowel Disease*, DOI 10.1007/978-3-319-49215-5_17

199

Table 17.1 Laboratory tests used to detect enteropathogens

Laboratory test	Organism suggested or identified
Microscopic stool examination	
Fecal leukocytes	Invasive or cytotoxin-producing bacteria
Trophozoïtes, cysts, oocysts, or spores	*Giardia lamblia, Entamoeba histolytica, Schistosoma mansoni*
Spiral or S-shaped Gram-negative bacilli	*Campylobacter*
Stool culture	
Standard	*Escherichia coli, Shigella, Salmonella, Campylobacter, Yersinia*
Specific selective medium (to be specified to the laboratory)	*Clostridium difficile,* E. coli O157:H7 *Aeromonas, Plesiomonas shigelloïdes, Klebsiella oxytoca, Vibrio parahemolyticus*
Stool cytotoxicity assay	*Clostridium difficile* (A or B toxin)
Culture of colonic biopsy sample	*Shigella, Salmonella, Campylobacter, Yersinia, Klebsiella oxytoca,* E. coli O157:H7
PCR on colonic biopsy sample	*Mycobacterium tuberculosis, Cytomegalovirus*
Circulating antibodies	*Shigella, Salmonella, Campylobacter, Yersinia, Entameoba histolytica*

Table 17.2 Main infectious agents responsible for IBD-like lesions during endoscopy

Microorganism	Possible ileal involvement	Crohn-like aspect	UC-like aspect
Aeromonas	N	+	++
Campylobacter	Y	++	+
Clostridium difficile	N	+	+
Escherichia coli	N	+	+
Klebsiella oxytoca	N	+	+
Mycobacterium tuberculosis	Y	+++	+
Plesiomonas shigelloides	N	+	+++
Salmonella enteritidis	Y	+	++
Shigella dysenteriae	Y	+	+++
Vibrio parahaemolyticus	N	+	+
Yersinia enterocolitica	Y	+++	+
Entamoeba histolytica	N	+	+++
Cytomegalovirus	Y	+	+++

N no, *Y* yes

ing 3 years, leading to a diagnosis of IBD, usually UC [5]. When the diagnosis is uncertain, one should avoid starting long-lasting anti-inflammatory treatment and be cautious when giving information to the family.

Food Allergy

Food proteins, usually milk or soy, may produce an allergic colitis which is typically encountered in infants under the age of 2 with a family history of atopy [6–8]. Rectosigmoidoscopy usually shows mucosal erythema and nodularity [9], but lesions may include aphthous ulcerations that mimic CD. The diagnosis of allergy is suspected if an eosinophilic infiltration of the mucosa is present on histology [9, 10]. Scratch tests using a panel of the main allergens responsible for food allergy in children can be used to direct the exclusion of the offending protein. A rapid disappearance of symptoms will then confirm the diagnosis [11].

Acute Appendicitis

Acute appendicitis may cause some diarrhea, associated with the classic right lower quadrant pain and tenderness. Imaging studies are an important component of the evaluation but may not be definitive. If there is any doubt regarding the possibility of appendicitis, or the abdominal tenderness worsens, a laparotomy should be performed to avoid gangrenous or perforated appendicitis. In some rare cases, CD will be discovered because of ileal involvement during operation [12, 13] or at the histological examination of the appendix [14].

Chronic or Recurrent Intestinal Symptoms

Chronic or recurrent intestinal symptoms represent the most frequent presentation of IBD in the pediatric population, and include symptoms such as abdominal pain and diarrhea lasting up to several months or years, especially in CD. This

Table 17.3 Useful investigations for differential diagnosis of IBD in children with chronic diarrhea

Blood	Polynuclear count and morphological features
	Lymphocyte count
	FACS enumeration of T and B lymphocytes
	Serum electrophoresis
	IgG, A, M
	Total hemolytic complement
	C_3, C_4 concentrations
	Antineutrophil cytoplasm antibody
	Anti-*Saccharomyces cerevisiae* antibody
	Antitransglutaminase antibody
	Specific IgE against food allergens
	Antibacteria antibody (*Shigella, Salmonella, Campylobacter, Yersinia, Entameoba histolytica*)
Stools	Fecal leukocytes
	Microscopic examination
	Standard and specific medium culture
	Clostridium difficile cytotoxin assay
Skin tests for	Tuberculosis
	Food allergens
Imaging of the abdomen	US examination
	MRI
Endoscopy	Esogastroduodenoscopy
	Biopsy for histology
	Ileocolonoscopy
	Biopsy for histology, bacterial culture, PCR
	Video capsule endoscopy

long delay until the diagnosis may be explained by the frequency in the general population of these nonspecific symptoms, as up to 10% of children between 7 and 11 years old seek medical attention for recurrent abdominal pain [15]. The periumbilical location of pain is not pathognomonic for functional abdominal pain, since it is present in most children with IBD. In patients with uncomplicated abdominal pain, constipation, lactose intolerance, peptic disease, food allergy, pathology of the urinary tract, or psychosocial causes should be considered and eliminated. The presence of fever, anorexia, weight loss or growth disturbance, perineal involvement, or blood in the stools suggests the possibility of IBD. This diagnosis is strengthened by laboratory investigations showing anemia and increased inflammatory markers (C-reactive protein, erythrocyte sedimentation rate), ultrasound examination of the abdomen showing a thickening of the intestinal wall, or elevated fecal calprotectin [16]. However, these features are not specific to IBD, and further investigations are useful to eliminate other diseases (Table 17.3).

Intestinal Infection

Even in case of chronic digestive manifestations, an infectious disease remains the most frequent differential diagnosis

to be considered [2, 17]. It is therefore important to collect stools for bacterial culture and parasitic pathogens at the initial evaluation of a patient with suspected IBD. Contrary to acute presentation, an antimicrobial treatment is generally not considered until laboratory tests have confirmed a specific infectious disease. Depending on the pathogen, the part of the gut involved and the symptoms may vary, leading to consideration of either CD or UC (Table 17.2).

Infection with *Yersinia enterocolitica* is usually associated with a mild illness in children [18], but subacute and chronic ileitis or ileocolitis have been reported [18, 19]. This can also be associated with erythema nodosum and polyarthritis. Endoscopic features include aphthoid lesions of the cecum and ileum with round or oval elevations with ulcerations. The ulcers are mostly uniform in size and shape, in contrast to CD [20]. US examination or magnetic resonance enterography (MRE) show mucosal thickening and nodular pattern of the terminal ileum and colon that can mimic CD, but also enlarged mesenteric lymph nodes [21]. In contrast to CD, fistula formation and fibrotic stenosis are not observed. Stool or biopsy sample cultures may require a specific enrichment medium, are time-consuming, and not always positive. The diagnosis can be made by serology, showing an increase (or a very high titer) of antibody in two successive sera. However, serology also has false-positives (antigenic cross-reaction with other bacteria), and false-negatives (serology is specific for only three serotypes: *Yersinia entero-colitica* 03 and 09, and *Yersinia pseudotuberculosis*).

Infection with enteropathogenic and enteroaggregative *Escherichia coli* (EPEC, EAEC) may be responsible for chronic diarrhea in children, especially when they live or travel in developing countries [22, 23].

Infection with *Clostridium difficile* leads to digestive disease ranging from self-limited diarrheal syndrome, to severe pseudomembranous colitis. Sometimes, sustained symptoms lead to consideration of the possibility of IBD. *Clostridium difficile* infection must be sought in children receiving antibiotics, especially beta-lactams, although it may occur without prior antibiotic therapy. Rectosigmoidoscopy, performed with care and minimal insufflation, reveals the presence of typical yellow-white pseudomembranes in approximately one-third of patients [24], and infection is confirmed by the presence of the toxin A or B in stool or by polymerase chain reaction. Nevertheless, *Clostridium difficile* infection can occasionally occur in patients with UC or CD, even without the use of antibiotics [25, 26], and stool toxin positivity has been reported in 5–25% of IBD patients with relapse, mostly after antibiotic exposure [24, 26]. Clinical symptoms are quite similar in both diseases, and it is recommended that stool assay for *Clostridium difficile* be obtained in children with IBD during acute relapses [24].

Giardia intestinalis infection can be associated with chronic diarrhea, abdominal pain, and weight loss [27], which may occasionally lead one to consider the possibility of IBD. Giardia is found in most countries in the world, the prevalence being highest in developing countries. Trophozoites or cysts of *Giardia intestinalis* can be found in fresh stool specimens or rectal biopsies. In some cases, it may be necessary to examine duodenal aspirations or biopsies. Jejunal morphology may be normal, although partial or even total villous atrophy has been reported [28, 29]. Failure to eradicate giardiasis can be due to hypogammaglobulinemia or deficit in secretory IgA.

Entamoeba histolytica infection occurs mostly in developing countries. Infection may be asymptomatic, or lead to a dysenteric syndrome. Demonstration of *Entamoeba histolytica* trophozoites and cysts in stools remains the mainstay of diagnosis. Chronic amoebic colitis could lead to clinical, radiological, and endoscopic findings that can be indistinguishable from those of IBD [30, 31]. However this differentiation is important because amoebiasis can become fulminant if the patient is treated with immunosuppressive agents for presumed IBD [32]. In these chronic manifestations, the parasite can be difficult to find in stool samples or in rectal biopsies, even using a concentration technique. The presence of high titers of antibodies in the serum may then be helpful in the diagnosis of chronic amoebiasis.

Intestinal tuberculosis remains a challenging diagnosis in developing countries, because treatments used for CD may adversely affect tuberculosis [33]. Intestinal tuberculosis involves the ileocecal region more frequently, isolated colonic location being present in only 10–25% of cases. Symptoms can be very similar to those of CD; these include diarrhea, abdominal pain, fever, weight loss, abdominal mass of the right iliac fossa, and even suppurative perineal lesions. The presence of intramural swelling, mesenteric thickness, stricture or fistula on US examination, or MRI can be encountered in both diseases [34], although the absence or minimal asymmetric thickening of colonic wall and the presence of enlarged necrotic lymph nodes favor the diagnosis of tuberculosis [35–38]. Nodules, ulcers, and strictures can be seen at ileocolonoscopy, or possibly at enteroscopy in the case of isolated jejunal lesions [39–42], but these lesions can be indistinguishable from those of CD. Usually, intestinal tuberculosis has less than four segments involved, a patulous ileocecal valve, transverse ulcers (longitudinal in CD), and more scars [43]. The characteristics of histological lesions may also be helpful, needing to perform multiple biopsies [44]: in tuberculosis, granuloma are typically bigger, often confluent, located beneath the ulcerations, and absent in noninflamed mucosa, and half of them contain caseum. Tuberculin skin test is positive in only 70–80% of patients with intestinal tuberculosis. The diagnosis may be facilitated by the presence of active pulmonary tuberculosis (but, this is only present in 20% of cases), or ascites, or large lymphadenopathy on imaging [35, 36]. Unfortunately, acid-alcohol resistant bacilli are very rarely present on direct examination of intestinal biopsies, and culture is positive in only 40% of cases. PCR for *Mycobacterium tuberculosis* on intestinal biopsies is better, showing an accuracy of >80% for the diagnosis of intestinal tuberculosis [45, 46]. Amplification of insertion element IS6110 that is specific for *M. tuberculosis* in the fecal samples [47] and the Quantiferon-TB gold, a blood test using an interferon-γ-release assay, look to be promising tools [48, 49], but their diagnostic value for the diagnosis of intestinal tuberculosis remains to be evaluated. In cases of persistent doubt, empiric treatment with antituberculosis drugs has been proposed in countries where the prevalence of tuberculosis is high, reconsidering diagnosis of CD if the patient's condition does not improve [50]. Nevertheless, this approach is not recommended by others who advise to make every effort to reach an accurate diagnosis before starting specific therapy [33].

Primary intestinal infection with *cytomegalovirus* (CMV) can occur in immunocompromised children, but it is exceptional in immunocompetent children [51]. Endoscopy reveals ulcerative and hemorrhagic colitis, and histological examination of the biopsy will confirm the infection with CMV by finding typical intranuclear inclusions in the colonic mucosa, associated with immunostaining with a specific antibody. PCR of colonic tissue can also be used to detect viral DNA in the colon, although the significance of a positive result remains unclear in the absence of histological features of CMV disease. The role of this virus in exacerbations of IBD remains under debate: is it only an opportunistic agent present in inflamed tissues, or active infection which really worsens colonic lesions? [52, 53]. CMV colitis is rare in CD or mild-moderate UC [53]. In patients with severe and/or refractory UC, local reactivation of CMV can be detected in inflamed colonic tissue in about 30% of cases, but does not influence the outcome in most studies [53]. Nevertheless, treatment with ganciclovir has allowed some patients with severe colitis to avoid colectomy despite poor response to conventional IBD therapies [54]. It is recommended to test for CMV reactivation via PCR and/or immunochemistry on colonic biopsies in all patients with severe colitis refractory to immunosuppressive therapy and treat with ganciclovir when CMV is detected [52, 55, 56].

Celiac Disease

Celiac disease is easily recognized in the classic mode of presentation of children who present with chronic diarrhea, anorexia, failure to thrive, and abdominal distension. Presentation is often less typical in older children who complain of abdominal pain, chronic diarrhea, anorexia, short stature, or iron-resistant anemia, symptoms that may also suggest IBD. In this situation, laboratory investigations should include specific antibodies against tissue transglutaminase, endomysium, or deamidated gliadin peptides. If these antibodies are positive, the diagnosis of celiac disease will be further confirmed by duodenal biopsy showing villous atrophy with increased number of intraepithelial lymphocytes [57].

Eosinophilic Gastroenteropathy

Eosinophilic gastroenteropathy is a rare condition characterized by infiltration of the gastrointestinal tract with eosinophils [58]. Most common symptoms are vomiting, abdominal pain, and growth failure. Diarrhea associated with rectal bleeding is present in 23% of cases, especially in infants, and symptoms of protein-losing enteropathy are present in 33–100% of cases [59, 60]. Endoscopic examination may show nodularity, erythema, friability, erosions, and ulcerations in the upper digestive tract and/or in the colon [9, 59, 61]. The diagnosis is strongly suggested by a context of food allergy or the association with hypereosinophilia in the blood, which is present in 70–100% of cases [59, 61]. The presence of excessive eosinophils in the digestive mucosa will confirm the diagnosis, although it may also be encountered in CD. Gastric biopsies may demonstrate eosinophilic gastroenteropathy more consistently, most patients having

more than 10 eosinophils per high-power field in the antral or duodenal mucosa [59, 62]. Allergic skin tests or serum-specific IgE against main food allergens are useful to guide dietary recommendations.

Primary or Acquired Immunodeficiency Diseases

The importance of the intestine as an immune barrier is highlighted by the proximity of gut-associated lymphoid tissue to the luminal surface of the gastrointestinal tract, an external environment which is rich in microbial pathogens and dietary antigens. Significant gastrointestinal disorders leading to chronic diarrhea, malabsorption, and failure-to-thrive are frequently present in primary or acquired immunodeficiency diseases [63]. In the recent years, a significant number of monogenic diseases, affecting the epithelial barrier, the inflammatory response, or the immune response, have been recognized as the cause of IBD-like manifestations (Table 17.4). These diseases should be sought after, especially in cases of very early (<6 years) or even infantile (<2 years) onset symptoms, and often present with a distinct phenotype, that is, indeterminate pancolitis or severe ulcerative or fistulizing perineal disease [64]. Although the frontier between these monogenic diseases (currently being discovered) and classic IBD is vague, the precise characterization of the genetic defect is of importance because therapeutic options may be different in some cases, like bone marrow transplantation, for example. This emphasizes the importance of a close collaboration between pediatric gastroenterologists, immunologists, and specialists in immunodeficiency syndromes for early efficient medical care and for active research to discover involved genes.

The most frequent manifestations of immunodeficiency syndromes are recurrent, persistent, and severe or unusual infections [65]. Disturbance of the immune system in the gut may also lead to autoimmune diseases, excessive production of IgE, or malignancies [66, 67].

Immunodeficient patients may present with chronic non-specific enterocolitis, characterized at small bowel biopsy by subtotal villous atrophy with acute and chronic inflammatory cell infiltration of the lamina propria [65, 68–79]. This chronic nonspecific enteropathy is not responsive to a gluten-free diet and occurs in several immunodeficiency disorders, affecting humoral response (X-linked agammaglobulinemia, IgA deficiency, common variable immunodeficiency), T-cell function (Wiskott-Aldrich syndrome, acquired immunodeficiency syndrome), or both (combined immunodeficiency). In some cases, strictures of the intestine may develop [68–71]. In these patients, it is important to rule out infection with opportunistic bacteria or parasites, and also with more common pathogens, such as rotavirus, adenovirus, picornavirus

[65]. In rare patients, the cause of the chronic enterocolitis is a disease affecting the epithelial barrier (Table 17.4).

Enterocolitis that resembles CD is mostly associated with neutropenia or defects of phagocytic function. Patients with chronic granulomatous disease may present with chronic colitis, perirectal abscesses and fistulae, and antral narrowing [72, 73]. The similarity with CD also includes endoscopic appearance, radiographic abnormalities, and even histologi-

Table 17.4 Gastrointestinal manifestations in genetic defects associated with immunodeficiency syndromes

Disease	Gastrointestinal manifestations	Gene
Epithelial barrier and epithelial response defects		
Dystrophic epidermolysis bullosa	Moderately severe colitis	COL7A1
Kindler syndrome	Hemorrhagic UC-like colitis	FERMT1
X-linked ectodermal dysplasia	Atypical CD-like enterocolitis, villous atrophy, and epithelial cell shedding	IKBKG (X-linked)
ADAM-17 deficiency	First week of life nonbloody, later bloody diarrhea	ADAM17
Familial diarrhea	Partially neonatal onset of familial watery diarrhea CD developed in adult age	GUCY2C
Neutropenia and defects in phagocyte bacterial killing		
Chronic granulomatous disease	Stomatitis, perineal abscesses, IBD-like enterocolitis	CYBB (X-linked), CYBA, NCF1, NCF2, NCF4
Glycogen storage disease type 1b	Perioral and perianal lesions, CD-like ileocolitis	SLC37A4
Congenital neutropenia	Stomatitis, CD-like colitis	G6PC3
Leukocyte adhesion deficiency 1	Stomatitis, ileocolitis, perianal abscess, fistulas, CD-like colitis	ITGB2
Hyper- and autoinflammatory disorders		
Mevalonate kinase deficiency	IBD-like enterocolitis	MVK
Phospholipase Cγ2 defects	UC-like colitis	PLCG2
Familial Mediterranean fever	UC-like colitis	MEFV
Familial hemophagocytic lymphohistiocytosis	IBD-like enterocolitis	STXBP2
X-linked lymphoproliferative syndrome 2	CD-like enterocolitis, fistulizing perianal disease	XIAP (X-linked)
X-linked lymphoproliferative syndrome 1	IBD-like enterocolitis, gastritis	SH2D1A (X-linked)
Hermansky–Pudlak syndrome	CD-like enterocolitis, perineal lesions	HPS1, HPS4, HPS6
B-cell and antibody defects		
Common variable immunodeficiency	Persistent intestinal infections, food allergies, autoimmune diseases, malignancies (gastric cancer, lymphoma), CD-like colitis	ICOS, LRBA
Agammaglobulinemia	Persistent intestinal infections, gastritis, malignancies (gastric cancer, lymphoma), CD-like colitis	BTK (X-linked) PIK3R1
Severe combined immunodeficiency	Severe persistent opportunistic infections, IBD-like enterocolitis	ZAP70, RAG2, IL2RG (X-linked), LIG4, ADA, CD3γ
Hyper-IgM syndrome	Oral ulcers, IBD-like	CD40LG (X-linked) AICDA
Wiskott–Aldrich syndrome	UC-like colitis	WAS (X-linked)
Omenn syndrome	Stomatitis, IBD-like enterocolitis	DCLRE1C
Hyper-IgE syndrome	Buccal granulomatous disease, UC-like colitis	DOCK8
Trichohepatoenteric syndrome	Intractable diarrhea, colitis	SKIV2L, TTC37
Regulatory T cells and immune regulation		
IPEX, IPEX-like	Autoimmune enteropathy, colitis	FOXP3 (X-linked), IL2RA, STAT1
IL-10 signaling defects	Stomatits, perianal abscesses and fistula, CD-like colitis	IL10RA, IL10RB, IL10

Adapted from Uhlig et al. [64]
Gene names were used according to HUGO gene nomenclature. *CD* Crohn's disease, *IBD* inflammatory bowel disease, *IPEX* X-linked immune dysregulation, polyendocrinopathy, enteropathy, *UC* ulcerative colitis

cal features showing granulomata and giant cells in the digestive mucosa. Nevertheless, a paucity of neutrophils, an increased number of eosinophils, eosinophilic crypt abscesses, pigmented macrophages, and nuclear debris suggest chronic granulomatous disease [74]. Patients with leukocyte adhesion molecule deficiency, a rare disorder of phagocytic function, also present with oral and perineal involvement that may be mistaken for CD. These manifestations include stomatitis with pharyngitis, gingivitis with periodontitis, ischiorectal abscesses, and distal ileocolitis [75]. Other disorders of neutrophils, such as congenital neutropenia, glycogen storage disease type 1b, and the Hermansky-Pudlak syndrome [76], are responsible for CD-like enterocolitis. The same presentation may be caused by T-cell or B-cell defects, IgA deficiency, and acquired immunodeficiency syndrome [63, 77].

Severe ulcerative or fistulizing perineal disease occurring in a very young child is suggestive of IL-10 signaling pathway defect [78–80] or X-linked lymphoproliferative syndrome 2 [81–83], and may also be encountered in phagocytic defects or Hermansky-Pudlak syndrome.

Autoimmune enteropathy is characterized by severe persistent diarrhea associated with circulating autoantibody against gut epithelial cell and/or another autoimmune disorder [84, 85]. An additional consideration is X-linked familial disease which includes polyendocrinopathy (IPEX syndrome) [86–88]. Although the colon is frequently involved [86, 89, 90], the lesions are predominant in the small intestine, with inflammatory cell infiltration of the mucosa, and subtotal or total villous atrophy [86, 87, 90], leading to secretory, protracted diarrhea in the first months of life [91, 92]. Nevertheless, antibodies to colonic epithelial cells have been also found in patients with UC [93], and 10% of IBD patients suffer from one or more autoimmune diseases [94], leading to some diagnostic difficulties in the older child.

Intestinal Neoplasm

Patients with *intestinal lymphoma* often present with chronic digestive symptoms, such as abdominal pain, distension, and/or diarrhea. Ultrasound examination shows a thickening of the intestinal wall, and/or narrowing of the lumen of the gut which can be very similar to CD [95]. Extent of the lesions is more precisely seen with a MRE, and upper digestive endoscopy and ileocolonoscopy are mandatory to provide histological confirmation. Nevertheless, if the lesions are limited to part of the small intestine, the biopsy may require an enteroscopy or even a surgical procedure, by laparoscopy or laparotomy. Predisposing conditions for intestinal lymphoma in children include inherited or acquired immunodeficiency syndromes, immunosuppressive therapy, and Epstein-Barr virus infection [96]. In developing coun-

tries, Mediterranean lymphoma is characterized by the proliferation of IgA-secreting B lymphocytes. The diagnosis is usually suspected because of the presence of alpha heavy chain in the serum [97].

Vasculitis Disorders

Henoch-Schonlein purpura (HSP) is a frequent vasculitis, involving the gut, skin, joints, and kidney. Diagnosis is easily made in a child presenting with typical skin purpura. Gastrointestinal symptoms, that is, colicky abdominal pain and bleeding, may precede the skin rash by a number of days, and some cases of isolated duodenojejunitis without purpura have been described [98].

In other less frequent systemic vasculitides, such as polyarteritis nodosa [99, 100], granulomatosis with polyangiitis (formerly known as Wegener granulomatosis) [101], Behcet's disease [102, 103], and lupus arteriosus [104], intestinal involvement can lead to chronic abdominal pain associated with bleeding. Endoscopic and histological findings may be very similar to CD, even with the presence of granuloma. Extradigestive manifestations, especially neurological, respiratory, renal, and cutaneous lesions, suggest systemic vasculitis [105] (Table 17.5). On the other hand, extraintestinal vasculitis can complicate IBD, involving the retina, brain, skin, muscle, joints, and lungs [106–111]. The differentiation between primary systemic vasculitis and IBD can be clinically challenging, but is important because their treatments and outcome are different [112]. The confirmation of the vasculitic process is more often evident on extraintestinal biopsies (skin, muscle, kidney) than on intestinal biopsies, and on angiography showing aneurysms and caliber variation of visceral arteries [100].

Abdominal Mass

The discovery of an abdominal mass has been found to reveal ileocolic CD in some adults and children [113–115]. Ultrasound examination and MRE are first-line investigations which will exclude extradigestive malignant tumors, such as lymphoma, sarcoma, nephroblastoma, or neuroblastoma. When the mass is developed from the digestive tract, glandular lymphoma or adenocarcinoma of the colon, although rare in children, can be suspected [116–118]. Radiological findings may be very similar in some benign lesions, like leiomyoma, pseudoinflammatory tumor, or tuberculosis [119, 120]. Nevertheless, surgical exploration is generally required, leading to correct diagnosis after histological examination of the excised tumor. Intestinal tuberculosis may be a challenging diagnosis, because histological findings may be very similar to those of CD, although granu-

Table 17.5 Extradigestive manifestations and useful investigations for the diagnosis of systemic vasculitis in children with digestive symptoms resembling Crohn's disease

Vasculitis	Extradigestive manifestations	Investigations
Polyarteritis nodosa	Multiple neuritis	Skin, muscle biopsy
	Myositis	Angiography
	Arterial hypertension	
	Skin ulcerations and gangrene	
Wegener granulomatosis	Epistaxis, sinusitis, otitis, hearing loss	Thoracic CT scan
	Stridor, hoarseness	c-ANCA
	Cough, wheezing, dyspnea, hemoptysis	Nasal mucosa biopsy
	Necrotizing glomerulonephritis	
	Skin ulcerations and gangrene	
	Conjunctivitis, uveitis, optic neuritis	
	Pseudotumor cerebri	
Behcet's disease	Serious buccal aphthous	HLA-B5
	Genital ulcers	
	Uveitis	
	Thrombophlebitis	
	Meningoencephalitis	
Lupus arteriosus	Typical facial erythema	Antinuclear antibody
	Myocarditis, pericarditis, endocarditis	Anti-DNA antibody
	Pleuropneumonitis	
	Glomerulonephritis	
	Thrombophlebitis	
	Hemolytic anemia and thrombopenia	
	Keratoconjunctivitis, retinitis	

lomata are typically larger and contain caseum in the case of tuberculosis [44]. Polymerase chain reaction for *Mycobacterium tuberculosis* should be systematically performed [45, 46].

Isolated Esophagogastroduodenal Involvement

Esophagogastroduodenal involvement is present in about 25% of children with CD, usually discovered during upper digestive endoscopy with systematic biopsies, performed at initial work-up [121–123]. More rarely, patients may present with symptoms suggestive of peptic disease, including epigastric burning pain and early satiety, these often being relieved by antacids or antisecretory treatment [124, 125]. Endoscopy can show heterogeneous lesions, but a bamboo-joint like appearance is suggestive of CD [122, 124, 126, 127]. Uncommonly, CD patients present with an isolated gastric or duodenal ulcer [125]. In the case of long-lasting symptoms or altered growth rate, the possibility of CD should be kept in mind, and a biopsy of the edge of the ulcer looking for the presence of granulomata should be performed [122, 124].

Isolated Perineal Disease

Skin tags, anal fissures, and perianal fistulae or abcesses are frequent in infants who are in diapers and/or have a history of constipation with hard stools.

Such perianal lesions also occur in half of the patients with CD, mostly in the context of colonic inflammation [128]. These lesions may precede other manifestations of intestinal disease in about one-third of these patients [129]. In adolescents, perianal lesions can be severe [130, 131], hidden, and unrecognized for several months. The diagnosis of CD should then be considered in the case of extensive or refractory perianal lesions occurring in older children. Confirmation of diagnosis will be obtained by pelvic magnetic resonance imaging (MRI) showing abscesses and fistulae and their relationship to the elevators, the presence of granuloma on biopsies of perianal lesions that required surgery, and/or colonoscopy that will show colitis [129, 131]. Severe ulcerative or fistulizing perineal disease occurring in a very young child is suggestive of monogenic diseases such as IL-10 signaling pathway defect [78–80], X-linked lymphoproliferative syndrome 2 [81–83], phagocytic defects [72], or Hermansky-Pudlak syndrome [76]. More rarely, perineal lesions can occur after trauma or sexual abuse [132, 133].

References

1. Schumacher G, Sandstedt B, Kollberg B. A prospective study of first attacks of inflammatory bowel disease and infectious colitis. Clinical findings and early diagnosis. Scand J Gastroenterol. 1994;29(3):265–74.
2. Rutgeerts P, Peeters M, Geboes K, et al. Infectious agents in inflammatory bowel disease. Endoscopy. 1992;24(6):565–7.
3. Surawicz CM, Belic L. Rectal biopsy helps to distinguish acute self-limited colitis from idiopathic inflammatory bowel disease. Gastroenterology. 1984;86(1):104–13.
4. Nostrant TT, Kumar NB, Appelman HD. Histopathology differentiates acute self-limited colitis from ulcerative colitis. Gastroenterology. 1987;92(2):318–28.
5. Notteghem B, Salomez JL, Gower-Rousseau C, et al. What is the prognosis in unclassified colitis? Results of a cohort study of 104 patients in the Northern-Pas-de-Calais region. Gastroenterol Clin Biol. 1993;17(11):811–5.
6. Goldman H, Proujansky R. Allergic proctitis and gastroenteritis in children. Clinical and mucosal biopsy features in 53 cases. Am J Surg Pathol. 1986;10(2):75–86.
7. Hill SM, Milla PJ, Phillips AD, et al. Colitis caused by food allergy in infants. Arch Dis Child. 1990;65(1):132–3.
8. Jenkins HR, Pincott JR, Soothill JF, et al. Food allergy: the major cause of infantile colitis. Arch Dis Child. 1984;59(4):326–9.
9. Odze RD, Bines J, Leichtner AM, et al. Allergic proctocolitis in infants: a prospective clinicopathologic biopsy study. Hum Pathol. 1993;24(6):668–74.
10. Rosekrans PC, Meijer CJ, van der Wal AM, et al. Allergic proctitis, a clinical and immunopathological entity. Gut. 1980;21(12):1017–23.
11. Boyce JA, Assa'a A, Burks AW, et al. Guidelines for the diagnosis and management of food allergy in the United States: report of the NIAID-sponsored expert panel. J Allergy Clin Immunol. 2010;126:S1–S58.
12. Fonkalsrud EW, Ament ME, Fleisher D. Management of the appendix in young patients with Crohn's disease. Arch Surg. 1982;117(1):11–4.
13. Yang SS, Gibson P, McCaughey RS, et al. Primary Crohn's disease of the appendix: report of 14 cases and review of the literature. Ann Surg. 1979;189(3):334–9.
14. Yokota S, Togashi K, Kasahara N, et al. Crohn's disease confined to the appendix. Gastrointest Endosc. 2010;72(5):1063–4.
15. McOmber ME, Shulman RJ. Recurrent abdominal pain and irritable bowel syndrome in children. Curr Opin Pediatr. 2007;19(5):581–5.
16. Diamanti A, Panetta F, Basso MS, et al. Diagnostic work-up of inflammatory bowel disease in children: the role of calprotectin assay. Inflamm Bowel Dis. 2010;16(11):1926–30.
17. Tedesco FJ, Hardin RD, Harper RN, Edwards BH. Infectious colitis endoscopically simulating inflammatory bowel disease: a prospective evaluation. Gastrointest Endosc. 1983;29(3):195–7.
18. Marks MI, Pai CH, Lafleur L, et al. Yersinia enterocolitica gastroenteritis: a prospective study of clinical, bacteriologic, and epidemiologic features. J Pediatr. 1980;96(1):26–31.
19. Abdel-Haq NM, Asmar BI, Abuhammour WM, et al. Yersinia enterocolitica infection in children. Pediatr Infect Dis J. 2000;19(10):954–8.
20. Matsumoto T, Iida M, Matsui T, et al. Endoscopic findings in Yersinia enterocolitica enterocolitis. Gastrointest Endosc. 1990;36(6):583–7.
21. Puylaert JB, Van der Zant FM, Mutsaers JA. Infectious ileocecitis caused by Yersinia, Campylobacter, and Salmonella: clinical, radiological and US findings. Eur Radiol. 1997;7(1):3–9.
22. Bhan MK, Raj P, Levine MM, et al. Enteroaggregative *Escherichia coli* associated with persistent diarrhea in a cohort of rural children in India. J Infect Dis. 1989;159(6):1061–4.
23. Fang GD, Lima AA, Martins CV, et al. Etiology and epidemiology of persistent diarrhea in northeastern Brazil: a hospital-based, prospective, case-control study. J Pediatr Gastroenterol Nutr. 1995;21(2):137–44.
24. Gryboski JD. Clostridium difficile in inflammatory bowel disease relapse. J Pediatr Gastroenterol Nutr. 1991;13(1):39–41.
25. Greenfield C, Aguilar Ramirez JR, Pounder RE, et al. Clostridium difficile and inflammatory bowel disease. Gut. 1983;24(8):713–7.
26. Meyers S, Mayer L, Bottone E, et al. Occurrence of Clostridium difficile toxin during the course of inflammatory bowel disease. Gastroenterology. 1981;80(4):697–700.
27. Pickering LK, Engelkirk PG. *Giardia lamblia*. Pediatr Clin North Am. 1988;35(3):565–77.
28. Ament ME, Rubin CE. Relation of giardiasis to abnormal intestinal structure and function in gastrointestinal immunodeficiency syndromes. Gastroenterology. 1972;62(2):216–26.
29. Levinson JD, Nastro LJ. Giardiasis with total villous atrophy. Gastroenterology. 1978;74(2 Pt 1):271–5.
30. Dunzendorfer T, Kasznica J. Amebic and/or ulcerative colitis? Gastrointest Endosc. 1998;48(4):450–1.
31. Ibrahim TM, Iheonunekwu N, Gill V, et al. Differentiating amoebic ulcero-haemorrhagic recto-colitis from idiopathic inflammatory bowel disease: still a diagnostic dilemma. West Indian Med J. 2005;54(3):210–2.
32. Gupta SS, Singh O, Shukla S, Raj MK. Acute fulminant necrotizing amoebic colitis: a rare and fatal complication of amoebiasis: a case report. Cases J. 2009;2:6557.
33. Almadi MA, Ghosh S, Aljebreen AA. Differentiating intestinal tuberculosis from Crohn's disease: a diagnostic challenge. Am J Gastroenterol. 2009;104(4):1003–12.
34. Jain R, Sawhney S, Bhargava DK, et al. Diagnosis of abdominal tuberculosis: sonographic findings in patients with early disease. AJR Am J Roentgenol. 1995;165(6):1391–5.
35. Malik A, Saxena NC. Ultrasound in abdominal tuberculosis. Abdom Imaging. 2003;28(4):574–9.
36. Makanjuola D. Is it Crohn's disease or intestinal tuberculosis? CT analysis. Eur J Radiol. 1998;28(1):55–61.
37. Sinan T, Sheikh M, Ramadan S, et al. CT features in abdominal tuberculosis: 20 years experience. BMC Med Imaging. 2002;2(1):3.
38. De Backer AI, Mortelé KJ, Deeren D, et al. Abdominal tuberculous lymphadenopathy: MRI features. Eur Radiol. 2005;15(10):2104–9.
39. Bhargava DK, Kushwaha AK, Dasarathy S, et al. Endoscopic diagnosis of segmental colonic tuberculosis. Gastrointest Endosc. 1992;38(5):571–4.
40. Das HS, Rathi P, Sawant P, et al. Colonic tuberculosis: colonoscopic appearance and clinico-pathologic analysis. J Assoc Physicians India. 2000;48(7):708–10.
41. Alvares JF, Devarbhavi H, Makhija P, et al. Clinical, colonoscopic, and histological profile of colonic tuberculosis in a tertiary hospital. Endoscopy. 2005;37(4):351–6.
42. Artru P, Lavergne-Slove A, Joly F, et al. Isolated jejunal tuberculosis mimicking Crohn disease. Diagnosis by push videoenteroscopy. Gastroenterol Clin Biol. 1999;23(10):1086–9.
43. Lee YJ, Yang SK, Byeon JS, et al. Analysis of colonoscopic findings in the differential diagnosis between intestinal tuberculosis and Crohn's disease. Endoscopy. 2006;38(6):592–7.
44. Pulimood AB, Peter S, Ramakrishna B. al. Segmental colonoscopic biopsies in the differentiation of ileocolic tuberculosis from Crohn's disease. J Gastroenterol Hepatol. 2005;20(5):688–96.

45. Amarapurkar DN, Patel ND, Amarapurkar AD, et al. Tissue polymerase chain reaction in diagnosis of intestinal tuberculosis and
Crohn's disease. J Assoc Physicians India. 2004;52:863–7.
46. Li JY, Lo ST, Ng CS, et al. Molecular detection of Mycobacterium
tuberculosis in tissues showing granulomatous inflammation
without demonstrable acid-fast bacilli. Diagn Mol Pathol.
2000;9(2):67–74.
47. Balamurugan R, Venkataraman S, John KR, et al. PCR amplification of the IS6110 insertion element of Mycobacterium tuberculosis in fecal samples from patients with intestinal tuberculosis.
J Clin Microbiol. 2006;44(5):1884–6.
48. Bartu V, Havelkova M, Kopecka E. QuantiFERON-TB Gold in the
diagnosis of active tuberculosis. J Int Med Res. 2008;36(3):
434–7.
49. Pai M, Zwerling A, Menzies D. Systematic review: T-cell-based
assays for the diagnosis of latent tuberculosis infection: an update.
Ann Intern Med. 2008;149(3):177–84.
50. Epstein D, Watermeyer G, Kirsch R. Review article: the diagnosis
and management of Crohn's disease in populations with high-risk
rates for tuberculosis. Aliment Pharmacol Ther. 2007;25(12):
1373–88.
51. Hinds R, Brueton MJ, Francis N, et al. Another cause of bloody
diarrhoea in infancy: cytomegalovirus colitis in an immunocompetent child. J Paediatr Child Health. 2004;40(9–10):581–2.
52. Kandiel A, Lashner B. Cytomegalovirus colitis complicating
inflammatory bowel disease. Am J Gastroenterol. 2006;101(12):
2857–65.
53. Lawlor G, Moss AC. Cytomegalovirus in inflammatory bowel disease: pathogen of innocent bystander ? Inflamm Bowel Dis.
2010;16(9):1620–7.
54. Papadakis KA, Tung JK, Binder SW, et al. Outcome of cytomegalovirus infections in patients with inflammatory bowel disease.
Am J Gastroenterol. 2001;96(7):2137–42.
55. Rahier JF, Ben-Horin S, Chowers Y, et al. European evidence-
based consensus on the prevention, diagnosis and management of
opportunistic infections in inflammatory bowel disease. J Crohns
Colitis. 2009;3(2):47–91.
56. Kornbluth A, Sachar DB. Ulcerative colitis practice guidelines in
adults (update): American College of Gastroenterology Practice
Parameters Committee. Am J Gastroenterol. 2004;99(7):
1371–85.
57. Rodrigues AF, Jenkins HR. Investigation and management of
coeliac disease. Arch Dis Child. 2008;93(3):251–4.
58. Talley NJ, Shorter RG, Phillips SF, et al. Eosinophilic gastroenteritis: a clinicopathological study of patients with disease of the
mucosa, muscle layer, and subserosal tissues. Gut. 1990;31(1):
54–8.
59. Whitington PF, Whitington GL. Eosinophilic gastroenteropathy in
childhood. J Pediatr Gastroenterol Nutr. 1988;7(3):379–85.
60. Kay MH, Wyllie R, Steffen RM. The endoscopic appearance of
eosinophilic gastroenteritis in infancy. Am J Gastroenterol.
1995;90(8):1361–2.
61. Khan S, Orenstein SR. Eosinophilic gastroenteritis: epidemiology,
diagnosis and management. Best Pract Res Clin Gastroenterol.
2005;19(2):177–98.
62. Kalach N, Huvenne H, Gosset P, et al. Eosinophil counts in upper
digestive mucosa of Western European children: variations with
age, organs, symptoms, Helicobacter pylori status, and pathological findings. J Pediatr Gastroenterol Nutr. 2011;52(2):175–82.
63. Agarwal S, Mayer L. Gastrointestinal manifestations in primary
immune disorders. Inflamm Bowel Dis. 2010;16(4):703–11.
64. Uhlig HH, Schwed T, Loletzko S, et al. The diagnostic approach
to monogenic very early onset inflammatory bowel disease.
Gastroenterology. 2014;147(5):990–1007.
65. Booth IW, Chrystie IL, Levinsky RJ, et al. Protracted Diarrhoea
Immunodeficiency and viruses. Eur J Pediatr. 1982;138(3):271–2.
66. Filipovich AH, Mathur A, Kamat D, et al. Primary immunodeficiencies: genetic risk factors for lymphoma. Cancer Res.
1992;52(19 Suppl):5465s–7s.
67. Washington K, Stenzel TT, Buckley RH, et al. Gastrointestinal
pathology in patients with common variable immunodeficiency
and X-linked agammaglobulinemia. Am J Surg Pathol.
1996;20(10):1240–52.
68. Teahon K, Webster AD, Price AB, et al. Studies on the enteropathy associated with primary hypogammaglobulinaemia. Gut.
1994;35(9):1244–9.
69. Bjarnason I, Sharpstone DR, Francis N, et al. Intestinal inflammation, ileal structure and function in HIV. AIDS. 1996;10(12):
1385–91.
70. Lim SG, Condez A, Poulter LW. Mucosal macrophage subsets of
the gut in HIV: decrease in antigen-presenting cell phenotype.
Clin Exp Immunol. 1993;92(3):442–7.
71. Abramowsky CR, Sorensen RU. Regional enteritis-like enteropathy in a patient with agammaglobulinemia: histologic and immu-
nocytologic studies. Hum Pathol. 1988;19(4):483–6.
72. Mulholland MW, Delaney JP, Simmons RL. Gastrointestinal complications of chronic granulomatous disease: surgical implications. Surgery. 1983;94(4):569–75.
73. Johnson FE, Humbert JR, Kuzela DC, et al. Gastric outlet obstruction due to X-linked chronic granulomatous disease. Surgery.
1975;78(2):217–23.
74. Schappi MG, Smith VV, Goldblatt D, et al. Colitis in chronic
granulomatous disease. Arch Dis Child. 2001;84(2):147–51.
75. Hawkins HK, Heffelfinger SC, Anderson DC. Leukocyte adhesion deficiency: clinical and postmortem observations. Pediatr
Pathol. 1992;12(1):119–30.
76. Hazzan D, Seward S, Stock H, et al. Crohn's-like colitis, enterocolitis and perianal disease in Hermansky-Pudlak syndrome.
Colorectal Dis. 2006;8(7):539–43.
77. Bernstein CN, Ament M, Artinian L, et al. Crohn's ileitis in a
patient with longstanding HIV infection. Am J Gastroenterol.
1994;89(6):937–9.
78. Glocker EO, Kotlarz D, Boztug K, et al. Inflammatory bowel disease and mutations affecting the interleukin-10 receptor. N Engl
J Med. 2009;361:2033–45.
79. Kotlarz D, Beier R, Murugan D, et al. Loss of interleukin-10 signaling and infantile inflammatory bowel disease: implications for
diagnosis and therapy. Gastroenterology. 2012;143:347–55.
80. Moran CJ, Walters TD, Guo CH, et al. IL-10R polymorphisms are
associated with very-early-onset ulcerative colitis. Inflamm Bowel
Dis. 2013;19:115–23.
81. Rigaud S, Fondaneche MC, Lambert N, et al. XIAP deficiency in
humans causes an X-linked lymphoproliferative syndrome.
Nature. 2006;444:110–4.
82. Worthey EA, Mayer AN, Syverson GD, et al. Making a definitive
diagnosis: successful clinical application of whole exome
sequencing in a child with intractable inflammatory bowel disease. Genet Med. 2011;13(3):255–62.
83. Yang X, Kanegane H, Nishida N, et al. Clinical and genetic characteristics of XIAP deficiency in Japan. J Clin Immunol.
2012;32:411–20.
84. Unsworth DJ, Walker-Smith JA, et al. Autoimmunity in diarrhoeal
disease. J Pediatr Gastroenterol Nutr. 1985;4(3):375–80.
85. Montalto M, D'Onofrio F, Santoro L, et al. Autoimmune enteropathy in children and adults. Scand J Gastroenterol. 2009;44(9):
1029–36.
86. Powell BR, Buist NR, Stenzel P. An X-linked syndrome of diarrhea, polyendocrinopathy, and fatal infection in infancy. J Pediatr.
1982;100(5):731–7.
87. Satake N, Nakanishi M, Okano M, et al. A Japanese family of
X-linked auto-immune enteropathy with haemolytic anaemia and
polyendocrinopathy. Eur J Pediatr. 1993;152(4):313–5.

88. Wildin RS, Smyk-Pearson S, Filipovich AH. Clinical and molecular features of the immunodysregulation, polyendocrinopathy, enteropathy, X linked (IPEX) syndrome. J Med Genet. 2002;39(8):537–45.
89. Hill SM, Milla PJ, Bottazzo GF, et al. Autoimmune enteropathy and colitis: is there a generalised autoimmune gut disorder? Gut. 1991;32(1):36–42.
90. Lachaux A, Loras-Duclaux I, Bouvier R. Autoimmune enteropathy in infants. Pathological study of the disease in two familial cases. Virchows Arch. 1998;433(5):481–5.
91. Catassi C, Fabiani E, Spagnuolo MI, et al. Severe and protracted diarrhea: results of the 3-year SIGEP multicenter survey. Working Group of the Italian Society of Pediatric Gastroenterology and Hepatology (SIGEP). J Pediatr Gastroenterol Nutr. 1999;29(1):63–8.
92. Ventura A, Dragovich D. Intractable diarrhoea in infancy in the 1990s: a survey in Italy. Eur J Pediatr. 1995;154(7):522–5.
93. Khoo UY, Bjarnason I, Donaghy A, et al. Antibodies to colonic epithelial cells from the serum and colonic mucosal washings in ulcerative colitis. Gut. 1995;37(1):63–70.
94. Ricart E, Panaccione R, Loftus EV, et al. Autoimmune disorders and extraintestinal manifestations in first-degree familial and sporadic inflammatory bowel disease: a case-control study. Inflamm Bowel Dis. 2004;10(3):207–14.
95. Sartoris DJ, Harell GS, Anderson MF, et al. Small-bowel lymphoma and regional enteritis: radiographic similarities. Radiology. 1984;152(2):291–6.
96. Isaacson PG. Gastrointestinal lymphomas of T- and B-cell types. Mod Pathol. 1999;12(2):151–8.
97. Martin IG, Aldoori MI. Immunoproliferative small intestinal disease: mediterranean lymphoma and alpha heavy chain disease. Br J Surg. 1994;81(1):20–4.
98. Gunasekaran TS, Berman J, Gonzalez M. Duodenojejunitis: is it idiopathic or is it Henoch-Schonlein purpura without the purpura? J Pediatr Gastroenterol Nutr. 2000;30(1):22–8.
99. Gundogdu HZ, Kale G, Tanyel FC, et al. Intestinal perforation as an initial presentation of polyarteritis nodosa in an 8-year-old boy. J Pediatr Surg. 1993;28(4):632–4.
100. Brogan PA, Malik M, Shah N, et al. Systemic vasculitis: a cause of indeterminate intestinal inflammation. J Pediatr Gastroenterol Nutr. 2006;42(4):405–15.
101. Radhakrishnan KR, Kay M, Wyllie R, et al. Wegener granulomatosis mimicking inflammatory bowel disease in a pediatric patient. J Pediatr Gastroenterol Nutr. 2006;43(3):391–4.
102. Akay N, Boyvat A, Heper AO, et al. Behcet's disease-like presentation of bullous pyoderma gangrenosum associated with Crohn's disease. Clin Exp Dermatol. 2006;31(3):384–6.
103. Stringer DA, Cleghorn GJ, Durie PR, et al. Behcet's syndrome involving the gastrointestinal tract – a diagnostic dilemma in childhood. Pediatr Radiol. 1986;16(2):131–4.
104. Sultan SM, Ioannou Y, Isenberg DA. A review of gastrointestinal manifestations of systemic lupus erythematosus. Rheumatology. 1999;38(10):917–32.
105. Gedalia A, Cuchacovich R. Systemic vasculitis in childhood. Curr Rheumatol Rep. 2009;11(6):402–9.
106. Nelson J, Barron MM, Riggs JE, et al. Cerebral vasculitis and ulcerative colitis. Neurology. 1986;36(5):719–21.
107. Garcia-Diaz M, Mira M, Nevado L, et al. Retinal vasculitis associated with Crohn's disease. Postgrad Med J. 1995;71(833):170–2.
108. Sargent D, Sessions JT, Fairman RP. Pulmonary vasculitis complicating ulcerative colitis. South Med J. 1985;78(5):624–5.
109. Speiser JC, Moore TL, Zuckner J. Ulcerative colitis with arthritis and vasculitis. Clin Rheumatol. 1985;4(3):343–7.
110. Weizman Z. Vasculitis involving muscle associated with Crohn's colitis. Gastroenterology. 1982;82(6):1483–4.
111. Saulsbury FT, Hart MH. Crohn's disease presenting with Henoch-Schonlein purpura. J Pediatr Gastroenterol Nutr. 2000;31(2):173–5.
112. Levine SM, Hellmann DB, Stone JH. Gastrointestinal involvement in polyarteritis nodosa (1986-2000): presentation and outcomes in 24 patients. Am J Med. 2002;112(5):386–91.
113. Gryboski JD, Fischer R. "Apple-core" lesion of the colon in Crohn's disease. Am J Gastroenterol. 1986;81(2):130–2.
114. Martinez CR, Siegelman SS, Saba GP, et al. Localized tumor-like lesions in ulcerative colitis and Crohn's disease of the colon. Johns Hopkins Med J. 1977;140(5):249–59.
115. Peterson IM, Milburn J, Reynolds M. Bowel obstruction and an apple-core lesion in an 18-year-old man. J Fam Pract. 1990;31(1):85–8.
116. Griffin PM, Liff JM, Greenberg RS, et al. Adenocarcinomas of the colon and rectum in persons under 40 years old. A population-based study. Gastroenterology. 1991;100(4):1033–40.
117. Karnak I, Ciftci AO, Senocak ME, et al. Colorectal carcinoma in children. J Pediatr Surg. 1999;34(10):1499–504.
118. Salas-Valverde S, Lizano A, Gamboa Y, et al. Colon carcinoma in children and adolescents: prognostic factors and outcome-a review of 11 cases. Pediatr Surg Int. 2009;25(12):1073–6.
119. Chaimoff C, Dintsman M, Lurie M. Lesions mimicking malignant tumors of the large bowel. Am J Proctol Gastroenterol Colon Rectal Surg. 1981;32(6):12–26.
120. Ciftci AO, Akcoren Z, Tanyel FC, et al. Inflammatory pseudotumor causing intestinal obstruction: diagnostic and therapeutic aspects. J Pediatr Surg. 1998;33(12):1843–5.
121. Lenaerts C, Roy CC, Vaillancourt M, et al. High incidence of upper gastrointestinal tract involvement in children with Crohn disease. Pediatrics. 1989;83(5):777–81.
122. Mashako MN, Cezard JP, Navarro J, et al. Crohn's disease lesions in the upper gastrointestinal tract: correlation between clinical, radiological, endoscopic, and histological features in adolescents and children. J Pediatr Gastroenterol Nutr. 1989;8(4):442–6.
123. Kirschner BS, Schmidt-Sommerfeld E, Stephens JK. Gastroduodenal Crohn's disease in childhood. J Pediatr Gastroenterol Nutr. 1989;9(2):138–40.
124. Rutgeerts P, Onette E, Vantrappen G, et al. Crohn's disease of the stomach and duodenum: a clinical study with emphasis on the value of endoscopy and endoscopic biopsies. Endoscopy. 1980;12(6):288–94.
125. Grubel P, Choi Y, Schneider D, et al. Severe isolated Crohn's-like disease of the gastroduodenal tract. Dig Dis Sci. 2003;48(7):1360–5.
126. Danzi JT, Farmer RG, Sullivan BH, et al. Endoscopic features of gastroduodenal Crohn's disease. Gastroenterology. 1976;70(1):9–13.
127. Kuriyama M, Kato J, Morimoto N, et al. Specific gastroduodenoscopic findings in Crohn's disease: comparison with findings in patients with ulcerative colitis and gastroesophageal reflux disease. Dig Liver Dis. 2008;40(6):468–75.
128. Markowitz J, Daum F, Aiges H, et al. Perianal disease in children and adolescents with Crohn's disease. Gastroenterology. 1984;86(5 Pt 1):829–33.
129. Galbraith SS, Drolet BA, Kugathasan S, et al. Asymptomatic inflammatory bowel disease presenting with mucocutaneous findings. Pediatrics. 2005;116(3):e439–44.
130. Shetty AK, Udall Jr J, Schmidt-Sommerfeld E. Highly destructive perianal Crohn's disease. J Natl Med Assoc. 1998;90(8):491–2.
131. Markowitz J, Grancher K, Rosa J, et al. Highly destructive perianal disease in children with Crohn's disease. J Pediatr Gastroenterol Nutr. 1995;21(2):149–53.
132. Porzionato A, Alaggio R, Aprile A, et al. Perianal and vulvar Crohn's disease presenting as suspected abuse. Forensic Sci Int. 2005;155(1):24–7.
133. Muram D. Anal and perianal abnormalities in prepubertal victims of sexual abuse. Am J Obstet Gynecol. 1989;161(2):278–81.

Laboratory Evaluation of Inflammatory Bowel Disease

Jennifer Strople and Benjamin D. Gold

Introduction

Although clinical history and physical exam may raise suspicion of Crohn disease (CD) or ulcerative colitis (UC), a focused laboratory evaluation can facilitate further differentiation between inflammatory bowel disease (IBD) and noninflammatory bowel disease – in particular, distinguishing between IBD, infectious processes, and functional bowel disorders (Table 18.1). These blood and stool studies, in combination with clinical presentation (thorough history, including family history of IBD or other autoimmune conditions, and physical examination), can help determine which child may require more extensive or invasive testing, such as radiological and endoscopic evaluation to definitively diagnose IBD and provide information to facilitate IBD phenotype. Moreover, the blood and stool evaluations may also provide insight into the severity of disease, if indeed IBD (i.e., prognostication). The first part of this review will focus on the evaluation of blood tests in the work-up of a child with suspected IBD. Initially, the nonspecific markers of disease (e.g., anemia) and inflammation (e.g., C-reactive protein (CRP) and erythrocyte sedimentation rate (ESR)) will be discussed. Subsequently, the more "specific" serological markers of IBD will be reviewed, and then, stool tests, which can be used to potentially delineate between IBD and non-IBD will be discussed.

J. Strople, MD (✉)
Division of Pediatric Gastroenterology, Hepatology and Nutrition, Ann and Robert H. Lurie Children's Hospital of Chicago, 225 E Chicago, Box 65, Chicago, IL 60611, USA
e-mail: Jstrople@luriechildrens.org

B.D. Gold, MD
Pediatric Gastroenterology, Hepatology and Nutrition, Children's Center for Digestive Healthcare, LLC, Atlanta, GA, USA

Blood Tests

Most clinicians, adult and pediatric, will agree that blood tests should be part of the initial screening process in children with symptoms compatible with UC or CD [1–6]. The specific blood evaluations performed should, at minimum, consist of a complete blood count, including white blood cell number with a differential, hemoglobin and hematocrit, and iron/red blood cell characteristics or indices such as mean corpuscular volume, as well as studies to further characterize iron deficiency including ferritin, total iron binding content (TIBC) and iron. In addition, liver biochemistries: alanine aminotransferase (ALT), aspartate aminotransferase (AST), alkaline phosphatase (ALP), gamma-glutamyl transpeptidase (GGT), albumin and total protein, and systemic inflammatory markers, such as ESR and CRP should be included in the initial laboratory evaluation of a child with suspected IBD [6, 7]. Although normal tests do not rule out the possibility of intestinal inflammation, if abnormalities are present, further diagnostic studies are generally warranted. In addition, serum biomarkers such as CRP and ESR can distinguish between quiescent and active disease and in some studies, elevations in these biomarkers have correlated with endoscopic evidence of mucosal disease [7]. As several of these parameters are included in the Pediatric Crohn Disease Activity Index (CDAI) (e.g., albumin, ESR), these blood tests may offer additional insight into disease activity, and potentially, severity [6, 8, 9].

Anemia

Anemia is a well-known complication of inflammatory bowel disease occurring in both UC[10] and CD [11–17]. Anemia is generally defined as a hemoglobin value <120 g/L. With respect to IBD, severe anemia is defined as a hemoglobin level <100 g/L. For reasons that are not well characterized, many patients with IBD are intolerant of oral iron replacement therapy or their anemia is refractory to such

© Springer International Publishing AG 2017
P. Mamula et al. (eds.), *Pediatric Inflammatory Bowel Disease*, DOI 10.1007/978-3-319-49215-5_18

Table 18.1 Laboratory tests for suspected inflammatory bowel disease

Test	Findings	Significance
Complete blood count and differential	Anemia (microcytic, macrocytic, normocytic), thrombocytosis, leukocytosis	*Anemia:* Assess severity of blood loss, evaluate for iron and other macronutrient deficiencies. Reported prevalence 16–77% in Crohn disease and 9–67% in ulcerative colitis [16, 17] *Thrombocytosis:* Acute phase reactant, nonspecific measure of inflammation. Reported prevalence variable, occurring in up to 85% of patients with Crohn disease and 70% patients with ulcerative colitis [37, 38]
ESR and CRP	Elevation	Nonspecific markers of inflammation, potential role in assessing disease activity, predicting disease relapse and monitoring therapeutic response [47, 61]
Liver function tests	Hypoalbuminemia Elevated transaminases Elevated alkaline phosphatase/GGT	*Hypoalbuminemia:* Surrogate marker of nutrition, possibly indicative of decreased liver production (negative acute phase reactant) or intestinal protein losses due to inflammation [23, 61] *AST/ALT/Alkaline phosphatase/GGT:* Role in evaluating for extra-intestinal complications of inflammatory bowel disease [66–68]
Stool Cultures – *E. Coli, Salmonella, Shigella, Campylobacter, Yersinia* species	Infection	Evaluate for primary infectious colitis, which may mimic inflammatory bowel disease and exclude co-infection, which may complicate disease [114, 115]
Clostridium difficile PCR	Infection	Evaluate for primary infection and co-infection. In patients with inflammatory bowel disease, *C. difficile* is the most common infectious agent identified [10, 116]
Stool calprotectin	Elevation	Alternative inflammatory marker, which appears to be a direct measure of intestinal inflammation. Potential role in assessing disease activity and predicting relapse in patients with inflammatory bowel disease [126, 127, 130]
Stool lactoferrin	Elevation	Another inflammatory marker that demonstrated in preliminary studies the potential of being utilized as a measure of intestinal inflammation. As with calprotectin, has the potential role of assessing response to therapy [126, 127, 130]
IBD serologies	Positive ASCA (IgA or IgG), pANCA, anti-OmpC, anti-CBir	May aid in classifying disease subtype and play a role in therapeutic decisions (prognostic factor). Inadequate screening tool due to low sensitivity compared to clinical history and routine laboratory tests [1, 95, 100, 101]

ESR erythrocyte sedimentation rate, *CRP* C-reactive protein, *IBD* inflammatory bowel disease, *AST* aspartate aminotransferase, *ALT* alanine aminotransferase, *GGT* Gamma glutamyl transpeptidase, *ASCA* Anti-Saccharomyces cerevisiae (ASCA), *pANCA* perinuclear antinuclear cytoplasmic antibody, *OmpC* outer membrane protein

supplementation [17]. In one recent, prospective treatment adult trial, parenteral iron therapy appears to be more efficient than oral iron therapy [18]. Further, there are some reports that suggest that oral iron therapy affects the gut microflora in a manner counter-productive to successfully treating the iron deficiency compared to those receiving parenteral therapy [19].

The reported prevalence of anemia is variable in IBD, but anemia appears to be more prevalent in CD compared to UC [20]. In one population-based adult Scandinavian study from Denmark, Norway and Sweden, the overall prevalence of anemia in IBD was 19% with iron deficiency and anemia of chronic disease being the primary etiologies [20]. Additionally, anemia may be more common in children compared to adolescents and adults [21]. Using the WHO age-adjusted definitions of anemia, Goodhand et al. [21] assessed the prevalence, severity, type, and response to treatment of anemia in patients attending pediatric, adolescent, and adult IBD clinics at a single center. These authors observed the prevalence of anemia to be 70% (41/59) in children, 42% (24/54) in adolescents, and 40% (49/124) in adults ($p < 0.01$). Overall, children (88% [36/41]) and adolescents (83% [20/24]) were more often iron-deficient than adults (55% [27/49]) ($p < 0.01$). In one study from Saudi Arabia, anemia was found in 86% of children affected by either ulcerative colitis or Crohn disease [22]. In other studies, anemia has been described occurring in 16–77% of patients with CD (16%, 58%, 70%, and 77% reported in pediatric cohorts) [14–17, 21, 23–26] and 9–67% of patients with ulcerative colitis (30% reported in one pediatric cohort) [17, 23, 26].

The cause of iron deficiency with or without frank anemia is likely multifactorial in both CD and UC [27]. In CD, anemia may result from iron, folate, or vitamin B12 micronutrient deficiencies from under or malnutrition which commonly accompanies extensive small bowel disease, particularly if the ileum is involved [27]. In addition, anemia may result from gross or occult gastrointestinal blood loss due to underlying intestinal inflammation. Finally, iron deficiency and/or anemia may be due to decreased overall iron stores due to chronic disease, and lack of appropriate dietary intake to replace iron stores [27]. The anemia observed in ulcerative colitis is generally the result of iron losses from chronic intestinal bleeding, but as with CD can be due to anemia of chronic disease. The assessment of iron status in IBD in many cases is rather difficult due to coexistent inflammation secondary to chronic disease [28]. For this assessment, several indices and markers have been suggested. Ferritin seems to play a central role in the definition and diagnosis of anemia in IBD and transferrin, transferrin saturation (Tsat), and soluble transferrin receptors have also been found to be useful markers in clinical practice. All these biochemical markers have limitations because they may be influenced by factors other than changes in iron balance. In addition, the iron metabolism regulators hepcidin and prohepcidin are still under investigation in IBD. Erythrocytes parameters like the red cell distribution width (RDW) and the percentage of hypochromic red cells as well as reticulocyte parameters such as hemoglobin concentration of reticulocytes, red blood cell size factor and reticulocyte distribution width could be useful markers for the evaluation of anemia.

Anemia of chronic disease that can be seen in IBD is also believed to be multifactorial in its etiopathogenesis. Three potential mechanisms leading to the anemia associated with chronic disease have been recently postulated, namely, (1) anemia results as a consequence of cytokine activation and subsequent alteration of iron homeostasis, (2) anemia occurs due to the inhibition of erythropoiesis, and (3) a shortened red blood cell half-life is associated with chronic disease and thereby results in the anemia [16, 29]. Additionally, the anemia of chronic disease such as that found in IBD involves erythropoiesis disturbance due to circulating inflammation mediators. In one study by Tsitsika et al., erythropoietin (Epo) levels in children and adolescents with IBD were investigated and correlated to disease activity [30]. In this particular study [30] 33 patients with IBD were evaluated (18 boys, 15 girls) ages 4–15 years (median 11 years). Patients were separated into two study groups related to their disease activity; those with active disease ($n = 21$), and those in remission ($n = 12$). Chronic disease-associated anemia was present only in patients with active disease, and, those patients also had a significantly higher possibility of low, altered Epo levels than expected compared with patients with inactive disease. Thus, it appears that impaired Epo production is another mechanism of anemia of chronic disease development.

Once the diagnosis of anemia is established, the etiology should be further investigated so treatment can be initiated. For macrocytic anemias, folate, vitamin B12, and methylmalonic acid levels should be obtained. Iron studies including ferritin, total iron binding content (TIBC), and iron levels should be evaluated in cases of microcytic anemia. However, the results of these studies may be difficult to interpret, as ferritin, a measure of iron stores, is also an acute phase reactant and may be falsely elevated in inflammatory conditions. Further in one recent retrospective pediatric study of 50 children with IBD compared to an equivalent number of celiac disease patients and controls demonstrated that serum hepcidin is increased in IBD children with active disease and it is responsible for iron malabsorption [31]. Thus, in patients with a microcytic anemia, obtaining a soluble transferrin receptor in addition to standard iron studies may be helpful in differentiating iron deficiency anemia and anemia of chronic disease [32–34]. Soluble transferrin receptor concentration, which is not affect by inflammation, is elevated in iron deficiency anemia, but remains normal in anemia of chronic disease [32–34]. In addition to soluble transferring receptor, intestinal ferroportin expression should be considered as a marker of anemia in relationship to inflammatory bowel disease and particularly Crohn disease in children. In a study performed by Burpee et al. [35], intestinal iron exporter ferroportin expression was studied in subjects with and without CD. In this investigation, the authors evaluated duodenal mucosal biopsies from 29 pediatric subjects, 19 of whom had CD and 10 were without CD. The authors observed that intestinal ferroportin protein was higher in anemic CD subjects than in nonanemic CD subjects, whereas ferroportin mRNA levels were not significantly different. Thus, intestinal ferroportin protein is upregulated in anemic CD subjects, suggesting yet another pathway for the iron deficiency and the anemia observed in children with CD [31, 35]. In a recent meta-analysis of studies comparing parenteral versus enteral iron therapy, IV iron demonstrated a higher efficacy in achieving a hemoglobin rise of >/=2.0 g/dL as compared to oral iron (OR: 1.57, 95% CI: 1.13, 2.18). Treatment discontinuation rates, due to adverse events or intolerance, were lower in the IV iron groups (OR: 0.27, 95% CI: 0.13, 0.59). The authors concluded that IV iron appears to be more effective and better tolerated than oral iron for the treatment of IBD-associated anemia, likely related to some of the pathways of iron malabsorption described above [36].

Acute Phase Reactants: Platelets

In inflammatory conditions such as CD and UC, there is a rise in acute phase reactant proteins as a result of chemokine stimulation. The assessment of acute phase reactants has been employed as laboratory tests in the standard work-up of the child with suspected IBD, as well as other inflammatory conditions in pediatric patients (e.g., juvenile rheumatoid arthritis) [37, 38]. Reactive thrombocytosis, a nonspecific marker of inflammation, is a result of this acute phase response. Since the first published paper describing the association of thrombocytosis with chronic IBD by Morowitz et al. [39], the characterization of platelet elevation in the peripheral blood has been a "standard" part of the work-up of patients for suspected IBD, and in the monitoring of their disease activity. Some studies of the pathogenesis of IBD have implicated platelets in the propagation of intestinal inflammation. In a murine model of intestinal inflammation, CD40–CD40L appears to be involved in the pathogenesis of intestinal inflammation, and suggest that modulation of leukocyte and platelet recruitment by activated, CD40-positive endothelial cells in colonic venules may represent a major action of this signaling pathway. In addition, Kayo et al. [40] evaluated the role of platelets in inflammation in peripheral blood and in the mucosa of a cohort of patients with active UC. These investigators compared the group of patients with active UC to patients with inactive UC and a small cohort of healthy controls. The authors observed a close association between activated platelets and neutrophils in both the affected colonic mucosa and peripheral blood of patients with active-phase UC compared to the normal volunteers (i.e., healthy controls) and those with inactive UC. The investigators inferred from their study results that a platelet-neutrophil association may play a role in the progression of inflammatory processes in UC [40]. There is also evidence that coagulation activation may mediate and amplify inflammatory cascades in IBD, especially via activating proteinase-activated receptor related pathways [41]. Patients with CD and UC are at least three to fourfold increased risk of developing thromboembolic (TE) complications compared to control patients [41]. Although the etiology is multifactorial, thromboembolic phenomena in IBD is largely attributable to coagulation activation and platelet aggregation during sys-temic inflammation [41]. Thus, it appears that platelets may in fact play more of a role in the propagation of intestinal inflammation and potentially some of the severe sequelae (e.g., thromboembolic processes) of the system inflammation of IBD, rather than being a simple "biomarker" of IBD [37, 41].

In children referred for endoscopy for evaluation of abdominal pain, diarrhea, rectal bleeding, weight loss, or mouth ulcerations, 85% of patients with CD and 70% of patients with UC had elevated platelet counts compared to 6% of children with normal endoscopic assessment [23]. The presence of thrombocytosis may be overestimated in this study, or a unique response in the child with IBD as a lower prevalence of increased platelets in IBD is reported in adults [42–44]. However, an elevated platelet count in a child with chronic intestinal symptoms should raise clinical suspicion of underlying intestinal inflammation. In one study evaluating pediatric patients with chronic abdominal complaints, the presence of an abnormal hemoglobin and/or elevated platelet count on a routine CBC was able to differentiate between IBD and healthy controls, with 90.8% sensitivity and 80.0% specificity [45]. Furthermore, the platelet count may help differentiate between IBD and infectious processes, as thrombocytosis is a relatively uncommon finding in diarrhea associated with enteric pathogens [42].

Mean platelet volume (MPV) is influenced by the degree and type of mucosal and system inflammation. One study analyzed overall accuracy of MPV in disease activity and compared MPV with other inflammatory markers in 61 UC patients and 27 healthy subjects [46]. MPV was compared to ESR, CRP, and white blood cell count. The authors found that MPV accuracy was roughly equivalent to standard acute phase reactants and was significantly lower in UC patients and particularly active UC patients than controls [46]. Thus MPV may be another indicator of intestinal inflammation and a useful marker in patients with symptoms concerning for IBD.

Acute Phase Reactants: Erythrocyte Sedimentation Rate (ESR) and C-reactive Protein (CRP) and Other Markers

ESR and CRP are two other nonspecific measures of inflammation which should be included in the evaluation of patients with suspected IBD [47]. Both ESR and CRP have been investigated in IBD for a number of reasons, namely, (1) diagnostic and differential diagnostic purposes, (2) assessment of disease activity (i.e., PDCAI) and risk of complications, (3) prediction of CD or UC relapse, and (4) for monitoring the effect of therapy. Under normal circumstances, CRP is produced by hepatocytes in low quantities but following an inflammatory stimulus, hepatocytes rapidly increase production of CRP under the influence of interleukin (IL)-6, tumor necrosis factor α, and IL-1β – all proinflammatory chemokines which are present in active IBD in both children and adults. CRP has a relatively short half-life (19 h) compared with other acute phase proteins and will therefore rise early after the onset of inflammation and rapidly decrease after the stimulus is resolved. Although it is still up for question, overall, CRP may be a better measure for assessing disease activity and predicting relapse. In CD in particular, CRP appears to correlates well with disease activity, and thus is one objective marker that may be helpful in distinguishing IBD from noninflammatory conditions [48]. Additionally, in clinical trials with biological therapies, elevated CRP levels prior to initiation of therapy are associated with higher response rate, whereas normal CRP levels are predictive of higher placebo response rates [48]. However, despite the advantages of CRP over other markers, it is still far from ideal. Not all IBD patients, CD or UC, mount a CRP response, and this must be kept in mind when measuring inflammatory markers in individual patients. It is unclear if this is due to differences in cytokine levels such as IL-6 or due to mucosal as compared to transmural disease differences among UC and CD, or whether this acute inflammatory marker elevation is genetically driven.

Both ESR and CRP can be elevated to varying degrees in IBD and therefore are helpful in distinguishing inflammatory from functional disorders. In a study of 91 children referred for chronic gastrointestinal symptoms the CRP was elevated in 100% of patients with CD and 60% UC, and ESR was elevated in 85% of patients with CD and 23% of patients with UC [23]. None of the patients with polyps or normal investigations had elevation of either marker. In adults with chronic abdominal symptoms, all patients with CD and 50% of patients with UC had elevated ESR and CRP, whereas none of the patients with functional disorders had elevation of both markers [49]. Therefore, using these markers in combination may increase the diagnostic yield [50].

Overall, the response of ESR and, in particular, CRP in UC appears to be less robust, with elevated values found in more extensive colitis compared to limited disease [51–54]. However, the development of highly sensitive CRP assays may improve the sensitivity of this test, even in patients with limited disease [55]. In a study by Poullis et al. [55], the authors evaluated 224 adult patients and determined the accuracy of the CRP in distinguishing IBD from functional GI disease. Using a newly developed enzyme-linked immunoassay approach to CRP measurement, the authors determined that a CRP cutoff value of 2.3 mg/L had a sensitivity of 100% and a specificity of 67% in differentiating functional bowel disease from new cases of IBD [55]. Compared to ESR, CRP has a shorter half-life and thus returns to baseline values more rapidly once the inflammatory stimulus has resolved. Because of this rapid decline, CRP may be a better

measure of remission and response to therapy than other inflammatory markers in patients with IBD [48].

Other laboratory markers, including leukocyte and platelet count, albumin, and 1-acid glycoprotein (orosomucoid), have been studied either less extensively in IBD, particularly in pediatric populations, or, have proven to be less useful than more traditional biomarkers such as CRP [48]. In a small cohort-sized study of adult UC patients (N = 28) before and after 8 week therapy for example, fecal samples were analyzed for myeloperoxidase (MPO), eosinophil protein X (EPX), mast cell tryptase, IL-1beta, and TNF-alpha using immunoassays [56]. Blood samples were analyzed for MPO, EPX, C-reactive protein, orosomucoid, and leucocyte counts. The investigators determined that fecal MPO and IL-1beta levels were elevated in all patients at inclusion despite different disease phenotypes (i.e., extent of disease). Striking reductions in fecal levels of MPO, EPX, tryptase, and IL-1beta were observed after 4 weeks of treatment in 20/28 patients [56]. Levels of fecal markers correlated with endoscopic scores, histological severity and circulating blood acute phase reactants; i.e., orosomucoid [56]. In one small study of Scandinavian adults with Crohn disease undergoing infliximab therapy, Crohn Disease Activity Index, the Harvey Bradshaw Index, C-reactive protein, as well as orosomucoid and albumin reached normal levels during infliximab treatment [57]. Orosomucoid was as sensitive as the more "traditional" inflammatory markers and correlated tightly with physician global assessment and CDAI [57]. Clearly as we learn more about the pathogenetics of IBD, CD, and UC, these types of novel biomarkers and others to be developed can serve as noninvasive, objective biomarkers for the diagnosis and monitoring of IBD.

Other Laboratory Evaluations

Liver function tests and electrolyte panels may add additional information to aid the clinician in differentiating IBD from non-IBD, in the determination of the IBD phenotype and, in particular, the presence or absence of extra-intestinal manifestations such as liver disease [58, 59]. Although severe liver disease can be the first presentation of IBD in pediatric patients, hypoalbuminemia, which may be due to liver parenchymal damage, decreased production and/or due to bowel injury accompanied by increased fecal loss, is a more frequent finding at diagnosis [59]. Hypoalbuminemia is observed in both CD and UC; however, overall decreased serum albumin appears to be present at a much higher frequency in CD. In pediatric cohorts, hypoalbuminemia has been reported in 35–64% of patients with CD and 15% of patients with UC [23, 24, 60–64]. In a relatively small-sized (N = 57) pediatric study of children with UC from Saudi Arabia, hypoalbuminemia was observed in over half (i.e.,

54%) of the cohort evaluated, with disease severity correlating with the degree of hypoalbuminemia [22]. In addition to being useful in the diagnosis of IBD compared to non-IBD, as well as a factor in the assessment of the child's overall nutritional status, hypoalbuminemia when present, may have value as a prognostic factor for surgical risk [60] as well as for osteopenia and decreased bone mineral density scores [62]. Albumin can also be used as a marker for response to therapy. In an adult multicenter clinical trial evaluating one of the biologics for therapy of CD, the authors investigated the effect of adalimumab on changes in laboratory values using data from CHARM trial [65]. In a total of 778 adult patients, adalimumab every-other-week ($N = 260$), adalimumab weekly ($N = 257$), or placebo ($N = 261$), the authors observed significant improvements in nutritional, hematologic, and inflammatory markers, including and specifically albumin, in moderately to severely active CD [65].

Similar to the pathobiology of anemia associated with IBD, the etiology of hypoalbuminemia in the child or adolescent with IBD is multifactorial, with protein loss from intestinal inflammation, decreased albumin production (negative acute phase response), and long-term poor nutrition all contributing to the overall low circulating levels of this important protein [52, 61, 63].

Elevation of AST and ALT may also be present on this initial screen in the evaluation of a patient with suspected IBD. In one study by Mendes et al. [66], the prevalence of abnormal hepatic biochemistries and chronic liver disease in a cohort of IBD patients was described in a retrospective case-control fashion. Patients with normal and abnormal liver biochemistries were compared, and in the cohort of 544 patients, abnormal hepatic biochemistries were present in nearly one-third of these adult patients. Contrary to what the investigators hypothesized, abnormal liver biochemistries in this single center cohort were not associated with IBD activity. These authors recommended that persistently abnormal hepatic biochemistries should be evaluated, but to use caution and not immediately attribute these abnormal liver biochemistries to IBD activity [66]. Abnormal liver biochemistries may also be primarily related to poor nutrition as a result of active disease, and thus spontaneous resolution of these transient elevations are common [67].

However, when AST/ALT are persistently elevated or seen in association with an elevated alkaline phosphatase, elevated direct bilirubin and/or γ-glutamyl transpeptidase, the extra-intestinal complication of primary sclerosing cholangitis (PSC) or autoimmune hepatitis/overlap syndrome should be considered. PSC is reported complication in 3–15% of children with IBD and can precede or occur coincident with diagnosis of IBD [68–71]. In a U.S. population-based health maintenance organization study, the prevalence of PSC in conjunction with IBD was characterized in addition to the demographic differences between racial/ethnic

groups in patients with PSC compared to non-IBD and non-liver disease controls. Using the Northern California Kaiser Permanente (KP) database, the authors identified 169 (101 males) cases fulfilling PSC diagnostic criteria with a mean age at diagnosis of 44 years (range 11–81); age-adjusted point prevalence was 4.15 per 100,000 on December 31, 2005 [72]. IBD was present in 64.5% (109/169) cases and was significantly more frequent in men than women with PSC (73.3% and 51.5%, respectively, $p = 0.005$) [72]. In another small-sized single center study ($N = 29$), the incidence of IBD in PSC patients was 68.9% (20/29) [73]. The investigators showed two peaks in the age distribution of PSC with male PSC patients demonstrated a first peak and female patients a second peak. Male PSC-IBD patients were in their teens and 20s making the first peak and female PSC-IBD patients were in their 50s and 60s making the second peak. Of note, the study demonstrated that PSC-IBD patents were significantly younger than the patients without IBD (33.6 vs. 58.9 years, $p < 0.001$) [73]. With regards to pediatric patients, Wilschanski et al. [70] demonstrated of 32 children with PSC, the majority were diagnosed in their second decade (median age: 13 years) and four children presented before the age of 2 years. Seventeen of the 32 patients had inflammatory bowel disease (IBD), all with colitis; 14 UC, and 3 CD [70]. Eight patients presented with chronic liver disease before clinical onset of IBD. Thus, of the hepatic pathologies reported associated with IBD in children and adults, PSC remains the more common presentation. In one longitudinal, cohort study by Feldstein et al. [68] 52 children with cholangiography-proven PSC were followed to determine the long-term outcome (mean follow-up was 16.7 years) of children with PSC diagnosed over a 20 year period (34 boys and 18 girls; mean age 13.8 ± 4.2 years; range, 1.5–19.6 years). Two thirds presented with symptoms and/or signs of PSC and 81% had concomitant IBD [68]. During follow-up, 11 children underwent liver transplantation for end-stage PSC and 1 child died with the median (50%) survival free of liver transplantation being 12.7 years. Compared with an age- and gender-matched U.S. population, survival was significantly shorter in children with PSC ($p < 0.001$). Using a statistical regression model for analysis, the authors determined that lower platelet count, splenomegaly, and older age were associated with shorter survival. Moreover, presence of autoimmune hepatitis overlapping with PSC ($p = 0.2$) or medical therapy ($p = 0.2$) did not affect survival. Thus, the authors concluded that PSC, whether associated with IBD or not, significantly decreases survival in this child population [68]. Furthermore, genotype–phenotype studies recently demonstrated that a continuum of disorders exists within inflammatory bowel disease, much better explained by placing patients into three groups (ileal Crohn disease, colonic Crohn disease, and ulcerative colitis) rather than simply by Crohn disease and ulcerative colitis as currently defined. The authors further observed that within these phenotypes "risk" can be determined with respect to those more likely to develop extra-intestinal manifestations such as PSC [74].

Renal as well as pancreatic disease may also be important extra-intestinal manifestations of IBD or can be adverse events associated with IBD pharmacotherapy [75–80]. In a multicenter study from Israel, both adults and children presenting with acute pancreatitis as the first symptom of IBD were retrospectively identified (10 years, 7 university hospitals) [80]. These authors demonstrated that 10 of 460 pediatric patients with IBD (2.17%), compared with only 2 in 3500 adults (0.06%) presented with pancreatitis. Eight children had colonic disease (four Crohn disease, four ulcerative colitis [three pancolitis]) with the mean amylase level being 1419 (range 100–1370) and three children (30%) having mildly elevated transaminases [80]. It is important to note was that median time between onset of the first episode of acute pancreatitis in relation to onset of IBD was 24 weeks (range 1–156) and the most common presentation in this cohort was abdominal pain.

Similarly, renal disease may precede diagnosis of IBD. Although small in sample size, Izzedine et al. [81] described four patients with severe interstitial nephritis demonstrated on histopathological examination of kidney biopsy specimens. Renal failure was discovered before or simultaneously with the diagnosis of CD, and patients were not treated with mesalamine. More importantly, impairment of renal function progressed to end-stage renal failure in three of the four patients [81]. A similar small case series of two pediatric patients with renal disease occurring concurrently with diagnosis of IBD has been reported [82]. Thus, with respect to appropriate adjunct or complementary lab tests to obtain in the work-up of a child with suspected IBD, given the reports of interstitial nephritis in patients with Crohn disease in the absence of 5-aminosalicylate exposure, a baseline comprehensive chemistry panel should be considered during the initial evaluation. Moreover, amylase and lipase should be considered at some point in the initial evaluation, during phenotyping once the diagnosis has been made, and in particular, where clinical signs and symptoms raise suspicion of pancreatic disease; prior to or after initiation of therapy particularly those medications with a predilection (e.g., 6MP, 5-ASA) for pancreatitis as a side effect.

The above paragraphs highlight the standard evaluation that is recommended for all children with history and physical exam findings suspicious for IBD. These diagnostic tests may aid the clinician in the differentiation of UC and CD from functional bowel disorders and infectious etiologies. However, because the clinical presentation of IBD is so diverse and symptoms can be nonspecific, at times, it may be difficult to distinguish between inflammatory and functional disorders. In fact, since May 13, 1932, when Dr.

Crohn and his colleagues, Oppenheimer and Ginzburg, presented a paper on terminal ileitis describing the features of Crohn disease to the American Medical Association, the average time from onset of symptoms to definitive diagnosis continues to be prolonged, ranging from 6 to 18 months [83–85].

Several other noninvasive studies have been proposed to aid in the diagnosis of inflammatory bowel disease including IBD serologies, fecal calprotectin, and lactoferrin. The following section reviews these tests including a brief overview of the use of IBD serology and the evidence to support or disprove their use in the preliminary evaluation of the child with suspected IBD. In addition, this section will describe the stool tests which are an essential part of the initial work-up of the child with suspected IBD, and includes a discussion of more novel markers of intestinal inflammation, fecal calprotectin, and fecal lactoferrin.

Specific Blood Tests: Inflammatory Bowel Disease Serologies

Anti-*Saccharomyces cerevisiae* (ASCA), an antibody response against *Saccharomyces cerevisiae* and perinuclear antinuclear cytoplasmic antibody (pANCA), an antibody response toward nuclear antigens with a perinuclear pattern, are two immunologic markers detected in IBD. There is much debate in both the pediatric and adult clinical settings regarding the proper use of these serologies in the evaluation of IBD, and there have been several studies assessing the accuracy and clinical utility of ASCA and pANCA in children with IBD [1, 5, 86–95]. Although these investigations differ in their study design and in some cases the type of serological profile obtained, overall, these markers appear to be reasonably specific for both CD and UC. In the reported studies, ASCA (IgG or IgA) specificity ranged from 88% to 97% for CD [88, 90–93] and pANCA specificity ranged from 65–95% for UC [87, 88, 90–93]. In children, the specificity of the combined serologies in differentiating IBD from non-IBD has been reported to range from 84% to 95% [1, 5, 88, 90, 94]. Unfortunately, the sensitivity of these serologies has been shown to be poor with overall sensitivity ranges reported between 55% and 78% [1, 5, 86, 88, 90, 94]. A meta-analysis of 60 adult and pediatric studies yielded similar findings and reported the sensitivity and specificity of ASCA IgG or IgA positive and pANCA negative for the detection of Crohn disease as 55% and 93%, respectively [96]. The sensitivity and specificity of positive pANCA for detection of UC were lower at 55.3% and 92.8%, respectively [96]. Therefore, a negative test result does not exclude the diagnosis of IBD, particularly in those patients with nonspecific symptoms such as abdominal pain and intermittent diarrhea. The addition of anti-OmpC, an antibody to the outer membrane porin of *Escherichia coli*, appears to add little to the diagnostic accuracy of this serologic panel in children [92, 93]. In two pediatric studies, the overall sensitivity of anti-OmpC for both CD and UC was very low [92, 93]. However, the use of the additional IBD serologies may help identify a small number of IBD patients who had negative ASCA and pANCA [92, 93, 97]. Younger children appear to have the greatest proportion of seronegativity to ASCA and ANCA and therefore these additional markers, particularly anti-cBir, may be most helpful in this population [97]. Moreover, with an increasing number of candidate genes being identified in patients with IBD, particularly CD, other serological markers have been identified that may increase the overall sensitivity of the assays [98]. For example, patients carrying the NOD2 mutations have an increased adaptive immune response to commensal organisms as measured by higher titers of antimicrobial antibodies, such as anti-CBir and ASCA [98]. Thus, use of a combination of serologic, genetic and inflammatory markers may further improve the diagnostic accuracy and utility of these tests for discriminating IBD from noninflammatory conditions [99].

Although their specificity is reasonable, overall ASCA and pANCA appear to be less sensitive than clinical history and routine laboratory tests (hemoglobin and ESR) in the evaluation of pediatric IBD. In a retrospective study, Khan et al. [94] evaluated 177 pediatric subjects who had pANCA and ASCA, hemoglobin, ESR and colonoscopy as part of their initial evaluation. In this study, 90 patients were diagnosed with IBD, and of those, 52 had UC and 39 were diagnosed with CD. Combining abnormal hemoglobin and/or ESR with rectal bleeding, the most distinguishing symptom for IBD in this study cohort, was more sensitive than positive ASCA and/or pANCA (86% versus 68%) and identified 86% of patients with IBD prior to endoscopy. A study by Sabery et al. [1] yielded similar findings. In this retrospective study which included 210 pediatric subjects, 40 with IBD, the sensitivity of ASCA and pANCA was again compared to hemoglobin and ESR [1]. The presence of an abnormal hemoglobin or ESR was the more sensitive screen, with a sensitivity of 83%, compared to 73% for the First Step® modified assay (Prometheus laboratories, San Diego, CA), and 60% for the confirmatory panel, which included anti-OmpC. In the subset of patients without rectal bleeding, a group whose symptoms may be more difficult to differentiate from functional disorders, the sensitivity of ASCA and pANCA decreased to 55% whereas the sensitivity of an abnormal hemoglobin or ESR remained high at 91%. In pediatric patients, the addition of antibodies to cBir flagellin to the serological panel does not appear to improve the diagnostic yield of this panel. A retrospective study of 304 pediatric patients with suspected IBD reported a sensitivity of 67% and specificity of 76% of the combined serological panel, and for anti-cBir specifically, the sensitivity and specificity were 50% and

53%, respectively [95]. As mentioned, combination of standard laboratory tests (hemoglobin, platelet count and ESR) had higher predictive value, with sensitivity of 72%, specificity of 94% and positive predictive value of 85% [95]. Additionally, as hemoglobin and ESR are both components of the PCDAI, they have added value as markers of disease severity and clinical response.

Given the cost of these tests and overall poor sensitivities documented in several pediatric studies, particularly compared to other clinical and laboratory parameters, currently, serology testing does not appear to have additive value as a screening test in the initial diagnostic work-up for patients with suspected IBD. However, these serologies may have a role in predicting disease course and identifying patients at risk for complicated disease. In a study by Targan et al. [100] 484 sera previously employed for a study evaluating other serological markers of IBD (namely, ASCA, pANCA, OmpC) were tested for anti-CBir1 by enzyme-linked immunosorbent assay. Interestingly, the authors observed that the presence and level of immunoglobulin G anti-CBir1 were associated with CD independently and were associated with a unique phenotype of CD, namely, small-bowel, internal-penetrating, and fibrostenosing disease. Papadakis et al. [101], also demonstrated that anti-CBir1 serum reactivity in CD patients is independently associated with fibrostenosing disease and complicated small bowel CD. Anti-OmpC and anti-IL2 have also been shown to be associated with more aggressive disease course in adult patients with CD [102]. As a single marker, ASCA may be most predictive of aggressive disease and several studies have demonstrated ASCA positivity (IgG or IgA) alone was associated with complicated disease behavior, perianal disease, and risk for surgery in both pediatric and adult cohorts [92, 103–105]. In children with CD, the presence of multiple serologic markers and degree of antibody elevation has been associated with more severe disease phenotypes, with frequency of internal-penetrating and fibrostenosing disease increasing with the number of antibodies present [106, 107]. Similar to adult data, anti-Omp C and anti-IL2 were independently associated with these complications [106]. A more recent cross-sectional study of adults with CD suggests that in addition to quantitative serologic markers, the presence of NOD2 genetic variants is associated with complicated disease [108]. Overall the data for pANCA and disease stratification/course is less robust, and a recent study demonstrated no correlation between disease severity and pANCA titers [109]; however, pANCA reactivity may be associated with primary nonresponse to anti-TNF therapy pediatric patients and absence of this marker may help predict long-term response to this medication [110, 111].

Approximately 10% of patients with IBD are diagnosed with IBD-unclassified (IBD-U), and this diagnosis may be higher in younger children as isolated colonic CD is more common [97]. There is interest in using these serologies to classify disease subtype in children with IBD-U and to assist in therapeutic decisions such as colectomy. In one longitudinal study of 406 children with Crohn's colitis, UC and IBD-U, ASCA + differentiated well between Crohn's colitis, IBD-U and UC (specificity 83%, PPV 96%); pANCA + had similar positive predictive value, but much lower sensitivity and specificity (65% and 66%, respectively) [112]. However, as the most common serologic profile in IBD-U is ASCA−/pANCA−, serology overall has lower utility in predicting subsequent disease type [112, 113]. Therefore, based on the above data, perhaps for now, the use of these serologies should be reserved as a potential prognosticator of disease course and assessment for risk for complicating disease.

Stool Evaluation

The presentation of pediatric inflammatory bowel disease can be markedly variable. However, those children who present with "classic" gastrointestinal complaints such as diarrhea and abdominal pain should have a thorough stool evaluation to rule out bacterial and parasitic etiologies of these symptoms. Standard stool cultures to look for entero-hemorrhagic *Escherichia. coli, Salmonella, Shigella, Yersinia,* and *Campylobacter* species, *Clostridium difficile* assay, preferably by PCR, and ova and parasite studies to look for *Entameoba histolytica* and other parasites are a necessary part of the work-up to differentiate infectious versus inflammatory enterocolitis and should be obtained prior to invasive procedures. In particular, *Yersinia enterocolitica* infections may mimic CD and thus specific emphasis should be placed on looking for this organism as isolation can be increased by using selective media [114, 115]. Also, defects in mucosal barrier function can predispose patients with IBD to infectious colitis, and *Clostridium difficile (C. difficile)* is the most common infectious agent identified [10, 116]. Overall *C. difficile* infection has been a growing problem and the rates of *C. difficile* infection have been increasing as have pediatric hospitalization due to this infection [117]. Clinical symptoms of *C. difficile* and IBD are similar and the prevalence of *C. difficile* is significantly greater in pediatric patients with IBD compared to children without this diagnosis [118, 119]. A positive stool test therefore does not rule out the possibility of IBD, and thus patients with a suspicious clinical history who do not improve with appropriate treatment of stool pathogens should have further diagnostic evaluations. In addition to differentiating between infectious colitis and IBD, there has been a lot of recent attention towards infectious agents in the etiopathogenesis of IBD; with focus either being on enteric microflora (i.e., commensals) as compared to infecting pathogens in the genetically susceptible host [4, 120].

Fecal Calprotectin

Calprotectin, a calcium binding protein in the S100 family, is an abundant protein in neutrophils, and to a lesser extent, macrophages and monocytes, accounting for approximately 60% of the cytosolic protein in neutrophils [121–123]. Calprotectin has bacterostatic and antifungal properties, and thus likely contributes to neutrophilic defenses [124]. In healthy individuals, concentrations of calprotectin are approximately six times higher in stool than plasma [123]. In IBD, a spot fecal calprotectin level correlates well with fecal excretion of [111] indium white cells, suggesting this protein can be an alternative marker of intestinal inflammation [125, 126]. Fecal calprotectin is easy to measure, resistant to proteolysis and stable in stool for 7 days, and thus has been proposed as a simple noninvasive investigative tool, which may help distinguish inflammatory from functional disorders [47, 123, 127–129].

Several studies have shown elevated fecal calprotectin levels in patients with both UC and CD compared to healthy controls and patients with irritable bowel syndrome (IBS) [47, 127–129]. In one large study of 602 new patient referrals who had symptoms compatible with either irritable bowel syndrome or organic disease, including 189 patients later diagnosed with IBD, fecal calprotectin levels of >10 mg/L had a sensitivity of 89% and specificity of 79% for organic diseases [130]. This test was more sensitive than either ESR or CRP and an abnormal fecal calprotectin had an odds ratio for disease of 27.8 [130]. A similar, but small cohort-sized study by Carroccio et al. [131] using the newer fecal calprotectin assay yielded a somewhat lower sensitivity for organic disease (sensitivity 66%), but similar specificity (84%). However, in the small subset of 9 adult patients with inflammatory bowel disease, the sensitivity and specificity of fecal calprotectin was 100% and 95%, respectively [131]. A subsequent meta-analysis of six prospective adult studies that assessed the diagnostic accuracy of fecal calprotectin in patients with suspected IBD revealed a pooled sensitivity and specificity of 93% and 96%, respectively [132]. A more recent meta-analysis of 8 prospective studies with combined 1062 patients found that patients with a fecal calprotectin level of </ = 40 μg/g had ≤1% chance of having IBD; however, the positive predictive value of this test was lower and a high calprotectin could not completely exclude IBS [133]. Other studies have demonstrated that fecal calprotectin may be superior to CRP in discriminating between IBD and irritable bowel syndrome with a diagnostic accuracy of 80–89% compared to 64–73% for CRP [134, 135].

There have also been several studies evaluating fecal calprotectin in the pediatric population. Carroccio et al. [131] study cohort included 50 children with chronic diarrhea, and the assay had a higher sensitivity (70%) and specificity (93%) in pediatric patients than in adults. Some pediatric studies have reported even higher sensitivity of the fecal calprotectin assay. Fagerberg et al. [127] obtained fecal cal-protectin levels in 36 pediatric patients with gastrointestinal symptoms who underwent colonoscopy for suspected inflammation. Using the standard upper reference limit of <50 μg/g for the modified assay, the test has a sensitivity and specificity for inflammation of 95% and 93%, respectively. Using the older assay, Bunn et al. [136] reported a sensitivity of 90% and specificity of 100% for identifying intestinal inflammation in 36 pediatric patients who underwent either colonoscopy or ^{99}Tc-labeled white blood scans for suspected inflammatory bowel disease. As there was a strong suspicion of IBD in these studies, there may be some selection bias, which resulted in these higher sensitivities and specificities. Other pediatric studies have reported similar sensitivities but lower specificities of the fecal calprotectin assay in differentiating IBD from other conditions [137, 138]. Two meta-analyses of prospective pediatric studies revealed a pooled sensitivity and pooled specificity of 92–97% and 70–76%, respectively [132, 139], whereas meta-analyses that also included respective pediatric case-control studies, which may introduce more bias, reported slightly lower pooled specificities (65–68%), with similar sensitivities [50, 140]. With relation to CD, disease location (small bowel versus colonic involvement) does not appear to limit the utility of this test [141, 142]. Based on these collective results, it appears fecal calprotectin correlates well with the presence of histologic inflammation in pediatric patients. In patients where symptoms overlap with both IBD and IBS, obtaining fecal calprotectin testing prior to endoscopy may be a cost effective screening strategy, particularly when the suspicion of IBD is low [143].

Fecal calprotectin may offer some insight into the severity of inflammation in children with IBD, with levels correlating with severity of mucosal disease, with a correlation superior to clinical activity indexes and CRP [141, 142, 144, 145]. As it correlates with mucosal disease, fecal calprotectin may be surrogate for mucosal healing. In one small prospective study of 24 newly diagnosed children with CD, a drop in fecal calprotectin of >50% after therapy had a specificity of 82% for predicting inactive endoscopic disease [146]. In adults, a level ≤250 μg/g predicted endoscopic remission in CD with 94.1% sensitivity and 62.2% specificity, whereas in UC a level >250 predicted active mucosal disease with a sensitivity of 71% and specificity of 100% [147]. Additionally, there have been several studies evaluating fecal calprotectin's role in predicting disease relapse. One prospective study of 32 children with IBD found that 90% of patients with fecal calprotectin > 400 μg/g experienced clinical relapse whereas 89% with fecal calprotectin below this threshold remained in clinical remission [148]. A larger prospective multicenter adult study also demonstrated that calprotectin concentrations in patients who relapsed where higher than those who did not, with a fecal calprotectin level of >150 μg/g

having a sensitivity of 69% and specificity of 69% to predict relapse [149]. Therefore, the assay offers an advantage over other nonspecific inflammatory markers as is appears to be a direct measure of intestinal inflammation and consequently may be followed prospectively in patients as a marker of disease activity and relapse. Although larger prospective pediatric clinical studies need to be performed, fecal calprotectin continues to offer promise in the evaluation of patients with suspected IBD and for monitoring disease activity prospectively.

Fecal Lactoferrin

Another potentially useful stool marker in patients with IBD is fecal lactoferrin. As with calprotectin, based on adult data, lactoferrin appears to be superior to CRP in differentiating between IBD and irritable bowel syndrome [134, 135]. In one adult study, this protein was shown to be the most useful of neutrophil-derived proteins in stool as a marker of intestinal inflammation [150]. In a large pediatric study in 148 children with CD, UC, irritable bowel syndrome, and healthy volunteers, fecal lactoferrin was shown to be a useful marker of inflammation in diagnosis and interval assessment, and it correlated well with the clinical activity indices and ESR [151]. Pfefferkorn et al. [152] similarly found fecal lactoferrin levels could be used to distinguish pediatric CD from non-IBD conditions, with sensitivity of 100%, specificity of 43% and negative predictive value of 100%. At higher cutoff values (≥60 μg/g), this marker could also be used to differentiate active from inactive disease with 84% sensitivity and 74% specificity [152]. In a meta-analysis of seven studies (n = 1012), four which included pediatric patients, fecal lactoferrin had a pooled sensitivity and specificity of 78% and 94%, respectively, in differentiating IBD from IBS [153]. Thus fecal lactoferrin appears to be another promising noninvasive marker of intestinal inflammation, and therefore a consideration in evaluation of patients with suspected inflammatory bowel disease. Similar to calprotectin, lactoferrin may also be useful to monitor response to therapy and predict clinical relapse [149, 154].

Summary

In the preceding paragraphs, we attempted to provide an overview of the laboratory tests, both blood and stool studies, available that can be used in the initial work-up of the child with suspected inflammatory bowel disease. Although a thorough clinical history and physical exam can raise suspicion of CD or UC it is important to include a focused laboratory evaluation. A combination of blood and stool tests may further differentiate between IBD and non-IBD in particular, inflammatory disease, compared to infectious processes and functional bowel disorders. Not only can a carefully chosen combination of blood and stool studies help determine which child may require more invasive testing, but they can also be used in the initial phenotyping of the disease, i.e., CD versus UC. Moreover, there are laboratory tests available, specifically IBD serologic markers such as ASCA and anti-CBir1, which can be employed to subtype CD and potentially provide the clinician with the ability to prognosticate disease severity. The definitive diagnosis of IBD is made by combining historical features, physical examination, radiological findings, and endoscopy and biopsy. However, laboratory investigations provide important information about inflammation and function of other organ systems that may or may not be involved in the child with IBD, which ultimately helps guide the clinician toward more invasive testing, making a definitive diagnosis and even phenotyping the IBD that facilitates the ability for the clinician to employ more precise targeted optimal therapies.

References

1. Sabery N, Bass D. Use of serologic markers as a screening tool in inflammatory bowel disease compared with elevated erythrocyte sedimentation rate and anemia. Pediatrics. 2007;119:e193–9.
2. Hait E, Bousvaros A, Grand R. Pediatric inflammatory bowel disease: what children can teach adults. Inflamm Bowel Dis. 2005;11:519–27.
3. Auvin S, Molinie F, Gower-Rousseau C, et al. Incidence, clinical presentation and location at diagnosis of pediatric inflammatory bowel disease: a prospective population-based study in northern France (1988-1999). J Pediatr Gastroenterol Nutr. 2005;41:49–55.
4. Oliva-Hemker M, Fiocchi C. Etiopathogenesis of inflammatory bowel disease: the importance of the pediatric perspective. Inflamm Bowel Dis. 2002;8:112–28.
5. Dubinsky MC, Ofman JJ, Urman M, Targan SR, Seidman EG. Clinical utility of serodiagnostic testing in suspected pediatric inflammatory bowel disease. Am J Gastroenterol. 2001;96:758–65.
6. Hyams J, Markowitz J, Otley A, et al. Evaluation of the pediatric Crohn disease activity index: a prospective multicenter experience. J Pediatr Gastroenterol Nutr. 2005;41:416–21.
7. Lewis JD. The utility of biomarkers in the diagnosis and therapy of inflammatory bowel disease. Gastroenterology. 2011;140:1817–26 e2.
8. Hyams JS, Ferry GD, Mandel FS, et al. Development and validation of a pediatric Crohn's disease activity index. J Pediatr Gastroenterol Nutr. 1991;12:439–47.
9. Griffiths AM, Otley AR, Hyams J, et al. A review of activity indices and end points for clinical trials in children with Crohn's disease. Inflamm Bowel Dis. 2005;11:185–96.
10. Mylonaki M, Langmead L, Pantes A, Johnson F, Rampton DS. Enteric infection in relapse of inflammatory bowel disease: importance of microbiological examination of stool. Eur J Gastroenterol Hepatol. 2004;16:775–8.
11. Roy CN, Weinstein DA, Andrews NC. 2002 E. Mead Johnson Award for Research in Pediatrics Lecture: the molecular biology of the anemia of chronic disease: a hypothesis. Pediatr Res. 2003;53:507–12.
12. Koutroubakis IE, Karmiris K, Kouroumalis EA. Treatment of anaemia in inflammatory bowel disease. Aliment Pharmacol Ther. 2006;23:1273–4. author reply 4-5
13. Wells CW, Lewis S, Barton JR, Corbett S. Effects of changes in hemoglobin level on quality of life and cognitive function in inflammatory bowel disease patients. Inflamm Bowel Dis. 2006;12:123–30.
14. Thayu M, Leonard MG, RN B, Mamula P. Prevalence of anemia in incident pediatric Crohn disease. J Pediatr Gastroenterol Nutr. 2005;41:547.
15. Thayu M, Mamula P. Treatment of iron deficiency anemia in pediatric inflammatory bowel disease. Curr Treat Options Gastroenterol. 2005;8:411–7.
16. Gasche C, Lomer MC, Cavill I, Weiss G. Iron, anaemia, and inflammatory bowel diseases. Gut. 2004;53:1190–7.
17. Wilson A, Reyes E, Ofman J. Prevalence and outcomes of anemia in inflammatory bowel disease: a systematic review of the literature. Am J Med. 2004;116(Suppl 7A):44S–9S.
18. Han YM, Yoon H, Shin CM, et al. Comparison of the efficacies of parenteral iron sucrose and oral iron sulfate for anemic patients with inflammatory bowel disease in Korea. Gut Liver. 2016;10:562–8.
19. Lee T, Clavel T, Smirnov K, et al. Oral versus intravenous iron replacement therapy distinctly alters the gut microbiota and metabolome in patients with IBD. Gut. 2016.
20. Bager P, Befrits R, Wikman O, et al. The prevalence of anemia and iron deficiency in IBD outpatients in Scandinavia. Scand J Gastroenterol. 2011;46:304–9.
21. Goodhand JR, Kamperidis N, Rao A, et al. Prevalence and management of anemia in children, adolescents, and adults with inflammatory bowel disease. Inflamm Bowel Dis. 2012;18:513–9.
22. Saadah OI. Ulcerative colitis in children and adolescents from the Western Region of Saudi Arabia. Saudi Med J. 2011;32:943–7.
23. Beattie RM, Walker-Smith JA, Murch SH. Indications for investigation of chronic gastrointestinal symptoms. Arch Dis Child. 1995;73:354–5.
24. Burbige EJ, Huang SH, Bayless TM. Clinical manifestations of Crohn's disease in children and adolescents. Pediatrics. 1975;55:866–71.
25. Dyer NH, Child JA, Mollin DL, Dawson AM. Anaemia in Crohn's disease. Q J Med. 1972;41:419–36.
26. Thomson AB, Brust R, Ali MA, Mant MJ, Valberg LS. Iron deficiency in inflammatory bowel disease. Diagnostic efficacy of serum ferritin. Am J Dig Dis. 1978;23:705–9.
27. Cronin CC, Shanahan F. Anemia in patients with chronic inflammatory bowel disease. Am J Gastroenterol. 2001;96:2296–8.
28. Murawska N, Fabisiak A, Fichna J. Anemia of chronic disease and iron deficiency anemia in inflammatory bowel diseases: pathophysiology, diagnosis, and treatment. Inflamm Bowel Dis. 2016;22:1198–208.
29. Oustamanolakis P, Koutroubakis IE, Kouroumalis EA. Diagnosing anemia in inflammatory bowel disease: beyond the established markers. J Crohns Colitis. 2011;5:381–91.
30. Tsitsika A, Stamoulakatou A, Kafritsa Y, et al. Erythropoietin levels in children and adolescents with inflammatory bowel disease. J Pediatr Hematol Oncol. 2005;27:93–6.
31. Martinelli M, Strisciuglio C, Alessandrella A, et al. Serum hepcidin and iron absorption in paediatric inflammatory bowel disease. J Crohns Colitis. 2016;10:566–74.
32. Margetic S, Topic E, Ruzic DF, Kvaternik M. Soluble transferrin receptor and transferrin receptor-ferritin index in iron deficiency anemia and anemia in rheumatoid arthritis. Clin Chem Lab Med. 2005;43:326–31.
33. Markovic M, Majkic-Singh N, Subota V. Usefulness of soluble transferrin receptor and ferritin in iron deficiency and chronic disease. Scand J Clin Lab Invest. 2005;65:571–6.

34. Baillie FJ, Morrison AE, Fergus I. Soluble transferrin receptor: a discriminating assay for iron deficiency. Clin Lab Haematol. 2003;25:353–7.

35. Burpee T, Mitchell P, Fishman D, et al. Intestinal ferroportin expression in pediatric Crohn's disease. Inflamm Bowel Dis. 2011;17:524–31.

36. Bonovas S, Fiorino G, Allocca M, et al. Intravenous versus oral iron for the treatment of anemia in inflammatory bowel disease: a systematic review and meta-analysis of randomized controlled trials. Medicine. 2016;95:e2308.

37. Matsumoto T. Platelets in inflammatory bowel disease. J Gastroenterol. 2006;41:91–2.

38. Danese S, Scaldaferri F, Papa A, et al. Platelets: new players in the mucosal scenario of inflammatory bowel disease. Eur Rev Med Pharmacol Sci. 2004;8:193–8.

39. Morowitz DA, Allen LW, Kirsner JB. Thrombocytosis in chronic inflammatory bowel disease. Ann Intern Med. 1968;68:1013–21.

40. Kayo S, Ikura Y, Suekane T, et al. Close association between activated platelets and neutrophils in the active phase of ulcerative colitis in humans. Inflamm Bowel Dis. 2006;12:727–35.

41. Stadnicki A. Involvement of coagulation and hemostasis in inflammatory bowel diseases. Curr Vasc Pharmacol. 2012;10:659–69.

42. Harries AD, Beeching NJ, Rogerson SJ, Nye FJ. The platelet count as a simple measure to distinguish inflammatory bowel disease from infective diarrhoea. J Infect. 1991;22:247–50.

43. Lam A, Borda IT, Inwood MJ, Thomson S. Coagulation studies in ulcerative colitis and Crohn's disease. Gastroenterology. 1975;68:245–51.

44. Talstad I, Rootwelt K, Gjone E. Thrombocytosis in ulcerative colitis and Crohn's disease. Scand J Gastroenterol. 1973;8:135–8.

45. Cabrera-Abreu JC, Davies P, Matek Z, Murphy MS. Performance of blood tests in diagnosis of inflammatory bowel disease in a specialist clinic. Arch Dis Child. 2004;89:69–71.

46. Yuksel O, Helvaci K, Basar O, et al. An overlooked indicator of disease activity in ulcerative colitis: mean platelet volume. Platelets. 2009;20:277–81.

47. Desai D, Faubion WA, Sandborn WJ. Review article: biological activity markers in inflammatory bowel disease. Aliment Pharmacol Ther. 2007;25:247–55.

48. Vermeire S, Van Assche G, Rutgeerts P. Laboratory markers in IBD: useful, magic, or unnecessary toys? Gut. 2006;55:426–31.

49. Shine B, Berghouse L, Jones JE, Landon J. C-reactive protein as an aid in the differentiation of functional and inflammatory bowel disorders. Clin Chim Acta. 1985;148:105–9.

50. Holtman GA, Lisman-van Leeuwen Y, Reitsma JB, Berger MY. Noninvasive tests for inflammatory bowel disease: a meta-analysis. Pediatrics. 2016;137

51. Sachar DB, Smith H, Chan S, Cohen LB, Lichtiger S, Messer J. Erythrocytic sedimentation rate as a measure of clinical activity in inflammatory bowel disease. J Clin Gastroenterol. 1986;8:647–50.

52. Solem CA, Loftus Jr EV, Tremaine WJ, Harmsen WS, Zinsmeister AR, Sandborn WJ. Correlation of C-reactive protein with clinical, endoscopic, histologic, and radiographic activity in inflammatory bowel disease. Inflamm Bowel Dis. 2005;11:707–12.

53. Fagan EA, Dyck RF, Maton PN, et al. Serum levels of C-reactive protein in Crohn's disease and ulcerative colitis. Eur J Clin Invest. 1982;12:351–9.

54. Saverymuttu SH, Hodgson HJ, Chadwick VS, Pepys MB. Differing acute phase responses in Crohn's disease and ulcerative colitis. Gut. 1986;27:809–13.

55. Poullis AP, Zar S, Sundaram KK, et al. A new, highly sensitive assay for C-reactive protein can aid the differentiation of inflammatory bowel disorders from constipation- and diarrhoea-predominant functional bowel disorders. Eur J Gastroenterol Hepatol. 2002;14:409–12.

56. Peterson CG, Sangfelt P, Wagner M, Hansson T, Lettesjo H, Carlson M. Fecal levels of leukocyte markers reflect disease activity in patients with ulcerative colitis. Scand J Clin Lab Invest. 2007;67:810–20.

57. Eivindson M, Gronbaek H, Skogstrand K, et al. The insulin-like growth factor (IGF) system and its relation to infliximab treatment in adult patients with Crohn's disease. Scand J Gastroenterol. 2007;42:464–70.

58. Maudgal DP, Ang L, Patel S, Bland JM, Maxwell JD. Nutritional assessment in patients with chronic gastrointestinal symptoms: comparison of functional and organic disorders. Hum Nutr Clin Nutr. 1985;39:203–12.

59. Kane W, Miller K, Sharp HL. Inflammatory bowel disease presenting as liver disease during childhood. J Pediatr. 1980;97:775–8.

60. Gupta N, Cohen SA, Bostrom AG, et al. Risk factors for initial surgery in pediatric patients with Crohn's disease. Gastroenterology. 2006;130:1069–77.

61. Ferrante M, Penninckx F, De Hertogh G, et al. Protein-losing enteropathy in Crohn's disease. Acta Gastroenterol Belg. 2006;69:384–9.

62. Semeao EJ, Jawad AF, Stouffer NO, Zemel BS, Piccoli DA, Stallings VA. Risk factors for low bone mineral density in children and young adults with Crohn's disease. J Pediatr. 1999;135:593–600.

63. Thomas DW, Sinatra FR. Screening laboratory tests for Crohn's disease. West J Med. 1989;150:163–4.

64. Heyman MB, Kirschner BS, Gold BD, et al. Children with early-onset inflammatory bowel disease (IBD): analysis of a pediatric IBD consortium registry. J Pediatr. 2005;146:35–40.

65. Rubin DT, Mulani P, Chao J, et al. Effect of adalimumab on clinical laboratory parameters in patients with Crohn's disease: results from the CHARM trial. Inflamm Bowel Dis. 2012;18:818–25.

66. Mendes FD, Levy C, Enders FB, Loftus Jr EV, Angulo P, Lindor KD. Abnormal hepatic biochemistries in patients with inflammatory bowel disease. Am J Gastroenterol. 2007;102:344–50.

67. Broome U, Glaumann H, Hellers G, Nilsson B, Sorstad J, Hultcrantz R. Liver disease in ulcerative colitis: an epidemiological and follow up study in the county of Stockholm. Gut. 1994;35:84–9.

68. Feldstein AE, Perrault J, El-Youssif M, Lindor KD, Freese DK, Angulo P. Primary sclerosing cholangitis in children: a long-term follow-up study. Hepatology. 2003;38:210–7.

69. Hyams JS. Extraintestinal manifestations of inflammatory bowel disease in children. J Pediatr Gastroenterol Nutr. 1994;19:7–21.

70. Wilschanski M, Chait P, Wade JA, et al. Primary sclerosing cholangitis in 32 children: clinical, laboratory, and radiographic features, with survival analysis. Hepatology. 1995;22:1415–22.

71. Fumery M, Duricova D, Gower-Rousseau C, Annese V, Peyrin-Biroulet L, Lakatos PL. Review article: the natural history of paediatric-onset ulcerative colitis in population-based studies. Aliment Pharmacol Ther. 2016;43:346–55.

72. Toy E, Balasubramanian S, Selmi C, Li CS, Bowlus CL. The prevalence, incidence and natural history of primary sclerosing cholangitis in an ethnically diverse population. BMC Gastroenterol. 2011;11:83.

73. Sano H, Nakazawa T, Ando T, et al. Clinical characteristics of inflammatory bowel disease associated with primary sclerosing cholangitis. J Hepatobiliary Pancreat Sci. 2011;18:154–61.

74. Cleynen I, Boucher G, Jostins L, et al. Inherited determinants of Crohn's disease and ulcerative colitis phenotypes: a genetic association study. Lancet. 2016;387:156–67.

75. Ridder RM, Kreth HW, Kiss E, Grone HJ, Gordjani N. Membranous nephropathy associated with familial chronic ulcerative colitis in a 12-year-old girl. Pediatr Nephrol. 2005;20:1349–51.

76. Siveke JT, Egert J, Sitter T, et al. 5-ASA therapy and renal function in inflammatory bowel disease. Am J Gastroenterol. 2005;100:501.

77. Van Staa TP, Travis S, Leufkens HG, Logan RF. 5-aminosalicylic acids and the risk of renal disease: a large British epidemiologic study. Gastroenterology. 2004;126:1733–9.

78. Margetts PJ, Churchill DN, Alexopoulou I. Interstitial nephritis in patients with inflammatory bowel disease treated with mesalamine. J Clin Gastroenterol. 2001;32:176–8.

79. De Broe ME, Stolear JC, Nouwen EJ, Elseviers MM. 5-Aminosalicylic acid (5-ASA) and chronic tubulointerstitial nephritis in patients with chronic inflammatory bowel disease: is there a link? Nephrol Dial Transplant. 1997;12:1839–41.

80. Broide E, Dotan I, Weiss B, et al. Idiopathic pancreatitis preceding the diagnosis of inflammatory bowel disease is more frequent in pediatric patients. J Pediatr Gastroenterol Nutr. 2011;52:714–7.

81. Izzedine H, Simon J, Piette AM, et al. Primary chronic interstitial nephritis in Crohn's disease. Gastroenterology. 2002;123: 1436–40.

82. Marcus SB, Brown JB, Melin-Aldana H, Strople JA. Tubulointerstitial nephritis: an extraintestinal manifestation of Crohn disease in children. J Pediatr Gastroenterol Nutr. 2008;46:338–41.

83. Perminow G, Brackmann S, Lyckander LG, et al. A characterization in childhood inflammatory bowel disease, a new population-based inception cohort from South-Eastern Norway, 2005-07, showing increased incidence in Crohn's disease. Scand J Gastroenterol. 2009;44:446–56.

84. Burgmann T, Clara I, Graff L, et al. The Manitoba Inflammatory Bowel Disease Cohort Study: prolonged symptoms before diagnosis–how much is irritable bowel syndrome? Clin Gastroenterol Hepatol. 2006;4:614–20.

85. Jelsness-Jorgensen LP, Bernklev T, Henriksen M, Torp R, Moum BA. Chronic fatigue is more prevalent in patients with inflammatory bowel disease than in healthy controls. Inflamm Bowel Dis. 2011;17:1564–72.

86. Canani RB, de Horatio LT, Terrin G, et al. Combined use of noninvasive tests is useful in the initial diagnostic approach to a child with suspected inflammatory bowel disease. J Pediatr Gastroenterol Nutr. 2006;42:9–15.

87. Olives JP, Breton A, Hugot JP, et al. Antineutrophil cytoplasmic antibodies in children with inflammatory bowel disease: prevalence and diagnostic value. J Pediatr Gastroenterol Nutr. 1997;25:142–8.

88. Ruemmele FM, Targan SR, Levy G, Dubinsky M, Braun J, Seidman EG. Diagnostic accuracy of serological assays in pediatric inflammatory bowel disease. Gastroenterology. 1998;115:822–9.

89. Dubinsky MC, Johanson JF, Seidman EG, Ofman JJ. Suspected inflammatory bowel disease – the clinical and economic impact of competing diagnostic strategies. Am J Gastroenterol. 2002;97:2333–42.

90. Hoffenberg EJ, Fidanza S, Sauaia A. Serologic testing for inflammatory bowel disease. J Pediatr. 1999;134:447–52.

91. Gupta SK, Fitzgerald JF, Croffie JM, Pfefferkorn MD, Molleston JP, Corkins MR. Comparison of serological markers of inflammatory bowel disease with clinical diagnosis in children. Inflamm Bowel Dis. 2004;10:240–4.

92. Zholudev A, Zurakowski D, Young W, Leichtner A, Bousvaros A. Serologic testing with ANCA, ASCA, and anti-OmpC in children and young adults with Crohn's disease and ulcerative colitis: diagnostic value and correlation with disease phenotype. Am J Gastroenterol. 2004;99:2235–41.

93. Elitsur Y, Lawrence Z, Tolaymat N. The diagnostic accuracy of serologic markers in children with IBD: the West Virginia experience. J Clin Gastroenterol. 2005;39:670–3.

94. Khan K, Schwarzenberg SJ, Sharp H, Greenwood D, Weisdorf-Schindele S. Role of serology and routine laboratory tests in childhood inflammatory bowel disease. Inflamm Bowel Dis. 2002;8:325–9.

95. Benor S, Russell GH, Silver M, Israel EJ, Yuan Q, Winter HS. Shortcomings of the inflammatory bowel disease Serology 7 panel. Pediatrics. 2010;125:1230–6.

96. Reese GE, Constantinides VA, Sim-illis C, et al. Diagnostic precision of anti-*Saccharomyces cerevisiae* antibodies and perinuclear

antineutrophil cytoplasmic antibodies in inflammatory bowel disease. Am J Gastroenterol. 2006;101:2410–22.

97. Markowitz J, Kugathasan S, Dubinsky M, et al. Age of diagnosis influences serologic responses in children with Crohn's disease: a possible clue to etiology? Inflamm Bowel Dis. 2009;15:714–9.

98. Young Y, Abreu MT. Advances in the pathogenesis of inflammatory bowel disease. Curr Gastroenterol Rep. 2006;8:470–7

99. Plevy S, Silverberg MS, Lockton S, et al. Combined serological, genetic, and inflammatory markers differentiate non-IBD, Crohn's disease, and ulcerative colitis patients. Inflamm Bowel Dis. 2013;19:1139–48.

100. Targan SR, Landers CJ, Yang H, et al. Antibodies to CBir1 flagellin define a unique response that is associated independently with complicated Crohn's disease. Gastroenterology. 2005;128: 2020–8.

101. Papadakis KA, Yang H, Ippoliti A, et al. Anti-flagellin (CBir1) phenotypic and genetic Crohn's disease associations. Inflamm Bowel Dis. 2007;13:524–30.

102. Mow WS, Vasiliauskas EA, Lin YC, et al. Association of antibody responses to microbial antigens and complications of small bowel Crohn's disease. Gastroenterology. 2004;126:414–24.

103. Amre DK, Lu SE, Costea F, Seidman EG. Utility of serological markers in predicting the early occurrence of complications and surgery in pediatric Crohn's disease patients. Am J Gastroenterol. 2006;101:645–52.

104. Solberg IC, Lygren I, Cvancarova M, et al. Predictive value of serologic markers in a population-based Norwegian cohort with inflammatory bowel disease. Inflamm Bowel Dis. 2009;15:406–14.

105. Zhang Z, Li C, Zhao X, et al. Anti-Saccharomyces cerevisiae antibodies associate with phenotypes and higher risk for surgery in Crohn's disease: a meta-analysis. Dig Dis Sci. 2012;57:2944–54.

106. Dubinsky MC, Lin YC, Dutridge D, et al. Serum immune responses predict rapid disease progression among children with Crohn's disease: immune responses predict disease progression. Am J Gastroenterol. 2006;101:360–7.

107. Dubinsky MC, Kugathasan S, Mei L, et al. Increased immune reactivity predicts aggressive complicating Crohn's disease in children. Clin Gastroenterol Hepatol. 2008;6:1105–11.

108. Lichtenstein GR, Targan SR, Dubinsky MC, et al. Combination of genetic and quantitative serological immune markers are associated with complicated Crohn's disease behavior. Inflamm Bowel Dis. 2011;17:2488–96.

109. Waterman M, Knight J, Dinani A, et al. Predictors of outcome in ulcerative colitis. Inflamm Bowel Dis. 2015;21:2097–105.

110. Dubinsky MC, Mei L, Friedman M, et al. Genome wide association (GWA) predictors of anti-TNFalpha therapeutic responsiveness in pediatric inflammatory bowel disease. Inflamm Bowel Dis. 2010;16:1357–66.

111. Arias MT, Vande Casteele N, Vermeire S, et al. A panel to predict long-term outcome of infliximab therapy for patients with ulcerative colitis. Clin Gastroenterol Hepatol. 2015;13:531–8.

112. Birimberg-Schwartz L, Wilson DC, Kolho KL, et al. pANCA and ASCA in Children with IBD-Unclassified, Crohn's Colitis, and Ulcerative Colitis-A Longitudinal Report from the IBD Porto Group of ESPGHAN. Inflamm Bowel Dis. 2016;22:1908–14.

113. Joossens S, Reinisch W, Vermeire S, et al. The value of serologic markers in indeterminate colitis: a prospective follow-up study. Gastroenterology. 2002;122:1242–7.

114. Fuchizaki U, Machi T, Kaneko S. Clinical challenges and images in GI. Yersinia enterocolitica mesenteric adenitis and terminal ileitis. Gastroenterology. 2006;131:1379. 659

115. Tuohy AM, O'Gorman M, Byington C, Reid B, Jackson WD. Yersinia enterocolitis mimicking Crohn's disease in a toddler. Pediatrics. 1999;104:e36.

116. Meyer AM, Ramzan NN, Loftus Jr EV, Heigh RI, Leighton JA. The diagnostic yield of stool pathogen studies during relapses of inflammatory bowel disease. J Clin Gastroenterol. 2004;38:772–5.

117. Zilberberg MD, Tillotson GS, McDonald C. Clostridium difficile infections among hospitalized children, United States, 1997-2006. Emerg Infect Dis. 2010;16:604–9.

118. Pascarella F, Martinelli M, Miele E, Del Pezzo M, Roscetto E, Staiano A. Impact of Clostridium difficile infection on pediatric inflammatory bowel disease. J Pediatr. 2009;154:854–8.

119. Martinelli M, Strisciuglio C, Veres G, et al. Clostridium difficile and pediatric inflammatory bowel disease: a prospective, comparative, multicenter, ESPGHAN study. Inflamm Bowel Dis. 2014;20:2219–25.

120. Sands BE. Inflammatory bowel disease: past, present, and future. J Gastroenterol. 2007;42:16–25.

121. Baldassarre ME, Altomare MA, Fanelli M, et al. Does calprotectin represent a regulatory factor in host defense or a drug target in inflammatory disease? Endocr Metab Immune Disord Drug Targets. 2007;7:1–5.

122. Bjerke K, Halstensen TS, Jahnsen F, Pulford K, Brandtzaeg P. Distribution of macrophages and granulocytes expressing L1 protein (calprotectin) in human Peyer's patches compared with normal ileal lamina propria and mesenteric lymph nodes. Gut. 1993;34:1357–63.

123. Roseth AG, Fagerhol MK, Aadland E, Schjonsby H. Assessment of the neutrophil dominating protein calprotectin in feces. A methodologic study. Scand J Gastroenterol. 1992;27:793–8.

124. Steinbakk M, Naess-Andresen CF, Lingaas E, Dale I, Brandtzaeg P, Fagerhol MK. Antimicrobial actions of calcium binding leucocyte L1 protein, calprotectin. Lancet. 1990;336:763–5.

125. Roseth AG, Schmidt PN, Fagerhol MK. Correlation between faecal excretion of indium-111-labelled granulocytes and calprotectin, a granulocyte marker protein, in patients with inflammatory bowel disease. Scand J Gastroenterol. 1999;34:50–4.

126. Tibble J, Teahon K, Thjodleifsson B, et al. A simple method for assessing intestinal inflammation in Crohn's disease. Gut. 2000;47:506–13.

127. Fagerberg UL, Loof L, Myrdal U, Hansson LO, Finkel Y. Colorectal inflammation is well predicted by fecal calprotectin in children with gastrointestinal symptoms. J Pediatr Gastroenterol Nutr. 2005;40:450–5.

128. Loftus Jr EV. Clinical perspectives in Crohn's disease. Objective measures of disease activity: alternatives to symptom indices. Rev Gastroenterol Disord. 2007;7(Suppl 2):S8–S16.

129. Angriman I, Scarpa M, D'Inca R, et al. Enzymes in feces: useful markers of chronic inflammatory bowel disease. Clin Chim Acta. 2007;381:63–8.

130. Tibble JA, Sigthorsson G, Foster R, Forgacs I, Bjarnason I. Use of surrogate markers of inflammation and Rome criteria to distinguish organic from nonorganic intestinal disease. Gastroenterology. 2002;123:450–60.

131. Carroccio A, Iacono G, Cottone M, et al. Diagnostic accuracy of fecal calprotectin assay in distinguishing organic causes of chronic diarrhea from irritable bowel syndrome: a prospective study in adults and children. Clin Chem. 2003;49:861–7.

132. van Rheenen PF, Van de Vijver E, Fidler V. Faecal calprotectin for screening of patients with suspected inflammatory bowel disease: diagnostic meta-analysis. BMJ. 2010;341:c3369.

133. Menees SB, Powell C, Kurlander J, Goel A, Chey WD. A meta-analysis of the utility of C-reactive protein, erythrocyte sedimentation rate, fecal calprotectin, and fecal lactoferrin to exclude inflammatory bowel disease in adults with IBS. Am J Gastroenterol. 2015;110:444–54.

134. Langhorst J, Elsenbruch S, Koelzer J, Rueffer A, Michalsen A, Dobos GJ. Noninvasive markers in the assessment of intestinal inflammation in inflammatory bowel diseases: performance of fecal lactoferrin, calprotectin, and PMN-elastase, CRP, and clinical indices. Am J Gastroenterol. 2008;103:162–9.

135. Schoepfer AM, Trummler M, Seeholzer P, Seibold-Schmid B, Seibold F. Discriminating IBD from IBS: comparison of the test performance of fecal markers, blood leukocytes, CRP, and IBD antibodies. Inflamm Bowel Dis. 2008;14:32–9.

136. Bunn SK, Bisset WM, Main MJ, Golden BE. Fecal calprotectin as a measure of disease activity in childhood inflammatory bowel disease. J Pediatr Gastroenterol Nutr. 2001;32:171–7.

137. Sidler MA, Leach ST, Day AS. Fecal S100A12 and fecal calprotectin as noninvasive markers for inflammatory bowel disease in children. Inflamm Bowel Dis. 2008;14:359–66.

138. Diamanti A, Panetta F, Basso MS, et al. Diagnostic work-up of inflammatory bowel disease in children: the role of calprotectin assay. Inflamm Bowel Dis. 2010;16:1926–30.

139. Degraeuwe PL, Beld MP, Ashorn M, et al. Faecal calprotectin in suspected paediatric inflammatory bowel disease. J Pediatr Gastroenterol Nutr. 2015;60:339–46.

140. Henderson P, Anderson NH, Wilson DC. The diagnostic accuracy of fecal calprotectin during the investigation of suspected pediatric inflammatory bowel disease: a systematic review and meta-analysis. Am J Gastroenterol. 2014;109:637–45.

141. Shaoul R, Sladek M, Turner D, et al. Limitations of fecal calprotectin at diagnosis in untreated pediatric Crohn's disease. Inflamm Bowel Dis. 2012;18:1493–7.

142. Henderson P, Casey A, Lawrence SJ, et al. The diagnostic accuracy of fecal calprotectin during the investigation of suspected pediatric inflammatory bowel disease. Am J Gastroenterol. 2012;107:941–9.

143. Yang Z, Clark N, Park KT. Effectiveness and cost-effectiveness of measuring fecal calprotectin in diagnosis of inflammatory bowel disease in adults and children. Clin Gastroenterol Hepatol. 2014;12:253–62. e2

144. Canani RB, Terrin G, Rapacciuolo L, et al. Faecal calprotectin as reliable non-invasive marker to assess the severity of mucosal inflammation in children with inflammatory bowel disease. Dig Liver Dis. 2008;40:547–53.

145. Aomatsu T, Yoden A, Matsumoto K, et al. Fecal calprotectin is a useful marker for disease activity in pediatric patients with inflammatory bowel disease. Dig Dis Sci. 2011;56:2372–7.

146. Zubin G, Peter L. Predicting endoscopic Crohn's disease activity before and after induction therapy in children: a comprehensive assessment of PCDAI, CRP, and fecal calprotectin. Inflamm Bowel Dis. 2015;21:1386–91.

147. D'Haens G, Ferrante M, Vermeire S, et al. Fecal calprotectin is a surrogate marker for endoscopic lesions in inflammatory bowel disease. Inflamm Bowel Dis. 2012;18:2218–24.

148. Walkiewicz D, Werlin SL, Fish D, Scanlon M, Hanaway P, Kugathasan S. Fecal calprotectin is useful in predicting disease relapse in pediatric inflammatory bowel disease. Inflamm Bowel Dis. 2008;14:669–73.

149. Gisbert JP, Bermejo F, Perez-Calle JL, et al. Fecal calprotectin and lactoferrin for the prediction of inflammatory bowel disease relapse. Inflamm Bowel Dis. 2009;15:1190–8.

150. Sugi K, Saitoh O, Hirata I, Katsu K. Fecal lactoferrin as a marker for disease activity in inflammatory bowel disease: comparison with other neutrophil-derived proteins. Am J Gastroenterol. 1996;91:927–34.

151. Walker TR, Land ML, Kartashov A, et al. Fecal lactoferrin is a sensitive and specific marker of disease activity in children and young adults with inflammatory bowel disease. J Pediatr Gastroenterol Nutr. 2007;44:414–22.

152. Pfefferkorn MD, Boone JH, Nguyen JT, Juliar BE, Davis MA, Parker KK. Utility of fecal lactoferrin in identifying Crohn disease activity in children. J Pediatr Gastroenterol Nutr. 2010;51:425–8.

153. Zhou XL, Xu W, Tang XX, et al. Fecal lactoferrin in discriminating inflammatory bowel disease from irritable bowel syndrome: a diagnostic meta-analysis. BMC Gastroenterol. 2014;14:121.

154. Buderus S, Boone J, Lyerly D, Lentze MJ. Fecal lactoferrin: a new parameter to monitor infliximab therapy. Dig Dis Sci. 2004;49:1036–9.

Fecal Biomarkers in Inflammatory Bowel Disease

19

Jennifer Damman and K.T. Park

Introduction

Inflammatory bowel diseases (IBDs), including ulcerative colitis (UC) and Crohn disease (CD), are chronic relapsing and remitting diseases due to intestinal inflammation. Endoscopic evaluation and histologic confirmation are required for diagnosis and are often used to monitor disease progression and response to therapy. After diagnosis of IBD, clinical disease remission is the goal of therapy; however, evidence suggests that mucosal healing is the outcome measure of choice [1–3]. While endoscopic confirmation is the gold standard in detecting mucosal healing [4], repeated endoscopy is costly and invasive. Because serial endoscopies to monitor disease activity is unrealistic, especially in children who require general anesthesia for endoscopic procedures, many gastroenterologists rely on surrogate markers of inflammation. These include serologic biomarkers (e.g. C-reactive protein (CRP), erythrocyte sedimentation rate (ESR)), clinical disease activity indices (e.g. CDAI, Pediatric Crohn's disease Activity Index (PCDAI)), and patient-reported symptoms. While these indices can be helpful in the diagnosis and monitoring of IBD, they have low specificity for accurate endoscopic correlation. Because inflamed mucosa contains a high number of neutrophils, fecal neutrophil-derived biomarkers such as fecal calprotectin (FC, structure shown in Fig. 19.1) and lactoferrin have emerged as promising tools to accurately assess mucosal-level inflammation to aid in the diagnosis and monitoring of IBD [6].

The goal of this chapter is to summarize current literature on the clinically available fecal biomarkers used in IBD practice. Of these biomarkers, FC and lactoferrin are the two most frequently studied. FC in particular has been extensively studied and shown to have sufficient sensitivity and specificity for detecting mucosal inflammation. This chapter will focus on FC because of the clinical utility and increasing use in clinical practice. This includes the diagnosis of IBD, monitoring of disease activity, response to pharmacologic therapy, detecting mucosal inflammation, and predicting relapse [7, 8–13]. We will also discuss the use of FC in distinguishing between symptoms caused by IBD and those due to other causes, such as irritable bowel syndrome (IBS) [11, 14–16]. Table 19.1 summarizes other available fecal biomarkers.

Fecal biomarkers play an important role in helping guide clinical decision making in patients with suspected or confirmed IBD. These surrogate markers of inflammation, with their ease of collection and relatively low cost, can be widely used in the diagnosis and long-term monitoring of IBD, with the potential to reduce the number of invasive and costly endoscopic procedures and improve patient outcomes.

Fecal Calprotectin Use in Distinguishing Irritable Bowel Syndrome from Inflammatory Bowel Disease

Irritable bowel syndrome (IBS) is a highly prevalent disorder, affecting an estimated 10–15% of the population [38], and accounts for up to 25% of a gastroenterologist's time in the outpatient setting [39]. IBS patients are also reported to utilize health care resources disproportionately to the seriousness of their symptoms [40]. In a study to estimate total costs for patients with IBS, functional diarrhea, functional constipation, and functional abdominal pain, Nyrop et al. found that the mean annual direct health care costs were $5049, $6140, $7522, and $7646, respectively [41]. There are many symptoms that overlap in patients with IBS and IBD (e.g., abdominal pain, bloating, diarrhea). Additionally, studies have found the prevalence of IBS in patients with IBD to be as high as 39% [42]. This overlap makes the treatment of IBD symptoms due to true intestinal inflammation difficult. Because IBD management relies on patient reported

J. Damman, MD • K.T. Park, MD, MS (✉)
Stanford Children's Inflammatory Bowel Disease Center,
Department of Pediatrics, Stanford, CA, USA
e-mail: ktpark@stanford.edu

© Springer International Publishing AG 2017
P. Mamula et al. (eds.), *Pediatric Inflammatory Bowel Disease*, DOI 10.1007/978-3-319-49215-5_19

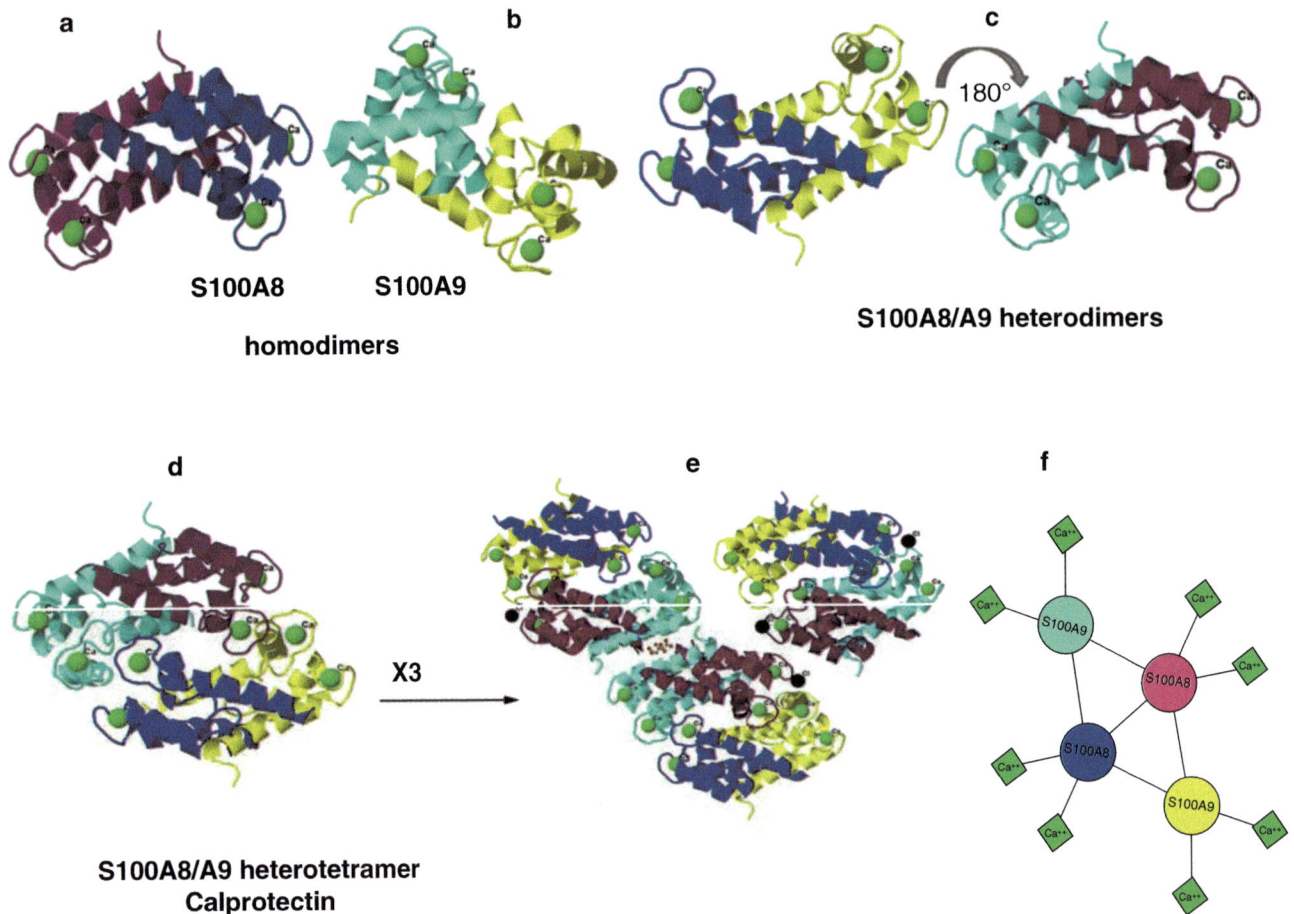

Fig. 19.1 Fecal calprotectin (Taken from Vogl et al. [5]) Tertiary and quaternary structures of S100A8 and S100A9 proteins presented by ribbon diagrams: (**a**) S100A8 homodimer; individual subunits are shown in *purple* and *dark blue*; (**b**) S100A9 homodimer; subunits are shown in *sea-blue* and *yellow*; (**c**) S100A8/A9 heterodimers shown in two projections rotated by 180°; (**d**) S100A8/A9 heterotetramer calprotectin and (**e**) S100A8/A9 dodecamer assembled from three calprotectins; (**f**) Schematic outline of the arrangements of S100SA8 and S100A9 in calprotectin. Subunits are presented in individual colors as in (**a**, **b**). Bound Ca^{2+} ions are shown by *green spheres* or *squares*, respectively

outcomes, this can lead to both overtreatment of IBS and undertreatment of IBD.

Given its ease of collection and analysis, low cost, and high sensitivity in detecting intestinal inflammation, FC is currently being used as a screening tool to differentiate between IBD and IBS, possibly decreasing the number of unnecessary diagnostic endoscopies. Because of the many overlapping symptoms between IBD and IBS, many patients with IBS undergo endoscopic evaluation, which is an invasive and costly evaluation [43]. Tibble et al. performed a prospective study to assess the value of FC in discriminating between patients with Crohn disease and IBS [10]. Results of this study showed that all patients with CD had increased FC (median 135 mg/L), which differed significantly from normal controls and patients with IBS. At a cutoff level of 30 mg/L, FC had a 100% sensitivity and 97% specificity in discriminating between active CD and IBS. FC was therefore found to be a useful biomarker to differentiate between symptoms due to IBD versus other noninflammatory states.

In a meta-analysis by van Rheenen et al. that included both adult and pediatric patients, quantitative FC was found to be a useful screening tool for identifying patients who warrant endoscopy for suspected IBD [11]. This meta-analysis showed that screening by measuring FC resulted in a 67% reduction in the number of adults requiring endoscopy, and a reduction of 35% in children. This study also highlighted a downside of using FC as a screening method in that it led to a delayed diagnosis in 6% of adults and 8% of children with IBD due to false negative results. This study also found that FC had a lower specificity in children when compared to adults [11]. However, in a more recent meta-analysis by Henderson et al. that included two newer pediatric studies, with the strict selection of only children undergoing their primary investigation for IBD, sensitivity was found to be increased,

Table 19.1 Mechanism of action

Fecal biomarker	Description
Calprotectin	Calprotectin is a member of the S100 family of calcium and zinc binding proteins that constitutes 60% of the neutrophil cytosolic protein [17]. When inflammatory epithelial cells die, calprotectin is released into the intestinal lumen in a non-degraded, calcium-bound form. Functions include antibacterial and antifungal activity, inhibition of metalloproteinases, and induction of apoptosis. It is resistant to bacterial degradation, reliably measured by ELISA, and has been shown to have a strong correlation with active inflammation in the gut [18]. Normal cut-off varies from 50 to 200 mcg/g. A rapid point-of-care (POC) test is available. FC is simple to collect and there are now in-home collection methods available. Samples can also be kept for up to 7 days in room temperature prior to laboratory measurement [19], making home collection more user-friendly for patients
S100A12	Like calprotectin, S100A12 is another member of the calcium and zinc-binding S100 protein family. It is expressed as a cytoplasmic protein in activated neutrophils [17], and contributes to leukocyte recruitment into inflamed mucosa [18]. Has been studied in adults and pediatric patients with UC, and studies have shown sensitivities up to 90% and specificity of 100% in discriminating IBD from IBS patients. It remains stable at room temperature for 7 days. Has not been widely used in clinical practice, likely because it has not been shown to be superior to the more commonly used calprotectin test [18]
Lactoferrin	An iron-binding 80-kD glycoprotein produced by secretory epithelium that is found in many body fluids, including milk, sputum, CSF and seminal fluid [17], and in intestinal epithelial cells. It is a major component of neutrophil secondary granules and is released during neutrophil degradation directly into the bloodstream or inflammatory areas [10]. It does not get digested in GI tract, is stable at room temperature for 7 days (although less stable than calprotectin [18]) and remains stable if frozen. Has bacteriostatic, bactericidal, antiviral and antifungal properties [20]. Cutoff level most commonly used is 7.25 mcg/g in adults and 29 mcg/g in children aged 2–9 years. A rapid POC test is available [18]
Pyruvate Kinase (M2-PK)	A heterodimer of pyruvate kinase (an enzyme of the glycolytic pathway) that is expressed in rapidly dividing cells in both serum and feces. It was originally used as a marker of cell turnover for the screening of colonic carcinoma, polyps and adenomas [21]. Has been studied as a potential biomarker of active IBD due to rapid cell turnover seen in IBD. Has been shown to accurately differentiate active inflammation versus inactive disease in patients with IBD, and can distinguish IBD from nonorganic disease in children [22]. Commercial feasibility is limited due to relatively short stability of 2 days [18]
Neopterin	A byproduct of the tetrahydropbiopterin (BH4) biosynthetic pathway [23]. Increased plasma neopterin is considered to be an early and sensitive biomarker of the inflammatory response for viral infections, certain malignancies, allograft rejection, autoimmune and neurodegenerative diseases. It is found in plasma and CSF [23–26]
Metalloproteinases	The human matrix metalloproteinases (MMPs) are a family of 24 zinc dependent endopeptides [27]. Recognized as key regulators of cell function through cleavage of cytokines, chemokines, receptors, proteases, and adhesion molecules to alter their function [27–29]. MMPs are released from neutrophils of the intestinal mucosa in patients with active IBD and has been shown to be elevated in colonic biopsies from patients with active UC [18]. Fecal MMP-9 levels have been reported to correlate with Mayo and endoscopic scores, serum CRP and FC in patients with UC [30]. Serum MMP-9 also has been found to correlate with disease activity in UC and CD, however there was a significant difference between UC and CD so further studies need to be done to determine usefulness as biomarkers for active IBD [27, 31]
Myeloperoxidases	Myeloperoxidase (MPO) plays an important role in the microbicidal activity of phagocytes. MPO is released into the phagosome from cytoplasmic granules of neutrophils and monocytes via degranulation. The primary function of MPO is to kill microorganisms but MPO can also be released to the outside of cells, where it can contribute to pathogenesis of disease [32]
Polymorphonuclear neutrophilic leukocyte elastase (PMN-e)	One of the serine proteases found in the azurophilic granules of neutrophils. Studies have suggested PMN-e is involved in pathologic processes of many inflammatory diseases due to their involvement in endothelial injury, inflammatory processes, and fibrosis [33–36]
Fecal immunochemical test (FIT)	Quantitative FITs measure fecal hemoglobin concentrations using an antibody specific for human hemoglobin. FIT has the advantage of rapid measurement of amount of blood in fecal samples, as it was originally used as a rapid screening test for colorectal cancer. It has low cost when compared to other fecal markers and has been shown to have as high sensitivity as FC for mucosal healing in UC patient. Inokuchi et al. found that both FIT and FC correlated with endoscopic features of CD patients, however FIT had very poor ability to detect disease limited to small bowel in CD patients [37]

whereas specificity was slightly decreased [14]. In this meta-analysis, which included a total of 715 pediatric patients, FC was found to have a very high sensitivity of 98% and a moderate specificity of 68% in the diagnosis of suspected pediatric IBD [14].

In a meta-analysis by von Roon et al. assessing the diagnostic precision of FC in IBD, FC was found to potentially discriminate between patients with IBD and those without IBD for both adult and pediatric populations [44]. A cutoff of 100 mcg/g was found to be more precise than a cutoff of

50 mcg/g. FC was found to have a good diagnostic precision in predicting relapse in IBD, and the precision of FC for the diagnosis of IBD was found to be superior to serological markers such as CRP, ESR, anti-saccharomyces cerevisiae antibodies (ASCA), anti-neutrophil cytoplasmic antibodies (ANCA), and outer membrane protein c (OmpC).

Park et al. compared the cost effectiveness of measuring FC before endoscopy in adult and pediatric patients with suspected IBD versus direct endoscopy alone, which is the current standard of care [45]. Results showed that screening adults and children to measure FC is effective and cost-effective in identifying patients with IBD when the pretest probability is <75% for adults and >65% in children. This analysis, using data from van Rheenen et al. [11], showed that in adults, FC screening saved $417 per patient but delayed diagnosis for 2 of the 32 patients who had IBD among 100 screened patients. In children, FC screening saved $300/patient but delayed diagnosis for 5 of the 61 patients who had IBD among 100 screened patients. If direct endoscopic evaluation remains standard of care for diagnosis of IBD, it would cost an additional $18,955 in adults and $6250 in children to avoid one false-negative result from FC screening [45]. These studies highlight that FC can be used to distinguish disorders of intestinal inflammation versus other noninflammatory disorders that may mimic IBD.

Fecal Calprotectin for Inflammatory Bowel Disease

Calprotectin Levels Correspond Directly with Endoscopic Activity

There is growing evidence to support mucosal healing as the outcome measure of choice in IBD [2, 46, 47–49, 50]. It has been shown that mucosal healing indicates better disease outcomes [1–3], reduced risk of relapse and reduced development of cancer and need for surgery in UC [49]. Evaluation of mucosal healing, however, requires endoscopy for direct visualization and histopathologic confirmation, which is costly and invasive. Targeting mucosal healing in children is particularly difficult given the invasive nature of frequent endoscopies that require general anesthesia. Given the impracticality of serial endoscopies, clinicians rely on other surrogate markers of clinical disease activity, including Clinical Disease Activity Index (CDAI), Pediatric Crohn's Disease Activity Index (PCDAI), Simple Clinical Colitis Activity Index, Mayo Clinic score, as well as serum and fecal biomarkers of inflammation such as CRP, ESR, FC, and lactoferrin. Because scoring mechanisms give substantive weight to subjective patient-reported symptoms, the use of these activity indices to guide therapy has recently been questioned since subjective patient reports do not always correlate with mucosal-level disease activity.

Serum surrogate markers such as CRP and ESR have been used to monitor disease activity in IBD; however, the relationship between these markers and disease activity is not fully understood [47, 51–57, 58]. Although widely used and readily available, a significant limitation of most biomarkers of inflammation is that they are nonspecific and can be elevated in many other non-intestinal diseases. CRP is a widely used marker and previous studies have examined the relationship between CRP and other clinical measures of disease activity in IBD [9, 47, 53, 54, 59, 60]. CRP has been found to be associated with clinical and endoscopic activity in IBD [7, 47, 61] but has been shown to have poor sensitivity for endoscopic activity in patients with IBD [62]. CRP also has been shown to be persistently normal in patients with CD despite active disease, making this a poor test to differentiate quiescent from active CD [52]. In a retrospective study examining the relationship between CRP and clinical, endoscopic, histologic, and radiographic activity in IBD, Solem et al. [62] found that CRP elevation was significantly associated with active clinical disease, other biomarkers of inflammation, and active disease at ileocolonoscopy in patients with CD. However, this study showed that 63% of CD patients with active clinical disease and a normal CRP had active disease by ileocolonoscopy. Furthermore, there was no association between CRP and radiographic activity. This study found that in patients with UC, while CRP elevation was significantly associated with clinical disease activity, biomarkers of inflammation and active disease at ileocolonoscopy, CRP concentrations were not associated with histologic activity in UC patients. In a review by Lewis et al. studying the role of several biomarkers in assessing endoscopic activity in IBD, FC showed the best correlation with endoscopic activity in both CD and UC [63]. Schoepfer et al. showed that FC correlated closest with the widely used Simple Endoscopic Score for Crohn's disease (SES-CD), followed by CRP, blood leukocytes, and the CDAI [9]. This study also showed that FC was the only biomarker that reliably discriminated inactive from mild, moderate, and highly active disease, highlighting the usefulness of FC in monitoring disease activity.

FC has also emerged as a potential surrogate marker that can be used to predict mucosal healing, which has become the outcome measurement of choice in monitoring IBD [1–3]. Lobaton et al. showed a significant correlation between FC levels and endoscopic activity in patients with UC [64]. In this study, a cutoff value of 250 mcg/g for Fecal Calprotectin ELISA (FC-ELISA) or a 280 mcg/g cutoff level for Fecal Calprotectin quantitative point of care test (FC-QPOCT) was found to be a more accurate marker of endoscopic activity than both clinical activity and measurement of other frequently used biomarkers. FC was shown to be an accurate biomarker of both "endoscopic remission" and "no endoscopic activity" (Mayo endoscopic subscore grade ≤1 and ≤ 0, respectively) [64]. In another study assessing the value of FC as a surrogate marker of mucosal inflammation, D'Haens et al. concluded that FC was the best available surrogate marker for the presence of mucosal inflammation and therefore should be considered a useful alternative to repeated endoscopic evaluations [46]. In this study, endoscopic scores correlated significantly with the level of fecal calprotectin in both CD and UC. Of note, this study reported median FC level of 465 mcg/g in UC patients, 175 mcg/g in CD patients, and 45 mcg/g in patients with IBS. In a recent study examining FC correlation with histologic remission and mucosal healing in IBD, Zittan et al. found that FC below 100 mcg/g was highly correlated with histologic remission and absence of basal plasmacytosis in both UC and CD, and a level <100 mcg/g had the highest sensitivity in terms of clinical and endoscopic remission for both CD and UC [65]. In a recent study by Langhorst et al., results showed that fecal biomarkers FC, lactoferrin, and Polymorphonuclear neutrophil (PMN)-elastase were able to distinguish between UC patients with mucosal healing from clinical remission and mild disease, showed significant correlations with endoscopy, and were predictive of flare [66]. These studies highlight the potential role of fecal biomarkers, FC in particular, in predicting endoscopic activity, which can potentially reduce the number of endoscopies performed for monitoring of mucosal healing.

Calprotectin Predicts IBD Relapse

Inflammatory bowel diseases are chronic diseases of inflammation that have a typical relapsing and remitting courses [67]. The primary goal of management is to prevent relapses and increase periods of remission. Because subclinical inflammation can lead to relapse [68], noninvasive biomarkers and clinical activity indices have been used in an attempt to predict relapses. Unfortunately, many widely used inflammatory markers have poor specificity and do not predict relapse [63, 47, 52, 62], and clinical disease indices (e.g., CDAI) have been shown to not correlate with disease activity [12]. FC has been proposed as the gold standard in noninvasive testing to evaluate intestinal inflammation in patients with IBD [10, 69–71] and has been shown to accurately predict relapse [12, 72–74].

The use of FC to predict relapse in patients with IBD could be particularly useful in initiating treatment in an earlier stage of relapse, even before onset of symptoms, to lessen severity of relapse and prolong periods between relapses. Many serum biomarkers, such as CRP, ESR, platelet count, white cell count, interleukin (IL)-1β, and tumor necrosis factor alpha (TNFα) have been used to help predict relapse in IBD. However, these markers are nonspecific and do not directly measure intestinal inflammation [72]. In a prospective study examining clinical, biologic, and histologic parameters as predictors of relapse in UC, Bitton et al. found that ESR, CRP, IL-β, IL-6, and IL-15 did not predict relapse in patients with quiescent

UC [47]. Tibble et al. found that FC predicts clinical relapse of disease activity in patients with both CD and UC [72]. Results of this study showed that a single FC level of >50 mg/L predicted clinical relapse with a 90% sensitivity and 83% specificity. In another prospective, randomized, controlled trial evaluating utility of serially measured FC, CRP, and CDAI in predicting endoscopic recurrence in CD patients after intestinal resection, Wright et al. showed that patients with endoscopic recurrence had higher FC values [12]. The study showed that 6- and 18-month FC levels correlated significantly with presence and severity of endoscopic recurrence, whereas CRP level and the CDAI did not. A FC cutoff of >100 mcg/g identified patients with endoscopic recurrence with an 89% sensitivity and 58% specificity [12].

Some studies have suggested that FC is less predictive of relapse in patients with CD compared to UC, or with ileal CD compared with colonic and ileocolonic CD [73–75]. Therefore, patients may need stratification based on phenotype to improve predictive value of FC in CD [74, 75]. In a study by Kallel et al. investigators showed when patients with CD confined to small bowel were excluded, FC levels above 340 μg/g had an almost 19-fold greater risk of relapse than those with lower concentrations [76]. Costa et al. found FC to be a stronger predictor of clinical relapse in UC than in CD [61]. In this study, investigators found that among IBD patients in clinical remission with a high FC >150 mcg/g, 50% of CD patients maintained remission compared with 19% of those with UC. This is in contrast to a study by Tibble et al. that showed FC was an equally reliable predictor of relapse in UC and CD [72]. Of note, in the study by Costa et al., it was also found that ESR and CRP did not prove to be useful predictors of clinical relapse in IBD as a whole [61].

Calprotectin Predicts Drug Responsiveness

FC has also been shown to predict response to medical therapy in patients with IBD [77]. De Vos et al. performed a study to evaluate the evolution of FC levels under infliximab induction therapy and its correlation with mucosal healing as compared to Mayo score in patients with UC [77]. Results showed that median FC levels decreased from 1260 mg/kg at baseline to 72.5 mg/kg at 10 weeks. After 10 weeks, infliximab therapy induced endoscopic remission and a decrease in FC to <50 mg/kg or at least 80% decrease from baseline level in 58% of patients. Furthermore, all patients with a FC level <50 mg/kg were found to be in endoscopic remission. This study highlighted the fast and sharp decrease in FC levels after Infliximab infusion, as well as showing the absence of this decrease identifies patients who may be nonresponders.

In a recent post hoc analysis by Sanborn et al., FC was found to correlate with clinical and endoscopic outcomes of patients with moderate to severe UC receiving tofacitinib (a JAK inhibitor) [8]. While this study found a strong correlation between FC and other clinical measurement outcomes at a population level, this was less strong at an individual level, likely due to high inter- and intrapatient variability in FC concentrations. These studies highlight the potential use of FC as a predictor of drug responsiveness, which could help guide therapeutic treatment options for patients with IBD.

On the Horizon: Monitoring

Although disease monitoring is common in clinical practice across specialties, the principles of monitoring are not well conceptualized, which can lead to suboptimal care [78]. In patients with IBD, disease monitoring strategies should focus on the judicious use of tests and procedures to accurately monitor disease progression, monitor response to medical therapy, reduce risk, prevent relapse, reduce costs, and improve patient care. The current outcome measure of choice in patients with IBD is mucosal healing [1, 2, 49], and direct endoscopic visualization and histologic evidence is gold standard in detecting mucosal healing.

Because repeated endoscopy is invasive and costly, IBD practitioners rely on non-invasive tools for disease monitoring, including physician-dependent global disease assessments, patient reported symptoms, clinical disease activity indices, and trends in serum biomarkers such as CRP and ESR to estimate mucosal-level inflammation. Fecal biomarkers have emerged as potentially superior surrogate markers to guide clinical decision making in patients with suspected or confirmed IBD. They are simple, non-invasive, low-cost, and many studies have shown superior accuracy and sensitivity when compared to other disease monitoring strategies. The most extensively studied and frequently used fecal biomarker in current clinical practice is FC. Although large-scale studies are required to definitively evaluate the role of FC in early and accurate detection of mucosal-level inflammation [79], FC has emerged as a superior marker that can be used for long-term monitoring in patients with IBD to accurately detect mucosal level healing and to guide clinical decision making without repeated invasive endoscopy.

References

1. Colombel JF, Rutgeerts P, Reinisch W, Esser D, Wang Y, et al. Early mucosal healing with infliximab is associated with improved long-term clinical outcomes in ulcerative colitis. Gastroenterology. 2011;141:1194–201.
2. KF F, Jahnsen J, BA M, MH V, Group I. Mucosal healing in inflammatory bowel disease: results from a Norwegian population-based cohort. Gastroenterol. 2007;133:412–22.
3. Meucci G, Fasoli R, Saibeni S, Valpiani D, Gullotta R, et al. Prognostic significance of endoscopic remission in patients with active ulcerative colitis treated with oral and topical mesalazine: a prospective, multicenter study. Inflamm Bowel Dis. 2012;18:1006–10.
4. Stange EF, Travis SP, Vermeire S, Beglinger C, Kupcinkas L, et al. European evidence based consensus on the diagnosis and management of Crohn's disease: definitions and diagnosis. Gut. 2006;55(Suppl 1):i1–15.
5. Vogl T, Gharibyan AL, Morozova-Roche LA. Pro-inflammatory S100A8 and S100A9 proteins: self-assembly into multifunctional native and amyloid complexes. Int J Mol Sci. 2012;13:2893–917.
6. Abraham BP, Kane S. Fecal markers: calprotectin and lactoferrin. Gastroenterol Clin N Am. 2012;41:483–95.
7. Schoepfer AM, Lewis JD. Serial fecal calprotectin measurements to detect endoscopic recurrence in postoperative Crohn's disease: is colonoscopic surveillance no longer needed? Gastroenterology. 2015;148:889–92.
8. Sandborn WJ, Panes J, Zhang H, Yu D, Niezychowski W, Su C. Correlation between concentrations of fecal calprotectin and outcomes of patients with ulcerative colitis in a phase 2 trial. Gastroenterology. 2016;150:96–102.
9. Schoepfer AM, Beglinger C, Straumann A, Trummler M, Vavricka SR, et al. Fecal calprotectin correlates more closely with the simple endoscopic score for Crohn's disease (SES-CD) than CRP, blood leukocytes, and the CDAI. Am J Gastroenterol. 2010;105:162–9.
10. Tibble J, Teahon K, Thjodleifsson B, Roseth A, Sigthorsson G, et al. A simple method for assessing intestinal inflammation in Crohn's disease. Gut. 2000;47:506–13.
11. van Rheenen PF, Van de Vijver E, Fidler V. Faecal calprotectin for screening of patients with suspected inflammatory bowel disease: diagnostic meta-analysis. BMJ. 2010;341:c3369.
12. Wright EK, Kamm MA, De Cruz P, Hamilton AL, Ritchie KJ, et al. Measurement of fecal calprotectin improves monitoring and detection of recurrence of Crohn's disease after surgery. Gastroenterology. 2015;148:938–47.e1.
13. Yang Z, Clark N, Park KT. Effectiveness and cost-effectiveness of measuring fecal calprotectin in diagnosis of inflammatory bowel disease in adults and children. Clin Gastroenterol Hepatol. 2014;12:253–62.e2.
14. Henderson P, Anderson NH, Wilson DC. The diagnostic accuracy of fecal calprotectin during the investigation of suspected pediatric inflammatory bowel disease: a systematic review and meta-analysis. Am J Gastroenterol. 2014;109:637–45.
15. Tibble JA, Sigthorsson G, Foster R, Forgacs I, Bjarnason I. Use of surrogate markers of inflammation and Rome criteria to distinguish organic from nonorganic intestinal disease. Gastroenterology. 2002;123:450–60.
16. Van de Vijver E, Schreuder AB, Cnossen WR, Muller Kobold AC, van Rheenen PF, North Netherlands Pediatric IBDC. Safely ruling out inflammatory bowel disease in children and teenagers without referral for endoscopy. Arch Dis Child. 2012;97:1014–8.
17. Wright EK, Kamm MA, De Cruz P, Hamilton AL, Ritchie KJ, et al. Comparison of fecal inflammatory markers in Crohn's disease. Inflamm Bowel Dis. 2016;22(5):1086–94.
18. Kopylov U, Rosenfeld G, Bressler B, Seidman E. Clinical utility of fecal biomarkers for the diagnosis and management of inflammatory bowel disease. Inflamm Bowel Dis. 2014;20:742–56.
19. RØseth AG, Fagerhol MK, Aadland E, Schjønsby H. Assessment of the neutrophil dominating protein calprotectin in feces: a Methodologic Study. Scand J Gastroenterol. 1992;27:793–8.
20. Klimczak K, Lykowska-Szuber L, Eder P, Krela-Kazmierczak I, Stawczyk-Eder K, et al. The diagnostic usefulness of fecal lactoferrin in the assessment of Crohn's disease activity. Eur J Intern Med. 2015;26:623–7.
21. Roszak D, Galecka M, Cichy W, Szachta P. Determination of faecal inflammatory marker concentration as a noninvasive method of evaluation of pathological activity in children with inflammatory bowel diseases. Adv Med Sci. 2015;60:246–52.

22. Chung-Faye G, Hayee B, Maestranzi S, Donaldson N, Forgacs I, Sherwood R. Fecal M2-pyruvate kinase (M2-PK): a novel marker of intestinal inflammation. Inflamm Bowel Dis. 2007;13:1374–8.
23. Ghisoni K, Martins Rde P, Barbeito L, Latini A. Neopterin as a potential cytoprotective brain molecule. J Psychiatr Res. 2015;71:134–9.
24. Parker DC, Mielke MM, Yu Q, Rosenberg PB, Jain A, et al. Plasma neopterin level as a marker of peripheral immune activation in amnestic mild cognitive impairment and Alzheimer's disease. Int J Geriatr Psychiatry. 2013;28:149–54.
25. Widner B, Leblhuber F, Fuchs D. Increased neopterin production and tryptophan degradation in advanced Parkinson's disease. J Neural Transm (Vienna). 2002;109:181–9.
26. Wirleitner B, Reider D, Ebner S, Bock G, Widner B, et al. Monocyte-derived dendritic cells release neopterin. J Leukoc Biol. 2002;72:1148–53.
27. O'Sullivan S, Gilmer JF, Medina C. Matrix metalloproteinases in inflammatory bowel disease: an update. Mediat Inflamm. 2015;2015:964131.
28. Rodriguez D, Morrison CJ, Overall CM. Matrix metalloproteinases: what do they not do? New substrates and biological roles identified by murine models and proteomics. Biochim Biophys Acta. 2010;1803:39–54.
29. Sternlicht MD, Werb Z. How matrix metalloproteinases regulate cell behavior. Annu Rev Cell Dev Biol. 2001;17:463–516.
30. Annahazi A, Molnar T, Farkas K, Rosztoczy A, Izbeki F, et al. Fecal MMP-9: a new noninvasive differential diagnostic and activity marker in ulcerative colitis. Inflamm Bowel Dis. 2013;19:316–20.
31. Matusiewicz M, Neubauer K, Mierzchala-Pasierb M, Gamian A, Krzystek-Korpacka M. Matrix metalloproteinase-9: its interplay with angiogenic factors in inflammatory bowel diseases. Dis Markers. 2014;2014:643645.
32. Klebanoff SJ. Myeloperoxidase: friend and foe. J Leukoc Biol. 2005;77:598–625.
33. Chua F, Laurent GJ. Neutrophil elastase: mediator of extracellular matrix destruction and accumulation. Proc Am Thorac Soc. 2006;3:424–7.
34. Doring G. The role of neutrophil elastase in chronic inflammation. Am J Respir Crit Care Med. 1994;150:S114–7.
35. Hara T, Ogawa F, Yanaba K, Iwata Y, Muroi E, et al. Elevated serum concentrations of polymorphonuclear neutrophilic leukocyte elastase in systemic sclerosis: association with pulmonary fibrosis. J Rheumatol. 2009;36:99–105.
36. Janoff A. Elastase in tissue injury. Annu Rev Med. 1985;36:207–16.
37. Inokuchi T, Kato J, Hiraoka S, Takashima S, Nakarai A, et al. Fecal immunochemical test versus fecal calprotectin for prediction of mucosal healing in Crohn's disease. Inflamm Bowel Dis. 2016;22(5):1078–85.
38. Saito YA, Schoenfeld P, Locke 3rd GR. The epidemiology of irritable bowel syndrome in North America: a systematic review. Am J Gastroenterol. 2002;97:1910–5.
39. Harvey RF, Salih SY, Read AE. Organic and functional disorders in 2000 gastroenterology outpatients. Lancet. 1983;1:632–4.
40. Russo MW, Wei JT, Thiny MT, Gangarosa LM, Brown A, et al. Digestive and liver diseases statistics, 2004. Gastroenterology. 2004;126:1448–53.
41. Nyrop KA, Palsson OS, Levy RL, Von Korff M, Feld AD, et al. Costs of health care for irritable bowel syndrome, chronic constipation, functional diarrhoea and functional abdominal pain. Aliment Pharmacol Ther. 2007;26:237–48.
42. Halpin SJ, Ford AC. Prevalence of symptoms meeting criteria for irritable bowel syndrome in inflammatory bowel disease: systematic review and meta-analysis. Am J Gastroenterol. 2012;107:1474–82.
43. Lasson A, Kilander A, Stotzer PO. Diagnostic yield of colonoscopy based on symptoms. Scand J Gastroenterol. 2008;43:356–62.
44. von Roon AC, Karamountzos L, Purkayastha S, Reese GE, Darzi AW, et al. Diagnostic precision of fecal calprotectin for inflammatory bowel disease and colorectal malignancy. Am J Gastroenterol. 2007;102:803–13.
45. Park KT, Colletti RB, Rubin DT, Sharma BK, Thompson A, Krueger A. Health insurance paid costs and drivers of costs for patients with Crohn's disease in the United States. Am J Gastroenterol 2016;111:15–23.
46. D'Haens G, Ferrante M, Vermeire S, Baert F, Noman M, et al. Fecal calprotectin is a surrogate marker for endoscopic lesions in inflammatory bowel disease. Inflamm Bowel Dis. 2012;18:2218–24.
47. Bitton A, Peppercorn MA, Antonioli DA, Niles JL, Shah S, et al. Clinical, biological, and histologic parameters as predictors of relapse in ulcerative colitis. Gastroenterology. 2001;120:13–20.
48. Schnitzler F, Fidder H, Ferrante M, Noman M, Arijs I, et al. Mucosal healing predicts long-term outcome of maintenance therapy with infliximab in Crohn's disease. Inflamm Bowel Dis. 2009;15:1295–301.
49. Peyrin-Biroulet L, Bressenot A, Kampman W. Histologic remission: the ultimate therapeutic goal in ulcerative colitis? Clin Gastroenterol Hepatol. 2014;12:929–34.e2.
50. Gheorghe C, Cotruta B, Iacob R, Becheanu G, Dumbrava M, Gheorghe L. Endomicroscopy for assessing mucosal healing in patients with ulcerative colitis. J Gastrointestin Liver Dis. 2011;20:423–6.
51. Boirivant M, Leoni M, Tariciotti D, Fais S, Squarcia O, Pallone F. The clinical significance of serum C reactive protein levels in Crohn's disease. Results of a prospective longitudinal study. J Clin Gastroenterol. 1988;10:401–5.
52. Fagan EA, Dyck RF, Maton PN, Hodgson HJ, Chadwick VS, et al. Serum levels of C-reactive protein in Crohn's disease and ulcerative colitis. Eur J Clin Investig. 1982;12:351–9.
53. Linskens RK, van Bodegraven AA, Schoorl M, Tuynman HA, Bartels P. Predictive value of inflammatory and coagulation parameters in the course of severe ulcerative colitis. Dig Dis Sci. 2001;46:644–8.
54. Moran A, Jones A, Asquith P. Laboratory markers of colonoscopic activity in ulcerative colitis and Crohn's colitis. Scand J Gastroenterol. 1995;30:356–60.
55. Niederau C, Backmerhoff F, Schumacher B, Niederau C. Inflammatory mediators and acute phase proteins in patients with Crohn's disease and ulcerative colitis. Hepato-Gastroenterology. 1997;44:90–107.
56. Nielsen OH, Vainer B, Madsen SM, Seidelin JB, Heegaard NH. Established and emerging biological activity markers of inflammatory bowel disease. Am J Gastroenterol. 2000;95:359–67.
57. Vermeire S, Van Assche G, Rutgeerts P. C-reactive protein as a marker for inflammatory bowel disease. Inflamm Bowel Dis. 2004;10:661–5.
58. Schoepfer AM, Trummler M, Seeholzer P, Seibold-Schmid B, Seibold F. Discriminating IBD from IBS: comparison of the test performance of fecal markers, blood leukocytes, CRP, and IBD antibodies. Inflamm Bowel Dis. 2008;14:32–9.
59. Gomes P, du Boulay C, Smith CL, Holdstock G. Relationship between disease activity indices and colonoscopic findings in patients with colonic inflammatory bowel disease. Gut. 1986;27:92–5.
60. Schunk K, Kern A, Oberholzer K, Kalden P, Mayer I, et al. Hydro-MRI in Crohn's disease: appraisal of disease activity. Investig Radiol. 2000;35:431–7.
61. Costa F, Mumolo MG, Ceccarelli L, Bellini M, Romano MR, et al. Calprotectin is a stronger predictive marker of relapse in ulcerative colitis than in Crohn's disease. Gut. 2005;54:364–8.
62. Solem CA, Loftus Jr EV, Tremaine WJ, Harmsen WS, Zinsmeister AR, Sandborn WJ. Correlation of C-reactive protein with clinical, endoscopic, histologic, and radiographic activity in inflammatory bowel disease. Inflamm Bowel Dis. 2005;11:707–12.

63. Lewis JD. The utility of biomarkers in the diagnosis and therapy of inflammatory bowel disease. Gastroenterology. 2011;140:1817–26.e2.

64. Lobaton T, Rodriguez-Moranta F, Lopez A, Sanchez E, Rodriguez-Alonso L, Guardiola J. A new rapid quantitative test for fecal calprotectin predicts endoscopic activity in ulcerative colitis. Inflamm Bowel Dis. 2013;19:1034–42.

65. Zittan E, Kelly OB, Kirsch R, Milgrom R, Burns J, et al. Low fecal calprotectin correlates with histological remission and mucosal healing in ulcerative colitis and colonic Crohn's disease. Inflamm Bowel Dis. 2016;22(3):623–30.

66. Langhorst J, Boone J, Lauche R, Rueffer A, Dobos G. Fecal lactoferrin, calprotectin, PMN-elastase, CRP and white blood cell count as an indicator for mucosal healing and clinical course of disease in patients with mild to moderate ulcerative colitis: post HOC analysis of a prospective clinical trial. J Crohns Colitis. 2016;10(7):786–94.

67. Langholz E, Munkholm P, Davidsen M, Binder V. Course of ulcerative colitis: analysis of changes in disease activity over years. Gastroenterology. 1994;107:3–11.

68. Riley SA, Mani V, Goodman MJ, Dutt S, Herd ME. Microscopic activity in ulcerative colitis: what does it mean? Gut. 1991;32:174–8.

69. Limburg PJ, Ahlquist DA, Sandborn WJ, Mahoney DW, Devens ME, et al. Fecal calprotectin levels predict colorectal inflammation among patients with chronic diarrhea referred for colonoscopy. Am J Gastroenterol. 2000;95:2831–7.

70. Roseth AG, Aadland E, Jahnsen J, Raknerud N. Assessment of disease activity in ulcerative colitis by faecal calprotectin, a novel granulocyte marker protein. Digestion. 1997;58:176–80.

71. Roseth AG, Schmidt PN, Fagerhol MK. Correlation between faecal excretion of indium-111-labelled granulocytes and calprotectin, a granulocyte marker protein, in patients with inflammatory bowel disease. Scand J Gastroenterol. 1999;34:50–4.

72. Tibble JA, Sigthorsson G, Bridger S, Fagerhol MK, Bjarnason I. Surrogate markers of intestinal inflammation are predictive of relapse in patients with inflammatory bowel disease. Gastroenterology. 2000;119:15–22.

73. D'Inca R, Dal Pont E, Di Leo V, Benazzato L, Martinato M, et al. Can calprotectin predict relapse risk in inflammatory bowel disease? Am J Gastroenterol. 2008;103:2007–14.

74. Gisbert JP, Bermejo F, Perez-Calle JL, Taxonera C, Vera I, et al. Fecal calprotectin and lactoferrin for the prediction of inflammatory bowel disease relapse. Inflamm Bowel Dis. 2009;15:1190–8.

75. Garcia-Sanchez V, Iglesias-Flores E, Gonzalez R, Gisbert JP, Gallardo-Valverde JM, et al. Does fecal calprotectin predict relapse in patients with Crohn's disease and ulcerative colitis? J Crohns Colitis. 2010;4:144–52.

76. Kallel L, Ayadi I, Matri S, Fekih M, Mahmoud NB, et al. Fecal calprotectin is a predictive marker of relapse in Crohn's disease involving the colon: a prospective study. Eur J Gastroenterol Hepatol. 2010;22:340–5.

77. De Vos M, Dewit O, D'Haens G, Baert F, Fontaine F, et al. Fast and sharp decrease in calprotectin predicts remission by infliximab in anti-TNF naive patients with ulcerative colitis. J Crohns Colitis. 2012;6:557–62.

78. Glasziou P, Irwig L, Mant D. Monitoring in chronic disease: a rational approach. BMJ. 2005;330:644–8.

79. Yamamoto T, Shimoyama T. Can fecal biomarkers detect ileal inflammation in inflammatory bowel disease? Am J Gastroenterol. 2015;110:1370.

Radiologic Evaluation of Pediatric Inflammatory Bowel Disease

20

Stephen M. Druhan and Benedict C. Nwomeh

Introduction

Radiologic imaging is a vital component of disease evaluation in the patient with inflammatory bowel disease (IBD). Imaging techniques are useful at initial presentation to help establish the diagnosis and to assess the location, extent, inflammatory activity, and severity of disease. These modalities are also very important for disease monitoring during and after treatment, in selecting appropriate treatment options, planning surgical strategies, and for assessing complications of disease and effects of therapeutic interventions.

Given current advances in imaging technology, conventional plain radiographs and contrast studies such as the upper gastrointestinal series and the small bowel follow-through study are utilized with less frequency; however, they are still important tools in the evaluation of IBD. In recent years, cross-sectional imaging techniques such as ultrasound, computer tomography, and, in particular, magnetic resonance imaging have added an extra dimension and a deeper perspective to our understanding of this disease.

Advances in imaging technology have brought newer generation CT scanners and MRI techniques that allow rapid acquisition of high-resolution images of diseased bowel with three-dimensional rendering. Imaging techniques have also enhanced our understanding of the various extraintestinal disease manifestations. This chapter will discuss the current role of these various modalities in the clinical management of pediatric patients with Crohn disease (CD) and ulcerative colitis (UC) and review some of the emerging techniques that may yield more detail and improve on the accuracy of current methods.

Crohn Disease

The hallmark of CD is segmental, transmural bowel involvement with a chronic relapsing course, and the propensity to affect any portion of the gastrointestinal tract. The disease may be limited to a single segment of bowel, commonly the terminal ileum. However, multiple segments may be affected, with intervening normal bowel, known as "skip lesions." Also, CD may be complicated by perianal disease, strictures, fistulas, and abscesses. This clinical pattern is closely mirrored by the radiologic findings. With several imaging modalities available, the clinical condition of the patient and the clinical question to be answered should determine which imaging techniques are employed.

Imaging Techniques

Plain Radiographs

Abnormalities in plain abdominal radiographs consistent with IBD are present in two-thirds of pediatric patients, but these are nonspecific findings such as mural thickening, dilatation, and abnormal pattern of gas and feces [1]. As such, the plain film has little role in the initial evaluation of the patient with CD. However, plain films remain the first-line investigation in the patient with an acute abdomen, in whom dilated bowel loops and air–fluid levels indicate acute intestinal obstruction, and pneumoperitoneum signifies intestinal perforation. For example, toxic megacolon affecting patients with Crohn colitis usually manifests as dilated colon.

S.M. Druhan, MD (✉)
Ohio State University School of Medicine,
Columbus, OH, USA

School of Medicine, University of Toledo Medical College,
Toledo, OH, USA

Nationwide Children's Hospital, Columbus, OH 43205, USA
e-mail: Stephen.Druhan@nationwidechildrens.org

B.C. Nwomeh, MD, MPH, FACS, FAAP
Pediatric Surgery Residency Program, The Ohio State University,
Columbus, OH, USA

Center for Pediatric and Adolescent IBD,
Nationwide Children's Hospital, Columbus, OH, USA

© Springer International Publishing AG 2017
P. Mamula et al. (eds.), *Pediatric Inflammatory Bowel Disease*, DOI 10.1007/978-3-319-49215-5_20

Contrast Studies

Despite the plethora of new imaging techniques, no radiologic test has replaced conventional contrast studies as the gold standard for the diagnosis of CD, although cross-sectional imaging (CT and MR enterography) does have the advantage for improved detection of extraenteric complication, with MR enterography having the potential to be used as a radiation-free alternative for the evaluation of patients with CD. Conventional contrast studies allow direct mucosal assessment in the hand of the experienced radiologist. The upper gastrointestinal (UGI) series is an excellent modality in which contrast is administered by mouth (or through a tube) for mucosal assessment of the stomach and duodenum. The small bowel follow-through (SBFT) is performed as a continuation of the UGI examination. Additional contrast is administered or ingested, and the contrast is followed through the jejunum and ileum into the right colon. Fluoroscopic compression images of the small intestine, specifically the terminal ileum, are obtained (Fig. 20.1). A small bowel enteroclysis examination involves direct injection of contrast and methylcellulose via a nasojejunal catheter placed under fluoroscopic guidance. A double contrast view of the small intestine is obtained, providing better distension and superior mucosal detail. However, the SBFT is often chosen instead of the enteroclysis study, because the latter is more unpleasant for the patient, involves a higher radiation dose, and is more difficult to perform. The barium enema (BE), using a single or double contrast technique, may be used to evaluate the colon. If reflux across the ileocecal valve is obtained, it also may provide a double contrast view of the terminal ileum. The ability to visualize the terminal ileum is critical, as it is frequently affected in CD. However, given the

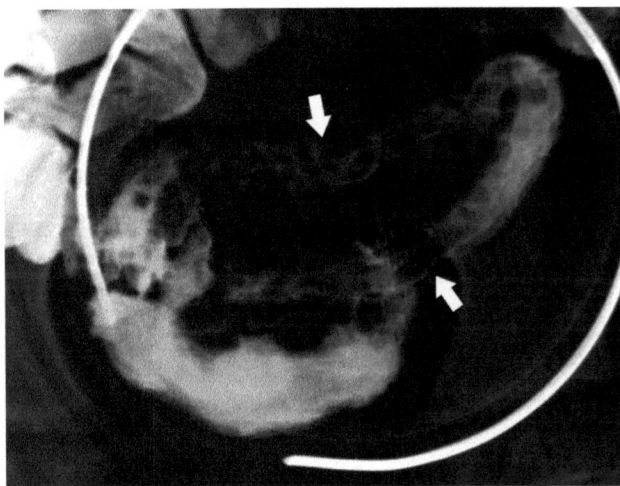

Fig. 20.1 Compression view of the right lower quadrant from SBFT demonstrates a long segment of narrowed, ulcerated, and nodular-appearing ileum giving the characteristic "cobblestone" appearance (*arrows*). Loop separation caused by thickening of bowel walls and mesentery inflammation

common availability of endoscopic assessment, patient discomfort with BE, and the risk for complications such as toxic megacolon, BE has been largely replaced by colonoscopy.

Early changes of CD include aphthous lesions, a coarse granular pattern, nodularity, and fold thickening, which may progress to deeper ulceration, cobblestoning, and fissuring. In the colon, ulceration occurs within a background of normal-appearing mucosa. Inflammatory edema produces mucosal elevations seen more commonly in the colon than the small bowel. In the patient with more severe CD, mucosal distortions and pseudopolyps may occur due to the elevation of submucosa at the margins of healing ulcers. As inflammation spreads in transmural and circumferential dimensions, the radiologic findings progress to strictures and shortening, with the most severe cases producing the characteristic "string sign." In addition, bowel may be noted to adhere to the adjacent loops or to other viscera, and deep ulcers may extend to create fistula. The finding of discontinuous, patchy, and asymmetric colonic mucosal changes is a hallmark of CD.

Unlike cross-sectional CT or MR studies, contrast studies are limited in their ability to image extraluminal extension of disease or extraintestinal manifestations. Only indirect assessment of bowel wall thickening or mesenteric involvement can be made. Mesenteric inflammation, thickening, and fibrosis may cause separation and shortening of bowel loops. Mesenteric lymphadenopathy may appear as extraluminal masses indenting the bowel wall.

Computer Tomography

Computed tomography (CT) still is the most widely used cross-sectional imaging modality in patients with CD given its wide availability. Its major role in children with CD is in the evaluation of disease extent and in assessing for complications, particularly in the acute situation. CT enteroclysis has been shown to be more accurate than SBFT in the diagnosis of CD, but neither is able to detect the early mucosal changes of CD [2]. Additionally, as with any enteroclysis study, this technique requires the introduction of a nasojejunal tube, generally not well accepted in the pediatric population. Changes readily detected by CT include bowel wall thickening, luminal narrowing, and mesenteric involvement. Mesenteric findings include thickening due to fibrofatty infiltration, lymphadenopathy, and fatty encroachment of the affected loop of bowel.

Patients with known CD, who present with new acute symptoms suspicious for complications or a deteriorating clinical course, are best imaged with CT to assess for progressive disease or the onset of complications such as obstruction, fistulae, abscesses, or malignant change (Fig. 20.2). Extraintestinal manifestations of CD in the hepatobiliary, pancreatic, urinary, and musculoskeletal systems are also readily assessed by CT. Specific CT findings of complications and extraintestinal manifestations of CD are discussed below.

The sensitivity of CT scan in patients with CD is increased by optimal opacification and distension of the bowel by administering oral contrast at an age- and weight-appropriate dose, or by the enteroclysis technique. Bowel wall thickening >3 mm in pediatric patients is generally considered abnormal [3]. Given that this young patient population frequently undergoes multiple studies, the current trend is moving toward MRI evaluation in the nonacute setting, thus minimizing exposure to ionizing radiation.

Magnetic Resonance Imaging

Magnetic resonance imaging (MRI) offers unique advantages to the pediatric patient because, in addition to being noninvasive, it avoids exposure to ionizing radiation. In many cases, MRI can replace or complement CT because its excellent soft tissue contrast and three-dimensional capabilities are ideal properties for imaging the bowel [4]. In the past, motion artifacts often limited MRI, but this problem has been largely overcome by the recent introduction of respiration-suspended sequences. Other technological advances, including improved coils, fat suppression, use of oral agents and intravenous gadolinium, powerful gradient systems, and ultrafast pulse sequences have led to overall improvement in gastrointestinal imaging. Optimal image quality depends greatly on adequate luminal distension with contrast medium. Without enteric contrast, MRI has produced inconsistent results in children with CD [5, 6].

The method of enteric contrast administration has proved to be a critical factor because oral ingestion of contrast agents that do not provide adequate bowel distension such as routine positive contrast agents or water, while patient-friendly, produces inadequate luminal distension, downgrades the

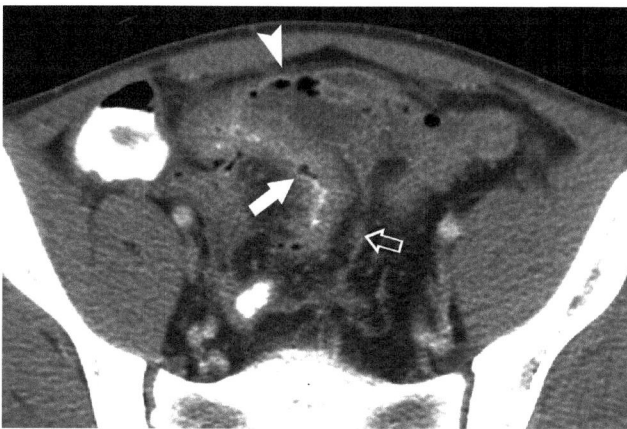

Fig. 20.2 Oral and intravenous contrast-enhanced CT image of the pelvis. A thickened loop of small bowel containing intraluminal contrast (*white arrow*) marginates an intraabdominal abscess containing fluid and air (*arrowhead*). An enhancing fistulous tract is seen extending to the base of the abscess cavity (*open arrow*)

image quality, and may limit the ability to detect early or minimal disease. The two techniques found to have the greatest success to evaluate for CD of the small bowel include MR enteroclysis and MR enterography utilizing a negative contrast agent that provides adequate bowel distension. The choice of oral contrast agent for MR enterography varies with institution. However, at our institution, we utilize VoLumen® (manufactured by E-Z-Em, Inc.), a low-concentration barium (0.1% weight/volume) that contains sorbitol to aid in bowel distension.

Magnetic resonance enteroclysis requires duodenal intubation to permit volume challenge, which causes reflex bowel atony and produces superb contrast for evaluating luminal, transmural, and extramural changes. It has been postulated that by combining the advantages of enteroclysis with three-dimensional cross-sectional imaging, MR enteroclysis has been touted as the only imaging modality that can provide comprehensive diagnostic information on small bowel CD [4]. However, routine use of MR enteroclysis in children has not been widely adopted because of the need to insert a duodenal tube fluoroscopically, entailing exposure to ionizing radiation, and the potential need for intravenous sedation.

Prospective comparison of MR enterography and CT enterography in the evaluation of small bowel Crohn disease has been performed [7] with the sensitivities for detecting active small bowel disease found to be similar (90.5% vs. 95.2%, respectively). Although MR enterography had a slightly lower sensitivity and specificity, this difference was not statistically significant for the 30 patients who underwent both imaging studies. However, image quality across the study cohort was better with CT enterography. In another study [8], MR enterography demonstrated good sensitivity in the detection of active CD and found good correlation between MR and CT enterography in the evaluation of wall thickening with mucosal hyperenhancement and the presence of the comb and halo signs. While CT enterography was found to be superior in the detection of fibrofatty proliferation and mesenteric lymph nodes, MR enterography was superior in the evaluation of fistulas. Currently, however, because MR enterography has a diagnostic effectiveness comparable to that of CT enterography [9], the trend is increasing toward MR enterography as a radiation-free alternative for the evaluation of patients with CD. Indeed, one study [10] concluded that MR enterography can be substituted for CT as the first-line imaging modality in pediatric patients with CD. This viewpoint is based on the ability of MR enterography to detect intestinal pathologic abnormalities in both small and large bowel as well as extraintestinal disease manifestations [11]. Furthermore, MR enterography provides an accurate noninvasive assessment of CD activity and mural fibrosis and can aid in formulating treatment strategies for symptomatic patients and assessing therapy response [10, 11].

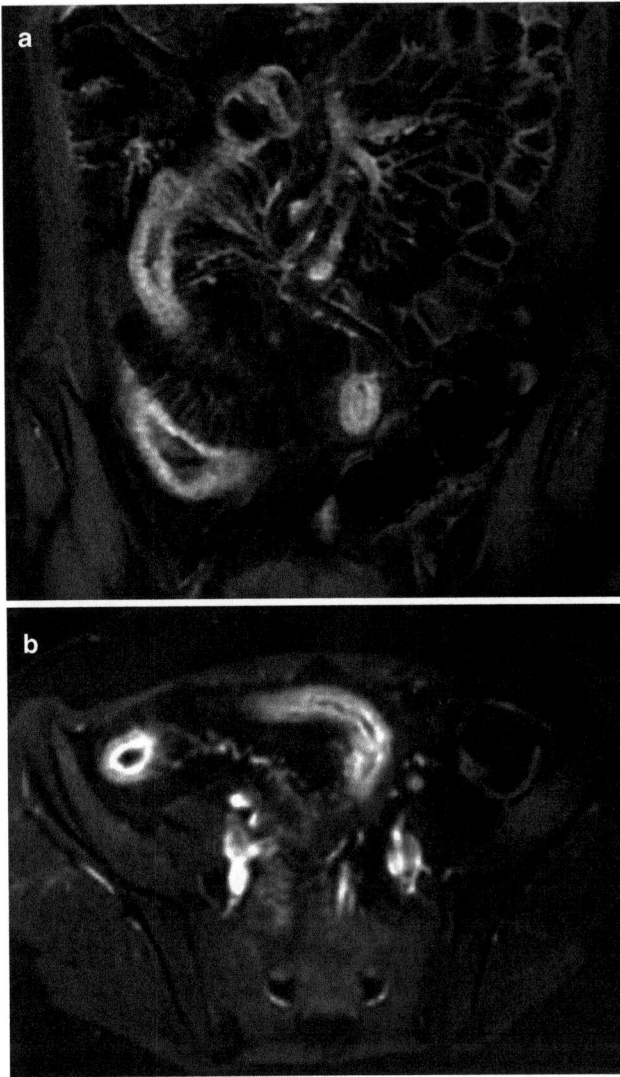

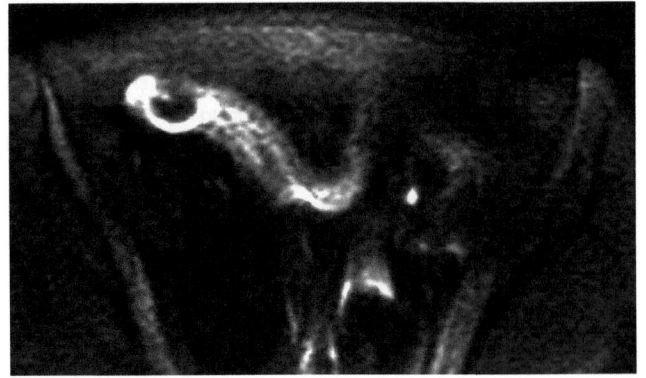

Fig. 20.4 Axial diffusion-weighted sequence demonstrates an area of restricted diffusion consistent with pathologic edema along a segment of affected bowel

Fig. 20.3 Coronal (**a**) and axial (**b**) post-gadolinium T1-weighted sequences illustrating mucosal hyperenhancement and wall thickening along a segment of bowel with active inflammation

The technique for MR enterography begins with the oral ingestion of contrast, but the type of oral contrast used again is controversial and is usually institution-specific. Again, at our institution, the utilization of VoLumen® has been well tolerated and shown to produce good-quality images. The patient is asked to ingest three 450 mL bottles over approximately 1–1 ½ h as tolerated, with each bottle being ingested over approximately 20 min. The field of view includes the abdomen and majority of the pelvis to evaluate the entirety of the small bowel. Imaging of the bowel begins with coronal T2 single-shot fast spin echo imaging, which is reviewed by

the radiologist to ensure adequate oral preparation with contrast reaching the colon. If adequate, the remainder of the MR enterography protocol is performed including axial T2-weighted axial diffusion-weighted sequence to evaluate for restricted diffusion in areas of pathologic edema, coronal pregadolinium T1-weighted, and dynamic steady-state free precession imaging in the coronal plane to evaluate for bowel peristalsis. The evaluation is enhanced utilizing intravenous glucagon to inhibit bowel motion in preparation for the longer postgadolinium sequences following the administration of IV contrast. These include axial, coronal, and sagittal T1-weighted sequences to evaluate enhancement pattern. Some institutions utilize additional 7-min delayed postcontrast T1-weighted sequences which are felt to aid in the evaluation of mural fibrosis as indicated by delayed enhancement. MR findings of active CD affecting the small bowel include mucosal hyperenhancement, wall thickening (Fig. 20.3a, b), restricted diffusion (Fig. 20.4), ulcers, mesenteric hypervascularity (Comb sign, Fig. 20.5), mesenteric inflammation, and reactive mesenteric nodes. Fibrostenotic lesions (Fig. 20.6a, b) may show homogenous T2 hyperintensity, although less than that in active inflammation, variable contrast enhancement, and minimal adjacent inflammatory changes. Again, delayed contrast-enhanced sequence has been utilized with some success to evaluate for delayed enhancement seen in mural fibrosis [11]. Often, there are components of both fibrosis and active inflammation present with the MRE evaluation, hopefully able to determine which predominates [11]. A true correlation between the degree of wall enhancement and amount of inflammatory change found histopathologically has not yet been established.

Complications of CD include penetrating disease and bowel obstruction, sinus tracts, fistulas, and abscess formation [12].

In addition to MR enterography in the assessment of IBD, we currently also use MRI of the pelvis for the evaluation of complex perianal disease, as discussed below.

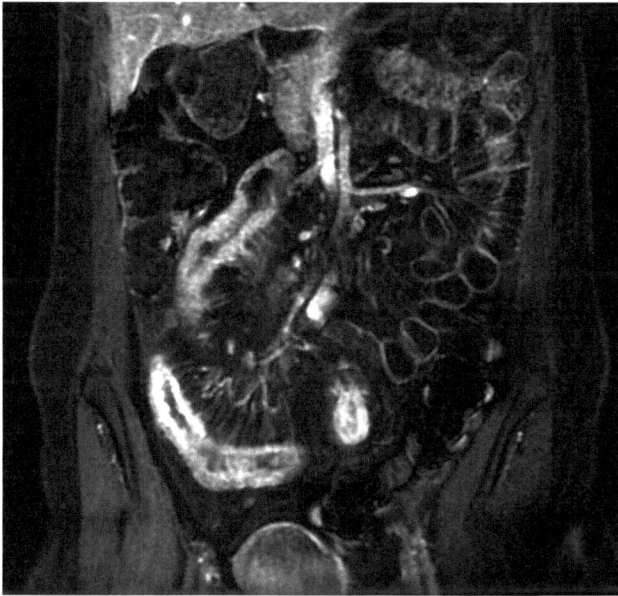

Fig. 20.5 Coronal post-gadolinium T1-weighted sequence demonstrates mesenteric hypervascularity consistent with prominent vasa recta subtending a segment of affected bowel (Comb sign)

Ultrasound

The lack of ionizing radiation and noninvasive nature of ultrasound (US) make it an ideal method of evaluation in children. In addition, for routine US imaging, bowel cleansing is not required, nor is enteric or intravenous contrast. However, because it is operator dependent, its role in patients with CD is currently generally limited to the evaluation of complications, particularly abscesses, and extraintestinal disease manifestations. It is rarely used for primary diagnosis. Affected bowel segments demonstrate wall thickening, lack of peristalsis, and poor stratification of the different layers (Fig. 20.7) [13]. Similar to adults, US findings in children with CD show good correlation with endoscopy [14]. The most promising use of US may be in the ongoing evaluation of disease activity as well as response to treatment. In children, the sonographic value of bowel wall thickening as an index of increased disease activity has been demonstrated [15, 16]. With moderate–severe disease, the predictive value of increased bowel wall thickening >2.5 mm in the ileum as an index of active disease was 88% (82% for colon >3 mm) [15]. Assessment of disease severity can also be enhanced by measuring the vessel density in the affected bowel segment using color Doppler US (Fig. 20.7) [17]. When incorporated into a clinical protocol, US may reduce the need for contrast studies [15, 18]. In expert hands, US has been used to assess fistulae and strictures, and also monitor postoperative disease recurrence [19].

There are a number of limitations to the use of US in CD. Although the assessment of terminal ileal disease with US is

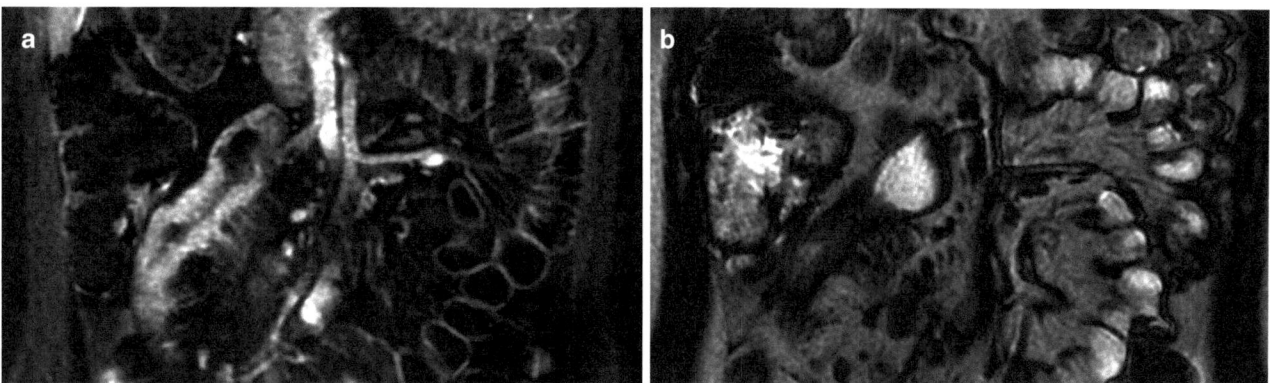

Fig. 20.6 Coronal post-gadolinium T1-weighted sequence revealing a fibrostenotic lesion showing homogenous T2 hyperintensity, uniform contrast enhancement, and minimal adjacent inflammatory changes. Dynamic sequences (not shown) showed non-peristalsis along this involved segment

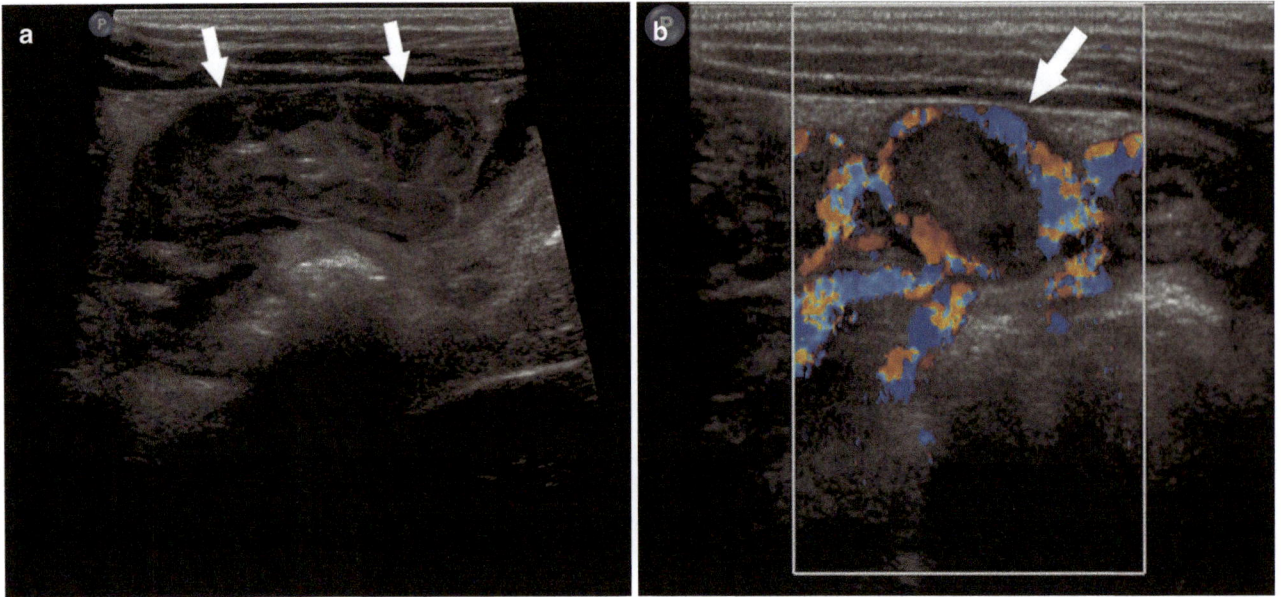

Fig. 20.7 (a) Longitudinal ultrasound of the right lower quadrant demonstrates a segmental region of thickened, hypoechoic small bowel (*arrows*). (b) Transverse Doppler image demonstrates hyperemia of bowel wall (*arrow*)

quite good, the proximal small bowel and distal portions of the colon are poorly imaged. In addition, superficial lesions as seen in early disease can be missed in both children and adults [14].

Ulcerative Colitis

Ulcerative colitis is a chronic, idiopathic, inflammatory disease of the rectal and colonic mucosa that is characterized by mucosal inflammation, edema, and ulceration. Several distinguishing features permit clinical and radiological distinction from CD. As a rule, UC nearly always affects the rectum and extends proximally to involve a variable length of colon in a contiguous fashion. Other than the occasional "backwash ileitis" of the terminal ileum, the small bowel is not affected. On rare occasions, variants with transmural involvement or without rectal inflammation also occur. Radiologic features of UC are quite distinct, although in the majority of cases, diagnosis is dependent on clinical presentation, laboratory tests and findings on colonoscopy and biopsy.

Imaging Techniques

Plain Radiographs

The nonspecific finding of mucosal edema occasionally noted on plain films is rarely helpful for diagnosis. However, in the patient presenting acutely with symptoms of toxic megacolon, the plain film shows marked colon dilatation and is adequate for monitoring response to treatment and the potential onset of bowel perforation.

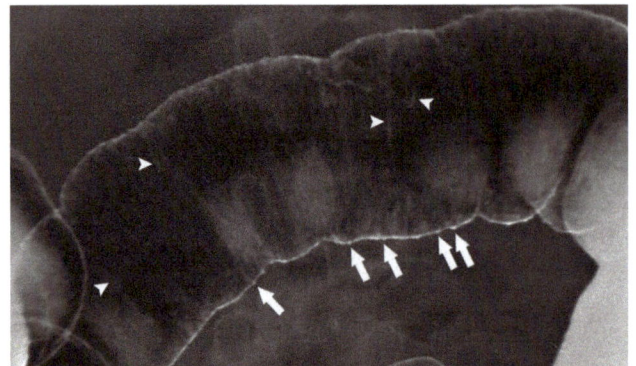

Fig. 20.8 Image (ACBE–UC). Anterior image of the transverse colon from ACBE demonstrating granular mucosa with early ulcerations seen in profile (*arrows*) and en face (*arrowheads*)

Contrast Enema

Given the availability of colonoscopy and its ability to obtain tissue for histologic assessment, as well as the discomfort of BE, contrast studies of the colon are less commonly performed than in the past. However, if needed, it can be used for confirming the diagnosis, evaluating extent and severity of disease, and detecting complications. The earliest change seen on the air-contrast study is a fine granular pattern of the colonic mucosa, which may be associated with blunting and broadening of the haustral folds due to mucosal edema. As the disease progresses, mucosal irregularity increases (Fig. 20.8). Subsequently, ulcers appear and begin to extend deeper, undermining the submucosa and forming flask-shaped or "collar-button" ulcers. Extensive mucosal ulceration may leave islands of residual inflamed mucosa that are recognized as "inflammatory pseudopolyps." In contrast to CD, these changes are contiguous, circumferential, and symmetric with no skip lesions. With long-standing disease, the colonic wall becomes rigid, shortened, and narrow due to fibrosis of the submucosa, giving the appearance of the "lead pipe" colon.

A contrast enema should be administered with extreme caution in the patient with an acute presentation. A physical examination to exclude peritoneal signs and a plain film to rule out toxic megacolon and free air should be performed prior to a BE, as any of these findings would be a contraindication.

CT

CT may be useful in differentiating UC from CD, and it has the advantage of being able to visualize bowel wall as well as adjacent structures [20]. Adequate preparation for the CT examination is important. When optimal colonic imaging is desired, oral contrast should be given sufficient time to opacify the entire small bowel and colon, and if necessary, additional rectal contrast should be administered. Early mucosal changes are difficult to detect on CT, but in chronic disease, bowel wall thickening and luminal narrowing are readily seen [21]. However, these rather nonspecific findings overlap with those of other colitides including Crohn colitis [20, 22]. Characteristic CT features in UC include a symmetric, contiguous wall thickening involving the rectum and extending proximally in a contiguous manner. Small bowel changes and skip lesions are absent. Thickening of the mesentery or mesenteric lymphadenopathy are rare, but proliferation of perirectal fat can occur.

MRI

Characteristic findings of MRI in the active stage of UC include loss of haustral markings, thickening, and contrast enhancement of the colonic wall [23, 24]. As with CT, these findings overlap those of CD. The few early pediatric studies available reveal inconsistencies in the ability of MRI to differentiate UC from CD [5, 6]. However, a diagnosis of UC was supported when disease progressed from the rectum proximally with mucosal enhancement and a low-signal submucosal stripe [5].

Recent advances in contrast-enhanced MRI among the pediatric population indicate that gadolinium-enhanced MRI favorably compares with endoscopy as a means to differentiate between CD and UC. However, endoscopy has the clear advantage in allowing tissue samples to be obtained for histologic evaluation, and thus cannot yet be replaced by MRI [6]. While MRI can detect the presence of colonic disease, at present, it seems more promising for characterizing small bowel disease related to IBD. Also, the ability of MRI to categorize disease into either CD or UC with high specificity remains a challenge.

US

As previously noted, US has the advantages of being cheap, noninvasive, and lacking in ionizing radiation, but its principal finding of increased bowel wall thickness is nonspecific and cannot distinguish between UC and CD. In addition, early mucosal changes are not detected with US, and the difficulty in visualizing the rectosigmoid limits its ability to evaluate the true extent of the disease. In the few pediatric studies, there appears to be a consensus that the appropriate role of US is in the monitoring of disease activity and assessing response to treatment [15, 25, 26]. With moderate–severe disease, the predictive value of increased bowel wall thickening >3 mm in the colon as an index of active disease was 82% [15].

Indeterminate Colitis

Patients with IBD whose clinical, endoscopic, pathologic, and radiologic presentation cannot easily be differentiated into CD or UC are assigned the diagnosis of indeterminate colitis (IC). Indeterminate colitis appears to be more common in children compared to adults, with a prevalence rate of nearly 30% recently reported in a cohort of 250 children with IBD [27].

One study has shown that the probability of making a definitive diagnosis of either CD or UC increases with age [12]. Careful radiologic evaluation may play a significant role in subsequent reclassification of patients with IC. The distinction between CD and UC may be important in selecting appropriate treatment and in determining prognosis.

Demonstration of small bowel inflammation, skip lesions, and mesenteric extension usually indicates CD, particularly in the absence of colonic disease. Patients classified as IC usually have normal small bowel imaging on the SBFT and CT. As noted previously, newer techniques such as US, radionuclide scans, and MRI may demonstrate small bowel disease, particularly in the distal ileum. Again, MR enterography is becoming a promising technique, and with recent advances in imaging, the detection of IBD has improved for both small bowel and colonic disease. However, in isolated colonic disease, the ability to distinguish UC and CD with high specificity remains a challenge. When extensive colonic disease is present, the finding of terminal ileal inflammation may be misleading because some patients with UC may have "backwash ileitis."

Although the colon is usually accessible for endoscopic evaluation, cross-sectional imaging with CT or MRI may demonstrate transmural involvement, extension into mesenteric fat, fistulae, or abscesses, which may prompt a more definitive reclassification as CD. Using US to differentiate between CD and UC has so far proved unreliable in children, although it may be useful for monitoring disease activity [14, 16, 28].

Other Radiologic Modalities in IBD

White Blood Cell (WBC) Scan

Radionuclide-labeled autologous WBC reinjected intravenously is taken up by inflamed tissues and can then be

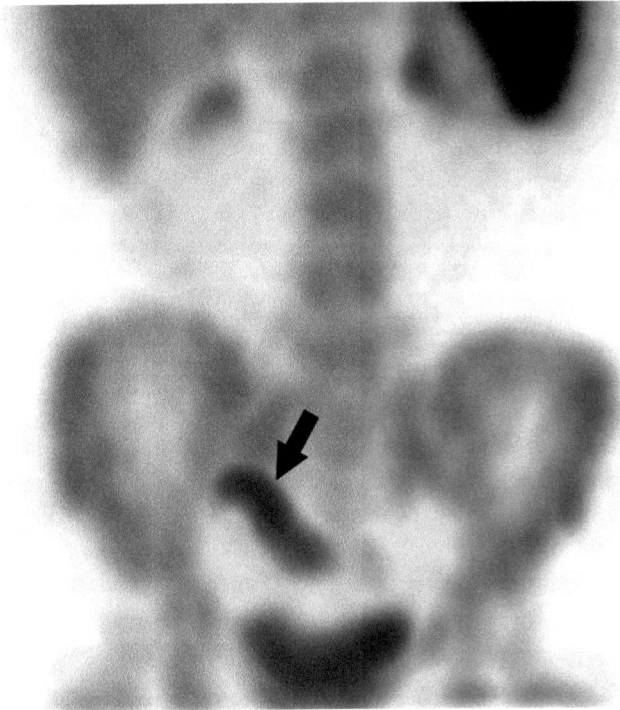

Fig. 20.9 3D volume rendered image from a Tc-HMPAO WBC scan of the abdomen demonstrates intense focal activity in the right lower quadrant (*arrow*) compatible with the diagnosis of active inflammatory bowel disease of the distal small bowel

detected by a gamma camera scan (Fig. 20.9). Within a few minutes of injection, the labeled WBC marginates in the inflamed bowel and usually increases in intensity over a period of 2–4 h. The WBC scan is a helpful diagnostic tool for the detection of inflammation and abscesses. Soon after it was introduced, the ^{111}In-labeled WBC scan was shown to be highly sensitive in patients with IBD [29]. Subsequently, Technetium-99 m hexamethyl propylene amine oxime (^{99m}Tc HMPAO)-labeled WBC scan was adopted because of ready availability, longer shelf life, lower radiation dose, and superior image resolution [30]. Most pediatric studies indicate that a positive WBC scan is highly predictive of IBD. However, false-negative studies can occur in very early disease or in patients who are in remission due to recent steroid treatment [30–32]. Negative scans have also been observed in children with proximal small bowel disease.

Localization of tracer activity can be a useful aid in differentiating children with CD from those with UC. Uptake localized to the small bowel or a more widespread but discontinuous bowel activity correlates highly with CD, whereas in UC, the characteristic finding is a continuous pattern of uptake involving the rectum with a variable proximal extension in the colon [30, 33–35]. The WBC scan can also be a reliable indicator of disease activity. A "scan score" calculated by comparing uptake of tracer in affected bowel segments with iliac crest bone marrow activity correlated much

better with clinical disease activity than did the erythrocyte sedimentation rate [36]. In the follow-up of patients with known IBD, a negative scan indicates remission and may prompt changes in treatment [30]. The WBC scan may be useful in several areas of clinical decision-making in children with known IBD. A positive WBC scan can identify ileal inflammation when ileoscopy is not feasible [37]. The finding of small bowel activity or skip areas of colonic involvement could help to establish the diagnosis of CD in patients previously assigned the diagnosis of indeterminate colitis [30]. In cases of luminal narrowing, a positive WBC scan may help distinguish active inflammation from fibrosis.

The WBC scan is attractive for children because it is associated with much less radiation exposure than contrast studies. However, scintigraphy has several limitations including false-positive studies in the presence of gastrointestinal bleeding and inability to define anatomic detail including strictures and fistulae [30, 31]. It is also time-consuming, and drawing sufficient blood for labeling can be a challenge in younger children.

Positron Emission Tomography

Positron emission tomography (PET) is a functional imaging technique that has been applied to the detection of inflamed areas of bowel. The high metabolic activity of inflamed tissue results in the uptake of the glucose analog, fluoro-2-deoxy-D-glucose (FDG), which has been radiolabeled with a positron-emitting isotope such as fluorine-18 (F-18). It is transported into cells at a rate proportional to the glycolytic activity of the cell. Within an hour of the intravenous injection of F-18 labeled FDG, the scan is performed, with a total image acquisition time of less than half an hour. PET scanning detects inflamed bowel in children with a reported accuracy similar to the WBC scan [38, 39]. As compared to the WBC scan, PET is faster and does not require blood to be drawn. However, PET scans depend on equipment and expertise that may not be generally accessible. Given the limited availability and the paucity of pediatric studies, PET has a minimal role in the evaluation of pediatric IBD at the present time.

Evaluation of Complications

Perianal Disease

Perianal disease occurs in over one-third of patients with CD but is not associated with UC. Diagnosis of external manifestations such as skin tags, fissures, ulcerations, and simple perianal abscesses requires only a careful inspection and digital rectal examination as appropriate. Additional information on complex abscesses, fistulae, and strictures can be obtained by performing an examination under anesthesia (EUA) with proctosigmoidoscopy and with imaging studies.

Anatomic classification of perianal disease is enhanced by use of modern imaging techniques, especially MRI and endoscopic ultrasound (EUS) [40–42]. Anal fistulography has been largely abandoned because of patient discomfort, poor accuracy, and inability to visualize the anal sphincter anatomy [43, 44]. CT is also unreliable in assessing perianal fistulae due to its poor intrinsic contrast resolution that limits its ability to define the anatomy of the levator muscle [45, 46]. Because CT entails exposure to ionizing radiation, it is also disadvantageous in children.

Both MRI and EUS appear to be highly accurate in demonstrating anal sphincter anatomy and in illustrating the relationship of abscesses and fistulae to the levators [40–42, 47–49]. Detailed and accurate demonstration of the anatomic relationships has significant implications for the surgical management of perianal disease [40, 50]. In patients with recurrent fistula-in-ano following initial operative intervention, subsequent surgery guided by MRI reduced further recurrence by 75% [51]. Similarly, among a group of patients undergoing infliximab therapy for fistula-in-ano, EUS was accurate in identifying a subset of patients who could discontinue treatment without recurrence of fistula drainage [52]. Both MRI and EUS have also been used to accurately define the perineal body and demonstrate anovaginal and rectovaginal fistulae [53–55]. While reports present conflicting accounts of the superiority of one technique over the other, the most accurate assessment of perianal disease has been obtained when any two out of the three techniques (EUA, MRI, and EUS) were combined [56]. However, the method chosen should take into account both the cost and the equipment and expertise available at individual institutions [57].

Enteric Fistula and Intraabdominal Abscesses

The incidence of enteric fistula and intraabdominal abscess in children with CD is approximately 10% each, with a cumulative incidence of up to 30% each in adult patients [58–60]. Intraabdominal abscesses are commonly evaluated with CT or US, and both modalities are also very effective in providing image guidance for percutaneous drainage of abscesses (Fig. 20.2) [61–63]. Abscesses frequently develop in the abdominal wall, peritoneal cavity, retroperitoneum or iliopsoas, and subphrenic region [60]. Abscesses occurring between loops of bowel (interloop abscesses) are common. In half of patients, the abscess cavity occurs near an anastomosis following surgical resection.

Radiologic demonstration of enteric fistula can be challenging. Fistula usually arises from the extension of primary small bowel or colonic disease into adjacent mesentery,

nearby bowel, skin, or the viscera of the genitourinary system. Fistula tracts can also extend into solid organs, muscle, or spine. Most commonly, fistulae arise from the terminal ileum and penetrate into the cecum or adjacent small bowel (Fig. 20.10a, b). These communications are difficult to define with standard contrast imaging due to overlap of bony structures and contrast-filled bowel, or because tissue edema prevents outlining of the fistulous tract with contrast. Enteroclysis is more sensitive for demonstrating fistula than the SBFT examination. CT is more useful for demonstrating fistula tracks, although it is only possible to determine whether a tract is patent when it has been opacified by contrast. The CT is also an excellent modality for evaluating fistulae with concomitant abscesses.

Other cross-sectional imaging modalities such as the MRI and US may also be useful in imaging enteric fistulae. MR is vastly superior for detecting enteric fistulae and intraabdominal abscesses compared to enteroclysis, and it appears to be at least as sensitive as CT scan (Fig. 20.11) [64, 65]. Although US is probably comparable to enteroclysis in detecting fistulae, there is insufficient experience with this technique to recommend its routine use at the present time [13].

One of the more dramatic manifestations of enteric fistula is involvement of the genitourinary tract. Most commonly, communication develops between the terminal ileum and the bladder, but may extend to involve the ureters, uterus, and vagina [66]. Bladder fistulae occur more frequently in males who do not have the protective shield of the uterus. Clinically, bladder fistulae present with pneumaturia and recurrent urinary tract infections. Bladder and vaginal fistulae are often difficult to visualize with conventional cystography or BE. The most sensitive imaging technique for bladder fistulae is CT with adequate oral contrast. The finding of air within the bladder in the absence of recent instrumentation is diagnostic of either a fistula or infection with a gas-forming organism. If the primary aim of the CT study is to detect fistulae, intravenous contrast should not be given so that any contrast material subsequently noted in the bladder or vagina confirms the diagnosis [66, 67].

Bowel Obstruction and Perforation

The radiologic hallmark of bowel obstruction is dilatation of proximal bowel with paucity of gas distally. Air–fluid levels may also be noted in proximal bowel. If contrast examination is performed, contrast progression to distal bowel is reduced according to the degree of the obstruction. It is important to distinguish between partial obstruction, where initial nonoperative treatment may be appropriate, and complete obstruction, where surgical intervention is often required. CT is helpful in evaluating the severity of intramural disease and any associated abscesses. The diagnosis of

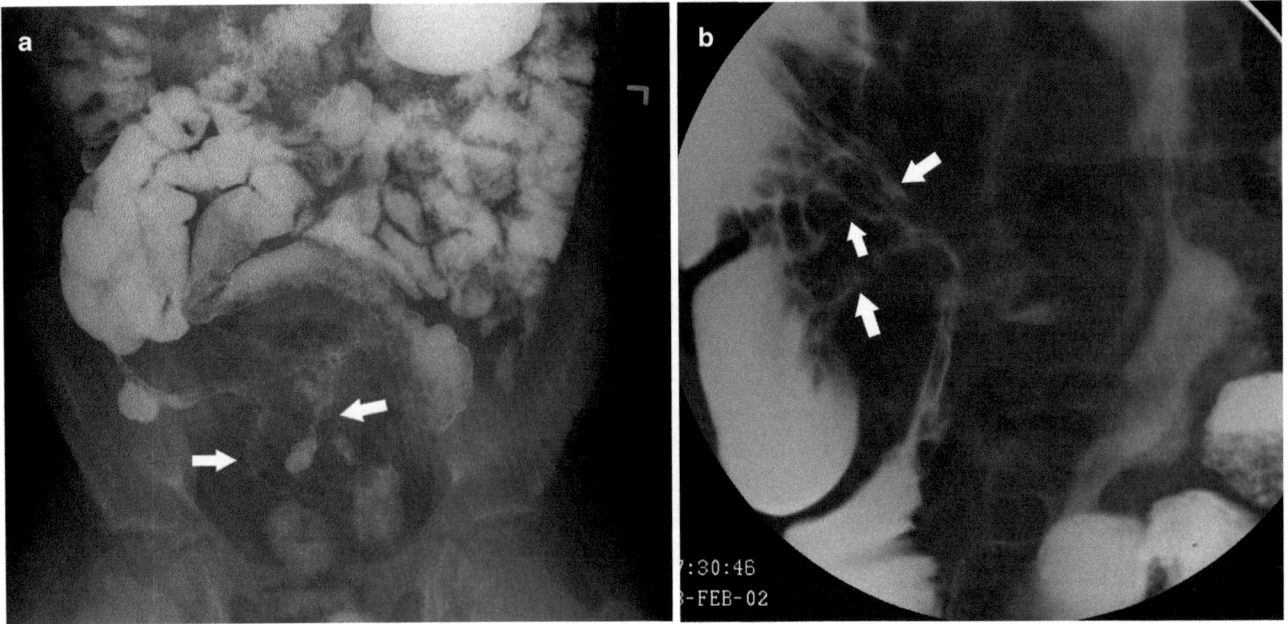

Fig. 20.10 (a) An overhead radiograph of the abdomen from a SBFT demonstrates narrowed segment of diseased small bowel from which arise multiple fistulae (*arrows*). Contrast is seen in the rectum consistent with enterocolic fistulae formation. (**b**) Image (SBFT—TI fistula). Coned view of the terminal ileum from SBFT demonstrates multiple fistulous tracts arising from the terminal ileum and extending to the cecum (*arrows*)

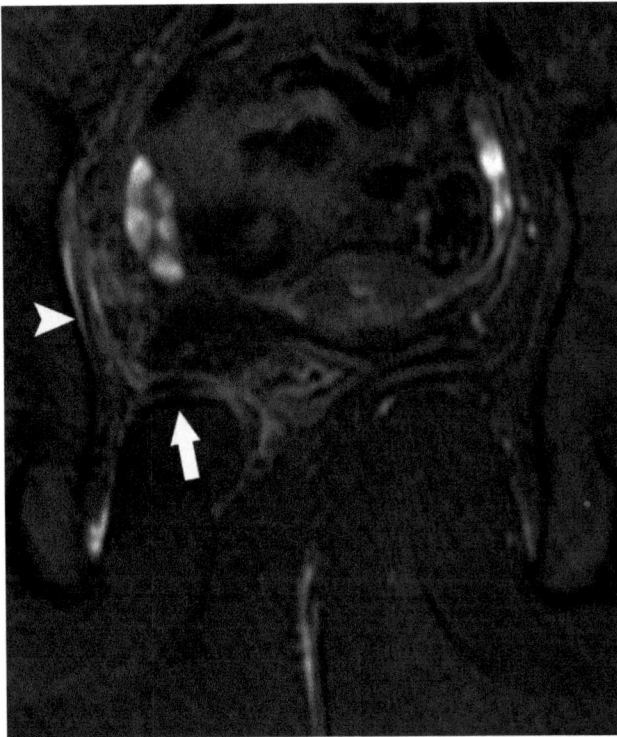

Fig. 20.11 Coronal T2-weighted fat-suppressed image of the pelvis demonstrates T2 bright linear fistulous tract arising from the right side of the rectum at the level of the levator musculature (*arrow*). T2 bright inflammatory changes are seen to extend deep into the pelvis along the obturator internus muscle (*arrowhead*)

intestinal perforation is made when free extraperitoneal gas is detected by either plain film or CT. The radiologic signs of bowel obstruction or perforation in patients with Crohn disease are similar to the findings in other patients, and further details will be found in most general radiology textbooks.

Toxic Megacolon

Toxic megacolon is a complication more frequently seen with UC, but may also occur in patients with severe CD. The clinical scenario is a patient with IBD presenting with an acute abdomen and signs of sepsis. Occasionally, toxic megacolon is the initial presentation of the patient with UC. The diagnosis should be made on a plain radiograph. Marked colonic dilatation with absent haustral pattern is seen, with the threshold for diagnosis depending on the child's age. In adolescents, the threshold is a colonic diameter >5 cm. Following initial medical treatment, serial films are obtained to monitor for progression and evidence of perforation. Colon contrast studies should be avoided as they increase the risk of perforation.

Extraintestinal Disease

Although IBD predominantly affects the gastrointestinal system, it is associated with a large number of extraintestinal manifestations that can significantly contribute to morbidity and affect the overall quality of life. Most commonly affected, as a direct pathophysiologic consequence of the disease, are the skin, eyes, and musculoskeletal and hepatobiliary systems. Ultimately, almost every organ system may be affected by either the secondary systemic effects of the disease or the adverse effects of treatment. Radiologic assessment of some of these systemic disorders is an important part of the comprehensive assessment of the patient with IBD. In addition to the brief account given below, detailed description of these systemic manifestations, including radiologic evaluation, will be found in the appropriate chapters in this book.

Hepatobiliary Disease

Gallstones

There is an overall increased incidence of gallstones in patients with IBD, but the association is far stronger with CD than UC. The best modality for detecting gallstones is US, although CT may be indicated in some situations.

Primary Sclerosing Cholangitis

Primary sclerosing cholangitis (PSC) is characterized by inflammatory fibrosis of the intrahepatic and extrahepatic biliary ducts with progression to stricture, cholestasis, and cirrhosis (Fig. 20.12). In contrast to gallstones, PSC is more strongly associated with UC than CD. Although endoscopic retrograde cholangiopancreatography (ERCP) has high sensitivity for detecting early biliary changes, in children, this procedure may require general anesthesia and depends on equipment and technical expertise that are not available to

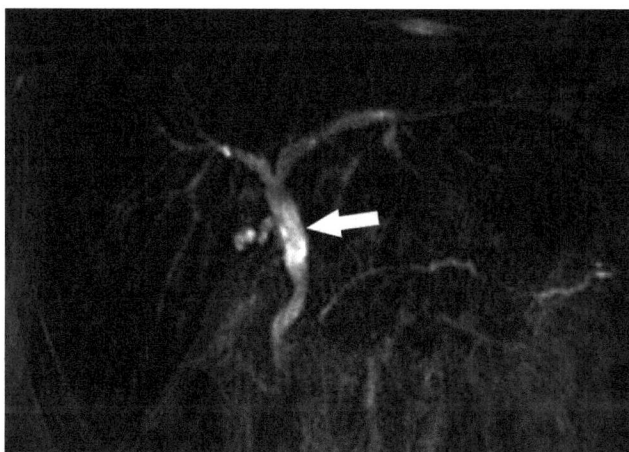

Fig. 20.12 MRCP maximum intensity projection (MIP) image of the biliary tree demonstrates common duct dilation (*arrow*) with patent left and right hepatic ducts

some pediatric centers. Magnetic resonance cholangiopancreatography (MRCP) is an alternative noninvasive method that produces similar cholangiographic images without exposure to ionizing radiation. However, due to lower sensitivity for detecting changes of PSC, ERCP should be considered when MRCP is negative but strong clinical suspicion persists [68].

Bone and Joint Disease

Osteopenia

Osteopenia and osteoporosis are well known complications of chronic IBD with several potential mechanisms including cytokines activation, malnutrition, malabsorption, delayed puberty, and treatment with corticosteroids [69, 70]. Reduced bone mineral density (BMD) causes skeletal fragility and increases the propensity for fractures in children with CD [71]. The most common method for the detection of reduced bone mineral density is the dual-energy X-ray absorptiometry (DXA) scan. The BMD measured by DXA scan of the lumbar spine, femoral neck, and radius is expressed as Z-scores, defined as the standard deviation of the measured BMD in relation to the mean for the child's age and sex. Presently, consensus is lacking on the normal ranges of Z-scores in children. In addition, when growth failure has occurred, correct assessment of BMD may require interpretation in terms of bone age or height age, rather than chronological age [72, 73]. The cost, limited availability, and difficult interpretation are some of the disadvantages to the use of DXA in children [74]. Unfortunately, alternative means of measuring BMD in children either have low sensitivity (quantitative ultrasound) or entail a higher radiation dose (quantitative computer tomography) [74, 75].

Future Trends

Emerging technological developments may soon alter the landscape for radiographic imaging of IBD. With advances in hardware and software leading to improved image resolution, cross-sectional imaging techniques may replace conventional contrast studies as the gold standard for small bowel evaluation in CD. While one of the most promising modalities is the MR enteroclysis combined with enteral contrast volume challenge [4], the MR enterography study is better tolerated in the pediatric population, and given its proven diagnostic effectiveness in the evaluation of CD, the trend is likely that MR enterography will substitute CT as the first-line imaging modality in the study of pediatric patients with CD. MRI will likely also play an increasing role in the differentiation of CD from UC, the follow-up of patients with indeterminate colitis, and the evaluation of disease activity and postoperative complications [24]. Increased use of pelvic MRI may also lead to the development a pediatric perianal disease index, similar to the one already described in adult patients with CD [76].

The now familiar technique of US may be put into increasing use as radiologists, and possibly gastroenterologists, begin to maximize its potential in the monitoring of disease activity and postoperative recurrence [13, 77].

One of the most exciting developments in the diagnostic assessment of IBD is the three-dimensional MRI and CT colonography, the so-called virtual endoscopy [78, 79].

Acknowledgments The authors would like to thank Dr. D. Gregory Bates for contributing to the images contained in this chapter.

References

1. Taylor GA, Nancarrow PA, Hernanz-Schulman M, Teele RL. Plain abdominal radiographs in children with inflammatory bowel disease. Pediatr Radiol. 1986;16(3):206–9.
2. Furukawa A, Saotome T, Yamasaki M, et al. Cross-sectional imaging in Crohn disease. Radiographics. 2004;24(3):689–702.
3. Jabra AA, Fishman EK, Taylor GA. Crohn disease in the pediatric patient: CT evaluation. Radiology. 1991;179(2):495–8.
4. Gourtsoyiannis NC, Papanikolaou N, Karantanas A. Magnetic resonance imaging evaluation of small intestinal Crohn disease. Best Pract Res Clin Gastroenterol. 2006;20(1):137–56.
5. Durno CA, Sherman P, Williams T, Shuckett B, Dupuis A, Griffiths AM. Magnetic resonance imaging to distinguish the type and severity of pediatric inflammatory bowel diseases. J Pediatr Gastroenterol Nutr. 2000;30(2):170–4.
6. Darbari A, Sena L, Argani P, Oliva-Hemker JM, Thompson R, Cuffari C. Gadolinium-enhanced magnetic resonance imaging: a useful radiological tool in diagnosing pediatric IBD. Inflamm Bowel Dis. 2004;10(2):67–72.
7. Siddiki HA, Fidler JL, Fletcher JG, et al. Prospective comparison of state-of-the-art MR enterography and CT enterography in small-bowel Crohn disease. AJR Am J Roentgenol. 2009;193(1):113–21.
8. Ippolito D, Invernizzi F, Galimberti S, Panelli MR, Sironi S. MR enterography with polyethylene glycol as oral contrast medium in the follow-up of patients with Crohn disease: comparison with CT enterography. Abdom Imaging. 2010;35(5):563–70.
9. Lee SS, Kim AY, Yang SK, et al. Crohn disease of the small bowel: comparison of CT enterography, MR enterography, and small-bowel follow-through as diagnostic techniques. Radiology. 2009;251(3):751–61.
10. Gee MS, Nimkin K, Hsu M, et al. Prospective evaluation of MR enterography as the primary imaging modality for pediatric Crohn disease assessment. AJR Am J Roentgenol. 2011;197(1):224–31.
11. Griffin N, Grant LA, Anderson S, Irving P, Sanderson J. Small bowel MR enterography: problem solving in Crohn's disease. Insights Imaging. 2012;3:251–63.
12. Allen PB, De Cruz P, Lee WK, Taylor S, Desmond PV, Kamm MA. Noninvasive imaging of the small bowel in Crohn disease: the final frontier. Inflamm Bowel Dis. 2011;17(9):1987–99.
13. Maconi G, Radice E, Greco S, Bianchi PG. Bowel ultrasound in Crohn disease. Best Pract Res Clin Gastroenterol. 2006;20(1):93–112.
14. Faure C, Belarbi N, Mougenot JF, et al. Ultrasonographic assessment of inflammatory bowel disease in children: comparison with ileocolonoscopy. J Pediatr. 1997;130(1):147–51.
15. Bremner AR, Griffiths M, Argent JD, Fairhurst JJ, Beattie RM. Sonographic evaluation of inflammatory bowel disease: a prospective, blinded, comparative study. Pediatr Radiol. 2006;36(9):947–53.
16. Haber HP, Busch A, Ziebach R, Stern M. Bowel wall thickness measured by ultrasound as a marker of Crohn disease activity in children. Lancet. 2000;355(9211):1239–40.
17. Spalinger J, Patriquin H, Miron MC, et al. Doppler US in patients with crohn disease: vessel density in the diseased bowel reflects disease activity. Radiology. 2000;217(3):787–91.
18. Bremner AR, Pridgeon J, Fairhurst J, Beattie RM. Ultrasound scanning may reduce the need for barium radiology in the assessment of small-bowel Crohn disease. Acta Paediatr. 2004;93(4):479–81.
19. Gasche C. Transabdominal bowel sonography in clinical decision-making. In: Mayless TM, Hanauer SB, editors. Advanced therapy of inflammatory bowel disease. Hamilton: B.C. Decker; 2001. p. 55–62.
20. Horton KM, Corl FM, Fishman EK. CT evaluation of the colon: inflammatory disease. Radiographics. 2000;20(2):399–418.
21. Jabra A, Fishman E, Taylor G. CT findings in inflammatory bowel disease in children. Am J Roentgenol. 1994;162(4):975–9.
22. Philpotts LE, Heiken JP, Westcott MA, Gore RM. Colitis: use of CT findings in differential diagnosis. Radiology. 1994;190(2):445–9.
23. Nozue T, Kobayashi A, Takagi Y, Okabe H, Hasegawa M. Assessment of disease activity and extent by magnetic resonance imaging in ulcerative colitis. Pediatr Int. 2000;42(3):285–8.
24. Maccioni F, Colaiacomo MC, Parlanti S. Ulcerative colitis: value of MR imaging. Abdom Imaging. 2005;30(5):584–92.
25. Maconi G, Ardizzone S, Parente F, Bianchi PG. Ultrasonography in the evaluation of extension, activity, and follow-up of ulcerative colitis. Scand J Gastroenterol. 1999;34(11):1103–7.
26. Ruess L, Blask AR, Bulas DI, et al. Inflammatory bowel disease in children and young adults: correlation of sonographic and clinical parameters during treatment. AJR Am J Roentgenol. 2000;175(1):79–84.
27. Carvalho RS, Abadom V, Dilworth HP, Thompson R, Oliva-Hemker M, Cuffari C. Indeterminate colitis: a significant subgroup of pediatric IBD. Inflamm Bowel Dis. 2006;12(4):258–62.
28. Miao YM, Koh DM, Amin Z, et al. Ultrasound and magnetic resonance imaging assessmentof active bowel segments in Crohn disease. Clin Radiol. 2002;57(10):913–8.
29. Segal AW, Ensell J, Munro JM, Sarner M. Indium-111 tagged leucocytes in the diagnosis of inflammatory bowel disease. Lancet. 1981;2(8240):230–2.
30. Del Rosario MA, Fitzgerald JF, Siddiqui AR, Chong SK, Croffie JM, Gupta SK. Clinical applications of technetium Tc 99 m hexamethyl propylene amine oxime leukocyte scan in children with inflammatory bowel disease. J Pediatr Gastroenterol Nutr. 1999;28(1):63–70.
31. Charron M, Di Lorenzo C, Kocoshis S. Are 99mTc leukocyte scintigraphy and SBFT studies useful in children suspected of having inflammatory bowel disease? Am J Gastroenterol. 2000;95(5):1208–12.
32. Fitzgerald PG, Topp TJ, Walton JM, Jackson JR, Gillis DA. The use of indium 111 leukocyte scans in children with inflammatory bowel disease. J Pediatr Surg. 1992;27(10):1298–300.
33. Charron M, del Rosario JF, Kocoshis S. Use of technetium-tagged white blood cells in patients with Crohn disease and ulcerative colitis: is differential diagnosis possible? Pediatr Radiol. 1998;28(11):871–7.
34. Alberini JL, Badran A, Freneaux E, et al. Technetium-99m HMPAO-labeled leukocyte imaging compared with endoscopy, ultrasonography, and contrast radiology in children with inflamma-

tory bowel disease. J Pediatr Gastroenterol Nutr. 2001;32(3): 278–86.

35. Charron M. Fernando del Rosario J, Kocoshis S. Distribution of acute bowel inflammation determined by technetium-labeled white blood cells in children with inflammatory bowel disease. Inflamm Bowel Dis. 1998;4(2):84–8.

36. Bhargava SA, Orenstein SR, Charron M. Technetium-99 m hexamethylpropyleneamine-oxime-labeled leukocyte scintigraphy in inflammatory bowel disease in children. J Pediatr. 1994;125(2): 213–7.

37. Charron M, Del Rosario F, Kocoshis S. Assessment of terminal ileal and colonic inflammation in Crohn disease with 99mTc-WBC. Acta Paediatr. 1999;88(2):193–8.

38. Skehan SJ, Issenman R, Mernagh J, Nahmias C, Jacobson K. 18F-fluorodeoxyglucose positron tomography in diagnosis of paediatric inflammatory bowel disease. Lancet. 1999;354(9181):836–7.

39. Lemberg DA, Issenman RM, Cawdron R, et al. Positron emission tomography in the investigation of pediatric inflammatory bowel disease. Inflamm Bowel Dis. 2005;11(8):733–8.

40. Morris J, Spencer JA, Ambrose NS. MR imaging classification of perianal fistulas and its implications for patient management. Radiographics. 2000;20(3):623–35; discussion 635–7.

41. deSouza NM, Hall AS, Puni R, Gilderdale DJ, Young IR, Kmiot WA. High resolution magnetic resonance imaging of the anal sphincter using a dedicated endoanal coil. Comparison of magnetic resonance imaging with surgical findings. Dis Colon Rectum. 1996;39(8):926–34.

42. Buchanan GN, Halligan S, Bartram CI, Williams AB, Tarroni D, Cohen CR. Clinical examination, endosonography, and MR imaging in preoperative assessment of fistula in ano: comparison with outcome-based reference standard. Radiology. 2004;233(3): 674–81.

43. Kuijpers HC, Schulpen T. Fistulography for fistula-in-ano. Is it useful? Dis Colon Rectum. 1985;28(2):103–4.

44. Pomerri F, Pittarello F, Dodi G, Pianon P, Muzzio PC. Radiologic diagnosis of anal fistulae with radio-opaque markers. Radiol Med (Torino). 1988;75(6):632–7.

45. Schratter-Sehn AU, Lochs H, Vogelsang H, Schurawitzki H, Herold C, Schratter M. Endoscopic ultrasonography versus computed tomography in the differential diagnosis of perianorectal complications in Crohn disease. Endoscopy. 1993;25(9):582–6.

46. Bartram C, Buchanan G. Imaging anal fistula. Radiol Clin N Am. 2003;41(2):443–57.

47. Hussain SM, Stoker J, Schouten WR, Hop WC, Lameris JS. Fistula in ano: endoanal sonography versus endoanal MR imaging in classification. Radiology. 1996;200(2):475–81.

48. West RL, Zimmerman DD, Dwarkasing S, et al. Prospective comparison of hydrogen peroxide-enhanced three-dimensional endoanal ultrasonography and endoanal magnetic resonance imaging of perianal fistulas. Dis Colon Rectum. 2003;46(10):1407–15.

49. Laniado M, Makowiec F, Dammann F, Jehle EC, Claussen CD, Starlinger M. Perianal complications of Crohn disease: MR imaging findings. Eur Radiol. 1997;7(7):1035–42.

50. Buchanan GN, Williams AB, Bartram CI, Halligan S, Nicholls RJ, Cohen CR. Potential clinical implications of direction of a transsphincteric anal fistula track. Br J Surg. 2003;90(10):1250–5.

51. Buchanan G, Halligan S, Williams A, et al. Effect of MRI on clinical outcome of recurrent fistula-in-ano. Lancet. 2002;360(9346): 1661–2.

52. Schwartz DA, White CM, Wise PE, Herline AJ. Use of endoscopic ultrasound to guide combination medical and surgical therapy for patients with Crohn perianal fistulas. Inflamm Bowel Dis. 2005;11(8):727–32.

53. Stewart LK, McGee J, Wilson SR. Transperineal and transvaginal sonography of perianal inflammatory disease. AJR Am J Roentgenol. 2001;177(3):627–32.

54. Stoker J, Rociu E, Schouten WR, Lameris JS. Anovaginal and rectovaginal fistulas: endoluminal sonography versus endoluminal MR imaging. AJR Am J Roentgenol. 2002;178(3):737–41.

55. Dwarkasing S, Hussain SM, Hop WC, Krestin GP. Anovaginal fistulas: evaluation with endoanal MR imaging. Radiology. 2004; 231(1):123–8.

56. Schwartz DA, Wiersema MJ, Dudiak KM, et al. A comparison of endoscopic ultrasound, magnetic resonance imaging, and exam under anesthesia for evaluation of Crohn perianal fistulas. Gastroenterology. 2001;121(5):1064–72.

57. Schwartz DA, Pemberton JH, Sandborn WJ. Diagnosis and treatment of perianal fistulas in Crohn disease. Ann Intern Med. 2001;135(10):906–18.

58. Gupta N, Cohen SA, Bostrom AG, et al. Risk factors for initial surgery in pediatric patients with Crohn disease. Gastroenterology. 2006;130(4):1069–77.

59. Michelassi F, Stella M, Balestracci T, Giuliante F, Marogna P, Block GE. Incidence, diagnosis, and treatment of enteric and colorectal fistulae in patients with Crohn disease. Ann Surg. 1993;218(5):660–6.

60. Yamaguchi A, Matsui T, Sakurai T, et al. The clinical characteristics and outcome of intraabdominal abscess in Crohn disease. J Gastroenterol. 2004;39(5):441–8.

61. Gervais DA, Hahn PF, O'Neill MJ, Mueller PR. Percutaneous abscess drainage in Crohn disease: technical success and short- and long-term outcomes during 14 years. Radiology. 2002;222(3): 645–51.

62. Jawhari A, Kamm MA, Ong C, Forbes A, Bartram CI, Hawley PR. Intra-abdominal and pelvic abscess in Crohn disease: results of noninvasive and surgical management. Br J Surg. 1998;85(3): 367–71.

63. Sahai A, Belair M, Gianfelice D, Cote S, Gratton J, Lahaie R. Percutaneous drainage of intra-abdominal abscesses in Crohn disease: short and long-term outcome. Am J Gastroenterol. 1997; 92(2):275–8.

64. Low RN, Francis IR, Politoske D, Bennett M. Crohn disease evaluation: comparison of contrast-enhanced MR imaging and single-phase helical CT scanning. J Magn Reson Imaging. 2000;11(2): 127–35.

65. Rieber A, Aschoff A, Nussle K, et al. MRI in the diagnosis of small bowel disease: use of positive and negative oral contrast media in combination with enteroclysis. Eur Radiol. 2000;10(9):1377–82.

66. Simoneaux S, Patrick L. Genitourinary complications of Crohn disease in pediatric patients. Am J Roentgenol. 1997;169(1):197–9.

67. Gore RM. CT of inflammatory bowel disease. Radiol Clin N Am. 1989;27(4):717–29.

68. Ferrara C, Valeri G, Salvolini L, Giovagnoni A. Magnetic resonance cholangiopancreatography in primary sclerosing cholangitis in children. Pediatr Radiol. 2002;32(6):413–7.

69. Semeao EJ, Jawad AF, Stouffer NO, Zemel BS, Piccoli DA, Stallings VA. Risk factors for low bone mineral density in children and young adults with Crohn disease. J Pediatr. 1999;135(5): 593–600.

70. Gokhale R, Favus MJ, Karrison T, Sutton MM, Rich B, Kirschner BS. Bone mineral density assessment in children with inflammatory bowel disease. Gastroenterology. 1998;114(5):902–11.

71. Semeao EJ, Stallings VA, Peck SN, Piccoli DA. Vertebral compression fractures in pediatric patients with Crohn disease. Gastroenterology. 1997;112(5):1710–3.

72. Herzog D, Bishop N, Glorieux F, Seidman EG. Interpretation of bone mineral density values in pediatric Crohn disease. Inflamm Bowel Dis. 1998;4(4):261–7.

73. Ahmed SF, Horrocks IA, Patterson T, et al. Bone mineral assessment by dual energy X-ray absorptiometry in children with inflammatory bowel disease: evaluation by age or bone area. J Pediatr Gastroenterol Nutr. 2004;38(3):276–80.

74. van Rijn RR, van der Sluis IM, Link TM, et al. Bone densitometry in children: a critical appraisal. Eur Radiol. 2003;13(4):700–10.

75. Levine A, Mishna L, Ballin A, et al. Use of quantitative ultrasound to assess osteopenia in children with Crohn disease. J Pediatr Gastroenterol Nutr. 2002;35(2):169–72.

76. Van Assche G, Vanbeckevoort D, Bielen D, et al. Magnetic resonance imaging of the effects of infliximab on perianal fistulizing Crohn disease. Am J Gastroenterol. 2003;98(2):332–9.

77. Canani RB, de Horatio LT, Terrin G, et al. Combined use of noninvasive tests is useful in the initial diagnostic approach to a child with suspected inflammatory bowel disease. J Pediatr Gastroenterol Nutr. 2006;42(1):9–15.

78. Guilhon de Araujo Sant'Anna AM, Dubois J, MC Miron, EG Seidman. Wireless capsule endoscopy for obscure small-bowel disorders: final results of the first pediatric controlled trial. Clin Gastroenterol Hepatol 2005;3(3):264-270.

79. Haykir R, Karakose S, Karabacakoglu A, Sahin M, Kayacetin E. Three-dimensional MR and axial CT colonography versus conventional colonoscopy for detection of colon pathologies. World J Gastroenterol. 2006;12(15):2345–50.

Endoscopy and Inflammatory Bowel Disease

21

Shishu Sharma, Krishnappa Venkatesh, and Mike Thomson

Introduction

Safe, informative, and effective endoscopy performed in a child-friendly situation with the minimum of distress to child and parent alike is a sine qua non of a unit adhering to best practice in the care of children and adolescents with pediatric inflammatory bowel disease (PIBD). The care of children and adolescents differs in important ways from that of adults. This is reflected in the emphasis placed on various aspects of endoscopy especially ileocolonoscopy (IC), such as the frequent use of general anesthesia, the number and location of mucosal biopsies, and the routine inclusion of ileal intubation during a complete examination. The question of who should conduct the procedure continues to receive attention among pediatric gastroenterologists. The current evidence and consensus recommends that endoscopy should be performed by a pediatric gastroenterologist or a gastroenterologist who has pediatric experience, under general anesthesia or deep sedation [1]. There can be few more satisfying experiences in medicine than making a clinical judgment and diagnosis in a child, confirming the nature and extent of the disease oneself by endoscopy, treating appropriately, and then visually demonstrating the success of such endeavors to child and parent by a follow-up procedure.

Endoscopy plays an important role in the initial diagnosis of inflammatory bowel disease (IBD), differentiation of IBD into Crohn disease (CD) and ulcerative colitis (UC), assessment of disease extent, monitoring of response to therapy, surveillance of cancer, and to perform endo-therapeutic procedures such as stricture dilatation [2].

S. Sharma • K. Venkatesh • M. Thomson (✉)
Sheffield Children's Hospital, Sheffield, UK
e-mail: mike.thomson@sch.nhs.uk

Endoscopy: Background History

The evolution of endoscopy in the diagnostic armamentarium was initially a slow process. Rigid esophagoscopes and sigmoidoscopes were introduced in the late nineteenth century and semiflexible endoscopes in the 1930s. They remained the only endoscopes in use until the 1960s. This was partly because of the lack of understanding about inflammatory bowel disease, which was for a long time thought to be a disease mainly confined to the rectosigmoid region. However, the invention of fiber optics in the 1950s heralded a new era leading to the development of the first flexible sigmoidoscope in 1963 and colonoscope in 1966. This made it possible to visualize, take biopsies, and perform endo-therapeutic procedures and reach the duodenum and the ileo-colon. The next major breakthrough was the arrival of video-chip technology in the 1980s. This allowed digital images to be displayed on a monitor and further to be stored, analyzed, and transmitted as necessary. Further advances have seen the development of Sonde enteroscopy [3], which was limited by lack of therapeutic potential, and then push enteroscopy, allowing the therapeutic endoscopist an access of up to 70–100 cm small bowel beyond the pylorus. Intraoperative endoscopy (IOE) appeared to be the only means available to access the whole of the small bowel at the turn of the century until the development of wireless capsule endoscopy (WCE). This technological breakthrough allowed the direct visualization of the entire small bowel without the need of external wires, fiber-optic bundles, or cables but as yet is limited to diagnostic input alone. Double balloon enteroscopy (DBE) is a more recent modality, which enables high-resolution endoscopic imaging of the entire small bowel, with the advantage over WCE of potential for mucosal biopsies and interventional endo-therapy.

© Springer International Publishing AG 2017
P. Mamula et al. (eds.), *Pediatric Inflammatory Bowel Disease*, DOI 10.1007/978-3-319-49215-5_21

Patient Preparation

Ideally, both the child and the parents should be offered a preparatory visit to the endoscopy unit to answer questions and defuse any potential concerns and anxieties regarding the procedure and admission. Children with greater knowledge of the procedure exhibit less distress and report less anxiety toward the procedure [4]. Younger children undoubtedly benefit from preadmission visits and the involvement of a play therapist to enable some understanding of what is to take place and why [5–7]. Diagrams may help in explanations to older children. Preparatory videotapes are also useful for informing the patient and parent regarding what to expect. Units can benefit from devising a sample videotape specific to their own facility. A reduction in anticipatory anxiety may even reduce the amount of intravenous sedation required [8].

A child-friendly decorated endoscopy room with age-appropriate videotapes and familiar faces is important at this time of high stress. Parents may stay to watch the procedure in some units when intravenous sedation is provided. Most anesthesiologists would object to having parents present during administration of a general anesthetic, beyond the initial induction. Improved medical compliance and belief in the treatment are potential advantageous consequences of allowing parents to directly view the initial disease and its remission at follow-up ileocolonoscopy [9]. Young children often request photographs or a videotape of the ileocolonoscopy, and older adolescents may view the procedure themselves.

A full screening is important to identify potential sedation or anesthetic risks. Although there is little correlation of mildly deranged peripheral coagulation indices with hemorrhage after mucosal biopsies, more pronounced bleeding diatheses may require forethought and appropriate blood product backup [10]. Properly informed consent should be obtained with an information sheet detailing potential complications and their incidence, and a separate consent should be signed in the event of research biopsies being requested.

Antibiotic Prophylaxis

Guidelines concerning antibiotic prophylaxis in children with lesions susceptible to endocarditis or in the immunocompromised child are available in the historical literature [11] but are now superseded by the American Society for Gastrointestinal endoscopy (ASGE) guidelines for antibiotic prophylaxis for gastrointestinal endoscopic procedure [12]. American Heart Association has also published new recommendations of antibiotic prophylaxis for infective endocarditis (IE) and do not advise antibiotics for routine diagnostic or therapeutic gastrointestinal endoscopic procedure, solely for prevention of IE [13]. AHA recommends antibiotic prophy-

laxis for patients undergoing gastrointestinal procedure with established gastrointestinal infections where Enterococcus is the suspected causative organism and with the following cardiac condition: (1) a prosthetic cardiac valve, (2) previous IE, (3) cardiac transplant recipients with valvulopathy, (4) unrepaired cyanotic CHD (including palliative shunts and conduits), (5) repaired CHD having residual defects at the site or adjacent to the site of a prosthetic device, and (6) completely repaired CHD with prosthetic device placed within the last 6 months of the gastrointestinal procedure. The recommended antibiotic regimen in the above situations should include ampicillin (50 mg/kg every 4–6 h, maximum 2 g every 4 h) or amoxicillin (50 mg/kg every 4–6 h, maximum 2 g every 4 h) in combination with gentamicin. Vancomycin or teicoplanin can be used in patients who are allergic to ampicillin/amoxicillin. The British Society of Gastroenterology recommends the above antibiotic prophylaxis in combination with metronidazole for patients with severe neutropenia ($<0.5 \times 109/l$) and/or who are profoundly immunocompromised (e.g., advanced hematological malignancy) and are undergoing procedures that are known to be associated with a high risk of bacteremia (Table 21.1) [14]. The preferred choice of antibiotics for biliary procedures is either ciprofloxacin or gentamicin or cephalosporins given intravenously just before the procedure. In our unit, prophylactic intravenous cefuroxime or co-amoxiclav is given for 24 h for percutaneous endoscopic gastrostomy (PEG) or jejunostomy (PEJ). The other condition where routine use of antibiotic prophylaxis is recommended is cirrhosis with acute GI bleed. The above recommendations are primarily based on evidence from adult studies but are also used for pediatric population.

Bowel Preparation

Poor bowel preparation is a major factor that may prevent or impede successful ileocolonoscopy. Although administration of regimens is not always easy, modern protocols can be remarkably effective in clearing the colon and ileum. Until 5 or 6 years ago, large volumes of oral electrolyte lavage solutions were used with variable success, coupled with the significant disadvantages of nasogastric administration and potential for fluid-electrolyte shifts in smaller children and infants. In one study, 40 mL/kg/hr. resulted in clear fecal effluent after a mean of 2.6 h [15]. Subsequently, more favorable results and compliance were reported with low-volume oral agents and enemas, along with decreased oral intake [16–19]. Use of sodium phosphate preparations was associated with a transient rise in mean serum sodium and phosphate, but with no change in serum calcium [17, 18]. Refinements were made to these oral and enema regimens as newer preparations, which were more acceptable to children, became available;

Table 21.1 Infection risk associated with various gastrointestinal procedures

High risk of bacteremia	High risk of infection unrelated to bacteremia	Low risk of infection
Dilatation of esophageal stricture	Endoscopic ultrasound with fine-needle aspiration (EUS-FNA)	Routine EGD, IC, or sigmoidoscopy
Sclerotherapy of esophageal varices	Percutaneous endoscopic gastrostomy (PEG) or jejunostomy (PEJ)	Polypectomy
ERCP in patients with: (i) Biliary disorders, e.g., cholangitis, primary sclerosing cholangitis (ii) Conditions where complete biliary drainage is difficult to achieve, e.g., cholangiocarcinoma (iii) Liver transplantation (iv) Pancreatic pseudocyst		

ERCP endoscopic retrograde cholangiopancreatography, *EGD* esophagogastroduodenoscopy, *IC* Ileocolonoscopy

Table 21.2 Successful low-volume regimens for the preparation of the bowel for colonoscopy

Study	Regimen	Diet	Success rate
Gremse et al. (1996) [17]	Oral sodium phosphate (45 ml/1.7 m^2) 6 pm and 6 am for am procedure	Clear liquid 24 h	18/19
Da Silva et al. (1997) [18]	Oral sodium phosphate (22.5 ml if <30 kg, 45 ml if >30 kg) pm and 5 am for am procedure	Clear liquid after first dose	10/14
Pinfield et al. (1999) [20]	Sodium picosulfate with magnesium citrate (2.5 g <2 years., 5 g 2–5 years., 10 g >5 years per dose) 24 and 18 h pre procedure	Clear liquid for 24 h	32/32 (3 vomited)
Dahshan et al. 1999 [21]	Magnesium citrate and X-prep	Clear liquid for 48 h	

Table 21.3 Bowel preparation for children undergoing colonoscopy

Medicine	<1 years	1–4 years	>4 years
Sodium picosulfate + Magnesium citrate (Picolax)	¼ sachet	½ sachet	1 sachet
Senna	1–2 mg/kg (maximum 30 mg)		

The above medications are repeated 10 h apart with a backup of enema 1 h before procedure (1/2 h for infants). One Picolax sachet contains sodium picosulfate 10 mg with magnesium citrate (K$^+$ 5 mmol, Mg^{2+} 87 mmol)

low-volume nonabsorbable polyethylene glycol preparations are becoming increasingly popular in pediatric units and are well tolerated, with no observable electrolytic disturbance [20, 21]. Table 21.2 outlines several low-volume regimens that have been used successfully in children. The regimen employed in our unit, shown in Table 21.3, combines the beneficial effects of oral low-volume administration of Senna and combination of sodium picosulfate with magnesium citrate, with the backup of an enema 1–2 h beforehand if no clear fecal effluent is observed [22]. No clinically significant fluid shifts or electrolyte imbalances have been observed in over 2,000 colonoscopies over a 5-year period in our unit.

The benefit of an antispasmodic agent administered directly before the ileocolonoscopy has recently been demonstrated in an adult study where hyoscyamine 0.5 mg was given intravenously [23]. An effective alternative could be hyoscine butylbromide 20 mg administered intravenously during the procedure. The use of such an agent given just prior to IC is determined by personal preference. The antispasmodic agents are certainly of benefit in spastic colonic situations as their use may facilitate ease of luminal visualization. On the other hand, these can turn out to be counterproductive, as they may also increase the compliance of the colon, theoretically allowing a greater chance of loop formation.

However, it should be remembered that the antispasmodic agents work only for a short period of time, perhaps as short as 5 min, and these may be readministered in certain situations, e.g., when one needs to relax a haustral fold to visualize a polyp which is just beyond and obscured by it or occasionally when one needs to relax a spastic ileocecal valve. Glucagon at a dose of 0.5 mg intravenously is also used as an alternative to Buscopan, especially while performing DBE.

Monitoring and Sedation

"Sedation and analgesia" comprise a continuum of states ranging from minimal sedation (anxiolysis) through general anesthesia. Moderate sedation is a medically controlled state of depressed consciousness that allows protective reflexes to be maintained and retains the patient's ability to maintain the airway independently and continuously. Deep sedation is a medically controlled state of depressed consciousness or unconsciousness from which the patient is not easily aroused and accompanied by a partial or complete loss of protective reflexes with inability to maintain a patent airway. General anesthesia is a controlled state of unconsciousness accompanied by a loss of protective reflexes [24, 25].

The aims of adequate sedation include patient safety, anxiolysis, analgesia, amnesia as well as adequate endoscopic examination, time, and cost-efficiency [26]. Debate has surrounded the relative merits and safety of sedation and general anesthesia for esophagogastroduodenoscopy (EGD) and IC in children for several years [27–29].

The risks of general anesthesia include those associated with intubation and administration of an anesthetizing agent, which can be minimized by proper preparation and good intubation technique. However, the benefits include complete amnesia and total avoidance of pain to the patient as well as freeing the endoscopist from managing airway, monitoring vital signs, and recovering the patient [27].

Intravenous sedation (IV-S) usually consists of a narcotic (meperidine or fentanyl) and a benzodiazepine (diazepam or midazolam), the former for analgesia and the latter for anxiolysis and amnesia. Ketamine and midazolam have also been used with reportedly lesser side effects [30]. Propofol is now being used increasingly as the preferred choice for controlled sedation. Table 21.4 lists some of the commonly used sedation regimens with the reversal agents. IV-S has been argued to be safe, effective, and less costly in comparison to general anesthesia with successful sedation achieved in more than 95% of elective procedures [32, 33]. However, careful monitoring of IV-S throughout the procedure is important [33–35]. In spite of the advantages of IV-S, pediatric gastrointestinal endoscopy has moved toward general anesthesia since it is now acknowledged that, to get the requisite cooperation, and therefore a properly conducted procedure with minimum distress to the child, deep sedation is usually necessary. It is further recognized that there are attendant safety issues of airway maintenance in this situation, and at the very least, a specific individual with appropriate advanced pediatric life support skills should be responsible for the child's cardiorespiratory welfare during such a procedure. The vast majority of pediatric gastrointestinal endoscopy in the United Kingdom, for instance, now occurs under general anesthesia.

Table 21.4 Sedation and reversal medications commonly employed in pediatric endoscopy

Ketamine: IV 1–2 mg/kg as a single dose [30]
Propofol: IV 1–2 mg/kg for induction and then 1.5–9 mg/kg/h using 1% injection for maintenance
Midazolam: IV initial dose 25–50 microgram/kg, if necessary titrate to maximum 6 mg (1 month to 6 years), 10 mg (6–12 years), or 7.5 mg (12–18 years) [30, 31]
Fentanyl: IV initial dose 0.5–1.0 μg/kg and then titrate to max 5 μg/kg
Meperidine/Pethidine: IV initial dose 0.5 mg/kg and then titrate to max 2 mg/kg or 75 mg whichever lower
Flumazenil: IV 0.02 mg/kg (max 0.2 mg) and repeat every minute to max of 0.05 mg/kg or max 1 mg
Naloxone: IV 0.1 mg/kg (max 2 mg) and repeat every 2–3 min to max 10 mg

When a child is sedated, resuscitation equipment should be easily accessible, and one or more people trained in pediatric advanced life support should be responsible for maintaining the airway and monitoring respiration, heart rate, blood pressure, and oxygen saturation [24, 36]. Sedation of younger children can be aided by environmental comforts such as a soothing voice or dimmed lights [37]. In all age groups, it is often necessary to use deep sedation because of the pain that can be associated with this procedure [38]. With deep sedation, it is clear that the risks are significant, including hypotension, respiratory compromise, and even respiratory arrest.

Recent studies examining the safety of general anesthesia for day-case IC in children refute the claims that there may be more risk of perforation because the operator cannot judge the degree of discomfort as a marker of impending traction injury [39, 40]. There is indeed a lack of evidence to support the contention that there is a higher complication rate with a general anesthetic than with sedation [41]. In fact, the airway is protected in a more effective and safer manner than with sedation, especially in upper endoscopy, with an improved operator satisfaction [42].

Pre-procedural medication with a benzodiazepine have been found to be useful in reducing patient anxiety and improve patient and parent acceptance of the procedure without any significant adverse effects [31].

Endoscopic Techniques in Inflammatory Bowel Disease

Upper Gastrointestinal Endoscopy

While it is generally accepted that ileocolonoscopy(IC) and biopsy have a central role in the initial diagnosis and differentiation of pediatric inflammatory bowel disease (PIBD) [43], it is now recommended that in nonemergency situations, the diagnostic workup for pediatric patients should start with a combined EGD and ileocolonoscopy [43–46] except in situations such as acute severe colitis, where a limited sigmoidoscopy is preferred over complete IC as the latter may increase the risk of perforation. However, a follow-up IC should be performed after the resolution of the acute attack.

Presence of upper gastrointestinal symptoms has been commonly considered as an indication to perform EGD [47]. Typically described upper gastrointestinal symptoms include dysphagia, nausea and/or vomiting, and aphthous lesions of the mouth. Diagnosis was often based on radiological changes [48], and EGD was reserved for those patients who had upper GI symptoms and/or uncertain diagnosis. However, several studies have shown a higher incidence of microscopic mucosal disease in the upper GI tract [47, 49–53] than previously thought even in the absence of any upper GI symptoms [44, 54]. Cameron et al. [49] in a prospective study described histological abnormalities on gastroduodenal biopsies in 71% of patients with CD. Histological abnormalities including granulomas are seen even when the gross appearance of the tissue is normal [43, 47, 53–55]. Therefore, it is important to take multiple biopsies (2 or more per section) from all sections of the visualized gastrointestinal tract, even in the absence of macroscopic lesions.

In a prospective 3-year study involving 420 patients with IBD from 27 centers, EGD was performed in 237 patients. Eighty percent of patients with CD had macroscopic and/or histologic changes in the upper GI tract, while in 9% of the patients, EGD was helpful in making a definitive diagnosis [56]. In another prospective single center study, 24/45 patients with CD had an upper GI involvement and presented at an younger age, had more severe disease, and were more likely to have extraintestinal manifestations [57].

Esophageal disease in CD (Fig. 21.1) can vary from small erosions to transmural involvement resulting in perforation and fistulization into adjacent organs [58]. Granulomas are reported in 20–39% of esophageal biopsies in patients with CD [59, 60]. Other findings include erythema, ulceration, polypoid lesions, pseudomembranous formations, strictures, and mucosal bridges [59, 61–64]. Endoscopic findings in the stomach and duodenum include linear and serpiginous ulcers, diffuse superficial ulcers, aphthous lesions, nodularity, cobblestone appearance, rigidity of the GI wall, and narrowing of the lumen [65].

Focal enhanced gastritis as an important feature of CD was first described by Schmitz-Moorman et al. [66] (Fig. 21.2). Further, several studies confirmed this finding with a positive predictive value of 71–94% [50, 52, 67, 68]. Parente et al. [68] found focal antral gastritis more frequently in *Helicobacter pylori*-negative adults with CD and then in those with UC or noninflammatory bowel conditions. Also, they reported focal antral gastritis to be specific in 84% of patients with CD. While the presence of focal antral gastritis is suggestive of Crohn disease, it is not pathognomonic of the condition.

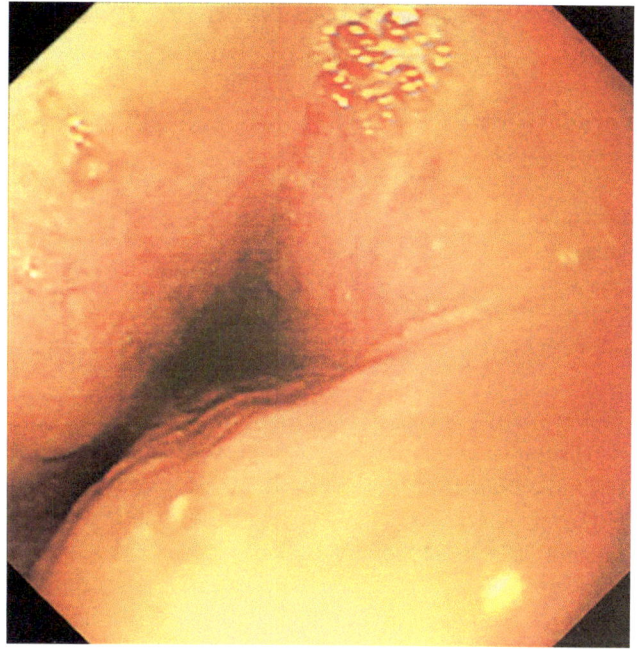

Fig. 21.1 Crohn disease of the esophagus showing discrete ulcers

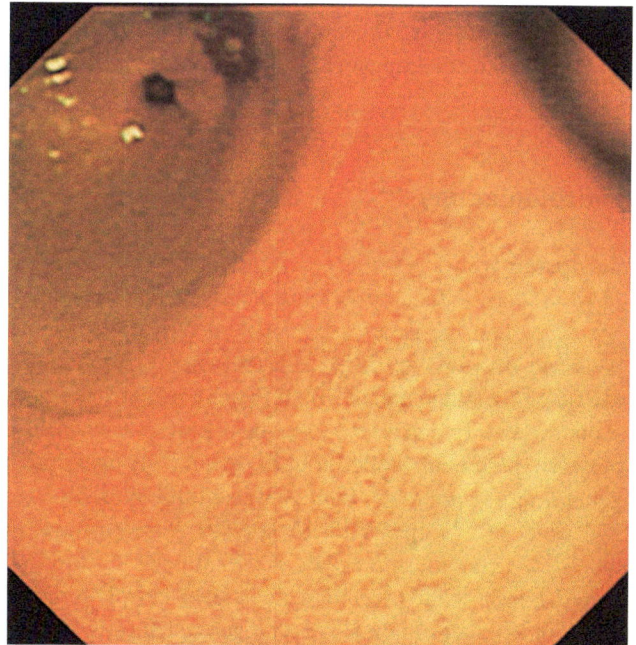

Fig. 21.2 Focal enhanced gastritis in Crohn disease

The presence of noncaseating granuloma is characteristic of CD. Granulomas are found in 7–68% of patients with CD in the upper GI tract [43, 47, 59, 65, 66] and often help in making a definitive diagnosis when none are found at other sites. Noncaseating granuloma in the upper gastrointestinal tract in the CD tends to occur in the superficial mucosa as compared to ileal CD where the muscularis or the serosal layers are primarily involved.

Table 21.5 Technical specifications of various pediatric colonoscopes

Parameter	Fujinon (EC-410 MP15)	Olympus (PCF 240 L/I)	Olympus variable stiffness (CF 240AL/I)	Pentax (EC-3440PK)
Angle of vision	140°	140°	140°	140°
Depth of field	6–100 mm	4–100 mm	3–100 mm	6–100 mm
Distal end	11 mm	11.3 mm	12.2 mm	11.5 mm
Insertion tube	11.1 mm	11.3 mm	12.0 mm	11.4 mm
Channel	2.8 mm	3.2 mm	3.2 mm	3.8 mm
Angle up/down	180°/180°	180°/180°	180°/180°	180°/180°
Angle right/left	160°/160°	160°/160°	160°/160°	160°/160°
Working length	1520 mm	1330 mm (I) 1680 mm (L)	1330 mm (I) 1680 mm (L)	1500 mm

Ulcerative colitis conventionally was thought to involve only the colon and possibly ileum (backwash ileitis). However, it is increasingly recognized that features of inflammation in the upper GI tract [44, 52, 53, 69, 70] are seen in UC. Ruuska et al. [53] in a prospective study reported either macroscopic or histological upper gastrointestinal lesions in 75% of patients with UC. Abdullah et al. [43] also reported an incidence of 70% of histological abnormalities in the upper GI tract in patients with UC. Tobin et al. [52] in a controlled blinded study described esophagitis in 72% and 50% of patients with CD and UC, respectively. Gastritis was, however, more common and seen in 92% of CD and 69% of UC.

Ileocolonoscopy

Equipment

Most modern units employ adult and pediatric videocolonoscopes, and the general technical specifications for the pediatric instruments differ little between manufacturers (Table 21.5). When and in whom to use a pediatric colonoscope is mainly a matter of personal preference. We use personal judgment based on age and/or body weight. In general terms, the lower limit for the adult colonoscope is 3–4 years of age and/or 12–15 kg. The extra stiffness of the adult versions diminishes the likelihood of forming sigmoid loops, but extra care must then be taken, especially in younger children and with general anesthesia, not to advance against undue resistance, to avoid the unlikely complication of colonic perforation. The larger diameter of the adult colonoscopes can also lead to problems of maneuverability within the smaller colonic lumen of a young child. The variable stiffness colonoscope (Table 21.5) may negotiate some of these problems. A control dial on the upper shaft of this small-diameter colonoscope (Olympus XCF-240AL/I, Olympus Inc., Tokyo, Japan) allows an increase in the stiffness of the insertion tube when passing through the sigmoid and transverse colon to avoid looping [71].

More recently, magnifying colonoscopes have been developed, and their value in combination with dye spray or chromoscopy in various gastrointestinal diseases has been described [72]. For instance, the decrease in the number of cryptal openings in ulcerative colitis can be observed and correlated to disease activity [73], but this does not substitute for histologic assessment.

For insufflation, there may be some advantage awarded by the use of carbon dioxide in place of air because it is more rapidly absorbed, leading to less patient discomfort and, theoretically, less risk of perforation [74, 75].

Ileocolonoscopy Basic Technique

Getting Started and Patient Positioning

The patient is usually positioned in the left lateral knee to chest position, although some operators prefer the right lateral position, citing easier sigmoid negotiation. Certainly, if the procedure is not subsequently allowing easy access to the splenic flexure, then patient repositioning from one side to the supine and then to the other side may be advantageous. In general, frequent turning of the patient is conducive to easier ileocolonoscopy as a whole and is to be advocated. An assistant stands on the operator's left to administer any abdominal pressure that may subsequently be deemed necessary to control, or try to prevent, loop formation in the sigmoid or transverse colon.

Practical Tips in Ileocolonoscopy

One important "trick" in learning ileocolonoscopy is to grasp the concept of the lumen and the positions of a clock face. For instance, if the lumen is at 9 o'clock, then to enter this requires anticlockwise rotation combined with upward deflection of the scope tip from the "neutral" position of 12 o'clock. Similarly, a combination of upward deflection of the tip with clockwise rotation of the colonoscope will allow entry of the lumen, suggested by a dark crescent, if seen at anywhere clockwise from 12 o'clock to 6 o'clock. Obviously, one may equally use downward tip deflection combined with the opposite rotatory control to that with upward tip deflection, and the execution and teaching of this concept are at personal discretion. With either approach, this is the most important maneuver that can be learned to assist in three-dimensional spatial orientation in the colon.

Prolonged "side viewing" of the bowel wall as it slides by should be avoided. Generally, the only place where, very temporarily, the lumen should be out of view is the occasional difficult negotiation of the splenic flexure. The patient's position may be changed throughout the procedure to facilitate removal of loops and to allow a better view of the lumen because the gravity-dependent material in the colonic lumen changes position. Relatively minimal insufflation of air is desirable in the sigmoid colon because excess air may increase the chance of sigmoid loop formation (carbon dioxide, provided by a specific commercially available delivery system attached to the colonoscope, as the insufflating gas of choice may be preferable because it is absorbed much more quickly, decreasing the pain sensation and the very unlikely chance of perforation; see "Complications."

In handling the colonoscope, it is good practice to have a flat unimpeded surface on which to place the remainder of the colonoscope that is not yet inserted; this is particularly important since any resistance encountered by the operator to forward advancement of the colonoscope can be attributed to colonic obstruction or loop formation within the child's colon. Hence, relatively quickly, the trainee can acquire a realization of the normal expected resistance to scope advancement. This, in turn, allows understanding of the likelihood of loop formation, without any external resistance to scope advancement, causing confusion with regard to the behavior of the colonoscope within the patient.

Generally, in ileocolonoscopy, gentle scope advancement with clear lumen visualization is desirable, and, usually, only the forefinger and thumb will be required to advance the colonoscope. If greater pressure is required, then the operator is not performing an optimum procedure, and loop formation is likely to have occurred.

Rectal Intubation

Prior to any colonoscopy, it is considered good practice to perform an anal and then a rectal digital examination, the latter to avoid missing, by colonoscopy, very low-lying rectal polyps (although, where possible, retroflexion of the colonoscope in the rectum should occur prior to removal of the instrument to avoid missing lesions close to the anal margin). Adequate water-soluble lubrication, avoiding the tip of the instrument, allows easy passage into the rectum, which can occur with or without digital guidance from the operator's index finger. The tip of the scope aimed posteriorly toward the spine combined with air insufflation allows visualization of the rectal mucosa and the three semilunar folds, or valves

of Houston, occurring on alternating sides of the lumen. Subsequently, direct visualization of the bowel lumen is mandatory, except in some circumstances at the splenic flexure. If, at any point, a maneuver results in loss of visualization of the lumen, then reversal of what the operator has just done will often return the lumen to view; if not, the gentle scope retraction combined with minor tip deflections using the wheels and minor rotation of the scope in both directions will usually result in reorientation in the lumen. Obviously, if luminal contents are blocking the view, then lens cleaning will help.

Sigmoid and Descending Colon

Gentle torquing of the shaft clockwise and anticlockwise combined with upward or downward tip deflection and scope advancement is ideal for negotiating the sigmoid colon, the so-called "torque-steering" technique. The initial sigmoid fold or valve can usually be passed by 90–120 of anticlockwise torsion. The different loops encountered in the sigmoid are demonstrated in Fig. 21.3. A so-called N loop may be overcome by transabdominal pressure by an assistant on the apex of the loop pushing toward the feet (see Fig. 21.3a). This often allows a so-called α loop to form, which can usually be tolerated as the instrument advances toward the splenic flexure (see Fig. 21.3b). Reducing an α loop is accomplished by initial clockwise rotation and then slow removal of the colonoscope, keeping the lumen in the center of the field of vision. This may not be possible until the transverse (or even ascending) colon has been entered, in which case, hooking the tip of the scope over the splenic flexure may assist it. Paradoxical movement of the tip forward may be observed as the instrument is withdrawn and the bowel "concertinas" over the colonoscope. Abdominal pressure in the left iliac fossa may be helpful. The sigmoid and descending colons are relatively featureless, with less haustral folds than more proximally in the colon.

Splenic Flexure and Transverse Colon

Non-looped colonoscope length used at this point might be 40 cm in older children and even 20–25 cm in those under the age of 3–4 years. This is valuable in determining whether a loop is present. At the splenic flexure, the spleen may then be seen as a dark blue transmural discoloration. When negotiating the splenic flexure, the most successful combination of tip maneuvers is that of clockwise, right, and up followed by anticlockwise after passing the flexure. Occasionally, placing the patient in the right decubitus position may assist. The transverse colon is recognized by the triangular haustral folds and is usually easily passed (Fig. 21.4). Supine or right decubitus positioning may ease this. A loop in the shape of a "U" may occur in a dependent transverse colon, which is supported by abdominal pressure. The more difficult γ loop may occur in a redundant transverse colon (Fig. 21.3c).

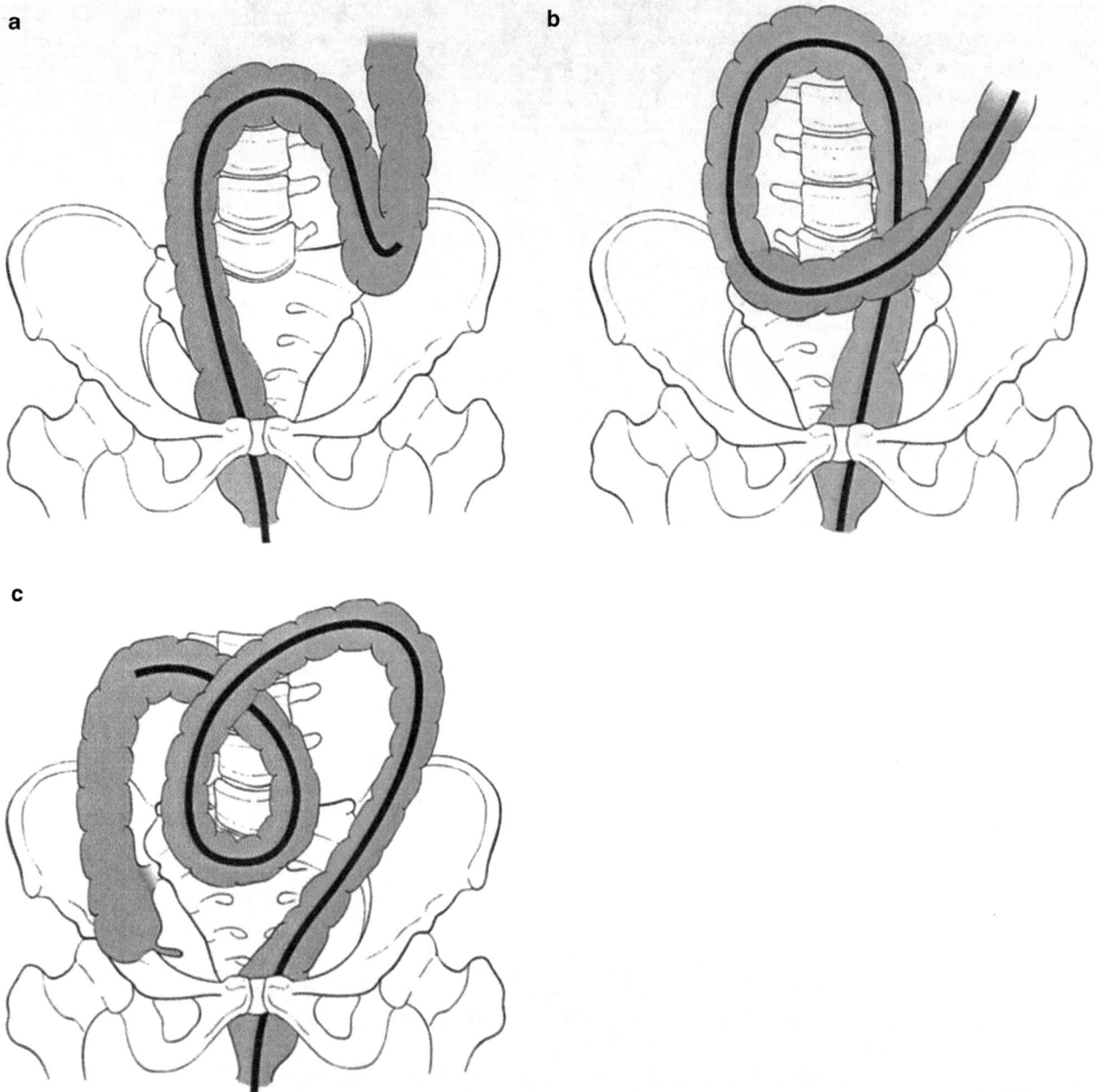

Fig. 21.3 Diagram of colonoscope sigmoid loops that may form (**a**) an N loop in the sigmoid colon, (**b**) an α loop in the sigmoid colon, and (**c**) a γ loop in a redundant transverse colon

In addition, a good bit of advice is to apply gentle suction as the tip is advanced in an attempt to concertina a potentially long dependent transverse colon over the colonoscope, thus maintaining a relatively short colonoscope and, hence, good control and maneuverability.

Hepatic Flexure and Ascending Colon
Non-looped colonoscope length used at this point might be 60 cm in older children and even 40 cm in those under the age of 3–4 years. This is valuable in determining whether a loop is present. The hepatic flexure is also recognized by

the dark, usually blue, discoloration seen through the bowel wall, and positional change to the supine or right decubitus may again facilitate identification of the lumen. The combination of right, up, and clockwise followed by anticlockwise rotation and suction down into the ascending colon once around the sharply angled hepatic flexure is usually the most effective maneuver, but various combinations, including position change and scope withdrawal, may be required. Another tip is to remember that it is easy to be too far advanced into the vault of the hepatic flexure, leading to advance into a blind end, and often slight

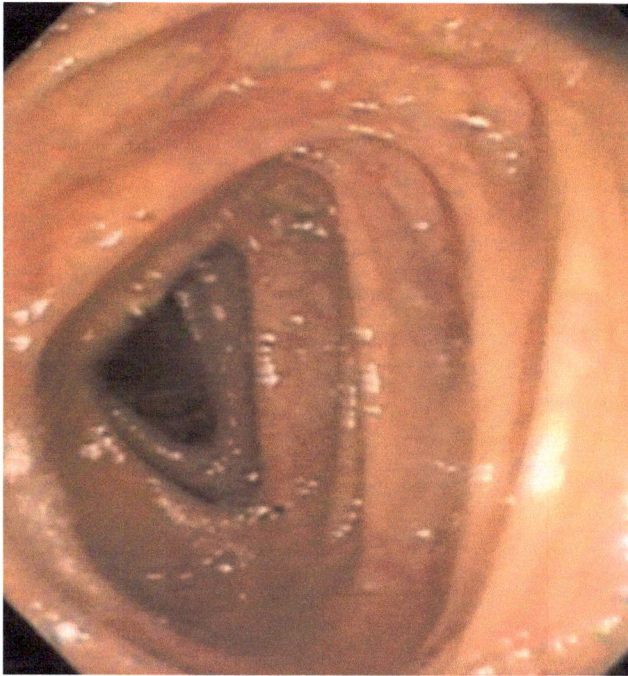

Fig. 21.4 Normal triangular appearance of transverse colon

withdrawal of the instrument may reveal the fact that one is trying to negotiate this blind-ended area. The two or three sharp folds then observed may then be most successfully negotiated by tip deflection using both up/down and left/right wheels with minimal advancement of the scope. This is most easily performed in the supine patient position, however.

Once the hepatic flexure is negotiated, the transverse colonic γ loop may be reduced with anticlockwise or clockwise rotation followed by withdrawal of the colonoscope and suction. Loop withdrawal is essentially informed guesswork initially. Studies with the colon map guider (ScopeGuide®, Olympus, Inc. Tokyo, Japan), based on using a colonoscope with an inbuilt electromagnetic loop that allows accurate real-time colonoscope three-dimensional positioning by detection using an external positioning device and displayed on a screen next to the patient, have shown that even expert colonoscopists get the type of loop present wrong in half of the cases [76–78]. Once one starts to remove the loop, using rotation only initially, a tip is to gently start to remove the colonoscope and try to determine whether within-patient resistance is increasing or whether the colonoscope is trying to push your hand away from the patient as the loop unfolds. Usually, trying clockwise or anticlockwise combined with instrument withdrawal will, with experience, allow early determination of which rotation direction is likely to be successful in "de-looping" the colonoscope. It is best to try to maintain good luminal vision during this procedure, but, not infrequently, the lumen is lost; however, if this loop removal

technique is effective, it is then not unusual to find oneself then looking at the appendiceal orifice and hence the cecum because the scope will have naturally traveled down the ascending colon. It is important to remember that the ascending colon, which in children is of variable length, may be as short as 5 cm in some younger patients.

Cecum

Three useful ways to ensure that one has reached the cecum are as follows:

1. Observing the colonoscopic illumination in the right iliac fossa (using the specific high-intensity light transillumination application available with some colonoscopes is not usually necessary in children, except with some obese adolescents, for whom it can be helpful when applied in a dark environment).
2. Digitally indenting the abdominal wall over the right iliac fossa and observing the corresponding effect on the colonic wall with the colonoscope.
3. Identifying the triradiate fold, appendiceal orifice, and (especially if gas bubbles and ileal effluent are being excreted from it) the typical two lips-like appearance of the ileocecal valve or Bauhin's valve.

A good maxim is that if there is any doubt in the operator's mind about having reached the cecum, then one is usually at the hepatic or even splenic flexure. Only about 80 cm of scope from the anus is needed when all loops are removed in an adult, and in smaller children, only 40–60 cm may be needed. This assumes normal anatomy of the ascending colon and cecum. Obviously, cecal strictures can confuse the picture.

Ileal Intubation and Its Importance

The Bauhin's valve is present approximately 1–4 cm distal to the appendiceal orifice opening into a smooth asymmetric fold and opens perpendicular to the axis of the colon. Figure 21.5 show the steps of the easiest technique for ileal intubation. Removal of any colonic loops is important to allow for a responsive scope with no paradoxical movement. Figures 21.5b and 21.6 show the valve maneuvered to the 6 o'clock position, usually after clockwise rotation of the scope and wheel-tip deflection to maintain a centered cecal view. Anticlockwise rotation can also be used but is less efficient. If too much gas is present, then the cecum may be "tented," and this should be suctioned prior to an ileal intubation attempt. Figures 21.5c and 21.7 show the insertion of the biopsy forceps such that just the tip or the first few millimeters are visibly exposed beyond the end of the scope. The scope is then inserted just beyond the fold (using the downward deflecting wheel with the scope as above already in the 6 o'clock position), and the tip is inclined downward so that

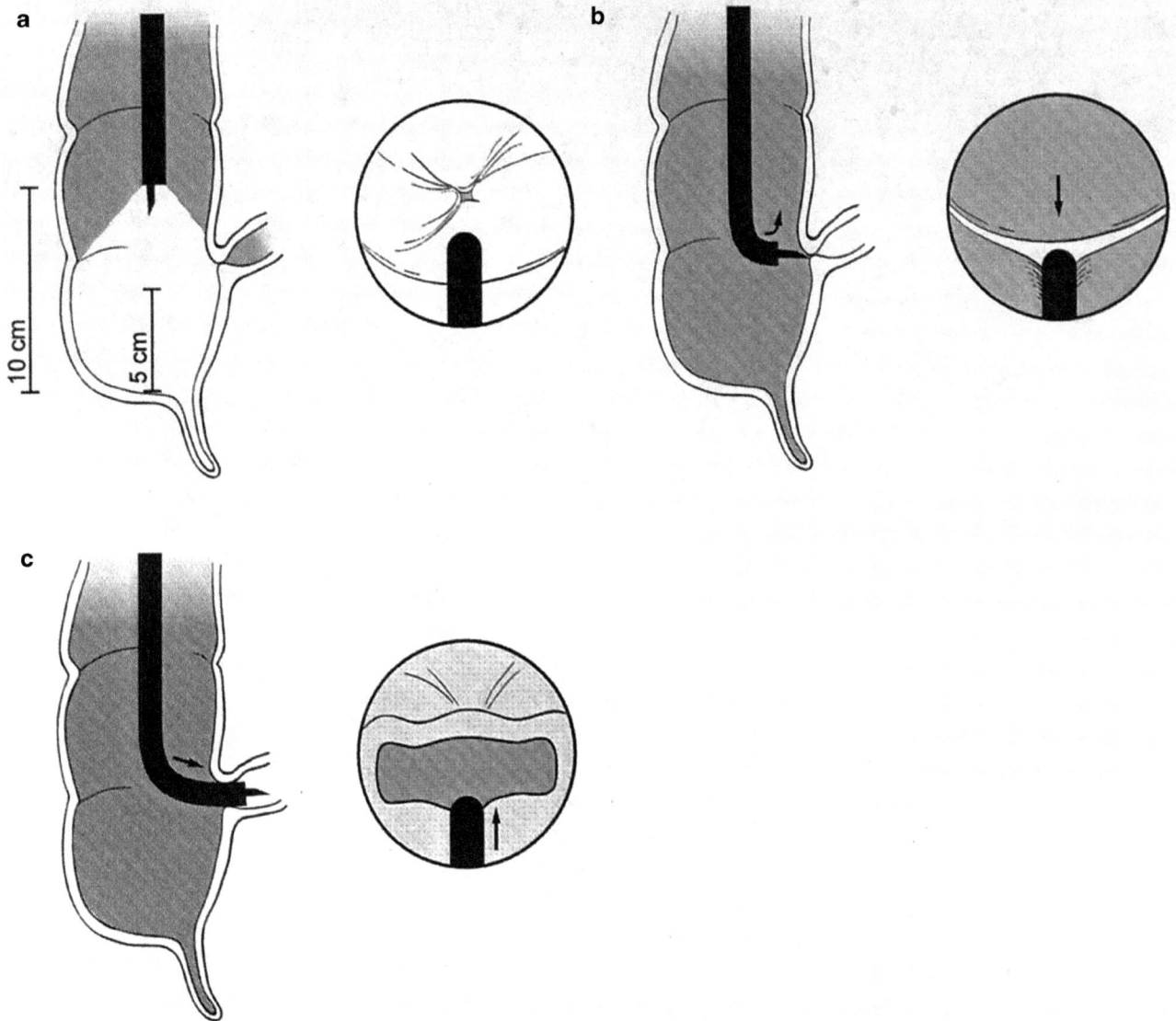

Fig. 21.5 (a) Identification of cecum with triradiate fold, appendiceal orifice, and ileocecal valve; (b) ileocecal valve at 6 o'clock position; (c) forceps opening up ileocecal valve with downward deflection of colonoscope tip

the forceps gently press into the wall. Slight left inclination may be required at this point to open the valve like a pair of lips on slight withdrawal of the scope (Fig. 21.5c). Once the valve is opened, the scope may be passed into the ileum with further downward deflection. Often this is facilitated by small right and left deflections with an assistant pressing on the abdomen over the transverse colon to support a dependent transverse and also prevent loop formation. In the absence of ileocecal valve strictures, and with practice, this technique will allow an ileal intubation rate of up to 100%. Perforation of the cecum or ileum with this technique is a theoretical concern raised by some observers unfamiliar with this technique, but this has not occurred in our experience of over 5,000 ileocolonoscopies and is extremely unlikely.

An alternative technique is "blind" intubation of the ileocecal valve. This involves the same positioning of the valve at 6 or 9 o'clock and then slowly withdrawing the scope back from just beyond the valve's fold while insufflating with air and deflecting the scope tip downward. The disadvantage of this technique is that it is not under direct vision.

Ileum

The ileal mucosa will have the typical velvetlike appearance of small bowel (Fig. 21.8), with the presence of smoother raised areas, which are Peyer patches, and, occasionally, lymphonodular hyperplasia of varying degrees (Fig. 21.9). Villi are more easily seen if the lumen is flooded with water. The ileal surface is shown in greater relief with a spray of standard blue or black ink (methylene blue in a 1:20 dilution

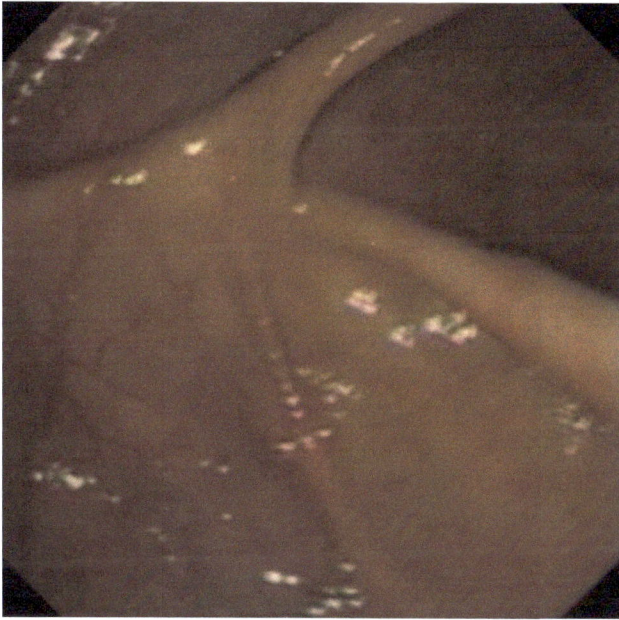

Fig. 21.6 Ileocecal valve at 6 o'clock

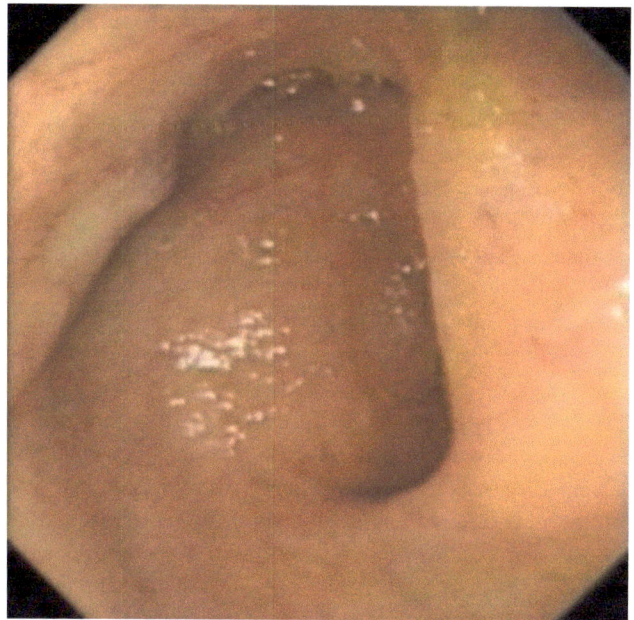

Fig. 21.8 Normal appearance of terminal ileum

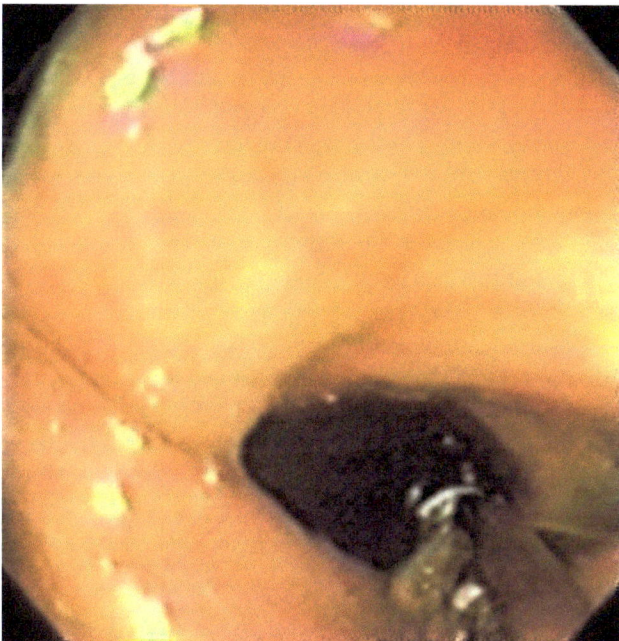

Fig. 21.7 Ileocecal entry using forceps

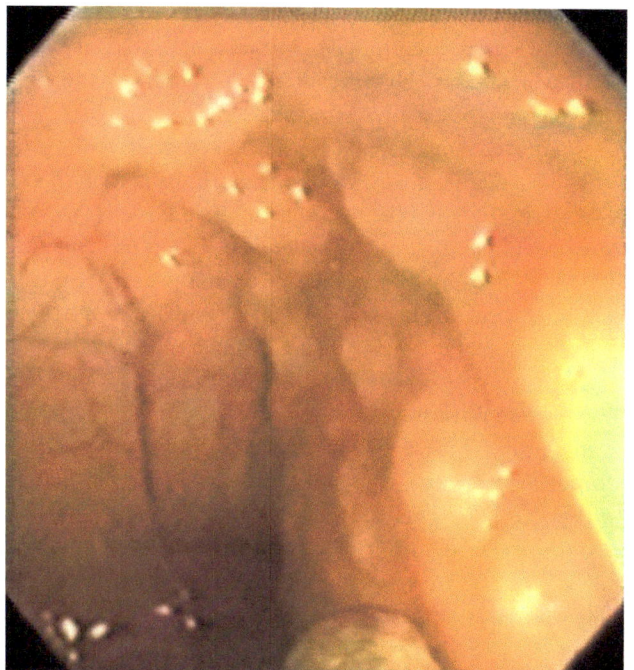

Fig. 21.9 Lymphonodular hyperplasia of the terminal ileum

may also be used); this is also useful in showing the detail of sessile polyps in the colon. Deeper intubation of the ileum by either technique is similar to duodenal negotiation during upper gastrointestinal endoscopy, and up to 40 cm of ileum can be observed.

It is pertinent here to discuss the diagnostic need for entering the ileum in children suspected of inflammatory bowel disease. Williams and colleagues, in 1982 [77], reported their experience of total ileocolonoscopy in children in which the terminal ileum was examined in 63 patients. In six children, ileitis detected by ileocolonoscopy was the sole finding of Crohn disease, which was previously unrecognized by radiologic contrast studies. Lipson and colleagues compared ileoscopy and barium studies, with an endoscopy specificity of 0.96 for diagnosis of Crohn disease in the terminal ileum [78]. In 14 of 46 children, ileoscopy revealed diagnosis, which would otherwise have been missed. This study also made clear that the endoscopic appearances could be completely normal, yet the diagnosis of Crohn disease could be made histologically by the presence of granulomata. Also, a pronounced lymphoid hyperplasia pattern was present radiologically in 24% of children and would have been a source of error in two cases had contrast radiographs been relied on to make the diagnosis without ileoscopy. More recently, Deere and colleagues showed that sigmoid, colonic, and rectal biopsies confirm the diagnosis of inflammatory bowel disease in only 60% of cases, and diagnosis based on morphologic criteria was possible in only 85% of cases when the cecum was reached without ileal intubation [79]. Geboes and colleagues assessed 300 patients, including adolescents and children, and found endoscopic and histologic ileal lesions in 123 and 125, respectively, of whom no colonic disease was present in 44 [80]. Ileal biopsies were essential for the diagnosis in 15 patients and contributory in 53. The Porto criteria now mandate terminal ileal intubation for diagnosis of IBD [1].

The Eurokids registry reports terminal ileal intubation (TII) rate of up to 79%. In individual center studies, TII rate has been reported up to 89%. In our center, the TII rate is 98%, which is probably because of an active training environment and the use of ScopeGuide®.

There are, of course, other indications apart from the principal one, that is, diagnosis of chronic inflammatory bowel disease, for entering the ileum in children. For instance, ileoscopy will facilitate diagnoses of other causes of ileitis such as infection with tuberculosis or Yersinia [81–83]. In addition, therapeutic dilatation of short terminal ileal strictures by per endoscopic balloon catheter may be attempted.

Endoscope Withdrawal

A more careful inspection of the colon is necessary on withdrawal of the scope, especially for the presence of polyps, which may have remained hidden behind a haustral fold during the initial insertion of the scope. Biopsies should be taken from all areas, including normal-looking mucosa to allow for accurate histological diagnosis. Biopsy technique is similar to EGD, with the exception that many colonoscopic biopsy forceps have a central barb, allowing more than one biopsy to be taken each time the biopsy forceps are passed.

Lastly, before removing the scope from the anus, a retroflexion maneuver obtained by maximum upward and right or left tip deflection and slight advancement of the scope into the rectal vault, followed by rotation clockwise and anticlockwise through 180°, completes the examination. This is necessary to observe the anorectal junction and distal rectum. Distal ulcers, inflammation, or even polyps can be missed if this is not done.

Dilatation of Strictures

Trans-endoscopic balloon dilators are appropriate for ileocolonic dilatation, employing the same concept and method as for upper gastrointestinal strictures, employing radiologic screening control. Long-term symptomatic relief can be afforded in some carefully selected patients, including adolescents in reported studies [84, 85]. Pressures of 35–50 psi in balloons of 12–18 mm are available. Theoretically, as for neoplastic or diverticulitis-associated strictures in adults, stent placement could be used as a last resort in inflammatory bowel disease-type strictures, but there are no reported cases of this occurring in childhood as yet.

Complications of Ileocolonoscopy

Complications, excluding those due to sedation, are summarized in Table 21.6. Complications are more common following therapeutic procedures. The literature to date reveals over 3,000 colonoscopies under 20 years of age reported, with five perforations—four post-polypectomy and one in a patient with severe ulcerative colitis. Ten procedure-related minor complications are noted, including four small post-polypectomy hemorrhages, three cases of post procedure abdominal pain with spontaneous resolution, one common peroneal nerve palsy secondary to peri-procedure positioning, and two with a post-procedure fever for more than 24 h [39, 40, 86, 87–91]. This equates to a complication rate owing to the procedure itself of approximately 0.3% and, without polypectomy, of about 0.05%. This is in keeping with the British definition of "minimal" risk and the American definition of "minor risk over minimal" [92].

A single case of a child with serosal surface tears owing to a rigid colonoscope and a large sigmoid loop was reported in 1974 [93]. Flexible pediatric colonoscopes or the new variable-stiffness colonoscopes may prevent this nowadays.

Table 21.6 Procedure-related and post-procedure complications in pediatric colonoscopy

Diagnostic procedure related
Vasovagal reactions
Hemorrhage
Perforation – traction serosal; direct transmural
Pancreatitis
Splenic trauma
Therapeutic procedure related
Perforation
Hemorrhage
Thermal injury – transmural
Post-procedure
Distension and discomfort (less if CO_2 insufflation used)
Delayed evidence of perforation or hemorrhage

The merits of conservative therapy of selected cases of colonic perforation have been discussed [94], and it would seem reasonable to adopt conservative management, for instance, in the case of silent asymptomatic perforations and those with localized peritonitis without signs of sepsis who continue to improve clinically without intervention [95]. In one study in adults, only 3 of 21 patients were managed nonsurgically, and there was no difference in the morbidity or mortality between primary repair and resection and anastomosis [96]. In another, conservative management was successful in 13 of 48 patients, and 12 of the 13 were postpolypectomy perforations [97].

In contradistinction to adults, bacteremia is not often detected in children, and only a low rate of bacteremia owing to bacterial translocation across the bowel wall has been demonstrated following pediatric ileocolonoscopy [98]. In addition, modern cleaning machines seem to largely prevent the glutaraldehyde-associated colitis reported in the past [99].

Splenic rupture is rarely seen and will present with hypovolemia and shoulder tip or abdominal pain within 24 h of the ileocolonoscopy [100]. Similarly, direct trauma to the tail of the pancreas is the proposed mechanism of injury in the rare case of pancreatitis reported [101].

Because of the rarity of complications in pediatrics, most pediatric endoscopists, when presented with such a clinical situation, will be unfamiliar with the etiology of the symptoms, and colleagues' opinions should often be sought [102].

Small Bowel Assessment

Wireless Capsule Endoscopy

The revised Porto criteria recommend small bowel imaging for completion of PIBD assessment and are essential in cases of CD, atypical UC, and IBD-U. Magnetic resonance enterography/enteroclysis (MRE) is a good tool to assess intestinal inflammation and damage, but there is no validated scoring tool for its use in PIBD [103]. Here we would like to discuss the role of wireless capsule endoscopy (WCE) as an effective and feasible tool for small bowel assessment.

In patients where endoscopy and MRE have failed to reach a conclusive diagnosis, WCE has been proven to be beneficial in reaching or refuting a diagnosis and describing disease distribution. WCE findings have been shown to be contributory toward change in the management of IBD, especially CD in about 75–92% of the cases [104, 105].

WCE is approved for use in children above 2 years of age, though there are case reports of this to be used in children as young as 8 months. It is usually delivered in the duodenum with the help of an age-appropriate upper GI endoscope. However, in children aged 6 years or more, this can be easily swallowed under direct supervision. Some centers use the same bowel preparation as for ileocolonoscopy. Simethicone (20 ml) before capsule deployment has been shown to improve luminal visualization [106].

We do not routinely use patency capsule before deploying the WCE. The patency capsule has dissolvable open ends and is easily expelled, if its passage through the bowel is delayed.

In our center, the child is allowed only clear fluids for at least 2 h post deployment of the capsule.

The capsule is usually expelled within next 24–48 h but can stay inside the bowel for up to 2 weeks. Capsule retention has been reported in the pediatric population but is more common in children with known small bowel pathology, malnutrition, or PIBD. In such situations, high-dose laxatives can be tried as a first resort to remove the capsule, and in PIBD, steroids and other anti-inflammatory agents are often successful as they reduce the inflammatory component of the stricture – double-balloon enteroscopy (DBE) can be used to retrieve a capsule, but if no symptoms are occurring, the capsule is usually left in situ – surgery is rarely if ever required and only with stricture symptoms when it would be required in any case.

Enteroscopy

Enteroscopy (ES) is now a standard and recently reviewed [107] endoscopic procedure in adult medicine. Though ES plays a role in examination of the small bowel and it has a place in PIBD that defies diagnosis by standard endoscopy and WCE, it is not routinely used. Indeed ES may be preferable to WCE if there is a clinical suspicion of obstruction, need for biopsy, or for a therapeutic procedure. It becomes a necessity when small bowel biopsy is required for differential diagnostic purpose or when both MRE and WCE fail to prove a strongly suspected small bowel pathology.

Push Enteroscopy

Sonde-type, intraoperative-assisted push enteroscopy [108–110] and more recently nonsurgical push enteroscopy [111] have been described in children. Sonde enteroscopy has largely been abandoned in favor of push enteroscopy [112, 113] given the desire for therapeutic capability. Push ES (PES) is endoluminal examination of the proximal jejunum using a long, flexible endoscope with or without an overtube.

The techniques of per oral push enteroscopy and laparoscopy-assisted enteroscopy continue to evolve and have been superseded by device-assisted enteroscopy (DAE).

Device-assisted ES (DAE) is either balloon-assisted or spiral. Single-balloon-assisted ES (SBE) uses an overtube equipped with balloon, and double-balloon-assisted ES (DBE) allows examination of the whole small bowel (via oral or anal route) due to assistance of balloons at the distal end of both endoscope and overtube. DBE usually requires two individuals (operator and assistant). Spiral ES uses assistance of single-use overtube, which has helical spirals at its distal end and rotates independently from the enteroscope.

The term intraoperative ES (IOE) is used when ES is performed during abdominal surgery (orally or via enterostomy). In such case, progression of the endoscope (gastroscope, colonoscope, pediatric colonoscope, or entero-scope) is manually assisted by the surgeon.

Instruments and Technique

Although a pediatric colonoscope can be used for enteros-copy, specifically designed enteroscopes up to 230 cm in length are now available. The Olympus SIF Q140 (Olympus, Center Valley, Pennsylvania, USA) has a diameter of 10.5 mm and is 250 cm long. A push enteroscope, like a colonoscope, allows four-way tip deflection to 160°–180°. An overtube, typically 60–100 cm in length with a soft Gore-Tex tapered tip, stiffens the enteroscope within the stomach and upper duodenum limiting looping, thereby allowing deeper advancement into the small bowel [112]. A push enteroscope can be introduced 120–180 cm beyond the liga-ment of Treitz, and with laparoscopic assistance, even the terminal ileum can be reached, allowing lesions such as a Meckel's diverticulum to be found [110].

Preparation for enteroscopy is the same as for EGD, although the procedure may be substantially longer and more uncomfortable. Therefore, it is the practice at our unit to use general anesthesia even in adolescents. Patients are positioned left lateral or semi-prone. After normal examina-tion of the esophagus and stomach, air is removed, and min-imal insufflation of the stomach allows deeper penetration into the small bowel when not using an overtube. At 60–80 cm in older children and adolescents, the ligament of Treitz is found, and extreme tip deflection is needed to find the lumen. The first jejunal loop is more readily identified because it is straighter and travels down to the pelvis. If using an overtube, which has been threaded over the entero-scope prior to oral insertion, this is deployed down the esophagus and into the second part of the duodenum; prepy-loric deployment will not aid in deeper small bowel penetra-tion. Some exponents use fluoroscopy to aid in overtube tip positioning [107]. When advancing the overtube, the entero-scope needs to be pulled back with clockwise rotation to straighten it, similar to the maneuver used to achieve the shortened scope position during endoscopic retrograde cholangiopancreatography.

A number of reports demonstrate the utility of push enter-oscopy in adults. One of few studies in children, using push enteroscopy, investigated the possibility of Crohn disease in children with growth retardation [114].

Double Balloon Enteroscopy

Double balloon enteroscopy (DBE) enables high-resolution endoscopic imaging of the entire small bowel. While push enteroscopy can aid in visualization of the proximal jeju-num, DBE goes a step further making it possible to examine, take biopsies, and perform therapeutic procedures such as hemostasis and balloon dilatation throughout the entire small bowel. The potential for mucosal biopsies and interventional endo-therapy provides significant advantage over WCE [115–117].

Instruments and Technique

The DBE system (Fujinon; Fujinon Inc., Japan) consists of a high-resolution video enteroscope (EN-450P5/20) with a flexible overtube. The video enteroscope has a working length of 200 cm and an outer diameter of 8.5 mm, while the flexible overtube has a length of 140 cm and outer diameter of 12 mm. The enteroscope has a 2.2 mm forceps channel that enables routine biopsy as well as other common thera-peutic interventions. The enteroscope as well as the over-tube are fitted with a balloon each at the tip. The overtube and balloons are disposable. The balloons can be inflated and deflated with air from a pressure-controlled pump sys-tem with maximum inflatable pressure of 45 mm (Figs. 21.10 and 21.11).

Both balloons are deflated at the start of the procedure. On reaching the duodenum, the overtube balloon is inflated to fix and stabilize the overtube within the lumen. Subsequently the enteroscope is advanced as far as possible. Then the enteroscope tip balloon is inflated, and the over-tube balloon is deflated. The overtube is now advanced to reach the enteroscope tip. The overtube is again inflated, and both enteroscope and overtube are gently withdrawn together in order to "concertina" the small bowel over both. The whole procedure is repeated, and each set of maneuvers

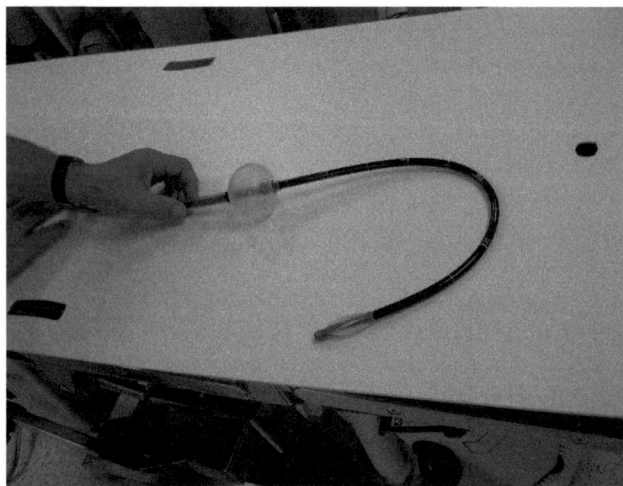

Fig. 21.10 Double balloon with balloon inflated

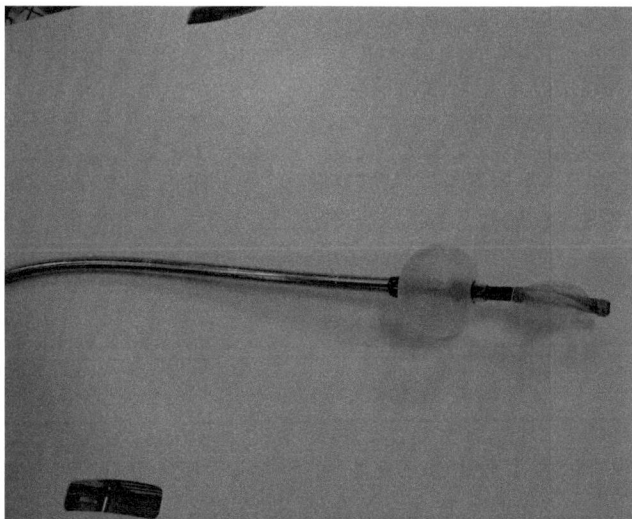

Fig. 21.11 Double balloon with balloon deflated

can allow up to 40 cm of small bowel to be examined, until the terminal ileum (TI) is reached. If the TI is not reached, then the distal most region reached is "tattooed" in the submucosal plane with an endo-needle. The DBE can then be repeated via the trans-anal route and retrograde movement from the TI proximally up the ileum allowing full examination of the whole small bowel. On withdrawal in either procedure, close examination of the mucosal surface occurs as with standard endoscopy, but lesions are dealt with as soon as found, whether this is on intubation or withdrawal. Bowel preparation is as for standard IC. The procedure is carried out under general anesthetic or deep sedation in the presence of an anesthetist.

DBE has been extensively evaluated in adults with obscure GI bleeding and to a lesser extent in CD. In a retrospective study involving 40 CD adult patients, active small bowel CD was found in 24 (60%) patients, leading to a change in therapy in 18 patients (75%). After a mean follow-up of 13 months, 83% of patients had persistent clinical improvement [118]. In another study of 37 patients with CD, the overall diagnostic yield of DBE was 59.4% [119]. In a pediatric study conducted by one of the authors, the diagnostic yield was 78.5%, and therapeutic success rate was 64.2%. None of the patient had any complication, suggesting that DBE is a safe and effective procedure in pediatric population [120].

Since CD can be confined to the small bowel alone, DBE has a definite role in the evaluation of patients with suspected CD with negative ileocolonoscopy and radiological investigations. In one study comparing DBE to small bowel follow through (SBFT) [121], DBE was able to detect early or faint lesions like aphthoid lesions, erosions, and small ulcers which were not found by SBFT. Also DBE was better in differentiating open and healed ulcers thus helpful in evaluation of response to treatment in CD. However, small strictures

were difficult to detect with DBE since they could be mistaken for an intestinal band. Complications reported in the literature include perforation, pancreatitis, bleeding, and aspiration pneumonia [122, 123].

Endoscopic Findings in Inflammatory Bowel Disease

It is important to recognize the normal appearance of the bowel macroscopically and histologically. The colonic mucosa when seen through an endoscope appears glistening salmon pink in color with a visible network of branching vessels seen beneath the mucosa. The smoothness of the mucosal surface is the hallmark of a healthy colon, and there is a lack of contact bleeding, friability, or exudates [124]. Microscopically the mucosa appears flat with normal crypt density, undistorted crypt architecture, intact surface epithelium, normal mucin content, and without any neutrophil infiltration [125].

Ulcerative Colitis

The earliest changes seen in UC are the presence of diffuse erythema and dull appearance of the vascular architecture consequent to the vascular congestion and edema. The engorged mucosa leads to contact bleeding and friability when touched with an endoscope. Progressively minute ulcers appear which coalesce to form large ulcers within a background of diffuse colonic inflammation with loss of vascular pattern and granularity [124]. The colonic mucosa is involved in a continuous fashion from the rectum extending further up the colon. Long-standing UC leads to the development of pseudopolyps (Fig. 21.12). The microscopic findings typical of UC include diffuse mucosal involvement from rectum up to cecum without granulomas. The presence of architectural distortion, basal plasmacytosis, cryptitis, and crypt abscesses are suggestive of chronicity. The severity of inflammation is worse distally, and reversal of this gradient should prompt for reconsideration of the diagnosis. However, there is no single set of microscopic or macroscopic findings for diagnosis of UC. At least five atypical phenotypes of UC have been described in the recently revised ESPGHAN Porto Criteria [103] (Table 21.7). The classic notion of noninvolvement of the upper GI tract in UC no longer holds true, as gastric erosions, ulcers, and microscopic features can be seen in 4–8% of patients with UC [126]. Therefore, the presence of focal gastritis or chronic gastric inflammation should not be a sole criterion to refute the diagnosis of UC. Besides, the EUROKIDS registry data suggests that rectal sparing can be seen in around 5% cases of pediatric UC [1].

Crohn Disease

Typical macroscopic findings of CD commence as mucosal aphthous lesions, which enlarge to form linear or transverse serpentine ulceration (Fig. 21.13). Characteristically the ulcers are focal with normal intervening mucosa, the so-called skip lesions (Fig. 21.14). As the disease progresses, it leads to nodularity, giving a cobblestone appearance (Fig. 21.15) and stenosis/stricturing (Fig. 21.16) of

bowel with pre-stenotic dilatation. Bowel wall thickening with luminal narrowing is typically seen on imaging, WCE, or during surgery. The other typical macroscopic findings are skip lesions and jejunal and ileal ulcers. The extraluminal findings include perianal fistulas, abscesses, anal stenosis, anal canal ulcers, and large and inflamed skin tags.

Nonspecific macroscopic findings of CD include edema, erythema, friability, and granularity. Terminal ileum is the

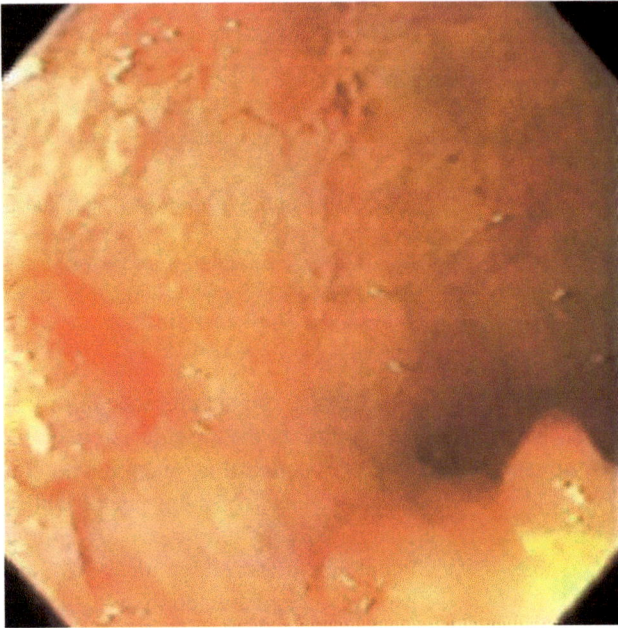

Fig. 21.12 Pseudopolyps in ulcerative colitis

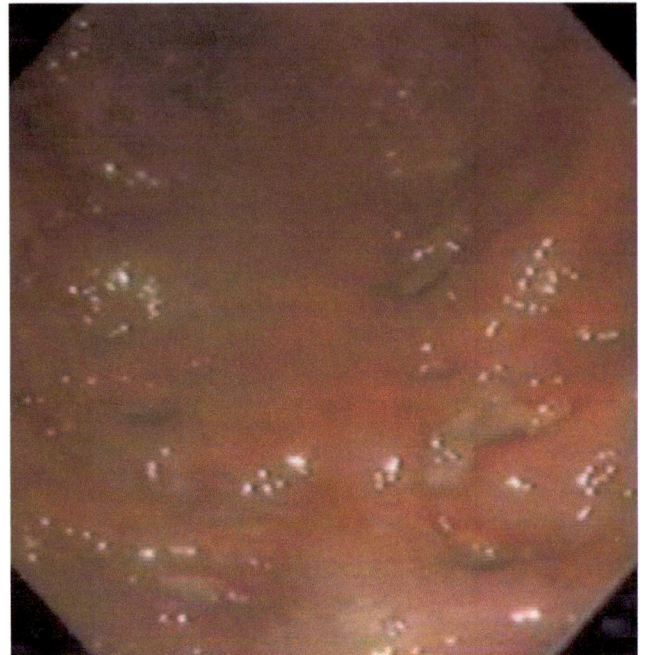

Fig. 21.13 Deep aphthous lesion in Crohn disease

Table 21.7 Phenotypes of pediatric UC at diagnosis

Presentation	Macroscopic	Microscopic
Typical	Contiguous disease from the rectum	Architectural distortion, basal lymphoplasmacytosis, disease most severe distally, no granulomas
Atypical		
1. Rectal sparing	No macroscopic disease in rectum or rectosigmoid	Same As typical, especially in the involved segment above sparing
2. Short duration	Contiguous disease from the rectum may also have rectal sparing	May have focal, plus signs of chronicity or architectural distortion may be absent; other features are identical. Usually occurs in young children with short duration of symptoms
3. Cecal patch	Left-sided disease from rectum with area of cecal inflammation and normal appearing segment between the two	Typical; biopsies from the patch may show nonspecific inflammation
4. UGI	Erosions or small ulcers in stomach, but are neither serpiginous nor linear	Diffuse or focal gastritis, no granuloma (except peri-cryptal)
5. Acute severe colitis	Contiguous disease from the rectum	May have transmural inflammation or deep ulcers, other features typical. Lymphoid aggregates are absent; ulcers are V-shaped fissuring ulcers

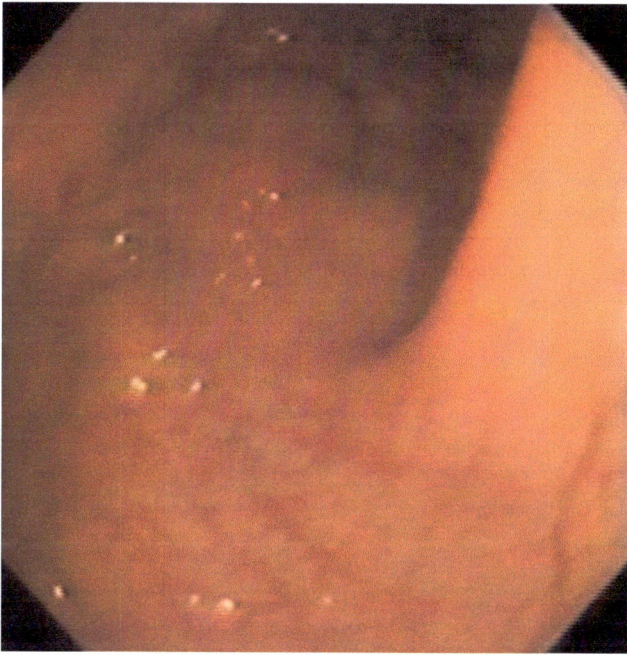

Fig. 21.14 Skip lesions in Crohn disease

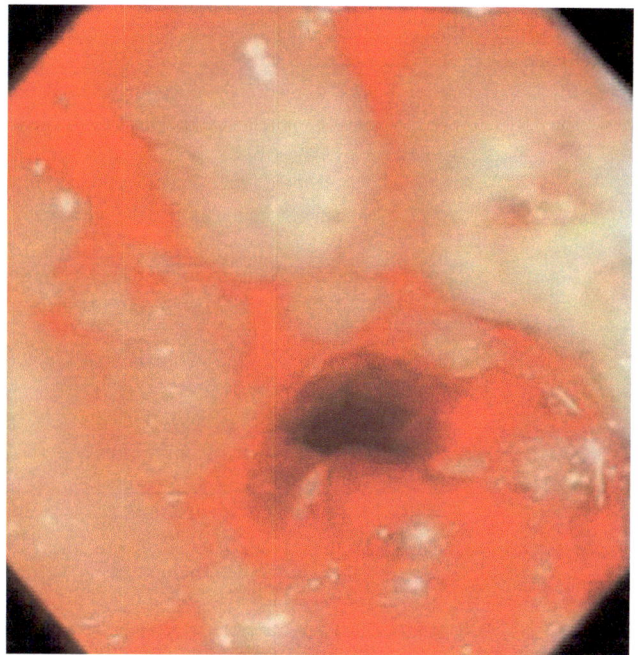

Fig. 21.16 Colonic stricture in Crohn disease

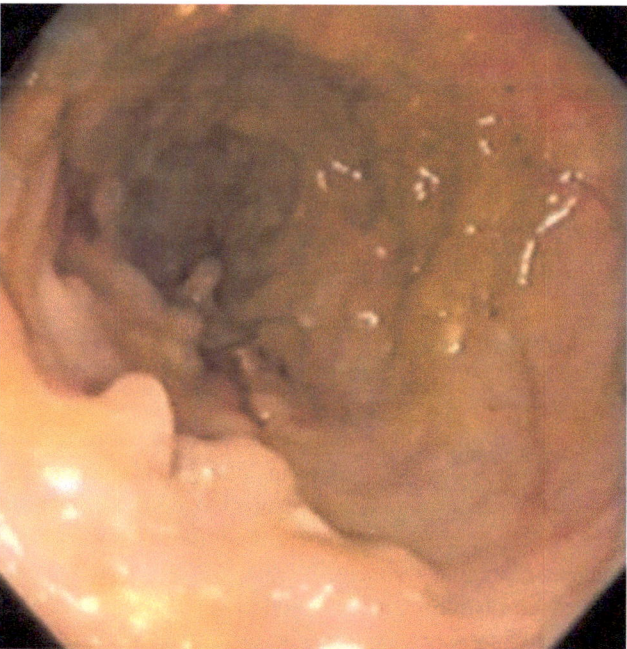

Fig. 21.15 Typical cobblestone appearance in Crohn disease

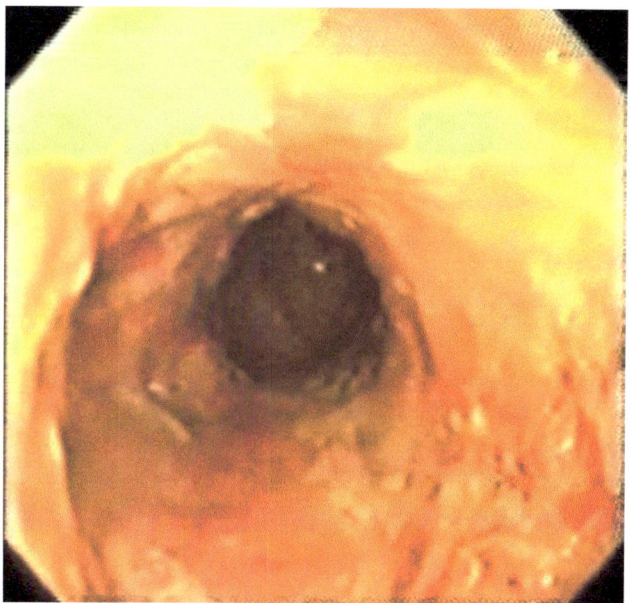

Fig. 21.17 Terminal ileal Crohn disease

most common site to be involved in CD (Fig. 21.17), hence, as has been stressed earlier; it is imperative that every attempt should be made to reach the terminal ileum at colonoscopy.

The presence of noncaseating granulomas on ileal biopsy is the classical histopathological finding in CD of the ileum.

The other typical microscopic findings of CD include focal chronic inflammation, transmural inflammatory infiltrate, and submucosal fibrosis.

Nonspecific microscopic findings of CD are granulomas adjacent to a ruptured crypt, mild nonspecific inflammatory infiltrate in the lamina propria, and mucosal ulceration/ero-

Table 21.8 UC v IBD-U v CD differentiation

Likelihood of UC	Features	Diagnostic approach
Class I: Nonexistent	Well-formed granulomas anywhere in the GI tract, remote from ruptured crypt	Diagnose as CD
	Deep serpentine ulcerations, cobblestoning, or stenosis anywhere in the small bowel or UGI tract	
	Fistulizing disease (internal or perianal)	
	Any ileal inflammation in the presence of normal cecum (i.e., incompatible with backwash ileitis)	
	Thickened jejunal or ileal bowel loops or other evidence of significant small bowel inflammation (more than a few scattered erosions) not compatible with backwash ileitis	
	Macroscopically and microscopically normal appearing skip lesions in untreated IBD (except with macroscopic rectal sparing and cecal patch)	
	Large inflamed perianal skin tags	
Class II: Rare with UC (<5%)	Combined (macroscopic and microscopic) rectal sparing, all other features are consistent with UC	IBD-U if at least 1 class II feature exists
	Significant growth delay (height velocity <2 standard deviation), not explained by other causes	
	Transmural inflammation in the absence of severe colitis, all other features are consistent with UC	
	Duodenal or esophageal ulcers, not explained by other causes (e.g., *Helicobacter pylori*, NSAIDs, and celiac disease)	
	Multiple aphthous lesions in the stomach, not explained by other causes (e.g., *H. pylori* and NSAIDs)	
	Positive anti-Saccharomyces cerevisiae antibody (ASCA) in the presence of negative pANCA	
	Reverse gradient of mucosal inflammation (proximal >distal) (except rectal sparing)	
Class III: Uncommon (5–10%)	Severe scalloping of the stomach or duodenum, not explained by other causes (e.g., celiac disease and *H. pylori*)	Diagnose as IBD-U if at least 2–3 features exists
	Focal chronic duodenitis on multiple biopsies or marked scalloping of the duodenum, not explained by other causes (e.g., celiac disease and *Helicobacter pylori*)	
	Focal active colitis on histology in more than one biopsy from macroscopically inflamed site	
	Non-bloody diarrhea	
	Aphthous lesion in the colon or UGI tract	

sions. The signs suggestive of chronicity are crypt architectural changes, colonic Paneth cell metaplasia, and goblet cell depletion. The presence of epithelioid granulomas is sufficient to make a diagnosis of CD even without classical macroscopic findings.

Inflammatory Bowel Disease-Undefined (IBD-U)

In the recently revised ESPGHAN Porto Criteria for the diagnosis of inflammatory bowel disease in children and adolescents, it is suggested that the term IBD-U is used for patients with colitis and clearly defined findings that are atypical for either CD or UC. Colitis features in children with untreated colitis are categorized in three classes, and patients with at least one class II and two to three class III features are diagnosed as IBD-U (Table 21.8).

Follow-Up and Surveillance Ileocolonoscopy

Intraluminal disease should be reassessed electively as guided by biochemical markers including fecal calprotectin. However, patients who do not respond to therapy or who are treatment dependent or who have doubtful diagnosis should have an early reassessment. It is the practice in many units to perform a follow-up ileocolonoscopy 2–3 months after the start of treatment in a newly diagnosed case of inflammatory bowel disease since Modigliani and colleagues showed that only 29% of adults with Crohn disease in clinical and biochemical remission actually achieved endoscopic remission [127]. It allows the physician to observe the mucosal efficacy of the therapy, because, in many instances, such as steroid use in colitis, the clinical improvement of the patient may not be mirrored by the mucosal improvement, which is regarded by most as the most important meter of a successful treatment regimen [9]. Ileocecal transcutaneous Doppler ultrasonography may be of benefit as a noninvasive alternative to repeat ileocolonoscopy in this situation, as noted above. In addition, the activity of mucosal inflammation may determine the long-term risk for carcinogenesis in the bowel.

Treatment Targets

The Selecting Therapeutic Targets in Inflammatory Bowel Disease (STRIDE) [128] program initiated by the International Organization for the Study of Inflammatory Bowel Diseases (IOIBD) has recommended treatment targets for IBD to be used for a "treat-to-target" clinical management strategy based on clinical/patient reported outcome (PRO) and endoscopic remission.

The clinical/PRO remission for Crohn disease is defined as resolution of abdominal pain and diarrhea/altered bowel habit, which should be assessed at a minimum of 3 months during active disease, and endoscopic remission defined as resolution of ulceration at ileocolonoscopy (or resolution of findings of inflammation on cross-sectional imaging in patients who cannot be adequately assessed with ileocolonoscopy), which should be assessed at 6–9-month interval during the active phase.

Similarly for ulcerative colitis, the clinical/PRO remission is defined as resolution of rectal bleeding and diarrhea/altered bowel habit, which should be assessed at a minimum of 3 months during active disease, and endoscopic remission defined as resolution of friability and ulceration at flexible sigmoidoscopy or colonoscopy, which should be assessed at 3-month interval during the active phase.

Though the CRP and fecal calprotectin are not the treatment targets, these can be used as adjunctive measures of inflammation for monitoring in CD. Failure of CRP or fecal calprotectin normalization should prompt further endoscopic evaluation, irrespective of symptoms.

Scoring Systems for Endoscopic PIBD Disease Activity

The focus is increasingly being shifted to mucosal healing as an important aspect of the treatment target of PIBD. This is further stressed upon by the STRIDE recommendations as above. There are various scoring systems currently in practice, namely, Mayo score, UCEIS, UCCIS, CDEIS, SES-CD, and Rutgeerts score. The standard scores used for Crohn disease are the Crohn's Disease Endoscopic Index of Severity (CDEIS) and the Simple Endoscopic Score for Crohn's Disease (SES-CD). Of these two, SES-CD seems to be more simplistic and also correlates well with CDEIS. The interobserver variability for SES-CD is less as compared to CDEIS [129–131]. The Rutgeerts score is primarily used in

postoperative patients. None of these scores are fully validated in the pediatric population.

For UC, the STRIDE Committee recommends the use of the Mayo score which, though not fully validated, has less inter- and intra-observer variation, is easy to use, and has well-established predictive values [132, 133]. The Ulcerative Colitis Endoscopic Index of Severity (UCEIS) also has less inter-observer variability but is not fully validated. The Ulcerative Colitis Colonoscopic Index of Severity (UCCIS) assesses four variables: vascular pattern, granularity, bleeding/friability, and ulceration. All are assessed in five segments throughout the colon. This index also needs further validation and cutoff values are not well defined.

Endosonography

Endoluminal ultrasonography of the rectum has been an established technique for years; however, more recently, an echocolonoscope has allowed combined examination of the mucosa and the bowel wall. This is a forward-viewing colonoscope with the transducer (7.5 MHz) situated in the rigid tip of the scope [134]. Alternatively, an ultrasound miniprobe can be introduced via the biopsy channel (7.5 or 12.5 MHz). A fluid interface is necessary for all endosonography, and this can be achieved either with a fluid-filled balloon or filling the relevant colonic segment with water. Because this may be time-consuming, it is easier to concentrate on the region of interest rather than attempt to examine the entire colon. In adult practice, staging of cancers is the major indication for endosonography. In children and adolescents, indications for this technique might include suspicion of early invasive cancer arising from an adenoma, assessment of the extent and depth of sessile polyps to guide reception technique, assessment of colonic strictures/fistulae/anastomoses, assessment of the extent and depth of inflammatory bowel disease, assessment of the extent and depth of vascular lesions, examination of rectal and colonic portal hypertension with varices, and suspicion of lymphoma.

Inflammatory bowel disease appears as wall thickening and subsequent loss of the normal layer structure of the colon with progressive inflammation. Although theoretical differentiation between ulcerative colitis and Crohn disease is possible owing to the transmural nature of Crohn disease, it has been shown recently that active ulcerative colitis can have echo-texture changes extending into the submucosa and that these changes correlate with disease activity [135]. Surgical decisions were made in one study of patients with Crohn disease in which endoscopic ultrasonography was used to differentiate between superficial and transmural involvement [136]. An ileo-anal pouch was undesirable when transmural disease was identified. Perirectal and pericolonic fistulae and abscesses have been seen using the rigid rectal ultrasound probe, and this is a potential application for endoscopic ultrasonography [137]. Catheter probe-assisted endoscopic ultrasonography in inflammatory bowel disease has advantages over an echocolonoscope, which may be technically difficult to use. One study recently showed that wall thickness was twice as great in active inflammatory bowel disease, but ulcerative colitis could not be differentiated from Crohn disease [138]. Loss of wall structure correlated with disease activity score in the Crohn disease group, and wall thickness correlated with disease activity in the ulcerative colitis group. Other parameters, such as superior mesenteric artery maximum flow velocity and increased Doppler ultrasonography demonstrating mural blood flow, are being examined as viable noninvasive substitutes for the determination of posttreatment ileocecal Crohn disease activity, thus potentially avoiding the need for follow-up ileocolonoscopy, as some units advocate.

New Endo-diagnostic Methods

High Magnification Chromoscopic Colonoscopy (HMCC)

Recent improvements in technology have led to the development of a generation of endoscopes with the ability to magnify endoscopic images. The high magnification endoscope allows conventional video imaging with the facility to increase magnification instantaneously up to 100 times by a thumb-activated lever. By pushing the lever downward, the magnified picture is obtained immediately, and by reverting back to the normal position, the image is returned to normal [139]. A topical dye-like indigo carmine 0.2–2% is sprayed on the mucosa helping further to delineate the pathology. During magnification chromoscopic colonoscopy, pit patterns are observed. These pit patterns are classified according to the modified Kudos' criteria [140], and based on the pit patterns, it is possible to predict the histology as well as take targeted biopsies.

This technique has been extensively used in cancer surveillance in adults [141, 142]. Matsumato et al. [73] observed that the presence or absence of network pattern (NWP) and crypt opening (CO) highly correlated with the severity of disease in ulcerative colitis both clinically and histologically. Fujiya et al. [143] devised a classification system based on minute findings. In a prospective study, they compared HMCC with the established Matt's criteria [144] and histopathological findings and found that while colonoscopy correlated well with histopathology and correctly identified normal and clearly defined abnormal mucosa, it was insufficient for the assessment of minute mucosal changes that reflect smoldering histopathological changes. HMCC on the

other hand not only helped to recognize distinctive features in such mucosa predicting the severity of the disease state, but it also helped in predicting relapses in those who were in a quiescent state. Further, in another prospective study, Sugano et al. [145] have found HMCC effective in the evaluation of minute mucosal changes in patients with UC in remission. HMCC has also been evaluated in cancer surveillance in UC [146] and has been shown to assist in taking targeted biopsies.

Confocal Laser Endomicroscopy

Confocal laser endomicroscopy (CLE) is an exciting new technology developed in the recent years. It is an adaptation of light microscopy, whereby a low power laser illumination is focused to a single point in a microscopic field of view. Light emanating from that specific point is focused to a pinhole detector. Light emanating from outside the focally illuminated spot is not focused to the pinhole and, therefore, is geometrically rejected from detection. The beam path is scanned in a raster pattern, and measurements of light returning to the detector from successive points are digitized to produce two-dimensional images. Each such image thus is an optical section representing one focal plane within the specimen [147–149].

The components of the confocal laser endomicroscope are based on the integration of a confocal laser microscope mounted in the tip of a conventional colonoscope (EC3870K; Pentax, Tokyo, Japan), which enables confocal microscopy in addition to standard videoendoscopy. The diameter of the distal tip and insertion tube is 12.8 mm. The distal tip contains an air and water jet nozzle, two light guides, a 2.8 mm working channel, and an auxiliary water jet channel. The water jet channel is used for the topical application of the contrast agent. During CLE, an argon ion laser delivers an excitation wavelength of 488 nm with a maximum laser output of <1 mw at the surface mucosa. Confocal images can then be collected at a scan rate of 0.8 frames/second (1024 × 1024 pixels) or 1.6 frames/second (1024 × 512 pixels). The optical slice thickness is 7 um with a lateral resolution of 0.7 um and z-axis range of 0–250 um below the surface layer. Sodium fluorescein is given intravenously at the time of the procedure as a contrast agent. Thus, it is possible to get cellular and subcellular microscopic images at the time of endoscopic procedure. Features of IBD seen at CLE include bifid crypts, crypt distortion and destruction, crypt abscess/cryptitis, goblet cell depletion, inflammatory cell infiltration, and enlarged tortuous vessel architecture [150]. In a recent prospective study involving 21 patients with IBD, CLE was able to identify intramucosal bacteria with a sensitivity of 89% and specificity of 100% using fluorescence in situ hybridization (FISH) as gold standard. The authors further performed a retrospective study in 113 patients with CD and UC and found intramucosal bacteria significantly more often than in control patients (66% vs 60% vs 14%, $p < 0.001$) [151].

The advantages of using CLE are that as it is less invasive, there are potentially significant time, histopathology input, materials, manpower, and consequent financial savings to institutions conducting pediatric endoscopic services. There is no doubt that this new technique will be useful in taking targeted biopsies in patients with IBD and reduce the need to take biopsies.

Therapeutic Endoscopy in IBD

Besides being essential for the diagnosis and reassessment of IBD, endoscopic expertise is also required for therapeutic procedures in PIBD. It is estimated that about half of pediatric Crohn disease patients require some kind of surgical intervention within a decade of diagnosis [152, 153], the common indications being structuring or penetrating disease of the terminal ileum and colon or at an anastomotic site [154–156].

Traditionally, the strictureplasty and bowel resection have been the mainstay of treatment for stricturing disease, but recently, endoscopic balloon dilatation (EBD) is emerging as a safe and effective alternative to the above surgical procedures in patients with Crohn disease with ileocecal and anastomotic strictures [157–163]. The decision to perform EBD depends on patient choice, endoscopist expertise/experience, procedural feasibility, and the stricture characteristics, e.g., number, nature, and length.

The success rate of EBD in adults has been reported to vary from 83 to 87% at 1 year to 64–58% at 5 years [157–163]. There is a lack of evidence and controlled trials to compare the recurrence rate post-EBD and postsurgical procedure.

A surgery-free outcome is reported to be highest when stricture length is <4 cm and when EBD is performed for anastomotic strictures [157, 164, 165]. There is an increased need of post-procedural surgery with prolonged Crohn disease duration and high C-reactive protein [157]. The success rate is demonstrated to be poor if the stricture is present at the Bauhin's valve [160, 166].

Though there is no reported use of EBD for duodenal strictures in PIBD, the authors have recently performed trans-endoscopic balloon dilatation of a duodenal stricture in an 11-year-old boy with Crohn disease.

The possible complications associated with EBD are bleeding and perforation. The presence of fistulizing disease and abscesses at or adjacent to the site stricture increases the risk of perforation and is thus considered to be a contraindication [167].

Intraluminal stenting has also been reported as a possible alternative to surgery to treat strictures, but current date does not suggest its routine or safe use.

Colon Capsule Endoscopy

Colon capsule endoscopy (CCE) is still in a nascent stage and is considered to be useful in situations where full colonoscopy could not be achieved or where patient is not compliant for an endoscopic procedure. The colon capsule when deployed goes into a sleep mode as it traverses through small bowel and gets reactivated as it reaches colon. It has been reported to have high specificity and sensitivity as compared to routine colonoscopy [106], but further randomized clinical trials are required to recommend its routine use.

Conclusions

Pediatric endoscopy differs significantly from their adult parallels in nearly every aspect, including patient and parent management and preparation, selection criteria for sedation and general anesthesia, bowel preparation, expected diagnoses, instrument selection, imperative for terminal ileal intubation, and requirement for biopsies from macroscopically normal mucosa.

The chapter has highlighted the importance of endoscopy in general and ileocolonoscopy in particular in the diagnostic and therapeutic management of IBD. Also, the role of other advanced diagnostic techniques like DBE has been discussed, while wireless capsule endoscopy is discussed in a separate chapter.

Endoscopy is a necessary and important investigation in the various stages of management of inflammatory bowel disease from diagnosis to surveillance of cancer. There is no dispute in the use of ileocolonoscopy in the initial assessment of patients with IBD. Recent data has shown that upper GI endoscopy also has an important role in the initial diagnosis and differentiation of IBD and hence is recommended as a part of initial investigation of all cases presenting with symptoms suggestive of IBD. Other endoscopic investigative modalities like WCE, DBE, HMCC, confocal endomicroscopy, and endosonography aid in further management of IBD. Apart from diagnosis, endoscopy also has an important role in the therapeutic management of IBD.

References

1. de Bie CI, Buderus S, Sandhu BK, de Ridder L, Paerregaard A, Veres G, Dias JA, Escher JC, EUROKIDS Porto IBD Working Group of ESPGHAN. Diagnostic workup of paediatric patients with inflammatory bowel disease in Europe: results of a 5-year audit of the EUROKIDS registry. J Pediatr Gastroenterol Nutr. 2012;54(3):374–80.
2. Leighton JA, Shen B, Baron TH, Adler DG, Davila R, Egan JV, Faigel DO, Gan SI, Hirota WK, Lichtenstein D, Qureshi WA, Rajan E, Zuckerman MJ, VanGuilder T, Fanelli RD, Standards of Practice Committee, American Society for Gastrointestinal Endoscopy.

ASGE guideline: endoscopy in the diagnosis and treatment of inflammatory bowel disease. Gastrointest Endosc. 2006;63: 558–65.

3. Foutch PG, Sawyer R, Sanowski RA. Push-enteroscopy for diagnosis of patients with gastrointestinal bleeding of obscure origin. Gastrointest Endosc. 1990;36:337–41.

4. Lewis Claar R, Walker LS, Barnard JA. Children's knowledge, anticipatory anxiety, procedural distress, and recall of esophagogastroduodenoscopy. J Pediatr Gastroenterol Nutr. 2002;34: 68–72.

5. Acharya S. Assessing the need for pre-admission visits. Paediatr Nurs. 1992;4:20–3.

6. Whiting M. Play and surgical patients. Paediatr Nurs. 1993;5: 11–3.

7. Glasper A, Stradling P. Preparing children for admission. Paediatr Nurs. 1989;85:18–20.

8. Mahajan L, Wyllie R, Steffen R, et al. The effects of a psychological preparation program on anxiety in children and adolescents undergoing gastrointestinal endoscopy. J Pediatr Gastroenterol Nutr. 1998;27:161–5.

9. Williams C, Nicholls S. Endoscopic features of chronic inflammatory bowel disease in childhood. In: Walker-Smith, editor. Baillieère's clinical gastroenterology. 8th ed; London: Baillière-Tindall, WB Saunders Company Ltd; 1994. p. 121–31.

10. Ewe K. Bleeding after liver biopsy does not correlate with indices of peripheral coagulation. Dig Dis Sci. 1981;26:388–93.

11. Rey JR, Axon A, Budzynska A, Kruse A, Nowak A. Guidelines of the European Society of Gastrointestinal Endoscopy (E.S.G.E.) antibiotic prophylaxis for gastrointestinal endoscopy. European Society of Gastrointestinal Endoscopy. Endoscopy. 1998;30:318–24.

12. ASGE Standards of Practice Committee, Khashab MA, Chithadi KV, et al. Antibiotic prophylaxis for GI endoscopy. Gastrointest Endosc. 2015;81:81.

13. Wilson W, Taubert KA, Gewitz M, et al. Prevention of infective endocarditis: guidelines from the American Heart Association: a guideline from the American Heart Association Rheumatic Fever, Endocarditis, and Kawasaki Disease Committee, Council on Cardiovascular Disease in the Young, and the Council on Clinical Cardiology, Council on Cardiovascular Surgery and Anesthesia, and the Quality of Care and Outcomes Research Interdisciplinary Working Group. Circulation. 2007;116:1736.

14. Allison MC, Sandoe JA, Tighe R, et al. Antibiotic prophylaxis in gastrointestinal endoscopy. Gut. 2009;58:869.

15. Sondheimer J, Sokol R, Taylor SF, et al. Safety, efficacy and tolerance of intestinal lavage in pediatric patients undergoing diagnostic ileo-colonoscopy. J Pediatr. 1991;119:148–52.

16. Abubakar K, Goggin N, Gormally S, et al. Preparing the bowel for ileo-colonoscopy. Arch Dis Child. 1995;73:459–61.

17. Gremse D, Sacks A, Raines S. Comparison of oral sodium phosphate to polyethylene glycol-based solution for bowel preparation for ileo-colonoscopy in children. J Pediatr Gastroenterol Nutr. 1996;23:586–90.

18. da Silva M, Brairs G, Patrick M, et al. Ileo-colonoscopy preparation in children: safety, efficacy, and tolerance of high versus low-volume cleansing methods. J Pediatr Gastroenterol Nutr. 1997;24:33–7.

19. Trautwein A, Vinitki L, Peck S. Bowel preparation before ileo-colonoscopy in the pediatric patient: a randomized study. Gastroenterol Nurs. 1996;19:137–9.

20. Pinfield A, Stringer M. Randomised trial of two pharmacological methods of bowel preparation for day case ileo-colonoscopy. Arch Dis Child. 1999;80:181–3.

21. Dahshan A, Lin C, Peters J, et al. A randomized, prospective study to evaluate the efficacy and acceptance of three bowel preparations for ileo-colonoscopy in children. Am J Gastroenterol. 1999;94:3497–501.

22. Chilton A, O'Sullivan M, Cox M, et al. A blinded, randomized comparison of a novel, low-dose, triple regimen with fleet phosphosoda: a study of colon cleanliness, speed and success of ileo-colonoscopy. Endoscopy. 2000;32:37–41.

23. Marshall J, Patel M, Mahajan R, et al. Benefit of intravenous antispasmodic (hyoscyamine sulfate) as premedication for ileo-colonoscopy. Gastrointest Endosc. 1999;49:720–6.

24. Committee on Drugs of the American Academy of Pediatrics. Guidelines for monitoring and management of pediatric patients during and after sedation for diagnostic and therapeutic procedures. Pediatrics. 1992;89:1110–5.

25. American Society of Anesthesiologists Task Force on Sedation and Analgesia by Non-Anesthesiologists. Practice guidelines for sedation and analgesia by non-anesthesiologists. Anesthesiology. 2002;96:1004–17.

26. Nowicki MJ, Vaughn CA. Sedation and anesthesia in children for endoscopy. Tech Gastrointest Endosc. 2002;4:225–30.

27. Hassall E. Should pediatric gastroenterologists be i.v. drug users? J Pediatr Gastroenterol Nutr. 1993;16:370–2.

28. Tolia V, Peters J, Gilger M. Sedation for pediatric endoscopic procedures. J Pediatr Gastroenterol Nutr. 2000;30:477–85.

29. Murphy S. Sedation for invasive procedures in paediatrics. Arch Dis Child. 1997;77:281–6.

30. Gilger MA, Spearman RS, Dietrich CL, Spearman G, Wilsey JMJ, Zayat MN. Safety and effectiveness of ketamine as a sedative agent for pediatric GI endoscopy. Gastrointest Endosc. 2004;59:659–63.

31. Liacouras CA, Mascarenhas M, Poon C, et al. Placebo-controlled trial assessing the use of oral midazolam as a premedication to conscious sedation for pediatric endoscopy. Gastrointest Endosc. 1998;47:455–60.

32. Chuang EM, Wenner WJ, Piccoli DA, et al. Intravenous sedation in pediatric upper gastrointestinal endoscopy. Gastrointest Endosc. 1995;42:156–60.

33. Squires R, Morriss F, Schluterman S, et al. Efficacy, safety and cost of intravenous sedation versus general anesthesia in children undergoing endoscopic procedures. Gastrointest Endosc. 1995;41: 99–104.

34. O'Connor KW, Jones S. Oxygen desaturation is common and is under-appreciated during elective endoscopic procedures. Gastrointest Endosc. 1990;36:S2–4.

35. Yaster M, Nicholson D, Deshpande JK. Midazolam-Fentanyl intravenous sedation in children:case report of respiratory arrest. Pediatrics. 1990;86:463–7.

36. Bendig D. Pulse oximetry and upper gastrointestinal endoscopy in infants and children. J Pediatr Gastroenterol Nutr. 1991;12: 39–43.

37. Gilger M. Conscious sedation for endoscopy in the pediatric patient. Gastroenterol Nurs. 1993;16:75–9.

38. Israel D, McLain B, Hassall E. Successful panileo-colonoscopy and ileoscopy in children. J Pediatr Gastroenterol Nutr. 1994;19:283–9.

39. Dillon M, Brown S, Casey W, et al. Ileo-colonoscopy under general anesthesia. Pediatrics. 1998;102:381–3.

40. Stringer M, Pinfield A, Revell L, et al. A prospective audit of paediatric ileo-colonoscopy under general anaesthesia. Acta Paediatr. 1999;88:199–202.

41. Hassall E. Who should perform pediatric endoscopic sedation? J Pediatr Gastroenterol Nutr. 1994;18:114–7.

42. Lamireau T, Dubrueil M, Daconceicao M. Oxygen saturation during esophagogastroduodenoscopy in children: general anesthesia versus intravenous sedation. J Pediatr Gastroenterol Nutr. 1998;27:172–5.

43. Abdullah BA, Gupta SK, Croffie JM. The role of esophagogastroduodenoscopy in the initial evaluation of childhood inflammatory bowel disease: a 7- year study. J Pediatr Gastroenterol Nutr. 2002;35:633–40.

44. Castellaneta SP, Afzal N, Srivistava A. Diagnostic role of upper gastrointestinal endoscopy in paediatric inflammatory bowel disease. J Pediatr Gastroenterol Nutr. 2004;39:257–61.
45. Haggitt RC, Meissner WA. Crohn's disease of the upper gastrointestinal tract. Am J Clin Pathol. 1973;59:613–22.
46. Griffiths AM, Alemayehu E, Sherman P. Clinical features of gastroduodenal crohn's disease in adolescents. J Pediatr Gastroenterol Nutr. 1989;8:166–71.
47. Lenaerts C, Roy CC, Vaillencourt M. High incidence of upper gastrointestinal tract involvement in children with crohn's disease. Pediatrics. 1989;83:771–81.
48. Fielding JF, Toye DKM, Beton DC, et al. Crohn's disease of the stomach and duodenum. Gut. 1970;11:1001–6.
49. Cameron DJS. Upper and lower GI endoscopy in children and adolescents with Crohn's disease: a prospective study. J Gastroenterol Hepatol. 1991;6:355–8.
50. Oberhuber G, Puspok A, Oesterreicher C, et al. Focally enhanced gastritis: a frequent type of gastritis in patients with crohn's disease. Gastroenterology. 1997;112:698–706.
51. Oberhuber G, Hirch M, Stolte M. High incidence of upper gastrointestinal tract involvement in Crohn's disease. Virchows Arch. 1998;432:49–52.
52. Tobin JM, Sinha B, Ramani P. Upper gastrointestinal mucosal disease in pediatric Crohn's disease and ulcerative colitis: a blinded controlled study. J Pediatr Gastroenterol Nutr. 2001;32: 443–8.
53. Ruuska T, Vaajalathi P, Arajarvi P. Prospective evaluation of upper gastrointestinal mucosal lesions in children with ulcerative colitis and Crohn's disease. J Pediatr Gastroenterol Nutr. 1994;19:181–6.
54. Mashako MN, Cezard J, Navarro J, et al. Crohn's disease lesions in the upper gastrointestinal tract – correlation between clinical, radiological, endoscopic and histological features in adolescents and children. J Pediatr Gastroenterol Nutr. 1989;8:442–6.
55. Kirschner BS. Gastroduodenal crohn's disease in childhood. J Pediatr Gastroenterol Nutr. 1989;9:138–40.
56. Kovacs M, Muller KE, Arato A, et al. Diagnostic yield of upper endoscopy in paediatric patients with Crohn's disease and ulcerative colitis. Subanalysis of the HUPIR registry. J Crohns Colitis. 2012;6:86–94.
57. Crocco S, Martelossi S, Giurici N, et al. Upper gastrointestinal involvement in paediatric onset Crohn's disease: prevalence and clinical implications. J Crohns Colitis. 2012;6:51–5.
58. Huchzermeyer H, Paul F, Seifert E, et al. Endoscopic results in five patients with Crohn's disease of the esophagus. Gastroenterology. 1976;8:75–81.
59. Ramaswamy K, Jacobson K, Jevon G. Esophageal Crohn disease in children: a clinical spectrum. J Pediatr Gastroenterol Nutr. 2003;36:454–8.
60. Rudolph I, Goldstein F, Di marino AJ, et al. Crohn's disease of the esophagus: three cases and literature review. Can J Gastroenterol. 2001;15:117–22.
61. Walker RS, Breuer RI, Victor T. Crohn's esophagitis: a unique cause of esophageal polyposis. Gastrointest Endosc. 1996;43: 511–5.
62. D'Haens G, Rutgeerts P, Geboes K, et al. The natural history of esophageal Crohn's disease: three patterns of evolution. Gastrointest Endosc. 1994;40:296–300.
63. Geboes K, Janssens J, Rutgeerts P, et al. Crohn's disease of the esophagus. J Clin Gastroenterol. 1986;8:31–7.
64. Hanai H, Honda S, Sugimoto K, et al. Endoscopic therapy for multiple mucosal bridges in the esophagus of a patient with Crohn's disease. Gastrointest Endosc. 1999;50:715–7.
65. Rutgeerts P, Onette E, Vantrappen G, et al. Crohn's disease of the stomach and the duodenum: a clinical study with emphasis on the value of endoscopy and endoscopic biopsies. Endoscopy. 1980;12: 288–94.
66. Schmitz-Moorman P, Malchow H, Pittner PM, et al. Endoscopic and biopsy study of the upper gastrointestinal tract in Crohn's disease patients. Pathol Res Pract. 1985;178:377–87.
67. Kundhal PS, Stormon MO, Zacho M, et al. Gastral antral biopsy in the differentiation of pediatric colitides. Am J Gastroenterol. 2003;98:557–61.
68. Parente F, Cercino C, Bollini S, et al. Focal gastric inflammatory infiltrates in inflammatory bowel disease. Am J Gastroenterol. 2000;95:705–11.
69. Kaufman SS, Vanderhoff J, Young R, et al. Gastroenteric inflammation in children with ulcerative colitis. Am J Gastroenterol. 1997;92:1209–12.
70. Sasaki M, Okada K, Koyama S, et al. Ulcerative colitis complicated by gastroduodenal lesions. J Gastroenterol. 1996;31:585–9.
71. Brooker J, Saunders B, Shah S, et al. A new variable stiffness colonoscope makes ileo-colonoscopy easier: a randomised controlled trial. Gut. 2000;46:801–5.
72. Tada M, Kawai K. Research with the endoscope. New techniques using magnification and chromoscopy. Clin Gastroenterol. 1986;15:417–37.
73. Matsumoto T, Kuroki F, Mizuno M, et al. Application of magnifying chromoscopy for the assessment of severity in patients with mild to moderate ulcerative colitis. Gastrointest Endosc. 1997;46:400–5.
74. Hussein A, Bartram CN, Williams C. Carbon dioxide insufflation for more comfortable ileo-colonoscopy. Gastrointest Endosc. 1984;30:68–70.
75. Stevenson G, Wilson J, Wilkinson J, et al. Pain following ileo-colonoscopy: elimination with carbon dioxide. Gastrointest Endosc. 1992;38:564–7.
76. Cirocco W, Rusin L. Fluoroscopy: a valuable ally during difficult ileo-colonoscopy. Surg Endosc. 1996;10:1080–4.
77. Latt T, Nicholl R, Domizio P, et al. Rectal bleeding and polyps. Arch Dis Child. 1993;69:144–7.
78. Williams C, Saunders B, Bell G, et al. Real-time magnetic three-dimensional imaging of flexible endoscopy. Gastrointest Endosc Clin N Am. 1997;7:469–75.
79. Williams C, Laage N, Campbell C, et al. Total ileo-colonoscopy in children. Arch Dis Child. 1982;57:49–53.
80. Lipson A, Bartram C, Williams CB, et al. Barium studies and ileoscopy compared in children with suspected Crohn's disease. Clin Radiol. 1990;41:5–8.
81. Deere H, Thomson M, Murch S, et al. Histological comparison of rectosigmoid and full colonoscopic biopsies in the assessment of inflammatory bowel disease in childhood. Gut. 1998;42:A55.
82. Geboes K, Ectors N, D'Haens G, et al. Is ileoscopy with biopsy worthwhile in patients presenting with symptoms of inflammatory bowel disease? Am J Gastroenterol. 1998;93:201–6.
83. Salvatore S, Thomson M. Crohn's disease or intestinal tuberculosis? Inflamm Bowel Dis Monitor. 1999;1:59–61.
84. Breysem Y, Janssons J, Coremans G, et al. Endoscopic balloon dilation of colonic and ileo-colonic Crohn's strictures: long-term results. Gastrointest Endosc. 1992;38:142–7.
85. Gevers A, Couckay H, Coremans G, et al. Efficacy and safety of hydrostatic balloon dilation of ileocolonic Crohn's strictures. A prospective long-term analysis. Acta Gastroenterol Belg. 1994;57: 320–2.
86. Hassall E, Barclay G, Ament ME. Colonoscopy in childhood. Pediatrics. 1984;73:594–9.
87. Gans S, Ament M, Cristie D. Pediatric endoscopy with flexible fiberscopes. J Pediatr Surg. 1975;10:375–80.
88. Howdle P, Littlewood J, Firth J, et al. Routine ileo-colonoscopy service. Arch Dis Child. 1984;59:790–3.
89. de la Torre ML, Vargas GM, Mora Tiscarreno M, et al. Angiodysplasia of the colon in children. J Pediatr Surg. 1995;30: 72–5.

90. Habr GA. Pediatric ileo-colonoscopy. Dis Colon Rectum. 1979; 22:530–5.

91. Jalihal A, Mishra SP, Arvind A, et al. Colonoscopic polypectomy in children. J Pediatr Surg. 1992;27:1220–2.

92. Nicholson R. Medical research with children: ethics law and practice. New York: Oxford University Press; 1986.

93. Livstone E, Cohen GM, Troncale FJ, et al. Diastatic serosal lacerations: an unrecognized complication of ileo-colonoscopy. Gastroenterology. 1974;67:1245–7.

94. Ho H, Burchell S, Morris P, et al. Colon perforation, bilateral pneumothoraces, pneumopericardium, pneumomediastinum, and subcutaneous emphysema complicating endoscopic polypectomy: anatomic and management considerations. Am Surg. 1996;62: 770–4.

95. Damore L, Rantis P, Vernava A, et al. Colonoscopic perforations. Etiology, diagnosis, and management. Dis Colon Rectum. 1996;39:1308–14.

96. Gedebou T, Wong R, Rappaport W, et al. Clinical presentation and management of iatrogenic colon perforations. Am J Surg. 1996;172:454–7.

97. Orsoni P, Berdah S, Verrier C, et al. Colonic perforation due to ileo-colonoscopy: a retrospective study of 48 cases. Endoscopy. 1997;29:160–4.

98. El-Baba M, Tolia V, Lin C, et al. Absence of bacteremia after gastrointestinal procedures in children. Gastrointest Endosc. 1996;44:378–82.

99. Rozen P, Somajan G, Baratz M, et al. Endoscope-induced colitis: description. Probable cause by glutaraldehyde, and prevention. Gastrointest Endosc. 1994;40:547–53.

100. Ong E, Bohlmer U, Wurbs D. Splenic injury as a complication of endoscopy: two case reports and a literature review. Endoscopy. 1991;23:302–4.

101. Thomas A, Mitre R. Acute pancreatitis as a complication of ileo-colonoscopy. J Clin Gastroenterol. 1994;19:177–8.

102. Rothbaum R. Complications of pediatric endoscopy. Gastrointest Endosc Clin N Am. 1996;6:445–59.

103. Levine A, Koletzko S, Turner D, Escher JC, Cucchiara S, de Ridder L, Kolho KL, Veres G, Russell RK, Paerregaard A, Buderus S, Greer ML, Dias JA, Veereman-Wauters G, Lionetti P, Sladek M, Martin de Carpi J, Staiano A, Ruemmele FM, Wilson DC, European Society of Pediatric Gastroenterology, Hepatology, and Nutrition. ESPGHAN revised porto criteria for the diagnosis of inflammatory bowel disease in children and adolescents. J Pediatr Gastroenterol Nutr. 2014;58(6):795–806. doi:10.1097/ MPG.0000000000000239.

104. Cohen SA, Gralnek IM, Ephrath H, Saripkin L, Meyers W, Sherrod O, Napier A, Gobin T. Capsule endoscopy may reclassify pediatric inflammatory bowel disease: a historical analysis. J Pediatr Gastroenterol Nutr. 2008;47:31–6.

105. Cohen SA, Gralnek IM, et al. The use of a patency capsule in pediatric crohn's disease: a prospective evaluation. Dig Dis Sci. 2011;56(3):860–5.

106. Oliva S, Di Nardo G, Hassan C, Spada C, Aloi M, Ferrari F, et al. Second-generation colon capsule endoscopy vs. colonoscopy in pediatric ulcerative colitis: a pilot study. Endoscopy. 2014;46(6): 485–92.

107. Lewis B. Enterosocopy. Giastrointest Endosc Clin N Am. 2000;10:101–6.

108. Duggan C, Shamberger R, Antonioli D, et al. Intraoperative enteroscopy in the diagnosis of partial intestinal enteroscopy in infancy. Dig Dis Sci. 1995;40:236–8.

109. Tada M, Misake F, Kawai K. Pediatric enteroscopy with a Sonde-type small intestine fiberscope (SSIF-type VI). Gastrointest Endosc. 1983;29:44–7.

110. Turck D, Bonnevalle M, Gottrand F, et al. Intraoperative endoscopic diagnosis of heterotopic gastric mucosa in the ileum causing recurrent acute intussusception. J Pediatr Gastroenterol Nutr. 1990;11:275–8.

111. Darbari A, Kalloo A, Cuffari C, et al. Diagnostic yield, safety, and efficacy of push enteroscopy in pediatrics. Gastrointest Endosc. 2006;64:224–8.

112. Barkin J, Lewis B, Reiner D, et al. Diagnostic and therapeutic jejunoscopy with a new, longer enteroscope. Gastrointest Endosc. 1996;38:55–8.

113. MacKenzie J. Push enteroscopy. Gastrointest Endosc Clin N Am. 1999;9:29–36.

114. Perez-Cuadrado E, Macenalle R, Iglesias J, et al. Usefulness of oral video push enteroscopy in Crohn's disease. Endoscopy. 1997;29:745–7.

115. Yamamoto H, Sekine Y, Sato Y, et al. Total enteroscopy with a non surgical steerable double balloon method. Gastrointest Endosc. 2001;53:216–20.

116. May A, Nachbar L, Wardek A, et al. Double balloon enteroscopy: preliminary experience with obscure gastrointestinal bleeding or chronic abdominal pain. Endoscopy. 2003;35:985–91.

117. Yamamoto H, Sugano K. A new method of enteroscopy: the double ballon method. Can J Gastroenterol. 2003;17:273–4.

118. Mensink PB, Groenen MJ, van Buuren HR, et al. Double-balloon enteroscopy in Crohn's disease patients suspected of small bowel activity: findings and clinical impact. J Gastroenterol. 2009;44: 271–6.

119. Manes G, Imbesi V, Ardizzone S, et al. Use of double-balloon enteroscopy in the management of patients with Crohn's disease: feasibility and diagnostic yield in a high-volume centre for inflammatory bowel disease. Surg Endosc. 2009;23:2790–5.

120. Thomson M et al. Double balloon enteroscopy in children: diagnosis, treatment and safety. World J Gastroenterol. 2010;16(1): 56–62.122.

121. Oshitani N, Yukawa T, Yamagami H, et al. Evaluation of deep small bowel involvement by Double balloon enteroscopy in Crohn's Disease. Am J Gastroenterol. 2006;101:1484–9.

122. Xin L, Liao Z, Jiang YP, et al. Indications, detectability, positive findings, total enteroscopy, and complications of diagnostic double-balloon endoscopy: a systematic review of data over the first decade of use. Gastrointest Endosc. 2011;74:563–70.

123. Moschler O, May A, Muller MK, et al. Complications in and performance of double-balloon enteroscopy (DBE): results from a large prospective DBE database in Germany. Endoscopy. 2011;43:484–9.

124. Chutkun RK, Waye J. Endoscopy in inflammatory bowel disease. In: Kirsner J, editor. Inflammatory bowel disease. Philadelphia: Saunders; 2000.

125. Jenkins D, Balsitis M, Gallivan MF. Guidelines for the initial biopsy diagnosis of suspected chronic idiopathic inflammatory bowel disease. the British society of Gastroenterology initiative. J Clin Pathol. 1997;50:93–105.

126. Robert ME, Tang L, Hao LM, et al. Patterns of inflammation in mucosal biopsies of ulcerative colitis: perceived differences in pediatric populations are limited to children younger than 10 years. Am J Surg Pathol. 2004;28:183–9.

127. Modigliani R, Mary J, Simon J, et al. Clinical, biochemical, and endoscopic picture of attacks in Crohn's disease: evolution on prednisolone. Gastroenterol. 1990;98:811–8.

128. Peyrin-Biroulet L et al. Selecting Therapeutic Targets in Inflammatory Bowel Disease (STRIDE): determining therapeutic goals for treat-to-target. Am J Gastroenterol. 2015;110:1324–40.

129. Adler DG, Chand B, Conway JD, Diehl DL, Kantsevoy SV, Kwon RS, et al. Capsule endoscopy of the colon. Gastrointest Endosc. 2008;68(4):621–3.

130. Daperno M, D'Haens G, Van Assche G, et al. Development and validation of a new, simplified endoscopic activity score for Crohn's disease: the SES-CD. Gastrointest Endosc. 2004;60:505–12.

131. Khanna R, Zou G, D'Haens G, et al. Reliability among central readers in the evaluation of endoscopic findings from patients with Crohn's disease. Gut. 2015;65(7):1119–25. Advance online publication.

132. Feagan BG, Reinisch W, Rutgeerts P, et al. The effects of infliximab therapy on health-related quality of life in ulcerative colitis patients. Am J Gastroenterol. 2007;102:794–802.

133. Sandborn WJ, Rutgeerts P, Feagan BG, et al. Colectomy rate comparison after treatment of ulcerative colitis with placebo or infliximab. Gastroenterology. 2009;137:1250–60.

134. Mallery S, van Dam J. Interventional endoscopic ultrasonography: current status and future direction. J Clin Gastroenterol. 1999;29:297–305.

135. Shimizu S, Tada M, Kawai K. Value of endoscopic ultrasonography in the assessment of inflammatory bowel diseases. Endoscopy. 1992;24:354–8.

136. Hildebrandt U, Kraus J, Ecker K, et al. Endosonographic differentiation of mucosal and transmucosal non-specific inflammatory bowel disease. Endoscopy. 1992;24:359–63.

137. Tio T, Mulder C, Wijers O, et al. Endosonography of peri-anal and peri-colorectal fistula and/or abscess in Crohn's disease. Gastrointest Endosc. 1990;36:331–6.

138. Soweid A, Chak A, Katz J, et al. Catheter probe assisted endoluminal US in inflammatory bowel disease. Gastrointest Endosc. 1999;50:41–6.

139. Togashi K, Konishi F. Magnification Chromo-colonoscopy. ANZ J Surg. 2006;76:1101–5.

140. Kudo S. Endoscopic mucosal resection of flat and depressed types of early colorectal cancer. Endoscopy. 1993;25:455–61.

141. Ohta A, Tominaga K, Sakai Y. Efficacy of magnifying colonoscopy for the diagnosis of colorectal neoplasia: comparison with histopathological findings. Dig Endosc. 2004;16:308–14.

142. Hurlstone DP, Fuji T, Lobo AJ. Early detection of colorectal cancer using high-magnification chromoscopic colonoscopy. Br J Surg. 2002;89:272–82.

143. Fujiya M, Saitoh Y, Nomura M, et al. Minute findings by magnifying colonoscopy are useful for the evaluation of ulcerative colitis. Gastrointest Endosc. 2002;56:535–42.

144. Matts SG. The value of rectal biopsy in the diagnosis of ulcerative colitis. Q J Med. 1961;30:393–407.

145. Sugano S, Fujinuma S, Sakai Y. Magnifying colonoscopy for the diagnosis of inflammatory changes in ulcerative colitis. Dig Endosc. 2006;18:173–80.

146. Matsumoto T, Nakamura S, Jo Y, et al. Chromoscopy might improve diagnostic accuracy in cancer surveillance for ulcerative colitis. Am J Gastroenterol. 2003;98:1827–33.

147. Delaney PM, Harris M. Fibroptics in confocal microscopy. In: Pawley JB, ed. Handbook of biological confocal microscopy; 1995. Boston: Springer: 515–523.

148. Kiesslich R, Goetz M, Vieth M, et al. Confocal laser endomicroscopy. Gastrointest Endosc Clin N Am. 2005;15:715–31.

149. Polglase AL, McLaren W, Skinner SA, et al. A fluorescence confocal endomicroscope for in vivo microscopy of the upper- and the lower-GI tract. Gastrointest Endosc. 2005;62:686–95.

150. Venkatesh K, Cohen M, Evans C, et al. Feasibility of confocal endomicroscopy in the diagnosis of pediatric gastrointestinal disorders. World J Gastroenterol. 2009;15:2214–9.

151. Moussata D, Goetz M, Gloeckner A, et al. Confocal laser endomicroscopy is a new imaging modality for recognition of intramucosal bacteria in inflammatory bowel disease in vivo. Gut. 2011;60:26–33.

152. Peyrin-Biroulet L, Loftus Jr EV, Colombel JF, Sandborn WJ. The natural history of adult Crohn's disease in population-based cohorts. Am J Gastroenterol. 2010;105:289–97.

153. Solberg IC, Vatn MH, Høie O, Stray N, Sauar J, Jahnsen J, Moum B, Lygren I, IBSEN Study Group. Clinical course in Crohn's disease: results of a Norwegian population-based ten-year follow-up study. Clin Gastroenterol Hepatol. 2007;5:1430–8.

154. Cosnes J, Cattan S, Blain A, Beaugerie L, Carbonnel F, Parc R, Gendre JP. Long-term evolution of disease behavior of Crohn's disease. Inflamm Bowel Dis. 2002;8:244–50.

155. Gupta N, Bostrom AG, Kirschner BS, Ferry GD, Gold BD, Cohen SA, Winter HS, Baldassano RN, Abramson O, Smith T, Heyman MB. Incidence of stricturing and penetrating complications of Crohn's disease diagnosed in pediatric patients. Inflamm Bowel Dis. 2010;16:638–44.

156. Yamamoto T, Watanabe T. Surgery for luminal Crohn's disease. World J Gastroenterol. 2014;20:78–90.

157. Bhalme M, Sarkar S, Lal S, Bodger K, Baker R, Willert RP. Endoscopic balloon dilatation of Crohn's disease strictures: results from a large United Kingdom series. Inflamm Bowel Dis. 2014;20:265–70.

158. Hagel AF, Hahn A, Dauth W, Matzel K, Konturek PC, Neurath MF, Raithel M. Outcome and complications of endoscopic balloon dilatations in various types of ileocaecal and colonic stenosis in patients with Crohn's disease. Surg Endosc. 2014;28:2966–72.

159. Hirai F, Beppu T, Takatsu N, Yano Y, Ninomiya K, Ono Y, Hisabe T, Matsui T. Long-term outcome of endoscopic balloon dilation for small bowel strictures in patients with Crohn's disease. Dig Endosc. 2014;26:545–51.

160. Endo K, Takahashi S, Shiga H, Kakuta Y, Kinouchi Y, Shimosegawa T. Short and long-term outcomes of endoscopic balloon dilatation for Crohn's disease strictures. World J Gastroenterol. 2013;19:86–91.

161. Nanda K, Courtney W, et al. Prolonged avoidance of repeat surgery with endoscopic balloon dilatation of anastomotic strictures in Crohn's disease. J Crohns Colitis. 2013;7:474–80.

162. de'Angelis N et al. Short- and long-term efficacy of endoscopic balloon dilation in Crohn's disease strictures. World J Gastroenterol. 2013;19:2660–7.

163. Gustavsson A, Magnuson A, et al. Endoscopic dilation is an efficacious and safe treatment of intestinal strictures in Crohn's disease. Aliment Pharmacol Ther. 2012;36:151–8.

164. Wibmer AG, Kroesen AJ, Grone J, Buhr HJ, Ritz JP. Comparison of strictureplasty and endoscopic balloon dilatation for stricturing Crohn's disease—review of the literature. Int J Colorectal Dis. 2010;25:1149–57.

165. Ajlouni Y, Iser JH, Gibson PR. Endoscopic balloon dilatation of intestinal strictures in Crohn's disease: safe alternative to surgery. J Gastroenterol Hepatol. 2007;22:486–90.

166. Mueller T, Rieder B, Bechtner G, Pfeiffer A. The response of Crohn's strictures to endoscopic balloon dilation. Aliment Pharmacol Ther. 2010;31:634–9.

167. Hassan C, Zullo A, De Francesco V, Ierardi E, Giustini M, Pitidis A, Taggi F, Winn S, Morini S. Systematic review: endoscopic dilatation in Crohn's disease. Aliment Pharmacol Ther. 2007;26:1457–64.

Pierre Russo

Preparation and Procedure-Induced Artifacts

Nondisease-related alterations in the colonic mucosa may be induced by certain enemas used in bowel preparation or by the procedure itself. For example, soap suds enemas may result in hyperemia and edema of the bowel, especially noted on endoscopy [1]. Oral sodium phosphate solutions (oral fleet) may cause aphthoid-like erosions endoscopically similar to Crohn's disease (CD) [2]. These correspond histologically to large lymphoid aggregates, although edema, hemorrhages, or mild acute inflammation have also been described [3] (Fig. 22.1). Mucin depletion and increased cell proliferation can be noted in the crypts [4, 5]. Hypertonic saline and biscodyl enemas can cause mucin depletion, focal disruption of surface epithelium, mild acute inflammation and edema, which usually resolve within 1 week [6]. Minor trauma to the mucosa may allow penetration of gas insufflated into the bowel during endoscopy, resulting in "pseudolipomatosis", characterized by the formation of numerous clear spaces in the mucosa [7] (Fig. 22.2). Cleansing solutions used to disinfect endoscopes, such as hydrogen peroxide, may produce adherent mucosal plaques, mucosal vacuolar changes, congestion, hemorrhage, and even pseudolipomatosis [8, 9] (Table 22.1).

Major Histologic Features Noted in Mucosal Specimens

Active colitis refers to the presence of neutrophils either in the lamina propria, in crypt epithelium (cryptitis) or within the lumen, forming small abscesses (crypt abscesses). Neutrophils confined to the lumen of mucosal vessels are not considered part of the process of active colitis. A predominantly neutrophilic infiltrate without significant architectural changes is generally a feature of diseases with a self-limiting course, such as infections and drug reactions. Neutrophils in these cases are frequently confined to the superficial portion of the mucosa, and may be associated with small erosions or ulcers (Fig. 22.3).

Focal active colitis (FAC) is observed in acute self-limited colitis and can be an early manifestation of idiopathic inflammatory bowel disease . In a recent report of 29 pediatric patients with FAC, 8 developed Crohn's disease, whereas the other patients had either infectious colitis or remained idiopathic [10].

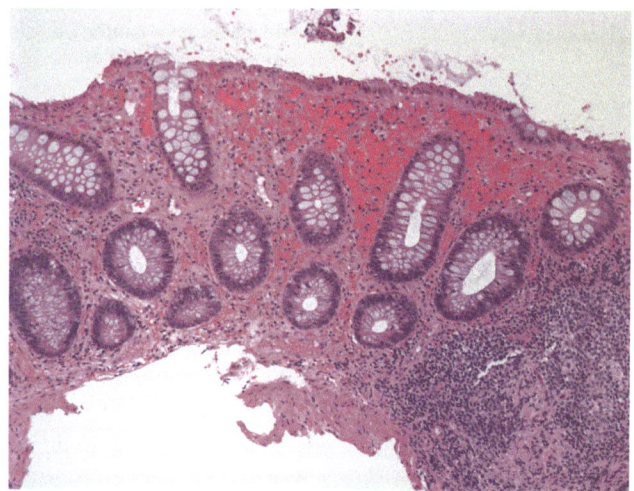

Fig. 22.1 Histologic features of phosphate enema effect. Superficial mucosal hemorrhage and focal mucin depletion of the colonic surface epithelium are noted. There is no inflammation of the crypts (hematoxylin-eosin (H+E), ×100)

P. Russo, MD
Department of Pathology and Laboratory Medicine,
Perelman School of Medicine at The University of Pennsylvania,
Philadelphia, PA, USA

Division of Anatomic Pathology, The Children's Hospital of
Philadelphia, Philadelphia, PA, USA
e-mail: russo@email.chop.edu

© Springer International Publishing AG 2017
P. Mamula et al. (eds.), *Pediatric Inflammatory Bowel Disease*, DOI 10.1007/978-3-319-49215-5_22

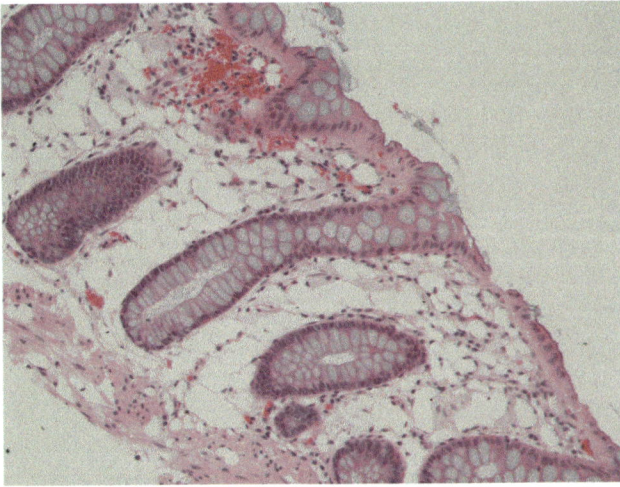

Fig. 22.2 Pseudolipomatosis. Numerous clear spaces in the lamina propria resulting from infiltration of the mucosa by insufflated gas during endoscopy suggests the presence of fat vacuoles (H+E, ×200)

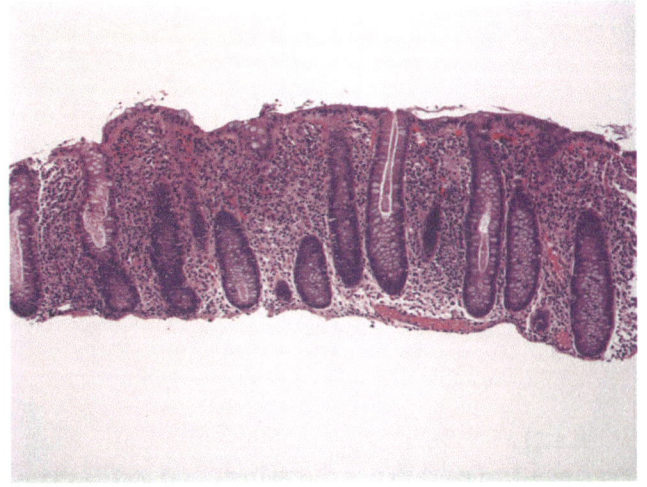

Fig. 22.3 Colitis in a 3-year-old due to Salmonella. There is a superficial, mild inflammatory infiltrate with small crypt microabscesses without significant crypt architectural changes, associated with superficial hemorrhages. Hematoxylin-eosin (H+E), ×100

Table 22.1 Differential diagnosis of colitis in infancy and childhood

Allergic	Eosinophilic colitis
Vascular	Necrotizing enterocolitis Henoch–Schönlein purpura Hemolytic uremic syndrome
Neuromuscular	Hirschsprung's disease Chronic pseudo-obstruction
Immunodeficiencies (congenital and acquired) Infectious	Bacterial, parasitic, viral
Chronic idiopathic	Ulcerative colitis Crohn's disease Lymphocytic colitis Collagenous colitis Autoimmune enterocolitis
Treatment related	Antibiotic-associated colitis Changes induced by other drugs Diversion colitis Neutropenic colitis Pouchitis Graft versus host disease Fibrosing colonopathy

Adapted and modified from Seidman (1995) #5234

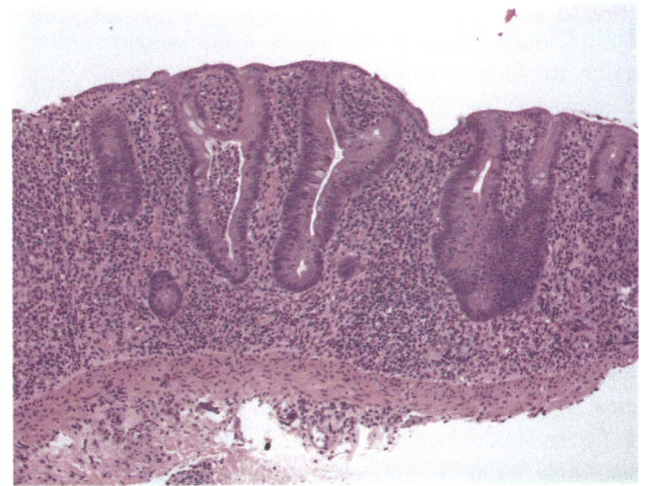

Fig. 22.4 Histologic features of IBD. Chronic mucosal damage is characterized by irregular branching of the crypts, increased intercryptal distance, and shortening of the crypts due to the presence of an inflammatory infiltrate in the deep mucosa separating the base of the crypts from the muscularis mucosa (basal plasmacytosis). In addition, there is goblet cell depletion and a microabscess. H+E, ×100

Eosinophilic colitis refers to a patchy or diffuse infiltrate dominated by eosinophils, usually with infiltration of the crypt or surface epithelium. Wide variations in the number of eosinophils in the normal colonic mucosa are due to differences in specimen site (greater numbers of eosinophils in the cecum as opposed to the rectum), age, and geography [11, 12]. In infants, the main consideration is milk allergy; parasitic infection and chronic inflammatory bowel disease (very early-onset IBD) are also possibilities.

The features of *chronic colitis* are based on the recognition of architectural changes in the mucosa, such as a "villiform" aspect of the surface epithelium, crypt destruction, and atrophy, and shortening of the crypts with irregular branching and loss of their regular outline. Shortening of the crypts is most often due to the presence of a basally situated chronic inflammatory infiltrate (basal plasmacytosis), which separates the base of the crypts from the muscularis mucosae (Fig. 22.4). Paneth cell metaplasia and pyloric metaplasia are

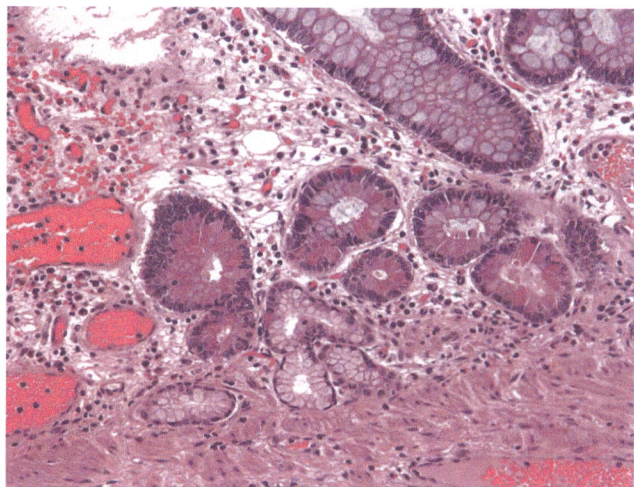

Fig. 22.5 Pyloric metaplasia and numerous crypts containing Paneth cells are noted in the deep mucosa of a patient with Crohn's disease

other useful findings (Fig. 22.5). In the normal colon, Paneth cells usually extend into the right colon, but their presence in the left colon is a feature of chronic damage, especially in the older child. Pyloric metaplasia is the presence of mucous glands normally present in the gastric antrum and pylorus. It is more frequently noted in Crohn's disease than ulcerative colitis (UC), but is also a useful feature of chronic damage. The presence of an increased mononuclear inflammatory cell infiltrate, usually an integral part of the process, is the least useful histologic parameter given the wide range in numbers of lymphocytes and plasma cells in normal specimens. Though considered a hallmark of chronic idiopathic inflammatory bowel disease, histologic features of chronicity may also be seen in other settings in pediatrics, such as immunodeficiency disorders, metabolic diseases such as glycogen storage disease type Ib, or result from mucosal injury due to ischemia or Hirschsprung's disease. *Chronic active colitis* refers to the presence of a neutrophilic infiltrate superimposed on the above changes, and is usually seen during exacerbations of IBD.

Acute Self-Limited Colitis and Its Distinction from IBD

Endoscopic features alone may not reliably distinguish acute self-limited colitis (ASLC) from IBD. Stool cultures and duration of diarrhea may help, as patients without an identifiable pathogen or in whom diarrhea lasts more than several weeks are more likely to have IBD. However, microbiologic investigations can reveal a colitis-causing pathogen such as *Salmonella*, *Campylobacter*, and *Yersinia* in up to 15% of patients with IBD [13]. ASLC is characterized by a predominantly neutrophilic infiltrate without significant crypt archi-

tectural changes. Neutrophils in these cases predominate in the superficial portion of the mucosa, and may be associated with small erosions or ulcers [14]. Neutrophils may also invade the crypt epithelium (cryptitis) or form small abscesses within the crypt lumen (crypt abscesses). Although numerous crypt abscesses suggest UC, they may be noted in CD as well as in infections and *Clostridium difficile*–related injury. The histologic diagnosis of IBD rests on the recognition of chronic mucosal damage, *chronic colitis*. Multiple biopsy studies of new-onset IBD in adults have shown that histologic features of chronic damage as noted above can reliably distinguish IBD from self-limited colitis [14–17].

Histologic Features of Early-Onset IBD

Despite the importance of recognizing chronic mucosal changes in the biopsies of patients with IBD, it has been well documented that initial colonic or rectal biopsies from 10% to 34% of pediatric patients ultimately shown to have UC lacked architectural distortion or other histologic features of chronic colitis [18–23]. This is seen particularly in younger patients (<10 years) and may be due to shorter duration of symptoms or longer progression to chronicity in children [24] (Fig. 22.6a,b). Focal active colitis may be a feature of self-limited colitis but may also be an early manifestation of IBD [10]. Close follow-up and repeat biopsies may be necessary in these cases. Increased mucosal eosinophils may be seen in the earliest biopsies of children eventually proven to have IBD, prompting a diagnosis of food allergy. In a recent case series of IBD diagnosed in 16 children less than 2 years of age, six children had an initial diagnosis of allergy [25]. On the other hand, histologic features similar to IBD may be seen in patients with primary immunodeficiencies and autoimmune enteropathy [26]. These conditions should always merit consideration when clinical manifestations of IBD occur in younger children. Histologic features that may point to a correct diagnosis in these patients include lack or paucity of plasma cells in the inflammatory infiltrate (as in Common Variable Immunodeficiency or Severe Combined Immunodeficiency), extensive crypt apoptotic activity, or absence of goblet and Paneth cells (as in autoimmune enteropathy). [27] An increasing number of rare monogenic diseases have been observed in patients with very early-onset inflammatory bowel disease [28] (Fig. 22.7).

Characteristic Features of Ulcerative Colitis and Crohn's Disease

The macroscopic and microscopic features which distinguish UC and Crohn's disease are, in most respects, similar in children and adults, and are outlined in Table 22.2. Biopsy

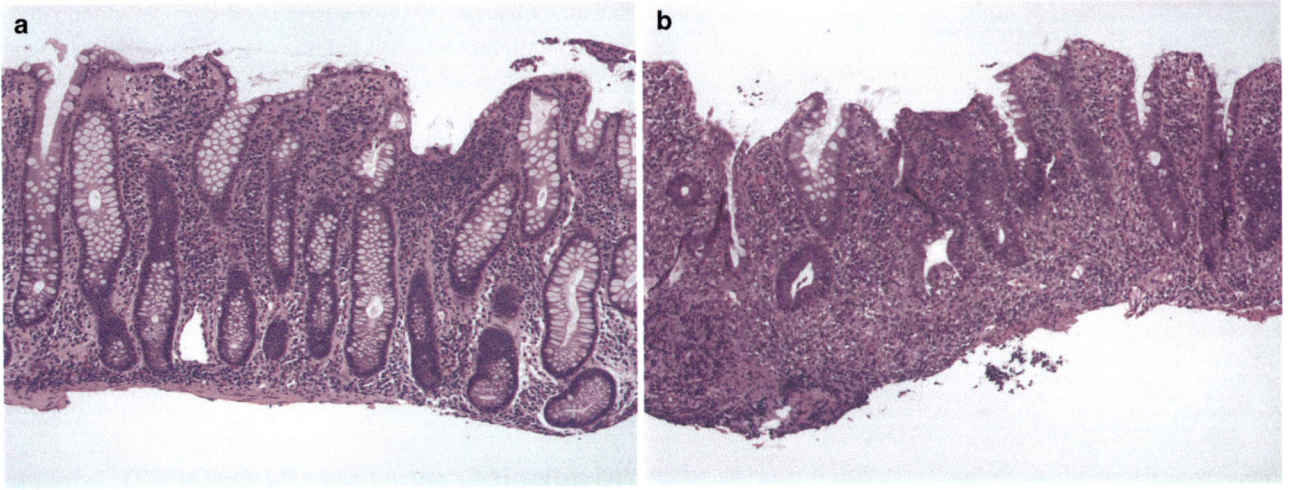

Fig. 22.6 (**a**) Colon biopsies of a 3-year-old girl with several months onset of diarrhea and abdominal pain. There is a lymphoplasmacytic inflammatory infiltrate with mild architectural distortion manifested by a slight irregularity in the outline of the crypts. (**b**) Follow-up biopsies several months later show more advanced disease with crypt atrophy and basal plasmacytosis (H+E, × 100)

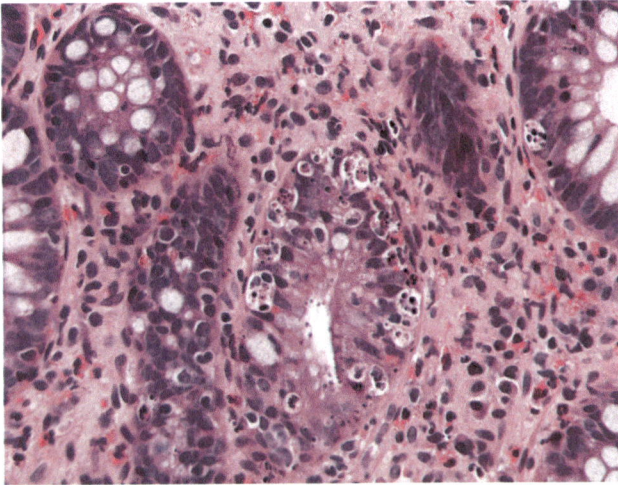

Fig. 22.7 Biopsy from a 3-year-old patient with a mutation in *DOCK8* and early-onset inflammatory bowel disease. Unusual features of this biopsy include extensive crypt apoptosis and numerous eosinophils

Table 22.2 Distinguishing features of ulcerative colitis and Crohn's disease

	Ulcerative colitis	Crohn's disease
Macroscopic		
Rectal involvement	Yes[a]	Variable
Distribution	Diffuse[a]	Segmental or diffuse
Terminal ileum	"Backwash" ileitis	Often thickened and stenosed
Serosa	Usually normal	"creeping fat"
Bowel wall	Normal thickness	Frequently thickened
Mucosa	Hemorrhagic	Cobblestone and ulcers linear
Pseudopolyps	Frequent	Less common
Strictures	No	Common
Fistulas	No	Common
Involvement of gut proximal to colon	No[b]	Common
Microscopic		
Inflammation	Confined to mucosa and superficial submucosa	Transmural
Lymphoid hyperplasia	Infrequent	common
Crypt abscesses	Extensive	Focal
Mucus depletion	Frequent	Infrequent
Deeply situated sarcoid-like granulomas	No	Yes
Fissures and sinuses	No	Yes
Villous surface transformation	Common	Infrequent
Submucosal fibrosis	Rare	Common
Neuromatous hyperplasia	Rare	Common

[a]Treatment may create the appearance of rectal sparing and discontinuous involvement
[b]See text

features helpful in differentiating these two entities in mucosal biopsies are outlined in Table 22.3. It should be noted, however, that, especially in early stages of disease, biopsies, even in combination with clinical and radiologic features, may not allow distinction between these two entities. Absence of ileal involvement does not rule out CD, and appears to be more frequent in younger patient with CD than older children or adults [29]. Similarly, diffuse colitis may be a manifestation of both CD and UC in children.

UC is classically defined as diffuse chronic mucosal inflammation limited to the colon, which invariably affects the rectum, and extends proximally in a symmetric uninterrupted pattern to involve part or all of the large intestine. The mucosa characteristically exhibits a diffuse hemorrhagic appearance (Fig. 22.8).

Table 22.3 Distinguishing features of ulcerative colitis and Crohn's disease in biopsies

	Ulcerative colitis	Crohn's disease
Distribution of inflammation	Diffuse	Frequently focal
Rectal involvement	Yes[a]	Variable
Proximal > distal colonic involvement	No[a]	Frequent
Crypt abscesses	Diffuse	Variable, often focal
Villous surface appearance	Common	Occasional
Pyloric metaplasia	Infrequent	Typical
Mucin depletion	Frequent	Infrequent
Granulomas	Superficial; foreign body	Deep; sarcoid-like

[a]See text

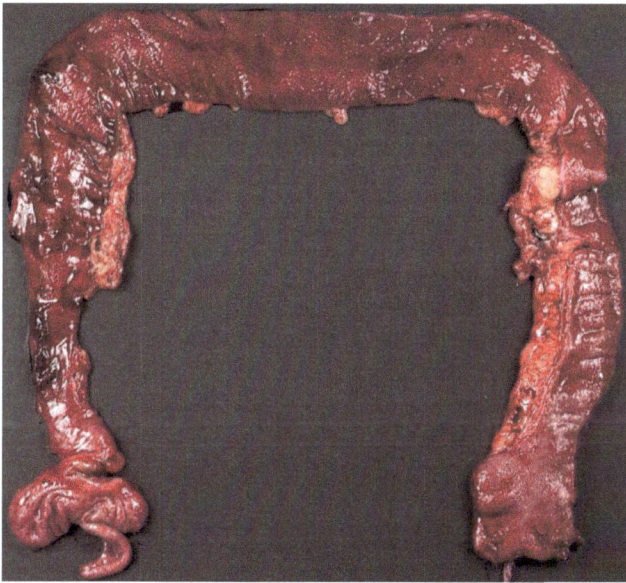

Fig. 22.8 Ulcerative colitis. Specimen from a total colectomy reveals a diffusely hemorrhagic granular mucosa from the rectum (*on the right*) to the ascending colon (*on the left*). The process is macroscopically continuous, without "skip" areas. Uninvolved appendix with a small amount of terminal ileum is also present

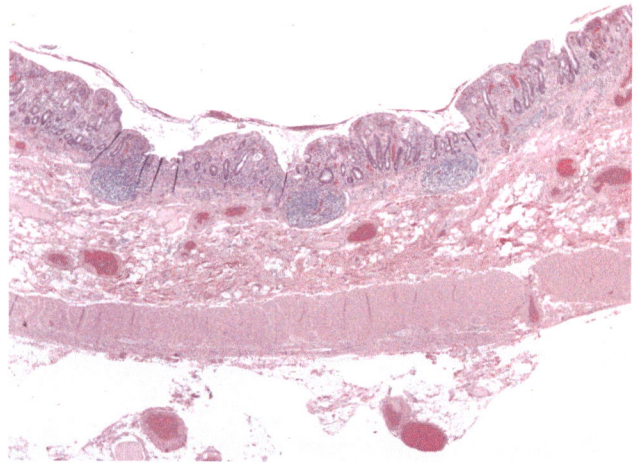

Fig. 22.9 Histologic section from the specimen in Fig. 22.6 is characterized by a diffuse inflammatory process limited to the mucosa and superficial portion of the submucosa. The colonic wall is of normal thickness

Microscopically, ulcerative colitis is characterized by inflammation limited to the mucosa and superficial submucosa (Fig. 22.9); deeper layers of the bowel are only exceptionally involved, as in toxic megacolon. Infiltration of the mucosa by neutrophils, with cryptitis, epithelial degeneration, goblet cell depletion, and crypt abscesses are characteristic though relatively nonspecific microscopic features of active UC. Chronicity, as previously defined, is characterized by crypt architectural changes such as irregular branching and atrophy, usually accompanied by a mononuclear inflammatory infiltrate. Increased crypt epithelial turnover in UC results in goblet cell depletion and Paneth cell metaplasia [30], less frequently observed in CD. The latter must be interpreted with caution in pediatric cases, as Paneth cells can be present in the distal colon in normal young children. Crypt abscesses are not specific, but when diffuse are suggestive of UC, whereas they tend to be more isolated in Crohn's disease [31]. Rupture of crypt abscesses into the lamina propria or erosions may result in collections of histiocytes which may simulate but should be distinguished from true granulomas (Fig. 22.10).

Pseudopolyps, more commonly found in UC than CD, are discrete areas resulting from surviving islands of mucosa or heaped-up granulation tissue. The latter are more accurately referred to as "inflammatory polyps". Occasionally, regenerating mucosa within such an inflammatory polyp may form irregular, dilated glands, which bear a marked resemblance to retention or "juvenile" polyps [31]. In contrast to adenomas, pseudopolyps have a short stalk and are generally smooth surfaced (Fig. 22.11). Extensive arborization and fusion of the polyps may result in mucosal bridging.

In contrast to UC, *CD* features segmental intestinal involvement, with thickening of the bowel wall consequent to transmural inflammation and fibrosis, resulting in obstructive strictures, especially in the ileocecal area. The serosa is typically congested,

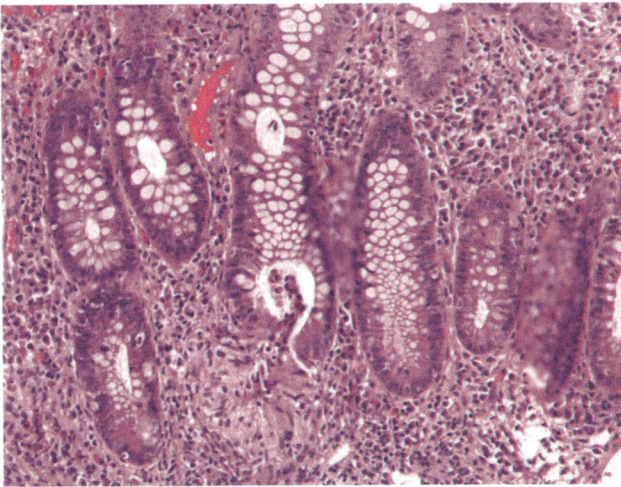

Fig. 22.10 Crypt microabscess with rupture resulting in a histiocytic reaction around the base of a crypt in a colonic biopsy from an 8-year-old girl with ulcerative colitis. H+E × 200

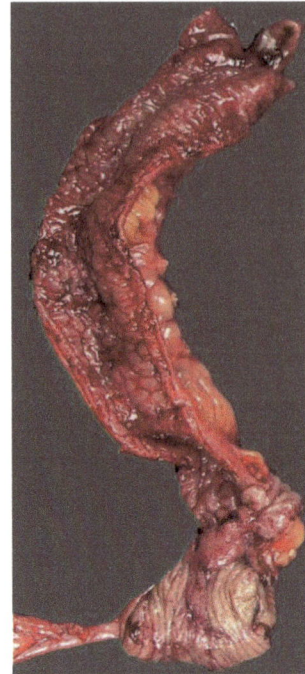

Fig. 22.12 Crohn's disease. Ileocecectomy specimen is characterized by a stricture in the area of the ileocecal valve. The mucosa has a "cobblestone" appearance, and the wall appears thickened with prominent and extensively adherent serosal fat. Contrast with Fig. 22.6

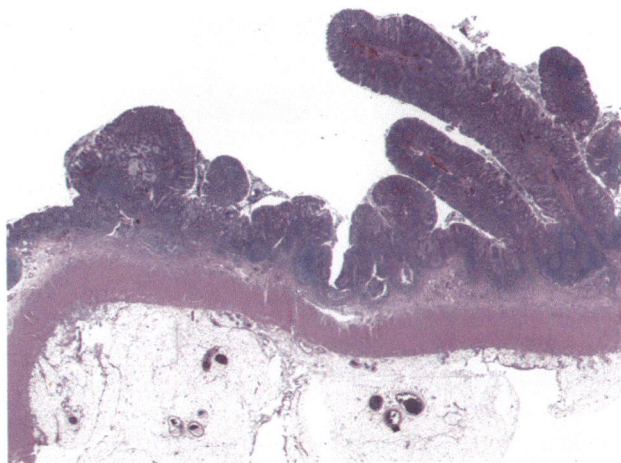

Fig. 22.11 Inflammatory "pseudopolyps" in a patient with ulcerative colitis. The base of the polyps are broad, and the polyps consist of heaped-up regenerating mucosa with an inflammatory infiltrate

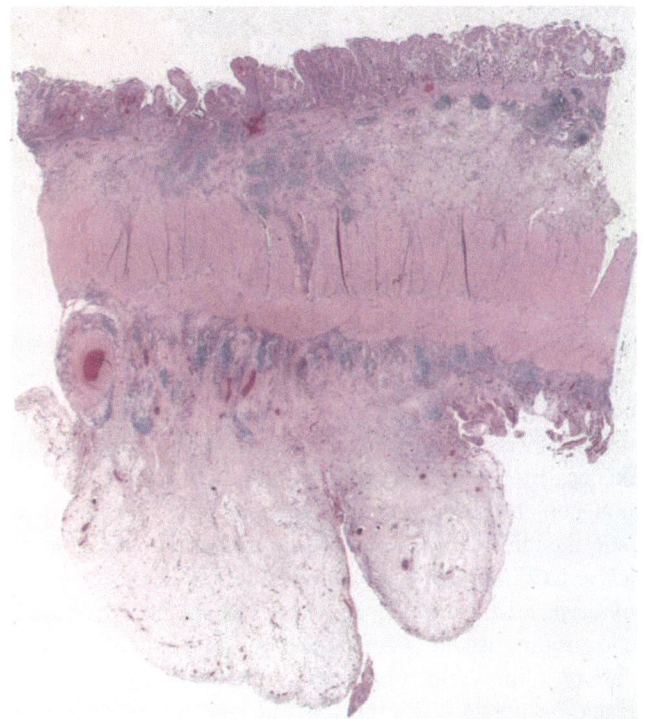

Fig. 22.13 Crohn's disease. Low power microscopic section demonstrates transmural involvement. Inflammation, in the form of lymphoid aggregates, extends through the muscularis propria into thickened serosal fat. Contrast with Fig. 22.9. H+E, × 10

with the presence of adhesions and fat wrapping, or "creeping fat". Mucosal involvement can be patchy and discontinuous. Aphthous ulcers overlying lymphoid tissue are among the earliest lesions observed endoscopically, but are nonspecific and may be seen in other conditions. Uneven involvement of the mucosa results in a typical "cobblestone" appearance (Fig. 22.12). Transmural involvement in resected specimens and the presence of granulomas are the major histologic features which distinguish CD from UC and other colitides. Transmural disease in CD usually results from submucosal edema, fibrosis and inflammation, typically in the form of lymphoid aggregates, also involving the muscle layers and the serosa (Fig. 22.13). Intramural abscesses are also noted, with fistulae, perforations and adhesions, which can involve multiple loops of bowel and

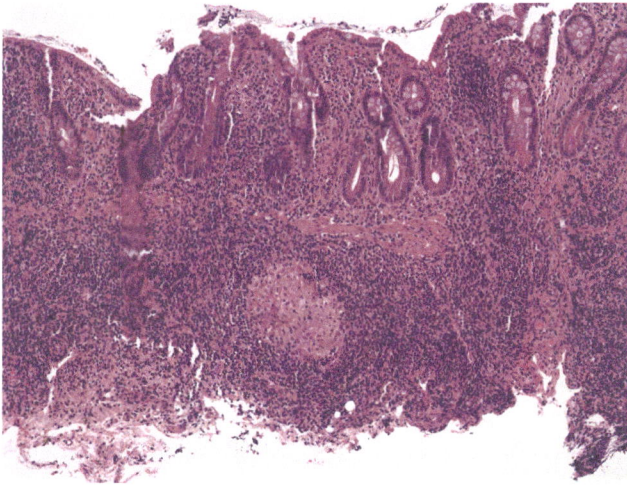

Fig. 22.14 Crohn's disease, terminal ileum. A well-formed, nonnecrotic granuloma is present in the superficial submucosa, away from any ruptured crypt. Contrast with Fig. 22.10. H+E, × 100

Table 22.4 Differential diagnosis of granulomas in colon specimens

Crohn's disease
Infections
Salmonella (microgranulomas)
Campylobacter (microgranulomas)
Mycobacteria (tuberculosis and avium-intracellulare)
Yersinia
Brucellosa
Tularemia
Schistosomiasis
Fungal infections
Mucin and foreign body granulomas
Chronic granulomatous disease
Pneumatosis intestinalis
Malakoplakia
Sarcoidosis

form a mass. The identification of pyloric metaplasia indicates chronic damage [32], and is seen more frequently with Crohn's disease than with UC. Lymphangiectasia, neural hyperplasia and vascular changes are frequently observed in CD and are almost never seen in UC.

Granulomas are virtually diagnostic of CD when they are well-formed, nonnecrotic, basally situated, and remote from areas of active inflammation (Fig. 22.14). Their presence in biopsies may predate radiologic evidence of disease, and prolonged follow-up is necessary when they are observed in the absence of grossly evident disease [33]. The likelihood of finding granulomas is clearly a function of the diligence with which they are sought, increasing with the number of biopsies and sections examined [34]. Granulomas appear to be more frequently observed in the pediatric age group. One large study in Germany found them in 26% of biopsy specimens from 42% of patients, twice as commonly as in adults [35]. Comparison of initial biopsies of children with and without rectosigmoid granulomas showed similar age of onset of disease in the two groups, though those with granulomas tended to have more extensive disease and perianal complications [36]. Shepherd and colleagues observed granulomas more frequently in their younger patients and those with a shorter clinical course, with an increased prevalence in the more distal portion of the gastrointestinal tract [37]. In a recent study at The Children's Hospital of Philadelphia, granulomas were identified in 61% of pediatric CD patients undergoing upper and lower endoscopy and were more frequent in untreated patients [38]. In nearly half of those patients, granulomas were present in the upper GI tract, in the terminal ileum, or both, but not in the colon.

Granulomas can also be seen, however, in a number of other conditions (Table 22.4). The granulomas seen in tuberculous infections of the gastrointestinal tract are typically multiple, large, and have caseous necrosis [39]. Those associated with yersiniosis are also necrotic and frequently present in mesenteric lymph nodes [40]. Chronic granulomatous disease (CGD) can present with a colitis similar to CD [41]. Numerous necrotizing granulomas may be observed; in noninflamed or quiescent cases, collections of pigmented macrophages may be noted in the mucosa (Fig. 22.15).

Colonic malignancy is a well-recognized long-term complication of UC. Recent evidence suggests that patients with Crohn's colitis incur a similar risk of colorectal cancer [42]. Duration of disease and pancolitis are well recognized as risk factors for the development of malignancy, with the risk of cancer increasing over that of the general population by 1% each year after 10 years of disease [43, 44]. Unfortunately, there is a paucity of prospective data describing long-term inflammatory bowel disease with early-onset ulcerative colitis and ultimate cancer risk in pediatric patients. Other less well-characterized risk factors include concomitant sclerosing cholangitis, an excluded, defunctionalized or bypassed segment and depressed red blood cell folate levels [43]. Children who develop colitis before the age of 10 years should undergo colonoscopy screening during their adolescence, and dysplasia and adenocarcinoma have been documented in adolescents and young adults with long-standing colitis [45]. Dysplasia in colitics is generally plaque-like or nodular, frequently referred to as the DALM (dysplasia-associated lesion or mass) lesion [46] (Fig. 22.16a, b). Epithelial dysplasia generally precedes carcinoma; therefore yearly surveillance colonoscopy is recommended. Since reliability and patient compliance of serial colonoscopy to detect dysplasia are not perfect, prophylactic colectomy should be considered in any individual who developed ulcerative colitis during childhood.

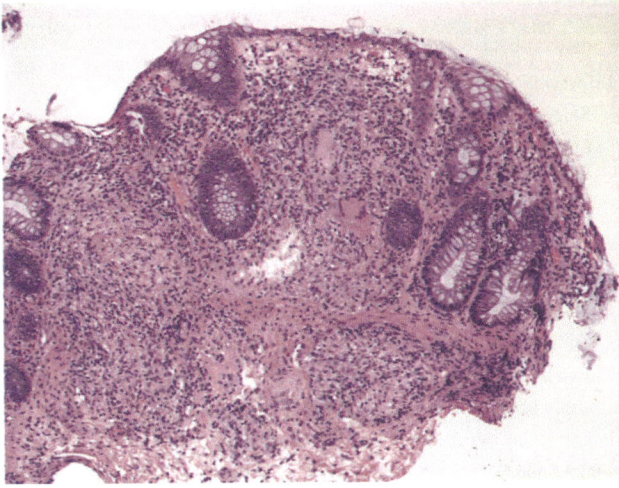

Fig. 22.15 Chronic granulomatous disease. Colon biopsy from a 5-year-old boy reveals numerous granulomas throughout the mucosa and submucosa. H+E ×100

"Atypical" Features in the Diagnosis of Ulcerative Colitis

Rectal Sparing and Patchiness

Although ulcerative colitis is traditionally considered to be a diffuse process that begins in the rectum and extends proximally in a continuous fashion, a number of studies suggest that initial rectal biopsies in children with UC may not demonstrate mucosal architectural changes as consistently as in adults or may even be "normal" (rectal sparing) (Fig. 22.17). An unequivocal diagnosis of IBD may be more difficult in these cases, as may be distinction between UC and CD.

Five of twelve children with untreated UC in one study were found to have mild patchy inflammation or normal histology in the rectum [21], whereas relative rectal sparing compared to adults was found in one study of 53 children [23]. In one study, "absolute" rectal sparing, in which evidence of both inflammation and chronicity is absent, is nonetheless infrequent in children with UC (4% of 73 pediatric cases), though "relative" rectal sparing, defined as the presence of inflammation without changes of chronicity, is more frequent, noted in 26% of cases [19]. Faubion et al. identified a 27% prevalence of rectal sparing in children with IBD and sclerosing cholangitis, suggesting the possibility that rectal sparing may be more common in this subset of patients [47]. Moreover, discontinuous involvement and rectal healing

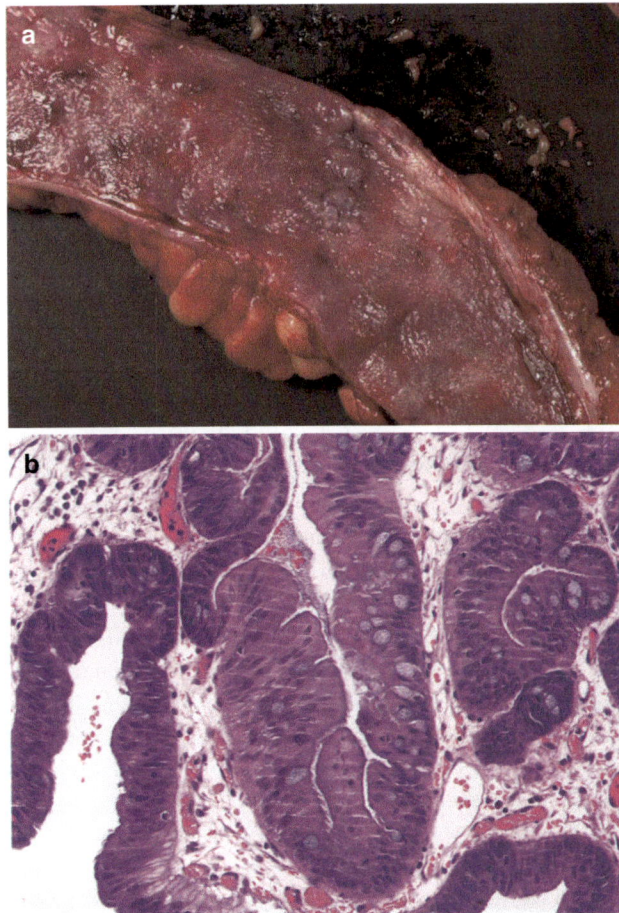

Fig. 22.16 Dysplasia in 16-year-old boy with 10 year history of ulcerative colitis. (**a**) plaque-like lesions present in the colon. (**b**) Histologic section through area of dysplasia in crypt and surface epithelium shows piled-up enterocytes with hyperchromatic nuclei and loss of polarity

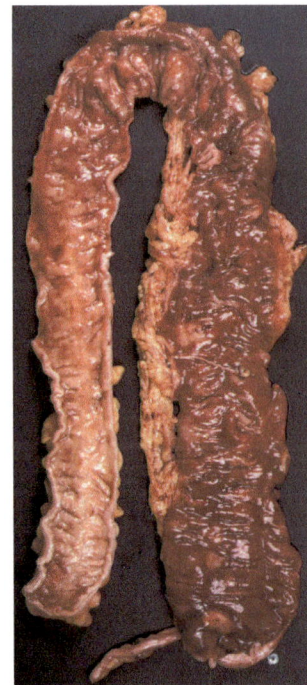

Fig. 22.17 Rectal sparing in ulcerative colitis. A 15-year-old female with several years history of ulcerative colitis which became refractory to medical therapy. The colectomy specimen reveals a diffuse colitis, much milder in the rectum than proximally

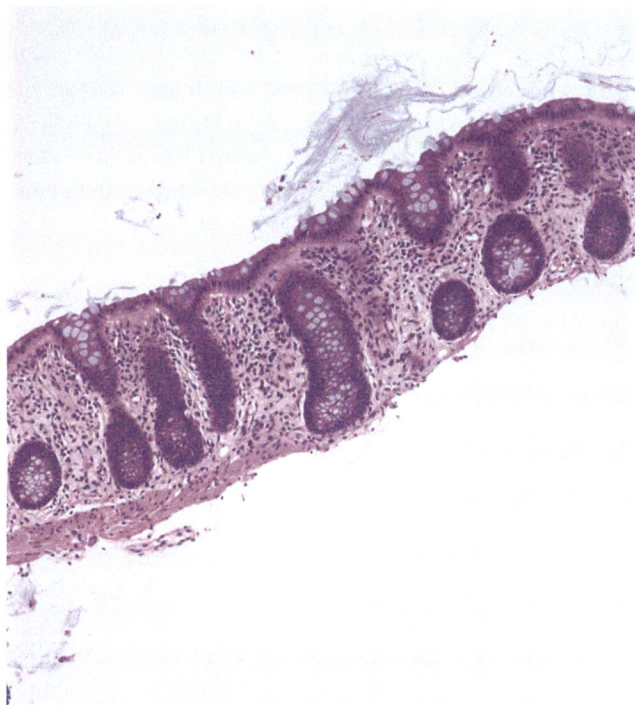

Fig. 22.18 "Quiescent" colitis. Rectal biopsy in an 11-year-old boy with history of ulcerative colitis while on therapy. Mild crypt architectural changes are present without active inflammation. H+E × 100

have been reported during the course of long-standing disease in adults, which likely results from treatment effect or natural variation in the course of disease and also reflects the current clinical practice of sampling multiple mucosal biopsies over time [48, 49]. *Medical therapy* can have a profound but variable effect on mucosal histology, ranging from decreased intensity of the inflammatory infiltrate to complete normalization of the mucosa, including discontinuity of mucosal disease in UC [50]. Quiescent colitis is characterized by mucosal atrophy and crypt architectural changes in the absence of the acute inflammation, ulceration, and mucus depletion seen in the active phase (Fig. 22.18).

Backwash Ileitis

"Backwash ileitis" refers to an abnormal radiologic or endoscopic appearance of the terminal ileum, usually in patients with an ulcerative pancolitis, which is postulated, as the name implies, to result from reflux of inflamed colonic contents into the terminal ileum. Strict morphologic criteria for this diagnosis, though not defined, rest mainly on a combination of length of involvement of the ileum (usually <10 cm), a normal ileocecal valve without radiologic and/or endoscopic signs of transmural disease or stenosis, and mild mucosal inflammation without granulomas. In a study by Heuschen, 22% of patients with pancolitis had evidence of

backwash at colectomy, whereas none of those with left sided colitis had evidence of backwash [51]. However, ileitis in UC may also represent primary ileal disease [52]. Recently, Haskell and colleagues found a 17% (34 of 200 patients) prevalence of inflammation in the terminal ileum of ileocolectomy specimens from patients with ulcerative colitis [53]. These changes were generally mild, consisting of villous atrophy, increased mononuclear cells in the lamina propria, and scattered crypt abscesses. Of these 34 patients, 32 had pancolitis, but in two patients colonic inflammation was subtotal or left sided. Furthermore, in the absence of granulomas, differentiating "backwash ileitis" from CD of the ileum can be problematic. Pyloric gland metaplasia has been suggested as a useful differentiating feature, if present [32]. "Backwash ileitis" is not believed to be a contraindication to the use of the ileum as a pouch nor to predispose to pouchitis after ileoanal anastomosis [54]. In one pediatric study, the presence of backwash ileitis, defined as a mild mixed inflammatory infiltrate of the lamina propria without crypt distortion, atrophy, or epithelial changes, and contiguous to active inflammation in the colon, did not increase the risk of pouch failure [52].

Upper GI Tract Involvement in UC

Disease of the upper intestinal tract in CD is well-documented and present in 30% of patients, in whom it may cause functional abnormalities such as delayed gastric emptying [55–58]. Endoscopic biopsies of the upper GI tract in children with IBD have revealed esophagitis, duodenal ulcers and villus atrophy, with a comparable prevalence in both CD and UC in some prospective studies [59, 60]. Upper GI tract disease with extensive duodenal involvement has been reported to occur concomitant with or many years after a well-established diagnosis of UC [61]. Whether upper GI tract disease reflects aberrant anatomic expression of UC, misdiagnosed CD or a coexisting illness is still debatable. In one study by Kundhal et al., granulomas were present on antral biopsy in 5 of 39 children with a diagnosis of ulcerative or intermediate colitis (14%), thus changing the diagnosis to CD [62]. On the other hand, conditions such as reflux esophagitis and *Helicobacter pylori*–associated gastritis are common, and may be coincidental in patients with UC [63], to which must be added the confounding effects of long-standing use of medications such as corticosteroids. Recent studies have reported that focally enhanced gastritis, defined as a perifoveolar or periglandular mononuclear or neutrophilic infiltrate around gastric crypts, is significantly more common in CD than in UC in patients without *H. pylori* [62, 63] (Fig. 22.19). In a retrospective study of 238 children with UGI biopsies, focal gastritis was present in 65% of patients with CD and in 20.8% of patients with UC, compared to

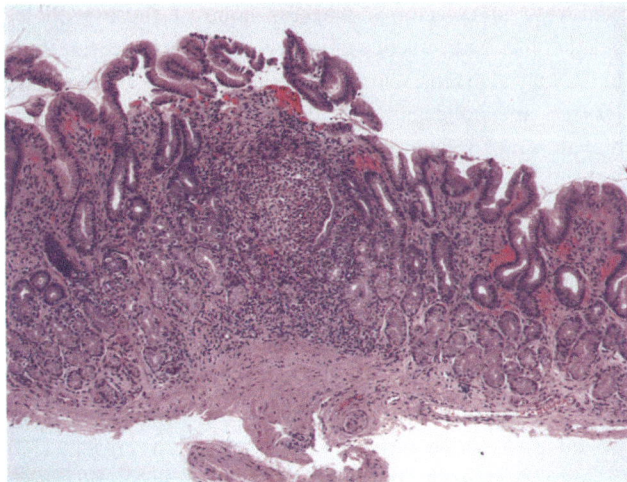

Fig. 22.19 Focal gastritis. Antral biopsy in a 14-year-old boy with IBD reveals a clustering of neutrophils and mononuclear inflammatory cells around several glands, in a background of diffuse mild chronic inflammation. H+E, × 200

2.3% of controls without IBD and one of 39 with *H. pylori* [64]. Pascasio reviewed 438 consecutive biopsies in children with gastritis looking for histologic markers for CD such as granulomas, and focal glandulitis [65]. Of 58 patients diagnosed as having CD by colonic biopsy and other standard criteria, 34 (77%) were predicted to have CD by gastric biopsy alone. Eosinophils were a significant component in many of the inflammatory foci. In their experience, none of the focal glandulitis biopsies had a history of UC.

Periappendiceal Inflammation in Ulcerative Colitis

Ulcerative colitis is classically regarded as a diffuse disease beginning in the rectum and extending proximally in a continuous fashion without skip areas. However, studies have documented *discontinuous mucosal disease*, or "skip" areas, in patients with ulcerative colitis: cecal involvement (cecal patch) separated by normal mucosa from distal colitis in 15–86% of patients undergoing surgery [66–70], and appendiceal involvement [71, 72]. D'Haens et al. found that 75% of patients had periappendiceal involvement at the time of diagnosis of distal UC, in whom inflammation was limited to the left side of the colon [67]. In a more recent study, 29 of 367 patients with UC who did not have a pancolitis and had no prior appendectomy were found to have periappendiceal inflammation, the severity of which paralleled that of the distal colon [73]. Yang et al. reported that involvement at the appendiceal orifice is not a consequence of therapy for extensive UC, but rather a distinctive "skip" lesion in patients with distal UC [74]. It has been suggested that the appendix may be a "priming" site for UC by acting as a reservoir for early

activating T cells [75]. One pediatric study examined appendices from resected intestinal specimens of patients with IBD who failed medical therapy and found that all the patients in the study (17 UC, 24 CD) had appendiceal involvement [76]. Appendiceal inflammation in these cases of UC is usually described as superficial, whereas inflammation in typical acute appendicitis is transmural.

Fulminant and Indeterminate Colitis

Severe fulminant colitis, also referred to as toxic megacolon, is a medical and surgical emergency, which, although reported to occur in up to 5% of all ulcerative colitis patients, is relatively uncommon in pediatric patients. Toxic megacolon usually occurs in the presence of severe pancolitis and results in profound dilatation of the colon secondary to severe intestinal inflammation with consequent disturbed intestinal motility. Under these conditions, disrupted mucosal integrity may allow entry of bacteria to submucosal tissues which may lead to necrosis, perforation and peritonitis. The use of antidiarrheal agents, a recent barium enema or colonoscopy have been implicated [77]. Histopathologic examination of these cases at presentation may not always adequately distinguish between UC and CD. Deep linear ulcers and fissuring with a "cobblestone" mucosa is commonly observed in these cases (Fig. 22.20a, b). Identification of small bowel involvement (other than "backwash ileitis"), deep lymphoid aggregates away from areas of mucosal ulceration and epithelioid granulomas are useful indicators in making a diagnosis of CD [78].

The term "indeterminate colitis" (IC) has been used for years to identify patients with IBD limited to the colon, but with features that do not allow distinction between UC and Crohn's disease. As originally used by Price, IC was applied to cases presenting as fulminant colitis with overlapping features of UC and CD [79]. An extended study by Wells et al. of the cohort of patients initially published by Price revealed that after histologic re-examination of 46 cases initially diagnosed as IC, 19 cases were considered to have CD, 11 cases were classified as probable UC, leaving 16 cases of IC. Four patients were further classified as UC or CD after a follow-up period of 2.5 years [80]. Thus, long-term follow-up studies of mostly adult patients initially classified with IC suggest that an eventual diagnosis of either UC or CD can be obtained in most patients. Silverberg et al., in a report of the Working Party of the 2005 World Congress of Gastroenterology, have suggested that the diagnosis of "indeterminate colitis" be rendered only in patients with suspected IBD after colectomy, and "unclassified IBD" for patients diagnosed after a biopsy that did not suggest UC or CD [81]. Epidemiologic studies cite a prevalence rate of IC of 5–10% in adults [82]. The outcome of ileal pouch procedures in patients with a

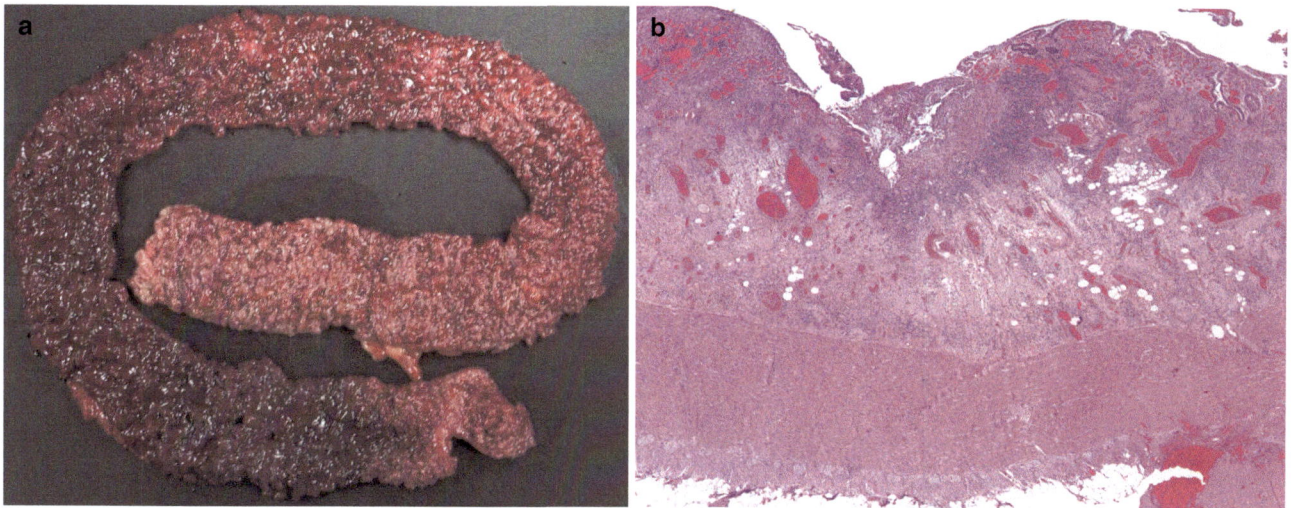

Fig. 22.20 Fulminant colitis. (**a**)Total colectomy specimen from a 17-year-old boy shows a granular diffusely hemorrhagic mucosa, predominantly towards the proximal portion of the colon (*left side* of the photograph). (**b**) Low power histologic section

diagnosis of IC (mainly adults) is also controversial, some studies reporting a higher rate of complications [83–85], others suggesting no difference in outcome between patients with IC and UC [86, 87]. The prevalence rate of IC may be higher in children, though there is a paucity of reliable epidemiologic data regarding that issue. In a Swedish study, 27% of cases of pediatric IBD were initially diagnosed as IC. During a 12-year period, diagnoses were changed in 32 of these 171 cases, 23 to UC [88]. One-fifth of cases of IBD in children less than 5 years of age were classified as IC in a study at the Children's Hospital of Philadelphia [89]. After a median follow-up of 7 years, 5 of 19 cases initially assigned to the IC group were reclassified as either CD or UC. Changes in diagnosis were made more frequently in those cases diagnosed before 1990, which could either be due to longer duration of follow-up, or to technical improvements in pediatric colonoscopy. A longitudinal study of 250 pediatric IBD patients reported that 74 (29%) were initially classified as IC, and only 29 were reclassified after a 7-year follow-up [90]. According to recent recommendations from a working group of the North American Society for Pediatric Gastroenterology, Hepatology and Nutrition, and the Crohn's and Colitis Foundation of America, a diagnosis of IC may be rendered in a pediatric patient with disease limited to the colon in cases where there is absolute rectal sparing, the presence of ileitis with disease limited to the left colon, severe focal gastritis or colitis with growth failure [91].

Pouchitis

In UC patients who undergo ileal pouch anal anastomosis (IPAA), the ileal mucosa commonly undergoes histologic modifications to a colon-like appearance resulting from changes in bacterial population, short-chain fatty acid and bile salt concentrations [92, 93]. Morphological similarity to an inflamed colon is reinforced by the detection of a mucin histochemical profile similar to that of colonic epithelium and by an inflammatory immunoprofile like that seen in ulcerative colitis [93]. At endoscopic examination, pouchitis may be mild, with mucosal hyperemia and edema, to severe, with ulcers, hemorrhage and pseudomembrane formation [94–96]. A minority of patients develop inflammation of the ileal limb proximal to the pouch, strictures (typically in the proximal pouch) and fistulas, and even extraintestinal disease which can mimic CD. Histologic examination of mucosal biopsy specimens obtained from these pouches typically demonstrate partial to complete villous blunting with crypt hyperplasia and increased mononuclear inflammatory cells and eosinophils in the lamina propria (Fig. 22.21). Areas of pyloric gland metaplasia may be present. Active inflammation, usually focal, is characterized by neutrophils in the lamina propria, cryptitis, crypt abscesses, and, in severe cases, erosions, or ulcers. Deep or transmural inflammation may be observed [93, 97–99]. Granulomas of the mucin or foreign body type may also be identified [93, 99]. Though these granulomas are not diagnostic of CD, as previously noted, they nonetheless cause concern; however, if such granulomas are found only in the pouch and not upon review of the colectomy specimen, it suggests that these granulomas may have arisen as a result of the abnormal luminal environment of the pouch and not from unrecognized CD. In addition, ischemic changes secondary to vascular compromise and pouch mucosal prolapse may occur, such as crypt hyperplasia, extension of smooth-muscle fibers from the muscularis mucosae into the lamina propria and superficial erosions with a fibrino-inflammatory exudate.

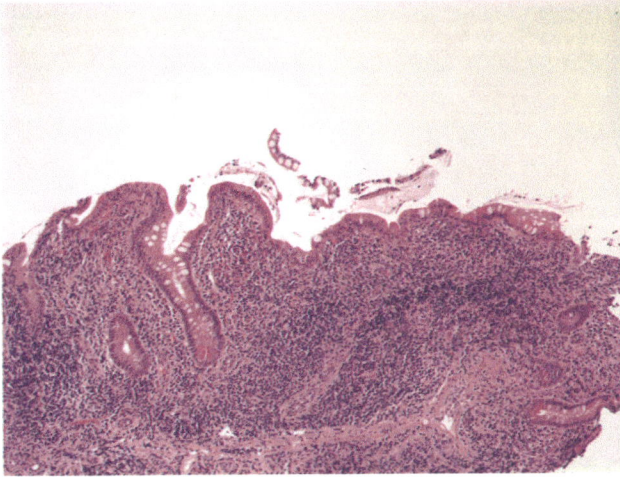

Fig. 22.21 Pouchitis. Biopsy from the neorectum in an 18-year-old female following an ileoanal pull-through reveals active chronic inflammation of the ileal mucosa with crypt loss and distortion

In view of the previous discussion, a diagnosis of CD should be considered only when review of the prior colectomy specimen reveals unequivocal features of CD, such as nonmucin granulomas, or when unequivocal CD develops in parts of the gastrointestinal tract distant from the pouch [97]. No single histologic feature in the colectomy samples of patients with UC or IC seems to be associated with pouch-related complications [100].

References

1. Withers GD, Scott RB. Drug-induced bowel injury. In: Walker WA et al., editors. Pediatric gastrointestinal disease. Hamilton: B C Decker; 2000. p. 788–95.
2. Zwas FR et al. Colonic mucosal abnormalities associated with oral sodium phosphate solution. Gastrointest Endosc. 1996;43(5):463–6.
3. Lam-Himlin D, Arnold CA, Montgomery EA. Histopathology of iatrogenic injury in the colorectum. Diagn Histopathol. 2011;17(9):404–8.
4. Driman DK, Preiksaitis HG. Colorectal inflammation and increased cell proliferation associated with oral sodium phosphate bowel preparation solution. Hum Pathol. 1998;29(9):972–8.
5. Watts DA et al. Endoscopic and histologic features of sodium phosphate bowel preparation-induced colonic ulceration: case report and review. Gastrointest Endosc. 2002;55(4):584–7.
6. Leriche M et al. Changes in the rectal mucosa induced by hypertonic enemas. Dis Colon Rectum. 1978;21(4):227–36.
7. Snover DC, Sandstad J, Hutton S. Mucosal pseudolipomatosis of the colon. Am J Clin Pathol. 1985;84(5):575–80.
8. Jonas G et al. Chemical colitis due to endoscope cleaning solutions: a mimic of pseudomembranous colitis. Gastroenterology. 1988;95(5):1403–8.
9. Ryan CK, Potter GD. Disinfectant colitis. Rinse as well as you wash. J Clin Gastroenterol. 1995;21(1):6–9.
10. Xin W, Brown PI, Greenson JK. The clinical significance of focal active colitis in pediatric patients. Am J Surg Pathol. 2003;27(8):1134–8.
11. Lowichik A, Weinberg AG. A quantitative evaluation of mucosal eosinophils in the pediatric gastrointestinal tract. Mod Pathol. 1996;9:110–4.
12. Pascal RR et al. Geographic variations in eosinophil concentration in normal colonic mucosa. Mod Pathol. 1997;10(4):363–5.
13. Schumacher G. First attack of inflammatory bowel disease and infectious colitis. A clinical, histological and microbiological study with special reference to early diagnosis. Scand J Gastroenterol Suppl. 1993;198:1–24.
14. Jenkins D et al. Guidelines for the initial biopsy diagnosis of suspected chronic idiopathic inflammatory bowel disease. The British Society of Gastroenterology Initiative. J Clin Pathol. 1997;50(2):93–105.
15. Dundas SA, Dutton J, Skipworth P. Reliability of rectal biopsy in distinguishing between chronic inflammatory bowel disease and acute self-limiting colitis. Histopathology. 1997;31(1):60–6.
16. Nostrant TT, Kumar NB, Appelman HD. Histopathology differentiates acute self-limited colitis from ulcerative colitis. Gastroenterology. 1987;92(2):318–28.
17. Tanaka M et al. Morphologic criteria applicable to biopsy specimens for effective distinction of inflammatory bowel disease from other forms of colitis and of Crohn's disease from ulcerative colitis. Scand J Gastroenterol. 1999;34(1):55–67.
18. Escher JC et al. Value of rectosigmoidoscopy with biopsies for diagnosis of inflammatory bowel disease in children. Inflamm Bowel Dis. 2002;8(1):16–22.
19. Glickman JN et al. Pediatric patients with untreated ulcerative colitis may present initially with unusual morphologic findings. Am J Surg Pathol. 2004;28(2):190–7.
20. Konuma Y et al. A study of the histological criteria for ulcerative colitis: retrospective evaluation of multiple colonic biopsies. J Gastroenterol. 1995;30(2):189–94.
21. Markowitz J et al. Atypical rectosigmoid histology in children with newly diagnosed ulcerative colitis. Am J Gastroenterol. 1993;88(12):2034–7.
22. Robert ME et al. Patterns of colonic involvement at initial presentation in ulcerative colitis: a retrospective study of 46 newly diagnosed cases. Am J Clin Pathol. 2004;122(1):94–9.
23. Washington K et al. Histopathology of ulcerative colitis in initial rectal biopsy in children. Am J Surg Pathol. 2002;26(11):1441–9.
24. Robert ME et al. Patterns of inflammation in mucosal biopsies of ulcerative colitis: perceived differences in pediatric populations are limited to children younger than 10 years. Am J Surg Pathol. 2004;28(2):183–9.
25. Cannioto Z et al. IBD and IBD mimicking enterocolitis in children younger than 2 years of age. Eur J Pediatr. 2009;168(2):149–55.
26. Daniels JA et al. Gastrointestinal tract pathology in patients with common variable immunodeficiency (CVID): a clinicopathologic study and review. Am J Surg Pathol. 2007;31(12):1800–12.
27. Glocker EO et al. Infant colitis – it's in the genes. Lancet. 2010;376(9748):1272.
28. Kelsen JR et al. Maintaining intestinal health: the genetics and immunology of very early onset inflammatory bowel disease. Cell Mol Gastroenterol Hepatol. 2015;1(5):462–76.
29. Guariso G et al. Inflammatory bowel disease developing in paediatric and adult age. J Pediatr Gastroenterol Nutr. 2010;51(6):698–707.
30. Tanaka M et al. Spatial distribution and histogenesis of colorectal Paneth cell metaplasia in idiopathic inflammatory bowel disease. J Gastroenterol Hepatol. 2001;16(12):1353–9.
31. Riddell R. Pathology of idiopathic inflammatory bowel disease. In: Kirsner J, editor. Inflammatory bowel disease. Philadelphia: WB Saunders; 2000. p. 427–50.
32. Koukoulis GK et al. Detection of pyloric metaplasia may improve the biopsy diagnosis of Crohn's ileitis. J Clin Gastroenterol. 2002;34(2):141–3.

33. Keller KM et al. Diagnostic significance of epithelioid granulomas in Crohn's disease in children. Multicenter Paediatric Crohn's Disease Study Group. J Pediatr Gastroenterol Nutr. 1990;10(1):27–32.

34. Schmitz-Moormann P, Pittner PM, Sangmeister M. Probability of detecting a granuloma in a colorectal biopsy of Crohn's disease. Pathol Res Pract. 1984;178(3):227–9.

35. Schmitz-Moormann P, Schag M. Histology of the lower intestinal tract in Crohn's disease of children and adolescents. Multicentric Paediatric Crohn's Disease Study. Pathol Res Pract. 1990;186(4):479–84.

36. Markowitz J, Kahn E, Daum F. Prognostic significance of epithelioid granulomas found in rectosigmoid biopsies at the initial presentation of pediatric Crohn's disease. J Pediatr Gastroenterol Nutr. 1989;9(2):182–6.

37. Shepherd NA. Granulomas in the diagnosis of intestinal Crohn's disease: a myth exploded? Histopathology. 2002;41(2):166–8.

38. Arts J et al. Efficacy of the long-acting repeatable formulation of the somatostatin analogue octreotide in postoperative dumping. Clin Gastroenterol Hepatol. 2009;7(4):432–7.

39. Pulimood AB et al. Endoscopic mucosal biopsies are useful in distinguishing granulomatous colitis due to Crohn's disease from tuberculosis. Gut. 1999;45(4):537–41.

40. El-Maraghi NR, Mair NS. The histopathology of enteric infection with Yersinia pseudotuberculosis. Am J Clin Pathol. 1979;71(6):631–9.

41. Isaacs D et al. Chronic granulomatous disease mimicking Crohn's disease. J Pediatr Gastroenterol Nutr. 1985;4(3):498–501.

42. Ullman T, Odze R, Farraye FA. Diagnosis and management of dysplasia in patients with ulcerative colitis and Crohn's disease of the colon. Inflamm Bowel Dis. 2009;15(4):630–8.

43. Ekbom A et al. Ulcerative colitis and colorectal cancer. A population-based study. N Engl J Med. 1990;323(18):1228–33.

44. Griffiths AM, Sherman PM. Colonoscopic surveillance for cancer in ulcerative colitis: a critical review. J Pediatr Gastroenterol Nutr. 1997;24(2):202–10.

45. Markowitz J et al. Endoscopic screening for dysplasia and mucosal aneuploidy in adolescents and young adults with childhood onset colitis. Am J Gastroenterol. 1997;92(11):2001–6.

46. Blackstone MO et al. Dysplasia-associated lesion or mass (DALM) detected by colonoscopy in long-standing ulcerative colitis: an indication for colectomy. Gastroenterology. 1981;80(2):366–74.

47. Faubion Jr WA et al. Pediatric "PSC-IBD": a descriptive report of associated inflammatory bowel disease among pediatric patients with psc. J Pediatr Gastroenterol Nutr. 2001;33(3):296–300.

48. Kim B et al. Endoscopic and histological patchiness in treated ulcerative colitis. Am J Gastroenterol. 1999;94(11):3258–62.

49. Kleer CG, Appelman HD. Ulcerative colitis: patterns of involvement in colorectal biopsies and changes with time. Am J Surg Pathol. 1998;22(8):983–9.

50. Geboes K, Dalle I. Influence of treatment on morphological features of mucosal inflammation. Gut. 2002;50(Suppl 3):III37–42.

51. Heuschen UA et al. Backwash ileitis is strongly associated with colorectal carcinoma in ulcerative colitis. Gastroenterology. 2001;120(4):841–7.

52. Alexander F et al. Fate of the pouch in 151 pediatric patients after ileal pouch anal anastomosis. J Pediatr Surg. 2003;38(1):78–82.

53. Haskell H et al. Pathologic features and clinical significance of "backwash" ileitis in ulcerative colitis. Am J Surg Pathol. 2005;29(11):1472–81.

54. Gustavsson S, Weiland LH, Kelly KA. Relationship of backwash ileitis to ileal pouchitis after ileal pouch-anal anastomosis. Dis Colon Rectum. 1987;30(1):25–8.

55. Gryboski JD et al. Gastric emptying in childhood inflammatory bowel disease: nutritional and pathologic correlates. Am J Gastroenterol. 1992;87(9):1148–53.

56. Kaufman SS et al. Gastroenteric inflammation in children with ulcerative colitis. Am J Gastroenterol. 1997;92(7):1209–12.

57. Lenaerts C et al. High incidence of upper gastrointestinal tract involvement in children with Crohn disease. Pediatrics. 1989;83(5):777–81.

58. Wright CL, Riddell RH. Histology of the stomach and duodenum in Crohn's disease. Am J Surg Pathol. 1998;22(4):383–90.

59. Abdullah BA et al. The role of esophagogastroduodenoscopy in the initial evaluation of childhood inflammatory bowel disease: a 7-year study. J Pediatr Gastroenterol Nutr. 2002;35(5):636–40.

60. Tobin JM et al. Upper gastrointestinal mucosal disease in pediatric Crohn disease and ulcerative colitis: a blinded, controlled study. J Pediatr Gastroenterol Nutr. 2001;32(4):443–8.

61. Valdez R et al. Diffuse duodenitis associated with ulcerative colitis. Am J Surg Pathol. 2000;24(10):1407–13.

62. Kundhal PS et al. Gastral antral biopsy in the differentiation of pediatric colitides. Am J Gastroenterol. 2003;98(3):557–61.

63. Parente F et al. Focal gastric inflammatory infiltrates in inflammatory bowel diseases: prevalence, immunohistochemical characteristics, and diagnostic role. Am J Gastroenterol. 2000;95(3):705–11.

64. Sharif F et al. Focally enhanced gastritis in children with Crohn's disease and ulcerative colitis. Am J Gastroenterol. 2002;97(6):1415–20.

65. Pascasio JM, Hammond S, Qualman SJ. Recognition of Crohn disease on incidental gastric biopsy in childhood. Pediatr Dev Pathol. 2003;6(3):209–14. Epub 2003 Mar 28.

66. Perry WB et al. Discontinuous appendiceal involvement in ulcerative colitis: pathology and clinical correlation. J Gastrointest Surg. 1999;3(2):141–4.

67. D'Haens G et al. Patchy cecal inflammation associated with distal ulcerative colitis: a prospective endoscopic study. Am J Gastroenterol. 1997;92(8):1275–9.

68. Goldblum JR, Appelman HD. Appendiceal involvement in ulcerative colitis. Mod Pathol Off J U S Can Acad Pathol Inc. 1992;5(6):607–10.

69. Groisman GM, George J, Harpaz N. Ulcerative appendicitis in universal and nonuniversal ulcerative colitis. Mod Pathol Off J U S Can Acad Pathol Inc. 1994;7(3):322–5.

70. Kroft SH, Stryker SJ, Rao MS. Appendiceal involvement as a skip lesion in ulcerative colitis. Mod Pathol Off J U S Can Acad Pathol Inc. 1994;7(9):912–4.

71. Matsumoto T et al. Significance of appendiceal involvement in patients with ulcerative colitis. Gastrointest Endosc. 2002;55(2):180–5.

72. Okawa K et al. Ulcerative colitis with skip lesions at the mouth of the appendix: a clinical study. Am J Gastroenterol. 1998;93(12):2405–10.

73. Arii R et al. How valuable is ductal plate malformation as a predictor of clinical course in postoperative biliary atresia patients? Pediatr Surg Int. 2011;27(3):275–7.

74. Yang SK et al. Appendiceal orifice inflammation as a skip lesion in ulcerative colitis: an analysis in relation to medical therapy and disease extent. Gastrointest Endosc. 1999;49(6):743–7.

75. Matsushita M et al. Appendix is a priming site in the development of ulcerative colitis. World J Gastroenterol. 2005;11(31):4869–74.

76. Kahn E, Markowitz J, Daum F. The appendix in inflammatory bowel disease in children. Mod Pathol. 1992;5(4):380–3.

77. Fazio VW. Toxic megacolon in ulcerative colitis and Crohn's colitis. Clin Gastroenterol. 1980;9(2):389–407.

78. Swan NC et al. Fulminant colitis in inflammatory bowel disease: detailed pathologic and clinical analysis. Dis Colon Rectum. 1998;41(12):1511–5.

79. Price AB. Overlap in the spectrum of non-specific inflammatory bowel disease – 'colitis indeterminate'. J Clin Pathol. 1978;31(6):567–77.

80. Besser RE et al. An outbreak of diarrhea and hemolytic uremic syndrome from Escherichia coli O157:H7 in fresh-pressed apple cider. JAMA. 1993;269(17):2217–20.

81. Silverberg MS et al. Toward an integrated clinical, molecular and serological classification of inflammatory bowel disease: report of a working party of the 2005 montreal world congress of gastroenterology. Can J Gastroenterol. 2005;19(Suppl A):5–36.

82. Shivananda S et al. Incidence of inflammatory bowel disease across Europe: is there a difference between north and south? Results of the European Collaborative Study on Inflammatory Bowel Disease (EC-IBD). Gut. 1996;39(5):690–7.

83. Atkinson KG, Owen DA, Wankling G. Restorative proctocolectomy and indeterminate colitis. Am J Surg. 1994;167(5):516–8.

84. Koltun WA et al. Indeterminate colitis predisposes to perineal complications after ileal pouch-anal anastomosis. Dis Colon Rectum. 1991;34(10):857–60.

85. Marcello PW et al. Evolutionary changes in the pathologic diagnosis after the ileoanal pouch procedure. Dis Colon Rectum. 1997;40(3):263–9.

86. Rudolph WG et al. Indeterminate colitis: the real story. Dis Colon Rectum. 2002;45(11):1528–34.

87. Yu CS, Pemberton JH, Larson D. Ileal pouch-anal anastomosis in patients with indeterminate colitis: long-term results. Dis Colon Rectum. 2000;43(11):1487–96.

88. Lindberg E et al. Inflammatory bowel disease in children and adolescents in Sweden, 1984–1995. J Pediatr Gastroenterol Nutr. 2000;30(3):259–64.

89. Mamula P et al. Inflammatory bowel disease in children 5 years of age and younger. Am J Gastroenterol. 2002;97(8):2005–10.

90. Romano C et al. Indeterminate colitis: a distinctive clinical pattern of inflammatory bowel disease in children. Pediatrics. 2008;122(6):e1278–81.

91. Bousvaros A et al. Differentiating ulcerative colitis from Crohn disease in children and young adults: report of a working group of the North American Society for Pediatric Gastroenterology, Hepatology, and Nutrition and the Crohn's and Colitis Foundation of America. J Pediatr Gastroenterol Nutr. 2007;44(5):653–74.

92. Antonioli D. Colitis in infants and children. In: Dahms B, Qualman S, editors. Gastrointestinal diseases. Basel: Karger; 1997. p. 77–110.

93. Apel R et al. Prospective evaluation of early morphological changes in pelvic ileal pouches. Gastroenterology. 1994;107(2):435–43.

94. Horton K, Jones B, Fishman E. Imaging of the inflammatory bowel diseases. In: Kirsner J, editor. Inflammatory bowel disease. 5th ed. Phildelphia: WB Saunders; 2000. p. 479–500.

95. Setti Carraro PG, Talbot IC, Nicholls JR. Patterns of distribution of endoscopic and histological changes in the ileal reservoir after restorative proctocolectomy for ulcerative colitis. A long-term follow-up study. Int J Color Dis. 1998;13(2):103–7.

96. Warren BF, Shepherd NA. The role of pathology in pelvic ileal reservoir surgery. Int J Color Dis. 1992;7(2):68–75.

97. Goldstein NS, Sanford WW, Bodzin JH. Crohn's-like complications in patients with ulcerative colitis after total proctocolectomy and ileal pouch-anal anastomosis. Am J Surg Pathol. 1997;21(11):1343–53.

98. Lohmuller JL et al. Pouchitis and extraintestinal manifestations of inflammatory bowel disease after ileal pouch-anal anastomosis. Ann Surg. 1990;211(5):622–7. discussion 627-9.

99. Sandborn WJ. Pouchitis following ileal pouch-anal anastomosis: definition, pathogenesis, and treatment. Gastroenterology. 1994;107(6):1856–60.

100. Nasseri Y et al. Rigorous histopathological assessment of the colectomy specimen in patients with inflammatory bowel disease unclassified does not predict outcome after ileal pouch-anal anastomosis. Am J Gastroenterol. 2010;105(1):155–61.

Video Capsule Endoscopy in Inflammatory Bowel Disease

23

Ernest G. Seidman, Che Yung Chao, and Ana Maria Sant'Anna

Introduction

Traditionally, ileocolonoscopy and biopsies along with radiological studies have served as the imaging "gold standards" for the evaluation of patients with suspected or known inflammatory bowel disease (IBD), both in adult and pediatric cases. Ideally, complete small bowel (SB) imaging should be included at the initial evaluation to establish the diagnosis and to assess the location, extent, and severity of disease. In pediatric-onset cases, we reported that esophagogastroduodenoscopy (EGD) with biopsies were of clinical value in order to ascertain the presence of findings suggestive of Crohn disease (CD) in the upper gastrointestinal tract [1]. This has long been incorporated in the diagnostic "Porto" guidelines of the European Society for Pediatric Gastroenterology Hepatology and Nutrition [2]. Realistically, it is uncommon to inspect the small bowel mucosa beyond 25 cm in either direction with bidirectional endoscopy. This translates to meters of small bowel mucosa not visualized endoscopically.

Other imaging techniques employed in IBD are extensively discussed elsewhere in this book. These include transabdominal ultrasound (US), with or without contrast enhancement (CEUS), endoscopic ultrasound (EUS), enterography by computed tomography (CTE), magnetic resonance imaging (MRE), balloon-assisted endoscopy, as well as nuclear scans and positron emission tomography. Despite these techniques, complete assessment of the small bowel has remained a challenge.

Whereas push enteroscopy surpasses EGD, it only affords visualization of the proximal jejunum and is relatively invasive in young children. Intraoperative enteroscopy is even more invasive, necessitating a laparotomy or laparoscopy. Potential complications that may ensue include prolonged ileus, obstruction, perforation, bleeding, or fistula formation. Ballon assisted enteroscopy (BAE) is a technique that can achieve diagnostic, as well as therapeutic, enteroscopy for the entire bowel, without requiring surgery [3]. However, BAE requires a long period of manipulation, and few centers have experience in pediatric patients. Early experience with BAE in pediatric patients dealt with biliary strictures, rarely IBD cases [4]. Data on the choice and timing of BAE vs. video capsule endoscopy (VCE) in pediatric IBD are discussed later in this chapter.

The small bowel had long been considered a relatively inaccessible "black box" for pediatric endoscopy specialists. All this changed rather dramatically with the development of VCE. This innovative technique is no longer considered an emerging technology [5]. It is now embraced as an essential small bowel imaging method that has truly revolutionized enteroscopy. VCE, more than any other test, provides a noninvasive method for the complete endoscopic evaluation of the small bowel mucosa [6–12].

The extremely short focal length of the lens permits incredibly precise imaging of the intestinal mucosa as the capsule transits along the lumen, without requiring insufflation of air. The astounding resolution of the lens yields extraordinarily detailed, high-quality images of the mucosa and offers the ability to visualize normal villi, easily identifying focal areas of villous edema or atrophy (Fig. 23.1). Other recent technological advances include longer battery

E.G. Seidman, MD, FRCPC, FACG (✉)
Division of Gastroenterology, McGill Faculty of Medicine,
McGill University Health Center, MGH Campus, C10.145,
1650 Cedar Avenue, Montreal,
QC, Canada, H3G 1A4
e-mail: ernest.seidman@mcgill.ca

C.Y. Chao, MBchB, FRACP
Advanced Clinical Fellow in IBD, Division of Gastroenterology,
Faculty of Medicine, McGill University, Montreal, QC, Canada

A.M. Sant'Anna, MD
Pediatric Capsule Endoscopy Lab, GI Division, Montreal
Children's Hospital, McGill Faculty of Medicine,
Montreal, QC, Canada

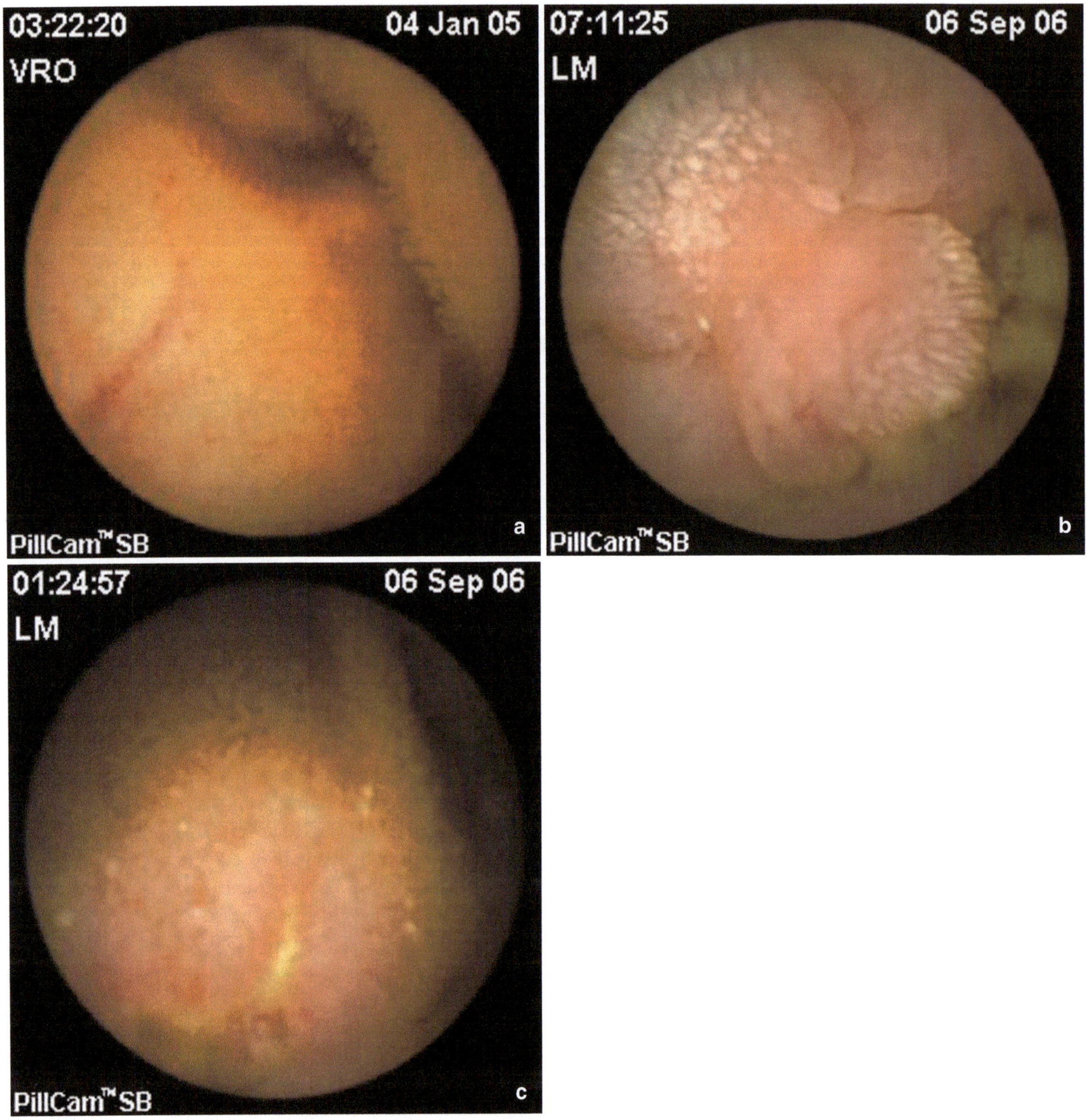

Fig. 23.1 Normal mucosal findings (**a**) in the mid-small bowel as seen by wireless capsule endoscopy in a child suspected of Crohn disease. The astonishing resolution of the capsule's lens (0.1 mm) affords visualization of normal villi and mucosal blood vessels. In contrast, subtle inflammatory changes of the small bowel mucosa that were not visualized radiologically can readily be seen focally by capsule endoscopy. These include areas of mucosal nodularity with focal villous atrophy and "white tipped villi, signifying inflammatory edema (**b**), as well as superficial linear ulcerations (**c**). Whereas these lesions detected by capsule endoscopy are typical of Crohn disease, they may be caused by other etiologies, including the use of medications such as nonsteroidal anti-inflammatory drugs

life, wider angle of vision, increased dynamic imaging speeds, and even real-time viewing to assure the capsule has traversed the pylorus [7]. The goals of this review are to provide an update on the clinical utility of VCE for IBD in the pediatric age group, as well as information on the practical applications of VCE in children.

Potential Uses of Capsule Endoscopy for Inflammatory Bowel Disease

The diagnosis of IBD entails the documentation of the extent as well as severity of the inflammation affecting segments of the gastrointestinal tract, as well as the exclusion of other

Table 23.1 Potential indications for small bowel capsule endoscopy in IBD

1. Diagnosis of suspected small bowel Crohn disease
2. Determination of the extent and severity of small bowel disease in established Crohn disease[a]
3. Evaluation of unexplained symptoms in established IBD
4. Evaluation of the presence of small bowel lesions in patients with colonic inflammatory bowel disease (ulcerative or indeterminate colitis, IBD-U)
5. Evaluation of mucosal healing of small bowel Crohn disease after treatment
6. Assessment of postoperative recurrence of small bowel Crohn disease
7. Incomplete colonoscopy
8. Assessment of pouchitis

[a]Particularly in cases of small bowel Crohn disease with symptoms potentially attributable to functional bowel disease

etiologies. There is no single test that is pathognomonic for ulcerative colitis (UC) or Crohn disease (CD). Bowel imaging techniques, whether endoscopic or radiological, are employed to support the diagnosis. The combination of ileocolonoscopy and EGD with multiple biopsies can usually differentiate between UC and CD based on the distribution and pattern of mucosal inflammation [2]. Endoscopic procedures provide invaluable information regarding the anatomic extent and severity of the mucosal inflammation. However, the vast majority of the small bowel is inaccessible to standard endoscopy or even enteroscopy. Over the past few years, several studies have established the utility of VCE to evaluate the small bowel in patients with IBD [6]. Whereas in adults, obscure bleeding is the most common indication for VCE, known or potential CD constitutes the majority (>60%) indication in children [13]. The potential uses of VCE in established or known IBD are summarized in Table 23.1, and discussed below.

Diagnostic Utility in Suspected Crohn Disease

Contrast small bowel radiography (SBR) and upper endoscopy (EGD and ileocolonoscopy) have long been the standard methods for evaluating known or suspected small bowel CD [2]. However, SBR has relatively low sensitivity for early and superficial lesions of CD in the small bowel [8, 11, 12]. Ileoscopy, when achieved, generally only affords examination of the distal and terminal ileum. Push enteroscopy can be employed to examine the proximal regions of the small bowel that cannot be examined by EGD. However, it too has a rather limited range. A recent Spanish consensus guideline recommends VCE as a far more promising tool for the evaluation of the small bowel in suspected IBD [14]. In cases where prior traditional investigations including EGD, ileocolonoscopy, and SBR were generally negative or nondiagnostic, VCE is vastly superior to establish, or exclude a diagnosis of "obscure" CD limited to the small bowel [6]. A meta-analysis reported a pooled odds ratio (OR) for VCE of 13.0

(95% confidence interval (CI) 3.2–16.3; $p < 0.0001$) compared with SBFT in detecting small-bowel abnormalities in patients with known or suspected CD [8]. The pooled OR for detecting lesions in known or suspected Crohn disease was 5.4 (95%CI 3.0–9.9) for VCE compared with enteroclysis. Another meta-analysis focused on 11 prospective comparative studies comparing VCE to other modalities for the diagnosis of established or suspected nonstricturing CD [15]. VCE was compared to multiple diagnostic modalities (ileoscopy, push enteroscopy, and small bowel radiography, including SBFT and enteroclysis, CT enterography, and small bowel MRI) in a total of 228 patients. The yield for VCE was significantly higher compared to barium small bowel radiography (63% vs. 23%, respectively). Similarly, the yield for VCE versus ileoscopy was 61% and 46%, whereas that for VCE versus CT was 69% and 30%, respectively. Subset analysis of patients with established CD showed that VCE had a higher yield compared to the other modalities. Ongoing issues include the lack of standardization between studies in terms of inclusion and exclusion criteria, as well as the widely variable capsule reading experience. Overall however, VCE is now established as more sensitive for small bowel mucosal lesions than other traditional imaging modalities. Moreover, a normal VCE examination has a very high negative predictive value, essentially ruling out small bowel CD.

Other techniques for small bowel imaging such as CT enterography (CTE) and MR enterography (MRE) are capable of evaluating bowel wall thickness and enhancement, supporting a diagnosis of CD. In addition, these techniques can also detect the presence of extraintestinal abnormalities, such as abscess formation. Also, CTE and MRE have been shown to correlate with disease activity. A small study compared VCE with MRE in 36 adults with known or suspected small bowel CD [17]. Among the 18 patients with known CD, VCE detected inflammatory lesions in the proximal and mid-small bowel (jejunum and ileum) in 12, compared to only one with MRI ($p = 0.016$). There was no significant difference in sensitivity between the two studies for terminal ileal involvement. The authors suggested that VCE is better

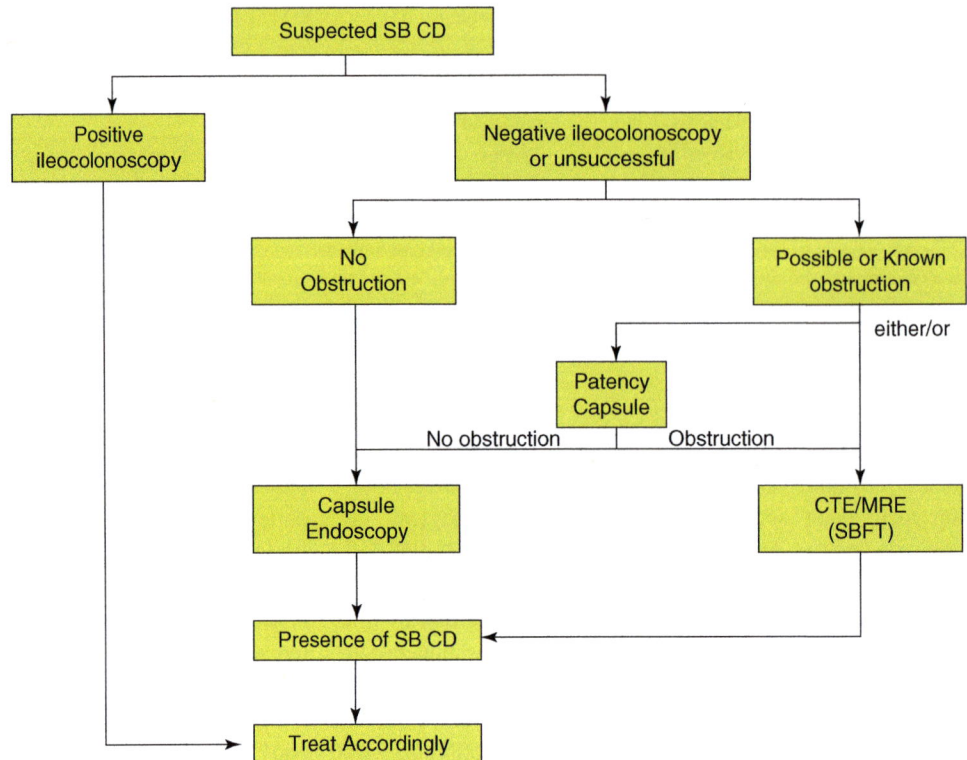

Fig. 23.2 Algorithm for the approach to suspected small bowel Crohn disease (CD). The absence of any mucosal lesions demonstrated by a complete assessment of the small bowel by capsule endoscopy essentially excludes active CD of the small bowel. Patients with symptoms suggestive of or known to have a stenosis should undergo either a patency capsule exam or evaluation by CTE or MRE prior to capsule endoscopy (From: Leighton et al. [12]; with permission). *Abbreviations*: *CD* small bowel Crohn disease, *CTE* CT enterography, *MRE* MR enterography, *SB* small bowel, *SBFT* small bowel follow through

to assess the severity and extent of small bowel inflammation. Another study compared MRE and VCE in 27 patients with established and 25 with suspected CD [10]. Among those with established CD, the yield for VCE was 93% compared to 79% with MRE. In those with suspected CD, VCE was more sensitive and specific (92%/100% vs. 77%/80%, respectively). Another small study (28 cases) used data analysis by consensus diagnosis, comparing VCE with CTE, SBFT, and ileocolonoscopy [11]. Although VCE had the highest sensitivity (83%) for CD, the specificity was lowest of the four modalities (53%).

A recent prospective study [16] in a tertiary pediatric center compared MRE, small intestine contrast US, and VCE in a cohort of 25 pediatric cases of known or suspected CD. The performance of each method was compared blinded to a reference standard for the upper small bowel and ileocolonoscopy. The authors concluded that all three methods were effective in assessing the small bowel. They recommended an integrated approach using more than one tool to achieve a complete assessment of the small bowel in known or suspected pediatric CD. Major limitations to the study are the limited cohort size (*n* = 25), combining known and suspected cases and the use of a consensus reference to the upper small bowel.

Additional prospective studies are required to define the roles of VCE vs. CTE or MRE in the diagnostic algorithm for known and suspected CD [6]. A recommended approach, based on available data [12], is illustrated in Fig. 23.2. An economic analysis comparing VCE to the traditional modalities for diagnosing CD [17] concluded that VCE was a less costly strategy if its diagnostic yield was 64% or greater, based on average diagnostic yields in the literature of 70% for VCE and 54% for SBFT and colonoscopy/ileoscopy. The authors suggested that VCE may also be less costly as a first-line test in this situation.

Detection of Postoperative CD Recurrence

The number of indications for VCE in established CD has been recently extensively reviewed [18]. Among them is to determine the presence of early postoperative recurrence of CD. Recurrence has been documented in the neo-terminal ileum in 73–93% of cases after resection [19]. A prospective comparison of VCE and ileocolonoscopy 6 months after surgery was carried out in 32 adult CD patients, 21 (68%) of whom had recurrent disease [20]. VCE was better able to identify proximal small bowel disease. However, ileocolonoscopy was more sensitive overall (90% vs. 62%). Other studies [19, 21] favored VCE or VCE and abdominal ultrasound. Overall, ileocolonoscopy remains the procedure of choice. However, in view of its noninvasive nature, VCE may be considered as an alternative approach in this clinical situation in the pediatric age group. VCE would be particularly helpful when the surgical anastomosis is not accessible by endoscopy [19].

Indeterminate Colitis

Indeterminate colitis (IC), referred to as IBD of undetermined type (IBD-U), may be defined as a chronic inflammatory bowel disease limited to the colon, without clear endoscopic or pathologic features diagnostic for either CD or UC. Pilot studies [18, 22] reported that VCE led to a change in diagnosis in 29–40% of patients. In a study involving 120 cases of UC and IBD-U, VCE revealed findings compatible with CD in 19 cases (15.8%), whereas barium small bowel imaging found just one case [23]. In a pediatric study in 26 cases of IBD-U [24], small bowel lesions typical of Crohn disease were detected by imaging in 7 and by VCE in 16 ($p < 0.05$). Overall, VCE appears to have utility as a diagnostic tool for CD in patients with IBD-U, as over 30% will be reclassified as CD (G). Larger prospective studies are needed to confirm the usefulness of VCE in this setting.

Use of VCE to Evaluate Mucosal Healing

Symptom assessment is a poor indicator of severity and extent of disease. Mucosal healing after treatment is predictive of reduced subsequent disease activity and decreased hospitalizations and surgery [25]. The high diagnostic precision of VCE can be useful to evaluate small bowel mucosal healing after treatment and thus impact upon disease management and clinical outcomes. Efthyemiou et al. [26] conducted a prospective, multicenter, case-series study. Forty patients with clinically active known or suspected CD were included, all with nonstricturing, nonpenetrating CD. All patients underwent VCE prior to the initiation of any treatment. Treatment was selected according to the treating physician. For the evaluation of mucosal healing, three endoscopic variables were collected: number of apthous ulcers, number of large ulcers, and period of time that any endoscopic lesion was visible (erythema, edema, ulcers). When patients achieved clinical response (after at least a month of treatment) they underwent a second VCE, with evaluation of the same parameters. The number of large ulcers before and after treatment were 8.3 ± 1.4 and 5 ± 0.8, respectively (mean ± SEM) (mean difference 3.3 ± 1.2, 95% confidence interval (CI) 0.8–5.9, $p = 0.01$).

Another pilot study aimed to determine the efficacy of infliximab in treatment of chronic refractory pouchitis complicated by ileitis, using capsule endoscopy [27]. VCE was repeated at week 10 and the Pouchitis Disease Activity Index score was determined. Clinical remission was achieved in 9/10 patients. At VCE and pouch endoscopy, a complete recovery of lesions was observed in eight patients.

In an ongoing study, we are evaluating VCE to assess mucosal healing of the small bowel in a cohort of adult patients with moderate to severe jejunal and or ileal CD [28]. After 6 months of adalimumab monotherapy a second VCE was carried out blinded to the initial severity score, using the Lewis Index [29]. The evaluation of the first ten cases showed complete mucosal healing in five and partial healing in four others (Lewis score decrease >50 %). Although promising, further study of the use of VCE to determine mucosal healing of the small bowel after therapy is needed. This concept is particularly appealing for pediatric onset disease, given the noninvasive nature of VCE.

Utility of VCE in "Obscure" Pediatric Onset CD

VCE was approved as a safe and beneficial in the pediatric population after the first trial [5]. Potential roles for VCE in suspected CD are substantiated by

- Isolated involvement of the small bowel in ~30% of CD cases.
- Normal findings on ileocolonoscopy and upper endoscopy are not sufficient to exclude jejunal or nonterminal ileal CD.
- Although cross-sectional imaging can detect transmural inflammation, superficial mucosal inflammatory lesions are frequently missed.

An early study used VCE in 12 adolescent patients with a clinical suspicion of CD despite negative EGD and colonoscopy [30]. Ileoscopy, achieved in 50% of the patients, was normal in all. Lesions suggestive of CD were identified by VCE in 7/12 (58%) cases. In our comparative and prospective, self-controlled pediatric trial, 30 patients from 10 to 18 years of age were evaluated for obscure small bowel disease [5]. Lesions consistent with a diagnosis of CD were found only by VCE in 10/20 (50%) patients suspected of CD, whereas the diagnosis was formally ruled out in 8. Two remaining cases were found to have eosinophilic gastroenteropathy (by histopathology obtained via subsequent enteroscopic assessment), for an overall VCE diagnostic yield of 60%. Other reports suggest that VCE is potentially useful in the evaluation of possible CD among young patients presenting with a protein-losing enteropathy [31] and/or growth failure when other studies are negative.

Specificity of VCE Findings

No gold standard test exists for the diagnosis of CD. The diagnosis is based on a compilation of clinical, endoscopic, histological, radiological, and biochemical findings. There is a justifiable concern that normal variant capsule findings in the small bowel may be overinterpreted. In adults, up to

13% of normal, asymptomatic individuals can have mucosal breaks and other minor lesions of the small bowel detected by VCE. Therefore, VCE findings of minor mucosal lesions of the small bowel are alone not sufficient for a diagnosis of CD. Other causes to be considered include celiac disease, infectious, ischemic, autoimmune as well as immunodeficiency-related, allergic and drug-induced etiologies. Nonsteroidal anti-inflammatory drug (NSAID) induced enteropathy is common and should be excluded, as it is generally conceded that lesions detected by VCE in NSAID enteropathy cannot be reliably distinguished from those due to CD. The chronicity of the lesions may assist is the differential diagnosis of CD and NSAID induced enteropathy [32].

A standard terminology system has been developed along with a VCE scoring index for small bowel inflammatory lesions such as seen for CD [29]. The parameters that were found to have the necessary inter- and intraobserver consistency were villous edema, mucosal ulcerations and the presence of stenotic lesions. This "Lewis Score" [29] provides an aid to diagnosis and a validated measure of mucosal damage:

- Combined with other clinical parameters the Lewis score could provide a threshold for establishing a positive exam and potentially for the diagnosis of CD.
- Provides an objective measure of assessing small bowel disease extent and severity, as well as the presence of stenotic lesions (whether or not ulcerated or traversed).
- Assists in determining appropriate patient management.
- Facilitates communication and standardization for assessing disease states.
- May be utilized to monitor drug therapy effectiveness.

In our experience, although scoring the mucosal lesions (villous edema, ulcers, strictures) to compile the "Lewis Score" are not specific for CD, they do accurately discriminate normal from a positive exam, and gauge the severity of mucosal inflammation (mild, moderate, severe) for each small bowel tertile [29]. Hopefully, such a standardized scoring system will be utilized by clinical investigators carrying out VCE so that the data from future trials are standardized and comparable. It is will also be important to develop a system for classifying the extent and severity of inflammatory lesions seen on VCE in normal individuals and to develop reliable criteria for the diagnosis of CD. Further validation studies in pediatric patients are needed.

An alternative, albeit more invasive endoscopic approach to VCE, is ballon assisted enteroscopy (BAE). Although used much less frequently in the pediatric age group, it has the distinct advantage to provide histological specimens for analysis [33]. A recent retrospective review examined the accuracy if BAE after VCE in 36 pediatric cases [34].

Overall, both VCE and BAE had a high sensitivity for histologically significant findings (100 vs. 87%, respectively). However, the specificity was higher for BAE (20% vs. 65%). Given the high diagnostic yield of both tests and in view of the high negative predictive value of VCE, the authors recommended carrying out VCE first [34].

Impact of VCE on Management

In the assessment of any diagnostic technology, a critical evaluation of the impact or added value of the test must be considered. A retrospective review of VCE in 83 children was reported by a single tertiary care center [35]. Among these approximately 60% were established CD, 20% IBD-U, and 20% suspected IBD. One year after VCE, patients with known CD had significant improvements in growth, higher body mass index, lower ESR and Harvey Bradshaw index. VCE also revealed more extensive disease extent in 43% of CD compared to other modalities used. The negative predictive value for suspected IBD was 94%. Moreover, 50% of IBD-U cases had their diagnosis changed to CD after VCE [35].

Practical Capsule Issues in Pediatric Patients

Capsule Retention

The major contraindication to VCE is the presence of a known or suspected gastrointestinal tract obstruction and/or small bowel strictures, because of the risk of capsule retention [6, 7, 13, 17]. The incidence of capsule retention varies widely between reports, from 0.75% to 5%. Most episodes of capsule retention are caused by NSAID, CD, or radiation induced strictures. In adult patients, tumors are more often implicated as a cause of capsule retention than in pediatrics. Most cases of retention are transitory and remain asymptomatic. However, it may rarely cause symptomatic small bowel obstruction and require endoscopic or surgical removal. To minimize the risk of capsule retention in the small bowel, a careful history should be taken regarding obstructive symptoms. Patients with established CD are generally at higher risk for stricture formation, and this risk increases with duration and severity of small bowel disease. The rate of capsule retention in patients with suspected CD appears to be quite low. In our pediatric prospective trial of VCE for suspected CD, capsule retention was seen in 10% (2/20) of cases, despite normal imaging by SBR [5]. In both cases, the capsule passed the unsuspected inflammatory stenosis subsequent to treatment with oral corticosteroids. The rate of capsule retention in patients with known CD is typically higher, in the range of 4–7% [18]. However, a retrospective review of over 1000 tests in pediatric patients reported retention in only 2.2% of CD cases, compared to 2.3% overall [13]. An example of a retained capsule is shown in Fig. 23.3.

Studies support the utility of a patency capsule to screen for the risk of retention in patients suspected of having a stricture or obstruction. The newer Agile Patency Capsule (Given Imaging Inc) has been approved in Europe, Canada as well as by the FDA in the United States for use in patients with suspected small or a known stricture. It is identical in size to the conventional imaging capsule, but rather than being inert, it is designed to dissolve spontaneously in the small bowel lumen. Its body is comprised of lactose with barium, a radiofrequency identification (RFID) tag, and two side timer plugs with exposed windows. It remains intact for a minimum of 30 h, and then begins to disintegrate. The system offers an RFID patency scanning device that can detect the RFID tag. If the patient witnesses excretion of the patency capsule intact or the scanner does not detect the RFID tag at or prior to 30 h, it is generally safe to proceed with the conventional VCE [36]. We employ an abdominal plain film at ~30 h to determine if the patency capsule has been excreted or is in the small vs. large bowel. If the patency scanner is contraindicated (due to a pacemaker or implanted cardiac

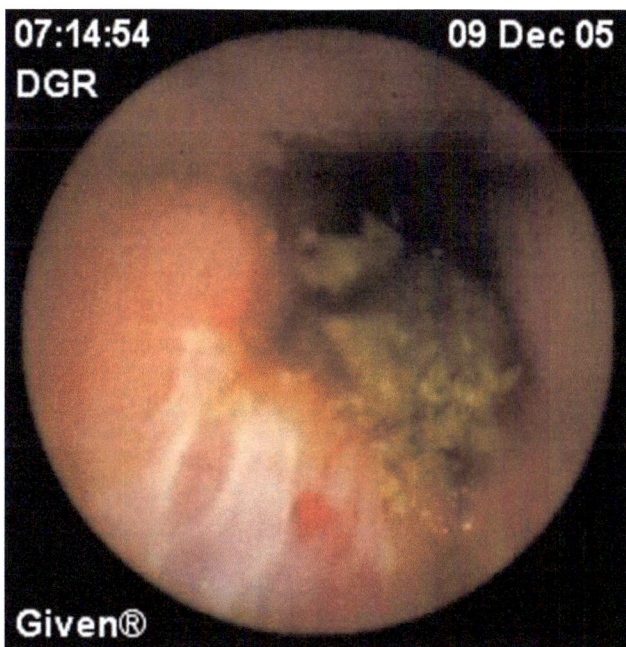

Fig. 23.3 Capsule endoscopy image of an ulcerated stricture in an adolescent patient with known Crohn disease. The patient had ongoing anemia and elevated markers of inflammation, despite a normal ileocolonoscopy and a barium small bowel follow through. The ulcerated stenosis of the mid-small bowel was seen only by capsule endoscopy. The patient presented with symptoms of partial bowel obstruction within 24 h of ingesting the capsule. All symptoms and radiological signs of bowel obstruction cleared promptly with intravenous corticosteroids, and the capsule was expelled shortly thereafter

defibrillator), fluoroscopy may be employed to check for the presence of the patency capsule or RFID tag. Although there have been rare cases of abdominal pain associated with the patency capsule, as well as exceptional episodes of temporary intestinal occlusion [37], it is generally very safe. In the unlikely event that a capsule is retained and induces symptoms, one can use ballon assisted enteroscopy (BAE) to dilate the stenosis and retrieve the capsule without surgery.

A recent multicenter study [38] evaluated the clinical utility of the systematic use of a patency capsule in known CD (our center) compared to selective use (only if obstructive symptoms, history of intestinal obstruction or surgery, or per treating physician's request). In this cohort of over 400 adult cases, the risk of retention was 1.5% without a prior patency capsule and 2.1% after a negative patency test ($p = 0.9$). However, 18 patients underwent VCE after a positive patency capsule test, with a retention rate of 11.1% ($p = 0.01$).

Preparations and Prokinetics

Given the inability to suction, wash, insufflate air or gas, the quality of the preparation is critical to adequately visualize the small bowel mucosa. Yet, the ideal preparation for VCE in the setting of IBD remains unknown. There is no universally accepted consensus on the "ideal" prep, or a validated scale with which to grade the utility of various preparations. Various trials have examined the use of oral sodium phosphate based or polyethylene glycol (PEG) based preparations, without reaching a firm conclusion. A consensus guideline for the use of bowel preparation in adults prior to colonoscopy and small bowel video capsule endoscopy was published [39]. In summary, the recommendations for VCE were to utilize a PEG-based regimen as first line (Grade A); sodium phosphate (NaP) based prep was not recommended in view of potential for renal damage and other adverse events (Grade B), unless PEG or sodium picosulfate is ineffective or not tolerated (Grade D); NaP should be avoided in chronic kidney disease, preexisting electrolyte disturbances, congestive heart failure, cirrhosis or a history of hypertension (Grade D). The authors furthermore stated [39] that there is insufficient evidence to support the use of prokinetics (Grade D) or simethicone (Grade D). No recommendation was made regarding timing of the dose (Grade D).

PEG-based regimens are generally recommended for children undergoing colonoscopy. A recent prospective, randomized single blinded pediatric study for preps in VCE was reported [40]. The effect of different preparation regimens was compared in 198 cases evaluated for bleeding or IBD by VCE. The primary outcome was the calculated percentage of visualized surface area. Patients were randomized to one of 5 groups: (A) 12 h liquid diet day prior to VCE; (B) high volume PEG (50 ml/kg up to 2 L; (C) low volume PEG (25 ml/kg up to 1 L0; (D) 3.76 mg simethicone; or (E) low dose PEG and simethicone as above. The highest visualization score achieved was for the combination preparation used in group E ($p < 0.01$). Overall diagnostic yield and tolerability were not different [40]. Inter-observer agreement was $\kappa = 0.89$; 95% CI 0.83 ± 0.71.

Two very recent studies examined the use of bowel preps prior to VCE in adults. A retrospective analysis of data from two tertiary care medical centers in Israel [41] compared 2-L PEG ($n = 360$) with a clear liquid diet plus 12-h fast protocol ($n = 500$). SB completion rates were higher in the PEG protocol (96% vs. 83%, $p < 0.001$) and SB passage time was significantly faster in the PEG protocol (mean 217 ± 73 vs. 238 ± 77 min, $p < 0.001$). However, bowel preparation quality was similar between groups (8% vs. 7% inadequate preparation). Overall positive SB findings were also similar between the two groups (57% vs. 51%, respectively, $p = 0.119$).

A randomized, blinded controlled trial comparing 3 prep regimens was reported by a Canadian group (42). Patients ($n = 198$) were randomized to clear fluids only, 2 sachets of Na picosulfate plus magnesium sulfate, or 2 L PEG the evening before VCE. No benefit was found for either prep compared to clear fluid diet in terms of visualization or diagnostic yield. Moreover, a significantly higher proportion of patients on clear fluids rated tolerance as easy or very easy ($p < 0.0001$).

In general, about 85% of VCE studies obtain images of the complete small bowel, including the terminal ileum and or cecum in large pediatric series [13]. However, in the randomized pediatric study on various preps described above, the cecum was seen in at least 95% for all five groups [40]. Some studies have thus examined the use of prokinetic agents to improve transit times and completeness of the small bowel evaluation [43]. In general, prokinetic agents may shorten gastric and/or small bowel transit times, but the ideal regimen remains controversial.

The adult consensus described above [39] did not support a prokinetic agent routinely. We recommend using a real-time viewer about an hour post capsule ingestion to determine whether it has exited the stomach. If not, we employ a single dose of erythromycin (2–4 mg/kg) to promote gastric motility. Rarely, if the capsule is still in the stomach 2 h after ingestion, we use gastroscopy to advance it into the duodenum.

One should routinely ascertain if there is any history suggestive of gastroparesis, if the patient is sedentary, or if medications are being used which may interfere with gastric emptying. Patients should be fasting for a minimum of 8 h prior to the test. We allow patients to drink clear fluids 1–2 h after the study has begun and to eat a light meal about 2 h after ingesting the capsule.

Endoscopic Placement of the Capsule

Patients of any age may be unable to swallow the capsule. This problem is very common in children under age 8. Patients can practice by swallowing similar sized jelly beans or other candies. If a parent has any doubt as to their child's ability to swallow the capsule, it is worthwhile having the child demonstrate that they are indeed capable of swallowing a similar sized object (vitamin tablet or jelly bean), prior to undergoing VCE.

For patients unable or unwilling to swallow the capsule, VCE can be safely performed by introducing the capsule into the proximal duodenum endoscopically, under direct vision. This can be accomplished by "front loading" the capsule on a gastroscope [42]. A specific capsule delivery device (Fig. 23.4) has been developed ("AdvanCE™", US Endoscopy, Mentor, Ohio, USA) which affords the secure delivery of the

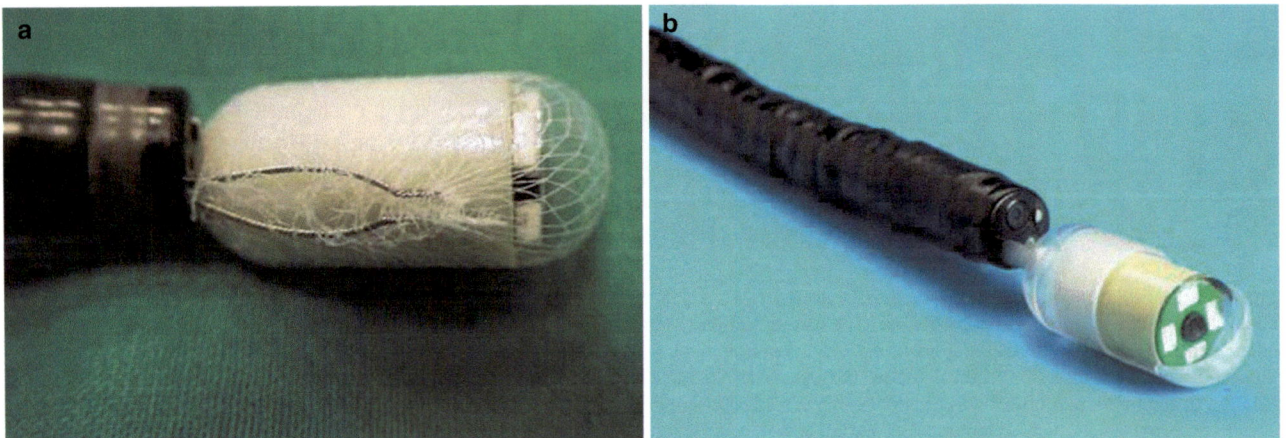

Fig. 23.4 Methods of "front loading" the capsule endoscope onto a gastroscope: (**a**) using a foreign body net, and (**b**) employing the US Endoscopy patency launching device (From: Keuchel et al. [44] (with permission))

capsule into the duodenum. As with the Roth net however, it may be difficult to launch the capsule into the duodenum in young children (Fig. 23.4). The same technique can be used in patients with severe gastroparesis.

Age and Size Limitations

Aside from swallowing issues, the capsule may be too large to cross the esophageal sphincters or pass through the pylorus and/or ileocecal valve. One study evaluated the feasibility of VCE in 83 children under age 8 [44]. It showed that VCE is feasible and safe to age 1.5 years. Overall, 24% swallowed the capsule (aged >4). Use of a foreign body net was associated with more mucosal trauma (50%) compared to the Advance™ capsule delivery device [45]. More recently a smaller retrospective study compared children unable to swallow the capsule (group A, $n = 11$) with those who were (group B, $n = 15$) [46]. Median ages [range] were 2 [10 months–9 years] and 12 [8–16 years]. The smallest child weighed 7.9 kg. Median [range] small bowel transit of 401 min [264–734] was significantly longer ($p = 0.0078$) for group A compared to group B's 227 min [56–512]. The authors attributed this to the effects of anesthetic agents. However, diagnostic yield was not different and no cases of capsule retention or adverse events occurred. Although the above study [44] did not employ endotracheal intubation, we caution to protect the child's airway, particularly for patients incapable of independently swallowing the capsule, or in those with neurological impairment.

Future Directions

After more than 15 years since small-bowel VCE was first reported, its use as a noninvasive tool that allows visualization of the entire small-intestinal mucosa has expanded momentously. In patients of all ages VCE has also been applied to other organs including the esophagus, stomach, and colon [47, 48]. The main indications for esophageal CE (ECE) are screening for gastroesophageal reflux disease/ Barrett's esophagus, and esophageal varices. However, the clinical benefit of ECE remains unconfirmed. Magnetically guided CE (MGCE), developed to visualize the gastric mucosa, is a new concept of capsule navigation and preparation protocol. First-generation colon CE (CCE) had moderate sensitivity and specificity compared with colonoscopy for colorectal neoplasia surveillance. To obtain higher accuracy, a second-generation CCE was developed with a high sensitivity for detecting clinically relevant polypoid lesions. Possible applications of CCE in pediatrics are IBD (or IBD-U) or polyposis syndromes.

A recent pediatric study prospectively enrolled 40 consecutive cases of established CD to evaluate the accuracy of CCE compared to MRE, CEUS, and ileocolonoscopy [49]. The sensitivity, specificity, positive, and negative predictive values for CCE were extremely high for colonic findings (89, 100, 100, and 97%, respectively). The accuracy was superior to MRE and CEUS. Similarly, the accuracy for small bowel findings exceeded for the other two modalities (90, 94, 95, and 90%, respectively) [49].

The results of the latter study along with the substantive evidence of the clinical accuracy of small bowel VCE raises the question as to whether we should consider reversing the investigative paradigm and screen the gastrointestinal tract using wireless capsules. Advantages include being less invasive and lower cost, anesthesia and radiation free [13]. In the not too distant future, VCE may include diagnostic and therapeutic functions such as magnifying endoscopy systems, targeted biopsy forceps, and drug delivery systems.

Conclusions
In summary, the advent of VCE has revolutionized the field of small bowel enteroscopy. It has led to improvements in the diagnosis and evaluation of small bowel disorders, including IBD, in a noninvasive manner and without exposing patients to radiation. Studies suggest that VCE is particularly useful in the evaluation of patients with small bowel CD and is considered to be superior to other imaging modalities. The availability of a standardized and validated scoring system is clinically useful to classify studies as normal or showing mucosal inflammation, and the severity of disease. Larger, prospective randomized controlled trials are still needed to further understand its role in the evaluation of pediatric IBD, reassessment of mucosal healing, and how it should be used in conjunction with other modalities, such as CT or MR cross-sectional imaging. In order to assure quality of care and interpretation, a more formalized approach to training will be required for credentialing pediatric trainees as has been initiated in adult GI programs [50].

References

1. Lenaerts C, Roy CC, Vaillancourt M, Weber AM, Morin CL, Seidman E. High incidence of upper GI tract involvement in children with Crohn disease. Pediatrics. 1989;83:777–81.
2. Levine A, Koletzko S, Turner D, Escher JC, Cucchiara S, de Ridder L, et al. ESPGHAN revised porto criteria for the diagnosis of inflammatory bowel disease in children and adolescents. J Pediatr Gastroenterol Nutr. 2014;58:795–806.
3. Yamamoto H, Kita H, Sunada K, et al. Clinical outcomes of double-balloon endoscopy for the diagnosis and treatment of small-intestinal diseases. Clin Gastroenterol Hepatol. 2004;2:1010–6.

4. Nishimura N, Yamamoto H, Yano T, et al. Safety and efficacy of double-balloon enteroscopy in pediatric patients. Gastrointest Endosc. 2008;71:287–94.

5. Guilhon de Araujo Sant'Anna AM, Dubois J, Miron MJ, Seidman EG. Wireless capsule endoscopy for obscure small bowel disorders: final results of the first pediatric controlled trial. Clin Gastroenterol Hepatol. 2005;3:264–270.

6. Kopylov U, Seidman EG. Role of capsule endoscopy in inflammatory bowel disease. World J Gastroenterol. 2014;20:1155–64.

7. Zeviit N, Shamir R. Wireless capsule endoscopy of the small intestine in children. J Pediatr Gastroenterol Nutr. 2015;60:696–701.

8. Marmo R, Rotondano G, Piscopo R, Bianco MA, Cipolletta L. Meta-analysis: capsule enteroscopy vs. conventional modalities in diagnosis of small bowel diseases. Aliment Pharmacol Ther. 2005;22:595–604.

9. Golder SK, Schreyer AG, Endlicher E, Feuerbach S, Scholmerich J, Kullmann F, Seitz J, Rogler G, Herfarth H. Comparison of capsule endoscopy and magnetic resonance (MR) enteroclysis in suspected small bowel disease. Int J Color Dis. 2006;21:97–104.

10. Albert JG, Martiny F, Krummenerl A, et al. Diagnosis of small bowel Crohn disease: a prospective comparison of capsule endoscopy with magnetic resonance imaging and fluoroscopic enteroclysis. Gut. 2005;54:1721–7.

11. Solem CA, Loftus Jr EA, Fletcher JG, et al. Small-bowel imaging in Crohn's disease: a prospective, blinded, 4-way comparison trial. Gastrointest Endosc. 2008;68:255–66.

12. Leighton J, Legnani P, Seidman EG. Role of capsule endoscopy in inflammatory bowel disease: where we are and where we are going. Inflamm Bowel Dis. 2007;13:331–7.

13. Cohen SA. Pediatric capsule endoscopy. Tech Gastrointest Endosc. 2013;15:32–5.

14. Arguelles-Arias F, Donat E, Fernandez-Urien I, Alberca F, Arguelles-Matin F, Marinez MJ, et al. Guideline for wireless capsule endoscopy in children and adolescents. Rev Esp Enferm Dig (Madrid). 2016;107:714–31.

15. Triester SL, Leighton JA, Leontiadis GI, et al. A meta-analysis of capsule endoscopy (CE) compared to other modalities in patients with non-stricturing small bowel Crohn disease. Am J Gastroenterol. 2006;101:954–64.

16. Aloi M, Di Naardo G, Romano G, Casciani E, Civitelli F, Oliva S, et al. Magnetic resonance enterography, small intestine contrast ultrasound, and capsule endoscopy to evaluate the small bowel in pediatric Crohn's disease: a prospective, blinded comparison study. Gastrointest Endosc. 2015;81:420–7.

17. Goldfarb NI, Pizzi LT, Fuhr Jr JP, et al. Diagnosing Crohn disease: an economic analysis comparing wireless capsule endoscopy with traditional diagnostic procedures. Dis Manag. 2004;7:292–304.

18. Kopylov U, Nemeth A, Koulaouzidis A, Makins R, Wild G, Afif W, et al. Small bowel capsule endoscopy in the management of established Crohn's disease: clinical impact, safety and correlation with inflammatory biomarkers. Inflamm Bowel Dis. 2015;21:93–100.

19. Pons Beltran V, Nos P, Bastida G, et al. Evaluation of postsurgical recurrence in Crohn's disease: a new indication for capsule endoscopy? Gastrointest Endosc. 2007;66:533–40.

20. Bourreille A, Jarry M, D'Halluin PN, et al. Wireless capsule endoscopy versus ileocolonoscopy for the diagnosis of postoperative recurrence of Crohn disease: a prospective study. Gut. 2006;55:978–83.

21. Biancone L, Calabrese E, Petruzziello C, et al. Wireless capsule endoscopy and small intestine contrast ultrasonography in recurrence of Crohn's disease. Inflamm Bowel Dis. 2007;13:1256–65.

22. Lo SK, Zaidel O, Tabibzadeh S, et al. Utility of wireless capsule enteroscopy (WCE) and IBD serology in re-classifying indeterminate colitis (IC). Gastroenterology. 2003;124:S1310.

23. Mehdizadeh S, Chen G, Enayati PJ, et al. Diagnostic yield of capsule endoscopy in ulcerative colitis and inflammatory bowel disease of unclassified type (IBDU). Endoscopy. 2008;40(1):30–5.

24. Di Nardo G, Oliva S, Ferrari F, et al. Usefulness of wireless capsule endoscopy in paediatric inflammatory bowel disease. Dig Liver Dis. 2011;43:220–4.

25. Bouguen G, Levesque BG, Pola S, Evans E, Sandborn WJ. Endoscopic assessment and treating to target increase the likelihood of mucosal healing in patients with Crohn's disease. Clin Gastroenterol Hepatol. 2014;12:978–85.

26. Efthymiou A, Viazis N, Mantzaris G, et al. Does clinical response correlate with mucosal healing in patients with Crohn's disease of the small bowel? A prospective, case-series study using wireless capsule endoscopy. Inflamm Bowel Dis. 2008;14:1542–7.

27. Calabrese C, Gionchetti P, Rizzello F, et al. Short-term treatment with infliximab in chronic refractory pouchitis and ileitis. Aliment Pharmacol Ther. 2008;27:759–6.

28. Seidman EG, Kopylov U, Chao CY, Girardin M, Starr M. Capsule endoscopy reveals small intestinal mucosal Crohn's disease healing after treatment with adalimumab: preliminary results of the SIMCHA Study. Gastroenterology. 2016;150:S996.

29. Gralnek I, Defranchis R, Seidman E, Leighton JA, Legnani P, Lewis BS. Development of a capsule endoscopy scoring index for small bowel mucosal inflammatory change. Aliment Pharmacol Ther. 2008;22:146–54.

30. Arguelles-Arias F, Caunedo A, Romero J, et al. The value of capsule endoscopy in pediatric patients with a suspicion of Crohn disease. Endoscopy. 2004;36:869–73.

31. Barkay O, Moshkowitz M, Reif S. Crohn disease diagnosed by wireless capsule endoscopy in adolescents with abdominal pain, protein-losing enteropathy, anemia and negative endoscopic and radiologic findings. Isr Med Assoc J. 2005;7:216–8.

32. Goldstein J, Eisen GM, Lewis B, et al. Video capsule endoscopy to prospectively assess small bowel injury with celecoxib, naproxen plus omeprazole, and placebo. Clin Gastroenterol Hepatol. 2005;3:133–41.

33. Nishimura N, Yamamoto H, Yano T, et al. Safety and efficacy of double-balloon enteroscopy in pediatric patients. Gastrointest Endosc. 2010;71:287–94.

34. Danialifar TF, Naon H, Liu QY. Comparison of diagnostic accuracy and concordance of video capsule endoscopy and double balloon enteroscopy in children. J Pediatr Gastroenterol Nutr. 2016;62(6):824–7.

35. Min SB, Le-Carlson M, Singh N, Nylund CM, Gebbia J, Haas K, et al. Video capsule endoscopy impacts decision making in pediatric inflammatory bowel disease: a single tertiary care center experience. Inflamm Bowel Dis. 2013;19:2139–49.

36. Cohen SA, Ephrath H, Lewis JD, Klevens A, Bergwek A, Liu S, et al. Pediatric capsule endoscopy: review of the small bowel and patency capsules. J Pediatr Gastroenterol Nutr. 2012;54:409–13.

37. Gay G, Delvaux M, Laurent V, et al. Temporary intestinal occlusion induced by a "patency capsule" in a patient with Crohn disease. Endoscopy. 2005;37:174–7.

38. Nemeth A, Kopylov U, Koulaouzidis A, Wurm Johansson G, Thorlacius H, Amre D, et al. Use of patency capsule in patients with established Crohn's disease. Endoscopy. 2016;16:373–9.

39. Mathus-Vliegen E, Pellisé M, Heresbach D, Fischbach W, Dixon T, Belsey J, et al. Consensus guidelines for the use of bowel preparation prior to colonic diagnostic procedures: colonoscopy and small bowel video capsule endoscopy. Curr Med Res Opin. 2013;29:931–45.

40. Oliva S, Cuccchiara S, Spada C, Hassan C, Ferrari F, Civitelli F, et al. Small bowel cleansing for capsule endoscopy in paediatric patients: a prospective random single-blind study. Dig Liver Dis. 2014;46:51–5.

41. Klein A, Dashkovsky M, Gralnek I, Peled R, Chowers Y, Khamaysi I, Har-Noy O, Levi I, Nadler M, Eliakim R, Kopylov U. Bowel preparation in "real-life" small bowel capsule endoscopy: a two-

center experience. Ann Gastroenterol. 2016;29(2):196–200. doi:10.20524/aog.2016.0012.

42. Hookey L, Louw J, Wiepjes M, Rubinger N, Van Weyenberg S, Day AG, Paterson W. Lack of benefit of active preparation compared with a clear fluid–only diet in small-bowel visualization for video capsule endoscopy: results of a randomized, blinded, controlled trial. Gastrointestinal Endoscopy. 2017;85(1):187–93.

43. Villa F, Signorelli C, Rondonotti E, et al. Preparations and prokinetics. Gastrointest Endosc Clin N Am. 2006;16:211–20.

44. Keuchel M, Dirks MH, Seidman EG. Swallowing and motility disorders, pacemakers & obesity. In: Keuchel M, Hagenmüller F, Fleischer D, editors. Atlas of video capsule endoscopy. Wurzburg: Springer; 2006. p. 24–9.

45. Fritscher-Raven A, Scherbakov P, Bufler P, et al. The feasibility of capsule endoscopy in detecting small intestinal pathology in children under age 8 years: a multicentre European study. Gut. 2009;58:1467–72.

46. Oikawa-Kawamoto M, Sogo T, Yamaguchi T, Tsunoda T, Kondo T, Komatsu H, et al. Safety and utility of capsule endoscopy for infants and young children. World J Gastroenterol. 2013;19:8342–8.

47. Hosoe N. Makoto Naganuma, Haruhiko Ogata. 2015. Current status of capsule endoscopy through a whole digestive tract. Dig Endosc. 2015;27:205–15.

48. Oliva S, Nardo GD, Cucchiara S, Gualdi G, Casciani E, Cohen SA. Capsule endoscopy in pediatrics: a 10-years journey. World J Gastroenterol. 2014;20:16603–8.

49. Oliva S, Cucchiara S, Civitelli F, Casciani E, Di Nardo G, Hassan C, et al. Colon capsule endoscopy compared with other modalities in the evaluation of pediatric Crohn's disease of the small bowel and colon. Gastrointest Endosc. 2016;83:975–83.

50. Hijaz NM, Septer SS, Attard TM. Present standard in pediatric gastroenterology fellowship training in the interpretation of capsule endoscopy. J Pediatr Gastroenterol Nutr. 2015;61:421–3.

Bone Health in Pediatric Inflammatory Bowel Disease

24

Dale Lee and Edisio Semeao

Introduction

Throughout childhood and adolescence, bone mineral accrual results in ethnic-, gender-, maturation-, and site-specific increases in bone dimensions and density. During the critical 2-year interval surrounding the time of peak height velocity, approximately 25% of skeletal mass is laid down and 90% of peak bone mass is established by 18 years of age [1]. This rapid accumulation of bone mass correlates with the rate of growth and requires the coordinated actions of growth hormone, insulin-like growth factor-I (IGF-I) and sex steroids in the setting of adequate biomechanical loading and nutrition. Individuals with higher peak bone mass in early adulthood have a protective advantage against fracture when the inexorable decline in bone mass associated with older age or menopause occurs. Accordingly, the National Institutes of Health (NIH) Consensus Statement on Osteoporosis Prevention, Diagnosis and Therapy concluded "bone mass attained early in life is perhaps the most important determinant of life-long skeletal health" [2]. Furthermore, the Consensus Statement specifically called for research to determine the impact of chronic diseases and glucocorticoid therapy on bone accrual in children and to determine the effects of bisphosphonates on the growing skeleton.

Children and adolescents with inflammatory bowel disease (IBD) have multiple risk factors for impaired bone development, including poor growth, delayed maturation, malnutrition, decreased weight-bearing activity, chronic inflammation, genetic susceptibility, and immunosuppressive therapies, such as glucocorticoids. The impact of these threats to bone health may be immediate, resulting in fragility fractures during childhood and adolescence [3–5], or delayed, due to suboptimal peak bone mass accrual [6]. Recent years have seen numerous studies on the effects of IBD on bone accrual during childhood and adolescence. Although the short- and long-term implications for fracture risk in pediatric IBD have not been characterized prospectively, a recent retrospective database study found that prepubertal children with IBD had an increased risk of fracture compared with controls [7].

This chapter summarizes the normal changes in bone density and structure during growth, as well as the risk factors for poor bone accrual in childhood IBD. The classification of bone health in children and adolescents is discussed, as are the advantages and disadvantages of available technologies for the assessment of bone in children and adolescents. The difficulties in assessing and interpreting bone measures in pediatric IBD are underscored in a review of selected studies, and an example is provided for a stepwise approach to identify discrete determinants of bone deficits in pediatric IBD [8]. Finally, potential therapies are described and discussed.

Skeletal Modeling and Bone Accrual During Childhood

Skeletal development is a complex process that is sensitive to the hormonal, mechanical, cytokine, and nutritional milieu of the bone. The bones are continuously modified and renovated by the two processes of modeling and remodeling: both result in the replacement of old bone with new bone. Remodeling is the major process in adults and does not result in a change of the bone shape. Remodeling takes place in the basic bone multicellular units on the trabecular surface and within the cortical bone. Normally, bone resorption by osteoclasts is followed by bone formation by osteoblasts; teams of

D. Lee, MD, MSCE (✉)
Department of Pediatrics, Seattle Children's Hospital, University of Washington, 4800 Sand Point Way NE, Seattle, WA 98105, USA
e-mail: dale.lee@seattlechildrens.org

E. Semeao, MD
Department of Pediatrics, The Children's Hospital of Philadelphia, University of Pennsylvania School of Medicine, 34th St and Civic Center Blvd, Philadelphia, PA 19104, USA

© Springer International Publishing AG 2017
P. Mamula et al. (eds.), *Pediatric Inflammatory Bowel Disease*, DOI 10.1007/978-3-319-49215-5_24

osteoclasts and osteoblasts are juxtaposed in the bone multi-cellular units and bone resorption and formation are tightly coupled. For example, treatment of postmenopausal women with bisphosphonates (an antiresorptive agent) resulted in significant reductions in bone resorption within 6 weeks, followed by a reduction in bone formation in 3 months [9, 10]. Skeletal remodeling is vital to microdamage repair. However, after mid-adulthood, the amount of resorption exceeds formation, resulting in a negative bone balance.

In contrast, modeling during growth and development results in new bone formed at a location different from the site of bone resorption; formation and resorption are not coupled within a bone multicellular unit. For example, a small study of bisphosphonate therapy in children reported significant reductions in bone resorption markers with no changes in formation markers [11]. Modeling results in an increase in bone diameter and modification of bone shape. Figure 24.1 summarizes the complex interplay of site-specific bone resorption and formation activities that are necessary to achieve bone growth from length A to B [12]. Growth in the diameter of the cortical shaft is the result of bone formation at the outer (periosteal) surface and bone resorption at the inner (endosteal) surface. Simultaneously, the growth plate moves upward and the wider metaphysis is reshaped into a diaphysis by continuous resorption by osteoclasts beneath the periosteum.

Changes in Cortical and Trabecular Bone with Growth

Cortical and trabecular bone do not respond in the same way to diseases, medications, or mechanical loading and should be considered two functional entities. Cortical bone forms the outer shell of most bones, while trabecular bone is more porous and filled with marrow and blood vessels. Trabecular volumetric bone mineral density (BMD), as measured by three-dimensional quantitative computed tomography (QCT), does not increase before puberty [13, 14]. During puberty trabecular BMD increases significantly in healthy children due to increases in trabecular thickness. The increase in BMD is comparable in girls and boys [15], but the increase is significantly greater in black adolescents than in white adolescents [16].

Sex differences in cortical dimensions are established during puberty (Fig. 24.2): [17] cortical width increases by periosteal bone formation in boys and by less periosteal bone formation but more endocortical apposition in girls. Androgens stimulate periosteal apposition, while estrogens inhibit periosteal apposition and stimulate endosteal apposition. These sex differences have important implications for

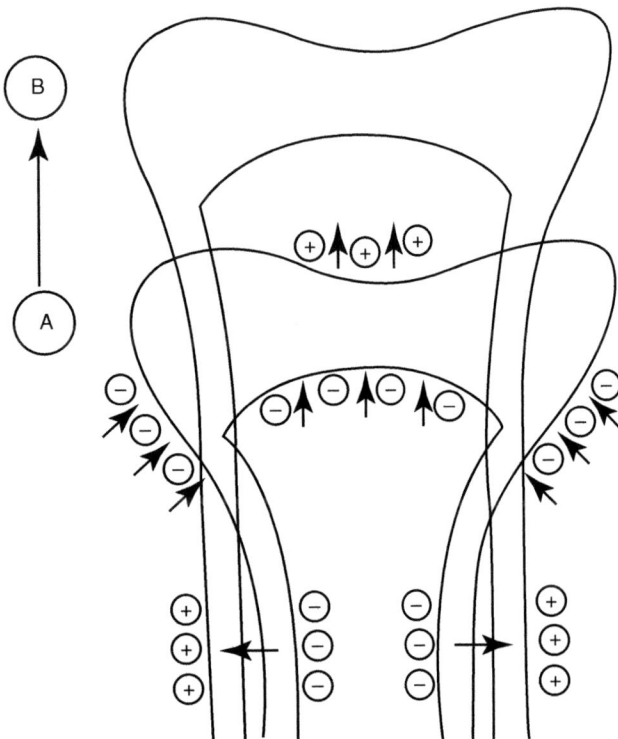

Fig. 24.1 Bone formation (+) and resorption (−) during growth (From: Baron [12])

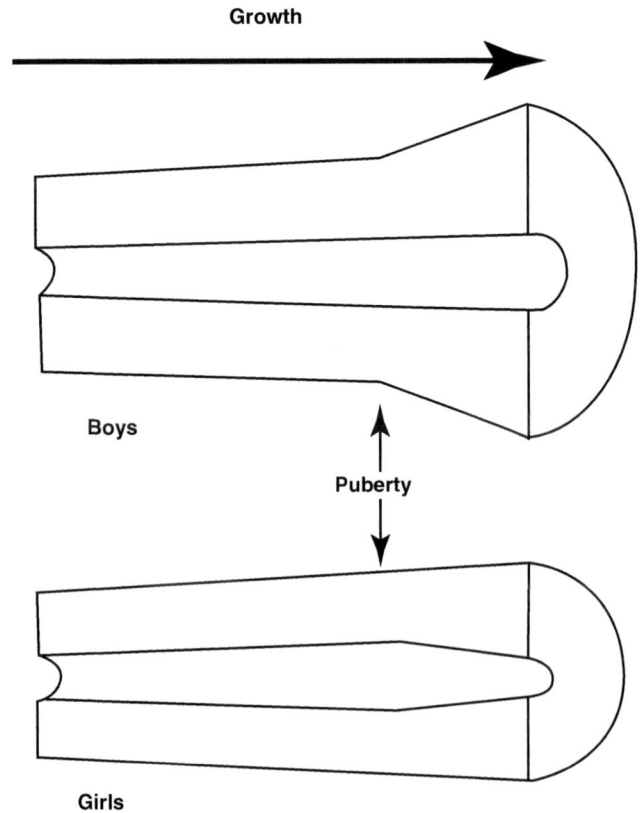

Fig. 24.2 Sex specific increases in cortical bone dimensions during growth and maturation (Adapted from: Seeman [17])

bone strength; the greater periosteal radius (R_p) in males results in greater bone strength. The long bones are tubular structures that are loaded mainly in bending. The resistance of long bones to bending (i.e. bone strength) is represented by the cross-sectional moment of inertia (CSMI) = $\pi/4$ (R_p^4 − R_e^4); R_p and R_e indicate the periosteal and endosteal radius, respectively [18]. These power relationships indicate that small increases in R_p result in marked increases in bone bending strength.

Because the patterns of modeling on the periosteal and endocortical envelopes during growth produce changes in cortical geometry that impact life-long fracture risk [19, 20], the long-term effects of chronic childhood diseases, such as IBD, likely depend on the stage of skeletal maturation at disease onset and the disease effects on the periosteal and endosteal surfaces. Children further from peak bone mass at Crohn disease onset may have irreversible deficits not seen in adult-onset Crohn disease.

Biochemical Markers of Bone Metabolism

Biochemical markers of bone metabolism are released into the circulation during the process of bone formation and resorption, providing information about the dynamic process of bone metabolism. Biomarkers of formation, such as bone-specific alkaline phosphatase (BSAP) and osteocalcin, are by-products of osteoblast activity. Biomarkers of bone resorption are related to collagen degradation products, including pyridinium cross-links and C-telopeptide of collagen cross-links (β-CTX) [21]. In adults, biochemical markers of bone turnover correlate well with formation and resorption, as measured by bone biopsy, and are independent predictors of fracture risk [22]. Further, bone biomarkers can be used to monitor the effectiveness of bone therapies [9]. Because formation and resorption are tightly coupled in adults, drugs that increase bone formation (e.g., teriparatide, which is a synthetic form of parathyroid hormone) increase markers of formation and resorption, while drugs that inhibit resorption (e.g., bisphosphonates) decrease markers of formation and resorption [23].

In adults, bone metabolism is primarily due to remodeling. However, in children biomarkers of bone metabolism in children represent the aggregate turnover due to (1) endochondral bone formation (longitudinal growth of bone), (2) increase in bone circumference, and (3) bone remodeling [24]. The pubertal growth spurt is reflected by marked increases in bone biomarkers [25]. Therefore, the use of bone biomarkers in children and adolescents requires consideration of gender, pubertal maturation, and growth velocity [25] and is most appropriately limited to short-term longitudinal studies to assess the impact of specific interventions [24].

Potential Threats to Bone Health in Pediatric IBD

Osteopenia has been well documented in children and adults with IBD [26–30]. Vertebral compression fractures have been reported in children with IBD [3–5], and hip, spine, and forearm fracture rates are significantly increased in adults with Crohn disease [31–36]. Kappelman et al. found that children with IBD <12 years of age had an increased risk of fracture (odds ratio [OR] 2.2, 95% confidence interval [CI] 1.2–3.8) and children with Crohn disease (CD) had a trend toward an increased risk of vertebral compression fracture, both compared with controls [7]. The osteopenia in IBD is multifactorial; likely etiologies include growth failure, delayed maturation, anorexia, malabsorption, cytokine effects on bone cells, and glucocorticoid therapies.

Malnutrition

Children with IBD are at risk for inadequate intake of calories as well as micronutrients including calcium, vitamin D, and zinc secondary to anorexia due to upper tract inflammation, malabsorption, increased metabolic demands, lactose intolerance, abdominal pain, or depression. Even in the setting of adequate caloric intake, malabsorption can cause deficiency states of the above micronutrients depending on location and severity of disease. Diarrhea can result in zinc deficiency, which has the potential to impact growth. Vitamin D deficiency may result from malabsorption as well as decreased exposure to sunlight due to disease flares. Vitamin K deficiency may result from malabsorption and altered bowel flora due to antibiotic use and IBD-associated dysbiosis, which may result in increased concentrations of under-carboxylated osteocalcin, which is associated with decreased bone turnover and fractures [37]. Nutrients that may contribute to impaired bone acquisition in pediatric IBD include calcium, vitamin D, vitamin K, and magnesium [38].

Multiple studies have reported that vitamin D deficiency frequently complicates pediatric IBD [39–42]. For example, Pappa et al. examined vitamin D levels in 130 children and young adults with IBD, 94 with Crohn disease, and 36 with ulcerative colitis. The prevalence of vitamin D deficiency (serum 25 (OH) vitamin D concentration ≤ 15 ng/mL) was 34.6%, and the mean serum 25 (OH) vitamin D concentration was similar in patients with Crohn disease and ulcerative colitis, 52.6% lower among patients with dark skin complexion, 33.4% lower during the winter months (December 22 to March 21), and 31.5% higher among patients who were taking vitamin D supplements. Patients with Crohn disease and upper gastrointestinal tract involvement were more likely to be vitamin D deficient than those without it. A similar study reported that 45% of children with IBD had vitamin D levels less than 20 ng/mL [39]. Of note, none of these studies detected a relation between vitamin D levels and spine BMD, as measured by dual energy x-ray absorptiometry (DXA) [39–41]. A recent study by Augustine et al. demonstrated an association between greater inflammatory burden and lower serum 1, 25 (OH) vitamin D concentration and higher PTH levels associated with higher 1, 25 (OH) vitamin D concentrations [43]. The authors suggest that inflammation may lower PTH and thereby decrease renal conversion of 25 (OH) vitamin D to 1,25 (OH) vitamin D.

Decreased Muscle Mass and Biomechanical Loading of the Skeleton

Bone adapts its strength in response to the magnitude and direction of the forces to which it is subjected. Mechanical forces on the skeleton arise primarily from muscle contraction. This capacity of bone to respond to mechanical loading with increased bone size and strength is greatest during growth, especially during adolescence [44]. Numerous studies have documented the beneficial effect of physical activity and biomechanical loading on bone geometry in healthy children [45–50]. These relationships dictate that studies of bone health in chronic childhood diseases consider the effects of alterations in muscle mass and strength.

Weight-bearing physical activity and biomechanical loading of bone are critical determinants of bone mass in growing normal children [51]. The influence of skeletal loading on bone accretion is illustrated in two exercise trials in healthy children. An easily implemented school-based jumping intervention augmented cortical thickness in the femoral neck of healthy children [52]. A randomized clinical trial of physical activity and calcium supplementation in prepubertal children resulted in a significant, positive interaction between calcium supplements and physical activity in both cortical thickness and cortical area [53]. Harpavat et al. reported that none of the subjects in a small series of children with IBD were participating in weight-bearing physical activities [54]. Werkstetter et al. compared 39 children with quiescent or mild IBD to 39 healthy controls and found decreased physical activity and lean mass in the children with IBD despite no differences in the measurements in quality of life or energy intake [55]. We recently reported that in children with incident Crohn disease, both muscle cross-sectional area and muscle strength are independently associated with cortical section modulus, a summary measure of cortical bone dimension and strength [56]. The reports of decreased lean mass and muscle strength in pediatric IBD suggest that decreased biomechanical loading of the skeleton may contribute to impaired bone accrual in this disorder, but additional studies are needed.

The relations between bone and muscle mass have been demonstrated in multiple studies in children and adolescents with Crohn disease. Burnham et al. reported that Crohn disease was associated with a 0.50 SD deficit ($p = 0.006$ compared with controls) in whole-body bone mineral content (BMC) relative to height in males, adjusted for age, race, and Tanner stage [8]. Adjustment for whole body lean mass attenuated this deficit to 0.19 SD ($p = 0.13$ compared with controls). The authors noted that the absence of a bone deficit after statistical adjustment for lean mass does not imply that the bones are normal or adequate. In a similar study, deficits in DXA estimates of femoral neck subperiosteal width were not statistically significant after adjustment for lean mass [57]. Our study of children with newly diagnosed Crohn disease found that cortical section modulus was 6.8% greater than predicted compared to healthy controls, given muscle cross-sectional area and strength deficits [56]. A prospective cohort study using tibia peripheral QCT in children with newly diagnosed Crohn disease reported that muscle mass improved significantly over 1 year following diagnosis, but cortical section modulus worsened significantly [58]. This apparent disconnect between changes in bone and muscle mass over time illustrates the limitations of the functional muscle bone unit paradigm in chronic inflammatory disease. In addition to lean mass and muscle strength, the role of inflammatory cytokines, physical activity, and therapeutic agents on bone outcomes must be further studied.

Glucocorticoid-Induced Osteopenia

Glucocorticoids are widely used in the treatment of IBD and impact bone formation and resorption. Decreased bone formation is the primary mechanism for bone loss in glucocorticoid-induced osteopenia [59]. Mesenchymal stems cells, which also give rise to adipocytes, myoblasts and chondrocytes, differentiate into osteoblasts. Glucocorticoids shift the cellular differentiation away from osteoblasts and towards adipocytes, and prevent the termination differentiation of osteoblasts [60]. Osteoblast numbers are decreased further by glucocorticoid-induced increases in osteoblast apoptosis [61]. In addition, glucocorticoids inhibit osteoblast production of bone matrix components [62]. Finally, glucocorticoids suppress the synthesis of insulin-like growth factor-I (IGF-1), a hormone important in bone formation [63]. The cellular response to glucocorticoids also includes an early phase of increased bone resorption, probably a result of the increased expression of receptor activator of nuclear factor-κ-B ligand (RANKL) and decreased osteoprotegerin (OPG) – increased RANKL and decreased OPG both promote osteoclastogenesis, as detailed below [64]. However, typically a more chronic state of decreased bone resorption develops due to loss of cell signaling to osteoclast progenitors and apoptosis [65].

Patients treated with glucocorticoids have an underlying disease, which frequently also carries a risk of osteoporosis. Therefore, the independent effects of glucocorticoids on bone turnover and bone structure during growth are not readily apparent from clinical studies. However, recent animal models demonstrate that glucocorticoid administration during growth resulted in decreased bone formation, decreased bone resorption, reductions in the age dependent increases in trabecular thickness, and reductions in linear growth and accrual of cortical thickness in the femur [66, 67]. These deficits were associated with decreased bone strength in the vertebrae and femur in mechanical testing [66, 67]. Of note, it is unclear if the reductions in femoral cortical thickness were proportionate to the significant reductions in bone length. That is, did the bones have normal cortical thickness and strength relative to the shorter length?

Inflammation and Bone Loss

Cellular inflammatory pathways in Crohn disease activate the protean transcriptional regulatory factor nuclear factor-κB with increased production of a variety of cytokines, such as interleukin-6 (IL-6) and tumor necrosis factor-α (TNF-α) [68]. Three groups of cytokines are particularly important in bone physiology: interleukin-6 (IL-6), TNF-α, and IL-1 [64]. Inflammatory cytokines promote osteoclastogenesis and accelerated bone resorption. TNF-α induces the expression of receptor activator of NF-κB ligand (RANKL). RANKL stimulates osteoclast differentiation and activation and inhibits osteoclast apoptosis, thereby dramatically prolonging osteoclast survival and increasing bone resorption [69, 70]. Additionally, TNF-α decreases expression of osteoprotegerin (OPG), a decoy receptor that blocks RANKL [71, 72]. Inflammatory mediators, including IL-1 and IL-6, also increase RANKL secretion and contribute to bone loss [73]. TNF-α also has direct effects on bone formation; it inhibits osteoblast differentiation, inhibits osteoblast collagen secretion, causes increased resorption by inducing osteoblasts secretion of IL-6, and induces osteoblast apoptosis [74, 75]. These effects on bone formation are strikingly similar to the effects of glucocorticoids [59, 60].

Assessment of Bone Status in Children and Adolescents

Classification of Bone Health and Relation to Fracture Risk

DXA is widely accepted as a quantitative measurement technique for assessing skeletal status. DXA scans involve the use of two x-ray beams and measurement of x-ray penetration through bone. The radiation exposure from a conventional DXA examination is less than 10 microsieverts (μSv), while a two-view chest x-ray would be 60 μSv, and a CT exam of the pelvis 5000 μSv [76]. In elderly adults, DXA BMD is a sufficiently robust predictor of osteoporotic fractures that it can be used to define the disease. The World Health Organization criteria for the diagnosis of osteoporosis in adults is based on a T-score, the comparison of a measured BMD result with the average BMD of young adults at the time of peak bone mass [77]. A T-score ≤−2.5 SD below the mean peak bone mass is used for the diagnosis of osteoporosis, and a T-score ≤ −2.5 SD with a history of a low-impact fracture is classified as severe osteoporosis. While the T-score is a standard component of DXA BMD results, it is clearly inappropriate to assess skeletal health in children through comparison with peak adult bone mass. Rather, children are assessed relative to age or body size, expressed as a Z-score. In adults, low impact fractures are defined as fractures that occur after a fall from standing height or less. This definition is often difficult to apply to fractures in children that occur during play or sports activities.

While there are no clear evidence-based guidelines for the definition of osteoporosis in children. The International Society for Clinical Densitometry has suggested that the diagnosis of osteoporosis in children and adolescents should include a history of clinically significant fracture and bone mineral content or density Z-score ≤ 2.0 (adjusted for age, sex, and bone size) [78]. Fractures occur commonly in otherwise healthy children with a peak incidence during early adolescence around the time of the pubertal growth spurt [21]. Faulkner et al. recently reported that peak gains in bone area preceded peak gains in BMC in a longitudinal sample of boys and girls, supporting the theory that the dissociation between skeletal expansion and skeletal mineralization results in a period of relative bone weakness [79]. This may be due to increased calcium demands during maximal skeletal growth.

Several studies have compared the DXA BMD of normal children and adolescents with forearm fractures to that of age-matched controls without fractures. Most [80–84], but not all [85, 86] found that mean DXA BMD was significantly lower in children with forearm fractures than in controls. One study reported that 69% of fractures in healthy children were due to low-energy falls at home [85]; illustrating the difficulties defining low-energy fractures in children. Studies using QCT or metacarpal morphometry to characterize cortical geometry showed that decreased cortical thickness was associated with significantly increased fracture risk [84, 87]. Finally, television, computer, and video viewing had a dose-dependent association with wrist and forearm fractures [88]. A recent prospective cohort study in over 6200 children in the United Kingdom reported a weak inverse relationship between whole body (less head) BMD at 9.9 years of age and subsequent fracture risk [odds ratio (OR) per SD decrease = 1.12; 95% CI, 1.02–1.25] [89]. The association between fracture risk and BMD was much stronger when adjusted for bone and body size; fracture risk was inversely related to BMC adjusted for bone area, height, and weight (OR = 1.89; 95% CI, 1.18–3.04).

These data suggest that low DXA BMD can be a contributing factor for pediatric fracture in healthy children; however, bone geometry and nonskeletal factors such as sports participation, body size, and sedentary activities may have an independent contribution to fracture risk. Importantly, the relationships between DXA BMD, bone geometry, and fracture risk in children with chronic diseases, such as IBD, may be different than those observed in healthy children.

Limitations of DXA in Children and Adolescents

DXA is, by far, the most commonly employed method for the assessment of bone health in children. However, DXA has several limitations that are pronounced in the assessment of children (Table 24.1). A study highlighting the importance of these limitations evaluated children referred for enrollment in a childhood osteoporosis protocol based on low DXA spine BMD and found 80% had at least one error in interpretation of the DXA scan [112]. The most common error was the use of T-scores, and ultimately, only 26% retained the diagnosis of low BMD.

The significant limitation of DXA is the reliance on measurement of areal rather than volumetric BMD. DXA provides an estimate of bone mineral density expressed as grams per anatomical region (e.g., individual vertebrae, whole body, or hip). Dividing the BMC within the defined anatomical region (g) by the projected area of the bone (cm^2) then derives "areal-BMD" (g/cm^2). This BMD is not a measure of volumetric density (g/cm^3) because it provides no information about the depth of bone. Bones of larger width and height also tend to be thicker. Since bone thickness is not factored into DXA estimates of BMD, reliance on areal-BMD inherently underestimates the bone density in individuals with short stature. Despite identical volumetric bone density, the child with smaller bones appears to have a mineralization disorder (decreased areal-BMD). This is clearly an important artifact in children with chronic diseases, such as IBD, that are associated with growth delay and short stature [113]. An analysis by Zemel et al. found that adjustment of age-specific BMC and BMD z-scores for age-specific height Z-scores were the least biased methods to correct for the confounding effect of height [114].

The confounding effect of skeletal geometry on DXA measures is now well recognized and multiple analytic strategies have been proposed to express DXA bone mass in a form that is less sensitive to differences in skeletal size [95, 96, 115–117]. The technique developed by Carter et al. is based on the observation that vertebral BMC scaled proportionate to the projected bone area to the 1.5 power [115]. Therefore, vertebral volume is estimated as (area)$^{1.5}$ and bone mineral apparent density (BMAD) is defined as BMC/(area)$^{1.5}$. Kroger et al. proposed an alternative estimate of vertebral volume: the lumbar body is assumed to have a cylindrical shape and volume of the cylinder is calculated as $(\pi)(\text{radius}^2)(\text{height})$, which is equivalent to $(\pi)((\text{width}/2)^2)(\text{area}/\text{width})$ [118, 119]. This approach was validated by comparison with MR measures of vertebral dimensions in 32 adults [116]; DXA-derived volumetric BMD correlated moderately well with BMD based on MR-derived estimates of vertebral volume ($R = 0.665$). Although these methods provide estimates of vertebral volume, the BMC includes the bone content of the superimposed cortical spinous processes.

A study by Wren et al. sought to evaluate the usefulness of DXA spine correction factors based on published geometric formula and anthropometric parameters, compared with three-dimensional QCT [120]. Subject height, weight, body mass index, skeletal age, and Tanner stage were assessed in 84 healthy children. While DXA and QCT measures of BMC

Table 24.1 Limitations of DXA techniques in infants and children

Scan acquisition	Fan beam results in magnification error with apparent differences in bone area and BMC as body size varies [90]
Scan analysis	Difficult to define landmarks and region of interest in the immature hip [91]
	Software developed to improve bone detection in the infant and child result in significantly different results for BMC and body composition [92–94]
Reference data [95–108]	Limited data in young children
	Analysis methods not standardized
	Variable hardware and software across published reference data sets
	Some are not gender-specific [109] Some presented relative to age, others relative to height, Tanner stage, and weight
Interpretation	Underestimates volumetric density in children with short stature [110, 111]
	Unable to distinguish between changes in bone dimensions and density
	Unable to distinguish between cortical and trabecular bone

were highly correlated ($r^2 = 0.94$), DXA areal BMD only moderately correlated with CT volumetric BMD ($r^2 = 0.39$), illustrating the potential confounding effects of bone size on DXA areal BMD. The correlations between QCT volumetric BMD and DXA estimates were particularly poor for subjects in Tanner stages 1–3 ($r^2 = 0.02$ for areal BMD), but multiple regression accounting for the anthropometric and developmental parameters greatly improved the agreement between the DXA and CT densities ($r^2 = 0.91$). These results suggest that DXA BMC is a more accurate and reliable measure than DXA BMD for assessing bone acquisition, particularly for prepubertal children and those in the early stages of sexual development. Use of DXA BMD would be reasonable if adjustments for body size, pubertal status, and skeletal maturity are made, but these additional assessments add significant complexity to research studies, and to clinical interpretation.

An additional shortcoming of DXA is that the integrated measure of bone mass in a given projected area does not allow distinction between cortical and trabecular bone. DXA-based measures provide no information on bone architecture and are limited in their usefulness to differentiate the spectrum of bone accrual during growth.

Comparisons to appropriate pediatric reference data are essential to describe accurately the clinical impact of childhood disease on bone development, to monitor changes in bone mineralization, and to identify patients for treatment protocols. Multiple sources of pediatric DXA reference data are now available for the calculation of DXA z-scores. These include varied approaches, such as gender-specific centile curves, age- and height- specific means and standard deviations, Tanner- and weight-specific percentiles, age-, sex-, weight- and height- adjusted curves, and Z-score prediction models [95–108]. Differences in reference data have a significant impact on the diagnosis of osteopenia in children with chronic disease [109]. For example, the use of reference data that are not gender-specific results in significantly greater misclassification of males as osteopenia [109]. In addition, the use of published pediatric reference ranges has been complicated by differences in scanner manufacturers, and frequent changes in hardware and software technology, including fan-beam technology, low-density software analysis modes and specialized pediatric software. These technical changes result in clinically significant alterations in DXA results [92]. The use of adequate reference data and validated classification schemes is important in the study of bone health in children.

Peripheral Quantitative Computed Tomography

A three-dimensional structural analysis of trabecular architecture and cortical bone dimensions can be obtained by computed tomography (CT). This technique offers an oppor-

tunity to overcome the limitations of two-dimensional imaging with DXA and advance our understanding of bone mineralization in children. CT provides an image unobscured by overlying structures [121]. The CT attenuation of different bone tissues provides quantitative information, referred to as quantitative CT (QCT). In contrast to DXA, this technique describes authentic volumetric BMD (vBMD), accurately measures bone dimensions, and distinguishes between cortical and trabecular bone. In order to minimize radiation exposure, special high-resolution scanners were developed for the peripheral skeleton (pQCT), specifically, the radius or tibia. The distal site is largely trabecular bone, while the midshaft is almost entirely cortical bone. The volume of each component is calculated from the scan thickness and cross-sectional area, and the density by attenuation of the x-ray beam. Bone strength can also be estimated by pQCT from the total bone area, and cortical thickness and density [122]. QCT studies of bone mineral accretion and bone strength demonstrated gender, maturation, and ethnic-specific patterns of development of bone strength during childhood and adolescence [123]. A study longitudinal in children with Crohn disease comparing QCT measured vBMD versus DXA-derived measures of BMD demonstrated greater BMD deficits at diagnosis and greater improvements over 12 months with the PQCT vBMD approach [124].

Clinical Studies of Bone Health in Pediatric IBD

Accounting for Body Size Differences

Numerous studies have reported decreased DXA BMD in children with IBD [39]. However, as detailed above, DXA studies are frequently confounded by disease effects of growth. For example, two studies reported that DXA BMD for age Z-scores were significantly correlated with height for age Z-scores in children with IBD [39, 125]. Furthermore, expression of DXA results as BMAD (an estimate of volumetric BMD) eliminated the correlation with height Z-scores [125]. Another study addressed the confounding effect of short stature by expressing the spine DXA results as percent predicted BMC for bone area for age and gender in 73 children with Crohn disease or ulcerative colitis [126]. The percent predicted bone area for age and gender was decreased in IBD, compared with controls, consistent with shorter stature. While the median BMD for age and gender Z-score was significantly decreased in IBD (mean Z-score in spine $= -1.6$, in whole body $= -0.9$), the percent predicated BMC for bone area, age, and gender was normal. The authors concluded that children with IBD have small bones for age due to growth retardation, but adequate bone mass relative to bone size. Finally, Herzog et al. reported that BMD Z-scores were less than −2.0 in 44% of children when expressed relative to chronologic age, but were less than −2.0 in only 26–30% when expressed relative to bone age of height age [127].

The above studies illustrate the varied approached used to adjust for the confounding effects of poor growth. Leonard et al. reported that whole body BMC relative to height predicted bone strength (estimate by stress-strain index) as measured by QCT [117]. From the same group, Burnham et al. assessed whole body BMC, lean mass and fat mass (as measured by DXA) relative to height in 104 children and young adults with established Crohn disease, and 233 healthy controls, 4–26 years of age. The studies demonstrated significant bone and muscle deficits [8, 128]. Individuals with Crohn disease had significantly lower height-for-age, body mass index (BMI)-for-age, and whole body lean mass-for-height Z-scores than healthy controls (all $p < 0.001$). Table 24.2 summarizes four sequential models in males and females. The least adjusted models assessed whole body BMC in Crohn disease, compared with controls, adjusted for age and race, and revealed substantial deficits. Assessment of BMC without consideration of the decreased skeletal size for age in subjects with Crohn disease group may overestimate bone deficits. Accordingly, the second model was also adjusted for height. Figure 24.3 demonstrates that the marked BMC deficits relative to age (A) are less pronounced when assessed relative to height (B). Adjustment for height attenuated the Crohn disease effect in the multivariate regression model; however, significant BMC deficits persisted in males and females with Crohn disease, compared with controls. In the third model in Table 24.2 Tanner stage was added to determine if delayed pubertal maturation for age contributed to the decreased BMC in Crohn disease. Adjustment for delayed pubertal maturation did not appreciably change the estimate of BMC deficits in Crohn disease. The fourth and final model, adjusted for lean mass, eliminated significant BMC deficits in Crohn disease.

None of the glucocorticoid measures were significantly correlated with BMC-for-height Z-scores. However, height Z-score was negatively and significantly associated with duration of glucocorticoid therapy ($r = −0.24$, $p = 0.02$), and cumulative (mg/kg) glucocorticoids ($r = −0.36$, $p < 0.001$). Parenteral nutrition, isolated upper tract disease, hypoalbu-minemia, nasogastric feeding, and decreased BMI Z-scores were associated with decreased BMC-for-height Z-scores, but these factors have the potential to be confounded by greater disease severity. Whereas BMC and BMD Z-scores for age may overestimate bone deficits, bone Z-scores for height have the potential to underestimate bone deficits. This can occur because children and adolescents with IBD may be of more advanced pubertal status than their comparators of similar height. As such, adjusting age-specific BMD or BMC z-scores for age-specific height Z-scores may be a more accurate approach [114].

Glucocorticoid Effect

Over 90% of the children and young adults in the prior study had a history of glucocorticoid exposure; therefore, it was not possible to distinguish between disease and glucocorticoid effects on bone. The impact of the underlying IBD process is best assessed in subjects with newly-diagnosed disease. The largest study of DXA BMD in newly diagnosed subjects was reported by Gupta et al. [129]; however, the study was complicated by the observation that BMD was markedly decreased in controls, compared with the DXA reference database. Overall, DXA spine BMD was comparable in the 41 children with ulcerative colitis and the controls, while results were significantly lower in the 82 subjects with Crohn disease. Laakso et al. reported on a longitudinal study of children and adolescents followed over a median of over 5 years and found greater lifetime glucocorticoid exposure to be associated with lower lumbar spine BMD [130]. The authors conclude that the findings may likely reflect both glucocorticoid effect and glucocorticoid exposure as a surrogate of more severe disease. In steroid-sensitive nephrotic syndrome, a condition without underlying inflammation but involving glucocorticoid therapy, no deficits in bone mineral content are seen, but this may be related to the increase in skeletal loading associated with increases in BMI [131]. This demonstrates the complex interaction between medication exposures, side effects of therapy, and underlying disease pathophysiology.

Table 24.2 Hierarchical models of whole body BMC Z-scores in Crohn disease [8]

Models	Males		Females	
	Z (95% CI)	p	Z (95% CI)	p
1. Age, race	−1.16 (−1.51, −0.82)	< 0.001	−0.61 (−0.95, −0.27)	0.001
2. Height, age, race	−0.63 (−0.95, −0.30)	< 0.001	−0.44 (−0.81, −0.06)	0.02
3. Height, age, race, tanner	−0.50 (−0.85, −0.15)	0.006	−0.35 (−0.72, 0.02)	0.06
4. Height, age, race, tanner, lean mass	−0.19 (−0.43, 0.06)	0.13	−0.05 (−0.34, 0.25)	> 0.2

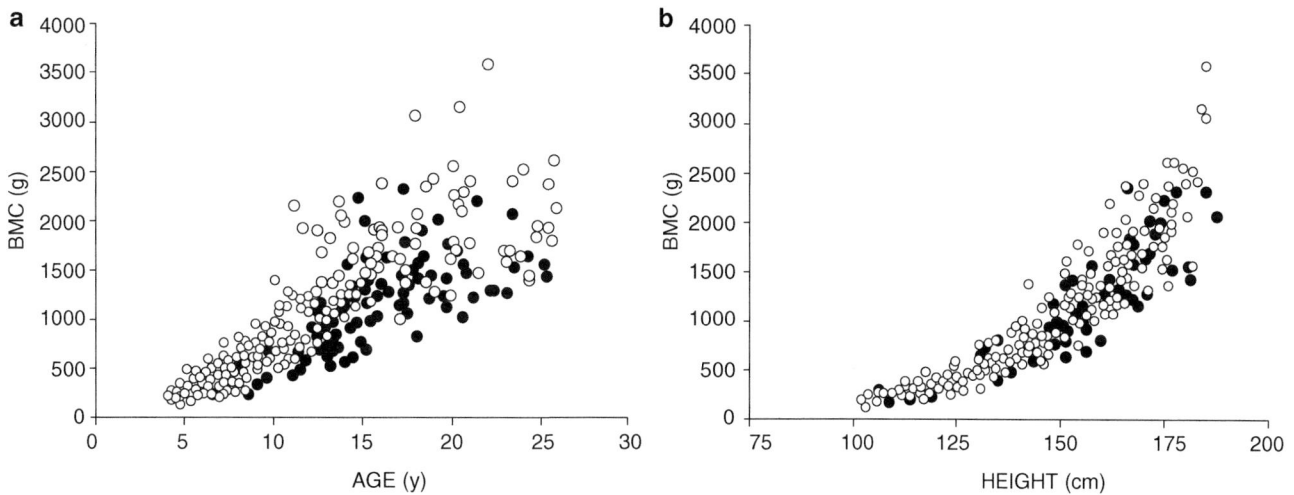

Fig. 24.3 Distribution of whole body BMC relative to age (**a**) and relative to height (**b**) in children and young adults with Crohn disease, compared with healthy controls (From Burnham et al. [8])

Impact of Disease Activity

Walther et al. recently compared lumbar spine BMAD Z-scores in 34 steroid-naïve and 53 steroid-treated children with IBD in order to obtain information about the influence of non-steroidal factors [125]. Overall, 56 had Crohn disease and 30 had ulcerative colitis. Reference data were obtained in 52 controls. The mean BMAD Z-scores in the subjects with Crohn disease were -0.76 ± 1.25 in females and -0.79 ± 0.92 in males. The mean BMAD Z-scores in the subjects with ulcerative colitis were -0.30 ± 0.75 in females and -1.08 ± 1.23 in males. Among the steroid-naïve subjects, the duration of treatment ranged from 0 to 8 years, but the majority (approximately 80%) were within the first 5 weeks of therapy. Among the steroid treated subjects, the cumulative steroid exposure averaged 4600 mg (range 0.05–25,000 mg) over the treatment duration of several days to 7.6 years. The mean BMAD Z-scores were comparable in steroid-naïve (-0.74 ± 1.08) and steroid-treated (-0.66 ± 1.08) subjects. The 19 subjects that had been treated with calcium and/or vitamin D supplements were all within the steroid-treated group. The study is limited by the small number of controls and the lack of data on disease activity between the steroid-naïve and steroid-treated groups. Nonetheless, these data demonstrate bone deficits in the absence of steroid therapy. The studies listed above were all based on DXA estimates of BMC and BMD and did not distinguish between cortical and trabecular bone.

Sylvester examined DXA BMD and bone biomarkers in 23 children with newly diagnosed Crohn disease [132]. Although BMD Z-scores did not differ between Crohn disease subjects and controls in this small sample, bone biomarkers were significantly lower in Crohn disease. This may be due to reduced bone remodeling, or reduced growth velocity. Importantly, activated T cells produced greater concentrations of interferon-γ, which may contribute to lower bone turnover.

Longitudinal Studies

Dubner et al. performed tibia pQCT in 78 CD subjects (ages 5–18 year) at diagnosis and followed them for 12 months [58]. At diagnosis, CD subjects had significant deficits in trabecular vBMD (Z-score: -1.32 ± 1.32, $p < 0.001$), section modulus (a summary measure of cortical bone dimensions and strength) (-0.44 ± 1.11, $p < 0.01$), and muscle cross-sectional area (-0.96 ± 1.02, $p < 0.001$), compared with controls. Over the first 6 months, trabecular vBMD and muscle Z-scores improved significantly (both $p < 0.001$); however, section modulus worsened ($p = 0.0001$) and all three parameters remained low after 1 year. Improvements in muscle were associated with improvements in section modulus and improvements in trabecular vBMD were greater in prepubertal subjects. Werkstetter et al. in a longitudinal study using forearm pQCT of 102 pediatric IBD patients (82 CD, 30 newly diagnosed) showed similar findings at diagnosis and median follow-up interval of 2.6 (0.9–5.8) years [133]. A study from Sweden following children with IBD over 2 years. At baseline, subjects had mean disease duration of 41.3 months and mean lumbar spine BMD Z-score of -0.9 ± 2.8 and this did not change significantly over the 2 year [134]. The authors note that corticosteroid and azathioprine exposures were not significantly associated with changes in BMD. Whereas the role of anti-TNF-alpha agents was not evaluated in the study from Sweden, Griffin et al. described the changes occurring over 12 months using QCT in children and adolescents initiating therapy with anti-TFN-alpha

[135]. In this study, 74 subjects with median disease duration of 2.1 years (range 0.2–9.7) had baseline trabecular BMD Z-score -1.44 ± 1.11, cortical BMD Z-score 0.19 ± 1.08, and cortical area Z-score -0.97 ± 1.35. After 12 months, trabecular BMD and cortical area increased significantly (0.45 ± 0.76 and 0.29 ± 0.65, respectively, both $p < 0.001$), but cortical BMD decreased. Bone biomarkers were significantly increased over the first 10 weeks of anti-TNF therapy and the authors hypothesize that the decline in cortical BMD is a consequence of rapid increase in periosteal bone formation necessary in catch-up growth. This study highlights the value of QCT distinction of cortical versus trabecular bone and also demonstrates the role of anti-TNF-alpha therapy in the bones of children with IBD.

Finally, the impact of childhood IBD on peak bone mass and risk of osteoporosis is not yet clear but has been described. Bernstein et al. assessed spine, proximal femur, and whole body BMD in 780 premenopausal adult women (age < 45 year) that were diagnosed with IBD prior to 20 years of age [136]. The mean BMD T-scores were normal in the spine (-0.14 ± 1.05), femoral neck (-0.15 ± 1.04) and whole body (0.09 ± 1.04) and results did not differ between the 12 subjects with disease onset before puberty, and the 58 subjects with disease onset after puberty. Alternatively, Azzopardi et al. recently described 83 adult subjects with Crohn disease and found that age of diagnosis <17 years was significantly associated with lower BMD ($p = 0.0006$) [137].

Potential Therapies for Bone Health in Pediatric IBD

Physical Activity

Physical activity is an important determinant of bone mass accretion during growth; simple loading exercises promote bone accretion in healthy children. Numerous studies have documented the beneficial effect of physical activity and biomechanical loading on bone geometry in healthy children [45–47, 49, 50, 138]. Bone adapts its strength in response to the magnitude and direction of the forces to which it is subjected. This capacity of bone to respond to mechanical loading with increased bone size and strength is greatest during growth, especially during adolescence [44]. Physical activity affects the skeleton via two distinct mechanisms, which function as osteogenic stimuli: (1) "muscle pull" involves the force of contracting muscles upon their bony attachments and (2) weight-bearing exercise results in the mechanical loading of the bone with compressive forces. A physical intervention trial in adults with CD utilizing a home-based program of low-impact dynamic muscle conditioning exercises did not show a statistically significant difference in bone mineral density of the lumbar spine and hip between cases and controls; however, analyses limited to those subjects achieving 100% adherence to the program did show a significant increase in trochanteric BMD [139]. A recent systematic review on the influence of physical activity on bone strength in children and adolescents concluded that physical activity has a significant positive impact on bone strength in the growing skeleton (36/37 studies) and that weight-bearing activity specifically enhances bone strength [140]. These findings were in healthy children, and the potential for physical activity to modulate the relationship between disease and bone metabolism will require further study. Based on existing evidence, a program consisting of resistance training (muscle-building) activity in addition to high-impact weight-bearing activity may result in positive impacts on skeletal health.

Vitamins and Minerals

Multiple prospective randomized double-blind intervention trials have documented that calcium supplementation promotes bone accretion in normal children and adolescents [141–146]. Subjects with Crohn disease involving the small bowel are at increased risk for calcium oxalate kidney stones. Normally dietary calcium binds with oxalate in the gut to form a complex that is poorly absorbed. In small bowel disease, fat malabsorption results in increased binding of fatty acids with calcium to form insoluble soaps, thereby increasing the soluble oxalate for absorption [147]. Calcium supplements result in decreased urinary oxalate without increasing urinary calcium above normal; therefore, calcium is recommended to prevent enteric hyperoxaluria [148]. To our knowledge, no calcium balance studies or calcium supplementation trials have been conducted in children with chronic illness.

Vitamin D is essential for the maintenance of adequate calcium levels for bone mineralization and functioning of the immune functioning and all pediatric IBD patients are at risk for vitamin D deficiency. In 1997, the Institute of Medicine concluded that the adequate intake of vitamin D in children and young adults in 200 IU per day [149]. However, in the years following the Institute of Medicine report, a series of publications have argued that 200 IU is not adequate in healthy children and adults [150–157]. A study of the serum 25-hydroxyvitamin D (25(OH)D) response to oral cholecalciferol reported that each additional 100 IU of cholecalciferol resulted in a 0.7 ng/mL increase in serum 25(OH)D over a 2–3 month period, then plateaued [152]. The exact dose required to achieve adequate serum 25(OH)D levels is children with IBD is unclear, but Weaver et al. reported that 863 IU/day would be required in healthy adolescent girls, on average to achieve a serum 25(OH)D of 32 ng/mL [154].

In 2011, the Institute of Medicine updated Recommended Daily Allowances (RDA) and Tolerable Upper Intake Levels (UL) for calcium and vitamin D, and these values are summarized in Table 24.3 [158]. These recommendations reflect the need for increasing calcium intake with age in order to accommodate the calcium needs for the rapidly growing skeleton, especially during the years of the adolescent growth spurt. A national dietary intake survey showed that calcium intake of children declines in all ethnic groups at the ages when calcium requirements increase [159]. Additional practice guidelines from the Endocrine Society propose that patients at risk for vitamin D deficiency require higher doses of vitamin D, specifically, 600–1000 IU/day for patients 4–18 years of age (UL 4000 IU) and 1500–2000 IU/day for patients 19–30 years of age (UL 10,000 IU) [160]. Serum 25-hydroxyvitamin D levels should be measured and optimized, especially in subjects at northern latitudes in the winter months. Future studies will need to further evaluate the role of inflammation on decreased PTH and decreased renal conversion of 25(OH)D to 1,25(OH)$_2$D as has been described by Augustine et al. [43].

Table 24.3 Institute of medicine 2011 dietary reference intakes for calcium and vitamin D

Age (year)	Calcium (mg/day)		Vitamin D (IU/day)	
	RDA	UL	AI	UL
4–8	1000	2500	600	3000
9–18	1300	3000	600	4000
19–30	1300	3000	600	4000

Bisphosphonates

The beneficial effects of bisphosphonates in adults with postmenopausal osteoporosis and corticosteroid-induced osteoporosis are well-recognized. However, concerns regarding the impact on the structure of the modeling skeleton initially tempered enthusiasm for these medications in children. Bisphosphonate therapy results in distinctive radiographic metaphyseal bands in children; the significance of these bands is unclear. Furthermore, some have suggested drug holidays for those receiving bisphosphonate therapy due to concern for over suppression of bone turnover and risk of avascular necrosis of the jaw [161]. Pamidronate proved effective in uncontrolled observational studies of children with osteogenesis imperfecta; bone density and size increased and the incidence of fractures decreased [162–164]. The treatment did not alter fracture healing, growth rate, or growth plate appearances. A report of osteopetrosis in a child treated with a cumulative pamidronate dose approximately seven fold greater than recommended raised concerns regarding the safety of this treatment in growing children [165, 166]. Similar complications have not been observed in children on lower doses [167].

Numerous case series and case reports have been published describing bisphosphonate therapy in children with disparate chronic diseases [168–176]. The two largest studies conducted in children with chronic inflammatory conditions are summarized in Table 24.4. Both of these studies demonstrated significant improvements in DXA BMD; however, only one was a randomized trial [11]. The trial had many important limitations.

Table 24.4 Bisphosphonate studies in children and adolescents with chronic inflammatory disease

Study/subjects	Intervention/outcome	Comments and results

Bianchi et al. [177] *Chronic rheum disorder and ↓ spine BMD* $N = 39^a$, age 5–18	*Design*: 12-month case series
	Oral alendronate
	  Weight <20 kg: 5 mg q day
	  Weight >20 kg: 10 mg q day
	  Instructed to ↑calcium to RDA
	Outcome:
	  DXA spine areal-BMD
		Serum alkaline phosphatase levels decreased by 16.5 ± 10.8%.
		Urinary excretion of NTX decreased by 17 ± 16.5%.
		Mean spine areal-BMD Z-scores (adjusted for sex, age, body surface area) increased from a mean of −2.7 at baseline to −1.9 at 6 months ($p < 0.01$ compared with baseline) and to −1.05 at 12 months ($p < 0.001$ compared with baseline).

Rudge et al. [11] *Chronic glucocorticoids* $N = 22^b$, age 4–17	*Design*: 12-month RCT
	Oral alendronate vs. placebo
	1–2 mg/kg weekly
	  No calcium supplements
	  Rx Vit D if level <20 ng/mL
	Outcome:
	  DXA of spine and femur shaft
		Baseline height Z-score significantly greater in placebo group (−0.2 vs. −2.0).
		18 completed study.
		Significant ↓ in bone resorption markers in alendronate group ($p < 0.01$)
		Lumbar spine: significant ↑ in BMAD in alendronate group ($p = 0.013$) compared with baseline, but not in placebo group ($p = 0.16$)
		Femur mid-shaft: marginal ↑in CSMI in alendronate group ($p = 0.08$) compared with baseline, but not in placebo group ($p = 0.18$)

[a]16 juvenile arthritis, 11 systemic lupus erythematosus (*SLE*), 6 dermatomyositis, 2 Behcet's syndrome, 2 granulomatosis with polyangiitis (formerly known as Wegener granulomatosis), and 2 undefined.
[b]7 juvenile arthritis, 6 SLE, 4 dermatomyositis, 2 IBD, 1 renal transplant, 1 autoimmune anemia, and 1 cystic fibrosis.

First, the study population included 22 children with highly disparate conditions, including juvenile arthritis, lupus, dermatomyositis, inflammatory bowel disease, renal transplantation, autoimmune anemia, and cystic fibrosis; only 18 completed the protocol. Second, baseline height Z-scores and subject age differed significantly between the intervention and placebo group. Third, the spine and femur BMD was assessed using DXA and was likely confounded by bone size. These data highlight the growing use of bisphosphonates in children, and the need for controlled trials using three-dimensional imaging techniques.

Insufficient data are available on the long-term effects of bisphosphonates to recommend its routine use in pediatric IBD, especially in patients at risk for low bone turnover due to cytokine effects [132, 178]. Furthermore, a recent study has demonstrated improvements in BMD and bone metabolism in IBD using anti-TNF-alpha therapy and controlling inflammation [135]. This suggests that addressing underlying inflammation should be the focus in addressing bone deficits in IBD. However, future studies may demonstrate an important role for bisphosphonate treatment in patients requiring long-term glucocorticoid therapy.

Summary

In conclusion, children with IBD are at risk for impaired bone mineral accrual. However, additional studies are needed to fully appreciate the magnitude of bone disease in pediatric IBD, as well as the implications for lifetime fracture risk and targeted therapies. Currently, the prevention of bone disease is best accomplished by controlling inflammation, providing adequate calcium and vitamin D supplementation, and encouraging physical activity. Prospective trials of therapeutic agents need to be performed to assess efficacy and safety in the developing skeleton.

References

1. Bailey DA, McKay HA, Mirwald RL, Crocker PR, Faulkner RA. A six-year longitudinal study of the relationship of physical activity to bone mineral accrual in growing children: the university of Saskatchewan bone mineral accrual study. J Bone Miner Res. 1999;14:1672–9.
2. NIH. Osteoporosis prevention, diagnosis, and therapy. NIH Consens Statement. 2000;17:1–36.
3. Semeao EJ, Stallings VA, Peck SN, Piccoli DA. Vertebral compression fractures in pediatric patients with Crohn's disease. Gastroenterology. 1997;112:1710–3.
4. Lucarelli S, Borrelli O, Paganelli M, et al. Vertebral fractures and increased sensitivity to corticosteroids in a child with ulcerative colitis: successful use of pamidronate. J Pediatr Gastroenterol Nutr. 2006;43:533–5.
5. Thearle M, Horlick M, Bilezikian JP, et al. Osteoporosis: an unusual presentation of childhood Crohn's disease. J Clin Endocrinol Metab. 2000;85:2122–6.
6. Sylvester FA. Cracking the risk of fractures in Crohn disease. J Pediatr Gastroenterol Nutr. 2004;38:113–4.
7. Kappelman MD, Galanko JA, Porter CQ, Sandler RS. Risk of diagnosed fractures in children with inflammatory bowel diseases. Inflamm Bowel Dis. 2011;17:1125–30.
8. Burnham JM, Shults J, Semeao E, et al. Whole body BMC in pediatric Crohn disease: independent effects of altered growth, maturation, and body composition. J Bone Miner Res Off J Am Soc Bone Miner Res. 2004;19:1961–8.
9. Garnero P, Darte C, Delmas PD. A model to monitor the efficacy of alendronate treatment in women with osteoporosis using a biochemical marker of bone turnover. Bone. 1999;24:603–9.
10. Prestwood KM, Pilbeam CC, Burleson JA, et al. The short-term effects of conjugated estrogen on bone turnover in older women. J Clin Endocrinol Metab. 1994;79:366–71.
11. Rudge S, Hailwood S, Horne A, Lucas J, Wu F, Cundy T. Effects of once-weekly oral alendronate on bone in children on glucocorticoid treatment. Rheumatology (Oxford). 2005;44:813–8.
12. Baron R. General principles of bone biology. In: Favus M, editor. Primer on the metabolic bone diseases and disorders of mineral metabolism. 5th ed. Philadelphia: Lippincott Williams & Wilkins; 2003. p. 1–8.
13. Gilsanz V, Roe TF, Mora S, Costin G, Goodman WG. Changes in vertebral bone density in black girls and white girls during childhood and puberty. N Engl J Med. 1991;325:1597–600.
14. Gilsanz V, Kovanlikaya A, Costin G, Roe TF, Sayre J, Kaufman F. Differential effect of gender on the sizes of the bones in the axial and appendicular skeletons. J Clin Endocrinol Metab. 1997;82:1603–7.
15. Gilsanz V, Gibbens DT, Roe TF, et al. Vertebral bone density in children: effect of puberty. Radiology. 1988;166:847–50.
16. Han ZH, Palnitkar S, Rao DS, Nelson D, Parfitt AM. Effect of ethnicity and age or menopause on the structure and geometry of iliac bone. J Bone Miner Res. 1996;11:1967–75.
17. Seeman E. Pathogenesis of bone fragility in women and men. Lancet. 2002;359:1841–50.
18. Burr DB, Turner CH. Biomechanics of bone. In: Flavus MJ, editor. Primer on the Metabolic bone diseases and disorders of mineral metabolism. 5th ed. Philadelphia: Lippincott Williams & Wilkins; 2003. p. 58–64.
19. Duan Y, Beck TJ, Wang XF, Seeman E. Structural and biomechanical basis of sexual dimorphism in femoral neck fragility has its origins in growth and aging. J Bone Miner Res. 2003;18:1766–74.
20. Duan Y, Turner CH, Kim BT, Seeman E. Sexual dimorphism in vertebral fragility is more the result of gender differences in age-related bone gain than bone loss. J Bone Miner Res. 2001;16:2267–75.
21. Khosla S, Melton 3rd LJ, Dekutoski MB, Achenbach SJ, Oberg AL, Riggs BL. Incidence of childhood distal forearm fractures over 30 years: a population-based study. JAMA. 2003;290:1479–85.
22. Garnero P, Hausherr E, Chapuy MC, et al. Markers of bone resorption predict hip fracture in elderly women: the EPIDOS Prospective Study. J Bone Miner Res. 1996;11:1531–8.
23. Black DM, Bilezikian JP, Ensrud KE, et al. One year of alendronate after one year of parathyroid hormone (1-84) for osteoporosis. N Engl J Med. 2005;353:555–65.
24. Schonau E, Rauch F. Biochemical markers of bone metabolism. In: Glorieux FH, editor. Pediatric bone: biology and diseases. San Diego: Academic Press; 2003. p. 339–57.
25. Szulc P, Seeman E, Delmas PD. Biochemical measurements of bone turnover in children and adolescents. Osteoporos Int. 2000;11:281–94.
26. Gokhale R, Favus MJ, Karrison T, Sutton MM, Rich B, Kirschner BS. Bone mineral density assessment in children with inflammatory bowel disease. Gastroenterology. 1998;114:902–11.

27. Fries W, Dinca M, Luisetto G, Peccolo F, Bottega F, Martin A. Calcaneal ultrasound bone densitometry in inflammatory bowel disease – a comparison with double x-ray densitometry of the lumbar spine. Am J Gastroenterol. 1998;93:2339–44.

28. Pollak RD, Karmeli F, Eliakim R, Ackerman Z, Tabb K, Rachmilewitz D. Femoral neck osteopenia in patients with inflammatory bowel disease. Am J Gastroenterol. 1998;93:1483–90.

29. Bischoff SC, Herrmann A, Goke M, Manns MP, von zur Muhlen A, Brabant G. Altered bone metabolism in inflammatory bowel disease. Am J Gastroenterol. 1997;92:1157–63.

30. Hyams JS, Wyzga N, Kreutzer DL, Justinich CJ, Gronowicz GA. Alterations in bone metabolism in children with inflammatory bowel disease: an in vitro study. J Pediatr Gastroenterol Nutr. 1997;24:289–95.

31. Semeao EJ, Jawad AF, Zemel BS, Neiswender KM, Piccoli DA, Stallings VA. Bone mineral density in children and young adults with Crohn's disease. Inflamm Bowel Dis. 1999;5:161–6.

32. van Staa TP, Cooper C, Brusse LS, Leufkens H, Javaid MK, Arden NK. Inflammatory bowel disease and the risk of fracture. Gastroenterology. 2003;125:1591–7.

33. Klaus J, Armbrecht G, Steinkamp M, et al. High prevalence of osteoporotic vertebral fractures in patients with Crohn's disease. Gut. 2002;51:654–8.

34. Vestergaard P, Krogh K, Rejnmark L, Laurberg S, Mosekilde L. Fracture risk is increased in Crohn's disease, but not in ulcerative colitis. Gut. 2000;46:176–81.

35. Bernstein CN, Blanchard JF, Leslie W, Wajda A, Yu BN. The incidence of fracture among patients with inflammatory bowel disease. A population-based cohort study. Ann Intern Med. 2000;133:795–9.

36. Loftus Jr EV, Crowson CS, Sandborn WJ, Tremaine WJ, O'Fallon WM, Melton 3rd LJ. Long-term fracture risk in patients with Crohn's disease: a population-based study in Olmsted County, Minnesota. Gastroenterology. 2002;123:468–75.

37. Szulc P, Chapuy MC, Meunier PJ, Delmas PD. Serum undercarboxylated osteocalcin is a marker of the risk of hip fracture in elderly women. J Clin Invest. 1993;91:1769–74.

38. Kleinman RE, Baldassano RN, Caplan A, et al. Nutrition support for pediatric patients with inflammatory bowel disease: a clinical report of the North American Society for Pediatric Gastroenterology, Hepatology And Nutrition. J Pediatr Gastroenterol Nutr. 2004;39:15–27.

39. von Scheven E, Gordon CM, Wypij D, Wertz M, Gallagher KT, Bachrach L. Variable deficits of bone mineral despite chronic glucocorticoid therapy in pediatric patients with inflammatory diseases: a Glaser Pediatric Research Network study. J Pediatr Endocrinol Metab. 2006;19:821–30.

40. Pappa HM, Gordon CM, Saslowsky TM, et al. Vitamin D status in children and young adults with inflammatory bowel disease. Pediatrics. 2006;118:1950–61.

41. Sentongo TA, Semaeo EJ, Stettler N, Piccoli DA, Stallings VA, Zemel BS. Vitamin D status in children, adolescents, and young adults with Crohn disease. Am J Clin Nutr. 2002;76:1077–81.

42. Pappa HM, Grand RJ, Gordon CM. Report on the vitamin D status of adult and pediatric patients with inflammatory bowel disease and its significance for bone health and disease. Inflamm Bowel Dis. 2006;12:1162–74.

43. Augustine MV, Leonard MB, Thayu M, et al. Changes in vitamin D-related mineral metabolism after induction with anti-tumor necrosis factor-alpha therapy in Crohn's disease. J Clin Endocrinol Metab. 2014;99:E991–8.

44. Parfitt AM. The two faces of growth: benefits and risks to bone integrity. Osteoporos Int. 1994;4:382–98.

45. Janz KF. Validation of the CSA accelerometer for assessing children's physical activity. Med Sci Sports Exerc. 1994;26:369–75.

46. Bass S, Pearce G, Bradney M, et al. Exercise before puberty may confer residual benefits in bone density in adulthood: studies in active prepubertal and retired female gymnasts. J Bone Miner Res. 1998;13:500–7.

47. Bass SL, Saxon L, Daly RM, et al. The effect of mechanical loading on the size and shape of bone in pre-, peri-, and postpubertal girls: a study in tennis players. J Bone Miner Res. 2002;17:2274–80.

48. Bass S, Pearce G, Young N, Seeman E. Bone mass during growth: the effects of exercise. Exercise and mineral accrual. Acta Univ Carol Med. 1994;40:3–6.

49. Lloyd T, Petit MA, Lin HM, Beck TJ. Lifestyle factors and the development of bone mass and bone strength in young women. J Pediatr. 2004;144:776–82.

50. Lloyd T, Chinchilli VM, Johnson-Rollings N, Kieselhorst K, Eggli DF, Marcus R. Adult female hip bone density reflects teenage sports-exercise patterns but not teenage calcium intake. Pediatrics. 2000;106:40–4.

51. Frost HM, Schonau E. The "muscle-bone unit" in children and adolescents: a 2000 overview. J Pediatr Endocrinol Metab. 2000;13:571–90.

52. Petit MA, McKay HA, MacKelvie KJ, Heinonen A, Khan KM, Beck TJ. A randomized school-based jumping intervention confers site and maturity-specific benefits on bone structural properties in girls: a hip structural analysis study. J Bone Miner Res. 2002;17:363–72.

53. Specker B, Binkley T. Randomized trial of physical activity and calcium supplementation on bone mineral content in 3- to 5-year-old children. J Bone Miner Res. 2003;18:885–92.

54. Harpavat M, Greenspan SL, O'Brien C, Chang CC, Bowen A, Keljo DJ. Altered bone mass in children at diagnosis of Crohn disease: a pilot study. J Pediatr Gastroenterol Nutr. 2005;40:295–300.

55. Werkstetter KJ, Ullrich J, Schatz SB, Prell C, Koletzko B, Koletzko S. Lean body mass, physical activity and quality of life in paediatric patients with inflammatory bowel disease and in healthy controls. J Crohns Colitis. 2012;6:665–73.

56. Lee DY, Wetzsteon RJ, Zemel BS, et al. Muscle torque relative to cross-sectional area and the functional muscle-bone unit in children and adolescents with chronic disease. J Bone Miner Res Off J Am Soc Bone Miner Res. 2015;30:575–83.

57. Burnham JM, Shults J, Petit MA, et al. Alterations in proximal femur geometry in children treated with glucocorticoids for Crohn disease or nephrotic syndrome: impact of the underlying disease. J Bone Miner Res. 2007;22:551–9.

58. Dubner SE, Shults J, Baldassano RN, et al. Longitudinal assessment of bone density and structure in an incident cohort of children with Crohn's disease. Gastroenterology. 2009;136:123–30.

59. Canalis E, Bilezikian JP, Angeli A, Giustina A. Perspectives on glucocorticoid-induced osteoporosis. Bone. 2004;34:593–8.

60. Pereira RC, Delany AM, Canalis E. Effects of cortisol and bone morphogenetic protein-2 on stromal cell differentiation: correlation with CCAAT-enhancer binding protein expression. Bone. 2002;30:685–91.

61. Weinstein RS, Jilka RL, Parfitt AM, Manolagas SC. Inhibition of osteoblastogenesis and promotion of apoptosis of osteoblasts and osteocytes by glucocorticoids. Potential mechanisms of their deleterious effects on bone. J Clin Invest. 1998;102:274–82.

62. Delany AM, Gabbitas BY, Canalis E. Cortisol downregulates osteoblast alpha 1 (I) procollagen mRNA by transcriptional and posttranscriptional mechanisms. J Cell Biochem. 1995;57:488–94.

63. Giustina A, Bussi AR, Jacobello C, Wehrenberg WB. Effects of recombinant human growth hormone (GH) on bone and intermediary metabolism in patients receiving chronic glucocorticoid treatment with suppressed endogenous GH response to

GH-releasing hormone. J Clin Endocrinol Metab. 1995;80: 122–9.

64. Kwan Tat S, Padrines M, Theoleyre S, Heymann D, Fortun Y. IL-6, RANKL, TNF-alpha/IL-1: interrelations in bone resorption pathophysiology. Cytokine Growth Factor Rev. 2004;15: 49–60.

65. Dempster DW, Moonga BS, Stein LS, Horbert WR, Antakly T. Glucocorticoids inhibit bone resorption by isolated rat osteoclasts by enhancing apoptosis. J Endocrinol. 1997;154:397–406.

66. Ikeda S, Morishita Y, Tsutsumi H, et al. Reductions in bone turnover, mineral, and structure associated with mechanical properties of lumbar vertebra and femur in glucocorticoid-treated growing minipigs. Bone. 2003;33:779–87.

67. Ortoft G, Andreassen TT, Oxlund H. Growth hormone increases cortical and cancellous bone mass in young growing rats with glucocorticoid-induced osteopenia. J Bone Miner Res. 1999;14: 710–21.

68. Podolsky DK. Inflammatory bowel disease. N Engl J Med. 2002;347:417–29.

69. Gilbert L, He X, Farmer P, et al. Inhibition of osteoblast differentiation by tumor necrosis factor-alpha. Endocrinology. 2000;141: 3956–64.

70. Lee SE, Chung WJ, Kwak HB, et al. Tumor necrosis factor-alpha supports the survival of osteoclasts through the activation of Akt and ERK. J Biol Chem. 2001;276:49343–9.

71. Kong YY, Feige U, Sarosi I, et al. Activated T cells regulate bone loss and joint destruction in adjuvant arthritis through osteoprotegerin ligand. Nature. 1999;402:304–9.

72. Walsh MC, Choi Y. Biology of the TRANCE axis. Cytokine Growth Factor Rev. 2003;14:251–63.

73. Kudo O, Sabokbar A, Pocock A, Itonaga I, Fujikawa Y, Athanasou NA. Interleukin-6 and interleukin-11 support human osteoclast formation by a RANKL-independent mechanism. Bone. 2003;32: 1–7.

74. Gilbert L, He X, Farmer P, et al. Expression of the osteoblast differentiation factor RUNX2 (Cbfa1/AML3/Pebp2alpha A) is inhibited by tumor necrosis factor-alpha. J Biol Chem. 2002;277: 2695–701.

75. Radeff JM, Nagy Z, Stern PH. Involvement of PKC-beta in PTH, TNF-alpha, and IL-1 beta effects on IL-6 promoter in osteoblastic cells and on PTH-stimulated bone resorption. Exp Cell Res. 2001;268:179–88.

76. Baim S, Wilson CR, Lewiecki EM, Luckey MM, Downs Jr RW, Lentle BC. Precision assessment and radiation safety for dual-energy X-ray absorptiometry: position paper of the International Society for Clinical Densitometry. J Clin Densitom Off J Int Soc Clin Densitom. 2005;8:371–8.

77. WHO. The WHO Study Group: Assessment of fracture risk and its application to screening for postmenopausal osteoporosis. Geneva: World Health Organization; 1994.

78. Rauch F, Plotkin H, DiMeglio L, et al. Fracture prediction and the definition of osteoporosis in children and adolescents: the ISCD 2007 Pediatric Official Positions. J Clin Densitom Off J Int Soc Clin Densitom. 2008;11:22–8.

79. Faulkner RA, Davison KS, Bailey DA, Mirwald RL, Baxter-Jones AD. Size-corrected BMD decreases during peak linear growth: implications for fracture incidence during adolescence. J Bone Miner Res. 2006;21:1864–70.

80. Chan GM, Hess M, Hollis J, Book LS. Bone mineral status in childhood accidental fractures. Am J Dis Child. 1984;138: 569–70.

81. Goulding A, Cannan R, Williams SM, Gold EJ, Taylor RW, Lewis-Barned NJ. Bone mineral density in girls with forearm fractures. J Bone Miner Res. 1998;13:143–8.

82. Goulding A, Jones IE, Taylor RW, Williams SM, Manning PJ. Bone mineral density and body composition in boys with dis-

tal forearm fractures: a dual-energy x-ray absorptiometry study. J Pediatr. 2001;139:509–15.

83. Goulding A, Jones IE, Taylor RW, Manning PJ, Williams SM. More broken bones: a 4-year double cohort study of young girls with and without distal forearm fractures. J Bone Miner Res. 2000;15:2011–8.

84. Ma D, Jones G. The association between bone mineral density, metacarpal morphometry, and upper limb fractures in children: a population-based case-control study. J Clin Endocrinol Metab. 2003;88:1486–91.

85. Ma DQ, Jones G. Clinical risk factors but not bone density are associated with prevalent fractures in prepubertal children. J Paediatr Child Health. 2002;38:497–500.

86. Cook SD, Harding AF, Morgan EL, et al. Association of bone mineral density and pediatric fractures. J Pediatr Orthop. 1987;7:424–7.

87. Skaggs DL, Loro ML, Pitukcheewanont P, Tolo V, Gilsanz V. Increased body weight and decreased radial cross-sectional dimensions in girls with forearm fractures. J Bone Miner Res. 2001;16:1337–42.

88. Ma D, Jones G. Television, computer, and video viewing; physical activity; and upper limb fracture risk in children: a population-based case control study. J Bone Miner Res. 2003;18: 1970–7.

89. Clark EM, Ness AR, Bishop NJ, Tobias JH. Association between bone mass and fractures in children: a prospective cohort study. J Bone Miner Res. 2006;21:1489–95.

90. Cole JH, Scerpella TA, van der Meulen MC. Fan-beam densitometry of the growing skeleton: are we measuring what we think we are? J Clin Densitom. 2005;8:57–64.

91. McKay HA, Petit MA, Bailey DA, Wallace WM, Schutz RW, Khan KM. Analysis of proximal femur DXA scans in growing children: comparisons of different protocols for cross-sectional 8-month and 7-year longitudinal data. J Bone Miner Res. 2000;15:1181–8.

92. Leonard MB, Feldman HI, Zemel BS, Berlin JA, Barden EM, Stallings VA. Evaluation of low density spine software for the assessment of bone mineral density in children. J Bone Miner Res. 1998;13:1687–90.

93. Shypailo RJ, Ellis KJ. Bone assessment in children: comparison of fan-beam DXA analysis. J Clin Densitom. 2005;8:445–53.

94. Koo WW, Hammami M, Shypailo RJ, Ellis KJ. Bone and body composition measurements of small subjects: discrepancies from software for fan-beam dual energy X-ray absorptiometry. J Am Coll Nutr. 2004;23:647–50.

95. Molgaard C, Thomsen BL, Prentice A, Cole TJ, Michaelsen KF. Whole body bone mineral content in healthy children and adolescents. Arch Dis Child. 1997;76:9–15.

96. Ellis KJ, Shypailo RJ, Hardin DS, et al. Z score prediction model for assessment of bone mineral content in pediatric diseases. J Bone Miner Res. 2001;16:1658–64.

97. Binkley TL, Specker BL, Wittig TA. Centile curves for bone densitometry measurements in healthy males and females ages 5–22 yr. J Clin Densitom. 2002;5:343–53.

98. Hannan WJ, Tothill P, Cowen SJ, Wrate RM. Whole body bone mineral content in healthy children and adolescents. Arch Dis Child. 1998;78:396–7.

99. Maynard LM, Guo SS, Chumlea WC, et al. Total-body and regional bone mineral content and areal bone mineral density in children aged 8-18 y: the Fels Longitudinal Study. Am J Clin Nutr. 1998;68:1111–7.

100. van der Sluis IM, de Ridder MA, Boot AM, Krenning EP, de Muinck Keizer-Schrama SM. Reference data for bone density and body composition measured with dual energy x ray absorptiometry in white children and young adults. Arch Dis Child. 2002;87:341–7. discussion -7.

101. Southard RN, Morris JD, Mahan JD, et al. Bone mass in healthy children: measurement with quantitative DXA. Radiology. 1991;179:735–8.
102. Henderson RC, Madsen CD. Bone density in children and adolescents with cystic fibrosis. J Pediatr. 1996;128:28–34.
103. Faulkner RA, Bailey DA, Drinkwater DT, McKay HA, Arnold C, Wilkinson AA. Bone densitometry in Canadian children 8-17 years of age. Calcif Tissue Int. 1996;59:344–51.
104. Glastre C, Braillon P, David L, Cochat P, Meunier PJ, Delmas PD. Measurement of bone mineral content of the lumbar spine by dual energy x-ray absorptiometry in normal children: correlations with growth parameters. J Clin Endocrinol Metab. 1990;70:1330–3.
105. Bonjour JP, Theintz G, Buchs B, Slosman D, Rizzoli R. Critical years and stages of puberty for spinal and femoral bone mass accumulation during adolescence. J Clin Endocrinol Metab. 1991;73:555–63.
106. del Rio L, Carrascosa A, Pons F, Gusinye M, Yeste D, Domenech FM. Bone mineral density of the lumbar spine in white Mediterranean Spanish children and adolescents: changes related to age, sex, and puberty. Pediatr Res. 1994;35: 362–6.
107. Plotkin H, Nunez M, Alvarez Filgueira ML, Zanchetta JR. Lumbar spine bone density in Argentine children. Calcif Tissue Int. 1996;58:144–9.
108. Braillon PM, Cochat P. Analysis of dual energy X-ray absorptiometry whole body results in children, adolescents and young adults. Appl Radiat Isot. 1998;49:623–4.
109. Leonard MB, Propert KJ, Zemel BS, Stallings VA, Feldman HI. Discrepancies in pediatric bone mineral density reference data: potential for misdiagnosis of osteopenia. J Pediatr. 1999;135:182–8.
110. Katzman DK, Bachrach LK, Carter DR, Marcus R. Clinical and anthropometric correlates of bone mineral acquisition in healthy adolescent girls. J Clin Endocrinol Metab. 1991;73:1332–9.
111. Prentice A, Parsons TJ, Cole TJ. Uncritical use of bone mineral density in absorptiometry may lead to size-related artifacts in the identification of bone mineral determinants. Am J Clin Nutr. 1994;60:837–42.
112. Gafni RI, Baron J. Overdiagnosis of osteoporosis in children due to misinterpretation of dual-energy x-ray absorptiometry (DEXA). J Pediatr. 2004;144:253–7.
113. Stephens M, Batres LA, Ng D, Baldassano R. Growth failure in the child with inflammatory bowel disease. Semin Gastrointest Dis. 2001;12:253–62.
114. Zemel BS, Leonard MB, Kelly A, et al. Height adjustment in assessing dual energy x-ray absorptiometry measurements of bone mass and density in children. J Clin Endocrinol Metab. 2010;95:1265–73.
115. Carter DR, Bouxsein ML, Marcus R. New approaches for interpreting projected bone densitometry data. J Bone Miner Res. 1992;7:137–45.
116. Kroger H, Vainio P, Nieminen J, Kotaniemi A. Comparison of different models for interpreting bone mineral density measurements using DXA and MRI technology. Bone. 1995;17:157–9.
117. Leonard MB, Shults J, Elliott DM, Stallings VA, Zemel BS. Interpretation of whole body dual energy X-ray absorptiometry measures in children: comparison with peripheral quantitative computed tomography. Bone. 2004;34:1044–52.
118. Kroger H, Kotaniemi A, Kroger L, Alhava E. Development of bone mass and bone density of the spine and femoral neck–a prospective study of 65 children and adolescents. Bone Miner. 1993;23:171–82.
119. Kroger H, Kotaniemi A, Vainio P, Alhava E. Bone densitometry of the spine and femur in children by dual-energy x-ray absorptiometry. Bone Miner. 1992;17:75–85.
120. Wren TA, Liu X, Pitukcheewanont P, Gilsanz V. Bone acquisition in healthy children and adolescents: comparisons of dual-energy x-ray absorptiometry and computed tomography measures. J Clin Endocrinol Metab. 2005;90:1925–8.
121. Gilsanz V. Bone density in children: a review of the available techniques and indications. Eur J Radiol. 1998;26.177–82.
122. Ferretti JL. Perspectives of pQCT technology associated to biomechanical studies in skeletal research employing rat models. Bone. 1995;17:353S–64S.
123. Leonard MB, Zemel BS. Current concepts in pediatric bone disease. Pediatr Clin North Am. 2002;49:143–73.
124. Tsampalieros A, Berkenstock MK, Zemel BS, et al. Changes in trabecular bone density in incident pediatric Crohn's disease: a comparison of imaging methods. Osteoporos Int J Established as Result Coop Eur Found Osteoporos Nat Osteoporos Found USA. 2014;25:1875–83.
125. Walther F, Fusch C, Radke M, Beckert S, Findeisen A. Osteoporosis in pediatric patients suffering from chronic inflammatory bowel disease with and without steroid treatment. J Pediatr Gastroenterol Nutr. 2006;43:42–51.
126. Ahmed SF, Horrocks IA, Patterson T, et al. Bone mineral assessment by dual energy X-ray absorptiometry in children with inflammatory bowel disease: evaluation by age or bone area. J Pediatr Gastroenterol Nutr. 2004;38:276–80.
127. Herzog D, Bishop N, Glorieux F, Seidman EG. Interpretation of bone mineral density values in pediatric Crohn's disease. Inflamm Bowel Dis. 1998;4:261–7.
128. Burnham JM, Shults J, Semeao E, et al. Body-composition alterations consistent with cachexia in children and young adults with Crohn disease. Am J Clin Nutr. 2005;82:413–20.
129. Gupta A, Paski S, Issenman R, Webber C. Lumbar spine bone mineral density at diagnosis and during follow-up in children with IBD. J Clin Densitom. 2004;7:290–5.
130. Laakso S, Valta H, Verkasalo M, Toiviainen-Salo S, Makitie O. Compromised peak bone mass in patients with inflammatory bowel disease – a prospective study. J Pediatr. 2014;164:1436–43. e1.
131. Leonard MB, Feldman HI, Shults J, Zemel BS, Foster BJ, Stallings VA. Long-term, high-dose glucocorticoids and bone mineral content in childhood glucocorticoid-sensitive nephrotic syndrome. N Engl J Med. 2004;351:868–75.
132. Sylvester FA, Davis PM, Wyzga N, Hyams JS, Lerer T. Are activated T cells regulators of bone metabolism in children with Crohn disease? J Pediatr. 2006;148:461–6.
133. Werkstetter KJ, Pozza SB, Filipiak-Pittroff B, et al. Long-term development of bone geometry and muscle in pediatric inflammatory bowel disease. Am J Gastroenterol. 2011;106:988–98.
134. Schmidt S, Mellstrom D, Norjavaara E, Sundh V, Saalman R. Longitudinal assessment of bone mineral density in children and adolescents with inflammatory bowel disease. J Pediatr Gastroenterol Nutr. 2012;55:511–8.
135. Griffin LM, Thayu M, Baldassano RN, et al. Improvements in bone density and structure during anti-TNF-alpha therapy in pediatric Crohn's Disease. J Clin Endocrinol Metab. 2015;100:2630–9.
136. Bernstein CN, Leslie WD, Taback SP. Bone density in a population-based cohort of premenopausal adult women with early onset inflammatory bowel disease. Am J Gastroenterol. 2003;98:1094–100.
137. Azzopardi N, Ellul P. Risk factors for osteoporosis in Crohn's disease: infliximab, corticosteroids, body mass index, and age of onset. Inflamm Bowel Dis. 2013;19:1173–8.
138. Bass S, Pearce G, Young N, Seeman E. Bone mass during growth: the effects of exercise. Exercise and mineral accrual. Acta Univ Carol Med (Praha). 1994;40:3–6.

139. Robinson RJ, Krzywicki T, Almond L, et al. Effect of a low-impact exercise program on bone mineral density in Crohn's disease: a randomized controlled trial. Gastroenterology. 1998;115:36–41.

140. Tan VP, Macdonald HM, Kim S, et al. Influence of physical activity on bone strength in children and adolescents: a systematic review and narrative synthesis. J Bone Miner Res Off J Am Soc Bone Mineral Res. 2014;29:2161–81.

141. Cadogan J, Eastell R, Jones N, Barker ME. Milk intake and bone mineral acquisition in adolescent girls: randomised, controlled intervention trial. BMJ. 1997;315:1255–60.

142. Chan GM, Hoffman K, McMurry M. Effects of dairy products on bone and body composition in pubertal girls. J Pediatr. 1995;126:551–6.

143. Johnston Jr CC, Miller JZ, Slemenda CW, et al. Calcium supplementation and increases in bone mineral density in children. N Engl J Med. 1992;327:82–7.

144. Lee WT, Leung SS, Wang SH, et al. Double-blind, controlled calcium supplementation and bone mineral accretion in children accustomed to a low-calcium diet. Am J Clin Nutr. 1994;60:744–50.

145. Lloyd T, Andon MB, Rollings N, et al. Calcium supplementation and bone mineral density in adolescent children. N Engl J Med. 1992;327:82–7.

146. Bonjour JP, Carrie AL, Ferrari S, et al. Calcium-enriched foods and bone mass growth in prepubertal girls: a randomized, double-blind, placebo-controlled trial. J Clin Invest. 1997;99:1287–94.

147. Stauffer JQ. Hyperoxaluria and intestinal disease. The role of steatorrhea and dietary calcium in regulating intestinal oxalate absorption. Am J Dig Dis. 1977;22:921–8.

148. Worcester EM. Stones from bowel disease. Endocrinol Metab Clin North Am. 2002;31:979–99.

149. Food and Nutrition Board, Institute of Medicine. Dietary reference intakes for calcium, phosphorus, magnesium, vitamin D, and fluoride. Washington, DC: National Academy Press; 1997.

150. Heaney RP. Long-latency deficiency disease: insights from calcium and vitamin D. Am J Clin Nutr. 2003;78:912–9.

151. Heaney RP. Functional indices of vitamin D status and ramifications of vitamin D deficiency. Am J Clin Nutr. 2004;80:1706S–9S.

152. Heaney RP, Davies KM, Chen TC, Holick MF, Barger-Lux MJ. Human serum 25-hydroxycholecalciferol response to extended oral dosing with cholecalciferol. Am J Clin Nutr. 2003;77:204–10.

153. Armas LA, Hollis BW, Heaney RP. Vitamin D2 is much less effective than vitamin D3 in humans. J Clin Endocrinol Metab. 2004;89:5387–91.

154. Weaver CM, Fleet JC. Vitamin D requirements: current and future. Am J Clin Nutr. 2004;80:1735S–9S.

155. Calvo MS, Whiting SJ, Barton CN. Vitamin D fortification in the United States and Canada: current status and data needs. Am J Clin Nutr. 2004;80:1710S–6S.

156. Calvo MS, Whiting SJ. Prevalence of vitamin D insufficiency in Canada and the United States: importance to health status and efficacy of current food fortification and dietary supplement use. Nutr Rev. 2003;61:107–13.

157. Looker AC, Dawson-Hughes B, Calvo MS, Gunter EW, Sahyoun NR. Serum 25-hydroxyvitamin D status of adolescents and adults in two seasonal subpopulations from NHANES III. Bone. 2002;30:771–7.

158. Institute of Medicine. Dietary reference intakes for calcium and vitamin D. Washington, DC: The National Academies Press; 2011.

159. Alaimo K, McDowell MA, Briefel RR, et al. Dietary intake of vitamins, minerals, and fiber of persons ages 2 months and over in the United States: Third National Health and Nutrition Examination Survey, Phase 1, 1988-91. Adv Data. 1994;258:1–28.

160. Holick MF, Binkley NC, Bischoff-Ferrari HA, et al. Evaluation, treatment, and prevention of vitamin D deficiency: an Endocrine Society clinical practice guideline. J Clin Endocrinol Metab. 2011;96:1911–30.

161. Ott SM. Long-term safety of bisphosphonates. J Clin Endocrinol Metab. 2005;90:1897–9.

162. Rauch F, Plotkin H, Zeitlin L, Glorieux FH. Bone mass, size, and density in children and adolescents with osteogenesis imperfecta: effect of intravenous pamidronate therapy. J Bone Miner Res. 2003;18:610–4.

163. Glorieux FH, Bishop NJ, Plotkin H, Chabot G, Lanoue G, Travers R. Cyclic administration of pamidronate in children with severe osteogenesis imperfecta. N Engl J Med. 1998;339:947–52.

164. Glorieux FH. Bisphosphonate therapy for severe osteogenesis imperfecta. J Pediatr Endocrinol Metab. 2000;13(Suppl 2):989–92.

165. Marini JC. Do bisphosphonates make children's bones better or brittle? N Engl J Med. 2003;349:423–6.

166. Whyte MP, Wenkert D, Clements KL, McAlister WH, Mumm S. Bisphosphonate-induced osteopetrosis. N Engl J Med. 2003;349:457–63.

167. Glorieux FH, Rauch F, Shapiro JR. Bisphosphonates in children with bone diseases. N Engl J Med. 2003;349:2068–71. author reply -71.

168. Steelman J, Zeitler P. Treatment of symptomatic pediatric osteoporosis with cyclic single-day intravenous pamidronate infusions. J Pediatr. 2003;142:417–23.

169. Gandrud LM, Cheung JC, Daniels MW, Bachrach LK. Low-dose intravenous pamidronate reduces fractures in childhood osteoporosis. J Pediatr Endocrinol Metab. 2003;16:887–92.

170. Cimaz R, Gattorno M, Sormani MP, et al. Changes in markers of bone turnover and inflammatory variables during alendronate therapy in pediatric patients with rheumatic diseases. J Rheumatol. 2002;29:1786–92.

171. Acott PD, Wong JA, Lang BA, Crocker JF. Pamidronate treatment of pediatric fracture patients on chronic steroid therapy. Pediatr Nephrol. 2005;20:368–73.

172. Stewart WA, Acott PD, Salisbury SR, Lang BA. Bone mineral density in juvenile dermatomyositis: assessment using dual x-ray absorptiometry. Arthritis Rheum. 2003;48:2294–8.

173. Rodd C. Bisphosphonates in dialysis and transplantation patients: efficacy and safety issues. Perit Dial Int. 2001;21(Suppl 3):S256–60.

174. Klein GL, Wimalawansa SJ, Kulkarni G, Sherrard DJ, Sanford AP, Herndon DN. The efficacy of acute administration of pamidronate on the conservation of bone mass following severe burn injury in children: a double-blind, randomized, controlled study. Osteoporos Int. 2005;16:631–5.

175. Ringuier B, Leboucher B, Leblanc M, et al. Effect of oral biphosphonates in patients with cystic fibrosis and low bone mineral density. Arch Pediatr. 2004;11:1445–9.

176. Hawker GA, Ridout R, Harris VA, Chase CC, Fielding LJ, Biggar WD. Alendronate in the treatment of low bone mass in steroid-treated boys with Duchennes muscular dystrophy. Arch Phys Med Rehabil. 2005;86:284–8.

177. Bianchi ML, Cimaz R, Bardare M, et al. Efficacy and safety of alendronate for the treatment of osteoporosis in diffuse connective tissue diseases in children: a prospective multicenter study. Arthritis Rheum. 2000;43:1960–6.

178. Gordon CM. Bone loss in children with Crohn disease: Evidence of "osteoimmune" alterations. J Pediatr. 2006;148:429–32.

5-Aminosalicylate Therapy

25

Michael Stephens and Michelle Gonzalez

Introduction

Aminosalicylates are a class of medications commonly used as first-line therapy for induction and maintenance of remission in mild to moderate inflammatory bowel disease (IBD) [1]. Although their use in ulcerative colitis (UC) is well established, their role in Crohn's disease (CD) remains controversial. Aminosalicylates were derived from sulfasalazine (SASP, salicylazosulfapyridine), a sulfa drug originally developed for the treatment of rheumatoid arthritis. The sulfasalazine molecule is comprised by two moieties with antimicrobial and anti-inflammatory properties, sulfapyridine and 5-aminosalicylic acid (5-ASA), respectively [2, 3]. In the colonic lumen, bacteria metabolize the azo bond that joins the subunits thereby releasing the therapeutically active 5-ASA and the inactive sulfapyridine [4]. Although effective for the treatment of IBD, the dose-related adverse effects and hypersensitivity reactions associated with sulfapyridine led to the development nonsulfa aminosalicylates. These modern formulations have similar efficacy as their predecessor and have improved side effect profiles.

Although the use of 5-ASAs in adults with IBD is well established, there is limited evidence for their safety and efficacy in the pediatric IBD population. This shortcoming is further accentuated by mounting evidence that suggests important differences between adult and pediatric IBD. Nonetheless, 5-ASAs are commonly used in pediatric IBD patients. Pending further studies of 5-ASAs in pediatric IBD, their use in this population remains mainly guided by the adult literature as detailed below.

Mechanism of Action

The exact mechanism of action of aminosalicylates in IBD remains unclear. The primary therapeutic effect of 5-ASA over the gastrointestinal mucosa is thought to be topical rather than systemic [5]. Colonic epithelial cells absorb 5-ASA and its effectiveness is in turn related to colonic mucosal concentrations. Systemic exposure remains low after oral and rectal administration. Current data suggest that 5-ASA induces the expression of a class of nuclear receptor genes, with resulting increased peroxisome proliferator-activated receptors (PPARs) in colonic epithelial cells. PPAR expression is particularly high in the colonic epithelium, and activation is largely driven by intestinal bacteria [6, 7]. PPAR-γ is involved in the control of inflammation, cell proliferation, apoptosis, and modulation of cytokine production. It has also been shown to have antitumorigenic effects [8]. As a result of these interactions, PPAR-γ may be the basis for future chemopreventive strategies against colorectal cancer (CRC) [9]. In turn, PPAR-γ expression has been shown to be down regulated in patients with active UC [10]. One randomized placebo controlled clinical trial of a PPAR-γ ligand (rosiglitazone) demonstrated efficacy in treating mild to moderate UC [11]. Cardiovascular side effects, however, have dampened enthusiasm for rosiglitazone. Other proposed mechanisms of action of 5-ASA have been described, including the inhibition of cyclooxygenase (COX) and 5-lipoxygenase pathways of arachidonic acid metabolism resulting in a decrease in pro-inflammatory prostaglandins and leukotrienes, and inhibition of interleukin-1, interleukin-2, and tumor necrosis factor-alpha [12]. 5-ASA has also been described as a potent antioxidant and free-radical scavenger [5, 12].

Pharmacokinetics

5-ASA is absorbed in the stomach and small intestine unless bound as a prodrug or combined with another delivery system [2]. As 5-ASA is thought to act topically, the clinical

M. Stephens, MD (✉) • M. Gonzalez, MD
Division of Pediatric Gastroenterology and Hepatology, Mayo Clinic Children's Center, 200 First Street SW, Rochester, MN 55905, USA
e-mail: stephens.michael@mayo.edu

© Springer International Publishing AG 2017
P. Mamula et al. (eds.), *Pediatric Inflammatory Bowel Disease*, DOI 10.1007/978-3-319-49215-5_25

Table 25.1 Preparations of 5-ASA

Drug	Formulation	Delivery system	Dosage form	Release location
Azo-bonded formulations				
Sulfasalazine (Azulfidine®)	Azo bond of 5-ASA to sulfapyridine	Broken down by colonic bacteria to release active 5-ASA moiety	Tablet 500 mg	Colon
Osalazine (Dipentum®)	Diazo bond of 5-ASA dimer	Broken down by colonic bacteria to release active 5-ASA moiety	Capsule 250 mg	Colon
Balsalazide (Colazal®)	Azo bond of 5-ASA and inactive carrier	Broken down by colonic bacteria to release active 5-ASA moiety	Capsule 750 mg	Colon
Mesalamine formulations				
Pentasa®	Controlled release	Time release	Capsules 250 mg, 500 mg	Small intestine, colon
Asacol®	Enteric coated; delayed release	pH-dependent (≥7)	Tablet 400 mg	Terminal ileum, colon
Asacol HD®	Enteric coated; delayed release	pH-dependent (≥7)	Tablet 800 mg	Terminal ileum, colon
Lialda®	Delayed release	pH-dependent (≥7)	Tablet 1200 mg	Terminal ileum, colon
Delzicol®	Delayed release	pH-dependent (≥7)	Capsule 400 mg	Terminal ileum, colon
Apriso®	Delayed and extended release	pH-dependent (≥6)	Capsule 375 mg	Terminal ileum, colon
Rowasa®	Topical		Rectal suspension 4 g/60 mL	Left colon
Canasa®	Topical		Suppository 1000 mg	Rectum

goal is to maximize delivery of the active drug to the site of inflammation in the colon while minimizing systemic absorption in the small intestine. Rectal gels, liquids, and foam enemas have been formulated to this effect [13]. However, these formulations have the undesirable side effects of leakage and abdominal bloating and many patients find them impractical. As a result, adherence to the dosing regimen is often poor, limiting their use as an adjunct therapy in many cases [14].

Oral 5-ASA agents are much better tolerated and are thought to be more practical and patient friendly. Sulfasalazine was the first prodrug that delivered 5-ASA to the colon via an azo-bond linked to sulfapyridine. This bond is cleaved by bacteria in the colon to release the active drug [2]. 5-ASA is primarily excreted in the stool, as it is poorly absorbed in the colon. The sulfapyridine component, however, is absorbed from the colon and then metabolized in the liver, with excretion through the urine. Due to the multiple dose-limiting side effects of sulfapyridine, newer formulations of 5-ASA have been created, with specific compositions to ensure delivery to the targeted area of inflammation. Some are bound to other prodrugs, while others are time-release preparations and pH-dependent release formulations [15–17]. The other prodrug formulations are olsalazine and balsalazide, which are bound by distinct azo bonds, and, like sulfasalazine, are then cleaved by intestinal bacteria, releasing the active medication into the colon. Olsalazine is a 5-ASA dimer linked by a diazo bond and balsalazide is 5-ASA linked to an inactive carrier molecule by a diazo bond.

pH-dependent delivery systems have been developed to target release of the active medication into the small bowel and colon. An acrylic-based resin, Eudragit, is used to coat these tablets. Asacol® and its newer bioequivalent, Delzicol® (mesalamine), are examples of such medications, and have been designed to release 5-ASA at a pH of 7 or higher in the terminal ileum and colon. Others have been formulated to release 5-ASA at a lower pH of 6 or greater, which are released more proximally in the ileum and through the colon.

Pentasa® (mesalamine) is a time-dependent release formulation in which the active drug is packaged into microgranules that are coated by ethylcellulose. The ethylcellulose coating dissolves when hydrated and the drug is released throughout the small intestine and colon.

Lialda® is a once-daily, high-strength formulation of mesalamine, utilizing Multi Matrix System (MMX) technology designed to deliver the active drug throughout the colon. The matrix is enclosed within a resistant coating which also disintegrates at a pH of 7.0 or greater, releasing the active medication within the terminal ileum and colon. Once the matrix is exposed to gut fluid, it expands and forms a viscous gel mass that is slowly released throughout the colon.

Most of the older formulations are limited by the amount of 5-ASA that can be delivered per capsule, which required that patients take multiple doses per day and several tablets per dose. However, the newer formulations allow for less frequent once to twice a day dosing and fewer amount of pills. Table 25.1 and Fig. 25.1 outline the formulations more commonly used in the United States, sites of action, and delivery system.

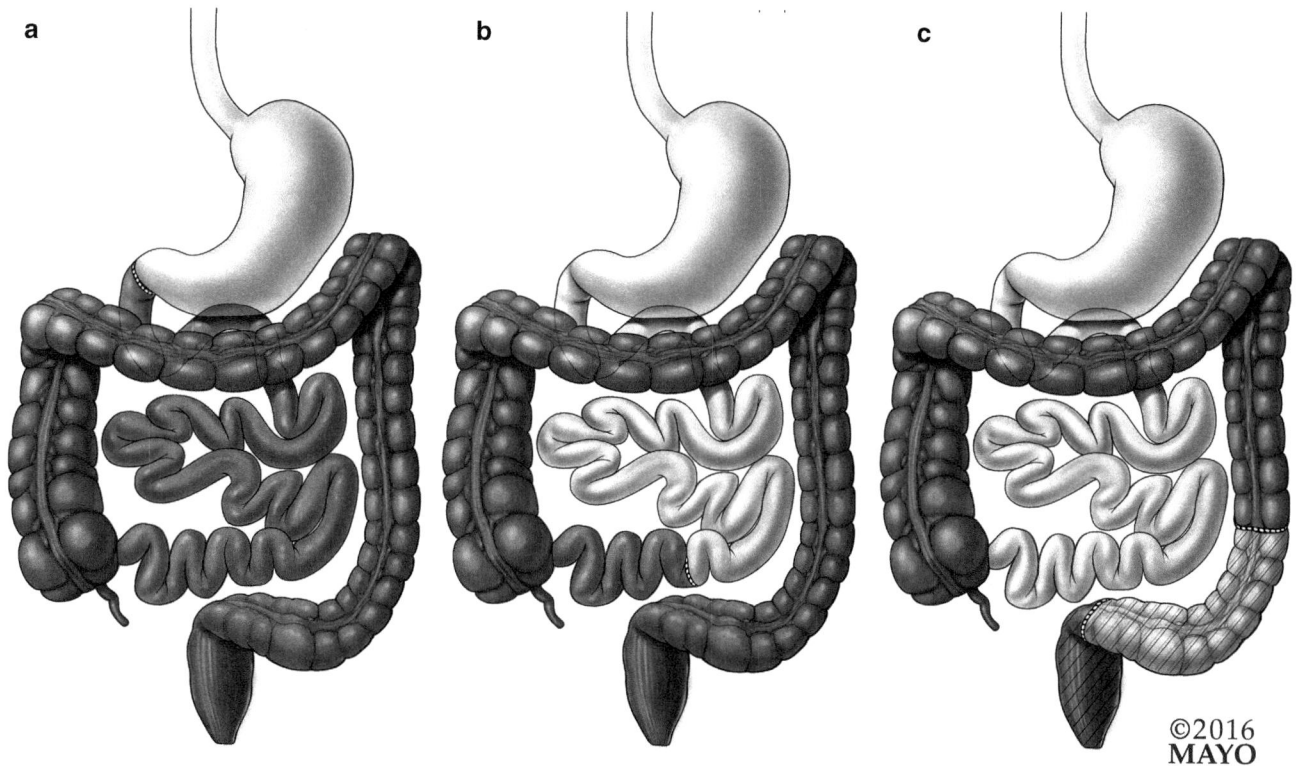

Fig. 25.1 (**a**) *Dark gray*: Pentasa. (**b**) *Dark gray*: Asacol, Asacol HD, Lialda, Apriso. (**c**) All three *shaded area*: Azulfidine, Colazal, Dipentum. *Light and dark striped*: Rowasa. *Dark striped only*: Canasa

Indications and Efficacy

Ulcerative Colitis

The efficacy of aminosalicylates for the induction and maintenance of remission of UC is well established in the adult literature and these medications remain the first-line treatment for mild to moderate disease [18, 19]. Although there is very little pediatric UC data, oral 5-ASA formulations are recommended as the first-line induction therapy for mild to moderately active pediatric UC as well [20].

In a recent systematic review and meta-analysis, both oral and rectal preparations of 5-ASAs were found to have modest efficacy at inducing remission in mild-to-moderate UC compared to placebo with no statistically significant difference between the preparations [21]. There is no standardized dosage or frequency of dosing for rectal preparations in inducing remission of UC. In the most recent Cochrane Review, rectal 5-ASA was superior to rectal steroids for inducing remission of UC [22]. There is improved efficacy with combined rectal and oral 5-ASA therapy compared with oral 5-ASA therapy alone [23]. Although there is no standard dosing of oral 5-ASA for inducing remission, doses of 1.5–4.8 g/day have been shown to be effective depending on disease severity. The result of the ASCEND I and II trials show a statistically significant higher rate of mucosal healing in

UC at 6 weeks with a dose of 4.8 g/day of delayed-release oral mesalazine over 2.4 g/day dosing [24]. However, a recent randomized control trial in pediatric UC patients showed equal effectiveness of high- and low-dose oral delayed-release mesalamine for achievement of clinical remission [25]. The reduction in fecal biomarkers, calprotectin and lactoferrin, was not statistically significant between the groups. Despite improved efficacy of combined oral and rectal 5-ASA therapy for inducing remission over oral 5-ASA alone, the remission rates are still significantly lower than with corticosteroids alone [22]. In UC, mesalamine has similar efficacy to sulfasalazine at equimolar doses.

Both oral and rectal mesalamine are more efficacious in preventing relapse of quiescent UC than placebo [19]. There are many randomized control trials that show topical 5-ASAs have comparable efficacy at preventing relapse of quiescent UC. On the other hand, in one recent meta-analysis, intermittent rectal mesalamine was superior to oral 5-ASAs with a number needed to treat (NNT) of 4 [23, 26]. In another recent meta-analysis, topical mesalamine was more effective at preventing relapse of quiescent UC compared to placebo with a NNT of 3 [27]. This study also showed a trend toward a greater effect size with continuous topical therapy compared with intermittent topical therapy. The analysis showed lower relapse rates when an overall higher total weekly dose of topical mesalamine was used, similar to the occurrence with higher doses of oral 5-ASA therapy for preventing relapse of quiescent UC. However, the majority of the patients in this study had only left-sided disease or proctitis.

In the adult population, oral 5-ASA has modest efficacy in maintaining remission of quiescent UC with good adherence but there is no standardized dosing regimen. Some of the more recent studies not only assessed efficacy in maintaining remission in UC, but also adherence to the prescribed treatment. In one recent study of MMX mesalamine at 2.4 g/day, there was only a 30% recurrence rate at 12 months for patients who were adherent to the medication more than 80% of the time, as compared to a 53% relapse rate at 12 months for patients who were less than 80% adherent to the medication regimen [28]. A meta-analysis showed that once-daily dosing of oral mesalamine was equally as effective as conventional dosing in preventing relapse in quiescent UC over 12 months of therapy [29, 30]. Although 5-ASA has proven to be effective in maintaining remission in quiescent ulcerative colitis, adherence must be considered when developing an individual's treatment plan.

There are a few studies evaluating the efficacy of 5-ASA for the treatment and maintenance of remission in pediatric UC. There is one recent study on the efficacy of mesalamine 500 mg suppositories for the treatment of ulcerative proctitis in children. For the 49 patients enrolled, there was a statistically significant decrease in the disease activity index at 3 weeks. 41 patients had a mild or an unrelated adverse event [31]. Another recent pediatric study compared the efficacy of oral beclomethasone dipropionate (BDP) to oral 5-ASA in the treatment of mild to moderate UC in the pediatric population. The results of the study showed clinical remission was achieved after 4 weeks in 12 of 15 patients treated with BDP but only 5 of 15 patients treated with 5-ASA, thus showing BDP more efficacious at inducing remission in mild to moderate pediatric UC than 5-ASA [32].

In general, the preparation of 5-ASA used is dependent on the location and the severity of disease. In addition, in pediatrics, particularly in the younger age groups who potentially have greater difficulty in swallowing pills, the mode of delivery is also crucial. There are currently no 5-ASA liquid formulations. However, certain capsule formulations, namely Pentasa® and Colazal®, may be opened and the content emptied into foods such as yogurt and peanut butter. Data on the efficacy of this practice, however, have not been published to date.

Rectal formulations are usually a reasonable starting choice in patients with mild disease limited to the rectum or left colon [33]. Adherence needs to be considered when using these formulations. Patients with more extensive disease involving the transverse and ascending colon may require the addition of an oral preparation.

Dosing of oral 5-ASA in the pediatric population is variable, but the dosages usually fall in the range of 30–100 mg/

kg/day. More recent guidelines established by ESPGHAN and the European Crohn's and Colitis Organisation (ECCO) suggest a dose of 60–80 mg/kg/day in 2 daily doses up to 4.8 g daily for mesalazine, and 40–70 mg/kg/day in 2 divided doses with a maximum of 4 g per day for sulfasalazine. Higher doses have been used, although it is not evidence based. For rectal dosing, 25 mg/kg up to a maximum of 1 g may be used once daily [20].

Crohn's Disease

The efficacy of 5-ASA in the induction and maintenance of remission in Crohn's disease (CD) is controversial. Currently, their use in treatment of pediatric CD is limited and only recommended in selected patients with very mild disease [34]. In a recent Cochrane review consisting of adult studies, sulfasalazine showed only a modest effect over placebo in inducing remission in mild to moderate CD at a dose of 3-6 g/day [35]. It showed a 38% higher chance of inducing remission compared to placebo-treated patients. However, this effect was limited to patients with Crohn colitis. Sulfasalazine was 34% less effective at inducing remission than corticosteroids alone and it was less effective than combination therapy with corticosteroids and sulfasalazine. Two studies, the Trial of Adjunctive Sulfasalazine (TAS) in Crohn's disease and the European Cooperative Crohn's Disease Study (ECCDS), showed that sulfasalazine was not a useful adjunct to corticosteroid therapy in achieving remission [36, 37].

A recent systematic review and meta-analysis of randomized controlled trials that excluded the Crohn's III trial data also suggests a modest effect of 5-ASA drugs inducing remission of active CD over placebo-treated patients with a NNT of 11 to prevent one patient's disease remaining active [38]. The effect was based on a mean reduction in CDAI scores. Had the data from the Crohn's III trial been available, the authors suspect there would have been no statistically significant difference between the 5-ASA treated group and the placebo-treated group. According to the latest Cochrane review, low-dose controlled-release mesalamine (1–2 g/day) was less effective at inducing remission in active CD compared to placebo-treated patients [35]. As with sulfasalazine, delayed-release mesalamine (2 g/day) was less efficacious than corticosteroids [39]. Trials evaluating higher doses of mesalamine (3–4.5 g/day) show inconsistent results. The majority of the studies show no difference in induction of remission in mild to moderately active CD relative to placebo [35]. Two of the studies showed statistically significant changes in CDAI scores, but they were found to be clinically insignificant. In a single trial, high dose mesalamine was less effective than budesonide [40]. Many of these studies were small and had several methodological weaknesses, which may limit the generalizability of the effects of mesalamine at inducing remission in mild to moderately active CD.

One pediatric study reviewed disease activity at diagnosis in 43 patients and compared the outcomes of single versus combination therapies. Ten of 25 patients in the mild group and 3 of 18 patients in the moderate to severe group received 5-ASA monotherapy immediately after diagnosis. These patients tended to have more exacerbations, shorter duration of the first remission, and longer total duration of systemic steroid use than patients receiving combination therapy, immunomodulators, or systemic steroids [41].

The role of 5-ASAs in maintaining remission in quiescent CD was also assessed in the review by Ford et al. No statistical significant benefit over placebo was found, although subgroup analysis of trials with low risk of bias showed mesalamine to be of benefit in preventing relapse with a NNT of 13 [38, 42]. This was the same result when a more conservative protocol analysis was completed, in which dropouts from individual studies were not considered treatment failures. There is one pediatric study evaluating maintenance of remission in CD patients after successful flare-up therapy with either nutrition or medications that showed that the relapse rate was similar with mesalazine and placebo [43].

Overall, evidence does not support the use of mesalamine for maintenance treatment in pediatric CD. Many gastroenterologists continue to use aminosalicylates in CD despite multiple studies showing at best a modest benefit over placebo [35]. The dosing of oral 5-ASA for pediatric CD is similar to that for pediatric UC with 50–80 mg/kg/day up to 4 g daily [34].

Surgically Induced Remission of Crohn's Disease and Prevention of Postoperative Recurrence

Surgical resection can induce remission in CD. However, endoscopic and clinical relapse of CD after surgical resection is common and has been reported to be as high as 75–90% and 20–30%, respectively, within 1 year [44, 45]. There is currently no standard therapy for preventing relapse post-operatively. Aminosalicylates in the postoperative setting have been extensively studied, but their effectiveness at preventing relapse after surgical resection remains controversial. In a systematic review and meta-analysis of 11 randomized controlled trials, the effect of mesalamine appears to be modest with a NNT of 13 compared to placebo or not treating after surgery [46]. In a Cochrane review, the effectiveness of mesalamine was even more modest with a NNT of 16–19 [47]. However, this effect seems to be limited to mesalamine only, as sulfasalazine demonstrated no advantage over the control therapy. There is heterogeneity in all of these studies including the dosage and preparation used, the length of treatment postsurgery, and the definition of remission. In a more recent network meta-analysis comparing different pharmacologic interventions in preventing relapse of CD after surgery, mesalamine was shown to reduce the risk of clinical relapse (relative risk or RR 0.60; 95% credible interval or CrI 0.37–0.88), but not endoscopic relapse (RR 0.67; 95% CrI 0.39–1.08) when compared to placebo [48].

Chemoprevention of Colorectal Carcinoma

Due to their structural similarity to aspirin, which has been shown to reduce the risk of CRC and adenomas in patients without IBD, it was believed that 5-ASAs had a similar effect on patients with a diagnosis of IBD [49]. However, more recent studies suggest that they may not provide much, if any, chemoprophylaxis for CRC. A population-based study including more than 8000 patients found that there was no protective effect of 5-ASA against CRC [50, 51]. This study evaluated the cumulative use of 5-ASA at 1, 5, and 7.5 years. Adherence to 5-ASA therapy was based on the frequency of prescription refills. It is possible that the cumulative use for longer than 7.5 years could be chemopreventive, but this has not been studied. In contrast, one small case-controlled study found that cumulative mesalamine doses decreased the risk of CRC in patients with IBD [52]. There are also several studies that have observed a significant chemopreventive effect of mesalamine compounds, especially at doses of >1.2 g/day. However, these studies been criticized because of the design, outcomes measured, and variables controlled for [53]. A more recent meta-analysis evaluating the nonreferral IBD patients suggested no protective effect of 5-ASA on CRC in IBD [54]. These results are, however, limited by the heterogeneity of the studies included. A chemopreventive effect was not seen in patients who received sulfasalazine regardless of setting (referral versus nonreferral).

As noted above, the exact mechanism of action of 5-ASA in the treatment of IBD is unknown, and the same can be said regarding chemoprophylaxis. One retrospective cohort study attempted to determine where in the dysplasia-carcinoma sequence they would exert their protective effect. The study identified patients with UC with no dysplasia, indefinite dysplasia, or flat low-grade dysplasia (LGD) and followed them for the development of high-grade dysplasia (HGD) or CRC. The data suggest that if mesalamine has any chemopreventive effect, it may act early in the neoplastic process before the development of LGD [53]. There are many in vivo and in vitro studies currently looking at the anti-inflammatory and antineoplastic effects on different proposed mechanism of action pathways, including inhibition of cyclooxygenase activity, enhanced apoptosis through inhibition of NF-κB and MAP kinases, improvement in the DNA replication process, inhibition of reactive oxygen species, and downregulation of oncogenes and transcription factors [49, 55]. 5-ASA is now thought to be involved in inhibition of protein synthesis, which may contribute to its anti-inflammatory and antineoplastic properties [56].

Side Effects

Sulfasalazine (SASP) therapy is usually accompanied with more side effects than the 5-ASA formulations due to the sulfapyridine moiety [2]. Up to 80–90% of patients who cannot tolerate sulfasalazine tolerate 5-ASA preparations [57]. In addition, patients who experience adverse reactions to a particular 5-ASA formulation often tolerate a different preparation.

Side effects of 5-ASA are listed in Table 25.2. The most common side effects of both SASP and 5-ASA are nausea, abdominal pain, diarrhea, dyspepsia, rash, and fever [58, 59]. Some of these effects, such as diarrhea, can be mitigated by a gradual increase in the dose [60]. Rare, but more serious side effects, include interstitial nephritis, pancreatitis, pericarditis, pneumonitis, hepatitis, neutropenia, and rarely, worsening colitis [57–59]. The risk of interstitial nephritis and pancreatitis is higher with 5-ASA, while the risk of hepatitis is higher

Table 25.2 Side effects of 5-ASA and sulfasalazine

5-ASA	Sulfasalazine
Common	*Common*
Headache	Headache
Diarrhea	Nausea
Nausea	Vomiting
Flatulence	Abdominal pain
Abdominal pain	Diarrhea
Rash	Anorexia
	Dyspepsia
	Rash
	Fever
Less common	*Less common*
Nephritis	Pancreatitis
Interstitial pneumonitis	Hepatitis
Worsening of colitis	Drug-induced connective tissue disease
Pancreatitis	Bone marrow suppression
Myopericarditis	Nephrotoxicity
	Interstitial nephritis
	Oligospermia
	Hemolytic anemia
	Folate deficiency
	Alveolitis

with SASP. Agranulocytosis, hemolytic anemia, and oligospermia have also been reported with SASP [59].

The safety profile of these medications in the pediatric literature is similar to that in adults [31, 61, 62]. As there are reports of hypersensitivity to 5-ASA causing worsening colitis, it can be challenging to clinically differentiate the gastrointestinal symptoms of diarrhea and abdominal pain as medication side effects from worsening underlying disease. There are no standard guidelines for monitoring these medications and the possible hypersensitivities. However, most studies and literature suggest regularly monitoring renal function.

5-ASA appears to be safe in pregnant and breastfeeding women [63–65]. Only a small amount of the drug is transferred to breast milk. There are reports of allergic reactions in nursing infants in the form of acute watery diarrhea [66, 67]. This usually resolves with cessation of the drug.

Adherence

Adherence to long-term 5-ASA therapy is of great concern in clinical practice. Approximately 40–60% of patients with UC do not take their oral 5-ASA therapy as prescribed [68]. Despite the benefits, the lowest adherence rates are in patients with quiescent UC, who may not understand the importance of continuing treatment when they are in clinical remission. Patients who are nonadherent have an increased risk of disease relapse than those patients who are adherent at least 80% of the time. Many factors contribute to nonadherence including dosing frequency, the number of pills, fear of side effects, and disease extent and duration [69, 70]. Before the introduction of delayed release and high dose formulations, 5-ASA was given in 3 to 4 divided doses per day. However, these newer formulations require twice daily or daily dosing with the same efficacy of conventional dosing. In a recent study looking at the persistency of oral 5-ASA therapy, patients receiving Lialda (MMX mesalamine) had significantly higher persistency at 12 months compared with patients receiving other oral 5-ASA formulations [71]. This study was from a large pharmacy database, but correlates with the understanding that simpler treatment plans lead to improved adherence in a number of chronic diseases, including UC [69]. There are few studies on adherence to medical regimens in the pediatric IBD population. Limited data suggest that patient age and emotional and behavioral functioning make a substantial contribution toward predicting adherence to oral 5-ASA [72]. Adolescents in the older age group (15–18 years old), for example, have been found to have lower rates of adherence than younger age groups.

A recent retrospective analysis on long-term mesalamine maintenance in adult patients with UC suggests that adherence, rather than daily dose, reduces long-term flare risk [73]. Thus, it is essential to take the time and discuss with each patient the importance of compliance and persistency.

Conclusion

5-ASA is a well-established first-line therapy for mild to moderate UC in the adult population. This remains an important option for children with mild to moderate UC. Its role in pediatric CD is limited given the lack of data supporting its efficacy. Few studies have addressed the use of 5-ASA in the pediatric population. An important step forward can be expected from the NIH-funded Predicting Response to Standardized Pediatric Colitis Therapy (PROTECT) Study. This will garner valuable efficacy, safety, and adherence data of 5-ASA in a large pediatric population. Also, robust phenotypic data will be paired with a comprehensive search for biomarkers (genetic, serologic, microbiome) that predict response and disease behavior.

References

1. Bergman R, Parkes M. Systematic review: the use of mesalazine in inflammatory bowel disease. Aliment Pharmacol Ther. 2006;23(7): 841–55.
2. Campregher C, Gasche C. Aminosalicylates. Best Pract Res Clin Gastroenterol. 2011;25(4–5):535–46.
3. Pithadia AB, Jain S. Treatment of inflammatory bowel disease (IBD). Pharmacol Rep. 2011;63(3):629–42.
4. Azadkhan AK, Truelove SC, Aronson JK. The disposition and metabolism of sulphasalazine (salicylazosulphapyridine) in man. Br J Clin Pharmacol. 1982;13(4):523–8.
5. Sandborn WJ. Treatment of ulcerative colitis with oral mesalamine: advances in drug formulation, efficacy expectations and dose response, compliance, and chemoprevention. Rev Gastroenterol Disord. 2006;6(2):97–105.
6. Desreumaux P, Ghosh S. Review article: mode of action and delivery of 5-aminosalicylic acid – new evidence. Aliment Pharmacol Ther. 2006;24(Suppl 1):2–9.
7. Egan LJ et al. Inhibition of interleukin-1-stimulated NF-kappaB RelA/p65 phosphorylation by mesalamine is accompanied by decreased transcriptional activity. J Biol Chem. 1999;274(37):26448–53.
8. Girnun GD et al. APC-dependent suppression of colon carcinogenesis by PPARgamma. Proc Natl Acad Sci U S A. 2002;99(21):13771–6.
9. Iacucci M, de Silva S, Ghosh S. Mesalazine in inflammatory bowel disease: a trendy topic once again? Can J Gastroenterol. 2010; 24(2):127–33.
10. Yamamoto-Furusho JK, Penaloza-Coronel A, Sánchez-Muñoz F, Barreto-Zuñiga R, Dominguez-Lopez A. Peroxisome proliferator-activated receptor-gamma (PPAR-γ) expression is downregulated in patients with active ulcerative colitis. Inflamm Bowel Dis. 2011; 17:680–1.
11. Lewis JD et al. Rosiglitazone for active ulcerative colitis: a randomized placebo-controlled trial. Gastroenterology. 2008;134(3):688–95.
12. MacDermott RP. Progress in understanding the mechanisms of action of 5-aminosalicylic acid. Am J Gastroenterol. 2000;95(12):3343–5.
13. Harris MS, Lichtenstein GR. Review article: delivery and efficacy of topical 5-aminosalicylic acid (mesalazine) therapy in the treatment of ulcerative colitis. Aliment Pharmacol Ther. 2011;33(9): 996–1009.

14. Prantera C, Rizzi M. 5-ASA in ulcerative colitis: improving treatment compliance. World J Gastroenterol. 2009;15(35):4353–5.
15. Baumgart DC, Sandborn WJ. Inflammatory bowel disease: clinical aspects and established and evolving therapies. Lancet. 2007; 369(9573):1641–57.
16. Sandborn WJ. Oral 5-ASA therapy in ulcerative colitis: what are the implications of the new formulations? J Clin Gastroenterol. 2008;42(4):338–44.
17. Cohen RD, Safdi AV. 5-ASA treatment for ulcerative colitis: what's on the horizon? Gastroenterol Hepatol. 2008;4(11):5–14.
18. Kornbluth A, Sachar DB. Ulcerative colitis practice guidelines in adults (update): American College of Gastroenterology, Practice Parameters Committee. Am J Gastroenterol. 2004;99(7):1371–85.
19. Sutherland L, Macdonald JK. Oral 5-aminosalicylic acid for induction of remission in ulcerative colitis. Cochrane Database Syst Rev. 2006;2:CD000543.
20. Turner D et al. Management of pediatric ulcerative colitis: joint ECCO and ESPGHAN evidence-based consensus guidelines. J Pediatr Gastroenterol Nutr. 2012;55(3):340–61.
21. Ford AC et al. Efficacy of 5-aminosalicylates in ulcerative colitis: systematic review and meta-analysis. Am J Gastroenterol. 2011; 106(4):601–16.
22. Marshall JK et al. Rectal 5-aminosalicylic acid for induction of remission in ulcerative colitis. Cochrane Database Syst Rev. 2010;1:CD004115.
23. Ford AC et al. Efficacy of oral vs. topical, or combined oral and topical 5-aminosalicylates, in Ulcerative Colitis: systematic review and meta-analysis. Am J Gastroenterol. 2012;107(2):167–76. author reply 177.
24. Lichtenstein GR, Ramsey D, Rubin DT. Randomised clinical trial: delayed-release oral mesalazine 4.8 g/day vs. 2.4 g/day in endoscopic mucosal healing – ASCEND I and II combined analysis. Aliment Pharmacol Ther. 2011;33(6):672–8.
25. Winter HS et al. High- and low-dose oral delayed-release mesalamine in children with mild-to-moderately active ulcerative colitis. J Pediatr Gastroenterol Nutr. 2014;59(6):767–72.
26. Mantzaris GJ et al. Intermittent therapy with high-dose 5-aminosalicylic acid enemas maintains remission in ulcerative proctitis and proctosigmoiditis. Dis Colon Rectum. 1994;37(1): 58–62.
27. Ford AC et al. Efficacy of topical 5-aminosalicylates in preventing relapse of quiescent ulcerative colitis: a meta-analysis. Clin Gastroenterol Hepatol Off Clin Pract J Am Gastroenterol Assoc. 2012;10(5):513–9.
28. Kane S et al. Strategies in maintenance for patients receiving long-term therapy (SIMPLE): a study of MMX mesalamine for the long-term maintenance of quiescent ulcerative colitis. Inflamm Bowel Dis. 2012;18(6):1026–33.
29. Ford AC et al. Once-daily dosing vs. conventional dosing schedule of mesalamine and relapse of quiescent ulcerative colitis: systematic review and meta-analysis. Am J Gastroenterol. 2011;106(12): 2070–7. quiz 2078.
30. Kamm MA et al. Randomised trial of once- or twice-daily MMX mesalazine for maintenance of remission in ulcerative colitis. Gut. 2008;57(7):893–902.
31. Heyman MB et al. Efficacy and safety of mesalamine suppositories for treatment of ulcerative proctitis in children and adolescents. Inflamm Bowel Dis. 2010;16(11):1931–9.
32. Romano C et al. Oral beclomethasone dipropionate in pediatric active ulcerative colitis: a comparison trial with mesalazine. J Pediatr Gastroenterol Nutr. 2010;50(4):385–9.
33. Regan BP, Bousvaros A. Pediatric ulcerative colitis: a practical guide to management. Pediatr Drugs. 2014;16(3):189–98.
34. Ruemmele FM et al. Consensus guidelines of ECCO/ESPGHAN on the medical management of pediatric Crohn's disease. J Crohns Colitis. 2014;8(10):1179–207.

35. Lim WC, Hanauer S. Aminosalicylates for induction of remission or response in Crohn's disease. Cochrane Database Syst Rev. 2010;12:CD008870.

36. Singleton JW et al. A trial of sulfasalazine as adjunctive therapy in Crohn's disease. Gastroenterology. 1979;77(4 Pt 2):887–97.

37. Malchow H et al. European Cooperative Crohn's Disease Study (ECCDS): results of drug treatment. Gastroenterology. 1984;86(2):249–66.

38. Ford AC et al. Efficacy of 5-aminosalicylates in Crohn's disease: systematic review and meta-analysis. Am J Gastroenterol. 2011;106(4):617–29.

39. Scholmerich J, Hartmann F, Dopper H. Oral 5-aminosalicylic acid versus 6-methylprednisolone in active Crohn's disease. Can J Gastroenterol. 1990;4:446–51.

40. Thomsen OO et al. A comparison of budesonide and mesalamine for active Crohn's disease. International Budesonide-Mesalamine Study Group. N Engl J Med. 1998;339(6):370–4.

41. Mesker T et al. Pediatric Crohn's disease activity at diagnosis, its influence on pediatrician's prescribing behavior, and clinical outcome 5 years later. Inflamm Bowel Dis. 2009;15(11):1670–7.

42. Akobeng AK, Gardener E. Oral 5-aminosalicylic acid for maintenance of medically-induced remission in Crohn's disease. Cochrane Database Syst Rev. 2005;1:CD003715.

43. Cezard JP et al. Prevention of relapse by mesalazine (Pentasa) in pediatric Crohn's disease: a multicenter, double-blind, randomized, placebo-controlled trial. Gastroenterol Clin Biol. 2009;33(1 Pt 1):31–40.

44. Rutgeerts P et al. Natural history of recurrent Crohn's disease at the ileocolonic anastomosis after curative surgery. Gut. 1984;25(6):665–72.

45. Rutgeerts P et al. Predictability of the postoperative course of Crohn's disease. Gastroenterology. 1990;99(4):956–63.

46. Ford AC et al. 5-aminosalicylates prevent relapse of Crohn's disease after surgically induced remission: systematic review and meta-analysis. Am J Gastroenterol. 2011;106(3):413–20.

47. Gordon M et al. Oral 5-aminosalicylic acid for maintenance of surgically-induced remission in Crohn's disease. Cochrane Database Syst Rev. 2011;1:CD008414.

48. Singh S et al. Comparative efficacy of pharmacologic interventions in preventing relapse of Crohn's disease after surgery: a systematic review and network meta-analysis. Gastroenterology. 2015;148(1):64–76. e2; quiz e14.

49. Wasan SK, Farraye FA. Do 5-ASAs prevent colorectal neoplasia in patients with ulcerative colitis? Still no answers COMMENT. Inflamm Bowel Dis. 2010;16(2):358–60.

50. Bernstein CN, Nugent Z, Blanchard JF. 5-aminosalicylate is not chemoprophylactic for colorectal cancer in IBD: a population based study. Am J Gastroenterol. 2011;106(4):731–6.

51. Terdiman JP et al. 5-aminosalicylic acid therapy and the risk of colorectal cancer among patients with inflammatory bowel disease. Inflamm Bowel Dis. 2007;13(4):367–71.

52. Tang J et al. Mesalamine protects against colorectal cancer in inflammatory bowel disease. Dig Dis Sci. 2010;55(6):1696–703.

53. Farraye FA et al. AGA technical review on the diagnosis and management of colorectal neoplasia in inflammatory bowel disease. Gastroenterology. 2010;138(2):746–U438.

54. Nguyen GC, Gulamhusein A, Bernstein CN. 5-aminosalicylic acid is not protective against colorectal cancer in inflammatory bowel disease: a meta-analysis of non-referral populations. Am J Gastroenterol. 2012;107(9):1298–305.

55. Munding J et al. The influence of 5-aminosalicylic acid on the progression of colorectal adenomas via the beta-catenin signaling pathway. Carcinogenesis. 2012;33(3):637–43.

56. Lyakhovich A et al. Interaction of mesalasine (5-ASA) with translational initiation factors eIF4 partially explains 5-ASA anti-inflammatory and anti-neoplastic activities. Med Chem. 2011;7(2):92–8.

57. Moum B. Which are the 5-ASA compound side effects and how is it possible to avoid them? Inflamm Bowel Dis. 2008;14:S212–3.

58. Baker DE, Kane S. The short- and long-term safety of 5-aminosalicylate products in the treatment of ulcerative colitis. Rev Gastroenterol Disord. 2004;4(2):86–91.

59. Ransford RA, Langman MJ. Sulphasalazine and mesalazine: serious adverse reactions re-evaluated on the basis of suspected adverse reaction reports to the Committee on Safety of Medicines. Gut. 2002;51(4):536–9.

60. Rao SS, Cann PA, Holdsworth CD. Clinical experience of the tolerance of mesalazine and olsalazine in patients intolerant of sulphasalazine. Scand J Gastroenterol. 1987;22(3):332–6.

61. Barden L et al. Mesalazine in childhood inflammatory bowel-disease. Aliment Pharmacol Ther. 1989;3(6):597–603.

62. DAgata ID, Vanounou T, Seidman E. Mesalamine in pediatric inflammatory bowel disease: A 10-year experience. Inflamm Bowel Dis. 1996;2(4):229–35.

63. Mogadam M et al. Pregnancy in inflammatory bowel disease: effect of sulfasalazine and corticosteroids on fetal outcome. Gastroenterology. 1981;80(1):72–6.

64. Habal FM, Hui G, Greenberg GR. Oral 5-aminosalicylic acid for inflammatory bowel disease in pregnancy: safety and clinical course. Gastroenterology. 1993;105(4):1057–60.

65. Bell CM, Habal FM. Safety of topical 5-aminosalicylic acid in pregnancy. Am J Gastroenterol. 1997;92(12):2201–2.

66. Ito S et al. Prospective follow-up of adverse reactions in breast-fed infants exposed to maternal medication. Am J Obstet Gynecol. 1993;168(5):1393–9.

67. Nelis GF. Diarrhea due to 5-aminosalicylic acid in breast-milk. Lancet. 1989;1(8634):383–3.

68. Moshkovska T et al. An investigation of medication adherence to 5-aminosalicylic acid therapy in patients with ulcerative colitis, using self-report and urinary drug excretion measurements. Aliment Pharmacol Ther. 2009;30(11–12):1118–27.

69. Higgins PDR et al. Systematic review: impact of non-adherence to 5-aminosalicylic acid products on the frequency and cost of ulcerative colitis flares. Aliment Pharmacol Ther. 2009;29(3):247–57.

70. Hommel KA, Davis CM, Baldassano RN. Medication adherence and quality of life in pediatric inflammatory bowel disease. J Pediatr Psychol. 2008;33(8):867–74.

71. Kane SV et al. Twelve-month persistency with oral 5-aminosalicylic acid therapy for ulcerative colitis: results from a large pharmacy prescriptions database. Dig Dis Sci. 2011;56(12):3463–70.

72. LeLeiko NS et al. Rates and predictors of oral medication adherence in pediatric patients with IBD. Inflamm Bowel Dis. 2013;19(4):832–9.

73. Khan N et al. Long-term mesalamine maintenance in ulcerative colitis: which is more important? Adherence or daily dose. Inflamm Bowel Dis. 2013;19(6):1123–9.

Antibiotic Therapy

26

Lindsey Albenberg, Howard Kader, and Adam Paul

Introduction

Treatment of inflammatory bowel disease (IBD) with antibiotics has been used for several decades. Such utilization was initially intuitive and over the past couple of decades shown to be effective. There is a triad relationship believed to be involved in the pathogenesis of IBD, genetic susceptibility – environmental antigen – host immune response. Given the exposure to foreign bacteria as well as host bacteria colonization, studies have shown that certain aspects of bacteria trigger an immune response that leads to intestinal mucosal inflammation. For reasons still not known, genetically susceptible patients lack the ability to turn off this immune system activation resulting in perpetual intestinal mucosal inflammation and clinical symptoms of IBD [1]. Additionally, patients with Crohn disease (CD) who have diverting ileostomies demonstrate a downstream decrease in disease activity when the fecal stream is interrupted and recurrence when placed back into continuity [2]. A specific infectious agent has yet to be identified, but more likely than not, it may not be any one organism but rather the process of the host's immune reaction to an infectious stimulus or to the commensal microbiota that ultimately results in the development of IBD in the susceptible individual. Antibiotics therefore pos-

sess the ability to change the course of inflammatory bowel disease in a variety of ways including reducing luminal bacterial content, changing the composition of the gut microbiota, reducing bacterial invasion of intestinal tissue, and limiting bacterial translocation [3]. An immunomodulatory effect has also been proposed [4].

Unfortunately, there are no randomized therapeutic antibiotic studies that have been performed in children with IBD to assess the efficacy and validity of their use. Most reported pediatric studies have at best mentioned that concurrent antibiotic use was permitted if already taking it during that specific study involving another medication intervention. Consequently, the pediatric gastroenterologist must extrapolate from and rely on adult evidence-based medicine clinical trials (class I or II studies) regarding the role of antibiotic therapy in the treatment of IBD.

The most frequently used maintenance antibiotics in management of adult IBD are metronidazole and ciprofloxacin. Ciprofloxacin has uniformly not been used in the treatment of children due to concerns regarding development of musculoskeletal disorders noted in studies of juvenile animals. To date, no long-term ciprofloxacin studies in children have been published, but short-term treatment of urinary tract infections and other infectious illnesses without adverse events can be found. Metronidazole has Food and Drug Administration's approval for the use in children for the treatment of infections and has been utilized in the chronic treatment of IBD.

L. Albenberg, DO (✉)
Perelman School of Medicine, The University of Pennsylvania, Philadelphia, PA, USA

Division of Pediatric Gastroenterology, Hepatology, and Nutrition, The Children's Hospital of Philadelphia, 3401 Civic Center Blvd, Philadelphia, PA 19104, USA
e-mail: albenbergl@email.chop.edu

H. Kader, MD
Department of Pediatrics, Division of Pediatric Gastroenterology and Nutrition, University of Maryland Children's Hospital, Baltimore, MD, USA

A. Paul, DO
Lehigh Valley Children's Hospital, Allentown, PA, USA

Antibiotic Use in Crohn Disease

Based on adult IBD trials, metronidazole and ciprofloxacin have shown significance in the management of mild to moderate Crohn disease involving the distal small bowel as well as perianal disease related to enterocutaneous fistula(e) and perhaps delay in recurrence after ileal resection [5, 6].

© Springer International Publishing AG 2017
P. Mamula et al. (eds.), *Pediatric Inflammatory Bowel Disease*, DOI 10.1007/978-3-319-49215-5_26

Active Crohn Disease

Several studies have been carried out over the last 30 years evaluating the use of antibiotics in active Crohn disease. While the results of many of these studies are conflicting, a recent meta-analysis of 15 randomized controlled trials demonstrated a small but statistically significant benefit of antibiotics in the treatment of Crohn disease [7]. In the only published prospective efficacy study in children, Hildebrand et al. evaluated the open-label use of oral metronidazole 10–35 mg/kg in 20 children between the ages of 7 and 18 years with active Crohn disease. This group demonstrated improvement in clinical symptoms in 15/20 patients (12 improved, three moderately improved) who were followed up for 6 months. Additionally, they reported that of 12 patients who were improved, nine discontinued the medication after 6 months with return of symptoms in seven patients within 11 months [8].

While pediatric studies evaluating the use of antibiotics in active Crohn disease are limited, several adult trials, both randomized and non-randomized, have been published. Ursing and Kamme described the use of metronidazole in five patients with Crohn disease and reported a response in four of them [9]. In the first double-blinded comparative study involving antibiotics, metronidazole was compared to sulfasalazine in active Crohn disease in 78 patients. Patients were randomized to receive either metronidazole or sulfasalazine for 4 months and then crossed over to receive the alternate drug for an additional 4 months. The authors found that metronidazole was slightly more effective than sulfasalazine in treating active Crohn disease based on improvements in the Crohn Disease Activity Index (CDAI) [3]. Further double-blinded studies, including one performed by Sutherland et al., evaluated two doses of metronidazole (20 and 10 mg/kg) versus placebo. One hundred and five patients were randomized, and 56 completed the 16-week study. The authors found significant reductions in disease activity index scores and serum orosomucoid levels among the groups receiving metronidazole versus those who received placebo. The authors also found that patients with both large and small disease responded better to therapy than those with isolated small bowel disease [10].

Few randomized trials have been published evaluating the use of ciprofloxacin as monotherapy in active Crohn disease. In a randomized study conducted by Colombel et al., 40 patients with mild to moderate active Crohn disease received either ciprofloxacin or mesalamine for 6 weeks. The authors found similar response rates 56 % versus 55 % among patients who received ciprofloxacin versus those who received mesalamine as assessed by improvements in CDAI scores [11]. Ciprofloxacin was also compared to placebo in a study conducted by Arnold et al. The authors randomized 47 patients with active, resistant moderate Crohn disease to receive ciprofloxacin or placebo in combination with their previously prescribed conventional therapies and followed the patients for 6 months. Significant decreases in CDAI were observed in the ciprofloxacin-treated group 187–112 versus 230–205 in the placebo-treated group [12].

Several studies conducted in adults have evaluated the use of combination therapy with ciprofloxacin and metronidazole in active Crohn disease. Response rates varied among the studies, but all demonstrated improvements ranging from 45 to 90 % in patients who used combined therapies, with the best responses among those patients with colonic involvement [13–15]. Interestingly, in one of these studies, ciprofloxacin and metronidazole in combination were compared to methylprednisolone among 41 adult patients with active Crohn disease. Similar reductions in symptoms and improvements in laboratory values (acute phase reactants, albumin, and hemoglobin) were seen in both groups [14]. Only one antibiotic combination study has been published in pediatric Crohn disease by Levine et al., and this was a limited 32-patient retrospective analysis of the combined use of azithromycin and metronidazole [16]. After 8 weeks of treatment, 66 % demonstrated clinical remission as defined by a Pediatric Crohn's Disease Activity Index (PCDAI) < 10. More severe disease with higher PCDAI and CRP values at baseline, presence of associated arthritis, and extensive disease (prominent upper intestinal disease or ileocolonic disease) were found to be associated with a lack of response.

Perianal Disease

Perianal Crohn disease including fistulae and abscesses occur in almost 50 % of patients with Crohn disease [17], and while a combination of surgical and medical treatment is preferred, antibiotics have shown some efficacy in several trials. Early reports by Ursing and Kamme noted improvements in perianal disease with the use of metronidazole [9]. In the first open-label study evaluating the use of metronidazole for perianal disease only, Bernstein et al. placed 21 consecutive patients with perianal Crohn disease on metronidazole. The authors reported that all 21 had a dramatic reduction in drainage, erythema, and induration and complete healing in ten of 18 patients maintained on the drug [18]. A follow-up study conducted by the same authors found continued efficacy of the drug in those patients maintained for longer periods of time including up to 1 year in 16 of 26 patients followed. The authors did however note that disease frequently returned when the drug dose was lowered or the drug was discontinued [19].

Topical metronidazole 10 % ointment has been evaluated as a means of minimizing adverse effects of systemic metronidazole in the treatment of perianal Crohn disease [20]. Maeda et al. performed a double-blind controlled trial comparing metronidazole ointment to placebo and showed no statistical reduction in PCDAI scores. However, metronidazole application three times daily for 4 weeks showed a significant reduction in perianal pain and discharge.

Antibiotics have also been investigated in conjunction with other medications including azathioprine and infliximab in the treatment of perianal Crohn disease. Dejaco et al. evaluated 52 adult patients with perianal fistulas in an open-labeled trial using ciprofloxacin and/or metronidazole [21]. Patients who were on azathioprine were allowed to continue (17 patients), and an additional 14 patients received azathioprine after 8 weeks of antibiotic therapy. The authors found that 50 % of patients had a clinical response to antibiotics at 8 weeks and 25 % continued to respond at week 20. They also found that patients who received azathioprine and antibiotics were more likely to respond than those who received antibiotics alone. They concluded that antibiotics may, therefore, offer a bridge to immunosuppression as there was a good short-term response. In a more recent randomized, controlled trial, West et al. evaluated ciprofloxacin versus placebo in conjunction with infliximab among 24 patients with perianal Crohn disease [22]. Although statistical significance was not achieved, the authors noted a trend toward improved response among patients who received ciprofloxacin and infliximab versus placebo and infliximab at week 18 (73 % versus 38 %). There is evidence to suggest that antibiotics reduce fistula drainage but less evidence to suggest that antibiotics lead to fistula healing [23]. Therefore, a recent global consensus on the treatment of perianal disease recommended that antibiotics should only be used as adjunctive therapy [23].

Postoperative Recurrence of Crohn Disease

A large proportion of patients with Crohn disease require surgery at some point during the course of their disease, and a majority of these patients will eventually develop recurrence of disease requiring additional surgery [24, 25]. Previous studies have suggested that bacteria may play a role in the recurrence of disease as inflammation recurs when the mucosa is reexposed to luminal contents and bacteria [26]. Based on this causal relationship, antibiotics may have a beneficial role in the prevention of postoperative recurrence of Crohn disease.

In a double-blind, placebo-controlled trial, Rutgeerts et al. evaluated the efficacy of metronidazole in the prevention of postoperative recurrence of Crohn disease following ileal resection [5]. Sixty adult patients were randomized to receive metronidazole or placebo for 3 months. While both groups demonstrated some endoscopic recurrence of disease at 3 months (75 % placebo group versus 52 % metronidazole group), the incidence of severe endoscopic disease recurrence was significantly reduced among the metronidazole-treated patients (13 % versus 43 %). The authors also found a statistically reduced recurrence rate among the metronidazole-treated group versus placebo at 1 year although no differences were seen at 2 and 3 years. A more recent study conducted with the use of ornidazole, a nitroimidazole antibiotic with fewer side effects than metronidazole (not available in the USA), has also been performed [27]. Eighty patients were randomized to receive ornidazole or placebo for 1 year beginning 1 week after ileal resection. Ornidazole significantly reduced the clinical recurrence rate at 1 year (7.9 % ornidazole group versus 37.5 % placebo group), although no significant difference in clinical recurrence was seen at 24 and 36 months. The endoscopic recurrence rate at 12 months was also lower among those patients who received ornidazole compared with placebo.

Taken together, available studies seem to indicate a reduction in postoperative recurrence among patients who receive antibiotics [28]. Optimal dosing and the duration of therapy needed to prevent recurrence are still unclear and will require future studies. Additionally, antibiotic selection may be critical. In a small randomized, double-blind, placebo-controlled pilot study, ciprofloxacin was not more effective than placebo for the prevention of postoperative recurrence in patients with Crohn disease [29].

Antibiotics in Ulcerative Colitis

There are few evidence-based studies demonstrating the utility of antibiotics in the treatment of ulcerative colitis aside from those involving colitis exacerbation secondary to *Clostridium difficile* superinfection. These patients were treated with antibiotics targeted for this organism or due to toxic megacolon, in which case treatment with antibiotics is employed until surgical resection can be performed. Dickinson et al. showed no significance in the use of vancomycin in patients with ulcerative colitis (UC) in 1985 [30], Chapman et al. also showed no advantage of intravenous metronidazole in 1986 [31], and Mantzaris et al. in 1997 showed no significance of ciprofloxacin use in mild to moderately active UC [32]. A subsequent study by Mantzaris et al. also showed no difference in response rates between patients with severe, acute colitis who were randomized to receive intravenous ciprofloxacin and hydrocortisone versus placebo and hydrocortisone [32]. Turunen et al. in a longer-term 6-month study of ciprofloxacin in active UC patients without improvement on steroids and mesalamine demonstrated a lower treatment failure rate, 21 % versus 44 % ($p < 0.002$), along with endoscopic and histologic improvement at 3 months but not at 6 months. The authors also found that at 12 months, there was no longer a significant difference in response rates between the two groups [33].

Antibiotics were compared with sulfasalazine in a double-blinded, controlled trial of patients with active, non-severe ulcerative colitis. Forty-six patients were randomized to receive metronidazole or sulfasalazine for 28 days [34]. The authors found that only six of 23 patients in the metronidazole group improved versus 13 of 19 patients in the sulfasalazine group and concluded that metronidazole was ineffective in the treatment of active ulcerative colitis.

Additional antibiotics including tobramycin, amoxicillin-clavulanic acid, amoxicillin, and tetracycline have also been studied in patients with active ulcerative colitis. Mixed results have been reported regarding the use of tobramycin. Burke et al. randomized 84 patients with acute relapse of their ulcerative colitis to receive tobramycin or placebo along with steroids for 7 days [35]. The authors found significant clinical improvements in the tobramycin group versus the placebo group after 3–4 weeks (74 % versus 43 %). Lobo et al. however reported that these response rates were short-lived as they followed up 81 of those previously followed up 84 patients for 2 years and found no difference in relapse rates between groups. A second study by Mantzaris et al. showed no difference in response rates in patients with severe active ulcerative colitis who received intravenous tobramycin and metronidazole in conjunction with corticosteroids versus placebo and corticosteroids alone [36, 37].

More recently, Ohkusa et al. reported some success in the treatment of active ulcerative colitis with the use amoxicillin, tetracycline, and metronidazole [38]. In this randomized, controlled trial, 20 patients with chronic, active ulcerative colitis were randomized to receive the above combination of antibiotics or placebo for 2 weeks. The antibiotics were selected based on their sensitivities toward *Fusobacterium varium* which has been proposed as a pathogenic factor in the development of UC in an experimental model [39]. The authors reported significant improvements in endoscopic/histologic scores as well as clinical symptoms at 3–5 months and 12–14 months. They also reported a significantly higher remission rate among the treatment group versus those who received placebo. In a follow-up study, Uehara et al. showed that antibiotic combination therapy with amoxicillin, tetracycline, and metronidazole was also useful in achieving remission in refractory and steroid-dependent cases of Crohn disease. Patients showed statistically significant reductions in their clinical activity indexes and histologic and endoscopic scores following 2 weeks of therapy. Moreover, 70.6 % of steroid-refractory or steroid-dependent patients were able to discontinue steroid therapy at 12 months [40]. In pediatrics, a recent study by Turner and colleagues retrospectively reported on their experiences using a 2–3-week course of combination oral antibiotics in children with moderate to severe, refractory UC or indeterminate colitis (IC) [41]. This regimen primarily consisted of metronidazole, amoxicillin, and doxycycline, with the addition of vancomycin in hospitalized patients. The antibiotic regimen was effective in 7/15 (47 %) of patients, inducing complete short-term remission and preventing the need for additional interventions.

Finally, patients who present with fever and a colitis exacerbation admitted to the hospital may also be treated with triple antibiotics, ampicillin, gentamicin, and metronidazole, until a bacterial superinfection triggering the disease exacerbation has been excluded, at which point the antibiotics are stopped after negative stool cultures and negative blood cultures. However, there is some suggestion that hospitalized patients with ulcerative colitis who receive both IV corticosteroids and antibiotics may have a decreased requirement for in-hospital rescue therapies than hospitalized patients with ulcerative colitis who receive IV corticosteroids alone [42]. This is a finding that needs to be further explored.

Emerging Therapies

More recently with the development of newer antimicrobials that have the majority of their action within the bowel lumen with minimal systemic absorption, researchers have started to study their effect in the management of IBD. Rifaximin (Xifaxan®) and nitazoxanide (Alinia®) are the two most recent potential therapeutic candidates.

Rifaximin comes in a tablet form to treat *Escherichia coli*-related traveler's diarrhea and also has effect against a broad range of small bowel bacteria covering most gram-positive and gram-negative bacteria, both aerobes and anaerobes. Side effects are minimal and may include headache, constipation, vomiting, and/or abdominal cramp/pain. Rifaximin has no bowel absorption but is not FDA approved for use in IBD or in children.

There are limited adult randomized controlled studies or placebo-controlled studies involving rifaximin reported in the treatment of Crohn disease. Shafran and Johnson first studied rifaximin in an open-label study among 29 adult patients with mild to moderate Crohn disease [43]. Patients received rifaximin for 16 weeks. The authors reported that 59 % of patients had a reduction in CDAI score of greater than or equal to 70 points at the end of 4 weeks and that 78 % had a reduction in CDAI score by greater than or equal to 70 points at the end of the 16-week treatment period. The authors concluded that rifaximin might show some promise in the treatment of Crohn disease. In a follow-up study, Shafran and Burgunder showed that rifaximin monotherapy led to clinical improvement in patients with Crohn disease. They reported that remission (CDAI less than 150) was achieved in 67 % of patients treated with rifaximin monotherapy, compared to 58 % in patients who received treatment with steroid [44].

One of the largest studies of the treatment of Crohn disease with rifaximin evaluated an extended release formulation, Rifaximin-EIR [45]. Rifaximin-EIR is coated with a gastric acid-resistant polymer and is designed to bypass the stomach and maximize delivery to the intestinal tract. In this study, 402 patients with moderately active Crohn disease received Rifaximin-EIR at different dosages versus placebo for 12 weeks. Patients could have active disease on stable dosages of mesalamine, thiopurines, or methotrexate, and recent steroid, anti-TNF, or antibiotic use was not allowed. Treatment with Rifaximin-EIR 800 mg twice daily was able to induce remission by CDAI (62 % compared to 43 % in the placebo group).

Rifaximin has also been evaluated in patients with ulcerative colitis. In 1999, Gionchetti et al. in their study of 28 moderate to severe ulcerative colitis patients showed no significant difference in clinical outcome in patients not responding to intravenous methylprednisolone after 7–10 days with the additional use of 400 mg bid of rifaximin [46]. The authors did, however, note a reduction in stool frequency, rectal bleeding, and sigmoidoscopy scores among the rifaximin group as compared to the placebo-treated group. Also, in an open-label pilot study of patients with left-sided ulcerative colitis who were experiencing a clinical relapse with maintenance therapy with mesalamine, the addition of rifaximin 400 mg twice daily induced clinical remission in 70 % [47]. An extension of this study adding an additional 20 patients (increasing total *n* to 30) demonstrated similar findings [48]. These data are encouraging, but larger, controlled studies are needed to confirm the results.

As opposed to the modest efficacy seen in Crohn disease and ulcerative colitis, antibiotics are very effective for the treatment of pouchitis following total proctocolectomy [49, 50]. Rifaximin has also been studied in this setting. In a study by Gionchetti and colleagues of patients with treatment-resistant pouchitis, the combination of rifaximin 2 g/day plus ciprofloxacin 1 g/day led to improvement in disease activity in ten out of 18 patients and remission in six out of 18 patients by Pouchitis Disease Activity Index (PDAI) [51]. A randomized, double-blind, placebo-controlled pilot study suggested that clinical remission was more likely in patients with active pouchitis treated with rifaximin as compared to placebo; however, the improvement did not reach statistical significance likely secondary to small sample size [52]. Rifaximin has also been evaluated as a maintenance of remission therapy in pouchitis once remission has been induced with other antibiotics [50]. The results were favorable and adverse events were rare.

Rifaximin may also be a promising treatment in pediatric IBD patients. Muniyappa et al. showed a significant improvement in symptoms following initiation of rifaximin during disease flares. Twenty-three patients (12 with CD and 11 with UC) with a median age of 15.1 years were given varying doses of rifaximin at onset of flare symptoms, which included diarrhea (87 %), abdominal pain (74 %), and bloody stools (65 %). Addition of rifaximin as the only treatment change resulted in symptom relief for 61 % of patients after 4 weeks of treatment. Of these patients, 80 % had resolution of all of their flare symptoms [53].

Nitazoxanide comes in both tablet and suspension forms making this ideal for pediatric use with FDA indications for parasitic infectious diarrhea (*Cryptosporidium parvum* and *Giardia lamblia* as well as helminths and tapeworms). The drug is metabolized by the cytochrome P450 mechanism in the liver with bile, feces, and urinary excretion. Its side effect profile is minimal with abdominal pain, diarrhea, headache, and nausea reported at similar rates as placebo. Some researchers have been studying its use to treat *Clostridium difficile* as well as in Crohn disease. To date, the only published data in inflammatory bowel disease is in patients with Crohn disease who have a concomitant cryptosporidial infection [54].

Both drugs, rifaximin and nitazoxanide, have shown some promise as primary therapies in inflammatory bowel disease. More rigorous testing including randomized, controlled trials are necessary before the drugs are accepted as appropriate mainstream treatment, however.

Limited data exist on the use of antibiotics for extra-intestinal manifestations associated with IBD. Oral vancomycin has shown some promise in treating the subset of pediatric IBD patients with primary sclerosing cholangitis (PSC). Davies et al. treated 14 IBD patients (11 ulcerative colitis) diagnosed with PSC with 50 mg/kg/day of oral vancomycin for 14 days. All showed significant improvement in their alanine aminotransferase, gamma-glutamyl transpeptidase, erythrocyte sedimentation rate, and clinical symptoms. Three patients who were rebiopsied demonstrated reversal of their fibrosis [55]. While this initial study was promising, further studies are needed to verify whether oral vancomycin is an effective long-term treatment in preventing the progression of PSC to cirrhosis in IBD patients.

Additional Considerations

When utilizing antibiotics in the acute or maintenance phase of therapy, careful consideration for which form of mesalamine treatment being used concurrently is especially necessary since medications such as olsalazine or sulfasalazine require the presence of bacteria to cleave their disulfide bond in order to permit action of the medication. Asacol requires a basic/neutral luminal pH to be effective such that with stenotic disease and the potential of bacterial overgrowth with a more locally acidic luminal pH, concurrent antimicrobial therapy theoretically may be beneficial.

While generally well tolerated, antibiotics can lead to side effects that may require discontinuation and should be monitored closely. As previously mentioned, ciprofloxacin has been noted to cause arthropathies in immature animals, and long-term use is generally avoided among very young children. There is also one pediatric study which evaluated the side effects associated with long-term metronidazole use. Duffy et al. reported on their experience among 13 pediatric Crohn disease patients who received metronidazole for 4–11 months [56]. The authors reported that 85 % (11 of 13) had peripheral neuropathies based on abnormal nerve conduction velocities or neurological examinations although only six of 11 were symptomatic. Complete resolution of the neuropathy occurred in five children, improvement occurred in three children, and there was no change in one child.

Summary

In summary, limited prospective studies investigating antibiotic use in pediatric inflammatory bowel disease are available. Based on available literature, some role for antibiotics including metronidazole and/or ciprofloxacin has been shown for acute exacerbations of Crohn disease and chronic penetrating Crohn disease. No available, objective evidence supports their use in acute ulcerative colitis. However, more recent reports of combination antibiotics in the treatment of severe ulcerative colitis are promising. Vancomycin may be useful in IBD patients with primary sclerosing cholangitis. Additional prospective studies are needed to evaluate the role of vancomycin and other antimicrobials including rifaximin and nitazoxanide.

References

1. Sartor RB. Pathogenesis and immune mechanisms of chronic inflammatory bowel diseases. Am J Gastroenterol. 1997;92(12 Suppl): 5S–11S.
2. Rutgeerts P, Goboes K, Peeters M, et al. Effect of faecal stream diversion on recurrence of Crohn's disease in the neoterminal ileum. Lancet. 1991;338(8770):771–4.
3. Perencevich M, Burakoff R. Use of antibiotics in the treatment of inflammatory bowel disease. Inflamm Bowel Dis. 2006;12(7): 651–64.
4. Sartor RB. Therapeutic manipulation of the enteric microflora in inflammatory bowel diseases: antibiotics, probiotics, and prebiotics. Gastroenterology. 2004;126(6):1620–33.
5. Rutgeerts P, Hiele M, Geboes K, et al. Controlled trial of metronidazole treatment for prevention of Crohn's recurrence after ileal resection. Gastroenterology. 1995;108(6):1617–21.
6. Ursing B, Alm T, Barany F, et al. A comparative study of metronidazole and sulfasalazine for active Crohn's disease: the cooperative Crohn's disease study in Sweden. II Result. Gastroenterology. 1982;83(3):550–62.
7. Su JW, Ma JJ, Zhang HJ. Use of antibiotics in patients with Crohn's disease: a systematic review and meta-analysis. J Dig Dis. 2015; 16(2):58–66.
8. Hildebrand H, Berg NO, Hoevels J, Ursing B. Treatment of Crohn's disease with metronidazole in childhood and adolescence. Evaluation of a six months trial. Gastroenterol Clin Biol. 1980; 4(1):19–25.
9. Ursing B, Kamme C. Metronidazole for Crohn's disease. Lancet. 1975;1(7910):775–7.
10. Sutherland L, Singleton J, Sessions J, et al. Double blind, placebo controlled trial of metronidazole in Crohn's disease. Gut. 1991;32(9):1071–5.
11. Colombel JF, Lemann M, Cassagnou M, et al. A controlled trial comparing ciprofloxacin with mesalazine for the treatment of active Crohn's disease. Groupe d'Etudes Therapeutiques des Affections Inflammatoires Digestives (GETAID). Am J Gastroenterol. 1999;94(3):674–8.
12. Arnold GL, Beaves MR, Pryjdun VO, Mook WJ. Preliminary study of ciprofloxacin in active Crohn's disease. Inflamm Bowel Dis. 2002;8(1):10–5.
13. Greenbloom SL, Steinhart AH, Greenberg GR. Combination ciprofloxacin and metronidazole for active Crohn's disease. Can J Gastroenterol. 1998;12(1):53–6.
14. Prantera C, Zannoni F, Scribano ML, et al. An antibiotic regimen for the treatment of active Crohn's disease: a randomized, controlled clinical trial of metronidazole plus ciprofloxacin. Am J Gastroenterol. 1996;91(2):328–32.
15. Prantera C, Berto E, Scribano ML, Falasco G. Use of antibiotics in the treatment of active Crohn's disease: experience with metronidazole and ciprofloxacin. Ital J Gastroenterol Hepatol. 1998;30(6): 602–6.
16. Levine A, Turner D. Combined azithromycin and metronidazole therapy is effective in inducing remission in pediatric Crohn's disease. J Crohns Colitis. 2011;5(3):222–6.
17. Schwartz DA, Pemberton JH, Sandborn WJ. Diagnosis and treatment of perianal fistulas in Crohn disease. Ann Intern Med. 2001; 135(10):906–18.
18. Bernstein LH, Frank MS, Brandt LJ, Boley SJ. Healing of perineal Crohn's disease with metronidazole. Gastroenterology. 1980; 79(3):599.
19. Brandt LJ, Bernstein LH, Boley SJ, Frank MS. Metronidazole therapy for perineal Crohn's disease: a follow-up study. Gastroenterology. 1982;83(2):383–7.
20. Maeda Y, Ng SC, Durdey P, et al. Randomized clinical trial of metronidazole ointment versus placebo in perianal Crohn's disease. Br J Surg. 2010;97(9):1340–7.
21. Dejaco C, Harrer M, Waldhoer T, Miehsler W, Vogelsang H, Reinisch W. Antibiotics and azathioprine for the treatment of perianal fistulas in Crohn's disease. Aliment Pharmacol Ther. 2003;18(11–12):1113–20.
22. West RL, van der Woude CJ, Hansen BE, et al. Clinical and endosonographic effect of ciprofloxacin on the treatment of perianal fistulae in Crohn's disease with infliximab: a double-blind placebo-controlled study. Aliment Pharmacol Ther. 2004;20(11–12):1329–36.
23. Gecse KB, Bemelman W, Kamm MA, et al. A global consensus on the classification, diagnosis and multidisciplinary treatment of perianal fistulising Crohn's disease. Gut. 2014;63(9):1381–92.
24. Baldassano RN, Han PD, Jeshion WC, et al. Pediatric Crohn's disease: risk factors for postoperative recurrence. Am J Gastroenterol. 2001;96(7):2169–76.
25. Penner RM, Madsen KL, Fedorak RN. Postoperative Crohn's disease. Inflamm Bowel Dis. 2005;11(8):765–77.
26. D'Haens GR, Geboes K, Peeters M, Baert F, Penninckx F, Rutgeerts P. Early lesions of recurrent Crohn's disease caused by infusion of intestinal contents in excluded ileum. Gastroenterology. 1998;114(2):262–7.
27. Rutgeerts P, Van Assche G, Vermeire S, et al. Ornidazole for prophylaxis of postoperative Crohn's disease recurrence: a randomized, double-blind, placebo-controlled trial. Gastroenterology. 2005;128(4):856–61.
28. Singh S, Garg SK, Pardi DS, Wang Z, Murad MH, Loftus EV, Jr. Comparative efficacy of pharmacologic interventions in preventing relapse of Crohn's disease after surgery: a systematic review and network meta-analysis. Gastroenterology. 2015;148(1):64–76.e62; quiz e14.
29. Herfarth HH, Katz JA, Hanauer SB, et al. Ciprofloxacin for the prevention of postoperative recurrence in patients with Crohn's disease: a randomized, double-blind, placebo-controlled pilot study. Inflamm Bowel Dis. 2013;19(5):1073–9.
30. Dickinson RJ, O'Connor HJ, Pinder I, Hamilton I, Johnston D, Axon AT. Double blind controlled trial of oral vancomycin as

adjunctive treatment in acute exacerbations of idiopathic colitis. Gut. 1985;26(12):1380–4.

31. Chapman RW, Selby WS, Jewell DP. Controlled trial of intravenous metronidazole as an adjunct to corticosteroids in severe ulcerative colitis. Gut. 1986;27(10):1210–2.

32. Mantzaris GJ, Archavlis E, Christoforidis P, et al. A prospective randomized controlled trial of oral ciprofloxacin in acute ulcerative colitis. Am J Gastroenterol. 1997;92(3):454–6.

33. Turunen UM, Farkkila MA, Hakala K, et al. Long-term treatment of ulcerative colitis with ciprofloxacin: a prospective, double-blind, placebo-controlled study. Gastroenterology. 1998;115(5):1072–8.

34. Gilat T, Suissa A, Leichtman G, et al. A comparative study of metronidazole and sulfasalazine in active, not severe, ulcerative colitis. An Israeli multicenter trial. J Clin Gastroenterol. 1987;9(4):415–7.

35. Burke DA, Axon AT, Clayden SA, Dixon MF, Johnston D, Lacey RW. The efficacy of tobramycin in the treatment of ulcerative colitis. Aliment Pharmacol Ther. 1990;4(2):123–9.

36. Lobo AJ, Burke DA, Sobala GM, Axon AT. Oral tobramycin in ulcerative colitis: effect on maintenance of remission. Aliment Pharmacol Ther. 1993;7(2):155–8.

37. Mantzaris GJ, Hatzis A, Kontogiannis P, Triadaphyllou G. Intravenous tobramycin and metronidazole as an adjunct to corticosteroids in acute, severe ulcerative colitis. Am J Gastroenterol. 1994;89(1):43–6.

38. Ohkusa T, Nomura T, Terai T, et al. Effectiveness of antibiotic combination therapy in patients with active ulcerative colitis: a randomized, controlled pilot trial with long-term follow-up. Scand J Gastroenterol. 2005;40(11):1334–42.

39. Ohkusa T, Okayasu I, Ogihara T, Morita K, Ogawa M, Sato N. Induction of experimental ulcerative colitis by Fusobacterium varium isolated from colonic mucosa of patients with ulcerative colitis. Gut. 2003;52(1):79–83.

40. Uehara T, Kato K, Ohkusa T, et al. Efficacy of antibiotic combination therapy in patients with active ulcerative colitis, including refractory or steroid-dependent cases. J Gastroenterol Hepatol. 2010;25(Suppl 1):S62–6.

41. Turner D, Levine A, Kolho KL, Shaoul R, Ledder O. Combination of oral antibiotics may be effective in severe pediatric ulcerative colitis: a preliminary report. J Crohns Colitis. 2014;8(11):1464–70.

42. Gupta V, Rodrigues R, Nguyen D, et al. Adjuvant use of antibiotics with corticosteroids in inflammatory bowel disease exacerbations requiring hospitalisation: a retrospective cohort study and meta-analysis. Aliment Pharmacol Ther. 2016;43(1):52–60.

43. Shafran I, Johnson LK. An open-label evaluation of rifaximin in the treatment of active Crohn's disease. Curr Med Res Opin. 2005;21(8):1165–9.

44. Shafran I, Burgunder P. Adjunctive antibiotic therapy with rifaximin may help reduce Crohn's disease activity. Dig Dis Sci. 2010;55(4):1079–84.

45. Prantera C, Lochs H, Grimaldi M, et al. Rifaximin-extended intestinal release induces remission in patients with moderately active Crohn's disease. Gastroenterology. 2012;142(3):473–81.e474.

46. Gionchetti P, Rizzello F, Ferrieri A, et al. Rifaximin in patients with moderate or severe ulcerative colitis refractory to steroid-treatment: a double-blind, placebo-controlled trial. Dig Dis Sci. 1999;44(6):1220–1.

47. Guslandi M, Giollo P, Testoni PA. Corticosteroid-sparing effect of rifaximin, a nonabsorbable oral antibiotic, in active ulcerative colitis: Preliminary clinical experience. Curr Ther Res Clin Exp. 2004;65(3):292–6.

48. Guslandi M, Petrone MC, Testoni PA. Rifaximin for active ulcerative colitis. Inflamm Bowel Dis. 2006;12(4):335.

49. Shen B, Achkar JP, Lashner BA, et al. A randomized clinical trial of ciprofloxacin and metronidazole to treat acute pouchitis. Inflamm Bowel Dis. 2001;7(4):301–5.

50. Shen B, Remzi FH, Lopez AR, Queener E. Rifaximin for maintenance therapy in antibiotic-dependent pouchitis. BMC Gastroenterol. 2008;8:26.

51. Gionchetti P, Rizzello F, Venturi A, et al. Antibiotic combination therapy in patients with chronic, treatment-resistant pouchitis. Aliment Pharmacol Ther. 1999;13(6):713–8.

52. Isaacs KL, Sandler RS, Abreu M, et al. Rifaximin for the treatment of active pouchitis: a randomized, double-blind, placebo-controlled pilot study. Inflamm Bowel Dis. 2007;13(10):1250–5.

53. Muniyappa P, Gulati R, Mohr F, Hupertz V. Use and safety of rifaximin in children with inflammatory bowel disease. J Pediatr Gastroenterol Nutr. 2009;49(4):400–4.

54. Smith S, Shaw J, Nathwani D. Nitazoxanide for cryptosporidial infection in Crohn's disease. Gut. 2008;57(8):1179–80.

55. Davies YK, Cox KM, Abdullah BA, Safta A, Terry AB, Cox KL. Long-term treatment of primary sclerosing cholangitis in children with oral vancomycin: an immunomodulating antibiotic. J Pediatr Gastroenterol Nutr. 2008;47(1):61–7.

56. Duffy LF, Daum F, Fisher SE, et al. Peripheral neuropathy in Crohn's disease patients treated with metronidazole. Gastroenterology. 1985;88(3):681–4.

Anthony R. Otley, Andrew S. Day, and Mary Zachos

Introduction

While similar in many respects, the inflammatory bowel diseases (IBD) can be classified based on certain distinctive endoscopic and histological characteristics. Clinical manifestations also vary between Crohn's disease (CD) and ulcerative colitis (UC), including their impact on nutritional status. A history of weight loss or poor weight gain is a very common symptom at presentation particularly with CD and severe UC [1, 2]. Linear growth impairment is reported even before the onset of intestinal symptoms in almost half of pediatric patients with CD [3]. Given the early age of onset, such impairment of growth is particularly problematic, with subsequent impact on onset of puberty, self-esteem, and quality of life.

In the treatment of IBD in children, nutrition and growth outcomes are critical indicators of overall well-being and therapeutic success in addition to other therapeutic targets of symptom resolution and mucosal healing. In addition to a multitude of pharmacologic approaches to therapy, there is extensive evidence supporting the efficacy of nutritional therapy in CD. Current guidelines support exclusive enteral nutrition (EEN) as the first-line therapy to induce remission in children with active CD [4]. Despite the obvious advantages including the direct impact on growth and nutrition and the avoidance of adverse drug effects, nutritional therapy has not been as widely accepted in North America as other parts of the world [5, 6].

Since linear growth and bone disease have been addressed in alternate chapters, this chapter will focus on nutritional deficiencies and the role of nutritional management in the treatment of IBD, highlighting updates since the last edition.

Nutritional Impairment in Pediatric Inflammatory Bowel Disease

Malnutrition is common in IBD. In a recent systematic review, the main nutritional consequences of pediatric IBD included growth stunting, slower pubertal development, underweight, and vitamin deficiencies. Nutritional impairments were more significant in CD, while overweight and obesity were more common in patients with UC [7]. Several cohort studies have demonstrated weight loss or poor weight gains at the time of initial diagnosis of CD. Griffiths et al. [8] reported that 80% of the 386 children diagnosed with CD over a period of 10 years had a history of weight loss. A registry cohort of 261 patients in northern France found that 27% of children were underweight and 32% had BMI below two standard deviations of normal at diagnosis. At maximal follow-up, 15% continued to suffer from malnutrition. A Danish prospective population-based cohort study reported that children with CD had poor nutritional status at diagnosis compared with the general pediatric population [9]. Among Australian children, a case-control study by Aurangzeb et al. [10] assessing nutritional status found that children with newly diagnosed IBD had lower mean body mass index (BMI) Z scores and weight-for-age percentiles than controls.

Weight loss is seen less commonly, particularly through the course of established UC, but has been seen in up to 65%

A.R. Otley, MD, MSc, FRCPC
Faculty of Medicine, Dalhousie University, Halifax, Canada

Division of Gastroenterology & Nutrition, IWK Health Centre, 5850 University Avenue, Halifax, NS, Canada, B3K 6R8
e-mail: arotley@dal.ca

A.S. Day, MB, MD, ChB, FRACP, AGAF
Pediatric Gastroenterology, Christchurch Hospital, Christchurch, New Zealand

Department of Pediatrics, University of Otago, Christchurch, New Zealand
e-mail: andrew.day@otago.ac.nz

M. Zachos, MD, FRCPC (✉)
Department of Pediatrics, McMaster University, McMaster Children's Hospital, 1200 Main St. West, Hamilton, ON L8N 3Z5, Canada
e-mail: mary.zachos@cogeco.ca

© Springer International Publishing AG 2017
P. Mamula et al. (eds.), *Pediatric Inflammatory Bowel Disease*, DOI 10.1007/978-3-319-49215-5_27

of children at diagnosis [1]. Kugathasan et al. [11] conducted a systematic review of 783 children with newly diagnosed IBD from two prospective inception cohorts to examine BMI status at presentation. Most children with CD and UC had a BMI in the normative range (5–84%). Low BMI (<5%) was seen in 22–24% of children with CD and 7–9% of children with UC.

Several interrelated factors contribute to growth impairment in IBD. Chronic suboptimal nutrition has long been implicated as a cause of growth retardation [1, 12–16]. In addition, direct growth-inhibiting effects of pro-inflammatory cytokines (such as TNF-α) released from the inflamed intestine have been more recently recognized for their role in growth impairment, as well as indirectly resulting in anorexic effects and early satiety [17]. Symptoms, including nausea, abdominal pain, or diarrhea in association with meals, also limit caloric intake. Localization of disease in the small bowel may lead to partial obstruction and early satiety. Small intestinal involvement may also lead to disaccharide intolerance resulting in shorter gut transit times, pain, and exacerbation of diarrhea. Malabsorption of food components and the diversion of calories to sites of gut inflammation may also lead to impaired weight gain and growth [18]. Thus, enhancement of growth is best achieved through control of intestinal inflammation and assurance of adequate nutrition [19, 20].

Dietary Intake and Body Composition in Children with IBD

Dietary Intake

The impact of CD on growth and body composition is determined by an interaction between the duration and severity of the inflammatory disease process, genetic predisposition, and the extent to which the demands for energy and nutrients are met. It is imperative that the management of children and adolescents with CD combines the control of inflammation while providing optimal nutrition support with adequate protein and sufficient calories to support growth.

The mean energy intake of patients with CD is less than age-matched controls particularly during symptomatic relapses [13] but also while asymptomatic [8]. Pons et al. [21] evaluated the dietary intake of 41 children with CD (18 active, 23 in remission) and compared them with the intakes of 22 age-matched control children without IBD. The energy intakes of the children with CD were less than the estimated energy requirements regardless of disease activity. Fat and carbohydrate intake were found to be lower in CD patients than in controls, while protein intake was similar in patient and control groups [21].

A recent study from Brazil found that total energy intake was lower than the daily recommended intake (DRI) in 50%

of the adolescents with active CD compared to 3.5% in inactive CD and 5.7% in the control group. Protein intake was found to be low in all three groups but significantly lower in the active CD group than in the inactive CD and control group (68.2% vs 17.2% and 14.3%, below the DRIs, respectively) [22].

Body Composition

A recent systematic review, reporting on a total of 1479 children with IBD (1123 Crohn's disease, 243 ulcerative colitis), attempted to define the alterations in non-bone tissue compartments in children with IBD [23]. Data were highly heterogeneous, in terms of methodology and patients. In this systematic review, six studies were prospective and 11 cross-sectional in design. Body composition methodologies included whole-body dual X-ray absorptiometry (DXA) most commonly, as well as peripheral quantitative computerized tomography (p-QCT), skinfold thickness, isotope dilutional studies, whole-body potassium measurement, total body potassium counting ($n = 30$), and bioelectrical impedance. Overall, the review concluded that almost all children with CD and half with UC have reduced lean mass; however, body fat alterations are not well defined.

Deficits in protein-related compartments were reported with lean mass deficits documented in 93.6% of CD and 47.7% of UC patients when compared with healthy control populations. Several studies have confirmed that children with CD have significant deficits in lean body mass (or fat-free mass), which is consistent with cachexia [24–27]. Wiskin [26] found that fat-free mass was related to disease activity regardless of changes in weight and concluded that weight or BMI may mask deficits in lean tissue in the presence of normal or increased proportions of body fat.

Body fat composition findings have been inconsistent [23]. Some studies report reductions in body fat in new diagnosis or active CD. For example, Boot et al. suggest proportional reductions in lean and fat mass, as shown by percentage body fat that did not differ significantly from zero in their combined IBD cohort [28]. In contrast, in an all CD cohort, Burnham et al. report that fat mass adjusted for age and fat mass adjusted for height were not significantly different from controls [24]. Similarly, in 42 children with CD, weight gain over a 2-year period was explained by gains in fat mass raising concerns regarding the long-term impact of disease on growth and bone health [29].

In addition to circulating inflammatory cytokines, there are several other factors that are likely to contribute to the reduction in protein compartments in IBD patients (Table 27.1).

Body composition studies have often been limited by the large proportion of participants that had received concomitant systemic corticosteroids at the time of body composition assessment. Glucocorticoids instigate remission but also promote muscle proteolysis and alter whole-body adiposity

Table 27.1 Factors affecting body composition

Circulating inflammatory cytokines
Medications, particularly glucocorticoids
Malnutrition
Resting energy expenditure
Height, weight, and pubertal status
Gender
Physical activity

[30]. Variations in the glucocorticoid treatment the participants received may have influenced some of the discrepancies in the fat-related data across the studies in this review. Future studies should attempt to differentiate between the effects of therapy and the disease process itself.

There is conflicting data from studies reporting resting energy expenditure (REE) in children with CD. Azcue et al. demonstrated that per unit of lean body mass, there was no difference between REE in patients with CD and controls, whereas patients with anorexia nervosa had significantly reduced REE [25]. In contrast, Zoli et al. [31] found elevated REE in growing children with CD. Surprisingly, the latter study did not reveal any further increase in REE with relapse of disease and suggested that energy may be "diverted" from growth to disease activity during relapse. Varille et al. showed that a lower fat-free body mass in pediatric IBD was associated with higher resting energy expenditure [32]. Thus, these energy imbalances may explain the cachectic changes seen in children with IBD even when disease is in remission. This resting energy expenditure imbalance is most likely driven by nutritional insufficiencies and chronic inflammation.

Height, age, and pubertal status may also influence body composition. Puberty affects fat and muscle compartments and should be accounted for in analysis of body composition. In children with IBD, height is reduced, and bone age and puberty are delayed when compared with healthy children of the same age, possibly explaining some of the body compositional deficits seen [23].

Gender can also influence body mass composition, as reported by Thayu et al., who studied the body composition of 74 children with CD at diagnosis. They found that boys with CD at diagnosis had significant fat-free mass deficits consistent with cachexia, whereas girls demonstrated both fat mass as well as fat-free mass deficits consistent with wasting [27]. In a recent systematic review, lower lean mass was common to both sexes in CD and UC, but deficits in females persisted for longer, possibly because males are known to accumulate lean tissue at puberty, while females reach peak lean mass before puberty [23].

The effect of malabsorption may lead to reduction in protein compartments due to protein-losing enteropathy that result in fluid shifts [25]. In addition, physical activity is important for muscle and bone strength in growing children and may be limited in pediatric IBD patients even when their disease is asymptomatic. Werkstetter compared 39 IBD patients in remission (or with only mild disease activity) with 39 healthy controls. Muscle function assessed by measuring handgrip strength was reduced in children with CD, which corresponded to deficits found in muscle cross-sectional area of the upper limb [33]. In addition, IBD patients tended to take fewer steps per day and engage in shorter periods of physical activity, particularly among females and patients with mild disease. Exercise studies in adolescents with CD have shown impaired fat metabolism during activity with a greater reliance on carbohydrates to meet the energy demands of submaximal exercise [34].

The clinical significance of muscle deficits in children with CD is not known; however, lean mass deficits may be associated with poor physical functioning and greater infection risk during childhood and compromised peak bone mass by young adulthood. Adult studies suggest that body fat composition predicts infectious complications following bowel resection in CD [35]. In adults, low muscle mass and sarcopenia are common and may be predictive of osteoporosis [36]. Further study of the long-term impact of altered body composition in children with IBD is required, as this may have clinical importance in terms of nutritional and pharmacological management, even when disease is in remission.

Because of the difficulty ensuring adequate energy and nutrient requirements of children with IBD, particularly during flares, active monitoring of nutritional status must be undertaken throughout childhood but especially in adolescence. Hannon et al. demonstrated that in stable adolescents with CD, enteral nutrition promotes anabolism by suppressing proteolysis and increasing protein synthesis [37]. Thus, where indicated, aggressive nutritional intervention should be initiated before puberty, whether disease is active or in remission, to correct the energy deficits and maximize growth potential.

Micronutrient Deficiencies

Low concentration of plasma micronutrients is commonly reported in IBD patients. Dietary intakes of children and adolescents with IBD may be compromised in micronutrient content in addition to protein and energy due to many factors including decreased food intake, intestinal losses, malabsorption, and drug effects [38].

Specific micronutrient and vitamin deficiencies are encountered more commonly with CD than with UC. Hendricks et al. [13] compared a group of adolescents with CD and growth failure with a control group of adolescents with CD who were growing normally. Mean serum ferritin levels were significantly decreased in both groups, and mean plasma zinc levels were borderline low in the growth failure group and low in the control group. Dietary zinc intake was below the recommended dietary allowance (RDA) in 88% of the group with growth failure and 44% of controls (64% combined) and less than 75% of the RDA in 41% of all adolescents with CD. Dietary iron intake was also below the RDA in 24% of all adolescents with CD, with one adolescent in the growth failure group consuming less than 75% of the RDA. One third of adolescents were consuming less than 75% of the RDA for calcium. In evaluation of 41 children with CD compared to age-matched controls, calcium intake was significantly less than the Australian recommended daily intake (RDI), and iron intake approached less than RDI [21]. Vitamin D is a key factor in both bone mineralization and immunomodulation. Levin et al. retrospectively assessed vitamin D in a group of 78 Australian children with IBD (70 CD, 5 UC, 3 IBDU) and explored associations between vitamin D status and clinical factors. Using a level of 50 nmol/l or less to indicate deficiency and 50–75 nmol/l to indicate insufficiency, 19% of children were vitamin D deficient and 38% were insufficient, respectively. Levels were not found to be associated with disease location or use of immunosuppressive drugs. Children with vitamin D deficiency had significantly greater corticosteroid exposure than those with normal status [39].

Alkhouri et al. investigated the prevalence of vitamin and zinc deficiencies in 61 children with newly diagnosed IBD (80% with ileal inflammation) compared to age- and sex-matched controls. Sixty-two percent had vitamin D deficiency (vs 75% in the controls). In contrast to other studies [40], Alkhouri et al. found no IBD patients with folate or vitamin B12 deficiency suggesting no reason for routine monitoring. However, vitamin A (16% deficient) and zinc (40% deficient) deficiencies were statistically more prevalent among the IBD patients than controls, suggesting that levels should be assessed at the time of diagnosis. In addition, since vitamin D deficiency was so common in the population tested, routine screening and supplementation are warranted [41].

Older studies of micronutrient intakes in CD have found mean intakes of zinc, copper, iron, calcium, folic acid, vitamin C, and vitamin D to be significantly ($P < 0.05$) lower than age-matched controls and RDAs [17]. Essential fatty acid status may also be altered, in association with low body mass index and disease activity [42]. Malabsorption of fat-soluble vitamins can be an issue in patients with ileal disease [43, 44]. Gerasimidis et al. looked at the impact of EEN on body composition and circulating micronutrients in plasma and erythrocytes of 17 children with active CD. At baseline, several children presented with suboptimal concentrations of carotenoids, trace elements, vitamins C and B6, and folate in plasma but not in erythrocytes [45]. The same group later reported anemia in 72% of children with IBD at diagnosis. Children with CD at diagnosis had significantly shorter

diagnostic delay and a lower BMI than those who were not. After EEN, the frequency of severe anemia decreased (32–9%; $P = 0.001$). Extensive colitis was associated with anemia in UC [46].

Despite recognition of the occurrence of potential nutritional deficiency in IBD patients, only ESPEN has recommended nutritional deficiency screening in this population [47]. The extent of micronutrient deficiency screening and whether or not to supplement a child's diet should be considered on an individual basis, following dietary assessment, as firm recommendations for vitamin and mineral supplementation await future studies [19]. Kleinman and colleagues [48] have suggested that patients should be recommended a multivitamin/mineral to meet 100–150% of the RDA when dietary intake is less than expected. Vitamin and mineral supplement adherence has been examined by two studies. In a cross-sectional study examining self-reported adherence to IBD maintenance medications as well as supplements, an average adherence rate of 80% was reported across all medications and supplements combined [49]. More recently, adherence specifically to vitamin and mineral supplements was assessed in 49 youth aged 11–18 years with IBD using a validated interview. Mean adherence rates ranged from 32 to 44% across supplements, which included multivitamins, calcium, or iron. Youth who did not know the reason for supplementation (approximately 25% of the sample) displayed substantially poorer adherence than did those with moderate or high levels of knowledge, across all supplements [50].

Elevated Body Mass Index in Inflammatory Bowel Disease

Although most emphasis of the nutritional aspects of IBD is focused upon impaired nutritional status, the increasing rate of childhood obesity is also relevant in children presenting with acute IBD. Several cohorts have observed that children with IBD are at comparable risk of overweight and obesity as the general population.

Sondike and colleagues [51] reported this phenomenon in a group of 166 children from Wisconsin, USA. Sixteen (12%) of a group of newly diagnosed children with CD were overweight (BMI >85%) or obese (BMI >95%). This feature was also evident in the children diagnosed with UC: 17.6% of these 34 children were overweight or obese. Observations by Kugathasan et al. from two large multicenter North American cohorts revealed that 10% of children with CD and 20–30% of children with UC had a BMI at diagnosis consistent with overweight or risk for overweight [11]. A large multicenter cohort of 1598 children with IBD found that approximately one in five children with CD and one in three with UC are overweight or obese [52]. Rates of obesity in UC are comparable to the general population. Attempts to evaluate whether overweight and obese status is associated with patient demographics or disease characteristics found that sociodemographic risk factors for obesity in the IBD population were similar to those in the general population. Prior IBD-related surgery was the only disease characteristic associated with overweight and obesity in children with CD (OR 1.73, 95% CI 1.07–2.82) [52].

Obesity is associated with a pro-inflammatory state that may be involved in the etiology of IBD. However, a prospective cohort study conducted on a sample of 300,724 participants recruited for the European Prospective Investigation into Cancer and Nutrition study found no association between obesity, as measured by the BMI with the onset of incident UC or CD [53].

General Management of Nutrition in Inflammatory Bowel Disease

Monitoring Nutritional Status

Assessment for under- (or over-)nutrition is an essential component of medical care of children with IBD. At a minimum, screening should include measurement of body weight and height for age, with calculation of BMI. Nutritional status can be expressed in terms of the degree of height deficit (shortness), weight deficit (underweight or lightness), or relative weight for height or BMI for age (thinness). Each component captures a different aspect of growth, and interpretation is further complicated during puberty when differences in measures for thinness can be driven by changes in lean muscle and/or fat [26]. Growth parameters should be routinely collected and graphically recorded on standardized charts. It is important to obtain information on familial growth patterns, particularly parental heights, as well as pre-illness measurements to assess growth potential and the impact of disease on growth, respectively.

Ongoing assessment of nutritional status includes history, physical examination, and laboratory testing. History should attempt to obtain information on appetite, weight changes, and dietary intake (often with the assistance of a registered dietician), as well as identification of medications and nutritional or herbal supplements, including vitamins and minerals. Review of psychosocial factors such as economic and cultural or environmental influences may be useful.

Physical examination, in addition to growth parameters and BMI, should include anthropometric assessment of body habitus along with recordings of sexual maturation by Tanner staging. Examination may reveal signs of generalized malnutrition or specific nutrient deficiencies.

Laboratory tests are valuable in assessment of specific nutrient deficiencies; however some measures of nutritional status can also be affected by inflammation (e.g., serum albumin and ferritin). Serum pre-albumin has a much shorter half-life (2 days) than albumin (18–20 days) and may be more useful in the assessment of nutritional status changes with nutritional support [54].

Other potential tests of nutritional status are urinary creatinine/height ratio or 3-methylhistidine determinations which reflect somatic (muscle) protein status and 24 h urine urea nitrogen which reflects protein catabolism. However due to the difficulty obtaining accurate specimens and assumptions required for interpretation, these lab tests are not used in routine clinical practice. Additional research techniques for assessment of nutritional status are dual-energy X-ray absorptiometry [24], bioelectric impedance analysis, and total body electrical conductance to determine total body water and fat mass and isotopic labeling of various molecules to determine energy expenditure and metabolic turnover rates [19].

Serum leptin may also have a role in nutritional assessment as a marker of fat stores [55–57] and has been found to be lower in children with severe protein energy malnutrition [58]. Controversy exists in the literature regarding the correlation of leptin levels with inflammation or whether it simply reflects nutritional status regardless of underlying disease. Hoppin et al. found no difference in serum leptin levels between children with IBD and controls and concluded that serum leptin levels depend on BMI and sex and not on disease activity or severity [59].

Aurangzeb et al. explored the relationship between leptin and BMI in newly diagnosed children with IBD in comparison to controls. Significantly lower mean serum levels were found in 28 newly diagnosed IBD patients compared to 56 controls (2.32 pg/ml +/−1.88 vs 5.09 pg/ml +/−4.86, p+0.009). In this group of children with IBD, leptin levels did not correlate with the degree of inflammation, as defined by serum markers of inflammation [10]. Further studies are required to elucidate the role of leptin in nutritional assessment of IBD patients.

Following diagnosis of IBD, there are numerous ongoing aspects of nutritional management to address. Nutritional issues relating to therapy may arise. The use of steroids often leads to increased appetite and commonly alters fluid balance with initial fluid retention and weight gain that only partially reflects improvements in underlying nutritional status. Steroids are clearly linked with impaired bone mineralization, with enhanced resorption, and with decreased new bone formation [60, 61]. Adequacy of calcium and vitamin D intake must be reviewed regularly. Inhibition of linear growth and altered final height, due to suppression of insulin-like growth factor-1 (IGF-1), is also a feature of daily corticosteroid therapy [62].

Other medications may interfere with the absorption of specific micronutrients. Sulfasalazine may interfere with folate metabolism by reducing absorption; however, daily supplementation does not appear necessary [63]. In contrast, folate supplementation is required when the immunosuppressive drug methotrexate is used, as this drug acts to inhibit the conversion of folate to the active moiety tetrahydrofolate [64].

Questions related to nutrition and which foods to avoid are among the commonest raised by families both at diagnosis and in routine follow-up. The current consensus from the North American Society for Pediatric Gastroenterology, Hepatology and Nutrition (NASPGHAN) is that diets of children with CD should be well balanced, based on the Food Guide Pyramid, and follow dietary reference intakes [19]. Brown et al. recently created a "global practice guideline," which attempted to consolidate the existing information regarding diet and IBD proposed by medical societies or dietary guidelines from patient-centered, IBD-related organizations. The dietary suggestions included nutritional deficiency screening, avoiding foods that worsen symptoms, eating smaller meals at more frequent intervals, eliminating dairy if lactose intolerant, limiting excess fat, reducing carbohydrates, and reducing high-fiber foods during flares. Enteral nutrition was recognized as being recommended for CD in some parts of the world more often than others (e.g., more in Japan than in the USA) [65].

Overall, CD, in contrast to UC, can have a tremendous and long-lasting impact upon nutritional status but can also be successfully treated with nutritional therapy. Minimal evidence exists for the treatment of UC with enteral nutrition. Wedrychowicz et al. recently evaluated the effect of EEN on endothelial growth factor (VEGF) and transforming growth factor beta 1 (TGF-β1) in both UC and CD [66]. However, due to the concomitant use of antibiotics and 5ASA in this study, the role of EEN in UC is impossible to determine from this study. Therefore, the remainder of this chapter will focus on the nutritional impact and management of CD.

History of the Use of EEN in CD

The effectiveness of elemental diets was originally identified in 1973 by Voitk when it was used in adult patients with CD to provide preoperative nutritional support [67]. The first controlled study of an elemental diet in adults with CD determined that an elemental diet was equally effective in the induction of remission as corticosteroids [68]. The role of EEN in pediatrics, where EEN had the important additional benefit of supporting growth, was first reported by Sanderson and colleagues in 1987 [69].

The type of EEN utilized has evolved from the initial use of elemental feeds by nasogastric tube toward using polymeric feeds, which have better palatability, lower cost, and the option of oral administration. Although still the subject of some debate, practice has moved toward the use of EEN for any disease location in the gastrointestinal tract. Ongoing

research continues to explore the mechanism of action of EEN and strategies to optimize acceptance and utility of nutritional therapy.

Postulated Mechanisms of Action of EEN in CD

Our understanding of the mechanisms by which the beneficial effects of EEN are achieved in active CD remains incomplete. Various mechanisms have been proposed over time including relative gut rest, avoidance of allergenic elements, nutritional mechanisms, alteration of the intestinal microflora, and specific anti-inflammatory effects. Gut rest does not appear to be a complete explanation as complete gut rest, with total parenteral nutrition and nil by mouth, does not lead to enhanced rates of remission. Avoidance of dietary protein allergens also does not seem to explain the effects of EEN fully as the benefits of EEN are shown to the same whether an elemental or polymeric formula is utilized. Recent studies have focused upon changes in the intestinal microbiota, direct anti-inflammatory activities, and effects upon gut barrier function.

The Intestinal Microbiota

The intestinal microbiota plays a central role in the pathogenesis of IBD, although current data does not indicate any one species as being causative on its own. The impact of EEN upon the intestinal microbiota has been examined in human settings and in an animal model of IBD.

Two early studies used molecular techniques to examine the impact of EEN upon the flora in the context of IBD [70, 71]. These reports illustrated changes in the flora consequent to the introduction of the enteral formula. A more recent study employed a more comprehensive molecular approach (denaturing gel gradient electrophoresis or DGGE) with a wider selection of probes, enabling a broader profile of the changes [72]. This study showed a reduction in the diversity of the bacterial species and changes within all the main bacterial groupings. These changes were sustained, with effects well beyond the period of EEN alone.

A subsequent study utilized 16S rRNA and whole genome high-throughput sequencing to ascertain additional understanding of the impact of EEN upon the microbiota [73]. All five children included in this study had dysbiosis at diagnosis of CD. EEN resulted in a prompt reduction of the number of operational taxonomic units (OTU), which correlated with induction of disease remission. Subsequent exacerbation of disease leads to an increase in the number of OTU. Furthermore, six specific *Firmicutes* families were shown to correlate closely with disease activity during and after exposure to EEN [73].

More recently, further studies from the UK [74] and the USA [75] have utilized advanced molecular tools to further define changes in the intestinal microbiota consequent to EEN. Although each of these reports indicates the impact of EEN, they do not yet illustrate whether these changes result solely from the difference in the nutrients supplied in the formulae or how these changes then influence mucosal inflammation.

Data from an animal model of CD complements these data. Using an IL-10 knockout model of gut inflammation, a Japanese group assessed changes after the administration of elemental formula [76]. The bacterial diversity and bacterial number were both reduced in those animals given the formula compared to a control group with normal mouse diet.

Two recent studies have also assessed patterns of the intestinal flora consequent to enteral feeding in non-IBD contexts. Smith et al. [77] assessed changes in bacterial composition in the stomach and duodenum of adults receiving enteral formulae via a gastrostomy for various noninflammatory indications. Higher levels of bacterial DNA were found in the upper gut after enteral feeding. The fecal flora was not examined in this patient group. A second study examined fecal microflora in a small group of adults requiring exclusive nasogastric feeding for a variety of medical indications [78]. Individuals with IBD were excluded from the study. The subjects provided stools at the start of, during, and at the end of a 14-day period of enteral feeds. Molecular methodology was employed to assess the flora (fluorescence in situ hybridization). Overall the investigators did not observe consistent changes in the microflora during this short period. However, they did note changes in particular groups of organisms in the individuals who developed diarrhea secondary to the enteral feeds. However, these effects differed to those seen consistently in individuals with IBD.

Anti-inflammatory Activities

Meister et al. [79] demonstrated in vitro anti-inflammatory activities of formulae in a series of experiments using explants (short-term culture of colonic tissue samples obtained endoscopically). These samples were incubated directly with an elemental formula or maintained in a control situation. The production of interleukin (IL)-1-β, IL-1-receptor antagonist (RA), and IL-10 was used as an indicator of cell responses. The cells incubated with formula lead to an increase in the ratio between IL-1RA and IL-1-β, compared to the control cells ($P < 0.05$). These changes were also evident when full protein-based formulae were employed. Further, these changes were not observed in biopsies taken from individuals with UC or with noninflamed IBD tissue.

More recently, an in vitro model of intestinal cells has been used to elucidate the anti-inflammatory effects of formulae [80]. These experiments utilized established colonic epithelial cells lines, which were stimulated with one or more pro-inflammatory cytokines to replicate intestinal inflammatory events. Polymeric formulae were then used to rescue or to prevent the cellular response to this inflammatory insult, with interleukin (IL)-8 utilized as an indicator of epithelial response. The effect of adding polymeric formula (PF) to this model was assessed in a series of different ways, with particular use of a two-compartment model, whereby the PF was separated from the inflammatory cytokine. Experiments using this model demonstrated that PF leads to alteration of the inflammatory effects of TNF-α (reduced levels of IL-8) and suggested alteration of cellular signal transduction pathways as a mechanism for this finding [80].

A similar model was utilized to show that the application of PF resulted in modulation of nuclear factor (NF)-κB activity, thereby modulating the production of pro-inflammatory cytokines [81].

Subsequent studies showed that vitamin D and two specific amino acids (arginine and glutamine) mediated the effects of PF in this setting [82]. These findings suggest that active components within the nutritional products used for EEN may explain the anti-inflammatory effects seen in vivo.

Epithelial Barrier Function

Disruptions to barrier function, measured as altered intestinal permeability, are demonstrated in individuals with CD [83]. It is unclear whether these are primary events or are consequent to inflammation. Data showing similar alterations in permeability in asymptomatic first-degree relatives of people with IBD suggests that these could be primary changes, which could thereby predispose to the development of inflammatory changes in some individuals [84]. Intestinal permeability improves with resolution of inflammation [85] including following EEN [86].

Recent in vitro studies have explored these mechanisms further [87]. These studies employed an in vitro model of inflammation similar to that described above, whereby intestinal epithelial cell monolayers were stimulated with pro-inflammatory stimuli and then rescued with PF. Using an Ussing chamber, these experiments demonstrated that EEN lead to complete reversal of cytokine-induced changes in transepithelial resistance, short-circuit current, and horseradish peroxidase flux. In addition, PF was shown to correct cytokine-induced changes in tight junction proteins and key mediators of tight junction function. A subsequent series of confirmatory experiments were conducted using an animal model of colitis. Colitis induced in interleukin-10 knockout mice resulted in altered barrier function. These changes were reversed by the administration of a PF to the affected animals. PF in this setting also had reversal of mucosal inflammatory changes [88].

Although the molecular mechanisms of these observations are not yet defined, these findings provide significant clues to the activity of EEN in vivo. More work is required to clearly define the molecular events behind these important observations and also to translate these findings to the in vivo situation.

Effectiveness of Exclusive Enteral Nutrition Therapy in Crohn's Disease

Induction of Remission

Multiple pediatric studies have indicated that approximately 60–90% of children fed an exclusive liquid diet will enter clinical remission. As shown in several studies and a meta-analysis [89] updated with the most recent randomized study [90], high remission rates with EEN are achieved irrespective of the type of enteral feed (14/15 93% achieved remission with elemental diet vs 15/19 73% on polymeric diet, n.s.).

In addition, there have been numerous open and comparative studies evaluating the use of EEN versus corticosteroids in adults [91–94] and children [69, 95, 96] with CD. Recently, patients enrolled at diagnosis into the growth relapse and outcomes with therapy in Crohn's disease (GROWTH CD) study were evaluated for disease activity, CRP, and fecal calprotectin for 1 year. Clinical remission at 12 weeks with EEN was superior to corticosteroids both when considering remission by PCDAI (OR, 2.07; 95% CI, 1.8–18.3) or combined normal PCDAI and CRP (OR 3.4; 95% CI, 1.3–9) [97].

In three meta-analyses investigating the use of EEN in CD, steroids were found to be more effective in the induction of remission [98–100]. The most recent Cochrane meta-analysis comparing induction of remission by corticosteroids (160 patients) versus EEN (192 patients) yielded a pooled odds ratio (OR) of 0.33 (95% CI: 0.21–0.53) favoring corticosteroid therapy [75]. However, these analyses involved predominantly adult studies of varying quality. A well-conducted pediatric randomized controlled study [101], added to the latest meta-analysis, allowed for a sensitivity analysis of high-quality studies based on the Jadad scale [102]. The two high-quality studies had conflicting results, one favoring steroid therapy [103] and one favoring EEN [101] though neither study demonstrated statistically significant differences. However, the more recent study demonstrated mucosal healing after 10 weeks of EEN in 14/19 (74%) of participants versus only 6/18 (33%) of those treated with steroid therapy. The question of equivalent or superior efficacy of steroids to EEN in children is also raised by Heuschkel et al. who combined in meta-analysis the data accrued in controlled trials conducted exclusively in children and adolescents [104]. They concluded that nutritional treatment and conventional corticosteroids are equally effective

in a pediatric population, even if not in adults. However, to reach this conclusion, their NNT was 182 patients to detect a 20% difference in treatment effects. The actual number they had from five randomized controlled trials was only 147 children, and hence, they included two nonrandomized trials to reach the desired sample size.

Day et al. have identified poor compliance resulting in inadequate volume of EEN received as a major reason why some patients did not achieve remission [105]. The effect of compliance was explored in a recently updated Cochrane meta-analysis by performing a sub-analysis of the data on a per-protocol basis, excluding patients who withdrew due to lack of acceptability of nasogastric tube feeding or palatability of the enteral feed. When comparing those who completed EEN therapy to the corticosteroid group, efficacy was equivalent for induction of clinical remission [89].

In addition, a number of pediatric retrospective studies have found that EEN is more effective than corticosteroids in improving disease severity and growth deficiency. Among these is a large retrospective study from Canada including 229 patients where EEN has been commonly used as induction therapy [106]. In addition, a recent retrospective study from China where the incidence of CD is much lower, EEN was also found to more effective than corticosteroids (90% vs 50% P < 0.05) [107]. Another large Canadian cohort found equal efficacy to corticosteroids [108].

In summary, existing studies and meta-analyses demonstrate high remission rates with EEN therapy depending on adherence. With efficacy to corticosteroids being similar, the advantages in mucosal healing, lack of corticosteroid side effects, and improvements in nutritional status strongly support the use of exclusive enteral nutrition over corticosteroid therapy for induction of remission. Current guidelines support EEN as the first-line therapy to induce remission in children with active CD [4]. Efforts to develop innovative palatable formulations to improve acceptance of this therapy among patients and strategies to improve geographic variability in utilization are required.

Comparative Effectiveness of Nutritional and Biological Therapy

In a recent prospective study of 90 children with CD, clinical outcomes of disease activity, quality of life, and mucosal healing estimated by fecal calprotectin were compared between partial enteral nutrition (PEN) (n = 16), EEN (n = 22), and anti-TNF therapy (n = 52). Clinical response (PCDAI reduction ≥15 or final PCDAI ≤10) was achieved by 64% on PEN, 88% EEN, and 84% anti-TNF (test for trend P = 0.08). FCP ≤250 µg/g was achieved with PEN in 14%, EEN 45%, and anti-TNF 62% (test for trend P = 0.001). Improvement in overall quality of life was not statistically significantly different between the three groups [109]. Further clinical and cost-effective studies are required to aid in the therapeutic decision pathway of pediatric CD.

Maintenance of Remission

Following the induction of remission, the use of EN as maintenance therapy may have additional benefits to prolonging remission, including delaying the requirement for further therapy (i.e., corticosteroids) and optimizing growth and nutrition. Most often maintenance EN is practiced in combination with maintenance medical therapy, but limitations of adherence may similarly impact enteral therapy as it does medical therapy.

To date the majority of the literature on maintenance of remission of CD with EN therapy has been in adult patients, mostly arising from multiple centers in Japan. There is a smaller and older body of work in pediatrics.

Maintenance of Remission with EN in Adults

Akobeng and Thomas [110] conducted a Cochrane review of enteral nutrition for maintenance of remission in Crohn's disease. They identified only two maintenance studies in adult patients which were randomized controlled studies, one where the comparison groups were two types of formula (elemental vs polymeric) [111] and another where a maintenance EN regimen was compared with regular diet [112]. Verma and colleagues studied 33 adult steroid-dependent CD patients in remission, who were randomized to elemental ($n = 19$) versus polymeric ($n = 14$) formula, and followed for maximum of 12 months. Fourteen or 43% of the total population remained in remission and off corticosteroid at 12 months, with no significant difference in relapse rates noted between the two formula groups [111]. They did not identify any disease- or patient-related factors that predicted response to enteral nutrition; however, their sample size was small limiting their ability to make meaningful comparisons. Although no "toxicity" was encountered per se, 6 (18%) of patients withdrew within 2 weeks of study start due to intolerance to feeds related to smell or taste problems.

Takagi [112] studied 51 adult patients in remission who were randomized to receive a half-elemental diet ($n = 26$) or a free diet group ($n = 25$). The half-elemental diet group was required to take half the daily caloric allowance as an elemental formula (either orally or via a nasogastric tube). While there were some restrictions placed on the caloric intake of the other "half" of their diet (aided through use of semi-weighed food diaries), there were no specifications for its composition. This was one of many Japanese studies which has looked at the question of maintenance EN how-

ever, and as such, the unrestricted free diet is likely different from the equivalent Western diet. The authors in the Takagi study chose a primary outcome of relapse over a 2-year period [112]. The study was stopped before achieving the 2-year follow-up for all participants because the relapse rate in the half-elemental diet group was significantly lower than that in the free diet group (34.6% vs 64%) after a mean follow-up of 11.9 months.

Yamamoto [113] carried out a systematic review examining EN for the maintenance of remission in Crohn's disease. They included studies where EN was compared with another therapy; thus the study by Takagi [112] was included, but not the study by Verma and colleagues [111]. They did not limit their review to RCTs, so three prospective nonrandomized trials [114–116] and six retrospective studies [117–121] were included. The number of patients included in most of these studies was small. One of the ten studies included pediatric patients alone [118]. Eight of ten studies were conducted in Japan. Knowledge of the country of origin for a study is important when interpreting the results and assessing generalizability. In Japan, EN has a central role in the management of CD. In all but one of the eight Japanese studies included in the systematic review, an elemental formula was used, and also in a majority of studies, the oral component of the diet was a low-fat diet. The impact of this dietary approach, compared with a maintenance polymeric formula and/or traditional Western diet, has not been directly studied. The contribution of the low-fat diet, and elemental formula with a relative low-fat component, may be a relevant factor in light of the work by Bamba et al. who suggested that a lower-fat diet may be an important factor related to the efficacy of EN in CD [122]. Another factor, when reviewing EN studies from Japan, is that virtually all participants with CD are on a 5ASA preparation, as this is viewed as a standard of care for maintenance [113]. Because all participants are exposed to this intervention, it would not be expected to bias the findings relative to the EN outcomes. Additionally azathioprine was used by a number of study participants, but as is the case with 5ASA, overall its use seemed to be balanced between the treatment and comparison groups in the studies, thereby limiting the bias this concomitant therapy might have introduced.

In the systematic review by Yamamoto [113], the authors broke down the studies by whether the patients had achieved a medically or surgically induced remission. Interestingly, different from what would be seen in studies conducted in North America, for those studies with patients who entered from a medically induced remission, the majority of patients went into remission with total parenteral nutrition or EEN. Regardless of the method of induction of remission (medical or surgical), the outcomes for the ten included studies showed benefit of EN for maintenance of remission (48–95%) over the non-EN comparison groups (21–65%)

[113]. In four studies the impact of dose of EN on remission rates was evaluated [117, 119, 121]. They found that higher amounts of enteral formula were associated with higher clinical remission rates. Another interpretation of these findings could be that patients with less active disease tolerated the enteral feeding better and, therefore, reached greater intakes than those with more active disease. Thus patients with milder disease may tolerate the nutrition better, rather than the higher intake being a predictor of maintenance of remission. As well, because there was no standard approach to "dosing" used in these studies, at this time no clear recommendations can be made regarding the minimum dose of EN required to optimally maintain remission.

Maintenance of Remission with EN in Pediatrics

Maintenance EN programs have been provided in various forms: overnight NG feeds in conjunction with normal daytime eating, short intervals of exclusive NG feeds every few months interspersed with regular diet, or as oral supplements in addition to oral eating through the day. Two Canadian groups have considered the first two approaches [118, 123]. Researchers at the Hospital for Sick Children in Toronto, Canada, reported on 28 children who after entering remission with EEN had subsequently continued overnight supplementary NG feeds in addition to normal diet in the daytime [118]. They were compared with 19 children in whom EEN successfully induced remission but who opted to discontinue nocturnal elemental feeding. At 12 months, 43% (12/28) of those receiving nocturnal EN had relapsed compared with 79% (15/19) who had discontinued supplemental elemental feedings ($P < 0.02$). A second group, from Montreal, Quebec, published a report utilizing a different approach to EN feeds, with intermittent intensive periods of nutritional therapy (EEN) [123]. This small study included eight children with CD and associated growth failure who were given intensive exclusive periods of formula for 1 month out of every 4 months. Disease activity markers fell in this group over time and in comparison to a control group who did not receive this intensive therapy. These eight children managed with intensive nutritional therapy also had significant catch-up growth [123].

EN in Combination with Medical Therapy

Thus far, the majority of studies investigating the role of EN with medical therapy have focused on concomitant use with infliximab. A meta-analysis of four adult studies, which were all from Japan, showed that specialized enteral nutrition therapy with infliximab resulted in 109 of 157 (69.4%) patients reaching clinical remission compared with 84 of 185 (45.4% with infliximab monotherapy [OR 2.73; 95% confidence interval 1.73–4.31, $P < 0.01$]. Maintenance of remission was also achieved in the combination treatment group [124].

In children, there have been minimal studies conducted to examine the use of immunomodulators and EEN in children with newly diagnosed CD, but Buchanan et al. reported that patients found it difficult to continue supplemental nutrition as maintenance or remission and therefore used a strategy of early introduction of azathioprine for maintenance of EEN-induced remission [125]. The relative importance of choice of initial induction therapy on 2-year outcomes in the setting of early thiopurine use was recently evaluated. In the setting of early thiopurine commencement, choice of EEN over corticosteroid induction was associated with reduced linear growth failure (7 vs 26%, $P = 0/02$), steroid dependency (7 vs 43%, $P = 0.002$), and improved primary sustained response to infliximab (86 vs 68%, $P = 0.02$) [126].

The effect of supportive short-term partial enteral nutrition (SPEN) on the treatment of children with severe CD along with unspecified conventional therapy was recently explored in a Korean cohort [127]. Patients with active CD were divided into mild, moderate, and severe categories according to PCDAI. The severe group was given the option of receiving SPEN, and 17 of 34 patients opted in. The remaining 17 patients were considered to be the non-SPEN group. Changes in nutritional status and PCDAI were significantly higher in the SPEN group ($P < 0.05$).

Further long-term study of the combination and synergistic effects of enteral nutrition and medical therapy particularly for maintenance of remission and mucosal healing is needed.

Repeated EEN and Long-Term Outcomes of Therapy

Despite the convincing results regarding immediate benefits of nutritional treatment, the efficacy of EEN for disease exacerbation and duration of remission is poorly studied.

The efficacy of repeated EEN therapy as a treatment for flares of disease tends to decrease with the second course. In a recent retrospective study, 26/52 patients received a second EEN course. The first compared to the second EEN tended to a higher remission rate (92% remission for the first course vs 77% n.s.). Duration of the second EEN therapy was shorter compared to the first (mean days 50 vs 43, $P < 0.05$). It was possible that nonadherence increased with the second course of EEN and contributed to the lower effectiveness. Disease activity measured by the mathematically weighted PCDAI (wPCDAI) was higher for the first course of EEN therapy (59 vs 40, $P < 0.0001$) [128]. Remission rates ranging from 57 to 80% have been reported by other retrospective studies evaluating a consecutive course of EEN [105, 129, 130].

In terms of 1–2-year outcomes, approximately half to two thirds of patients will relapse [128, 130, 131]. Predictors of higher relapse rates include the type of induction therapy (corticosteroids have higher relapse rates than EEN induction) [130, 131] and the type of NOD2 genotypes (92% R702W or G908R vs 50% 1007 fs vs 60% wild type, $P < 0.01$) [128].

Additional Effects and Proof of Efficacy of EEN

EEN and Mucosal Healing

For some time the treatment goals for the management of active CD have focused on the induction of remission, judged clinically (resolution of symptoms) and biochemically (normalization of altered inflammatory markers). More recently it has become clear that the goal of treatment should be the achievement of mucosal healing. Mucosal healing in both CD and UC is clearly associated with improved long-term outcomes [132]. Persisting inflammatory changes are likely to contribute to poor growth in children and are also associated with an increased risk of subsequent disease relapse [133]. Mucosal healing may also influence disease progression and extraintestinal disease patterns.

Both EEN and infliximab lead to high rates of mucosal healing in CD: more so than other therapies used to induce remission (such as corticosteroids) [134].

At the turn of the century, Fell and colleagues [135] undertook a prospective assessment of mucosal healing in a group of children treated with EEN. These 29 children with active CD were treated with a polymeric formula. In addition to baseline endoscopic assessment, repeat colonoscopy was completed after 6–8 weeks time in order to judge endoscopic and histologic changes. EEN lead to clinical remission in 79% of these children. Overall there was significant endoscopic improvement in these children. A one-point improvement in the colonoscopy grading score was seen in the ileum and colon ($P < 0.0001$ and $P < 0.001$, respectively). Eight of the children achieved mucosal healing in the ileal region, while eight also had colonic mucosal healing.

More recently the results of two prospective Italian studies and an Australian study show the enhanced rates of mucosal healing following EEN comparing to corticosteroids [101, 136, 137]. Berni-Canani and colleagues [101] evaluated the responses in children managed with EEN or corticosteroids. Thirty-seven children were treated nutritionally for 8 weeks with various different formulae (polymeric, semi-elemental, and elemental), while ten received corticosteroids. Clinical remission rates were similar in the two groups (86.5% vs 90%, respectively), but mucosal healing rates were quite different. Twenty-six of the 37 children

treated nutritionally had mucosal improvements, and seven of them had complete mucosal healing. In contrast, just four of the steroid group had improvement noted, and none had mucosal healing.

In a second Italian study, children with active CD were allocated to receive either EEN (polymeric formula) or corticosteroids. Baseline colonoscopic assessment was followed by repeat colonoscopy at 10 weeks. Fourteen (74%) of the 19 children treated with EEN had mucosal healing. In contrast, mucosal healing was achieved in just six (33%) of the 18 children treated with corticosteroids ($P < 0.05$). Grover et al. evaluated the effects of 6 weeks of EEN in a cohort of 26 children. Paired endoscopic assessments showed that 58% of the group had complete or near-complete MH following EEN [137]. Subsequent work by this group in a larger group of children demonstrated that complete MH (seen in 18 of 54 children) after EEN resulted in sustained remission for up to 3 years [138].

Data from adult patients also clearly demonstrates high rates of mucosal healing consequent to EEN. Yamamoto et al. [139] assessed the mucosal changes following an elemental formula in 28 adults with active CD. In this series of patients treated with EEN, clinical remission was seen in 71%. Furthermore, endoscopic healing or improvements were documented in 44% and 78% of patients, respectively.

Mucosal healing with EEN does not appear to be dependent on the type of formula utilized. Benefits have been documented with elemental [101, 139, 140] or polymeric formulae [135, 136].

Coincident with promoting healing of the inflamed mucosa, EEN is also shown to lead to changes in levels of inflammatory mediators. Several reports published in the final decade of the last century demonstrated that EEN lead to reduced mucosal production of pro-inflammatory cytokines (especially TNF-α and interleukin-2) [140, 141] and prompted downregulation of pro-inflammatory genes measured within the intestinal mucosa [135, 142]. In addition, Fell et al. [135] also demonstrated increased levels of TGF-β mRNA, consistent with increased production of this anti-inflammatory cytokine. Yamamoto and colleagues [139] also showed that the mucosal levels of multiple pro-inflammatory cytokines fell to control levels consequent to treatment with an elemental formula. The ratio between IL-1β and IL-1ra within the mucosa was also normalized.

Overall these data clearly show alterations in levels of inflammatory mediators within the mucosa following treatment with EEN. The full implications of achieving mucosal healing with EEN in children are not yet well defined. Maintenance EN may have a role in maintaining the levels of mucosal healing. It is also not clear if mucosal healing with one therapy (such as EEN) is different to that achieved by another agent (e.g., steroids). Furthermore, treatment protocols have not yet evolved to stratify maintenance therapy upon the level of mucosal healing.

EEN and Changes in Fecal Markers of Inflammation

Various proteins measured in the stool are valid markers of the level and extent of gut inflammation [143]. The most well-known markers are calprotectin and lactoferrin, but others include S100A12 and osteoprotegerin.

In a study by Gerasimidis et al., fecal calprotectin (FC) levels were measured on multiple occasions during and following a course of EEN in 15 children [144]. The children received a polymeric formula, and clinical disease activity was defined by determination of PCDAI scores, with a score of 10 or less being judged as clinical remission. FC levels fell only in the children who were in clinical remission by the end of the period of EEN, but FC levels were normalized in only one child. Interestingly, the FC level after 1 month of EEN was associated with clinical response at the end of EEN, suggesting a predictive value at this time. In a study comparing partial EN (PEN), EEN, and anti-TNF therapy, FC ≤ 250 µg/g was achieved with PEN in 14%, EEN in 45%, and anti-TNF in 62% (test for trend $P = 0.001$).

The levels of S100A12 (a protein related to calprotectin) were evaluated in a small group of Australian children managed with EEN for active CD [145]. Levels fell in the subset of children who achieved clinical remission and normal CRP.

Recent work showed that EEN treatment also led to reductions in levels of another fecal inflammatory marker, osteoprotegerin (OPG) [146]. Levels of OPG fell to around 25% in response to 6–8 weeks of EEN (1994 ± 2289 pg/g at baseline to 406 ± 551 pg/g after EEN: $P = 0.002$). The value of this marker in predicting response to EEN or in correlating with mucosal healing has not yet been determined.

EEN: Nutritional Status and Growth

Along with improvements in disease activity, weight and growth improvements are also commonly seen with EEN. Numerous studies show improved weight gains, while some have illustrated changes in specific nutritional markers. Several studies have suggested that nutritional improvements occur at different times to changes in specific inflammatory markers. These studies demonstrate that improvements in nutrition do not correlate with the timing of normalizing inflammatory markers [54, 147]. It is not clear whether the nutritional changes are essential to achieve anti-inflammatory improvements. However, satisfactory weight gains are associated with response to EEN, illustrating the importance of these events [105].

Insulin-like growth factor (IGF)-1 is a key mediator of growth hormone signaling. Alterations in this protein occur due to the effects of cytokines (reduced hepatic production secondary to interleukin-6) and are commonly observed in active CD. A number of studies illustrate early increases in IGF-1 and its related binding protein (IGF-BP3) after commencement of EEN [148]; unpublished data, Day et al. [105]. IGF-1 levels rose after just 7 days of EEN in a small group of 12 children [147].

Detailed nutritional assessments, including body composition analysis, have been conducted in individuals receiving EEN. One key study evaluated body composition using multiple direct methods to define fat, water, total body protein, and potassium [149]. A group of 30 individuals with CD were assessed before and after 3 weeks of EEN. Within this short time, increased weight was linked with proportionate increases in body fat, protein, and water. Another study documented changes in body compartments in a group of Canadian children [25]. Body water, lean body mass, and height increases were observed in the children who had received EEN, but not in a comparison group treated with corticosteroids. EEN has been shown by other authors to promote anabolism consequent to suppression of proteolysis and enhanced protein synthesis [18, 37].

These changes in nutrition manifest in weight gains during EEN. The average weight gain in a group of Australian children treated with 6–8 weeks of EEN was 4.7 ± 3.5 kg [105]. In addition, weight Z scores increased over the duration of EEN from −0.2767 ± 0.9707 to 0.1866 ± 0.8024 ($P = 0.0016$). Weight standard deviation scores increased after 8 and 16 weeks ($P < 0.05$) in a small cohort of 14 UK children with a mean age of 12.5 years [148]. However, studies do report variable weight gains [136, 150].

EEN is also noted to have a positive benefit upon linear growth, with improved height velocity even within a short period of time [17, 69]. In a meta-analysis, Newby and colleagues [151] illustrated a significant improvement in height velocity Z scores with EEN compared to outcomes after treatment with corticosteroids. In the aforementioned Australian study, children receiving EEN gained up to 3 cm during the 8-week course of EEN; however there was no change in height Z scores across the whole group [105].

EEN and Bone Health

CD is associated with reductions in bone mineral density, which can lead to osteopenia and increased fracture risk. EEN appears to have benefits upon bone health. Whitten et al. [152] evaluated serum markers of bone turnover in a group of children with active newly diagnosed CD who were treated with polymeric formula as sole therapy to induce remission. Serum levels of bone resorption and bone production were measured at baseline and then again after 6–8 weeks of EEN. Control data was obtained from a group of children without IBD with normal growth patterns. Serum levels of C-terminal telopeptides of type-1 collagen (CTX), a marker of bone resorption, were elevated at baseline and fell during therapy ($P = 0.002$). In addition, levels of bone-specific alkaline phosphatase (BAP), a marker of new bone formation, were low at baseline but rose significantly during therapy ($P = 0.02$). This study did not include evaluation of other aspects of bone health or bone densitometry.

A more recent study has evaluated the impact of EEN upon vitamin D, an important factor involved in bone health [39]. This study retrospectively evaluated levels of vitamin D in 78 children with CD. A subgroup ($n = 38$) had been treated with EEN at diagnosis. These children treated with EEN had higher levels of vitamin D than a comparison group of 17 children treated with corticosteroids after diagnosis ($P = 0.04$), suggesting that EEN provided a protective effect for this aspect of bone health.

Further information supporting the role of EEN in bone health was shown in a small German study. In this report, ten children with CD managed with EEN had repeated assessments of bone densitometry. The administration of EEN lead to improved trabecular and cortical density by 3 months after starting EEN, although further improvements were not seen subsequently [153].

Altogether, these data suggest that EEN provides significant beneficial effects upon bone metabolism in children with CD. However, further confirmatory studies are required.

EEN and Quality of Life

Impaired QOL is well recognized in children with CD. The IMPACT questionnaire was developed and validated several years ago as a disease-specific tool to measure QOL in pediatric IBD [154]. Given the importance of eating and food in many cultures and the disruption of these usual patterns during treatment with EEN, there has been some concern that EEN could further impair QOL in these children. The influence of EEN upon QOL has been examined in just a small number of studies in children and adults.

An initial report on the effects of EEN upon QOL and functioning was published by a French group [155]. This study involved 30 children with active CD: half of the group was treated with EEN via an NG tube, while the other half of the group was given corticosteroids. The children were assessed by an adaptation of the IBD Questionnaire and underwent a series of psychological assessments, including a psychological interview. A disease-specific pediatric scoring tool was not utilized in this cohort. The authors showed that the children managed with EEN overall had improvements in their well-being. Several reported concerns about feeling different, disruptions to family routines, and the cosmetic effects of the NG tube itself. The children managed with EEN had better scores of anxiety and depression measures than those treated with corticosteroids. Both groups had

disruptions to daily activities such as school absences. A study from the UK looked specifically at QOL in a group of 26 children with active CD who were all managed with EEN [156]. This study reported remission rates and measured QOL using the IMPACT II questionnaire. Almost 90% of these children entered remission with EEN. Overall, 24 of the 26 children had improved QOL scores during this therapy. In this group of English children, the use of NG tubes to provide the formula did not impact adversely upon QOL.

In contrast to these findings, Hill et al. [157] found that the use of EEN was associated with lower QOL scores in their evaluation of children in their Australian center. This study involved the repeated assessment of various variables, including QOL and disease activity, at diagnosis and then six-monthly in 41 children (with 186 assessments in total). Nine children had assessments while receiving EEN: these children were noted to have lower QOL scores than other children on no treatments or those on other medical therapies. However, the group treated with EEN was also those with the highest disease activity scores and lowest nutritional parameters. Furthermore, multiple regression analyses showed that the only independent factor for prediction of QOL in the overall group was disease activity.

These data relate to the use of EEN as therapy for active disease. The ongoing influence of maintenance EN upon QOL has also been assessed in a large group of Japanese adults with known CD [158]. Ninety-five of the 126 patients included were receiving EN as maintenance therapy at the time of the assessment. The investigators used the adult IBD Questionnaire to assess QOL scores. In addition to QOL, other parameters were evaluated. Overall, this study showed that disease activity affected QOL, while nutritional treatment improved QOL. Overall scores and subscores for bowel and systemic symptoms were better in the patients with long-standing disease who were receiving maintenance EN.

In the PLEASE study discussed above, comparing anti-TNF therapy, EEN, and PEN, with assessment of outcomes at 8 week of therapy, a secondary outcome of QOL was assessed [109]. While clinical response (PCDAI reduction ≥ 15 or final PCDAI ≤ 10) was obtained in 64% of PEN, 88% EEN, and 84% anti-TNF, improvement in overall QOL was not statistically different between the three groups ($P = 0.86$). However, QOL improvement in the body image domain was greatest in the EEN group ($P = 0.03$) and with anti-TNF in the emotional functioning domain ($P = 0.04$).

At present, the overall impression of the available data is that the net benefits of EEN upon QOL are positive, likely consequent to improved energy and improved disease control. However, these data are not yet comprehensive, and further study is required to more fully understand the relationships between nutritional therapies and QOL in children with CD.

Pre-/Postoperative Effects

Two recent adult studies from China have examined the role of EEN in the preoperative setting. Li G et al. retrospectively reviewed the influence of preoperative 3-month EEN on the incidence of intra-abdominal septic complications (IASCs) after bowel resections for enterocutaneous fistulas (ECFs). The EEN group had a significantly higher serum albumin level and lower CRP at operation and suffered a lower risk of IASCs (3.6% vs 17.6%, P < 0.05) [159]. In addition, Li Y et al. demonstrated that preoperative optimization of CD following immunosuppressive therapy by EEN prolongs the immunosuppressant-free interval, reduces the risk of urgent surgery and reoperation, and decreases complications after abdominal surgery [160].

There is limited data from Japan on the impact of enteral nutrition on postoperative recurrence of CD. Initial intraoperative enteroscopic evaluation by Esaki suggested prophylactic effects of enteral nutrition on postoperative recurrence of small intestinal CD [121]. Yamamoto et al. studied the impact of long-term enteral nutrition on the clinical and endoscopic recurrence rates in a prospective, nonrandomized, parallel, controlled study of 40 adults who underwent resection for ileal or ileocolonic CD. Twenty patients continuously received enteral nutritional therapy (EN group) overnight via nasogastric tube and had a low-fat diet during the day. The 20 controls had neither nutritional therapy nor food restriction (non-EN group). Six months after operation, five patients (25%) in the EN group and eight (40%) in the non-EN group developed endoscopic recurrence, but the difference did not achieve significance. At 1 year a significant difference was found in both clinical recurrence (5% in the EN group vs 35% in the non-EN group) and endoscopic recurrence rates (30% in the EN group vs 70% in the non-EN group) [116]. This preliminary work in the postoperative setting supports the effectiveness of enteral nutrition, but additional studies are required to replicate this effect or determine regimens of postoperative EN use that would optimize long-term compliance and outcomes.

Adverse Effects of Enteral Nutrition

There are very few adverse effects associated with the use of EN. Loose stools may be reported, particularly in those with predominantly colonic disease distribution. Nausea and constipation are less commonly reported [135].

A cross-sectional Japanese study in adults has reported a risk of selenium deficiency in patients with CD being treated with EN. Selenium concentrations were measured and compared in 29 patients with CD treated by EN, 24 patients with CD who were not being treated with EN, and 21 healthy controls. Selenium levels were only decreased in CD patients receiving EN and were inversely correlated to the duration and daily dose of EN. Clinical manifestations of selenium deficiency were only found in one patient [161]. A European study examining the effect of exclusive EN on antioxidant concentrations in childhood CD reported conflicting results with respect to selenium. Mean selenium concentrations of the cohort increased significantly from 0.82 μmol/l to 1.14 mmol/L (P < 0.001). There were, however, significant reductions in mean concentrations of vitamins C and E [162]. A recent study on the impact of EEN on circulating micronutrients resulted in improved concentration for several nutrients, but interestingly, more than 90% of patients had depleted concentrations of all carotenoids, which later improved on normal diet [163]. Multiple factors including differences in age groups, disease activity, nutritional status, and EN formulae may all impact on vitamin and antioxidant levels and the disparate results of the above studies. Further investigation of potential adverse effects at the micronutrient level is required.

Another potential biochemical side effect reported to occur with EEN is transient elevation of transaminase enzymes. Schatorjé et al. [164] performed prospective follow-up of liver enzymes in 11 new consecutive children who were primarily treated with total enteral nutrition (TEN) for 6 weeks. Liver enzymes were measured before starting TEN and after 3, 6, and 12 weeks. Overall, nine of 11 patients developed a marked elevation of aspartate transaminase (AST), and ten had an elevated alanine transaminase (ALT) peaking at 3 and 6 weeks. GGT was slightly elevated in three patients during therapy, including two boys with either pre-existing or persistent raised transaminases. Alkaline phosphatase and bilirubin remained normal. The mean follow-up period was 2.1 years (1.0–3.5 years). None of the patients developed liver disease during follow-up, and liver biopsy was therefore not performed [164]. However, subsequent to this publication, a letter to the editor by Lemberg et al. reviewing transaminase results in their published cohort of 12 children with newly diagnosed CD managed with 8 weeks of EEN showed conflicting data. ALT levels were borderline elevated in only two of their patients at 3 weeks of EEN and one patient at 8 weeks of EEN therapy [165]. At diagnosis, all of the markers were within normal ranges. After 2–3 weeks of EEN, the average AST levels were 26.2. Subsequent means were 25 at 8 weeks and 16.8 at 1–2 months after EEN. Average ALT levels rose initially to 21.9 U/L and were subsequently 21.2 at 8 weeks and 14.2 at 1–2 months after EEN. ALT levels were above the upper range of normal (45 U/L) at 2–3 weeks in only two children (51 and 48, respectively) and at 8 weeks in one child (48 U/L). GGT levels did not change and liver disease did not develop in any of the patients. Thus, the effect of EEN on the liver is unclear from existing data. Further prospective investigation is required to clarify the effects of EEN on transaminase levels.

Severe adverse events related to EN are rare. To date there are three case reports of refeeding syndrome consequent to the use of EEN in CD [166, 167]. The two cases reported by Akobeng et al. occurred within days of starting EEN in severely malnourished children [167]. Although rare, it is important for clinicians to be aware of refeeding syndrome and to identify and monitor patients at risk.

Factors Affecting Response to EEN

Disease-Related Factors

Disease Duration

Several studies suggest higher efficacy of EEN in children with newly diagnosed CD over those with established disease duration. A multicenter North American study using a semi-elemental formula showed a remission rate of 83% in children newly diagnosed with CD [168], compared to a response rate of 50% in children with previously diagnosed CD. An Australian retrospective study found 12 of 15 (80%) children with newly diagnosed CD entered remission, defined by PCDAI, compared to 7 of 12 (58%) children, who had been diagnosed with CD for a mean of 3.2 years [105]. The latter study also showed that although some children in this group did not enter remission, each had reductions in PCDAI scores and each had nutritional improvements.

As previously discussed, the efficacy of repeated EEN therapy as a treatment for flares of disease tends to decrease with the second course [128], but the contribution of nonadherence in this setting versus disease duration is unclear.

Disease Location

Disease location has often been considered to potentially influence the effectiveness of EEN. Several early reports suggested increased efficacy when there is small bowel involvement [119, 129] and a trend toward earlier relapse in those with isolated colonic involvement [129]. Yet, Afzal et al. [150] demonstrated, in a prospective study of 65 children with acute intestinal CD treated with exclusive polymeric diet, that even the patients with disease limited to the colon had remission rates of 50%, albeit much lower than those with ileocolonic (82% remission rate) or ileal disease (91.7% remission rate).

Buchanan and colleagues [125], using carefully defined phenotypic classification in 110 patients on EEN, found no significant differences in the remission rates based on disease location. This is supported by a retrospective study by Rubio et al. who recently compared remission rates according to route of administration and found that the site of disease

activity had no impact on response to nutritional therapy [169]. Disease location could not be examined by the meta-analysis by Narula and Zachos et al. due to insufficient data [89, 100]. The most recent randomized trial evaluating elemental versus polymeric formula also did not identify any difference in remission rates based on disease location [90]. Thus, until the influence of disease location on response to EEN is more clearly delineated, it is reasonable to recommend it for all patients with CD regardless of disease site.

EEN-Related Factors

Polymeric Versus Elemental/Semi-elemental Diets

Nutritional therapy is classified by the nitrogen source derived from the amino acid or protein component of the formula. Elemental diets are created by mixing of single amino acids and are entirely antigen-free. Oligopeptide or semi-elemental diets are made by protein hydrolysis and have a mean peptide chain length of four or five amino acids, which is too short for antigen recognition or presentation. Polymeric diets contain whole protein from sources such as milk, meat, egg, or soy. They can be classified more simply as elemental (amino acid-based), semi-elemental (oligopeptide), and polymeric (whole-protein) diets.

Although elemental diets were used in the initial studies focusing upon the nutritional treatment of CD, subsequent studies in both children and adults have compared these elemental diets to polymeric diets [90, 103, 135, 170, 171]. Comparisons between any combination of the different protein sources when combined in meta-analysis [89, 100] have shown no significant difference in effectiveness. Similarly, one study comparing polymeric diets differing in glutamine enrichment showed no difference in remission rates [172].

Fat Composition

Several trials have been conducted to investigate the importance of fat composition [122, 173–175], building on the hypothesis that the proportion or type of fat in an enteral feed could affect the production of pro- or anti-inflammatory mediators. Two trials, Leiper et al. [174] and Sakurai et al. [175], investigated the effect of low versus high long-chain triglyceride (LCT) content and differing amounts of medium-chain triglycerides, respectively, in adult patients and showed no difference in effect. Another study by Bamba et al. [122] comparing diets of low (3.06 g/day), medium (16.56 g/day), or high fat (30.06 g/day) contents showed higher remission rates in the lowest fat group. By intention to treat analysis, remission was achieved in eight of 11 patients (72.7%) of the low-fat group, four of 13 (30.8%) in the medium-fat group, and two of 12 (16.7%) of the high-fat group. However, all of these studies were flawed by either small sample sizes, high dropout rates, or unvalidated activity indices used to define remission. When studies evaluating fat composition were combined by meta-analysis [89, 100], a nonsignificant trend favoring very low-fat and low LCT content has been demonstrated. However, these results should be interpreted with caution due to statistically significant heterogeneity and small size, which may have lacked statistical power to show differences should they exist. In addition, subgroup analyses could not be performed based on the n6 or n9 fatty acid composition in the feeds due to significant heterogeneity. The possibility that fat composition influences immunomodulatory or anti-inflammatory effect in active CD warrants further exploration with larger trials. In summary, no specific formula composition of EN diets has been conclusively shown to influence induction of remission in active CD.

Exclusive Versus Partial EN

The question of whether supplementary EN could be considered instead of EEN was explored in a randomized controlled pediatric trial by Johnson et al. [176]. This study showed that the combination of partial EN (50% of energy requirements) with normal diet leads to a substantially lower rate of remission compared to the use of EEN (100% of energy requirements) (15% in PEN vs 42% in EEN; $P < 0.035$).

Gupta et al. [177] recently retrospectively examined a novel protocol providing patients with 80–90% of caloric needs by EN and allowing consumption of remaining calories from a normal diet. Fifteen of twenty-three (65%) of the patients receiving the novel partial EN protocol achieved remission [177]. However, subsequent work from this group, as part of the PLEASE study [109], would suggest that although patients/families are instructed to consume 10–20% of calories from a normal diet, it would seem that in many what actually occurs is that overall caloric consumption is increased. Close monitoring of intake by dietitians revealed that the PEN group consumed 150.8% +/− 36.2 of their estimated energy requirement from a combination of formula (77.7% +/− 14.2) and food (72.9% +/− 25.5) so that 47.0% +/− 13.5 of their caloric intake was from food. While PEN plus ad lib diet improved clinical symptoms in this study, EEN and anti-TNF therapies were superior for inducing remission. These data suggest that EEN is effective due to the exclusion or at least a significant reduction of certain components of normal diets. Emerging data and further efforts are underway to study the effect of restricted table food-based diets on CD.

Duration of Therapy

The duration of EEN therapy ranges from 2 to 12 weeks in the literature and varies substantially in different parts of the world. The early effects of EN have been achieved over the first 4 weeks of therapy. Additional later effects in the fourth to eighth week of therapy may include further anti-inflammatory and nutritional benefits [105].

Delivery of EEN

Route of Administration of EEN

EEN can be administered by various different routes, such as oral and nasogastric (NG), or via a gastrostomy tube. The choice of route of administration will often be dependent on clinical judgment and reflects local practice, tolerance of formulae, and patient choice. Elemental or semi-elemental formulae may be more difficult to take orally. Since polymeric formulae have the same clinical benefits, lower cost, and better palatability (allowing for oral administration), they may be associated with increased interest, tolerance, and compliance of EN therapy, which remains the greatest challenge of this form of therapy. However, while, generally, children will accept the oral route more than the NG route, oral feeding may lead to greater difficulties over time as the child tries to maintain sufficient volume over a longer period of time. Rubio et al. [169] retrospectively reviewed 106 patients treated with either fractionated oral or continuous enteral feedings and found that both routes were efficacious in inducing remission and mucosal healing. After 8 weeks of EEN, 34/35 (75%) achieved remission in the oral group and 52/61 (85%) in the enteral nutrition group ($P = 0.157$). All patients showed a significant decrease in disease severity assessed by PCDAI and significant improvements in anthropometric measures and inflammatory indices. Weight gain was greater in the enteral group ($P = 0.041$) [169].

Some reports refer to the practice of routine placement of a NG tube at the start of the course of EEN and then encouragement of oral intake so that children end up with removal of the tube and ongoing oral feeds [90]. On the other hand, children who struggle with tolerance soon after commencing a period of EEN orally can subsequently be switched to NG administration [125].

Approach to Reintroduction of Normal Diet

Following the completion of the course of EEN, the next step will be the recommencement of normal regular diet. An international review of protocols in different units illustrated the range of approaches [178]. Overall, the time taken to reintroduce a normal diet (following a 6–8 week period of EEN) at these pediatric units varied from 1 to 12 weeks.

One of the most accepted approaches to reintroduce normal diet is a gradual introduction of food quantity, while formula volume is progressively decreased [178]. This approach entails the introduction of a meal every 2–3 days while reducing the volume of formula with the introduction of each meal, so that the adjustment takes place over 7–10 days time [105, 125]. Although not formally evaluated in this setting, this approach has been well accepted with very few children having disruptions to the reintroduction of normal diet [personal observations, A. Day].

One group has reported the immediate introduction of food, while formula volume is decreased to overnight feeds [179]. A further approach has involved the use of a low-allergen diet, with new low-allergen foods (initially lamb, potato, chicken, or rice) introduced every 2 or 3 days, followed by the progressive reintroduction of other foods and food groups [180]. This method of returning to a normal diet was evaluated by Shergill-Bonner et al. in 100 patients, and no clear benefits were demonstrated [181]. Similarly Faiman et al. reported a retrospective cohort study where 20 patients had reintroduction of food using the low-allergen approach, while a comparison group ($n = 19$) followed a low-residue diet for 3 days before reestablishing their usual unrestricted diet, with their EEN being weaned over a 2-week period. As with other studies which have looked at this issue, no significant differences were noted between the two groups with respect to relapse rate and duration of remission [182].

Geographic Variability and Barriers to Utilization of EEN

There is significant geographic variation in the practice and recommendations for EEN as primary therapy in the management of children with CD [65]. In Europe and Japan, guidelines recommend EEN as the first-line therapy for induction of remission in children with CD [183, 184]. The variation in use is noted between and within different countries across the world [5, 185–187]. In an early study by Levine et al. [5], significant variations in the use of EEN were reported in a trans-Atlantic survey of 167 physicians from the USA, Canada, Western Europe, and Israel. In that study, while 4% of North American pediatric gastroenterologists used EEN regularly, 62% of European practitioners reported regular use. These European numbers were echoed in a report from a survey of Swedish pediatric GI units, which showed that 65% of the units used EEN as their primary therapy in newly diagnosed CD [185]. The variation in practice among North American pediatric gastroenterologists was revisited in a survey of 326 NASPGHAN members from North America (86% USA, 14% Canada) [187]. They reported that 31% of respondents never used EN, 55% reported sparse use, and 12% reported regular use. Physicians in Canada reported significantly more use than in America ($P < 0.001$). Variations in EN use within a country were also demonstrated in a study of Australian pediatric gastroenterologists by Day et al. [186]. In both the North American and Australian studies, currently working and previously working in a center where EEN was used were important factors for both the perceived appropriateness of EEN and the regularity of its use. North American pediatric gastroenterologists reported that concerns about adherence were the main disadvantage of EEN and provided a barrier to wider usage. Australian respondents also commented that adherence was a concern but cited other issues including cost and resource demands. Both of these surveys noted that experience with EEN during gastroenterology training related to current use and confidence with EEN.

While this preliminary work has attempted to explore physician factors to explain the use of EEN, currently only one pilot study has been published which assesses factors influencing patient or parent acceptance [188]. Individual qualitative interviews were conducted with 11 pediatric Crohn's disease patients and their parents from various clinics across Canada to explore the experience of choosing (or not choosing) a treatment option. Of the 11 patients, seven had received some form of EN as part of their initial treatment. Issues raised during the qualitative interviews were grouped into six themes, and for each of these themes, considerations and impacts on practice were derived (see Table 27.2). Patient, family, and societal/cultural factors undoubtedly play a role in the acceptance and use of EEN. The fear of corticosteroid-related side effects, the cost of EEN (which is rarely covered by insurance plans in many countries), concerns over giving up conventional foods, poor palatability of formulae, and fear of tube feedings are some of the reasons patients and/or parents give for not choosing EEN [189].

Another potential barrier to the incorporation of EN as a realistic therapeutic option is adequate resources to support an EN program. There are no published studies which have delineated the optimal resources required. A recent clinical report on EN as primary therapy in pediatric Crohn's disease from the NASPGHAN highlighted several issues of importance [189]. Attitudes among the health-care staff that promote the use of EN and the center's experience appear to play a large role [187]. Dedicated dieticians are fundamental to an EN program, determining appropriate nutrient intake, and in administration of the program. Nursing support with experience in administering and teaching care of tube feedings and use of the feeding pumps is necessary for those who are unable to tolerate oral formula. Formula cost is also an important consideration, particularly when semi-elemental or elemental formulae are chosen, and they are providing sole-source nutrition during the period of exclusive EN feeding. Also, formula costs may not be covered by the relevant health system or drug insurance plans. In some jurisdictions, coverage may be obtained if formula is delivered by a tube, either NG or gastrostomy tube. The high cost is likely to be a barrier to utilization of this therapy.

Table 27.2 Thematic summary of patient and family interviews

Factor/themes (with examples)	Considerations and impact on practice after discussion in workshop
Messaging from healthcare team	
"Pharmacist said incidence of most side effects from steroids was 10% or lower" Family opted for the steroid because they did not feel the efficacy of the EEN was explained	Need for multidisciplinary education and conviction; ensure accurate and consistent messaging Written information to ensure accurate recall by families
Parental assumptions and expectations	
"At 14, no way would she do that" "12 is a difficult, in-between age. Maybe if he was younger or older, he would (been convinced to) have tried the [formula]."	Importance of connecting parents with experienced parents Involve social work or health psychology
Social concerns	
Integration into school, activities, not eating "EEN would be socially isolating" "Patient became emotional about not eating (worried about missing the food he like, being different from his friends)"	Importance of connecting patients to youth with EEN experience; use available resources (videos, camp/social experience)
Guilt	
Parents felt that he had already been through so much that they did not want to upset him further "At 10 or 11, it was hard to imagine that he could only drink, when his friends were eating"	Focus on benefits of EEN, not only challenges Importance of connecting parents with experienced parents Involve social work or health psychology
Child as the decision maker	
"Parents have to respect the wishes of their children (even very young children). The option of a steroid was the only one our son wanted to look at, so we had to go with his wishes." (patient was 10 years old when EEN was offered) "You can't make your teen do what they don't want to do"	Be sure child is present and actively engaged in discussions regarding treatment The child is a key player in the decision making, but they are not the only player – parental involvement is also important; it is a difficult decision to make alone Engage supports – such as peers – and connect with patient who has been on EEN
Adaptation	
"It seems so traumatic at first, but you have to look ahead. There are so many possibilities for a good outcome." "It is hard, but it will get a lot better" "Nervous but relieved [at decision to place NG tube]." "The tube was in for 10½ weeks, stayed in, and was changed three times. Very successful. She gained weight."	Have families share their experiences and strategies

Taken from Johan Van Limbergen et al. [188]
EEN exclusive enteral nutrition, *NG* nasogastric

Conclusion

Nutrition is an important component of the management of IBD in children and adolescents. Successful use of EEN as a form of therapy, specifically for CD, requires a dedicated multidisciplinary team of nurses, dieticians, social workers, and medical staff to support children and families during therapy. Pediatric gastroenterologists must consider EEN in the therapeutic decision process since it yields all of the target outcomes of interest in the management of CD including alleviation of symptoms, mucosal healing, correction of nutritional deficiencies, optimization of growth, and normalization of quality of life, without adverse effects encountered with most pharmacologic therapies.

With a renewed interest in the role of nutrition in the treatment of IBD, a remaining challenge is the difficulty in maintaining remission as many patients do not welcome repeated restrictions on normal eating. The combination of enteral and drug therapy with immunomodulators, or other therapies, to maintain remission requires further study.

Avenues of investigation will likely include exploration of specific oral diets and nutrients that have pharmacologic properties, such as the ability to induce immunomodulation. Although the influence of nutrition on the pathogenesis of IBD and the role of nutrition in the therapy of IBD remain unclear, future investigation of the potential interactions among nutrition and the genome, microbiome, and immune system will enhance our understanding of pathogenesis and have an important clinical impact on the treatment of pediatric IBD.

References

1. Seidman E, LeLeiko N, Ament M, Berman W, Caplan D, Evans J, et al. Nutritional issues in pediatric inflammatory bowel disease. J Pediatr Gastroenterol Nutr. 1991;12(4):424–38.
2. Alhagamhmad MH, Day AS, Lemberg DA, Leach ST. An update of the role of nutritional therapy in the management of Crohn's disease. J Gastroenterol. 2012;47(8):872–82.

3. Kanof ME, Lake AM, Bayless TM. Decreased height velocity in children and adolescents before the diagnosis of Crohn's disease. Gastroenterology. 1988;95(6):1523–7.
4. Ruemmele FM, Veres G, Kolho KL, Griffiths A, Levine A, Escher JC, et al. Consensus guidelines of ECCO/ESPGHAN on the medical management of pediatric Crohn's disease. J Crohns Colitis. 2014;8(10):1179–207.
5. Levine A, Milo T, Buller H, Markowitz J. Consensus and controversy in the management of pediatric Crohn disease: an international survey. J Pediatr Gastroenterol Nutr. 2003;36(4):464–9.
6. Ruemmele FM, Hyams JS, Otley A, Griffiths A, Kolho KL, Dias JA, et al. Outcome measures for clinical trials in paediatric IBD: an evidence-based, expert-driven practical statement paper of the paediatric ECCO committee. Gut. 2015;64(3):438–46.
7. dos Santos GM, Silva LR, Santana GO. Nutritional impact of inflammatory bowel diseases on children and adolescents. Rev Paul Pediatr. 2014;32(4):403–11.
8. Griffiths A. Inflammatory bowel disease; Chapter 41. In: WADPHJe, editor. Pediatric gastrointestinal disease. 3rd ed. Hamilton: BC Decker; 2000.
9. Jakobsen C, Paerregaard A, Munkholm P, Faerk J, Lange A, Andersen J, et al. Pediatric inflammatory bowel disease: increasing incidence, decreasing surgery rate, and compromised nutritional status: a prospective population-based cohort study 2007-2009. Inflamm Bowel Dis. 2011;17(12):2541–50.
10. Aurangzeb B, Leach ST, Lemberg DA, Day AS. Assessment of nutritional status and serum leptin in children with inflammatory bowel disease. J Pediatr Gastroenterol Nutr. 2011;52(5):536–41.
11. Kugathasan S, Nebel J, Skelton JA, Markowitz J, Keljo D, Rosh J, et al. Body mass index in children with newly diagnosed inflammatory bowel disease: observations from two multicenter North American inception cohorts. J Pediatr. 2007;151(5):523–7.
12. Kelts DG, Grand RJ, Shen G, Watkins JB, Werlin SL, Boehme C. Nutritional basis of growth failure in children and adolescents with Crohn's disease. Gastroenterology. 1979;76(4):720–7.
13. Kirschner BS, Klich JR, Kalman SS, deFavaro MV, Rosenberg IH. Reversal of growth retardation in Crohn's disease with therapy emphasizing oral nutritional restitution. Gastroenterology. 1981;80(1):10–5.
14. Kirschner BS, Voinchet O, Rosenberg IH. Growth retardation in inflammatory bowel disease. Gastroenterology. 1978;75(3):504–11.
15. Motil KJ, Altchuler SI, Grand RJ. Mineral balance during nutritional supplementation in adolescents with Crohn disease and growth failure. J Pediatr. 1985;107(3):473–9.
16. Motil KJ, Grand RJ, Maletskos CJ, Young VR. The effect of disease, drug, and diet on whole body protein metabolism in adolescents with Crohn disease and growth failure. J Pediatr. 1982;101(3):345–51.
17. Thomas AG, Taylor F, Miller V. Dietary intake and nutritional treatment in childhood Crohn's disease. J Pediatr Gastroenterol Nutr. 1993;17(1):75–81.
18. Shamir R, Philip M, Levine A. Growth retardation in pediatric Crohn's disease: pathogenesis and interventions. Inflamm Bowel Dis. 2001;13:620–8.
19. Kleinman RE, Baldassano RN, Caplan A, Griffiths AM, Heyman MB, Issenman RM, et al. Nutrition support for pediatric patients with inflammatory bowel disease: a clinical report of the North American Society for Pediatric Gastroenterology, Hepatology And Nutrition. J Pediatr Gastroenterol Nutr. 2004;39(1):15–27.
20. Thayu M, Denson LA, Shults J, Zemel BS, Burnham JM, Baldassano RN, et al. Determinants of changes in linear growth and body composition in incident pediatric Crohn's disease. Gastroenterology. 2010;139(2):430–8.
21. Pons R, Whitten KE, Woodhead H, Leach ST, Lemberg DA, Day AS. Dietary intakes of children with Crohn's disease. Br J Nutr. 2009;102(7):1052–7.
22. Costa CO, Carrilho FJ, Nunes VS, Sipahi AM, Rodrigues M. A snapshot of the nutritional status of Crohn's disease among adolescents in Brazil: a prospective cross-sectional study. BMC Gastroenterol. 2015;15:172.
23. Thangarajah D, Hyde MJ, Konteti VK, Santhakumaran S, Frost G, Fell JM. Systematic review: body composition in children with inflammatory bowel disease. Aliment Pharmacol Ther. 2015;42(2):142–57.
24. Burnham JM, Shults J, Semeao E, Foster BJ, Zemel BS, Stallings VA, et al. Body-composition alterations consistent with cachexia in children and young adults with Crohn disease. Am J Clin Nutr. 2005;82(2):413–20.
25. Azcue M, Rashid M, Griffiths A, Pencharz PB. Energy expenditure and body composition in children with Crohn's disease: effect of enteral nutrition and treatment with prednisolone. Gut. 1997;41(2):203–8.
26. Wiskin AE, Wootton SA, Hunt TM, Cornelius VR, Afzal NA, Jackson AA, et al. Body composition in childhood inflammatory bowel disease. Clin Nutr (Edinburgh, Scotland).
27. Thayu M, Shults J, Burnham JM, Zemel BS, Baldassano RN, Leonard MB. Gender differences in body composition deficits at diagnosis in children and adolescents with Crohn's disease. Inflamm Bowel Dis. 2007;13(9):1121–8.
28. Boot AM, Bouquet J, Krenning EP, de Muinck Keizer-Schrama SM. Bone mineral density and nutritional status in children with chronic inflammatory bowel disease. Gut. 1998;42(2):188–94.
29. Sylvester FA, Leopold S, Lincoln M, Hyams JS, Griffiths AM, Lerer T. A two-year longitudinal study of persistent lean tissue deficits in children with Crohn's disease. Clin Gastroenterol Hepatol Off Clin Pract J Am Gastroenterol Assoc. 2009;7(4):452–5.
30. Mitch WE, Goldberg AL. Mechanisms of muscle wasting. The role of the ubiquitin-proteasome pathway. N Engl J Med. 1996;335(25):1897–905.
31. Zoli G, Care M, Falco F, Parazza M, Spano CG. Effect of oral elemental diet on nutritional status, intestinal permeability and disease activity in Crohn's patients. Gastroenterology. 1996;110(4):A1054.
32. Varille V, Cezard JP, de Lagausie P, Bellaiche M, Tounian P, Besnard M, et al. Resting energy expenditure before and after surgical resection of gut lesions in pediatric Crohn's disease. J Pediatr Gastroenterol Nutr. 1996;23(1):13–9.
33. Werkstetter KJ, Ullrich J, Schatz SB, Prell C, Koletzko B, Koletzko S. Lean body mass, physical activity and quality of life in paediatric patients with inflammatory bowel disease and in healthy controls. J Crohns Colitis. 2012;6(6):665–73.
34. Nguyen T, Ploeger HE, Obeid J, Issenman RM, Baker JM, Takken T, et al. Reduced fat oxidation rates during submaximal exercise in adolescents with Crohn's disease. Inflamm Bowel Dis. 2013;19(12):2659–65.
35. Li Y, Zhu W. Body fat composition predicts infectious complications after bowel resection in Crohn's disease. Inflamm Bowel Dis. 2015;21(8):E19.
36. Bryant RV, Ooi S, Schultz CG, Goess C, Grafton R, Hughes J, et al. Low muscle mass and sarcopenia: common and predictive of osteopenia in inflammatory bowel disease. Aliment Pharmacol Ther. 2015;41(9):895–906.
37. Hannon TS, Dimeglio LA, Pfefferkorn MD, Denne SC. Acute effects of enteral nutrition on protein turnover in adolescents with Crohn disease. Pediatr Res. 2007;61(3):356–60.
38. Hwang C, Ross V, Mahadevan U. Micronutrient deficiencies in inflammatory bowel disease: from A to zinc. Inflamm Bowel Dis. 2012;18(10):1961–81.
39. Levin AD, Wadhera V, Leach ST, Woodhead HJ, Lemberg DA, Mendoza-Cruz AC, et al. Vitamin D deficiency in children with inflammatory bowel disease. Dig Dis Sci. 2011;56(3):830–6.
40. Yakut M, Ustun Y, Kabacam G, Soykan I. Serum vitamin B12 and folate status in patients with inflammatory bowel diseases. Eur J Intern Med. 2010;21(4):320–3.

41. Alkhouri RH, Hashmi H, Baker RD, Gelfond D, Baker SS. Vitamin and mineral status in patients with inflammatory bowel disease. J Pediatr Gastroenterol Nutr. 2013;56(1):89–92.

42. Trebble TM, Wootton SA, May A, Erlewyn-Lajeunesse MD, Chakraborty A, Mullee MA, et al. Essential fatty acid status in paediatric Crohn's disease: relationship with disease activity and nutritional status. Aliment Pharmacol Ther. 2003;18(4):433–42.

43. Driscoll Jr RH, Meredith SC, Sitrin M, Rosenberg IH. Vitamin D deficiency and bone disease in patients with Crohn's disease. Gastroenterology. 1982;83(6):1252–8.

44. Geerling BJ, Badart-Smook A, Stockbrugger RW, Brummer RJ. Comprehensive nutritional status in patients with long-standing Crohn disease currently in remission. Am J Clin Nutr. 1998;67(5): 919–26.

45. Gerasimidis K, Talwar D, Duncan A, Moyes P, Buchanan E, Hassan K, et al. Impact of exclusive enteral nutrition on body composition and circulating micronutrients in plasma and erythrocytes of children with active Crohn's disease. Inflamm Bowel Dis. 2012;18(9):1672–81.

46. Gerasimidis K, Barclay A, Papangelou A, Missiou D, Buchanan E, Tracey C, et al. The epidemiology of anemia in pediatric inflammatory bowel disease: prevalence and associated factors at diagnosis and follow-up and the impact of exclusive enteral nutrition. Inflamm Bowel Dis. 2013;19(11):2411–22.

47. Van Gossum A, Cabre E, Hebuterne X, Jeppesen P, Krznaric Z, Messing B, et al. ESPEN guidelines on parenteral nutrition: gastroenterology. Clin Nutr (Edinburgh, Scotland). 2009;28(4):415–27.

48. Kleinman RE, Balistreri WF, Heyman MB, Kirschner BS, Lake AM, Motil KJ, et al. Nutritional support for pediatric patients with inflammatory bowel disease. J Pediatr Gastroenterol Nutr. 1989;8(1):8–12.

49. Kitney L, Turner JM, Spady D, Malik B, El-Matary W, Persad R, et al. Predictors of medication adherence in pediatric inflammatory bowel disease patients at the Stollery Children's Hospital. Can J Gastroenterol. 2009;23(12):811–5.

50. Greenley RN, Stephens KA, Nguyen EU, Kunz JH, Janas L, Goday P, et al. Vitamin and mineral supplement adherence in pediatric inflammatory bowel disease. J Pediatr Psychol. 2013;38(8):883–92.

51. Sondike S. Weight status in pediatric IBD patients at the time of diagnosis: effects of the obesity epidemic. J Pediatr Gastroenterol Nutr. 2004;39(Suppl 1):S317.

52. Long MD, Crandall WV, Leibowitz IH, Duffy L, del Rosario F, Kim SC, et al. Prevalence and epidemiology of overweight and obesity in children with inflammatory bowel disease. Inflamm Bowel Dis. 2011;17(10):2162–8.

53. Chan SS, Luben R, Olsen A, Tjonneland A, Kaaks R, Teucher B, et al. Body mass index and the risk for Crohn's disease and ulcerative colitis: data from a European Prospective Cohort Study (The IBD in EPIC Study). Am J Gastroenterol. 2013;108(4):575–82.

54. Teahon K, Pearson M, Smith T, Bjarnason I. Alterations in nutritional status and disease activity during treatment of Crohn's disease with elemental diet. Scand J Gastroenterol. 1995;30(1): 54–60.

55. Grinspoon S, Gulick T, Askari H, Landt M, Lee K, Anderson E, et al. Serum leptin levels in women with anorexia nervosa. J Clin Endocrinol Metab. 1996;81(11):3861–3.

56. Hassink SG, Sheslow DV, de Lancey E, Opentanova I, Considine RV, Caro JF. Serum leptin in children with obesity: relationship to gender and development. Pediatrics. 1996;98(2 Pt 1):201–3.

57. Singhal A, Farooqi IS, O'Rahilly S, Cole TJ, Fewtrell M, Lucas A. Early nutrition and leptin concentrations in later life. Am J Clin Nutr. 2002;75(6):993–9.

58. Soliman AT, ElZalabany MM, Salama M, Ansari BM. Serum leptin concentrations during severe protein-energy malnutrition: correlation with growth parameters and endocrine function. Metab Clin Exp. 2000;49(7):819–25.

59. Hoppin AG, Kaplan LM, Zurakowski D, Leichtner AM, Bousvaros A. Serum leptin in children and young adults with inflammatory bowel disease. J Pediatr Gastroenterol Nutr. 1998;26(5):500–5.

60. Gokhale R, Favus MJ, Karrison T, Sutton MM, Rich B, Kirschner BS. Bone mineral density assessment in children with inflammatory bowel disease. Gastroenterology. 1998;114(5):902–11.

61. Compston JE. Management of bone disease in patients on long term glucocorticoid therapy. Gut. 1999;44(6):770–2.

62. Hyams JS, Carey DE. Corticosteroids and growth. J Pediatr. 1988;113(2):249–54.

63. Franklin JL, Rosenberg HH. Impaired folic acid absorption in inflammatory bowel disease: effects of salicylazosulfapyridine (Azulfidine). Gastroenterology. 1973;64(4):517–25.

64. Feagan BG, Rochon J, Fedorak RN, Irvine EJ, Wild G, Sutherland L, et al. Methotrexate for the treatment of Crohn's disease. The North American Crohn's Study Group Investigators. N Engl J Med. 1995;332(5):292–7.

65. Brown AC, Rampertab SD, Mullin GE. Existing dietary guidelines for Crohn's disease and ulcerative colitis. Exp Rev Gastroenterol Hepatol. 2011;5(3):411–25.

66. Wedrychowicz A, Kowalska-Duplaga K, Jedynak-Wasowicz U, Pieczarkowski S, Sladek M, Tomasik P, et al. Serum concentrations of VEGF and TGF-beta1 during exclusive enteral nutrition in IBD. J Pediatr Gastroenterol Nutr. 2011;53(2):150–5.

67. Voitk AJ, Echave V, Feller JH, Brown RA, Gurd FN. Experience with elemental diet in the treatment of inflammatory bowel disease. Is this primary therapy? Arch Surg. 1973;107(2):329–33.

68. O'Morain CA, Segal AW, Levi AJ. Elemental diet as primary treatment of acute Crohn's disease: a controlled trial. Br Med J (Clin Res Ed). 1984;288(6434):1859–62.

69. Sanderson IR, Udeen S, Davies PS, Savage MO, Walker-Smith JA. Remission induced by an elemental diet in small bowel Crohn's disease. Arch Dis Child. 1987;62(2):123–7.

70. Lionetti P, Callegari ML, Ferrari S, Cavicchi MC, Pozzi E, de Martino M, et al. Enteral nutrition and microflora in pediatric Crohn's disease. JPEN J Parenter Enteral Nutr. 2005;29(4 Suppl):S173–5. discussion S5-8, S84-8.

71. Pryce-Millar E, Murch SH, Heuschkel RB. Enteral nutrition therapy in Crohn's disease changes the mucosal flora [abstract]. JPGN J Pediatr Gastroenterol Nutr. 2004;39(Suppl 1):289.

72. Leach ST, Mitchell HM, Eng WR, Zhang L, Day AS. Sustained modulation of intestinal bacteria by exclusive enteral nutrition used to treat children with Crohn's disease. Aliment Pharmacol Ther. 2008;28(6):724–33.

73. Kaakoush NO, Day AS, Leach ST, Lemberg DA, Nielsen S, Mitchell HM. Effect of exclusive enteral nutrition on the microbiota of children with newly diagnosed Crohn's disease. Clin Trans Gastroenterol. 2015;6:e71.

74. Quince C, Ijaz UZ, Loman N, Eren AM, Saulnier D, Russell J, et al. Extensive modulation of the fecal metagenome in children with Crohn's disease during exclusive enteral nutrition. Am J Gastroenterol. 2015;110(12):1718–29. quiz 30.

75. Lewis JD, Chen EZ, Baldassano RN, Otley AR, Griffiths AM, Lee D, et al. Inflammation, antibiotics, and diet as environmental stressors of the gut microbiome in pediatric Crohn's disease. Cell Host Microbe. 2015;18(4):489–500.

76. Kajiura T, Takeda T, Sakata S, Sakamoto M, Hashimoto M, Suzuki H, et al. Change of intestinal microbiota with elemental diet and its impact on therapeutic effects in a murine model of chronic colitis. Dig Dis Sci. 2009;54(9):1892–900.

77. Smith AR, Macfarlane S, Furrie E, Ahmed S, Bahrami B, Reynolds N, et al. Microbiological and immunological effects of enteral feeding on the upper gastrointestinal tract. J Med Microbiol. 2011;60(Pt 3):359–65.

78. Whelan K, Judd PA, Tuohy KM, Gibson GR, Preedy VR, Taylor MA. Fecal microbiota in patients receiving enteral feeding are

highly variable and may be altered in those who develop diarrhea. Am J Clin Nutr. 2009;89(1):240–7.

79. Meister D, Bode J, Shand A, Ghosh S. Anti-inflammatory effects of enteral diet components on Crohn's disease-affected tissues in vitro. Dig Liver Dis Off J Ital Soc Gastroenterol Ital Assoc Study Liver. 2002;34(6):430–8.

80. de Jong NS, Leach ST, Day AS. Polymeric formula has direct anti-inflammatory effects on enterocytes in an in vitro model of intestinal inflammation. Dig Dis Sci. 2007;52(9):2029–36.

81. Nahidi L, Corley SM, Wilkins MR, Wei J, Alhagamhmad M, Day AS, et al. The major pathway by which polymeric formula reduces inflammation in intestinal epithelial cells: a microarray-based analysis. Genes Nutr. 2015;10(5):479.

82. Alhagamhmad MH, Day AS, Lemberg DA, Leach ST. Exploring and enhancing the anti-inflammatory properties of polymeric formula. JPEN J Parenter Enteral Nutrition. 2016. PMID: 26826259. [Epub ahead of print].

83. Hollander D. The intestinal permeability barrier. A hypothesis as to its regulation and involvement in Crohn's disease. Scand J Gastroenterol. 1992;27(9):721–6.

84. Teahon K, Smethurst P, Levi AJ, Menzies IS, Bjarnason I. Intestinal permeability in patients with Crohn's disease and their first degree relatives. Gut. 1992;33(3):320–3.

85. Suenaert P, Bulteel V, Lemmens L, Noman M, Geypens B, Van Assche G, et al. Anti-tumor necrosis factor treatment restores the gut barrier in Crohn's disease. Am J Gastroenterol. 2002;97(8): 2000–4.

86. Guzy C, Schirbel A, Paclik D, Wiedenmann B, Dignass A, Sturm A. Enteral and parenteral nutrition distinctively modulate intestinal permeability and T cell function in vitro. Eur J Nutr. 2009;48(1):12–21.

87. Nahidi L, Day AS, Lemberg DA, Leach ST. Differential effects of nutritional and non-nutritional therapies on intestinal barrier function in an in vitro model. J Gastroenterol. 2011;47(2):107–17.

88. Nahidi L, Leach ST, Mitchell HM, Kaakoush NO, Lemberg DA, Munday JS, et al. Inflammatory bowel disease therapies and gut function in a colitis mouse model. Biomed Res Int. 2013; 2013:909613.

89. Narula N, Tondeur M, Sherlock M, Zachos M. Enteral nutritional therapy for induction of remission in Crohn's disease. Update. Cochrane Database Syst Rev. 2015;CD000542.

90. Grogan JL, Casson DH, Terry A, Burdge GC, El-Matary W, Dalzell AM. Enteral feeding therapy for newly diagnosed pediatric Crohn's disease: a double-blind randomized controlled trial with two years follow-up. Inflamm Bowel Dis. 2012;18(2):246–53.

91. Gorard DA, Hunt JB, Payne-James JJ, Palmer KR, Rees RG, Clark ML, et al. Initial response and subsequent course of Crohn's disease treated with elemental diet or prednisolone. Gut. 1993;34(9):1198–202.

92. Lindor KD, Fleming CR, Burnes JU, Nelson JK, Ilstrup DM. A randomized prospective trial comparing a defined formula diet, corticosteroids, and a defined formula diet plus corticosteroids in active Crohn's disease. Mayo Clin Proc. 1992;67(4):328–33.

93. Lochs H, Steinhardt HJ, Klaus-Wentz B, Zeitz M, Vogelsang H, Sommer H, et al. Comparison of enteral nutrition and drug treatment in active Crohn's disease. Results of the European Cooperative Crohn's Disease Study. IV. Gastroenterology. 1991;101(4):881–8.

94. Malchow H, Ewe K, Brandes JW, Goebell H, Ehms H, Sommer H, et al. European Cooperative Crohn's Disease Study (ECCDS): results of drug treatment. Gastroenterology. 1984;86(2):249–66.

95. Seidman EG, Griffiths AM, Jones A, Issenman R. Semi-elemental diet versus prednisone in pediatric Crohn's disease. Gastroenterology. 1993;104:A778.

96. Seidman EG, Lohoues MJ, Turgeon J, Bouthillier L, Morin CL. Elemental diet versus prednisone as initial therapy i Crohn's disease: early and long-term results. Gastroenterology. 1991;100:150A.

97. Levine A, Turner D, Pfeffer Gik T, Amil Dias J, Veres G, Shaoul R, et al. Comparison of outcomes parameters for induction of remission in new onset pediatric Crohn's disease: evaluation of the porto IBD group "growth relapse and outcomes with therapy" (GROWTH CD) study. Inflamm Bowel Dis. 2014;20(2):278–85.

98. Fernandez-Banares F, Cabre E, Esteve-Copmans M, Gassull MA. How effective is enteral nutrition in inducing clinical remission in active Crohn's disease? A meta-analysis of the randomized clinical trials. J Parenter Enter Nutr. 1995;19:1056–64.

99. Messori A, Trallori G, D'Albrasio G, Milla M, Vanozzi G, Pacini F. Defined-formula diets versus steroids in the treatment of active Crohn's disease. A Meta-Analysis. Scand J Gastroenterol. 1996;31:267–72.

100. Zachos M, Tondeur M, Griffiths AM. Enteral nutritional therapy for induction of remission in Crohn's disease. Cochrane Database Syst Rev. 2007(1):CD000542.

101. Berni Canani R, Terrin G, Borrelli O, Romano MT, Manguso F, Coruzzo A, et al. Short- and long-term therapeutic efficacy of nutritional therapy and corticosteroids in paediatric Crohn's disease. Dig Liver Dis Off J Ital Soc Gastroenterol Ital Assoc Study Liver. 2006;38(6):381–7.

102. Jadad AR, Moore RA, Carroll D, Jenkinson C, Reynolds DJ, Gavaghan DJ, et al. Assessing the quality of reports of randomized clinical trials: is blinding necessary? Control Clin Trials. 1996;17(1):1–12.

103. Gonzalez-Huix F, de Leon R, Fernandez-Banares F, Esteve M, Cabre E, Acero D, et al. Polymeric enteral diets as primary treatment of active Crohn's disease: a prospective steroid controlled trial. Gut. 1993;34(6):778–82.

104. Heuschkel RB, Menache CC, Megerian JT, Baird AE. Enteral nutrition and corticosteroids in the treatment of acute Crohn's disease in children. J Pediatr Gastroenterol Nutr. 2000;31(1):8–15.

105. Day AS, Whitten KE, Lemberg DA, Clarkson C, Vitug-Sales M, Jackson R, et al. Exclusive enteral feeding as primary therapy for Crohn's disease in Australian children and adolescents: a feasible and effective approach. J Gastroenterol Hepatol. 2006;21(10): 1609–14.

106. Otley A, Grant A, Giffin N, Mahdi G, Rashid M, Van Limbergen J. Steroids no more! Exclusive Enteral nutrition therapy in pediatric patients with Crohn's disease results in long term avoidance of corticosteroid therapy. J Crohns Colitis. 2015;9(Supplement 1):S393.

107. Luo Y, Yu J, Zhao H, Lou J, Chen F, Peng K, et al. Short-term efficacy of exclusive enteral nutrition in pediatric Crohn's disease: practice in China. Gastroenterol Res Pract. 2015;2015:428354.

108. Soo J, Malik BA, Turner JM, Persad R, Wine E, Siminoski K, et al. Use of exclusive enteral nutrition is just as effective as corticosteroids in newly diagnosed pediatric Crohn's disease. Dig Dis Sci. 2013;58(12):3584–91.

109. Lee D, Baldassano RN, Otley AR, Albenberg L, Griffiths AM, Compher C, et al. Comparative effectiveness of nutritional and biological therapy in North American children with active Crohn's disease. Inflamm Bowel Dis. 2015;21(8):1786–93.

110. Akobeng AK, Thomas AG. Enteral nutrition for maintenance of remission in Crohn's disease. Cochrane Database Syst Rev. 2007;3:CD005984.

111. Verma S, Holdsworth CD, Giaffer MH. Does adjuvant nutritional support diminish steroid dependency in Crohn disease? Scand J Gastroenterol. 2001;36(4):383–8.

112. Takagi S, Utsunomiya K, Kuriyama S, Yokoyama H, Takahashi S, Iwabuchi M, et al. Effectiveness of an 'half elemental diet' as maintenance therapy for Crohn's disease: a randomized-controlled trial. Aliment Pharmacol Ther. 2006;24(9):1333–40.

113. Yamamoto T, Nakahigashi M, Umegae S, Matsumoto K. Enteral nutrition for the maintenance of remission in Crohn's disease: a systematic review. Eur J Gastroenterol Hepatol. 2010;22(1):1–8.

114. Verma S, Kirkwood B, Brown S, Giaffer MH. Oral nutritional supplementation is effective in the maintenance of remission in Crohn's disease. Dig Liver Dis Off J Ital Soc Gastroenterol Ital Assoc Study Liver. 2000;32(9):769–74.

115. Yamamoto T, Nakahigashi M, Saniabadi AR, Iwata T, Maruyama Y, Umegae S, et al. Impacts of long-term enteral nutrition on clinical and endoscopic disease activities and mucosal cytokines during remission in patients with Crohn's disease: a prospective study. Inflamm Bowel Dis. 2007;13(12):1493–501.

116. Yamamoto T, Nakahigashi M, Umegae S, Kitagawa T, Matsumoto K. Impact of long-term enteral nutrition on clinical and endoscopic recurrence after resection for Crohn's disease: a prospective, non-randomized, parallel, controlled study. Aliment Pharmacol Ther. 2007;25(1):67–72.

117. Hirakawa H, Fukuda Y, Tanida N, Hosomi M, Shimoyama T. Home elemental enteral hyperalimentation (HEEH) for the maintenance of remission in patients with Crohn's disease. Gastroenterol Jpn. 1993;28(3):379–84.

118. Wilschanski M, Sherman P, Pencharz P, Davis L, Corey M, Griffiths A. Supplementary enteral nutrition maintains remission in paediatric Crohn's disease. Gut. 1996;38(4):543–8.

119. Esaki M, Matsumoto T, Nakamura S, Yada S, Fujisawa K, Jo Y, et al. Factors affecting recurrence in patients with Crohn's disease under nutritional therapy. Dis Colon Rectum. 2006;49(10 Suppl): S68–74.

120. Ikeuchi H, Yamamura T, Nakano H, Kosaka T, Shimoyama T, Fukuda Y. Efficacy of nutritional therapy for perforating and non-perforating Crohn's disease. Hepato-Gastroenterology. 2004;51(58):1050–2.

121. Esaki M, Matsumoto T, Hizawa K, Nakamura S, Jo Y, Mibu R, et al. Preventive effect of nutritional therapy against postoperative recurrence of Crohn disease, with reference to findings determined by intra-operative enteroscopy. Scand J Gastroenterol. 2005;40(12):1431–7.

122. Bamba T, Shimoyama T, Sasaki M, Tsujikawa T, Fukuda Y, Koganei K, et al. Dietary fat attenuates the benefits of an elemental diet in active Crohn's disease: a randomized, controlled trial. Eur J Gastroenterol Hepatol. 2003;15(2):151–7.

123. Belli DC, Seidman E, Bouthillier L, Weber AM, Roy CC, Pletincx M, et al. Chronic intermittent elemental diet improves growth failure in children with Crohn's disease. Gastroenterology. 1988;94(3):603–10.

124. Nguyen DL, Palmer LB, Nguyen ET, McClave SA, Martindale RG, Bechtold ML. Specialized enteral nutrition therapy in Crohn's disease patients on maintenance infliximab therapy: a meta-analysis. Ther Adv Gastroenterol. 2015;8(4):168–75.

125. Buchanan E, Gaunt WW, Cardigan T, Garrick V, McGrogan P, Russell RK. The use of exclusive enteral nutrition for induction of remission in children with Crohn's disease demonstrates that disease phenotype does not influence clinical remission. Aliment Pharmacol Ther. 2009;30(5):501–7.

126. Grover Z, Lewindon P. Two-year outcomes after exclusive enteral nutrition induction are superior to corticosteroids in pediatric Crohn's disease treated early with thiopurines. Dig Dis Sci. 2015;60(10):3069–74.

127. Kang Y, Kim S, Kim SY, Koh H. Effect of short-term partial enteral nutrition on the treatment of younger patients with severe Crohn's disease. Gut Liver. 2015;9(1):87–93.

128. Frivolt K, Schwerd T, Werkstetter KJ, Schwarzer A, Schatz SB, Bufler P, et al. Repeated exclusive enteral nutrition in the treatment of paediatric Crohn's disease: predictors of efficacy and outcome. Aliment Pharmacol Ther. 2014;39(12):1398–407.

129. Knight C, El-Matary W, Spray C, Sandhu BK. Long-term outcome of nutritional therapy in paediatric Crohn's disease. Clin Nutr (Edinburgh, Scotland). 2005;24(5):775–9.

130. Cameron FL, Gerasimidis K, Papangelou A, Missiou D, Garrick V, Cardigan T, et al. Clinical progress in the two years following a course of exclusive enteral nutrition in 109 paediatric patients with Crohn's disease. Aliment Pharmacol Ther. 2013;37(6):622–9.

131. Lambert B, Lemberg DA, Leach ST, Day AS. Longer-term outcomes of nutritional management of Crohn's disease in children. Dig Dis Sci. 2012;57(8):2171–7.

132. Froslie KF, Jahnsen J, Moum BA, Vatn MH, Group I. Mucosal healing in inflammatory bowel disease: results from a Norwegian population-based cohort. Gastroenterology. 2007;133(2):412–22.

133. Tibble JA, Sigthorsson G, Bridger S, Fagerhol MK, Bjarnason I. Surrogate markers of intestinal inflammation are predictive of relapse in patients with inflammatory bowel disease. Gastroenterology. 2000;119(1):15–22.

134. Modigliani R, Mary JY, Simon JF, Cortot A, Soule JC, Gendre JP, et al. Clinical, biological, and endoscopic picture of attacks of Crohn's disease. Evolution on prednisolone. Groupe d'Etude Therapeutique des Affections Inflammatoires Digestives. Gastroenterology. 1990;98(4):811–8.

135. Fell JME, Paintin M, Arnaud-Battandier F, Beatties RM, Hollis A, Kitching P, et al. Mucosal healing and a fall in mucosal pro-inflammatory cytokine mRNA induced by a specific oral polymeric diet in paediatric Crohn's disease. Aliment Pharmacol Ther. 2000;14:281–9.

136. Borrelli O, Cordischi L, Cirulli M, Paganelli M, Labalestra V, Uccini S, et al. Polymeric diet alone versus corticosteroids in the treatment of active pediatric Crohn's disease: a randomized controlled open-label trial. Clin Gastroenterol Hepatol Off Clin Pract J Am Gastroenterol Assoc. 2006;4(6):744–53.

137. Grover Z, Muir R, Lewindon P. Exclusive enteral nutrition induces early clinical, mucosal and transmural remission in paediatric Crohn's disease. J Gastroenterol. 2014;49(4):638–45.

138. Grover Z, Burgess C, Muir R, Reilly C, Lewindon PJ. Early mucosal healing with exclusive enteral nutrition is associated with improved outcomes in newly diagnosed children with luminal Crohn's disease. J Crohns Colitis. 2016;10(10):1159–64.

139. Yamamoto T, Nakahigashi M, Umegae S, Kitagawa T, Matsumoto K. Impact of elemental diet on mucosal inflammation in patients with active Crohn's disease: cytokine production and endoscopic and histological findings. Inflamm Bowel Dis. 2005;11(6):580–8.

140. Breese EJ, Michie CA, Nicholls SW, Williams CB, Domizio P, Walker-Smith JA, et al. The effect of treatment on lymphokine-secreting cells in the intestinal mucosa of children with Crohn's disease. Aliment Pharmacol Ther. 1995;9(5):547–52.

141. Breese EJ, Michie CA, Nicholls SW, Murch SH, Williams CB, Domizio P, et al. Tumor necrosis factor alpha-producing cells in the intestinal mucosa of children with inflammatory bowel disease. Gastroenterology. 1994;106(6):1455–66.

142. Ferguson A, Glen M, Ghosh S. Crohn's disease: nutrition and nutritional therapy. Baillieres Clin Gastroenterol. 1998;12(1): 93–114.

143. Judd TA, Day AS, Lemberg DA, Turner D, Leach ST. Update of fecal markers of inflammation in inflammatory bowel disease. J Gastroenterol Hepatol. 2011;26(10):1493–9.

144. Gerasimidis K, Nikolaou CK, Edwards CA, McGrogan P. Serial fecal calprotectin changes in children with Crohn's disease on treatment with exclusive enteral nutrition: associations with disease activity, treatment response, and prediction of a clinical relapse. J Clin Gastroenterol. 2011;45(3):234–9.

145. de Jong NS, Leach ST, Day AS. Fecal S100A12: a novel noninvasive marker in children with Crohn's disease. Inflamm Bowel Dis. 2006;12(7):566–72.

146. Nahidi L, Leach ST, Sidler MA, Levin A, Lemberg DA, Day AS. Osteoprotegerin in pediatric Crohn's disease and the effects of exclusive enteral nutrition. Inflamm Bowel Dis. 2011;17(2): 516–23.

147. Bannerjee K, Camacho-Hubner C, Babinska K, Dryhurst KM, Edwards R, Savage MO, et al. Anti-inflammatory and growth-stimulating effects precede nutritional restitution during enteral feeding in Crohn disease. J Pediatr Gastroenterol Nutr. 2004; 38(3):270–5.

148. Beattie RM, Camacho-Hubner C, Wacharasindhu S, Cotterill AM, Walker-Smith JA, Savage MO. Responsiveness of IGF-I and IGFBP-3 to therapeutic intervention in children and adolescents with Crohn's disease. Clin Endocrinol. 1998;49(4):483–9.

149. Royall D, Greenberg GR, Allard JP, Baker JP, Jeejeebhoy KN. Total enteral nutrition support improves body composition of patients with active Crohn's disease. JPEN J Parenter Enteral Nutr. 1995;19(2):95–9.

150. Afzal NA, Davies S, Paintin M, Arnaud-Battandier F, Walker-Smith JA, Murch S, et al. Colonic Crohn's disease in children does not respond well to treatment with enteral nutrition if the ileum is not involved. Dig Dis Sci. 2005;50(8):1471–5.

151. Newby EA, Sawczenko A, Thomas AG, Wilson D. Interventions for growth failure in childhood Crohn's disease. Cochrane Database Syst Rev. 2005;3:CD003873.

152. Whitten KE, Leach ST, Bohane TD, Woodhead HJ, Day AS. Effect of exclusive enteral nutrition on bone turnover in children with Crohn's disease. J Gastroenterol. 2010;45(4):399–405.

153. Werkstetter KJ, Schatz SB, Alberer M, Filipiak-Pittroff B, Koletzko S. Influence of exclusive enteral nutrition therapy on bone density and geometry in newly diagnosed pediatric Crohn's disease patients. Ann Nutr Metab. 2013;63(1–2):10–6.

154. Otley A, Smith C, Nicholas D, Munk M, Avolio J, Sherman PM, et al. The IMPACT questionnaire: a valid measure of health-related quality of life in pediatric inflammatory bowel disease. J Pediatr Gastroenterol Nutr. 2002;35(4):557–63.

155. Gailhoustet L, Goulet O, Cachin N, Schmitz J. Study of psychological repercussions of 2 modes of treatment of adolescents with Crohn's disease. Arch Pediatr. 2002;9(2):110–6.

156. Afzal NA, Van Der Zaag-Loonen HJ, Arnaud-Battandier F, Davies S, Murch S, Derkx B, et al. Improvement in quality of life of children with acute Crohn's disease does not parallel mucosal healing after treatment with exclusive enteral nutrition. Aliment Pharmacol Ther. 2004;20(2):167–72.

157. Hill R, Lewindon P, Muir R, Grange I, Connor F, Ee L, et al. Quality of life in children with Crohn disease. J Pediatr Gastroenterol Nutr. 2010;51(1):35–40.

158. Kuriyama M, Kato J, Morimoto N, Fujimoto T, Kono H, Okano N, et al. Enteral nutrition improves health-related quality of life in Crohn's disease patients with long disease duration. Hepato-Gastroenterology. 2009;56(90):321–7.

159. Li G, Ren J, Wang G, Hu D, Gu G, Liu S, et al. Preoperative exclusive enteral nutrition reduces the postoperative septic complications of fistulizing Crohn's disease. Eur J Clin Nutr. 2014;68(4):441–6.

160. Li Y, Zuo L, Zhu W, Gong J, Zhang W, Gu L, et al. Role of exclusive enteral nutrition in the preoperative optimization of patients with Crohn's disease following immunosuppressive therapy. Medicine. 2015;94(5):e478.

161. Kuroki F, Matsumoto T, Iida M. Selenium is depleted in Crohn's disease on enteral nutrition. Dig Dis. 2003;21(3):266–70.

162. Akobeng AK, Richmond K, Miller V, Thomas AG. Effect of exclusive enteral nutritional treatment on plasma antioxidant concentrations in childhood Crohn's disease. Clin Nutr (Edinburgh, Scotland). 2007;26(1):51–6.

163. Gerasimidis K, Talwar D, Duncan A, Moyes P, Buchanan E, Hassan K, et al. Impact of exclusive enteral nutrition on body composition and circulating micronutrients in plasma and erythrocytes of children with active Crohn's disease. Inflamm Bowel Dis. 2011;18(9):1672–81.

164. Schatorje E, Hoekstra H. Transient hypertransaminasemia in paediatric patients with Crohn disease undergoing initial treatment with enteral nutrition. J Pediatr Gastroenterol Nutr. 2010;51(3): 336–40.

165. Lemberg DA, Leach ST, Day AS. Transient hypertransaminasemia in pediatric patients with Crohn disease. J Pediatr Gastroenterol Nutr. 2011;53(2):229.

166. Afzal NA, Addai S, Fagbemi A, Murch S, Thomson M, Heuschkel R. Refeeding syndrome with enteral nutrition in children: a case report, literature review and clinical guidelines. Clin Nutr (Edinburgh, Scotland). 2002;21(6):515–20.

167. Akobeng AK, Thomas AG. Refeeding syndrome following exclusive enteral nutritional treatment in Crohn disease. J Pediatr Gastroenterol Nutr. 2010;51(3):364–6.

168. Seidman E. Relapse prevention/growth enhancement in pediatric Crohn's disease: multicentre randomized controlled trial of intermittent enteral nutrition versus alternate day prednisone. J Pediatr Gastroenterol Nutr. 1996;23:A344.

169. Rubio A, Pigneur B, Garnier-Lengline H, Talbotec C, Schmitz J, Canioni D, et al. The efficacy of exclusive nutritional therapy in paediatric Crohn's disease, comparing fractionated oral vs. continuous enteral feeding. Aliment Pharmacol Ther. 2011;33(12): 1332–9.

170. Beattie RM, Schiffrin EJ, Donnet-Hughes A, Huggett AC, Domizio P, MacDonald TT, et al. Polymeric nutrition as the primary therapy in children with small bowel Crohn's disease. Aliment Pharmacol Ther. 1994;8(6):609–15.

171. O'Sullivan MA, O'Morain CA. Nutritional therapy in Crohn's disease. Inflamm Bowel Dis. 1998;4(1):45–53.

172. Akobeng AK, Miller V, Stanton J, Elbadri AM, Thomas AG. Double-blind randomized controlled trial of glutamine-enriched polymeric diet in the treatment of active Crohn's disease. J Pediatr Gastroenterol Nutr. 2000;30(1):78–84.

173. Gassull MA, Fernandez-Banares F, Cabre E, Papo M, Giaffer MH, Sanchez-Lombrana JL, et al. Fat composition may be a clue to explain the primary therapeutic effect of enteral nutrition in Crohn's disease: results of a double blind randomised multicentre european trial. Gut. 2002;51(2):164–8.

174. Leiper K, Woolner J, Mullan MM, Parker T, van der Vliet M, Fear S, et al. A randomised controlled trial of high versus low long chain triglyceride whole protein feed in active Crohn's disease. Gut. 2001;49(6):790–4.

175. Sakurai T, Matsui T, Yao T, Takagi Y, Hirai F, Aoyagi K, et al. Short-term efficacy of enteral nutrition in the treatment of active crohn's disease: a randomized, controlled trial comparing nutrient formulas. J Parenter Enteral Nutr. 2002;26(2):98–103.

176. Johnson T, Macdonald S, Hill SM, Thomas A, Murphy MS. Treatment of active Crohn's disease in children using partial enteral nutrition with liquid formula: a randomised controlled trial. Gut. 2006;55(3):356–61.

177. Gupta K, Noble AJ, Baldassano RN, Sreedharan R, Grossman AB. A novel enteral nutritional therapy protocol for the treatment of pediatric Crohn's disease. JPGN J Pediatr Gastroenterol Nutr. 2010;51(Suppl 2):E87.

178. Whitten KE, Rogers P, Ooi CK, Day AS. International survey of enteral nutrition protocols used in children with Crohn's disease. J Dig Dis. 2012;13(2):107–12.

179. Otley A, Murray A, Crhistensen B, Williams T, Rashid M, Ste-Marie M. Primary enteral nutrition induces and maintains remission and reduces steroid exposure in a paediatric Crohn's

disease population. Gastroenterology. 2005;128(4(Suppl 2)):W1053.

180. Riordan AM, Hunter JO, Cowan RE, Crampton JR, Davidson AR, Dickinson RJ, et al. Treatment of active Crohn's disease by exclusion diet: East Anglian multicentre controlled trial. Lancet. 1993;342(8880):1131–4.

181. Shergill-Bonner R, Brennan M, Torrente F, Heuschkel R. Food reintroduction after exclusive enteral nutrition – a clinical experience. JPGN J Pediatr Gastroenterol Nutr. 2007;44:E36.

182. Faiman A, Mutalib M, Moylan A, Morgan N, Crespi D, Furman M, et al. Standard versus rapid food reintroduction after exclusive enteral nutritional therapy in paediatric Crohn's disease. Eur J Gastroenterol Hepatol. 2014;26(3):276–81.

183. Konno M, Kobayashi A, Tomomasa T, Kaneko H, Toyoda S, Nakazato Y, et al. Guidelines for the treatment of Crohn's disease in children. Pediatr Int. 2006;48(3):349–52.

184. Lochs H, Dejong C, Hammarqvist F, Hebuterne X, Leon-Sanz M, Schutz T, et al. ESPEN guidelines on enteral nutrition: gastroenterology. Clin Nutr (Edinburgh, Scotland). 2006;25(2):260–74.

185. Grafors JM, Casswall TH. Exclusive enteral nutrition in the treatment of children with Crohn's disease in Sweden: a questionnaire survey. Acta Paediatr. 2011;100(7):1018–22.

186. Day AS, Stephenson T, Stewart M, Otley AR. Exclusive enteral nutrition for children with Crohn's disease: use in Australia and attitudes of Australian paediatric gastroenterologists. J Paediatr Child Health. 2009;45(6):337–41.

187. Stewart M, Day AS, Otley A. Physician attitudes and practices of enteral nutrition as primary treatment of paediatric Crohn disease in North America. J Pediatr Gastroenterol Nutr. 2009;52(1):38–42.

188. Van Limbergen J, Haskett J, Griffiths AM, Critch J, Huynh H, Ahmed N, et al. Toward enteral nutrition for the treatment of pediatric Crohn disease in Canada: a workshop to identify barriers and enablers. Can J Gastroenterol Hepatol. 2015;29(7):351–6.

189. Critch J, Day AS, Otley A, King-Moore C, Teitelbaum JE, Shashidhar H. Use of enteral nutrition for the control of intestinal inflammation in pediatric Crohn disease. J Pediatr Gastroenterol Nutr. 2012;54(2):298–305.

Probiotic Therapy

28

David R. Mack

Introduction

The term probiotic was first used as an antithesis to the term antibiotic and, thus, used to describe substances that promote the growth of another microorganism produced by another microorganism [1]. However, the definition most commonly accepted is that developed by a joint Food and Agricultural Organization of the United Nations/World Health Organization task force, namely, "live microorganisms that confer a health benefit when administered in adequate amounts" [2]. Currently, most microorganisms used as probiotics are bacteria that have been derived from human, animal, and food sources. Most species belong to the *Lactobacillus* and *Bifidobacterium* genus, but other bacterial strains with the genera *Enterococcus*, *Streptococcus*, and *Escherichia* are also in usage. The most common nonbacterial probiotic is the fungus *Saccharomyces boulardii* that is derived from the lychee fruit and has a unique property of being intrinsically resistant to antibiotics.

The use of probiotics to provide health benefits has been proposed for a long time. In recent years there is increased study, awareness, and interest for their use in a number of gastrointestinal conditions in children including IBD [3]. Indeed, probiotics are being ingested by patients with IBD sometimes through the advice of the physician but mostly self-prescribed as a form of alternative medicine [4, 5]. Recent reports compared to even a few years ago suggest an increase in their usage such that up to 50 % of patients with IBD are at least trying probiotics if not taking them on a regular basis [5–9]. The reasons for using probiotics is most

often related to worse disease severity, adverse effects of treatments, and health beliefs [4–6].

This interest is being generated as a result of a number of interrelated fields of study. For instance, careful epidemiological studies have demonstrated that IBD is increasing in some Western countries and includes a rise in younger children [10] implicating an environmental factor. The environmental influence on the intestinal immune system is particularly relevant as the luminal contents of the intestinal system represent an exposure to the outside world as well as its own perpetuated microenvironment of the intestinal microbiota.

Some of the best evidence that the gut microbiota play a key role in IBD comes from animal model studies. Although the experimental animal models of IBD do not exactly mimic human UC and poorly mimic CD, these studies have shown that the development of intestinal inflammation is dependent on the presence of resident bacteria. A key finding is that in a number of distinct animal models with induced, spontaneous, or genetically engineered disease, chronic colonic inflammation is initiated and perpetuated in the presence of resident enteric bacteria, whereas germ-free (sterile) conditions prevent or dramatically attenuate the development of disease [11, 12]. For instance, the loss of the transcriptional factor T-bet in mice, which regulates the differentiation and function of immune system cells, was shown to promote the bacterial community to become colitogenic [13]. Moreover, the induced colitis could be communicated to other genetically intact hosts by vertical transfer of the colitogenic microbiota [13] demonstrating that the composition of the microbial community could directly be involved in the pathogenesis of colitis.

In children there is indirect evidence suggesting the role of the intestinal microbiota in the pathogenesis of IBD. The number of immune responses and the magnitude of immune response of antibodies to the *Escherichia coli* outer-membrane porin C (OmpC), *Saccharomyces cerevisiae* (ASCA), and anti-flagellin antibodies (anti-CBir1) are predictive of aggressive Crohn's disease phenotypes [14]. Exposure to antibiotics increases the odds of being newly

D.R. Mack, MD, FRCPC
Department of Paediatrics, Faculty of Medicine,
University of Ottawa, Ottawa, ON, Canada

CHEO IBD Centre, Ottawa, ON, Canada

Pediatric Gastroenterology, Hepatology and Nutrition,
Children's Hospital of Eastern Ontario,
401 Smyth Road, Ottawa, ON K1H 8L1, Canada
e-mail: dmack@cheo.on.ca
© Springer International Publishing AG 2017
P. Mamula et al. (eds.), *Pediatric Inflammatory Bowel Disease*, DOI 10.1007/978-3-319-49215-5_28
357

diagnosed with CD [OR 1.74, 95 % CI 1.35–2.23] and markedly so in children [OR 2.75, 95 % CI 1.72–4.38] [15]. Moreover, in a small number (13 %) of new-onset CD patients entered into the RISK study (N = 447), antibiotics were being administered. Compared to CD patients not on antibiotics at the time of study entry, antibiotics were found to amplify the dysbiosis with the greatest impact on noninflammatory microbes [16].

The human gastrointestinal tract is colonized with a complex ecosystem of bacteria, Archaea, and fungi [17]. Some 400 different bacterial species have been cultured [18], but of the more than 1000 bacterial species, most remain unculturable [18, 19]. Most of the intestinal bacteria belong to two phyla, the *Bacteroidetes* and *Firmicutes*, with less abundance of *Actinomycetes*, *Proteobacteria*, and *Fusobacteria* [18–20] although in an individual the diversity is much lower consisting of around 160 different bacterial species [18]. Comparing the microbiota between 124 individuals, only 18 species were common to all individuals and 57 species common to > 90 % of individuals but with variability in relative abundance of core phylotypes [19]. Of interest to IBD, differences in the intestinal microbiota between of CD and UC have been described [16, 21, 22], and new-onset pediatric CD may have a distinct microbial profile as compared to adults and post-treatment cohorts [23].

It is becoming clear that the complex interactions between microbial, genetic, immune, and environmental factors are critical in the pathogenesis of IBD. It remains unknown whether the human gut microbiome triggers are altered as a secondary response to the intestinal inflammation or maintains the chronicity of intestinal mucosal inflammation that is the hallmark of IBD. Nevertheless, as the majority of IBD susceptibility genes identified are involved in regulation of innate and adaptive immunity or maintenance of the intestinal mucosal barrier, it is apparent that the microbiome may play an integral role in the development and natural history of disease. Potential for effects on the immunologic reaction of the host or mucosal barrier function to lessen interaction with the host immune system, displaced pathobionts from luminal-mucosal interface, and persistence of benefit or altered metabolic consequences of the microbiome should be considered in the role of probiotics in the complex microbiome of the intestinal tract. The aim of this chapter is to review the clinical data with respect to probiotic use in IBD and their comorbidities that are currently available and provide speculation for future potential.

Ulcerative Colitis

Induction of Remission

A Cochrane review [24] published in 2007 analyzed the first trials involving probiotics for induction of remission for UC. A formal meta-analysis was not performed due to the significant differences in probiotics, outcomes, and trial methodology, and all were small trials with mild-to-moderate disease. The probiotics were given as single and blends of microorganisms, probiotic in combination with a prebiotic fructooligosaccharide/inulin mixture and combined with allopathic medicine. It was concluded that addition of a probiotic did not improve overall remission rates in patients with mild-to-moderate UC, but their addition may have reduced disease activity. The data were analyzed using intention to treat for the three studies that measured proportion of patients achieving remission [25–27].

For the three included studies:

- Probiotics (Yakult™) + 5-ASA had similar effectiveness [40 %] to placebo + 5-ASA [30 %] for induction of remission [25]: OR 0.64 (95 % CI: 0.10–4.10).
- Probiotics (*E. coli* Nissle 1917) + steroids had similar effectiveness [68.4 %] as mesalazine + steroids [74.6 %] for induction of remission [26]: OR 1.35 (95 % CI: 0.6–3.04).
- Probiotics (VSL#3™) + balsalazide had similar effectiveness [80 %] to placebo + balsalazide [70 %] for induction of remission [27]: OR 0.58 (95 % CI: 0.18–1.91).

As a comparison, in a trial of 268 UC patients with moderate severity, 4.8 grams of delayed release oral mesalamine was found to have clinical benefit in 70 % and superior to a response rate of 59 % for those using a lower dose of 2.4 grams of a delayed release oral mesalamine for moderate UC disease activity [28].

There have been some additional larger randomized placebo-controlled trials studies since the Cochrane systematic review and some studies in children. One such study is the Miele et al. [29] trial that recruited children with moderate-to-severe disease. VSL#3™ or placebo was administered along with corticosteroids and mesalamine. The corticosteroid dose (1 mg/kg/day to a maximum of 40 mg/day) and mesalamine (50 mg/kg/day) dose were those commonly used. The corticosteroids were tapered after a month if subjects were in remission. In this study, remission was achieved in 13 of 14 participants (92.8 %) treated with VSL#3™ and IBD therapy and in 4 of 15 patients (36.4 %) treated with placebo and IBD therapy (p < 0.001). This result must take in context the response rate to corticosteroids and mesalamine in the placebo-treated group. As a comparison, in a multicenter North American registry reporting the outcome of children with newly diagnosed UC, 60 % of those treated with corticosteroids were in remission at 3 months [30].

Another larger study by Fujimori and colleagues [31] utilized a quality of life measure to study patients on stable doses of aminosalicylates and/or prednisolone for at least 4 weeks while in remission or with mildly active UC. The probiotic was taken once daily and the prebiotic twice daily and the study was not double dummy controlled. The only measure of disease activity was C-reactive protein on a small number from each group. Only those patients taking a combination of a prebiotic and *B. longum* had an improvement ($p = 0.03$), whereas those subjects on the individual components (either prebiotic alone or probiotic individually) did not.

In a multicenter, randomized, double-blind, placebo-controlled trial from India, Sood et al. [32] studied the blend probiotic VSL#3™ in adults with mild-to-moderate UC. Participants were assigned randomly to groups that were given 3.6×10^{12} CFU VSL#3 ($N = 77$) or placebo ($n = 70$) twice daily for 12 weeks. A primary end point of 50 % decrease in the Ulcerative Colitis Disease Activity Index (UCDAI) at 6 weeks was achieved in a greater number of those receiving probiotic (32.5 %) than the group given placebo (10 %) ($p = 0.001$). A secondary end point of remission by 12 weeks was achieved in 33 subjects given probiotic (42.9 %) compared with 11 subjects given placebo (15.7 %, $p = 0.001$).

The response to rectal enemas of *E. coli* Nissle in subjects with distal proctitis of moderate activity was studied by Matthes et al. [33]. The concentration of the probiotic was 10^8 CFU/mL, and subjects with mild-to-moderate disease activity were randomized to receive enemas once daily containing either 10 mL, 20 mL, 40 mL, or placebo that was volume matched to the three different enema volumes used in the *E. coli* Nissle groups. Permissible concomitant therapies included loperamide drops to improve retention capacity for enemas and oral UC maintenance treatment with aminosalicylates or steroids at a constant level for at least 2 weeks prior to the study. A disease activity index was used to measure response, and if there was no response at 2 weeks, they were classified as nonresponders but otherwise could continue up to 8 weeks of therapy. In contrast to per-protocol analyses, intention to treat analysis revealed the number of responders was not significantly higher in the *E. coli* Nissle group than in the placebo group ($p = 0.4430$) in this Phase II study. In another *E. coli* Nissle study, Petersen et al. [34] randomized 100 patients with active UC to ciprofloxacin or placebo for 1 week followed by *E. coli* Nissle 1917 or placebo for 7 weeks as add-on treatments. In the per-protocol analysis, the group receiving placebo followed by *E. coli* Nissle 1917 fewer patients (54 %) reached remission compared to the group receiving placebo/placebo (89 %, $p < 0.05$).

In children with active distal colitis, significant improvement was seen in those receiving rectal administration of 1×10^{10} CFU of *L. reuteri* ATCC 55730 with concomitant mesalazine for 8 weeks compared to controls as determined by the Mayo Disease Activity Index [35]. Oral and rectal administration of 8 weeks of *L. casei* (8×10^8 CFU) was found to have equal beneficial effects on histological disease severity scores for those with mild left sided compared to 5-aminosalicylate alone [36].

In another of the larger trials, Tursi and colleagues [37] also evaluated VSL#3 in adults with relapsing mild-moderate UC as additional therapy to their usual 5-aminosalicylate and/or immunomodulator therapy. A total of 3.6×10^9 CFU/day (two sachets twice a day) of the blend of probiotics were ingested for the 8-week study period. The primary outcome was a 50 % decrease in the Ulcerative Colitis Disease Activity index. Newly described in the manuscript were weighted parameters for stool frequency, amount of rectal bleeding, mucosal appearance, and physician's rating for disease activity. There is no information with regard to the validation of this scale, and it is significantly different from the validated Pediatric Ulcerative Disease Activity Index [38]. A greater percentage of those receiving the probiotics achieved the primary outcome (63.1 vs. 40.8, intention to treat $p = 0.031$, 95 % CI 0.47–0.69). However, secondary outcomes of stool frequency, physician's assessment of disease activity, and endoscopic scores were similar between the two groups.

Subsequent to the Cochrane meta-analysis, Shen et al. [39] did a larger meta-analysis of probiotics in IBD that included nine trials of patients with UC. In the trials, probiotics were used largely as add-on therapy, and the analyses suggested a significant benefit in favor of probiotics ($p = 0.01$, RR=1.51) although there was significant heterogeneity ($p = 0.004$, I2=65 %). The beneficial effect appeared to be present only with VSL#3 [40], with higher remission rates when added to conventional therapy as compared to conventional therapy alone (43.8 % vs. 24.8 %; OR 2.4; 95 % CI 1.48–3.88; $p = 0.001$). The quality of evidence precluded a recommendation supporting the agent. With this information, however, the Toronto Consensus on clinical practice guidelines for the medical management of nonhospitalized UC patients recommended against probiotics to induce remission outside of clinical trials [41]. Similarly, there is no recommendation for the use of probiotics from the second European evidence-based consensus on the diagnosis and management of ulcerative colitis [42]. Furthermore, it must be remembered that the studies evaluated mild and moderate UC and the use of probiotics has not been studied in severe disease. While there have been no increased adverse events reported in studies, there continue to be case reports of bacteremia in those with severe colitis taking probiotics [43].

Maintenance of Remission

Naidoo and colleagues performed a Cochrane review on probiotics for maintenance of remission in ulcerative colitis [44]. There were four studies [45–48] included, and those excluded were those where subjects were followed for less than 3 months, where patients were not in remission at the start of the study, or studies that were not a randomized control trial. As detailed in Table 28.1, the total number of subjects

Table 28.1 Randomized controlled trials of probiotics used as ulcerative colitis maintenance therapy for a minimum of 3 months

Participants [# Treated]	Trial design	Probiotic (strains)	Dosing (CFU/day)	Trial length (months)	Ref.
103 [50]	DBRDD	Single strain (*E. coli* Nissle)	5×10^{10}	3	[45]
327 [162]	DBRDD	Single strain (*E. coli* Nissle)	5×10^{9}	12	[46]
187 [127]	R	Single strain (*L. rhamnosus* GG)	1.8×10^{10}	12	[47]
32 [20]	DBRPC	Blend (*L. acidophilus* LA-5, *B. animalis* BB-12)	1.5×10^{11}	13	[48]
29 [14]	DBRPC	Blend (VSL#3™)	$4.5\text{-}18 \times 10^{9}$	12	[29]

Legend: *DBRPC* Double-blind randomized placebo-controlled, *R* Randomized, *DBRDD* Double-blind, randomized, double-dummy, *Blend* combination of two or more probiotic organisms

receiving probiotic treatment is 409 among these 4 studies with 3 different probiotic preparations being used along with differing doses of probiotics being administered. Relapse rate was similar between those receiving probiotics compared to controls who received mesalamine ($n = 555$; 40.1 % vs. 34.1 %; OR 1.33; 95 % CI 0.94–1.90). In the Wildt study [48], there was no difference in the relapse rate at 1 year comparing the blend probiotic preparation (*L. acidophilus* LA-5 + *B. animalis* BB-12) with placebo ($n = 32$; 75 % vs. 92 %; OR 0.27; 95 % CI 0.03–2.68). Given the number of patients studied, study bias, and event number, the authors concluded there was insufficient evidence to make conclusions about efficacy of probiotics for maintenance in UC.

Miele et al. [29] randomized VSL#3 or placebo as add-on therapy in 29 consecutive children and reported 3 of 14 (21.4 %) patients treated with VSL#3 and IBD therapy relapsed within 1 year of therapy, compared to 11 of 15 (73.3 %) patients treated with placebo and IBD therapy ($p = 0.014$; RR=0.32; CI=0.025–0.773; NNT=2). This study was included in the meta-analysis of Shen et al. [39] of clinical relapse in maintaining therapy in UC. Analysis for the five included studies did not show significant advantage in maintaining treatment with probiotics compared with control group ($p = 0.47$, RR=0.89), and heterogeneity was not significant ($p = 0.19$, I2=35 %). Similar to induction of remission, the Toronto Consensus on clinical practice guidelines for the medical management of nonhospitalized UC patients recommended against probiotics for maintenance outside of clinical trials [41].

Pouchitis

Pouchitis is the most common complication of ileal pouch-anal anastomosis surgery for ulcerative colitis, and although the exact etiology is not clear, host genetic factors, local pouch issues, and the microbiota contained within the pouch

are thought to be involved (see chapter on Pouchitis). Most patients will develop this problem in the first year after the operation, and antibiotics can be an effective form of therapy in many [49, 50] although some patients are antibiotic-resistant and others improve on antibiotics but relapse following the discontinuation of antibiotics. As antibiotics can provide relief for most with pouchitis, a basic assumption has been that the microbiota of the pouch play an important role in the development and chronicity of pouchitis. Therefore, alteration/modulation of the pouch reservoir microbiota by addition of probiotics has been studied for both prevention and treatment of pouchitis.

Probiotics as Treatment of Pouchitis

There are few trials for treating mild-moderate pouchitis with small numbers of adult participants. Kuisma et al. [51] recruited 20 patients (10 intervention arm) for a DBRPC trial of *L. rhamnosus* GG 2×10^{10} CFU/day for 3 months. Patients with chronic, active pouchitis were excluded. The Pouchitis Disease Activity Index [52] was utilized for evaluation of clinical effect and prior to study entry, the mean PDAI was in the mild range (8.0 ± 0.8). There was no difference following the intervention period with clinical response (defined as a PDAI score reduction of ≥ 3) occurring in 1/10 (10 %) patients in the probiotic group and 0/10 (0 %) patients in the placebo group (10 % vs. 0 %, $p = 0.32$).

In an open-label trial of 51 UC patients with ileal pouch-anal anastomosis using a fermented milk product with a blend of probiotic strains (*L. acidophilus* strain La5 + *B. lactis* strain Bb12) containing 5×10^{10} CFU/day [53] there was a reported improvement in endoscopic evaluation. In another open-label trial [54], 16 of 23 patients (69 %) with mild pouchitis were in remission after treatment with VSL#3, and the median total Pouchitis Disease Activity Index scores reported before therapy improved following therapy (10 versus 4, $p < 0.01$).

Thus, there is limited evidence for a role of probiotics as monotherapy for mild-moderate pouchitis at the present time. Limiting access of microbiota to the mucosa of the pouch may be a mechanism, whereby probiotics provide benefit. Alternatively, changing the composition of the pouch microbiota may be important, although it is interesting that no long-term colonization of probiotic strains is achieved [55]. Thus, it may not be surprising that once the deleterious microbiota have colonized the pouch, probiotic monotherapy can do little to alter the situation.

Prevention of Initial Postoperative Onset of Pouchitis

Two trials have studied whether there is an advantage to initiate probiotics immediately following ileal pouch-anal anastomosis, and both found there to be benefit based on delayed onset of pouchitis. In a placebo-controlled trial [56], only 2 of 20 (10 %) subjects in the probiotic arm had developed pouchitis at the end of 1 year as compared to 8 of 20 (40 %, no episodes 80 % vs. 60 %, $p = 0.03$) in the control arm. The Peto odds ratio for prevention of pouchitis by the probiotic (VSL#3™) compared with placebo was 4.76, (95 % CI 1.16–19.56). Singh et al. [57] concluded for this part of their Cochrane review that low-quality evidence suggests that VSL#3 may be more effective than placebo for prevention of pouchitis.

Maintenance of Pouchitis Remission

The initial controlled trial for maintenance of remission of pouchitis was in the year 2000 using the blend probiotic product VSL#3™ and reported an outstanding effect in the prevention of recurrence in patients with antibiotic-dependent pouchitis. Prior to the administration of the blend probiotic, participants in his trial were successfully treated with a combination of antibiotics (ciprofloxacin + rifaximin). At the end of the 9-month study period, only 3 of 20 (15 %) subjects had developed pouchitis in the intervention group, whereas all 20 participants in the control group had a recurrence of pouchitis within 4 months of cessation of antibiotics [58]. A similar result was noted in another European trial of VSL#3™ also evaluating prevention of recurrence in relapsing or chronic pouchitis patients [55]. Remission of the pouchitis was induced in these participants by administering 4 weeks of a combination of antibiotics (metronidazole + ciprofloxacin) followed by either VSL#3™ or a placebo. In the probiotic treatment group, remission was maintained in 17 of 20 (85 %) subjects, but only 1 of 16 (6 %, $p < 0.0001$) receiving placebo. The pooled Peto odds ratio for these two studies for the combined rate of maintenance of remission with probiotic

bacteria compared to placebo (97 % versus 3 %, $p < 0.0001$) was 25.39 (95 % CI 10.37–62.17). The number needed to treat with oral probiotic therapy to prevent one additional relapse was 2 [59]. However, a GRADE analysis indicated that the quality of the evidence supporting this outcome was low due to very sparse data [57].

In contrast, an open-label trial by Shen and colleagues [60] reported a poor response for prevention of pouchitis recurrence using the same probiotic. In their trial, 31 subjects were prescribed a 2-week treatment of a single antibiotic (ciprofloxacin) followed by VSL#3™. In contrast to the other studies, the VSL#3™ was bought by patients rather than supplied through the study. Probiotic therapy was stopped by 9 of 31 (29 %) 7 weeks into therapy and 25 of 31 (81 %) by 8 months because of either failure to prevent pouchitis ($n = 23$) or side effects of the probiotic administration ($n = 2$). Only 6 of 31 (19 %) subjects did not develop clinical evidence of pouchitis by the end of the 8-month trial period. Even among these six subjects, endoscopy revealed some level of pouch inflammation. In contrast to other studies, in this trial [60], there was a single antibiotic administered, and endoscopy was not performed prior to probiotic administration to ensure pouch inflammation had completely resolved.

For those with poor pouch function, pouch-related dysfunction was not improved in a study [61] of 33 patients randomized to receive probiotics (*L. plantarum 299v* + *B. infantis CURE 21*) or placebo as measured by the pouch functional score ($p = 0.119$), pouch disease activity index ($p = 0.786$), or any of the fecal biomarkers tested (calprotectin, lactoferrin, myeloperoxidase, and eosinophilic cationic protein).

A recent clinical practice guideline on management of pouchitis [50] did not recommend probiotics as sole therapy for acute treatment of pouchitis but did suggest VSL#3 (or chronic use of antibiotics) for patients with prompt recurrence of pouchitis following antibiotic usage or multiple recurrences of pouchitis despite antibiotics. Table 28.2 lists randomized trials of probiotics in prevention of onset or recurrence of pouchitis.

Crohn's Disease

Induction of Remission

There is a paucity of studies investigating the use of probiotics to treat active inflammation. In two open-label studies [63, 64], probiotics (using combination of *B. breve* + *L. casei* + *B. longum* + prebiotics or *L. rhamnosus* GG, respectively) were added as adjuvant therapy to immunomodulators and corticosteroids. In the former study [55], seven of ten patients were reported to respond as determined by Crohn's Disease

Activity Index scores with the most noticeable improvement in diarrhea. However, there was no improvement in inflammation as measured by erythrocyte sedimentation rate (ESR) and C-reactive protein (CRP). In the open-label trial using *L. rhamnosus* GG [64], three of the four children were reported to have improved Pediatric Crohn's Disease Activity Index (PCDAI) scores or serial determinations over the 6 months of the trial. Specifics with regard to ESR or CRP are not reported although the ESR is a component of the PCDAI [62].

A placebo-controlled trial using *L. rhamnosus* GG was the sole study included in a Cochrane review of efficacy of probiotic supplementation for the induction of remission in CD [65]. Four of five patients in the probiotic group achieved remission compared to five of six in the placebo group (OR 0.80, 95 % CI 0.04–17.20). Subjects received antibiotics and concurrent therapy of corticosteroids raising some methodological concerns. Thus, although this one small study did not show that probiotics had any effect in treating active CD, at most, one could conclude there is insufficient evidence regarding the effectiveness of probiotics for treatment of active CD. Subgroup analysis by Shen et al. [39] of three studies including patients with CD did not determine a significant benefit in favor of probiotics for inducing a remission or clinical response in CD ($p = 0.35$, RR=0.89).

Maintenance of Remission

Randomized trials (see Table 28.3) studying probiotics as maintenance therapy in CD have been performed, using probiotics as monotherapy or in combination with 5-aminosalicylates [66–69]. Among these studies [70–72], there were no differences in the number of relapses in patients receiving *E. coli* Nissle compared to placebo ($p = 0.11$), *Saccharomyces boulardii* (1 g/day) plus mesalazine (2 g/day) compared to mesalazine alone (3 g/day) ($p = 0.08$), or patients receiving *L. rhamnosus* GG ($p = 0.77$).

In the largest maintenance trial in children, Bousvaros et al. [66] reported no difference in relapse rate for subjects receiving *L. rhamnosus* strain GG 2×10^{10} CFU/day (31 %, 12 of 39) or placebo (17 %, 6 of 36, $p = 0.18$). The time to relapse is shown in Fig. 28.1, and although there was a trend to a shorter time to relapse in those receiving probiotics, the results were not statistically different ($p = 0.10$) in this study.

In a subgroup meta-analysis [(39)] there was no significant difference in clinical relapse ($p = 0.71$, RR=1.09; 7 studies) or endoscopic relapse ($p = 0.75$, RR=1.08) with the use of probiotics.

Table 28.2 Randomized trials of probiotics in prevention of onset or recurrence of pouchitis

Participants [# Treated]	Trial design	Probiotic (strains)	Dosing (CFU/day)	Trial length (months)	Ref.
40 [20]	DBRPC	Blend (VSL#3™)	9×10^{11}	12	[55]
40 [20]	DBRPC	Blend (VSL#3™)	1.8×10^{12}	9	[60]
36 [20]		Blend (VSL#3™)	9×10^{11}	12	[61]
21 [17]	DBRPC	Blend (*L. plantarum 299 + B. infantis Cure21*)	5×10^{9} (each)	0.75	[62]

Legend: *DBRPC* Double-blind randomized placebo-controlled, *Blend* combination of two or more probiotic organisms

Table 28.3 Randomized trials of probiotics for maintenance of remission of Crohn's disease

Participants [# Treated]	Trial design	Probiotic (strains)	Dosing (CFU/day)	Trial length (months)	Ref.
28 [16]	DBRPC	Single strain (*E. coli Nissle 1917*)	5×10^{10}	12	[66]
32 [16]	R	Single strain (*S. boulardii*)	N/A	6	[67]
11 [5]	DBRPC	Single strain (*L. rhamnosus* strain GG)	2×10^{9}	6	[68]
75 [39]	DBRPC	Single strain (*L. rhamnosus* strain GG)	2×10^{10}	24	[69]

Legend: *DBRPC* Double-blind randomized placebo-controlled, *R* Randomized

Prevention of Postoperative Recurrence

Another aspect of CD that has been studied is prevention of recurrence of disease following surgical resection. Details of the trials are included in Table 28.4. Three of the trials involved a single probiotic strain and two trials included a blend of probiotics. In the *L. rhamnosus* GG trial [67], 9 of 15 (60 %) in *L. rhamnosus* GG group in clinical remission had endoscopic recurrence, and 6 of 17 (35 %) in placebo group in clinical remission had endoscopic recurrence (*p* = 0.297). In the first *L. johnsonii* LA1 trials [68], endoscopic recurrence was seen in 21 of 43 (43 %) in the

L. johnsonii LA1 group and 30 of 47 (64 %) in the placebo group at 6 months (*p* = 0.15). The second *L. johnsonii* LA1 trial [69] showed similar overall endoscopic scores between the probiotic and placebo groups (*p* = 0.48) and similar numbers of endoscopic recurrence (21 % of those taking *L. johnsonii* LA1 versus 15 % taking placebo (*p* = 0.33)). None of the secondary outcomes (clinical recurrence, histological score, C-reactive protein) showed any difference, either. Similarly, the two studies using a blend of probiotics failed to reveal any differences in endoscopic recurrence between treatment and placebo groups [73, 74]. A Cochrane meta-analysis [75] that combined all the studies failed to find

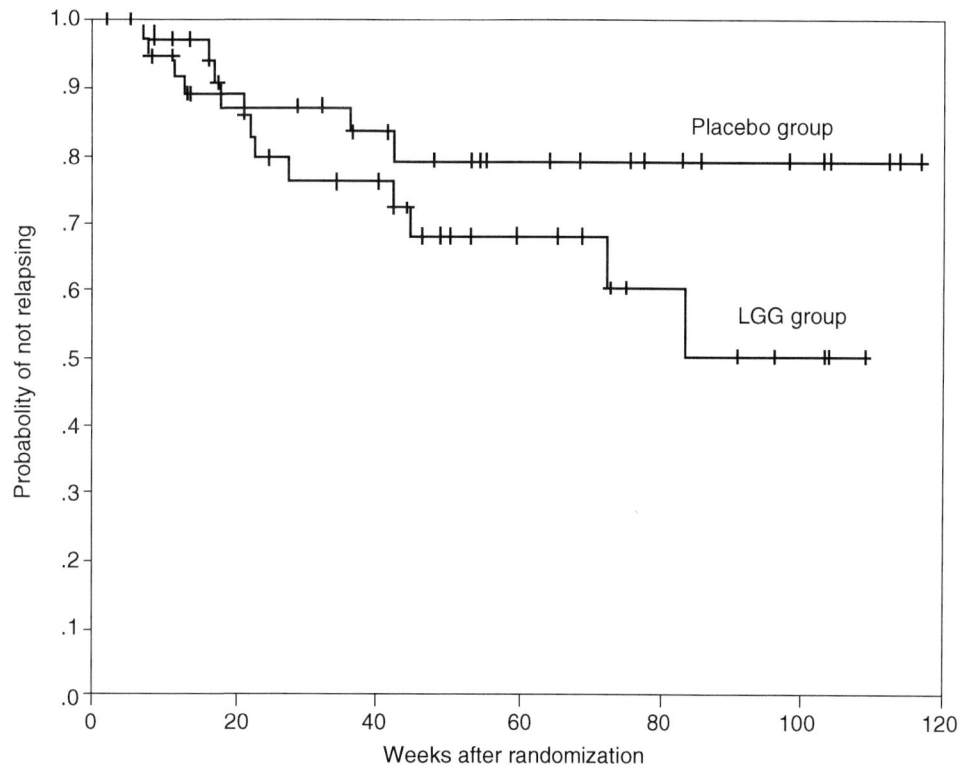

Fig. 28.1 Kaplan-Meier survival curve showing the probability of staying relapse-free during the duration of the study treatment duration for participants administered *L. rhamnosus* GG or placebo (*Source:* Figure reproduced from Bousvaros et al. [66]. Permission from Copyright Clearance Center (Danvers, MA))

Table 28.4 Randomized placebo-controlled trials of probiotics for prevention of recurrence of postoperative Crohn's disease

Participants [# Treated]	Probiotic (strains)	Dosing (CFU/day)	Trial length (months)	Ref.
45 [23]	Single strain (*L. rhamnosus* GG)	1.2×10^9	12	[73]
98 [48]	Single strain (*L. johnsonii* LA1)	4×10^9	6	[74]
70 [34]	Single strain (*L. johnsonii* strain LA1)	10^{10}	3	[75]
30 [2]	Blend probiotics + prebiotics (Synbiotic 2000™)	10^{10}	24	[76]
120 [58]	Blend probiotics (VSL#3™)	1.8×10^{12}	12	[77]

Legend: *CFU* colony-forming units, Synbiotic 2000™ organisms: *P. pentosaceus, L. raffinolactis, L. paracasei* subsp. paracasei 19 and *L. plantarum* 2362 VSL#3™ organisms: *L. acidophilus, L. plantarum, L. paracasei, L. bulgaricus, B. breve, B. longum, B. infantis,* and *S. thermophilus*

efficacy for postoperative prophylaxis. The relative risk of clinical recurrence with any probiotic relative to placebo (n = 213) was 1.41 (95 % CI 0.59–3.36), any endoscopic recurrence (n = 333) was 0.98 (95 % CI 0.74–1.29), and severe endoscopic recurrence (n = 213) was 0.96 (95 % CI 0.58–1.59). In another meta-analysis [76] that reviewed the effect of *Lactobacillus* alone for maintenance of remission induced by medical or surgical intervention [(67–69, 73, 74)] no difference was found vs. placebo. However, for the trials that compared placebo specifically with *L. rhamnosus* GG, pooled estimates showed a significant benefit in placebo (RR 1.68; 05 % CI 1.07–2.64) compared to subjects receiving *L. rhamnosus* GG.

Subsequent to this analysis but consistent with these previous studies, a randomized trial of VSL#3 (9×10^{11} CFU daily) for 90 days versus placebo (given within 30 days of ileocolic resection and reanastomosis) was performed. For those with no or mild endoscopic recurrence at day 90, VSL#3 was continued until day 365 [78]. At 90 days, a similar number of patients in each group had severe endoscopic lesions (9.3 % vs. 15.7 %, p = 0.19). At day 365, a similar number of patients that took the probiotic for all 365 days versus those that only took the probiotic from day 90 through 365 had severe endoscopic lesions (10.0 % vs. 26.7 %, p = 0.09).

Associated Conditions

Arthralgia

In an open-label trial, 16 patients with either Crohn's disease or ulcerative colitis completed a 3-month course of 9×10^{11} CFU/day of a blend probiotic (VSL#3™) to assess whether there was clinical improvement in arthralgia [79]. Participants had quiescent IBD at entry and no clinical or laboratory evidence of arthritis and were not taking nonsteroidal anti-inflammatory medications, and other medications were unchanged. An improvement in peripheral but not axial arthralgia was reported using an articular index score. There was no joint pain improvement as reported using a patient-completed visual analog scale. Notably, this study had a dropout rate of 45 %.

Sclerosing Cholangitis

With the reported benefit of antibiotics in pilot clinical studies of primary sclerosing cholangitis [80], interest has extended to the potential benefits of probiotics in this condition. Fourteen participants with concurrent IBD were randomized to the treatment with a blend probiotic (*L. acidophilus, L. casei, L. salivarius, L. lactis, B. bifidum, and B lactis*; total

daily dose of 10^{10} CFU/day) or placebo during 3 months in a double-blind crossover design that included a 1-month washout period [77]. The subjects remained on ursodeoxycholic acid during the trial. The results of this study showed no evidence of benefit from the probiotics on PSC-related symptoms, serum liver biochemistry, or liver function.

Summary

The evidence for efficacy for probiotics for treatment of IBD has to date been relatively disappointing considering the current theories regarding the importance of the intestinal microbiota in the development and chronicity of IBD. For CD, there is no aspect of the disease that has definitively responded to this form of therapy, be it induction of remission, maintenance of medical remission, or postoperatively. In fact, it may be that *L. rhamnosus* GG has a deleterious effect on maintaining CD remission [76]. For UC, there may be modest benefit for probiotics as an adjuvant to traditional therapy. VSL#3™ has now been included in clinical practice guidelines for recurrent and relapsing antibiotic sensitive pouchitis [50]. However, cost-effectiveness for adding probiotics to conventional therapy has been questioned [81].

It remains to be seen why the evidence so far is generally disappointing. Much like one cannot extrapolate the benefits that a single strain may possess in cell culture to humans or a particular proven health benefit for a particular probiotic strain to all other probiotics, it is too early to dismiss the potential for probiotics to modulate the intestinal microbiome for health benefits in IBD. There remain questions about the effective dosing and length of treatment. It is unknown whether the inclusion of prebiotics with a probiotic enhances the activity of the selected probiotic or whether active cultures may offer advantages over freeze-dried probiotics, the latter of which need to become metabolically active in the luminal environment of the host. Route of delivery may be particularly relevant when discussing distal colonic disease. In animal models, rectal administration of a probiotic has been found to be superior to oral administration to enhance mucosal epithelial cell-derived protective mechanisms in the distal colon [82]. In human studies of ulcerative colitis, oral and rectal administration of 5-aminosalicylates combined has been shown to be superior to the use of oral 5-aminosalicylates in the treatment of pancolitis [83]. Stability of the intestinal microbiota that leads to its resilience to short-term interventions [84] and persistence of functional capacity [85] are other important factors.

Another important issue may be related to the probiotics under study. Many of the studies have been conducted using strains of bacteria that are relatively inexpensive to produce in mass quantities, namely, *Lactobacilli* strains. *Lactobacilli* strains make up only a very small fraction of the microbiota of the human gastrointestinal tract and are likely allochthonous to the intestinal tract and therefore raise questions about utility for treating medical conditions [86]. It may be that a wider variety of strains (and those normally colonizing the intestinal tract) will be of importance, as well as the route of delivery and variety of organisms, as seen in the preliminary work of fecal transplantation therapy [87]. In addition, as detailed in the introduction, there are specific bacterial species that have now been identified to be altered in patients with CD [16, 23]. Taken together, it suggests that more effective strains exist than are currently available.

The high diversity of the intestinal microbiota [19] between individuals raises the question as to whether there is too much emphasis placed on individual bacterial species. The high human diversity explanation may lie within the realm of the presence of a range of bacterial species that share common functions that would help in the adaptation to different host-derived selective pressure and diet. This functional redundancy is being further maintained between phylogenetically related intestinal microbiota through horizontal gene transfer of mobile elements, promoted by high density and close proximity of members of the gut microbiota [88–90]. Thus, greater emphasis may need to be placed on studying the functional aspects of the intestinal microbiome rather than individual bacterial species. Newer techniques are allowing for these types of study [91, 92]. Perhaps delivering functional units rather than a given strain, combining specific microbes with a specific host genotype might be necessary as genetics is an integral part of the pathogenesis of CD; the genetic makeup of the human host has not been explored in probiotic trials nor has delivering genetically altered microorganisms in order to deliver specific genes to the mucosal microbiome. This approach might also provide a health benefit [93, 94], albeit administration of genetically modified microbes to humans will require significant safety measures.

Given the current situation of parental and self-prescribing of alternative care products including those described as probiotics, it behooves those providing care for IBD patients to ask about all prescription and nonprescription items being administered to their IBD patients. Among the most serious clinical scenarios to consider is that in which a patient is initiating immunosuppressive therapy. Most patients undergo the initiation of immunomodulators without incident, and most studies of probiotic administration have not uncovered significant risks [44, 76]. However, severely ill patients do have an increased risk with the use of probiotics. The most serious example to date involved the use of a combination of probiotics in severe pancreatitis where there was a significantly increased risk of death in patients receiving probiotics as compared to controls [95]. Furthermore, ill patients in ICU settings developed fungemia from the use of *S. boulardii* as probiotic [96] with bacteremia [43] and sepsis from a *Lactobacillus* strain also reported in a UC patient [97]. There is no evidence

to support the use of probiotics for severe IBD and little clinical experience in the use of probiotics in severely immunocompromised IBD patients. With commercialization of probiotics ahead of scientific and clinical investigation, as practitioners we should demand that the various aspects of IBD care are critically appraised before encouraging patients to ingest undocumented probiotic products as therapy in IBD.

References

1. Lilley DM, Stillwell RH. Probiotics: growth factors produced by microorganisms. Science. 1965;147:747–8.
2. FAO/WHO. Evaluation of health and nutritional properties of powder milk and live lactic acid bacteria. Food and Agriculture Organization of the United Nations and World Health Organization Expert Consultation Report, 2001. http://www.fao.org.
3. Thomas DW, Greer FR, American Academy of Pediatrics Committee on Nutrition; American Academy of Pediatrics Section on Gastroenterology, Hepatology and Nutrition. Probiotics and prebiotics in pediatrics. Pediatrics. 2010;126:1217–31.
4. Li FX, Verhoef MJ, Best A, et al. Why patients with inflammatory bowel disease use or do not use complementary and alternative medicine: a Canadian national survey. Can J Gastroenterol. 2005;19:567–73.
5. Quattropani C, Ausfeld B, Straumann A, et al. Complementary alternative medicine in patients with inflammatory bowel disease: use and attitudes. Scand J Gastroenterol. 2003;38:277–82.
6. Heuschkel R, Afzal N, Wuerth A, et al. Complementary medicine use in children and young adults with inflammatory bowel disease. Am J Gastroenterol. 2002;97:382–8.
7. Day AS, Whitten KE, Bohane TD. Use of complementary and alternative medicines in children and adolescents with inflammatory bowel disease. J Paediatr Child Health. 2004;40:681–4.
8. Hilsden RJ, Verhoef MJ, Best A, et al. Complementary and alternative medicine use in Canadian patients with inflammatory bowel disease: results of a national survey. Am J Gastroenterol. 2003;98:1563–8.
9. Joos SS, Rosemann TT, Szecsenyi JJ, et al. Use of complementary and alternative medicine in Germany – a survey of patients with inflammatory bowel disease. BMC Complement Altern Med. 2006;6:19. doi:10.1186/1472-6882-6-19.
10. Benchimol EI, Guttmann A, Griffiths AM, et al. Increasing incidence of pediatric inflammatory bowel disease in Ontario, Canada: evidence from health administrative data. Gut. 2009;58:1490–7.
11. Sartor RB. Mechanisms of disease: pathogenesis of Crohn disease and ulcerative colitis. Nat Clin Pract Gastroenterol Hepatol. 2006;3:390–407.
12. Clavel T, Haller D. Bacteria- and host-derived mechanisms to control intestinal epithelial cell homeostasis: implications for chronic inflammation. Inflamm Bowel Dis. 2007;13:1153–64.
13. Garrett WS, Lord GM, Punit S, et al. Communicable ulcerative colitis induced by T-bet deficiency in the innate immune system. Gut. 2007;131:33–45.
14. Dubinsky MC, Kugathasan S, Mei L, et al. Increased immune reactivity predicts aggressive complicating Crohn disease in children. Clin Gastroenterol Hepatol. 2008;6:1105–11.
15. Ungaro R, Bernstein CN, Gearry R, et al. Antibiotics associated with increased risk of new-onset Crohn's disease but not ulcerative colitis: a meta-analysis. Am J Gastroenterol. 2014;109:1728–38.
16. Gevers D, Kugathasan S, Denson LA, et al. The treatment-naïve microbiome in new-onset Crohn's disease. Cell Host Microbe. 2014;15:382–92.

17. Gerritsen J, Smidt H, Rijkers GT, de Vos WM. Intestinal microbiota in human health and disease: the impact of probiotics. Genes Nutr. 2011;3:209–40.

18. Rajiliic-Stojanovic M, Smidt H, de Vos WM. Diversity of the human gastrointestinal tract microbiota revisited. Environ Microbiol. 2007;9:2125–36.

19. Qin J, Li R, Raes J, et al. A human microbial gene catalogue established by metagenomic sequencing. Nature. 2010;464:559–65.

20. Mariat D, Firmesse O, Levenez F, et al. The Firmicutes/ Bacteroidetes ratio of the human microbiota changes with age. BMC Microbiol. 2009;9:123.

21. Frank DN, St Amand AL, Feldman RA, et al. Molecular-phylogenetic characterization of microbial community imbalances in human inflammatory bowel disease. Proc Natl Acad Sci U S A. 2007;104:13780–5.

22. Sokol H, Seksik P, Rigottier-Gois L, et al. Specificities of the fecal microbiota in inflammatory bowel disease. Inflamm Bowel Dis. 2006;12:106–11.

23. Assa A, Butcher J, Li J, et al. Mucosa-associated ileal microbiota in new-onset pediatric Crohn's disease. Inflamm Bowel Dis. 2016; 22:1533–9.

24. Mallon PT, McKay D, Kirk SJ, Gardiner K. Probiotics for induction of remission in ulcerative colitis. Cochrane Database Syst Rev. 2007;(4):CD005573.

25. Kato K, Mizuno S, Umesaki Y, et al. Randomized placebo-controlled trial assessing the effect of bifidobacteria-fermented milk on active ulcerative colitis. Aliment Pharmacol Ther. 2004;20: 1133–41.

26. Rembacken BJ, Snelling AM, Hawkey PM, et al. Non-pathogenic *Escherichia coli* versus mesalazine for the treatment of ulcerative colitis: a randomized trial. Lancet. 1999;354:635–9.

27. Tursi A, Brandimarte G, Giorgetti GM, et al. Low-dose balsalazide plus a high-potency probiotic preparation is more effective than balsalazide alone or mesalazine in the treatment of acute-mild-to-moderate ulcerative colitis. Med Sci Monit. 2004;10:Pl126–31.

28. Hanauer SB, Sandborn WJ, Kornbluth A, et al. Delayed-release oral mesalamine at 4.8 g/day (800 mg tablet) for the treatment of moderately active ulcerative colitis: the Ascend II trial. Am J Gastroenterol. 2005;100:2478–85.

29. Miele E, Pascarella F, Giannetti E, et al. Effect of a probiotic preparation (VSL#3) on induction and maintenance of remission in children with ulcerative colitis. Am J Gastroenterol. 2009;104:437–43.

30. Hyams J, Markowitz J, Lerer T, et al. The natural history of corticosteroid therapy for ulcerative colitis in children. Clin Gastroenterol Hepatol. 2006;4:1118–23.

31. Fujimori S, Gudis K, Mitsui K, et al. A randomized controlled trial on the efficacy of synbiotic versus probiotic or prebiotic treatment to improve the quality of life in patients with ulcerative colitis. Nutrition. 2009;25:520–5.

32. Sood A, Midha V, Makharia GK, et al. The probiotic preparation, VSL#3 induces remission in patients with mild-to-moderately active ulcerative colitis. Clin Gastroenterol Hepatol. 2009;7:1202–9.

33. Matthes H, Krummenerl T, Giensch M, et al. Clinical trial: probiotic treatment of acute distal ulcerative colitis with rectally administered *Escherichia coli* Nissle 1917 (EcN). BMC Complement Altern Med. 2010;10:13.

34. Petersen AM, Mirsepasi H, Hallkjaer SI, et al. Ciprofloxacin and probiotic *Escherichia coli* Nissle add-on treatment in active ulcerative colitis: a double-blind randomized placebo controlled clinical trial. J Crohns Colitis. 2014;8:1498–505.

35. Oliva S, Di Nardo G, Ferrari F, et al. Randomised clinical trial: the effectiveness of *Lactobacillus reuteri* ATCC 55730 rectal enema in children with active distal ulcerative colitis. Aliment Pharmacol Ther. 2012;35:327–34.

36. D'Inca R, Barollo M, Scarpa M, et al. Rectal administration of *Lactobacillus casei* DG modifies flora composition and Toll-like receptor expression in colonic mucosa of patients with mild ulcerative colitis. Dig Dis Sci. 2011;56:1178–87.

37. Tursi A, Brandimarte G, Papa A, et al. Treatment of relapsing mild-to-moderate ulcerative colitis with the probiotic VSL#3 as adjunctive to a standard pharmaceutical treatment: a double-blind, randomized, placebo-controlled study. Am J Gastroenterol. 2010; 105:2218–27.

38. Turner D, Otley AR, Mack D, et al. Development, validation, and evaluation of a pediatric ulcerative colitis activity index: a prospective multicenter study. Gastroenterology. 2007;133:423–32.

39. Shen J, Zuo ZX, Mao AP. Effect of probiotics on inducing remission and maintaining therapy in ulcerative colitis, Crohn's disease, and pouchitis: meta-analysis of randomized controlled trials. Inflamm Bowel Dis. 2014;20:21–35.

40. Mardini HE, Grigorian AY. Probiotic mix VSL#3 is effective adjuvant therapy for mild to moderately active ulcerative colitis: a meta-analysis. Inflamm Bowel Dis. 2014;20:1562–7.

41. Bressler B, Marshall JK, Bernstein CN, et al. Clinical practice guidelines for the medical management of nonhospitalized ulcerative colitis: the Toronto consensus. Gastroenterology. 2015;148: 1035–58.

42. Dignass A, Lindsay JO, Sturm A, et al. Second European evidence-based consensus on the diagnosis and management of ulcerative colitis Part 2: current management. J Crohns Colitis. 2013;7:1–33.

43. Meini S, Laureano R, Fani L, et al. Breakthrough *Lactobacillus rhamnosus GG* bacteremia associated with probiotic use in an adult patient with severe active ulcerative colitis: case report and review of the literature. Infection. 2015;43:777–81.

44. Naidoo K, Gordon M, Fagbemi AO, et al. Probiotics for maintenance of remission in ulcerative colitis. Cochrane Database Syst Rev. 2011;(12):CD007443.

45. Kruis W, Schutz E, Fric P, et al. Double-blind comparison of an oral *Escherichia coli* preparation and mesalazine in maintaining remission of ulcerative colitis. Aliment Pharmacol Ther. 1997;11:853–8.

46. Kruis W, Fric P, Pokrotnieks J, et al. Maintaining remission of ulcerative colitis with the probiotic *Escherichia coli* Nissle 1917 is as effective as with standard mesalazine. Gut. 2004;53:1617–23.

47. Zocco MA, dal Verme LZ, Cremonini F, et al. Efficacy of Lactobacillus GG in maintaining remission of ulcerative colitis. Aliment Pharmacol Ther. 2006;23:1567–1564.

48. Wildt S, Nordgaard I, Hansen U, et al. A randomized double-blind placebo-controlled trial with Lactobacillus acidophilus La-5 and Bifidobacterium animalis subsp. lactis BB-12 for maintenance of remission in ulcerative colitis. J Crohn Colitis. 2011;5:115–21.

49. Elahi B, Nikfar S, Derakhshani S, et al. On the benefit of probiotics in the management of pouchitis in patients underwent ileal pouch anal anastomosis: a meta-analysis of controlled clinical trials. Dig Dis Sci. 2008;53:1278–84.

50. Pardi DS, D'Haens G, Shen B, et al. Clinical guidelines for the management of pouchitis. Inflamm Bowel Dis. 2009;15:1424–31.

51. Kuisma J, Mentula S, Jarvinen H, et al. Effect of Lactobacillus rhamnosus GG on ileal pouch inflammation and microbial flora. Aliment Pharmacol Ther. 2003;17:509–15.

52. Sandborn WJ, Tremaine WJ, Batss KP, et al. Pouchitis following ileal pouch-anal anastomosis: a pouchitis disease activity index. Mayo Clin Proc. 1994;69:409–15.

53. Laake KO, Bjorneklett A, Aamodt G, et al. Outcome of four weeks' intervention with probiotics on symptoms and endoscopic appearance after surgical reconstruction with a J-configuration ileal-pouch-anal-anastomosis in ulcerative colitis. Scand J Gastroenterol. 2005;40:43–51.

54. Gionchetti P, Rizzello F, Morselli C, et al. High-dose probiotics for the treatment of active pouchitis. Dis Colon Rectum. 2007;50: 2075–8.

55. Mimura T, Rizzello F, Helwig U, et al. Once daily high dose probiotic therapy (VSL#3) for maintaining remission in recurrent or refractory pouchitis. Gut. 2004;53:108–14.

56. Gionchetti P, Rizzello F, Helwig U, et al. Prophylaxis of pouchitis onset with probiotic therapy: a double-blind, placebo-controlled trial. Gastroenterology. 2003;124:1202–9.

57. Singh S, Stroud AM, Holubar SD, et al. Treatment and prevention of pouchitis after ileal pouch-anal anastomosis for chronic ulcerative colitis. Cochrane Database Syst Rev. 2015;(11):CD001176.

58. Gionchetti P, Rizzello F, Venturi A, et al. Oral bacteriotherapy a maintenance treatment in patients with chronic pouchitis: a double-blind, placebo-controlled trial. Gastroenterology. 2000;119:305–9.

59. Holubar SD, Cima RR, Sandborn WJ, Pardi DS. Treatment and prevention of pouchitis after ileal pouch-anal anastomosis for chronic ulcerative colitis. Cochrane Database Syst Rev. 2010;(6):CD001176.

60. Shen B, Brzezinski A, Fazio VW, et al. Maintenance therapy with a probiotic in antibiotic-dependent pouchitis: experience in clinical practice. Aliment Pharmacol Ther. 2005;22:721–8.

61. Bengtsson J, Aderlath I, Ostblom A, et al. Effect of probiotics (*Lactobacillus plantarum 299v* plus *Bifidobacterium CURE21*) in patients with poor iléal pouch function: a randomised controlled trial. Scand J Gastroenterol. 2016;51:1087–92.

62. Turner D, Griffiths AM, Walters TD, et al. Appraisal of the Pediatric Crohn Disease Activity Index (PCDAI) on four prospectively collected datasets: recommended cutoff values and clinimetric properties. Am J Gastroenterol. 2010;105:2085–92.

63. Fujimori S, Tatsuguchi A, Gudis K, et al. High dose probiotic and prebiotic co therapy for remission induction of active Crohn disease. J Gastroenterol Hepatol. 2007;22:1199–204.

64. Gupta P, Andrew H, Kirschner BS, Guandalini S. Is Lactobacillus GG helpful in children with Crohn disease? Results of a preliminary, open-label study. J Pediatr Gastroenterol Nutr. 2000;31:453–7.

65. Butterworth AD, Thomas AG, Akobeng AK. Probiotics for induction of remission in Crohn disease. Cochrane Database Syst Rev. 2008;(3):CD006634.

66. Bousvaros A, Guandalini S, Baldassano RN, et al. A randomized, double-blind trial of Lactobacillus GG versus placebo in addition to standard maintenance therapy for children with Crohn disease. Inflamm Bowel Dis. 2005;11:833–9.

67. Prantera C, Scribano ML, Falasco G, et al. Ineffectiveness of probiotics in preventing recurrence after curative resection for Crohn disease: a randomized controlled trial with Lactobacillus GG. Gut. 2002;51:405–9.

68. Marteau P, Lemann M, Seksik P, et al. Ineffectiveness of Lactobacillus johnsonii LA1 for prophylaxis of postoperative recurrence in Crohn disease: a randomized, double blind, placebo controlled GETAID trial. Gut. 2006;55:842–7.

69. Van Gossum A, Dewitt O, Louis E, et al. Multicenter randomized-controlled clinical trial of probiotics (Lactobacillus johnsonii, LA1) on early endoscopic recurrence of Crohn disease after ileo-cecal resection. Inflamm Bowel Dis. 2007;13:135–42.

70. Malchow H. Crohn disease and *Escherichia coli*: a new approach in therapy to maintain remission of colonic Crohn disease. J Clin Gastroenterol. 1997;25:653–8.

71. Guslandi M, Mezzi G, Sorghi M, Testoni PA. Saccharomyces boulardii in maintenance treatment of Crohn disease. Dig Dis Sci. 2000;45:1462–4.

72. Schultz M, Timmer A, Herfarth HH, et al. Lactobacillus GG in inducing and maintaining remission of Crohn disease. BMC Gastroenterol. 2004;4:5.

73. Chermesh I, Tamir A, Reshed R, et al. Failure of Synbiotic 2000 to prevent postoperative recurrence of Crohn disease. Dig Dis Sci. 2007(52):385–9.

74. Madsen K, Backer JL, Leddin D, et al. A randomized trial of VSL#3 for the prevention of endoscopic recurrence following surgery for Crohn disease. Gastroenterology. 2008;134(Suppl 1):A361.

75. Doherty G, Bennett G, Patil S, et al. Interventions for prevention of post-operative recurrence of Crohn disease. Cochrane Database Syst Rev. 2009;(4):CD006873.

76. Shen J, Ran Z, Yin MH, et al. Meta-analysis: the effect and adverse events of Lactobacilli versus placebo in maintenance therapy for Crohn disease. Intern Med J. 2009;39:103–9.

77. Vleggaar FP, Monkelbaan JF, van Erpecum KJ. Probiotics in primary sclerosing cholangitis: a randomized placebo-controlled crossover pilot study. Eur J Gastroenterol Hepatol. 2008;20:688–92.

78. Fedorak RN, Feagan BG, Hotte N, et al. The probiotic VSL#3 has anti-inflammatory effects and could reduce endoscopic recurrence after surgery for Crohn's disease. Clin Gastroenterol Hepatol. 2015;13:928–35.

79. Karimi O, Pena S, van Bodegraven AA. Probiotics (VSL#3) in arthralgia in patients with ulcerative colitis and Crohn disease: a pilot study. Drugs Today. 2005;41:453–9.

80. Ali HA, Carey EJ, Lindor KD. Current research on the treatment of primary sclerosing cholangitis. Intractable Rare Dis Res. 2015;4:1–6.

81. Park KT, Perez F, Tsai R, et al. Cost-effectiveness analysis of adjunct VSL#3 therapy versus standard medical therapy in pediatric ulcerative colitis. J Pediatr Gastroenterol Nutr. 2011;53:489–96.

82. Dykstra NS, Hyde L, Adawi D. Pulse probiotic administration induces ongoing small intestinal Muc3 expression in rats. Pediatr Res. 2011;69:206–11.

83. Marteau P, Probert CS, Lindgren S, et al. Combined oral and enema treatment with Pentasa (mesalazine) is superior to oral therapy alone in patients with extensive mild/moderate active ulcerative colitis: a randomized, double blind, placebo controlled study. Gut. 2005;54:960–5.

84. Berg D, Clemente JC, Colombel JF. Can inflammatory bowel disease be permanently treated with short-term interventions on the microbiome? Expert Rev Gastroenterol Hepatol. 2015;9:781–95.

85. Smith MI, Yatsunenko T, Manary MJ, et al. Gut microbiomes of Malawian twin pairs discordant for kwashiorkor. Science. 2013;339:548–54.

86. Walter J. Ecological role of Lactobacilli in the gastrointestinal tract: implications for fundamental and biomedical research. Appl Environ Microbiol. 2008;74:4895–6.

87. Landy J, Al-Hassi HO, McLaughlin SD, et al. Review article: faecal transplantation therapy for gastrointestinal disease. Aliment Pharmacol Ther. 2011;34:409–15.

88. Jones BV, Marchesi JR. Accessing the mobile metagenome of the human gut mjicrobiota. Mol BioSyst. 2007;3:749–58.

89. Jones BV. The human gut mobile metagenome: a metazoan perspective. Gut Microbes. 2010;1:415–31.

90. Jones BV, Marchesi JR. Transposon-aided capture (TRACA) of plasmids resident in the human gut mobile metagenome. Nat Methods. 2007;4:55–61.

91. Braat H, Rottiers P, Hommes DW, et al. A phase 1 trial with transgenic bacteria expressing interleukin-10 in Crohn disease. Clin Gastroenterol Hepatol. 2006;4:754–9.

92. Starr AE, Deeke SA, Ning Z, et al. Proteomic analysis of ascending colon biopsies from a paediatric inflammatory bowel disease inception cohort identifies protein biomarkers that differentiate Crohn's disease from UC. Gut. 2016; doi:10.1136/gutjnl-2015-310705.

93. Zhang X, Ning Z, Mayne J, et al. In vitro metabolic labeling of intestinal microbiota for quantitative metaproteomics. Anal Chem. 2016;88:6120–5.

94. Loos M, Remaut E, Rottiers P, De Creus A. Genetically engineered Lactococcus lactis secreting murine IL-10 modulates the functions of bone marrow-derived dendritic cells in the presence of LPS. Scand J Immunol. 2009;69:130–9.

95. Besselink MG, van Santvoort HC, Buskens E, et al. Probiotic prophylaxis in predicted severe acute pancreatitis: a randomised, double-blind, placebo-controlled trial. Lancet. 2008;371:651–9.

96. Munoz P, Bouza E, Cuenca-Estrella M, et al. *Saccharomyces cerevisiae* fungemia: an emerging infectious disease. Clin Infect Dis. 2005;40:1625–34.

97. Farina C, Arosio M, Mangia M, Moioli F. Lactobacillus casei subsp. rhamnosus sepsis in a patient with ulcerative colitis. J Clin Gastroenterol. 2001;33:251–2.

Corticosteroids

Charles M. Samson and Johanna C. Escher

Introduction

Glucocorticosteroids have been around for about 60 years as a first-line treatment to induce remission in Crohn disease and ulcerative colitis in children and adults. The first randomized trial demonstrating their efficacy in active IBD was conducted in 1965 by Truelove et al. [1]. Systemic corticosteroid treatment may cause disfiguring cosmetic side effects during short-term use and bone demineralization as well as growth failure in long-term treatment, therefore limiting its use in children and adolescents. In addition to the side effects, corticosteroid resistance and dependence are common. The current trend is to minimize or even avoid corticosteroid use in pediatric as well as adult inflammatory bowel disease (IBD). In pediatric Crohn disease, enteral nutrition as primary therapy is a safe and effective alternative to prednisolone, whereas introduction of immune modulating therapy and biological treatment early in the course of disease is a successful steroid-sparing strategy [2]. In this chapter, the working mechanism, efficacy, side effects, and pharmacokinetics of "classic" (systemic) as well as topical corticosteroids such as budesonide will be reviewed.

The Working Mechanism of Corticosteroids

Under homeostatic conditions, activation of the innate and adaptive immune system is counteracted by endogenous glucocorticoids [3, 4]. At lower dosages, steroids may well follow these physiological pathways, whereas at higher concentrations other mechanisms may be involved.

Upon binding of the high-affinity glucocorticoid receptor, a cascade of events takes place starting with the dissociation of molecular chaperones followed by nuclear translocation. At this location, specific DNA sequences in the promoter region of steroid-responsive genes (glucocorticoid response elements) are bound leading to suppression of the genes encoding for the transcription of inflammatory proteins such as those involved in the mitogen-activated protein kinase (MAPK) pathway. Subsequently, the production of inflammatory mediators such as prostaglandins is reduced. The major anti-inflammatory effects of glucocorticoids appear to be due largely to interaction between the activated glucocorticoid receptor and transcription factors, notably nuclear factor-kappaB (NF-kappaB) and activator protein 1 (AP-1), that mediate the expression of inflammatory genes [5]. Inflammation may also become suppressed by increasing the synthesis of the anti-inflammatory mediators such as interleukin 10 and of inhibitor of kappa Ba (IκBa), which is regarded as an inhibitor of the key inflammatory transcription factor NF-κB. Inhibition of nongenomic mechanisms may also be involved. An example is the activation of endothelial nitric oxide synthase by glucocorticoids leading to the production of nitric oxide (NO). NO is an important modulator of the inflammatory cascade in IBD by affecting leukocyte-endothelial interactions, leukocyte infiltration, and vasodilatation. In summary, it has become clear that glucocorticoids interact with a wide range of molecules and therefore exert their immunosuppression by affecting various inflammatory pathways.

C.M. Samson, MD
Gastroenterology, Hepatology and Nutrition, Department of Pediatrics, Washington University School of Medicine,
1 Children's Place, CB 8116, St Louis, MO 63110, USA
e-mail: samson_c@kids.wustl.edu

J.C. Escher, MD, PhD (✉)
Department of Pediatric Gastroenterology, Erasmus MC-Sophia Children's Hospital, University Medical Center,
Dr Molewaterplein 60, 3015 GJ Rotterdam, The Netherlands
e-mail: j.escher@erasmusmc.nl

Systemic Corticosteroids

Placebo-controlled trials on the safety and efficacy of prednisolone have not been performed in children with Crohn disease or ulcerative colitis. Multiple studies, however, as reviewed by Heuschkel et al. [6], have compared the results

© Springer International Publishing AG 2017
P. Mamula et al. (eds.), *Pediatric Inflammatory Bowel Disease*, DOI 10.1007/978-3-319-49215-5_29

of enteral nutrition versus a course of steroids in the treatment of active Crohn disease in children and reported clinical remission in 85% of children treated with predniso(lo)ne. In children with severe acute ulcerative colitis, current guidelines recommend intravenous methylprednisolone as first-line treatment [7], with response rates of 71% as reported from a prospective trial in this group of patients [8].

One of the major drawbacks of corticosteroids is the range of side effects that may emerge during treatment, being cosmetic (acne, moon face, weight gain), psychological (mood swings, insomnia, depression), metabolic (bone demineralization, diabetes), or a risk of infections as a result of immune suppression. In children, the effect of systemic corticosteroids on growth is a special concern [9]. Moreover, it has long been known that corticosteroids do not heal the mucosa in IBD [10] and are not effective for the maintenance of remission [11–13]. From recent excellent data, drawn from a multicenter observational registry in the USA, we are now informed about the natural history of corticosteroid therapy in children with Crohn disease [14] as well as ulcerative colitis [15]. Despite the use of immunomodulators, 31% of children with CD and 45% of children with UC were found to be corticosteroid dependent at 1 year after diagnosis [14, 15]. This is in accordance with data from adults [16–18].

Topical Corticosteroids

Targeting local and systemic inflammatory processes in IBD therapeutic agents of first choice (e.g., aminosalicylates, corticosteroids) have been developed in special galenic forms to accomplish the topical delivery of the active compounds to the terminal ileum (Crohn disease) and/or the colon (Crohn disease and ulcerative colitis).

For over 10 years, nonsystemic corticosteroids such as budesonide, beclomethasone dipropionate, fluticasone, and hydrocortisone thiopivalate have been of interest for the targeted therapy of IBD. Budesonide is a glucocorticosteroid with a weak mineralocorticosteroid activity. It has a favorable ratio between anti-inflammatory activity and systemic glucocorticosteroid effect. This is explained by a high local glucocorticosteroid activity and an extensive first-pass hepatic degradation to metabolites with very low glucocorticosteroid activity. Due to these circumstances, the well-known glucocorticosteroid adverse effects are less frequent than with the conventional corticosteroids.

Pharmacokinetics

The absolute bioavailability of budesonide is very low, which results from gastrointestinal afflux mediated by P-glycoprotein, the product of the multidrug resistance 1 (MDR1) gene, and from biotransformation via cytochrome p450 3A (CYP3A) in the gut and liver. After this extensive first-pass metabolism, the metabolites 6β-hydroxybudesonide and 16α-hydroxyprednisolone are formed. Glucocorticoid activity of these metabolites amounts to only 1–10% of the parent drug.

Two pharmacokinetic studies have been performed in children with Crohn disease [19, 20]. Absolute bioavailability of budesonide (Entocort®) was found to be similar in children (9 ± 5%) compared to healthy adults (11 ± 7%) [20]. Consistently, overall systemic elimination of budesonide (Budenofalk®) reflected by clearance and half-life was not different in children and adults [19]. Conversion to 6β-hydroxybudesonide was shown to be 1.5-fold higher in children than in adults, suggesting enhanced biotransformation via CYP3A enzymes in children [19]. Corrections in dosing of budesonide based on body weight or body surface may not adequately reflect differences in pharmacodynamics. Therefore, the dose of budesonide (9 mg, once daily) decided on in both pediatric clinical trials [21, 22] was the same as used in adults with Crohn disease.

Topical Steroid Formulations

There are two oral formulations of budesonide used for treatment of Crohn disease: controlled ileal release (Entocort®) and pH-dependent release (Budenofalk®). Budenofalk is available in the EU but not in the USA. The controlled ileal release capsules contain 3 mg of budesonide distributed in approximately 100 pellets that have an outer coating of Eudragit L100–55 that dissolves at pH of 5.5 or higher. Absorption of Entocort® in the ileocaecal region ranges from 52 to 79%. The pH-dependent Budenofalk® capsules also contain 3 mg of budesonide in 400 pellets of 1 mm diameter and are coated with Eudragit, resistant to pH below 6.

For rectal treatment of left-sided ulcerative colitis, budesonide is available as enemas containing 2 mg per 100 ml of enema (Entocort® enema), and recently a new budesonide foam containing 2 mg per 25 ml of enema (Uceris® enema) has been developed with a goal of optimizing drug retention and providing uniform drug delivery to the rectum and distal colon with a mean spread of 25 cm [23]. Also, an oral controlled release system, MMX® extended-release budesonide 9 mg tablets (Uceris®; Cortiment®), characterized by a multi-matrix structure, has been developed. This new formulation has a gastric-resistant outer layer that dissolves as the luminal pH increases over 7.0 [24, 25]. It aims at a homogenous distribution of budesonide through the ascending, transverse, and descending colon, in order to treat colonic IBD, more specifically ulcerative colitis.

Efficacy of Oral Budesonide Treatment in Crohn Disease

Two randomized clinical trials have been performed comparing safety and efficacy of budesonide versus prednisolone in children with active ileocecal Crohn disease [21, 22]. In the non-blinded study by Levine et al., 33 patients (mean age 14.3 years) with active mild-to-moderate pediatric Crohn disease were randomized to 12 weeks of treatment with pH-modified release budesonide (Budenofalk® 9 mg, once daily) or prednisone (40 mg, once daily) [26]. The groups treated with budesonide and prednisone did not differ by age, onset of disease, location of disease, or disease activity. Remission (defined as Pediatric Crohn Disease Activity Index PCDAI $\leq$ 10) at 12 weeks was reported in 9/19 patients (47%) of the budesonide treatment group and in 7/14 patients (50%) of the prednisone treatment group (difference not statistically significant). Side effects occurred in 32% and 71% of patients treated with budesonide and prednisone, respectively ($p < 0.05$). Severity of cosmetic side effects was significantly lower in patients treated with budesonide ($p < 0.01$).

The study by Escher et al. was a randomized, double-blind, double-dummy, controlled multicenter clinical trial. In a joined effort by the IBD working group of the European Society of Paediatric Gastroenterology, Hepatology and Nutrition (ESPGHAN), 36 centers located in eight European countries took part [22]. Planned sample size was 120, but the study was terminated prematurely due to low enrolment numbers, with 48 patients (mostly new patients) with active Crohn disease involving ileum and/or ascending colon completing the 12-week study. Patients (mean age 13 years) were randomized to budesonide (Entocort 9 mg, once daily for 8 weeks, tapered to 6 mg for 4 weeks) or prednisolone (1 mg per kg bodyweight, once daily for 4 weeks, followed by 4 week tapering down to a 2.5 mg daily dose). Primary outcome parameter was clinical remission (modified Crohn's Disease Activity Index (CDAI $\leq$ 150)) at 8 weeks. Clinical remission was reported within 2 weeks of treatment in about 50% of the patients in both groups. At week 8, 12/22 patients in the budesonide group (55%) and 17/24 patients in the prednisolone group (71%) were in clinical remission ($p = 0.25$). The observed 16% difference in remission rate in favor of prednisone was statistically not significant. In case of planned enrolment of 120 patients, the extrapolated difference in remission rates would still not have reached significance. Mean CDAI of the patients was 239 (budesonide group) and 268 (prednisolone), representing mild-to-moderate disease. It is unknown whether prednisolone may be more effective than budesonide in patients with severe disease. Data from the North American prospective Pediatric IBD Collaborative Research Group Registry show that oral budesonide was used in 13% of children with newly diagnosed Crohn disease, mostly combined with 5-ASA (in 77%) or immunomodulators (43%). Despite the fact that oral budesonide is designed for controlled ileal release, less than 50% of these patients had disease located in the terminal ileum and/or ascending colon [27].

In adults, a Cochrane systematic review demonstrated that budesonide is more effective than placebo, though inferior to conventional corticosteroids in mild-to-moderate active Crohn disease in the terminal ileum and/or ascending colon. However, the likelihood of adverse events and adrenal suppression with budesonide is lower [28]. Four trials comparing budesonide versus prednisolone in adults showed less corticosteroid-related adverse events in the budesonide group [29–32]. Based on the above evidence, ECCO guidelines state that oral budesonide (9 mg once daily) for mild-to-moderate ileocaecal Crohn disease is an alternative to systemic corticosteroids for induction of remission in children [33] and a preferred treatment in adults [34].

Side Effects of Budesonide in Children

Glucocorticosteroid (GCS)-associated side effects such as moon face and acne were shown to occur significantly less in children treated with budesonide compared to prednisolone [22]. In the randomized clinical trial by Escher et al., moon face was almost three times as common in the prednisolone group. All short-term GCS-associated side effects of budesonide versus prednisolone are listed in Table 29.1. Adrenal suppression, expressed as a decrease in mean morning plasma cortisol levels, was evident during budesonide remission induction but significantly less compared to prednisolone treatment. Headache was reported in both treatment groups in 4/22 (budesonide group) and 4/26 patients (prednisolone group) and may be associated with benign intracranial hypertension as reported by Levine et al. [35].

A retrospective review of six prepubertal children with Crohn disease showed linear growth to be subnormal (2 cm/year) during budesonide maintenance treatment [36]. It remains unclear, however, whether impaired growth in these children (with PCDAI's of 15–27.5, indicating active disease) was due only to budesonide treatment or to ongoing mucosal inflammation.

Maintenance Treatment in Crohn Disease

Maintenance treatment with budesonide has not been studied prospectively in children. Systemic corticosteroids however have not been shown to be effective in prolonging clinical remission. A Cochrane review based on four placebo-controlled randomized trials in adults with Crohn disease [31, 37–39] concluded that maintenance treatment with oral budesonide at 6 mg/day is not effective in preventing relapses

Table 29.1 Glucocorticosteroid-associated side effects of budesonide versus prednisolone in children with ileocaecal Crohn disease

	Budesonide n = 22	Prednisolone n = 26[a]	p-value
Moon face	5	15	0.01
Buffalo hump	0	1	NS
Acne	1	7	0.033
Hirsutism	2	3	NS
Skin striae	0	1	NS
Bruising easily	1	1	NS
Swollen ankles	0	1	NS
Hair loss	1	3	NS
Mood swings	3	2	NS
Depression	2	1	NS
Insomnia	5	4	NS
Any such sign[b]	11	20	0.030

RCT by Escher et al. [22], with permission
NS not statistically significant
[a]One of these had no on-treatment data regarding possible glucocorticosteroid side effects
[b]Some patients had more than one sign

of Crohn disease in adults [40]. In addition, a recent meta-analysis demonstrated that there is no statistically significant benefit of oral budesonide over placebo in the prevention of relapse in adults with quiescent Crohn disease, while glucocorticosteroid-related side effects were significantly more common with budesonide [11]. In light of this evidence, and the concerns on longitudinal growth in children, maintenance treatment with budesonide should not be recommended.

Budesonide in Ulcerative Colitis

No studies have been performed in children. In adults, topical steroid treatment with budesonide foam enemas is more efficacious than placebo in inducing remission in patients with mild-to-moderate left-sided colitis as demonstrated in two randomized, double-blinded studies [41] and has demonstrated a favorable safety profile [42]. However, budesonide enema was less effective in left-sided UC compared to 5-ASA [43]. In adults with mild-to-moderate active left-sided colitis, three studies have each shown a modest effect of budesonide MMX formulation for inducing remission compared to placebo, and the drug is well tolerated [44–47]. The role of these mediations in maintenance of remission in ulcerative colitis has not been studied.

Conclusion

Corticosteroids have been the first-line treatment in Crohn disease for many years. Disfiguring acute and serious long-term side effects, such as growth retardation and bone demineralization, limit their use. The current trend in pediatric as well as adult Crohn disease is to minimize and avoid repeated corticosteroid use by introducing immunomodulators early in the course of disease. In Europe, primary treatment of active Crohn disease by a 6–8 week course of enteral nutrition is favored over remission induction by prednisolone. Systemic or topical corticosteroids are not effective as maintenance treatment.

Adrenal suppression is less severe during budesonide treatment compared to prednisolone, and glucocorticosteroid-associated side effects such as acne and moon face occur less frequently.

Corticosteroids do not heal the mucosa, do not prevent relapse, and do not alter the course of disease. In the current era, confidence with early immunomodulator and biological treatment is growing, with a tendency toward step-down instead of step-up treatment. While this strategy needs to be substantiated by prospective studies, it is clear that corticosteroids are losing their position as first-line treatment of pediatric IBD.

References

1. Truelove SC, Witts LJ. Cortisone in ulcerative colitis; preliminary report on a therapeutic trial. Br Med J. 1954;2(4884):375–8.
2. Markowitz J, Grancher K, Kohn N, Lesser M, Daum F. A multicenter trial of 6-mercaptopurine and prednisone in children with newly diagnosed Crohn's disease. Gastroenterology. 2000;119(4):895–902.
3. Barnes PJ, Adcock IM. How do corticosteroids work in asthma? Ann Intern Med. 2003;139(5 Pt 1):359–70.
4. Rhen T, Cidlowski JA. Antiinflammatory action of glucocorticoids–new mechanisms for old drugs. N Engl J Med. 2005;353(16):1711–23.
5. Hayashi R, Wada H, Ito K, Adcock IM. Effects of glucocorticoids on gene transcription. Eur J Pharmacol. 2004;500(1–3):51–62.
6. Heuschkel RB, Menache CC, Megerian JT, Baird AE. Enteral nutrition and corticosteroids in the treatment of acute Crohn's disease in children. J Pediatr Gastroenterol Nutr. 2000;31(1):8–15.
7. Turner D, Travis SP, Griffiths AM, Ruemmele FM, Levine A, Benchimol EI, et al. Consensus for managing acute severe ulcerative colitis in children: a systematic review and joint statement from ECCO, ESPGHAN, and the Porto IBD Working Group of ESPGHAN. Am J Gastroenterol. 2011;106(4):574–88.
8. Turner D, Mack D, Leleiko N, Walters TD, Uusoue K, Leach ST, et al. Severe pediatric ulcerative colitis: a prospective multicenter study of outcomes and predictors of response. Gastroenterology. 2010;138(7):2282–91.
9. Pappa H, Thayu M, Sylvester F, Leonard M, Zemel B, Gordon C. Skeletal health of children and adolescents with inflammatory bowel disease. J Pediatr Gastroenterol Nutr. 2011;53(1):11–25.
10. Beattie RM, Nicholls SW, Domizio P, Williams CB, Walker-Smith JA. Endoscopic assessment of the colonic response to corticosteroids in children with ulcerative colitis. J Pediatr Gastroenterol Nutr. 1996;22(4):373–9.
11. Ford AC, Bernstein CN, Khan KJ, Abreu MT, Marshall JK, Talley NJ, et al. Glucocorticosteroid therapy in inflammatory bowel disease: systematic review and meta-analysis. Am J Gastroenterol. 2011;106(4):590–9. quiz 600
12. Steinhart AH, Ewe K, Griffiths AM, Modigliani R, Thomsen OO. Corticosteroids for maintenance of remission in Crohn's disease. Cochrane Database Syst Rev. 2003;(4):CD000301.

13. Lennard-Jones JE, Misiewicz JJ, Connell AM, Baron JH, Jones FA. Prednisone as maintenance treatment for ulcerative colitis in remission. Lancet. 1965;1(7378):188–9.
14. Markowitz J, Hyams J, Mack D, Leleiko N, Evans J, Kugathasan S, et al. Corticosteroid therapy in the age of infliximab: acute and 1-year outcomes in newly diagnosed children with Crohn's disease. Clin Gastroenterol Hepatol. 2006;4(9):1124–9.
15. Hyams J, Markowitz J, Lerer T, Griffiths A, Mack D, Bousvaros A, et al. The natural history of corticosteroid therapy for ulcerative colitis in children. Clin Gastroenterol Hepatol. 2006;4(9):1118–23.
16. Faubion Jr WA, Loftus Jr EV, Harmsen WS, Zinsmeister AR, Sandborn WJ. The natural history of corticosteroid therapy for inflammatory bowel disease: a population-based study. Gastroenterology. 2001;121(2):255–60.
17. Ho GT, Chiam P, Drummond H, Loane J, Arnott ID, Satsangi J. The efficacy of corticosteroid therapy in inflammatory bowel disease: analysis of a 5-year UK inception cohort. Aliment Pharmacol Ther. 2006;24(2):319–30.
18. Targownik LE, Nugent Z, Singh H, Bernstein CN. Prevalence of and outcomes associated with corticosteroid prescription in inflammatory bowel disease. Inflamm Bowel Dis. 2014;20(4):622–30.
19. Dilger K, Alberer M, Busch A, Enninger A, Behrens R, Koletzko S, et al. Pharmacokinetics and pharmacodynamic action of budesonide in children with Crohn's disease. Aliment Pharmacol Ther. 2006;23(3):387–96.
20. Lundin PD, Edsbacker S, Bergstrand M, Ejderhamn J, Linander H, Hogberg L, et al. Pharmacokinetics of budesonide controlled ileal release capsules in children and adults with active Crohn's disease. Aliment Pharmacol Ther. 2003;17(1):85–92.
21. Levine A, Weizman Z, Broide E, Shamir R, Shaoul R, Pacht A, et al. A comparison of budesonide and prednisone for the treatment of active pediatric Crohn disease. J Pediatr Gastroenterol Nutr. 2003;36(2):248–52.
22. Escher JC. Budesonide versus prednisolone for the treatment of active Crohn's disease in children: a randomized, double-blind, controlled, multicentre trial. Eur J Gastroenterol Hepatol. 2004;16(1):47–54.
23. Brunner M, Vogelsang H, Greinwald R, Kletter K, Kvaternik H, Schrolnberger C, et al. Colonic spread and serum pharmacokinetics of budesonide foam in patients with mildly to moderately active ulcerative colitis. Aliment Pharmacol Ther. 2005;22(5):463–70.
24. Fiorino G, Fries W, De La Rue SA, Malesci AC, Repici A, Danese S. New drug delivery systems in inflammatory bowel disease: MMX and tailored delivery to the gut. Curr Med Chem. 2010;17(17):1851–7.
25. Brunner M, Ziegler S, Di Stefano AF, Dehghanyar P, Kletter K, Tschurlovits M, et al. Gastrointestinal transit, release and plasma pharmacokinetics of a new oral budesonide formulation. Br J Clin Pharmacol. 2006;61(1):31–8.
26. Levine A, Broide E, Stein M, Bujanover Y, Weizman Z, Dinari G, et al. Evaluation of oral budesonide for treatment of mild and moderate exacerbations of Crohn's disease in children. J Pediatr. 2002;140(1):75–80.
27. Otley A, Leleiko N, Langton C, Lerer T, Mack D, Evans J, et al. Budesonide use in pediatric crohn's disease. J Pediatr Gastroenterol Nutr. 2012;55(2):200–4.
28. Rezaie A, Kuenzig ME, Benchimol EI, Griffiths AM, Otley AR, Steinhart AH, et al. Budesonide for induction of remission in Crohn's disease. Cochrane Database Syst Rev. 2015;(6):CD000296.
29. Rutgeerts P, Lofberg R, Malchow H, Lamers C, Olaison G, Jewell D, et al. A comparison of budesonide with prednisolone for active Crohn's disease. N Engl J Med. 1994;331(13):842–5.
30. Bar-Meir S, Chowers Y, Lavy A, Abramovitch D, Sternberg A, Leichtmann G, et al. Budesonide versus prednisone in the treatment of active Crohn's disease. Israeli Budesonide Study Group. Gastroenterology. 1998;115(4):835–40.
31. Gross V, Andus T, Ecker KW, Raedler A, Loeschke K, Plauth M, et al. Low dose oral pH modified release budesonide for maintenance

of steroid induced remission in Crohn's disease. The Budesonide Study Group. Gut. 1998;42(4):493–6.
32. Campieri M, Ferguson A, Doe W, Persson T, Nilsson LG. Oral budesonide is as effective as oral prednisolone in active Crohn's disease. The Global Budesonide Study Group. Gut. 1997;41(2):209–14.
33. Ruemmele FM, Veres G, Kolho KL, Griffiths A, Levine A, Escher JC, et al. Consensus guidelines of ECCO/ESPGHAN on the medical management of pediatric Crohn's disease. J Crohns Colitis. 2014;8(10):1179–207.
34. Dignass A, Van Assche G, Lindsay JO, Lemann M, Soderholm J, Colombel JF, et al. The second European evidence-based Consensus on the diagnosis and management of Crohn's disease: current management. J Crohns Colitis. 2010;4(1):28–62.
35. Levine A, Watemberg N, Hager H, Bujanover Y, Ballin A, Lerman-Sagie T. Benign intracranial hypertension associated with budesonide treatment in children with Crohn's disease. J Child Neurol. 2001;16(6):458–61.
36. Kundhal P, Zachos M, Holmes JL, Griffiths AM. Controlled ileal release budesonide in pediatric Crohn disease: efficacy and effect on growth. J Pediatr Gastroenterol Nutr. 2001;33(1):75–80.
37. Greenberg GR, Feagan BG, Martin F, Sutherland LR, Thomson AB, Williams CN, et al. Oral budesonide as maintenance treatment for Crohn's disease: a placebo-controlled, dose-ranging study. Canadian Inflammatory Bowel Disease Study Group. Gastroenterology. 1996;110(1):45–51.
38. Lofberg R, Rutgeerts P, Malchow H, Lamers C, Danielsson A, Olaison G, et al. Budesonide prolongs time to relapse in ileal and ileocaecal Crohn's disease. A placebo controlled one year study. Gut. 1996;39(1):82–6.
39. Ferguson A, Campieri M, Doe W, Persson T, Nygard G. Oral budesonide as maintenance therapy in Crohn's disease–results of a 12-month study. Global Budesonide Study Group. Aliment Pharmacol Ther. 1998;12(2):175–83.
40. Kuenzig ME, Rezaie A, Seow CH, Otley AR, Steinhart AH, Griffiths AM, et al. Budesonide for maintenance of remission in Crohn's disease. Cochrane Database Syst Rev. 2014;(8):CD002913.
41. Sandborn WJ, Bosworth B, Zakko S, Gordon GL, Clemmons DR, Golden PL, et al. Budesonide foam induces remission in patients with mild to moderate ulcerative proctitis and ulcerative proctosigmoiditis. Gastroenterology. 2015;148(4):740–50.e2.
42. Rubin DT, Sandborn WJ, Bosworth B, Zakko S, Gordon GL, Sale ME, et al. Budesonide foam has a favorable safety profile for inducing remission in mild-to-moderate ulcerative proctitis or proctosigmoiditis. Dig Dis Sci. 2015;60(11):3408–17.
43. Hartmann F, Stein J, BudMesa-Study G. Clinical trial: controlled, open, randomized multicentre study comparing the effects of treatment on quality of life, safety and efficacy of budesonide or mesalazine enemas in active left-sided ulcerative colitis. Aliment Pharmacol Ther. 2010;32(3):368–76.
44. D'Haens GR, Kovacs A, Vergauwe P, Nagy F, Molnar T, Bouhnik Y, et al. Clinical trial: preliminary efficacy and safety study of a new Budesonide-MMX(R) 9 mg extended-release tablets in patients with active left-sided ulcerative colitis. J Crohns Colitis. 2010;4(2):153–60.
45. Travis SP, Danese S, Kupcinskas L, Alexeeva O, D'Haens G, Gibson PR, et al. Once-daily budesonide MMX in active, mild-to-moderate ulcerative colitis: results from the randomised CORE II study. Gut. 2014;63(3):433–41.
46. Sandborn WJ, Danese S, D'Haens G, Moro L, Jones R, Bagin R, et al. Induction of clinical and colonoscopic remission of mild-to-moderate ulcerative colitis with budesonide MMX 9 mg: pooled analysis of two phase 3 studies. Aliment Pharmacol Ther. 2015;41(5):409–18.
47. Sandborn WJ, Travis S, Moro L, Jones R, Gautille T, Bagin R, et al. Once-daily budesonide MMX(R) extended-release tablets induce remission in patients with mild to moderate ulcerative colitis: results from the CORE I study. Gastroenterology. 2012;143(5):1218–26.e1–2.

6-Mercaptopurine Therapy

30

Carmen Cuffari

Introduction

6-Mercaptopurine (6-MP) and its parent drug azathioprine (AZA) are well known for their immunosuppressive and lymphocytotoxic properties [1, 2]. These antimetabolite drugs have been shown to suppress disease activity in up to 70% of children with moderate to severe Inflammatory Bowel Disease (IBD); among these patients, 50% will achieve a clinical response after 4 months of continuous maintenance 6-MP therapy [3, 4], suggesting that inherent differences in drug metabolism or immunomodulation may influence clinical responsiveness to therapy [5]. Moreover, although the overall risk of 6-MP-induced toxicity is low [6], these same presumed pharmogenomic determinants can only explain in part susceptibility to untoward antimetabolite-associated side effects [7], including the risk of malignancy [8]. The risk of EBV-associated lymphoma among patients with leukemia on maintenance 6-MP therapy is well known and now has also been shown in patients with IBD on long-term antimetabolite therapy. Although the absolute risk for lymphoma remains low [9], many pediatric gastroenterologists have now been compelled to consider alternate forms of immunosuppression. Unfortunately, the commercial availability of drug monitoring has not provided pediatricians any reassurance on potentially further minimizing the overall risk of antimetabolite-associated toxicity. Herein, we will review the use of AZA and 6-MP in the management of pediatric patients with IBD. Furthermore, the application of pharmacogenetic and 6-MP metabolite testing will also be discussed based on an analysis of the literature. Several recommendations will also be provided on applying this technology in clinical practice.

C. Cuffari, MD
Division of Pediatric Gastroenterology and Nutrition, Department of Pediatrics, The Johns Hopkins University School of Medicine, 600 N. Wolfe St. CMSC 2-123, Baltimore, MD 21287, USA

The Johns Hopkins Hospital, Department of Pediatrics, Division of Gastroenterology, 600 N. Wolfe St. CMSC 2-123, Baltimore, MD 21287, USA
e-mail: ccuffari@jhmi.edu

Clinical Indication

Maintenance Therapy

6-MP and AZA are often considered the immunosuppressant drugs of choice in the management of patients with steroid-dependent IBD. Pearson and coworkers published a meta-analysis of nine controlled clinical trials in adult patients with CD that showed clinical responsiveness to either 6-MP or AZA therapy was largely dependent on duration of therapy. In that study, 40–70% of patients successfully achieved corticosteroid withdrawal after a median delay in clinical response time of 16 weeks [10]. On account of this delay in clinical response time, many clinicians are either reluctant to prescribe these slow-acting agents or will prematurely discontinue antimetabolite drug therapy in favor of the more rapid onset biological therapies [11].

Although the delay in clinical response precludes the use of 6-MP as an induction therapy, the notion of using prednisone as a bridge to antimetabolite therapy was first studied by Markowitz and coworkers. In that study, 55 children with newly diagnosed (<6 weeks) CD were randomized in a prospective placebo controlled clinical trial to receive corticosteroids either with or without 6-MP therapy. All patients were placed on a corticosteroid weaning schedule. Patients on combination 6-MP and corticosteroid therapy had achieved clinical remission more effectively, and with a lower cumulative dose of corticosteroids than patients on placebo. Indeed, 92% of patients on 6-MP, and just 6% of patients on placebo, maintained clinical remission after 12 months of follow-up [12]. Interestingly, these investigators chose not to use mesalamine in either treatment arm, despite a probable therapeutic benefit in using slow released 5-ASA formulations in patients with mild to moderate CD [13]. Although, this study would support the notion of initiating antimetabolite as a first line therapy in patients with severe and aggressive disease phenotypes, most pediatric gastroenterologist will try to determine steroid dependency prior to instituting antimetabolite therapy. Future studies are

© Springer International Publishing AG 2017
P. Mamula et al. (eds.), *Pediatric Inflammatory Bowel Disease*, DOI 10.1007/978-3-319-49215-5_30

375

needed to improve our understanding of genotype-phenotype correlations in clinical practice. This would allow clinicians to identify aggressive disease phenotypes and tailor medical therapy more effectively while minimizing the overall need for corticosteroids [14].

Adjunct Therapy

It has been the practice in many institutions, including our own, to initiate maintenance anti-TNF alpha therapy in patients that have proven refractory to either long-term 6-MP or AZA therapy. In a double blind randomized control trial of maintenance infliximab therapy over a 54 weeks trial period (ACCENT 1), 41% of all adult patients with CD achieved and maintained a favorable clinical response. Patients on maintenance infliximab therapy were also more likely to discontinue corticosteroids (29%) and sustain a protracted clinical response than patients on placebo (9%). This study was the first large multicentered study to have shown that retreatment with infliximab was more effective than placebo for maintaining clinical remission in patients with CD. Although 29% of all the patients recruited into the study were on concurrent immunosuppressive therapy, it should be noted that most patients had previously been unsuccessful in achieving disease remission on either 6-MP or AZA [15].

Several important questions come to mind when reviewing the ACCENT I study, including whether all individuals with CD who are treated with infliximab should receive concurrent immunosuppressive therapy despite having not benefited from them in the past. The answer to this question is best addressed by the apparent need for some form of adjunct immunosuppressive therapy in order to prevent antibody against infliximab formation (HACA). The concurrent use of immunosuppressive therapy has in the past been shown by Rutgeerts and coworkers to maintain a favorable clinical response to maintenance infliximab therapy, presumably due to the prevention of HACA antibody formation. In that study, 75% (12/16) of patients on concurrent 6-mercaptopurine maintained a favorable clinical response, compared to 50% (9/18) on no concurrent immunosuppressive therapy [16]. In the ACCENT 1 study, only 18% of the patients on neither concurrent prednisone nor immunosuppressive drug therapy developed HACA, compared to just 10% of patients on concurrent azathioprine or methotrexate therapy [15].

The SONIC [17] and SUCCESS [18] studies have clearly shown an improved overall maintenance of clinical response to combination anti-TNF and antimetabolite therapy in patients with moderate to severe Crohn's disease and ulcerative colitis, respectively. In both double-blinded clinical trials, the efficacy of infliximab monotherapy was compared to AZA and combination AZA and infliximab in patients that were naïve to either immunosuppression or biologic therapy.

Overall, the combination of AZA and infliximab showed an improved corticosteroid free remission (26 wks: SONIC [17]; 16 wks: SUCCESS [18]) compared to monotherapy alone.

Despite an evidence-based improvement in overall clinical response with combination therapy, the increased risk of lymphoma has precluded the concurrent use of antimetabolites with anti-TNF therapy. A recent meta-analysis showed a standardized incidence ratio of about 5, ranging from 2.8 in the analysis of 8 population studies to >9 in 10 referral studies. The risk was most noteworthy among ongoing users of antimetabolite therapy, but not former users. The most noteworthy risk was among patients after 1 year of exposure and less than 30 years of age. It is important to note that although the relative risks of lymphoma in active users was high, there remains a very low absolute risk of malignancy. Among patients <30 years, the risk was shown to remain 1:2000 patient years [9].

The notion of using methotrexate in lieu of either 6-MP or AZA has been downplayed on account of its limited usefulness in patients with UC [19], and its limited effectiveness when used in combination with infliximab compared to infliximab alone in achieving an overall improvement in steroid free clinical remission in patients with Crohn's disease [20]. Although the risk of teratogenicity in males is low, the concern for birth defects among our adolescent female patients with IBD on methotrexate therapy must be underscored [21].

Although these results of SONIC and SUCCESS clearly demonstrate the steroid-sparing effects of a "top down" therapeutic approach to patients with severe active disease, physicians must appreciate that CD is a lifelong disease, and the risk for lymphomas and other neoplasia with combination immunosuppression must be considered [22, 23]. This is of critical importance, especially in a pediatric population who would be anticipated to receive maintenance infliximab therapy for many years. Albeit low, the risk of hepatosplenic T-cell lymphoma in pediatric patients on combination infliximab and 6-MP remains most disconcerting [24, 25].

Postoperative Prophylaxis

In patients with ileocolonic disease, the reoperation rate after surgical correction ranges from 25–60% after 5 years to up to 91% after 15 years. The recurrence risk after colocolic reanastomosis is much less. A good predictor of disease recurrence is disease behavior. Patients with perforating disease are twice more likely than patients with nonperforating disease to require subsequent surgeries [26]. It still remains difficult to accurately predict the course of disease in any particular patient with CD, and the clinical value of prophylactic therapy remains unclear.

Hanauer et al. described 131 adult patients with CD who underwent intestinal resection and ileocolonic anastomosis and were randomized to receive either placebo, 6-MP (50mmg/day) or mesalamine (3 g/day) as prophylactic therapy. Patients were evaluated prospectively with serial colonoscopies and small bowel barium enemas. In that study, 6-MP was shown to significantly ($p <0.05$) lower the clinical (50%) and endoscopic recurrence (43%) of CD compared to the mesalamine (clinical (58%); endoscopic (63%)) and placebo (clinical (77%); endoscopic (64%)) treatment groups. Although the dose of 6-MP used in this study was lower than that used for maintenance therapy, a well-defined prophylactic dose has yet to be defined. Despite the fact that clinical recurrence was similar between the 6-MP and mesalamine treatment groups, this study may support the continued use of antimetabolite drugs postoperatively in patients with aggressive disease phenotypes [27]. However, more recently Savarino et al. described 51 adult patients who were randomized to receive adalimumab (ADA), AZA, or mesalamine after ileocolonic resection. At 2 years, rate of endoscopic occurrence was lower in the ADA group (6.3%) compared with AZA (64.7%) or mesalamine (83.3%), with clinical recurrence also less frequent with ADA compared to AZA or mesalamine. There is no prospective pediatric data regarding the use of these medications for postoperative prevention [54].

Drug Monitoring

Most often, pediatricians will measure drug efficacy based on either an improvement in their patients' clinical symptoms and quality of life or their ability to maintain remission while weaning off of corticosteroid therapy. In general, most physicians will tend to rely on their clinical judgment and experience in determining the dosage of AZA (2–2.5 mg/kg/day) [28, 29] or 6-MP (1–1.5 mg/kg/day) [30, 31] in treating patients with IBD. However, not all patients achieve clinical remission with this treatment approach despite presumed therapeutic drug dosing. This has led some physicians to adopt a dose escalation treatment strategy beyond traditional dosages. In these patients, 6-MP-induced leukopenia is used as a clinical end point to gauge drug dosing. Although Colonna and coworkers have shown that clinical response time is less in those patients with 6-MP-induced leukopenia, overall clinical response to therapy is independent of either 6-MP dose or total leukocyte count. In that study, none of their patients developed clinical signs of bone marrow suppression, required hospitalization for concurrent infection or required transfusions despite total leukocyte counts <5000 [32]. A true separation between immunosuppression [1] and cytotoxicity [2] has yet to be defined since the dosing of 6-MP and AZA has been based largely on clinical outcome. Indeed, the wide range in antimetabolite drug doses used in clinical practice would suggest that a safe and established therapeutic

dose has yet to be determined [29–32]. As a consequence, the clinician must always remain aware of potential adverse effects, including allergic reactions, hepatitis, pancreatitis, bone marrow suppression, and lymphoma while attempting to achieve an optimal therapeutic response [6].

In comparison, the pediatric oncologist will effectively tailor the dose of either 6-MP or AZA based on the measure of erythrocyte 6-MP metabolite levels. Indeed, the notion of a therapeutic window of clinical efficacy and toxicity based on the measurement of AZA therapy has now become the standard of care in most pediatric practices treating patients with leukemia [33–35].

6-Mercaptopurine Metabolism

6-MP and its prodrug AZA are by themselves inactive, and must be transformed into their active ribonucleotides that function as purine antagonists. These antimetabolites are then incorporated into DNA, thereby interfering with ribonucleotide replication [36, 37]. The metabolism of 6-MP and AZA occurs intracellularly along the competing routes catalyzed by hypoxanthine phosphoribosyl transferase and thiopurine S-methyltransferase (TPMT), giving rise to 6-thioguanine nucleotides (6-TGn), and 6-methyl-mercaptopurine (6-MMP), respectively (Fig. 30.1) [5]. 6-TGn is the active ribonucleotide of 6-MP that functions as a purine antagonist inducing lymphocytotoxicity and immunosuppression [1, 2].

An apparent genetic polymorphism has been observed in TPMT activity in both the Caucasian and African-American populations. Negligible activity was noted in 0.3%, and low levels (<5 U/mL of blood) in 11% of individuals [5]. TPMT enzyme deficiency is inherited as an autosomal recessive trait, and to date, 10 mutant alleles and several silent and intronic mutations have been described [38]. In patients with

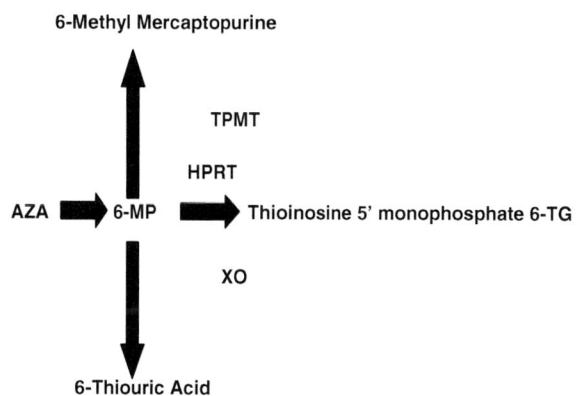

Fig. 30.1 The metabolism of azathioprine. *AZA* azathioprine; 6-MP, 6-mercaptopurine, *TPMT* thiopurine methyl transferase, *XO* xanthine oxidase, *HPRT* hypoxanthine phosphoribosyl transferase, *5-ASA* mesalamine

the heterozygous TPMT genotype, 6-MP metabolism is shunted preferentially into the production of 6-TG nucleotides. Although 6-TG nucleotides are thought to be lymphocytotoxic, and beneficial in the treatment of patients with leukemia and lymphoma, patients with low (<5) TPMT activity are at risk for bone marrow suppression by achieving potentially toxic erythrocyte 6-TGn levels on standard doses of 6-MP [39]. Despite low TPMT enzyme activity levels, therapeutic erythrocyte 6-TGn metabolite levels can still be achieved without untoward cytotoxicity by lowering the dose of 6-MP by about 50% [40].

6-MP Metabolite Monitoring in IBD

The measurement of the erythrocyte 6-MP metabolites 6-TGn and 6-MMP have been proposed as a useful clinical tool for measuring clinical efficacy, documenting patient compliance to therapy and explaining some drug-induced toxicity in patients with IBD. In our preliminary study in 25 adolescent patients with CD on long-term 6-MP therapy, high performance liquid chromatography measurement of erythrocyte 6-TG metabolite levels showed an inverse correlation with disease activity. Although a wide range of metabolite levels was associated with a favorable clinical response, patients with high 6-TGn levels (>250 pmoles/8 × 10 [8] RBCs) were uniformly asymptomatic [41]. Similar results have been reported in 93 pediatric and 45 adult patients with IBD in whom disease remission correlated well with erythrocyte 6-TGn levels between 230 and 260 pmoles/8 × 10 [8] RBCs, respectively [42, 43]. Although these studies and others would support the notion of a therapeutic index of clinical responsiveness based on the measurement of erythrocyte 6-TGn levels [44], several studies have shown no clinical correlation with metabolite monitoring (Table 30.1) [45–48]. This lack of consensus may in part be due to the heterogeneous nature of CD and ulcerative colitis, and may also be dependent on disease severity. Moreover, erythrocyte 6-TGn metabolite levels have not correlated with

Table 30.1 Clinical responsiveness to 6-MP and AZA therapy based on threshold (235–250[a]) erythrocyte 6-TGn metabolite levels

| Study patients | 6-TGn response threshold | | | |
	(Response)	Above	Below	Odds ratio
Dubinsky [42]	92 (30)	.78	.40	5.0
Gupta [45]	101 (47)	.56	.43	1.7
Belaiche [46]	28 (19)	.75	.65	1.6
Cuffari [49]	82. (47)	.86	.35	11.6
Achar [43]	60 (24)	.51	.22	3.8
Lowry [47]	170 (114)	.64	.68	0.9
Goldenberg [48]	74 (14)	.24	.18	1.5

[a]pmoles/8 × 10[8] RBCs

either lean body mass, adiposity, or surface to volume differences in children (personal observation). As a consequence, conventional weight-based drug therapy has been neither reliable nor predictive. Despite all of its limitations, 6-MP metabolite monitoring still remains the only objective means of monitoring patient compliance, toxicity, and clinical responsiveness to antimetabolite therapy.

In a study of adult patients with CD, high (>290) erythrocyte 6-TGn level showed a positive predictive value of 86% of obtaining a favorable clinical response to induction AZA therapy in patients with steroid refractory CD [49].

TPMT Activity

Genetic polymorphism in TPMT enzyme activity can be quantitatively measured by TPMT phenotype testing. One in 300 patients have absent TPMT enzyme activity, and are at risk for severe bone marrow suppression [39]. There have been a number of cases of irreversible bone marrow suppression both in patients with IBD and in patients with leukemia on standard doses of 6-MP or AZA therapy (personal communications). 6-MP metabolism is clearly influenced by inherent differences in TPMT activity present within the population. In a prospective open-labeled study in patients with IBD, the response rate to induction AZA therapy was highest in patients with less than average (<12 U/mL blood) TPMT activity. Clinical response also correlated well with achieving high erythrocyte (>250) 6-TGn metabolite levels. Indeed, the knowing of the low (<5) TPMT activity before initiating AZA therapy in two patients led to a low dosing strategy (1 mg/kg/day) with a favorable clinical response without untoward side effects [39]. Moreover, Kaskas and coworkers suggested that an effective low (0.25 mg/kg/day) treatment approach can be safely and effectively adopted in patients with the homozygous recessive genotype [40]. Both of these studies would support the contention that a low dose treatment strategy may be used to treat those patients with low TPMT activity.

In comparison, 10% of the population is considered to be rapid metabolizers' of 6-MP, and in theory would require larger than standard doses of drug in order to achieve any therapeutic drug benefit. In these patients, 6-MP metabolism is shunted away from 6-TGn production and into the formation of 6-MMP. A study in children with IBD showed that a subgroup of these patients remain refractory to therapy despite a dose optimizing treatment strategy [50]. This may in part be due to high hepatic TPMT activity that may draw most of the 6-MP from the plasma, thereby limiting the amount of substrate available for the bone marrow and peripheral leukocytes. A similar study in adult patients with IBD was also able to identify these rapid metabolizers based on the measure of erythrocyte TPMT activity levels. In that study, patients with above average (>12) TPMT activity levels were less likely to respond to AZA therapy, and more likely to require higher dosages (2 mg/kg/day) of AZA from the outset in order to optimize erythrocyte 6-TGn metabolite levels. Moreover, patients with above average (>12) TPMT activity had a mean erythrocyte 6-TGn level that leveled off below a presumed therapeutic (<250) treatment level after 8 weeks of continuous AZA therapy. Sixty-nine % patients with TPMT activity levels ≤12 U/mL blood achieved a clinical response compared to just 30% of patients with above average (>12) TPMT activity after 4 months of continuous therapy. This study was the first to suggest that the pretreatment knowledge of TPMT activity may allow physicians to predict clinical response, and effectively dose AZA in order to maximize efficacy while minimizing the risk of toxicity. Indeed, in that study, patients with a TPMT enzyme activity less than 15 U/mL of blood were six times (OR: 6.2) more likely to show a favorable response to AZA therapy [49]. A recent study exploited the use of allopurinol, a potent inhibitor of xanthine oxidase, in patients with high (>16) TPMT activity who shunt 6-MP metabolism away from the production of 6-TGn metabolites, and remain refractory to presumed therapeutic antimetabolite drug dosing. In that study, the concomitant use of allopurinol with either AZA or 6-MP (reduced to 25–50% of the initial dose) in patients with presumed high TPMT activity levels achieved a significant increase in erythrocyte 6-TGn metabolite levels and the subsequent induction of disease remission. Although this treatment strategy led to a decrease in total leukocyte count, no patient developed clinical signs of toxicity [51].

6-MP Toxicity

Many pediatricians have been reluctant to prescribe 6-MP on account of potential drug related toxicity including pancreatitis 3%, bone marrow depression 2%, super-infection 7%, and hepatitis 0.3% [52]. Severe side effects are either idiosyncratic or related to generic polymorphism as described above. Although Black and coworkers suggested the notion that pharmacogenetic differences in 6-MP metabolism influence a patient's risk of drug toxicity [7], TPMT polymorphism accounts for only 25% of all 6-MP-induced side effects [53]. However, genetic polymorphisms may play a role in determining the long-term risk for malignancy. In several pediatric oncology studies, the risk for secondary malignancies, including acute myeloblastic leukemia and myelodysplasia was higher in those children with low TPMT activity levels with acute lymphocytic leukemia on maintenance 6-MP therapy [54]. Recent studies in IBD have now shown that past exposure to thiopurines also increases the risk of myeloid disorders 7 fold compared to patients with IBD naïve to antimetabolite therapy [8].

Conclusion

6-MP and AZA have proven efficacy in the maintenance of disease remission in children with IBD. The application of pharmacogenomic and metabolite testing in clinical practice has helped to improve the overall clinical response to antimetabolite therapy in children with IBD and reduce the risk of antimetabolite-induced side effects. The careful monitoring of complete blood counts, and erythrocyte 6-TG metabolite levels are indicated in patients with either low (<5) or above average (>12) TPMT levels; relying on either total leukocyte counts or mean corpuscular volume as the sole measure of dosing adequacy should be used with caution [53].

References

1. Tiede I, Fritz G, Strand S, et al. CD28-dependent Rac1 activation is the molecular target of azathioprine in primary human CD4+ T lymphocytes. J Clin Invest. 2003;111:1122–4.
2. Carvalho RS, Mahoney JA, Oliva-Hemker MM, et al. Inherent resistance to 6-thioguanine induced apoptosis correlates with disease activity in children with IBD. Gastroenterology. 2006;265:A203.
3. Markowitz J, Rosa J, Grancher K, Aiges H, Daum F. Long-term 6-mercaptopurine treatment in adolescents with Crohn's disease. Gastroenterology. 1990;99:1347–51.
4. Verhave M, Winter HS, Grand RJ. Azathioprine in the treatment of children with inflammatory bowel disease. J Pediatr. 1990;117:809–14.
5. Weinshilboum RN, Sladek S. Mercaptopurine pharmacogenetics: monogenic inheritance of erythrocyte thiopurine methyl transferase activity. Am J Hum Genet. 1980;32:651–62.
6. Present DH, Meltzer SJ, Krumholz MP, et al. 6-mercaptopurine in the management of inflammatory bowel disease: short and long-term toxicity. Ann Intern Med. 1995;111:641–9.
7. Black AJ, McLeod HL, Capell HA. Thiopurine methyl transferase predicts therapy-limitingsever toxicity from azathioprine. Ann Intern Med. 1998;129:716–8.
8. Lopez A, Mounier M, Bouvier AM, et al. Increased risk of acute myeloid leukemia and myelodysplastic syndromes in patients who received thiopruine treatment for inflammatory bowel disease. Clin Gastroenterol Hepatol. 2014;12:1324–9.
9. Kotlyar DS, Lewis JD, Beaugerie L, et al. Risk of lymphoma in patients with inflammatory bowel disease treated azathioprine and 6-mercaptopurine: a meta-analysis. Clin Gastroenterol Hepatol. 2015;13:847–58.
10. Pearson DC, May GR, Fick GH, Sutherland SR. Azathioprine and 6-mercaptopurine in Crohn's disease: a meta-analysis. Ann Intern Med. 1995;122:132–42.
11. Markowitz J, Hyams J, Mack D, et al. Corticosteroid therapy in the age of infliximab: acute and 1-year outcomes in newly diagnosed children with Crohn's disease. Clin Gastroenterol Hepatol. 2006;4:1124–9.
12. Markowitz J, Grancher K, Kohn N, et al. A multi-center trial of 6-mercaptopurine and prednisone therapy in children with newly diagnosed Crohn's disease. Gastroenterology. 2000;119:895–902.
13. Camma C, Giunta M, Rosselli M, Cottone M. Mesalamine in the maintenance treatment of Crohn's disease: a meta-analysis adjusted for confounding variables. Gastroenterology. 1997;113:1465–73.
14. Brant SR, Panhuysen CI, Bailey-Wilson JE, et al. Linkage heterogeneity for the IBD1 locus in Crohn's disease pedigrees by disease onset and severity. Gastroenterology. 2000;119:1483–90.

15. Hanauer SB, Feagan BG, Lichtenstein GR, et al. Maintenance infliximab for Crohn's disease: the ACCECT I randomized trial. Lancet. 2002;359:1541–9.
16. Rutgeerts P, D'Haens G, Targan S, et al. Efficacy and safety of retreatment with anti-tumor necrosis factor antibody (infliximab) to maintain remission in Crohn's disease. Gastroenterology. 1999; 117:761–9.
17. Colombel JF, Sandborn WJ, Reinisch W, et al. Infliximab, azathioprine, or combination therapy for Crohn's disease. N Engl J Med. 2010;362:1383–95.
18. Panaccione R, Ghosh S, Middleton S, et al. Combination therapy with infliximab and azathioprine is superior to monotherapy with either agent in ulcerative colitis. Gastroenterology. 2014;146: 392–400.
19. Carbonnel F, Colombel JF, Filippi J, et al. Methotrexate is not superior to placebo for inducing steroid-free remission, but induces steroid-free clinical remission in a larger proportion of patients with ulcerative colitis. Gastroenterology. 2016 Feb;150(2):380–8.
20. Feagan BG, McDonald JW, Panaccione R, et al. Methotrexate in combination with infliximab is no more effective than infliximab alone in patients with Crohn's disease. Gastroenterology. 2014; 146(3):681–8.
21. Weber-Schoendorfer C, Hoeltzenbein M, Wacker E, Meister R, Schaefer C. No evidence for an increased risk of adverse pregnancy outcome after paternal low-dose methotrexate: an observational cohort study. Rheumatology. 2014;53:757–63.
22. Siegel CA, Hur C, Korzenik JR, et al. Risks and benefits of infliximab for the treatment of Crohn's disease. Clin Gastroenterol Hepatol. 2006;8:1017–24.
23. Thayu M, Markowitz JE, Mamula P, et al. Hepatosplenic T-cell lymphoma in an adolescent patient after immunomodulator and biologic therapy for Crohn disease. J Pediatr Gastroenterol Nutr. 2005;2:220–2.
24. Mamula P, Markowitz JE, Cohen LJ, et al. Infliximab in pediatric ulcerative colitis: two-year follow-up. J Pediatr Gastroenterol Nutr. 2004 Mar;38(3):298–301.
25. Baldassano RN, Han PD, Jeshion WC, et al. Pediatric Crohn's disease: risk factors for postoperative recurrence. Am J Gastroenterol. 2001;7:2169–76.
26. Hanauer SB, Korelitz BI, Rutgeerts P, et al. Post-operative maintenance of Crohn's disease remission with 6-mercaptopurine, mesalamine or placebo: a 2 year trial. Gastroenterology. 2004;127: 723–9.
27. Ewe K, Press AG, Singe CC, et al. Azathioprine combined with prednisolone or monotherapy with prednisolone in active Crohn's disease. Gastroenterology. 1993;105:367–72.
28. Candy S, Wright J, Gerber M, Adams G, Gerig M, Goodman R. A controlled double blind study of azathioprine in the management of Crohn's disease. Gut. 1995;37:674–8.
29. Korelitz BI, Adler DJ, Mendelsohn RA, et al. Long-term experience with 6-mercaptopurine in the treatment of Crohn's disease. Am J Gastroenterol. 1993;88:1198–205.
30. Present DH, Korelitz BI, Wisch N, et al. Treatment of Crohn's disease with 6-mercaptopurine. A long-term, randomized, double-blind study. N Engl J Med. 1980;302:981–7.
31. Colonna T, Korelitz BI. The role of leukopenia in 6-mercaptopurine-induced remission of refractory Crohn's disease. Am J Gastroenterol. 1993;89:362–6.
32. Lennard L, Rees CA, Lilleyman JS, et al. Childhood leukemia: a relationship between intracellular 6-mercaptopurine metabolites and neutropenia. Br J Clin Pharmacol. 1993;16:359–63.
33. Zimm S, Collins JM, Riccardi R, et al. Variable bioavailability of oral mercaptopurine Is maintenance chemotherapy in acute lymphoblastic leukemia being optimally delivered. N Engl J Med. 1983;308:1005–9.
34. McLeod HL, Relling MV, Liu Q, Pui CH, Evans WE. Polymorphic thiopurine methyl transferase in erythrocytes is indicative of activity in leukemic blasts from children with acute lymphoblastic leukemia. Blood. 1995;85:1897–902.
35. Christie NT, Drake S, Meyn RE. 6-thioguanine induced DNA damage as a determinant of cytotoxicity in cultured hamster ovary cells. Cancer Res. 1986;44:3665–71.
36. Fairchild CR, Maybaum J, Kennedy KA. Concurrent unilateral chromatid damage and DNA strand breaks in response to 6-thioguanine treatment. Biochem Pharmacol. 1986;35:3533–41.
37. Alves S, Prata MJ, Ferreira F, Amorim A. Screening of thiopurine methyl s-transferase mutations by horizontal conformation-sensitive gel electrophoresis. Hum Mutat. 2000;15:246–53.
38. Evans WE, Horner M, Chu YQ, et al. Altered mercaptopurine metabolism, toxic effects, and dosage requirements in a thiopurine methyltransferase deficient child with acute lymphoblastic leukemia. J Pediatr. 1991;119:985–9.
39. Kaskas BA, Louis E, Hinderof U, et al. Safe treatment of thiopurine S-transferase deficient Crohn's disease patients with azathioprine. Gut. 2003;52:140–2.
40. Cuffari C, Theoret Y, Latour S, et al. 6-mercaptopurine metabolism in Crohn's disease: correlation with efficacy and toxicity. Gut. 1996;39:401–6.
41. Dubinsky MC, Lamothe S, Yang HY, Targan SR, Sinnett D, Theoret Y, Seidman EG. Pharmacogenomics and metabolite measurement for 6-mercaptopurine therapy in inflammatory bowel disease. Gastroenterology. 2000;118:705–13.
42. Achar JP, Stevens T, Brzezinski A, Seidner D, Lashner B. 6-Thioguanine levels versus white blood cell counts in guiding 6-mercaptopruine and azathioprine therapy. Am J Gastroenterol. 2000;95:A272.
43. Cuffari C, Hunt S, Bayless TM. Utilization of erythrocyte 6-thioguanine metabolite levels to optimize therapy in IBD. Gut. 2001;48:642–6.
44. Gupta P, Gokhlae R, Kirschner BS. 6-mercaptopurine metabolite levels in children with inflammatory bowel disease. J Pediatr Gastroenterol Nutr. 2001;33:450–4.
45. Belaiche J, Desager JP, Horsman Y, Louis E. Therapeutic drug monitoring of azathioprine and 6-mercaptopurine metabolites in Crohn's disease. Scand J Gastroenterol. 2001;36:71–6.
46. Lowry PW, Franklin CL, Weaver AL, Szumlanski C, Mays DC, Loftus EV, Tremaine WJ, Lipsky JJ, Weinshilboum RM, Sandborn WJ. Leukopenia resulting from a drug interaction between azathioprine or 6-mercaptopurine and mesalamine, sulphasalazine or balsalazide. Gut. 2001;49:656–64.
47. Goldenberg BA, Rawsthorne P, Berstein CN. The utility of 6-thioguanine metabolite levels in managing patients with inflammatory bowel disease. Am J Gastroenterol. 2004;99:1744–8.
48. Cuffari C, Dassoupolus T, Bayless TM. Thiopurine methyl-transferase activity influences clinical response to azathioprine therapy in patients with IBD. Clin Gastroenterol Hepatol. 2004;2:410–7.
49. Dubinsky MC, Yang H, Hassard PV, Seidman EG, Kam LY, Abreu MT, Targan SR, Vasiliauskas E. 6-MP metabolite profiles provide a biochemical explanation for 6-MP resistance in patients with inflammatory bowel disease. Gastroenterology. 2002;122:904–15.
50. Sparrow MP, Hande SA, Friedman S, et al. Allopurinol safely and effectively optimizes thioguanine metabolites in inflammatory bowel disease patients not responding to azathioprine and mercaptopurine. Aliment Pharmacol Ther. 2005;22:441–6.
51. Markowitz J, Grancher K, Mandel F, Daum F. Immunosuppressive therapy in pediatric inflammatory bowel disease: results of a survey of the North American Society for pediatric Gastroenterology and Nutrition. Subcommittee on immunosuppressive use of the pediatric IBD collaborative research forum. Am J Gastroenterol. 1993;88: 44–8.

52. Colombel JF, Ferrari N, Debuysere H, et al. Genotypic analysis of thio-purine S-methyltransferase in patients with Crohn's disease and severe myelosuppression during azathioprine therapy. Gastroenterology. 2000 Jun;118(6):1025–30.

53. Garza A, Sninsky CA. Changes in red cell mean corpuscular volume (MCV) during azathioprine or 6-mercaptopurine therapy for Crohn's disease may indicate optimal dose titration. Gastroenterology. 2001;120:A3166.

54. Savarino E, Bodini G, Dulbecco P, et al. Adalimumab is more effective than azathioprine and mesalamine at preventing postoperative recurrence of Crohn's disease: a randomized controlled trial. Am J Gastroenterol. 2013;108(1):1731–42.

Methotrexate

31

Joel R. Rosh

Introduction

The inflammatory bowel diseases (IBDs) are characterized by chronic gastrointestinal inflammation in association with ongoing and inappropriate activation of the mucosal immune system [1]. In the correct clinical setting, pharmacologic treatment can include locally acting anti-inflammatory therapies, immune-modifying agents and now, biologic therapies. The short-term goal of therapy remains the relief of clinical symptoms, while the long-term goal is to improve quality of life while changing the natural history of the disease by decreasing the incidence of adverse outcomes such as the need for hospitalization and surgical intervention. The long-term goals have undergone a paradigm shift over the last decade, embracing a model that emphasizes the induction and then maintenance of not only a clinical but a biologic remission marked by mucosal healing [2].

Glucocorticosteroids have both anti-inflammatory as well as immunomodulatory effects. As such, steroids are still the most commonly used immune-modifying agent and have the longest history of use as induction agents. At a year after diagnosis, more than 30% of pediatric Crohn's patients will remain dependant on glucocorticosteroids and almost 10% will already have undergone surgery, demonstrating steroids' inability to alter the course of Crohn's disease [3]. In addition to this lack of long-term efficacy, chronic corticosteroid use is associated with a legion of side effects mandating the identification of more effective, steroid-sparing agents. Concordantly, approximately 60% of pediatric Crohn's disease patients will be placed on immunomodulatory therapy within the first year of diagnosis [4].

J.R. Rosh, MD
Pediatric Gastroenterology, Clinical Development and Research Affairs, Goryeb Children's Hospital/Atlantic Health, 100 Madison Avenue, Morristown, NJ 07962, USA

Icahn School of Medicine at Mount Sinai, New York, NY, USA
e-mail: joel.rosh@atlantichealth.org

The thiopurines, 6-mercaptopurine (6MP) and azathioprine (AZA), have been shown to be efficacious as well as steroid sparing and are covered in more detail in Chap. 30. Using the Harvey-Bradshaw Index (HBI) as end-point, the prospective multicenter trial by Markowitz, et al., showed that 91% of pediatric Crohn's patients who underwent successful induction remain in remission on 6MP/AZA at 18 months [5]. With the subsequent advent and pediatric validation of the Pediatric Crohn's Disease Activity Index (PCDAI), more recent studies of thiopurines have demonstrated a lower long-term efficacy closer to 30–40% [6]. Additionally, pancreatitis and idiosyncratic reactions including gastrointestinal toxicity, fever and idiopathic pancreatitis are seen in 5–10% of patients. Increasing concerns related to potential toxicity from thiopurine therapy, especially with regard to hemophagocytic lymphohistiocytosis (HLH) and lymphoma, especially hepatosplenic T-cell lymphoma (HSTCL), have driven clinicians to look for other potential immune-modifying agents [7].

Methotrexate has emerged as an effective and overall well-tolerated alternative to the thiopurines [8]. Controlled trials have confirmed methotrexate as an effective agent in inducing as well as maintaining clinical remission in adult patients with Crohn's disease [9, 10]. While a prospective pediatric trial has not yet been performed, there is now ample published data regarding the efficacy of this agent in pediatric Crohn's disease [11].

Mechanism of Action

Methotrexate is a folic acid derivative originally designed as an analogue of dihydrofolic acid. As a competitive antagonist of folic acid, methotrexate inhibits folate-dependent enzymes such as dihydrofolate reductase (DHFR) which is critical to both purine and pyrimidine synthesis. In relatively high doses, methotrexate inhibits DNA production and exerts antiproliferative as well as cytotoxic effects [12].

© Springer International Publishing AG 2017
P. Mamula et al. (eds.), *Pediatric Inflammatory Bowel Disease*, DOI 10.1007/978-3-319-49215-5_31

383

Table 31.1 Effects of adenosine-related pathways on adaptive immune response

Increased interleukin (IL)-10
Increased IL-2
Inhibition of neutrophil chemotaxis
Decreased leukotriene B$_4$ (LTB$_4$)
Decreased tumor necrosis factor alpha
Decreased IL-6
Decreased IL-8
Decreased selective adhesion molecules (SAM)

When given for immune mediated diseases, low-dose methotrexate is used. At these doses, methotrexate does not exert such a profound antimetabolite effect. This is an important clinical distinction since at low dose, there is a relative absence of otherwise common side effects such as hair loss and folate supplementation may decrease the toxicity but not the apparent of efficacy of low-dose methotrexate [13].

The mechanism of action of low-dose methotrexate still needs to be fully elaborated. While not antiproliferative, low-dose methotrexate may induce T-cell apoptosis [14, 15], although there are studies that do not agree with this finding [16]. Other potential mechanisms of action include methotrexate's effect on intracellular and extracellular concentrations of adenosine and the effects of adenosine on the adaptive immune response [17] (see Table 31.1). Methotrexate has also been shown to have a more direct effect on a variety of regulatory cytokines [18, 19].

Improved understanding of methotrexate's mechanism of action and pharmacokinetics may also affect the recommended dosing. As has become appreciated with the thiopurines, metabolites of the parent drug may be the more clinically important compounds. There is now evidence that intracellular methotrexate polyglutamates are the active immune-modifying compounds [20] and that there are genetic polymorphisms that have been shown to affect intracellular methotrexate polyglutamate levels. Therefore, pharmacokinetics and pharmacogenetics may play a large role in the efficacy and potential toxicity of methotrexate in any individual [21]. The importance of methotrexate polyglutamate levels in IBD patients has not yet been studied. Such studies may lead to dosing recommendations based upon pharmacogenomics rather than weight-based dosing. For now, however, dosing is based upon weight or body surface area measurements (see Table 31.2).

Efficacy

In 1995, Feagan et al. published their 16-week induction study demonstrating that 25 mg of intramuscular methotrexate delivered weekly is an effective, steroid-sparing,

Table 31.2 Methotrexate (MTX):dosing and monitoring

Supplemental oral folic acid 1 mg/day to be given to all patients
Consider pretreatment with ondansetron for first 4–8 doses of MTX and then as needed
Dose (subcutaneous injection on a weekly basis)
15 mg/m^2 (body surface area) to a maximum dose of 25 mg once a week
Maintenance
Consider conversion to oral dosing if stable > 3 months
If clinical remission for > 3–6 months consider decreasing dose to 10 mg/m^2 to a maximum of 15 mg once a week
Patient Monitoring
Complete blood count with differential and platelets (CBC), erythrocyte sedimentation rate (ESR) and/or C-reactive protein (CRP), Hepatic Function Panel weekly for the first month and then every 2–3 months if stable
The dose should be reduced by 50% for elevation in alanine aminotransferase (ALT) > twice baseline
The dose should be reduced by 50% for white blood count (WBC) <4000, absolute neutrophil count (ANC) <1500 or platelet <120,000 and held for 2 weeks for WBC <3000, ANC <1000 or platelets <100,000.

MTX should be held for 2 weeks for nonproductive cough >1 week, and discontinued for pneumonitis or serious infections

induction strategy in adult patients with active Crohn's disease [9]. This study of 141 patients showed that 39% were in a steroid-free remission at 16 weeks compared to 19% of placebo patients. Those who achieved remission with methotrexate were then offered enrollment in a 40-week double-blind placebo-controlled maintenance trial of 15 mg of methotrexate administered intramuscularly on a weekly basis. Seventy-six patients participated and demonstrated a methotrexate remission rate of 65% compared to 39% with placebo. No serious adverse events were noted [10]. In addition, there have been head-to-head trials suggesting that the effect of methotrexate is similar to that seen with thiopurines [22, 23]. Data on the use of methotrexate to treat ulcerative colitis has been variable [24, 25]. Two prospective studies are nearing completion which will hopefully help further knowledge on this question.

There is now a fairly robust published experience with methotrexate in pediatric IBD, especially Crohn's disease [26–35]. Mack et al. [28] first reported on 14 patients with a mean age of 10.6 years who had active Crohn's disease and were intolerant or unresponsive to 6-mercaptopurine. Subcutaneous (SQ) administration of methotrexate was used and 64% of the patients showed clinical improvement by as early as 4 weeks. Steroid sparing was also demonstrated.

Another single center experience [30] demonstrated a 12-month steroid-free remission rate of about 33% which is similar to that seen in reports of adult patients with Crohn's disease. Good tolerance of the methotrexate therapy was reported. Two larger, multicenter retrospective reports [27, 29] demonstrated a 40–45% 1-year steroid-free remission rate with methotrexate as a second line immune modulator in pediatric Crohn's disease patients. No difference in effect was seen whether the indication for the methotrexate was lack of thiopurine efficacy or intolerance. Again, overall good drug tolerance was demonstrated as were a steroid-sparing effect and a positive effect on linear growth [27]. Similar retrospective reports have been published from several European countries showing a 12-month remission rate of 25–52% and these studies are well summarized elsewhere [11]. Along with this growing evidence of the efficacy of methotrexate as monotherapy in treating pediatric Crohn's disease, there has been an increasing level of concern regarding the potential toxicities of thiopurine therapy, especially in the pediatric population. These two effects have likely led to a much higher rate of methotrexate use in this setting. In fact, a multicenter report from the Pediatric IBD Collaborative Research Group demonstrated that the number of patients exposed to methotrexate quadrupled from 2002 to 2010 (14–60%) [34].

In addition to its use as monotherapy, there is a growing experience of using methotrexate in combination with monoclonal antibodies directed against tumor necrosis factor alpha (TNF). While the prospective COMMIT trial did not show improved efficacy of infliximab dosed in combination with methotrexate compared to infliximab monotherapy in adults with Crohn's disease [36], many factors including high rates of corticosteroid use at baseline may have been critically confounding [37]. More recently, retrospective data from the Pediatric IBD Collaborative Research Group demonstrated improved infliximab durability when administered in combination with methotrexate [38]. It has been shown that the methotrexate dose may be critical to fully achieve this effect and a weekly dose of 12.5–15 mg weekly may be optimal when methotrexate is used as a concomitant agent [39, 40].

Dose and Administration

Methotrexate is administered once a week. The route of administration can be parenteral (subcutaneous or intramuscular) or oral. Since there are no head-to-head prospective trials comparing the efficacy of oral and parenteral methotrexate for IBD, it remains controversial whether there is a preferred route of administration. Retrospective reports have provided some data relative to this question. Two uncontrolled, observational studies published within a year of each other differed in their conclusions with one showing no difference between oral and parenteral methotrexate [41] and the other showing clear advantage to the parenteral route [42].

Pharmacokinetic studies have been performed to see if there is a clinically significant difference in absorption between the two routes as it is recognized that oral absorption is individually variable and subject to a saturation effect with decreasing rates of absorption at higher doses [43].

In IBD, studies of adult [41] as well as pediatric patients [42] have demonstrated a wide individual range of methotrexate bioavailability. Interestingly, a study in adult patients showed the oral route to provide about 73% of the bioavailability that was seen with the parenteral route, while no such difference was seen in the pediatric study. Both of these pharmacokinetic studies were performed on subjects who were clinically stable on methotrexate maintenance therapy. Therefore, neither provides bioavailability data on patients being induced with methotrexate and there is retrospective data to suggest the parenteral route may induce a more rapid remission [26]. Additionally, it has recently been pointed out that any difference in bioavailability between these two routes of administration still falls within the FDA's definition of bioequivalence [44].

The question as to whether there is a clinically important difference in efficacy based upon the route of administration was investigated in a more direct, albeit retrospective manner, in the 2015 study by Turner et al. who used a propensity score analysis to look at outcomes in pediatric CD patients treated with oral vs. parenteral (subcutaneous) methotrexate [27]. This study demonstrated that any superiority of SQ over an oral route of administration was quite modest and the authors suggest that a change to oral MTX can be considered in those patients successfully induced with parenteral MTX. It is notable that a recent meta-analysis of the use of MTX in rheumatoid arthritis patients offered a different approach. This study demonstrated that efficacy and toxicity are related to an individual's absorbed dose rather than route of administration and the authors concluded that it is best to start patients on a relatively high oral dose and convert to the parenteral route in those who fail to respond [45].

In addition to the ongoing questions with regard to the optimal route of administration, the actual ideal dose of methotrexate for pediatric IBD patients has not been studied. The usual recommended dose is 15 mg/m^2 once weekly to a maximum weekly dose of 25 mg [46]. All patients are supplemented daily with folic acid 1 mg orally to avoid the development of medication-related nausea and subsequent anticipatory intolerance [47]. It has also been shown to be beneficial to recommend oral ondansetron as premedication before each of the first eight doses to prevent drug-associated nausea [48].

Toxicity and Monitoring

In patients with inflammatory bowel disease, low-dose methotrexate has been shown to be a well-tolerated agent with more than 90% of clinical trial patients able to complete study drug [19, 49]. Reported side effects are usually transient or respond to dose reduction and, less commonly, drug withdrawal (the potential side effects of low-dose methotrexate are summarized in Table 31.3).

Table 31.3 Side effects and toxicities of low-dose methotrexate

Teratogenicity
Contraindicated in women of child-bearing potential
Contraindicated in breastfeeding women
Gastrointestinal—folate related
Nausea and behavioral/anticipatory intolerance—most common
Abdominal pain, diarrhea
Stomatitis including esophagitis
Bone Marrow Suppression
Monitor with CBC (Table 31.2 for schedule)
Increased with trimethoprim-sulfamethoxazole
Hepatic
Monitor with routine liver chemistries (Table 31.2 for schedule)
Increased risk with obesity, concomitant hepatotoxic medications
Routine liver biopsy not recommended
Possible role for elastography
Infections
Upper respiratory most common
Rarely herpetic as well
Rarely clinically serious
Pneumonitis
Immune-mediated
Rare
Suspect if prolonged nonproductive cough
Preliminary evaluation = chest radiograph and pulmonary function tests
Dermatologic
Hypersensitivity reactions

There were early reports from the rheumatology literature that pediatric patients may have fewer methotrexate-induced side effects compared to adult patients [50]. An exception to this may be the development of learned associations and anticipatory intolerance to the medication [47]. Nausea has been correlated with inhibition of folate-dependant enzymes. As a result, folic acid supplementation may help limit this side effect, which has been reported in more than 20% of the adult patients who participated in clinical IBD trials [51]. Use of ondansetron as a premedication for the first 4–8 weeks can effectively mitigate against the development of nausea [48]. Other gastrointestinal side effects include abdominal pain, diarrhea and stomatitis that may even evolve into mucositis involving the esophagus [52].

In light of the potential for hepatic toxicity with high-dose methotrexate, liver-related complications have been well studied with low-dose methotrexate. There may be a disease-related rate of liver complications following therapy with low-dose methotrexate. Patients with psoriasis were shown to have a 7% rate of hepatic fibrosis [53] as compared to the 1% rate in rheumatoid arthritis [54]. The low rate of hepatic fibrosis and cirrhosis in RA has led to the official recommendation of the American College of Rheumatology that routine, surveillance liver biopsies not be performed [54].

Studies in juvenile idiopathic arthritis (JIA) patients have shown at least as good hepatic tolerance [55]. Similarly, negligible rates of drug-related hepatotoxicity have been seen in adult IBD patients treated with prolonged low-dose methotrexate [56]. This may actually occur at a higher rate in pediatric patients with a meta-analysis demonstrating a rate of elevated liver chemistries as high as 10% with 6% requiring dose reduction [57].

Rather than biopsy, routine liver chemistry monitoring should be performed as shown in Table 31.2. Elastography is a promising tool to noninvasively monitor for drug-induced hepatic fibrosis and it may be more sensitive than measuring liver chemistries [58].

Bone marrow suppression leading to leukopenia or thrombocytopenia occurs in about 1% of low-dose methotrexate treated patients [19]. This is usually transient and responds to dose reduction or holding of the drug. Routine monitoring of complete blood counts should be performed to look for bone marrow suppression (Table 31.2). Concomitant medications, especially antifolate agents such as trimethoprim-sulfamethoxazole should be avoided with methotrexate therapy as these can exacerbate potential bone marrow suppression. Theoretically, this may be true of sulfasalazine as well although the combination of low-dose methotrexate and sulfasalazine has been utilized without increased toxicity [59].

An immunologically mediated pneumonitis can also rarely be seen with methotrexate therapy. Screening asymptomatic pediatric patients does not seem warranted [50] and in fact, the rarity of this condition when methotrexate is used for inflammatory disease has recently been further characterized [60]. Clinically, a persistent cough or other symptoms should prompt a chest radiograph and pulmonary function studies with suspension of methotrexate therapy until clarification of the clinical picture is achieved.

The most important toxicity of methotrexate is related to its teratogenicity. Methotrexate is completely contraindicated in pregnancy as well as during breastfeeding. All patients and their families must be educated about this prior to starting methotrexate therapy.

References

1. de Souza HSP, Fiocchi C. Immunopathogenesis of IBD:current state of the art. Nat Rev Gastroenterol Hepatol. 2016;13:13–27.
2. Neurath MF, Travis SP. Mucosal healing in inflammatory bowel diseases: a systematic review. Gut. 2012;61:1619–35.
3. Markowitz J, Hyams J, Mack D, et al. Corticosteroid therapy in the age of infliximab: acute and 1-year outcomes in newly diagnosed children with Crohn disease. Clin Gastroenterol Hepatol. 2006;4:1124–9.
4. Jacobstein DA, Mamula P, Markowitz JE, Leonard M, Baldassano RN. Predictors of immunomodulatory use as early therapy in pediatric Crohn disease. J Clin Gastroenterol. 2006;40:145–8.

5. Markowitz J, Grancher K, Kohn N, et al. A multicenter trial of 6-mercaptopurine and prednisone in children with newly diagnosed Crohn disease. Gastroenterology. 2000;119:895–902.

6. Riello L, Talbotec C, Garnier-Lengline H, et al. Tolerance and efficacy of azathioprine in pediatric Crohn disease. Inflamm Bowel Dis. 2011;17:2138–43.

7. Kotlyar DS, Lewis JD, Beaugerie L, et al. Risk of lymphoma in patients with inflammatory bowel disease treated with azathioprine and 6-mercaptopurine: a meta-analysis. Clin Gastroenterol Hepatol. 2015;13:847–58.

8. Panaccione R. Methotrexate: lessons from rheumatology. Can J Gastroenterol. 2005;9:541–2.

9. Feagan BG, Rochon J, Fedorak RN, et al. Methotrexate for the treatment of Crohn disease. The North American Crohn study group investigators. N Engl J Med. 1995;332:292–7.

10. Feagan BG, Fedorak RN, Irvine EJ, et al. A comparison of methotrexate with placebo for the maintenance of remission in Crohn disease. North American Crohn study group investigators. N Engl J Med. 2000;342:1627–32.

11. Scherkenbach LA, Stumpf JL. Methotrexate for the management of Crohn's disease in children. Ann Pharmacother. 2016;50:60–9.

12. Chabner BA, Allegra CJ, Curt GA, et al. Antineoplastic agents. In: Hardman JG, Limbird LE, Molinoff PB, et al., editors. Goodman and Gilman's the pharmacological basis of therapeutics. 9th ed. New York: McGraw-Hill; 1996. p. 1243–7.

13. Shea B, Swinden MV, Ghogomu ET, et al. Folic acid and folinic acid for reducing side effects in patients receiving methotrexate for rheumatoid arthritis. J Rheumatol. 2014;41:1049–60.

14. Paillot R, Genestier L, Fournel S, et al. Activation-dependent lymphocyte apoptosis induced by methotrexate. Transplant Proc. 1998;30:2348–50.

15. Genestier L, Paillot R, Quemeneur L, et al. Mechanisms of action of methotrexate. Immunopharmacology. 2000;47:247–57.

16. Johnston A, Gudjonsson JE, Sigmundskottir H, et al. The anti-inflammatory action of methotrexate is not mediated by lymphocyte apoptosis, but by the suppression of activation of adhesion molecules. Clin Immunol. 2005;114:154–63.

17. Cronstein BN. The mechanism of action of methotrexate. Rheum Dis Clin North Am. 1997;23:739–55.

18. van Dieren JM, Kuipers EJ, Samsom JN, Nieuwenhuis EE, van der Woude J. Revisiting the immunomodulators tacrolimus. Methotrexate, and mycophenolate mofetil: their mechanisms of action and role in the treatment of IBD. Inflamm Bowel Dis. 2006;12:311–27.

19. Schroder O, Stein J. Low dose methotrexate in inflammatory bowel disease: current status and future directions. Am J Gastroenterol. 2004;98:530–7.

20. Ranganathan P. An update on methotrexate pharmacogenetics in rheumatoid arthritis. Pharmacogenomics. 2008;9:439–51.

21. Herrlinger KR, Cummings JR, Barnardo MC, Schwab M, Ahmad T, Jewell DP. The pharmacogenetics of methotrexate in inflammatory bowel disease. Pharmacogenet Genomics. 2005;15:705–11.

22. Ardizzone S, Bollani S, Manzionna G, et al. Comparison between methotrexate and azathioprine in the treatment of chronic active Crohn disease: a randomized, investigator-blind study. Dig Liver Dis. 2003;35:619–27.

23. Mate-Jimenez J, Hermida C, Canter-Perona J, et al. 6-mercaptopurine or methotrexate added to prednisone induces and maintains remission in steroid-dependent inflammatory bowel disease. Eur J Gastroenterol Hepatol. 2000;12:1227–33.

24. Chande N, Wang Y, MacDonald JK, McDonald J. Methotrexate for induction of remission in ulcerative colitis. Cochrane Database Syst Rev. 2014;(8): CD006618. doi:10.1002/14651858.CD006618. pub3.

25. Khan N, Abbas AM, Moehlen M, Balart L. Methotrexate in ulcerative colitis: a nationwide retrospective cohort from the Veterans Affairs Health Care System. Inflamm Bowel Dis. 2013;19:1379–83.

26. Turner D, Grossman AB, Rosh JR, Kugathasan S, Gilman AR, Baldassano R, Griffiths AM. Methotrexate following unsuccessful thiopurine therapy in pediatric Crohn disease. Am J Gastroenterol. 2007;102:2804–12.

27. Turner D, Doveh E, Cohen A, Wilson ML, Grossman AB, Rosh JR, Lu Y, Bousvaros A, Deslandres C, Noble A, Baldassano RN, Levine A, Lerner A, Wilson DC, Griffiths AM. Efficacy of oral methotrexate in paediatric Crohn's disease: a multicentre propensity score study. Gut. 2015;64:1898–904.

28. Mack DR, Young R, Kaufman SS, Ramey L, Vanderhoof JA. Methotrexate in patients with Crohn disease after 6-mercaptopurine. J Pediatr. 1998;132:830–5.

29. Uhlen S, Belbouab R, Narebski K, et al. Efficacy of methotrexate in pediatric Crohn disease: a French multicenter study. Inflamm Bowel Dis. 2006;12:1053–7.

30. Boyle B, Mackner L, Ross C, Moses J, Kumar S, Crandall W. A single-center experience with methotrexate after thiopurine therapy in pediatric Crohn disease. J Pediatr Gastroenterol Nutr. 2010; 51:714–7.

31. Ravikumara M, Hinsberger A, Spray CH. Role of methotrexate in the management of Crohn disease. J Pediatr Gastroenterol Nutr. 2007;44:427–30.

32. Weiss B, Lerner A, Shapiro R, et al. Methotrexate treatment in pediatric Crohn disease patients intolerant or resistant to purine analogues. J Pediatr Gastroenterol Nutr. 2009;48:526–30.

33. Willot S, Noble A, Deslandres C. Methotrexate in the treatment of inflammatory bowel disease: an 8-year retrospective study in a Canadian pediatric IBD center. Inflamm Bowel Dis. 2011;17:2521–6.

34. Sunseri W, Hyams JS, Lerer T, et al. Retrospective cohort study of methotrexate use in the treatment of pediatric Crohn's disease. Inflamm Bowel Dis. 2014;20:134–5.

35. Haisma S-M, Lijftogt T, Kindermann A, et al. Methotrexate for maintaining remission in paediatric Crohn's patients with prior failure or intolerance to thiopurines: a multicenter cohort study. J Crohns Colitis. 2015;9:305–11.

36. Feagan BG, McDonald JW, Panaccione R, et al. Methotrexate in combination with infliximab is no more effective than infliximab alone in patients with Crohn's disease. Gastroenterology. 2014;146:681–8.

37. Narula N, Peyrin-Biroulet L, Colombel JF. Combination therapy with methotrexate in inflammatory bowel disease: time to COMMIT? Gastroenterology. 2014;146:608–11.

38. Grossi V, Lerer T, Griffiths A, et al. Concomitant use of immunomodulators affects the durability of infliximab therapy in children with Crohn's disease. Clin Gastroenterol Hepatol. 2015;13: 1748–56.

39. Vahabnezhad E, Rabizadeh S, Dubinsky MC. A 10-year, single tertiary care center experience on the durability of infliximab in pediatric inflammatory bowel disease. Inflamm Bowel Dis. 2014;20: 606–13.

40. Colman RJ, Rubin DT. Optimal doses of methotrexate combined with anti-TNF therapy to maintain clinical remission in inflammatory bowel disease. J Crohns Colitis. 2015;9:312–7.

41. Kurnik D, Loebstein R, Fishbein E, Almog S, Halkin H, Bar-Meir S, Chowers Y. Bioavailability of oral vs. subcutaneous low-dose methotrexate in patients with Crohn disease. Aliment Pharmacol Ther. 2003;18:57–63.

42. Stephens MC, Baldassano RN, York A, Widemann B, Pitney AC, Jayaprakash N, Adamson PC. The bioavailability of oral methotrexate in children with inflammatory bowel disease. J Pediatr Gastroenterol Nutr. 2005;40:445–9.

43. Balis FM, Mirro J, Reaman GH, et al. Pharmacokinetics of subcutaneous methotrexate. J Clin Oncol. 1988;6:1882–6.

44. Wilson A, Patel V, Chande N, Ponich T, Urquhart B, Asher L, Choi Y, Tirona R, Kim RB, Gregor JC. Pharmacokinetic profiles for oral and subcutaneous methotrexate in patients with Crohn's disease. Aliment Pharmacol Ther. 2013;37:340–5.

388

J.R. Rosh

45. Goodman SM, Cronstein BN, Bykerk VP. Outcomes related to methotrexate dose and route of administration in patients with rheumatoid arthritis: a systematic literature review. Clin Exp Rheumatol. 2015;33:272–8.

46. Ruemmele FM, Veresd G, Kolhoe KL, et al. Consensus guidelines of ECCO/ESPGHAN on the medical management of pediatric Crohn's disease. J Crohns Colitis. 2014;8:1179–207.

47. Bulatovic M, Heijstek MW, Verkaaik M, et al. High prevalence of methotrexate intolerance in juvenile idiopathic arthritis: development and validation of a methotrexate intolerance severity score. Arthritis Rheum. 2011;63:2007–13.

48. Kempinska A, Benchimol E, Mack A, Barkey J, Boland M, Mack DR. Short-course ondansetron for the prevention of methotrexate-induced nausea in children with Crohn disease. J Pediatr Gastroenterol Nutr. 2011;53:389–93.

49. Lemann M, Zenjari T, Bouhnik Y, et al. Methotrexate in Crohn disease: long-term safety and toxicity. Am J Gastroenterol. 2000;95:1730–4.

50. Graham LD, Myones BL, Rivas-Chacon RF, Pachman LM. Morbidity associated with long-term methotrexate therapy in juvenile rheumatoid arthritis. J Pediatr. 1992;120:468–73.

51. Chong RY, Hanauer SB, Cohen RD. Efficacy of parenteral methotrexate in refractory Crohn disease. Aliment Pharmacol Ther. 2001;15:35–44.

52. Batres LA, Gabriel CA, Tsou VM. Methotrexate-induced esophagitis in a child with crohn disease. J Pediatr Gastroenterol Nutr. 2003;37:514–6.

53. Roenigk Jr HH, Auerbach R, Maibach H, et al. Methotrexate in psoriasis: revised guidelines. J Am Acad Dermatol. 1988;19:145–56.

54. Kremer JM, Alarcon GS, Lightfood Jr RW, et al. Methotrexate for rheumatoid arthritis. Suggested guideline for monitoring liver toxicity. Arthritis Rheum. 1994;37:316–28.

55. Kugathasan S, Newman AJ, Dahms BB, Boyle JT. Liver biopsy findings in patients with juvenile rheumatoid arthritis receiving long-term weekly methotrexate therapy. J Pediatr. 1996;128:149–51.

56. Khan N, Abbas AM, Whang N, Balart LA, Bazzano LA, Kelly TN. Incidence of liver toxicity in inflammatory bowel disease patients treated with methotrexate: a meta-analysis of clinical trials. Inflamm Bowel Dis. 2012;18:359–67.

57. Valentino PL, Church PC, Shah PS, Beyene J, Griffiths AM, Feldman BM, Kamath BM. Hepatotoxicity caused by methotrexate therapy in children with inflammatory bowel disease: a systematic review and meta-analysis. Inflamm Bowel Dis. 2014;20:47–59.

58. Laharie D, Zerbib F, Adhoute X, Boué-Lahorgue X, Foucher J, Castéra L, Rullier A, Bertet J, Couzigou P, Amouretti M, de Lédinghen V. Diagnosis of liver fibrosis by transient elastography (Fibro Scan) and non-invasive methods in Crohn's disease patients treated with methotrexate. Aliment Pharmacol Ther. 2006;23: 1621–8.

59. Rains CP, Noble S, Faulds D. Sulfasalazine. A review of its pharmacological properties and therapeutic efficacy in the treatment of rheumatoid arthritis. Drugs. 1995;50:137–56.

60. Conway R, Low C, Coughlan RJ, O'Donnell MJ, Carey JJ. Methotrexate use and risk of lung disease in psoriasis, psoriatic arthritis, and inflammatory bowel disease: systematic literature review and meta-analysis of randomised controlled trials. BMJ. 2015;350:h1269.

Infliximab Therapy for Pediatric Crohn Disease and Ulcerative Colitis

Philip Minar, Dana MH. Dykes, Ana Catalina Arce-Clachar, and Shehzad A. Saeed

Introduction

Both Crohn disease (CD) and ulcerative colitis (UC) are chronic inflammatory conditions of the gastrointestinal tract characterized by relapsing and remitting course over a period of time. The goal of therapy in pediatric inflammatory bowel disease (IBD) should be to induce and maintain clinical remission, prevent delays in growth and puberty, and improve quality of life, while minimizing the adverse effects of medications [1]. Since the onset of IBD peaks in early adolescence in children, there exists a very narrow window of opportunity before growth retardation, and developmental deficiencies become permanent. These goals are often not achieved with conventional therapeutic strategies (sulfasalazine, 5-aminosalicylates, and corticosteroids). The short-term complete response is only 60% in children with IBD with 17% steroid resistance, and 1-year outcomes are even more concerning with steroid dependency noted in 30–45% of children with IBD [2, 3]. They are also associated with significant side effects [4, 5]. For maintenance of remission, immunomodulators (IMM), including thiopurines (TP) and methotrexate (MTX), have long been the mainstay of therapy but the long-term response rates are variable, ranging from 49 to 80% for TPs and 27% for MTX [6–8]. Besides, most of these medications have slow onset of action. Relapsing or continuously active disease often leads to complications necessitating surgery, but it is well known that resection of the inflamed bowel, at least in CD, does not cure the disease and that recurrence occurs in most patients. Enteral nutrition has an important role in the management of IBD, especially in CD, including prevention and correction of malnutrition, prevention of osteoporosis, and the promo-

tion of optimal growth and development [9, 10], but long-term adherence has been less than ideal.

Keeping in mind these special circumstances, the advent of biologic therapies has dramatically changed the landscape for treatment of both adult and pediatric IBD. Infliximab was the first anti-TNF medication approved for usage in children in 2006, with recent approval of adalimumab for treatment of moderate to severe pediatric CD (discussed in Chap. 33). Infliximab is a chimeric monoclonal IgG1 antibody to TNFα and is the first biological therapy that was approved for IBD. It is composed of a (± 75%) human constant and (± 25%) murine variable region. TNFα is a prominent pro-inflammatory cytokine. The number of TNF-producing cells is greatly increased in the lamina propria in the bowel of patients with CD, and increased concentrations of TNF have been found in the stool of children with CD [11–13]. Besides neutralization of TNF, infliximab also blocks leukocyte migration and induces apoptosis of T lymphocytes and monocytes, one of the key mechanisms of action of this drug [14–18]. A third mechanism of action involves complement fixation and complement-dependent cytotoxicity (CDC) and antibody-dependent cellular cytotoxicity (ADCC) [19].

In this chapter, we will review the current evidence for the role of effectiveness of biologic therapies, specifically infliximab, in pediatric CD and UC, its early use affecting outcomes, combination therapy vs. monotherapy, and review the role of therapeutic drug monitoring in optimizing treatment and effect of infliximab on surgery and hospitalizations.

Crohn Disease

Infliximab in Pediatric Crohn Disease (PCD)

Current evidence suggests CD develops as the result of a dysregulated immune response to the intestinal microbial flora in a genetically susceptible host [20]. Targan et al.

P. Minar, MD • D.MH. Dykes, MD • A.C. Arce-Clachar, MD
S.A. Saeed, MD (✉)
Division of Gastroenterology, Hepatology and Nutrition,
Cincinnati Children's Hospital Medical Center,
Cincinnati, OH, USA
e-mail: saeeds@childrensdayton.org

© Springer International Publishing AG 2017
P. Mamula et al. (eds.), *Pediatric Inflammatory Bowel Disease*, DOI 10.1007/978-3-319-49215-5_32

showed that more than 80% of adult Crohn patients had a clinical response 4 weeks after a single infusion (5 mg/kg) of infliximab [21]. This study was followed by ACCENT 1 in which 58% of adult patients (335/573) had a clinical response after the first infusion and randomized to either placebo or infliximab (dosed as 5 or 10 mg/kg) [22]. Both doses of infliximab were more effective in achieving clinical remission at week 54 compared to placebo with no statistical difference in clinical response or remission between the 5 and 10 mg/kg groups. Early pediatric studies [23, 24] also demonstrated clinical response (94%) and remission (48%) after a single dose of infliximab. These small clinical reports along with the landmark adult studies paved the way for the first randomized clinical trial with infliximab in PCD.

Infliximab Is Within REACH for Pediatric CD

The Randomized, Multicenter, Open Label Study to Evaluate the Safety and Efficacy of Anti-TNF Chimeric Monoclonal Antibody in Pediatric Subjects with Moderate to Severe Crohn Disease (REACH) enrolled PCD patients with a Pediatric Crohn Disease Activity Index (PCDAI) >30 [25]. Notably, all children enrolled were receiving concurrent, stable doses of an immunomodulator (thiopurine). All subjects received the same induction regimen of 5 mg/kg at 0, 2, and 6 weeks with clinical response (decrease in PCDAI by 15 points from baseline) evaluated at week 10. Subjects meeting clinical response criteria were randomized to receive infliximab every 8 or 12 weeks. One hundred twelve children were enrolled and 103 (92%) were randomized. Hyams et al. found that 88.4% had a clinical response by week 10 with 55% in clinical remission (PCDAI ≤ 10). By week 54, 63.5% of subjects allocated to every 8 week infusions had a clinical response with 55.8% in clinical remission compared to a clinical remission rate of 23.5% for those who received infliximab every 12 weeks ($p < 0.001$). Not only did the subjects receiving infusions every 8 weeks improved clinically, they also had dramatic improvements in their mean height z-score by week 54 as well.

While REACH established infliximab efficacy and set the precedent for maintenance dosing in pediatric CD, this landmark study may not reflect current practices in PCD treatment algorithm with infliximab. As discussed, all children in REACH were receiving and continued concomitant thiopurine therapy throughout the trial. While REACH demonstrated efficacy of combination infliximab/thiopurine therapy, there is legitimate concern with this dual therapy approach given the association of hepatosplenic T-cell lymphoma (HSTCL) in patients receiving this combination, especially in young (<35 years old) males [26].

Early Use of Infliximab

In contrast to UC, CD-specific phenotypes (severe growth failure, fistula formation) and poor response to 5-aminosalicylates present unique challenges toward the successful management of this progressive disease. The pivotal studies by Markowitz et al. [6] showed that early induction with thiopurines improved rates of sustained clinical remission and reduced steroid use compared to placebo in PCD; however, there was no effect on linear growth with early thiopurine use, and subsequent studies have not replicated these results. With the success of REACH in children, and the Study of Biological and Immunomodulator Naïve Patients in Crohn Disease [27] (SONIC) in adult CD, many pediatric gastroenterologists started to adopt early introduction of anti-TNF therapy with/without an immunomodulator (IMM) in a select group of patients who were judged to be at increased risk of disease complications. The speculation was that early anti-TNF would improve mucosal healing and result in less structural damage leading to fewer complications and the need for surgery.

Walters et al. [28] evaluated the practice of early anti-TNF therapy in a well-defined inception cohort of PCD subjects who were enrolled in the Crohn and Colitis Foundation of America sponsored RISK Stratification study (RISK; Risk Stratification and Identification of Immunogenetic and Microbial Markers of Rapid Disease Progression in Children with Crohn Disease). RISK is an ongoing, prospective observational research program starting in 2008 and includes 552 children <17 years of age with newly diagnosed, inflammatory (nonpenetrating and nonstricturing) CD. In this study, the authors separated the cohort into triads (those who initiated anti-TNF therapy within the first 3 months of diagnosis, subjects who received an IMM within 3 months, and a group who did not receive either an IMM or anti-TNF therapy within the first 3 months of diagnosis) and evaluated the 1-year clinical outcomes. The physician global assessment (PGA) and PCDAI were used to document response. Patients receiving a combination of anti-TNF and IMM ($n = 12$) were not included in the analysis. Sixty-eight of the 552 subjects received anti-TNF within the first 3 months of the initial diagnosis; therefore, the authors performed a propensity score analysis to match the subjects in each triad and reduce the risk of selection bias. Sixty-seven of 68 early anti-TNF subjects received infliximab. The IMM group ($n = 68$) included 14/68 patients on azathioprine, 40/68 on 6-mercaptopurine, and 14/68 on methotrexate. Overall, there was no difference in complete response (as defined by the PGA) at 3 months (50% anti-TNF, 45.5% IMM, 42.5% no IMM/anti-TNF). However, at 1 year, 85.3% of those receiving early anti-TNF were in remission compared to 60.3% with an IMM ($p = 0.0003$) and 54.4% in the no IMM/anti-TNF group. The authors did not find any patient specific characteristics (age, gender, albumin, C-reactive protein) or disease phenotype (deep ulcerations at diagnostic colonoscopy) that affected the probability of surgery-free remission. Similar to REACH, they found the mean height z-score increased by 0.14 in the early anti-TNF triad compared to the other two triads.

Combination Therapy Versus Infliximab Monotherapy

The hallmark studies of infliximab, such as REACH and SONIC, demonstrated efficacy of combination therapy, while SONIC also showed superiority of combination therapy compared to monotherapy, as 56.8% of infliximab & thiopurine subjects achieved corticosteroid-free clinical remission at week 26 compared to 44.4% of those receiving infliximab monotherapy ($p < 0.02$). Although combination therapy was associated with higher rates of clinical remission compared to infliximab monotherapy in SONIC, there was a trend but not statistically significant difference in mucosal healing at week 26 between the two groups (43.9% vs 30.1%, $p = 0.06$). With a growing, concerning list of IBD patients diagnosed with HSTCL, especially in young, male patients who had received combination thiopurine and anti-TNF therapy, many pediatric gastroenterologists are hesitant to prescribe this combination.

Grossi et al. [29] evaluated the real-world experience of concomitant use of IMM and infliximab in PCD. The study population included 502 Crohn disease patients in the Pediatric Inflammatory Bowel Disease Collaborative Research Group Registry who had received infliximab. They included all children with CD younger than 15 who had received a minimum of three induction doses of infliximab. The primary outcome was continuation of infliximab after initiation of therapy. The probability of remaining on infliximab was evaluated using the Kaplan-Meier curve analysis. They found 84% of patients remained on infliximab at 1 year, 76% at 2 years, 69% at 3 years, and 60% at 5 years (Fig. 32.1). Overall, they found that clinical factors including disease extent, age at diagnosis, perirectal involvement, or starting anti-TNF within 2 years of diagnosis did not affect durability of anti-TNF response. They further showed that patients receiving concomitant IMM for >6 months were much more likely to remain on infliximab over time (Fig. 32.2) as compared to both no IMM exposure or IMM use <6 months. Overall, 47% of patients receiving infliximab required an intensification (increased dose or frequency), which was delayed if infliximab was combined with IMM for greater than 6 months ($p < 0.05$).

An additional significant finding from this registry is that male patients receiving MTX for more than 6 months demonstrated a significant greater likelihood of remaining on infliximab (similar for females but a smaller cohort size). Furthermore, they showed that a combination of MTX and infliximab durability was superior to TP/infliximab. For comparison, in an adult trial that evaluated rates of clinical remission with a combination of MTX and infliximab therapy, Feagan et al. failed to show any differences in 1-year clinical outcomes compared to infliximab monotherapy. However, the combination group had a lower likelihood of developing immunogenicity (4% vs. 20%, $p = 0.01$) and had

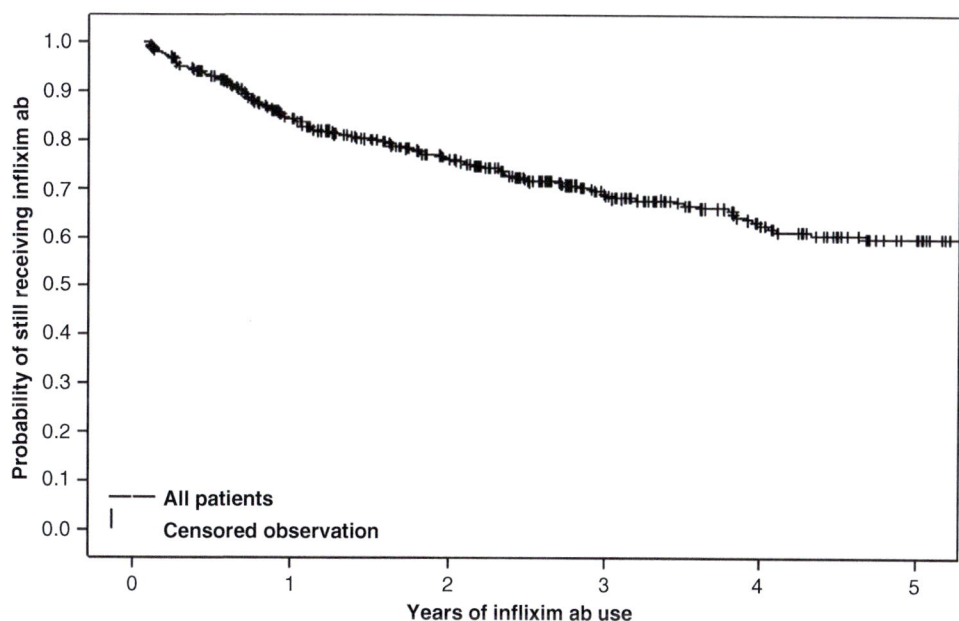

Fig. 32.1 Likelihood of remaining on infliximab treated (monotherapy + combination) over 5 years in 502 pediatric Crohn's patients. At 1 year, the probability of remaining on infliximab was 0.84 (± 0.02) with probability rates of 0.69 (± 0.03) and 0.6 (± 0.03) at 3 and 5 years, respectively, after starting infliximab (Printed with permission)

Fig. 32.2 Effect of concomitant immunomodulator (either thiopurine or methotrexate) use on the likelihood of remaining on infliximab. The probability of remaining on infliximab at 5 years after infliximab starts in patients with more than 6 months of concomitant immunomodulator use was 0.70 (± 0.04) compared with 0.48 (± 0.08) in patients with no immunomodulator and 0.55 (± 0.06) for those with <6 months of immunomodulator use (Printed with permission)

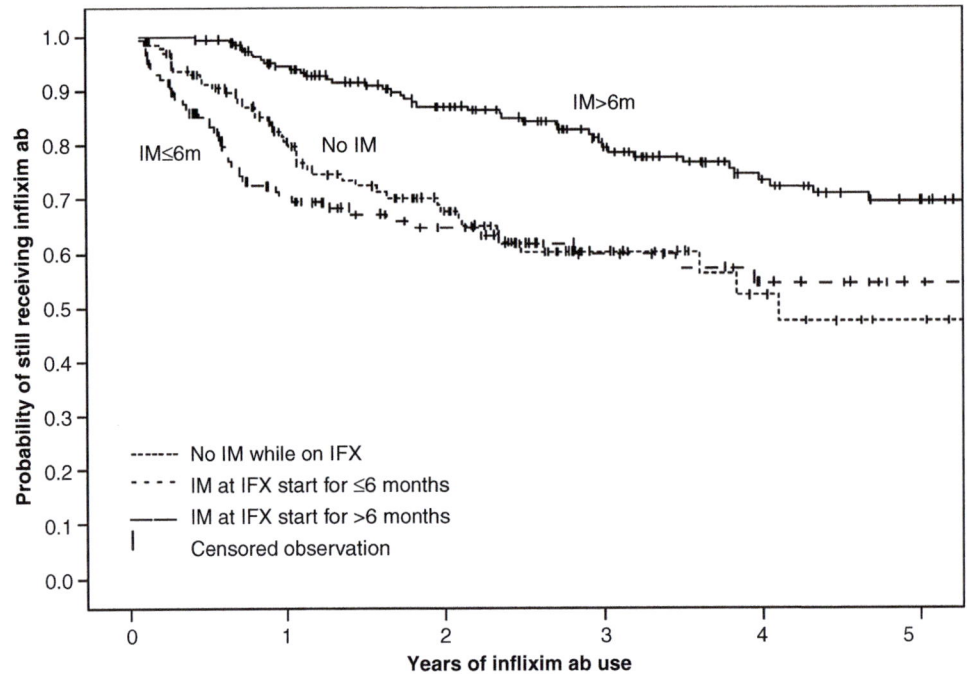

a higher median serum trough infliximab concentration (6.35 mcg/ml) compared to those on infliximab monotherapy (3.75 mcg/ml, $P = 0.08$) [30]. In terms of safety, Grossi et al. reported one case of malignancy and two deaths in the study population. While more long-term pediatric safety studies are needed, it is noteworthy that Osterman et al. found that continuation of IMM after stepping up to infliximab did not improve rates of surgery and hospitalization but was associated with increased risk of opportunistic infections including herpes zoster [31].

Proactive Therapeutic Drug Monitoring and Treat-To-Target in CD

The defining feature of CD is its relapsing and remitting course. The overarching treatment goal is to induce and sustain remission while minimizing secondary complications. SONIC and other studies have shown that infliximab heals the intestinal lining (absence of ulcerations), and mucosal healing has evolved as a "target" of Crohn management [27, 32]. Although the United States Food and Drug Administration (FDA) will mandate documentation of intestinal healing in future drug trials, in clinical practice, pediatric gastroenterologists are left to debate the safety and utility of repeat endoscopy to document mucosal healing versus using surrogate biomarkers or disease activity scores to guide treatment strategies. Until surrogate markers are further validated and cut-off values are better established (such as for fecal calprotectin) in those receiving infliximab, pediatric gastroenterologists will need to

develop best practices to utilize therapeutic drug monitoring (TDM) as multiple studies have found that a detectable serum trough concentration correlates with clinical response and mucosal healing [33–36], while loss of response to infliximab largely results from increased clearance of the drug (high inflammatory burden, diarrhea) and/ or presence of antibodies to the drug [37, 38].

Similar to TDM for TP metabolite concentrations, regular monitoring of infliximab serum concentrations is predicted to improve drug efficacy by tailoring dosing regimens to an individual's pharmacokinetics [39, 40]. Recent evidence suggests that proactive TDM, as an alternative to reactionary TDM (testing with clinical symptoms), may be associated with improved clinical outcomes as proactive drug monitoring allows for dosing adjustments to a target range when the patient is asymptomatic [41]. In a large retrospective study of 90 adults who had 1,232 consecutive serum IFX trough and ATI levels drawn, an IFX trough level at week 14 < 2.2 µg/ml predicted IFX discontinuation due to persistent loss of response (LOR) or hypersensitivity reactions, even in patients who had clinically responded to induction dosing [42]. While the target range to achieve this has been controversial, Ungar et al. showed in adults that an infliximab trough of 6–10 mcg/ml is associated with mucosal healing [43]. An intriguing hypothesis is that anti-TNF monotherapy with proactive TDM may minimize the need for combination therapy with IMM and infliximab; Vaughn et al. showed that proactive TDM with infliximab monotherapy may be more beneficial and safer than combination therapy with an IMM [41]. Arguments for proactive TDM include preventing undetectable or subtherapeutic trough concentration (subsequently decreasing risk of immunogenicity) and potentially preventing future morbidity via intensification of therapy before the patient is symptomatic. In their retrospective review, Vaughn et al. showed that in adult CD patients, with a strategy of proactive therapeutic concentration monitoring vs a standard of care group (where drug level monitoring was symptom based), achieving an infliximab trough of ≥ 5 mcg/ml resulted in >90% probability of maintaining infliximab over 5 years. They found during the proactive monitoring that only 29% were in the target range of 5–10 mcg/ml, which is similar to the pediatric study of CD patients in which 24% had undetectable levels and 38% were <3 mcg/ml [34, 41]. Interestingly, Vaughn et al. found that small-dose adjustments (median escalation of 100 mg, range 50–250 mg) were enough to improve the trough levels in contrast to common methods of infliximab intensification in clinical practice of doubling from 5 to 10 mg/kg or decreasing the frequency of infusions from 8 to 6 weeks [41].

TDM in pediatric CD is in its infancy; however, future studies will need to address the ideal infliximab concentration following induction and during maintenance therapy in children. In a study of pediatric Crohn and ulcerative colitis patients, Singh et al. found that a week 14 infliximab level (first maintenance dose) of ≥ 5 µg/ml had a positive predictive value of 83% and a negative predictive value of 53% for long-term remission [40].

TDM Methods Multiple assays have been developed to improve the monitoring for circulating infliximab levels including the enzyme-linked immunosorbent assay (ELISA), the radioimmunoassay (RIA), and the homogenous mobility shift assay (HMSA) offered by Prometheus® (Prometheus Laboratories Inc., San Diego CA) [44–46]. Infliximab serum concentrations can be determined quickly and at low cost with the ELISA technique. However, due to infliximab drug interference, the ELISA does not detect the presence of antibodies to infliximab if circulating drug is present. Newer technologies have afforded additional commercial laboratories to offer novel assays that can detect both infliximab concentration and antibody to infliximab in the presence of a drug using HMSA or the electrochemiluminescence immunoassay (ECLIA).

Incidence of Primary and Repeat Abdominal Surgeries in the Infliximab Era

The cumulative incidence of surgery 10 years after diagnosis in Crohn disease ranges from 40 to 70% in adults, although it is not yet clear if earlier use of anti-TNF therapy will reduce this risk. In a large pediatric cohort of 989 CD patients, Gupta et al. noted that 13% of children required

intestinal resection after a median of 2.8 years, with 17% at 5 years and 28% at 10 years [47]. In a univariate regression analysis, infliximab use was associated with decreased risk of surgery (hazard ratio = 0.42, 95% confidence interval 0.23–0.76, $p < 0.004$). Park et al. [48] reported similar decreased risk of abdominal surgery in children receiving anti-TNF therapy (OR 0.57, 95% confidence interval 0.46–0.7) in a large utilization review of anti-TNF therapy. Prospective studies to evaluate whether anti-TNF therapy has reduced the overall rates of surgery in PCD are ongoing.

The postoperative recurrence of endoscopic inflammation following abdominal resection in pediatric patients with CD has been shown to be as high as 50%, 73%, and 77% at 1, 5, and 10 years, respectively [49]. The ECCO 2010 guidelines advocate for use of thiopurines in high-risk patients (smokers, previous intestinal surgery, penetrating disease, perianal disease, or extensive small bowel resection) following abdominal surgery [50]. There have been multiple studies (randomized controlled, prospective, and retrospective observations) that overall have shown inconclusive evidence to support TP use following the primary resection in adults with Crohn disease [49, 51].

Prophylactic anti-TNF use following abdominal surgery is limited in both adult and pediatric CD; however, early results are promising. Regueiro et al., in a randomized, double-blind, placebo-controlled trial, found that the 11 patients who were randomized to receive infliximab within 4 weeks of ileal resection had a significant reduction in endoscopic recurrence at 12 months compared to the 13 patients assigned to placebo (9% recurrence in infliximab treated vs. 84% in placebo group) [52]. The established risk factors for subsequent intestinal resection are a history of penetrating disease, cigarette smoking, and postoperative endoscopic recurrence of intestinal inflammation. Postoperative surveillance and prophylaxis are discussed in more detail in Chap. 43.

Ulcerative Colitis

In active UC, T cells (Th1 and Th2 producing IFNγ and IL-5, respectively) play an important role by producing cytokines and chemokines which stimulate macrophages to secrete tumor necrosis factor (TNFα), IL-1β, and IL-6 [53]. The Active Ulcerative Colitis Trials 1 and 2 (ACT 1 and ACT 2) were the first multicenter trials that evaluated efficacy of infliximab in adult UC patients [54, 55]. These studies showed that infliximab was superior to placebo in achieving induction and remission in patients with moderate to severe UC. These studies served as the impetus for several single-center and retrospective studies in pediatric UC.

Infliximab in Moderate-to-Severe UC

Acute severe UC has a mortality rate of 1% in children [56]. To assess disease severity in UC, a pediatric index known as Pediatric UC Activity Index (PUCAI) was developed and validated [56–58]. Since the initial use of infliximab in the treatment of moderate-to-severe ulcerative colitis in 2005 in adults with the ACT1 and ACT2 studies, six studies have been conducted in children, four retrospectively and two prospectively [59–62]. The first four retrospective studies were single center with small cohorts and short follow-up. Hyams et al. published the first of the prospective studies in 2010 [63]. A total of 52 children were treated with infliximab. Of these, 63% were corticosteroid (CS) refractory and 35% CS dependent. At the initiation of therapy with infliximab, 51% of patients were on 5-aminosalicylates, 63% on IMM, and 87% on CS. The study showed that 38% of the patients had CS-free inactive disease at 1 year and 21% at 2 years, and 61% did not require colectomy by 2 years. Turner et al. reported the second prospective study [57]. They evaluated the short-term response (clinical improvement based on the PUCAI score, improved laboratory parameters: CBC, ESR, CRP, albumin at day 3 and 5 of admission) to intravenous corticosteroids in 128 children hospitalized with acute severe colitis. Based on the PUCAI score, they showed that 29% (37 patients) did not respond to CS treatment. Of these patients, 33 received infliximab, from which 55% maintained good response at 12 months follow-up. Hyams et al. [64] reported an 8-week infliximab-induced response rate of 73.3% and remission rate of 28.6% by week 54 in patients who were unresponsive to conventional treatment.

Infliximab in Refractory UC

Even though treatment with infliximab in moderate-to-severe UC has been widely proven, there are still many patients who fail to respond or unable to maintain remission. These patients represent a therapeutic challenge. In the prospective study conducted by Turner et al., of CS refractory patients treated with infliximab, 12% still remained steroid dependent at 12 months follow-up, and almost half (52%) required a colectomy [57].

This poor response raises a question – should hospitalized patients with severe colitis be treated with an escalated dosing schedule to capture response and minimize risk of surgery? Data from adults [65] suggests as such, and a pediatric study by Falaiye et al. hints at this approach while describing their single center retrospective experience in 29 patients who required hospitalization for active colitis and were treated with infliximab [66]. All of the patients were anti-TNF naïve at the initiation of the treatment. Their results showed that 62% (18 patients) needed infliximab dose esca-

lation, 62% (18 patients) had infliximab failure (33% to side effects and 67% ineffective despite the dose escalation), and 41% (12 patients) required colectomy. They also demonstrated that there was a relationship between the need for dose escalation and lower body mass index (BMI) z-score, low serum albumin (median of 3.0 g/dl), and elevated ESR (median of 53 mm/hr) from baseline. Of the 29 patients in the study, 15 had UC, 12 CD, and 2 IBD unspecified (IBD-U); there was no statistically significant difference in the rates of steroid-free clinical remission, failure of infliximab, dose escalation, or colectomy between these phenotypes. They concluded that this population may be at increased risk of infliximab failure, and early dose escalation is needed, especially if they have low BMI z-score, low albumin, and high ESR, although dose escalation does not guarantee a response to anti-TNF.

Therapeutic Drug Monitoring

Several studies in adults have demonstrated that fecal calprotectin as well as infliximab trough levels in addition to clinical symptoms have an impact in the decision to optimize the therapy. Huang et al. concluded in their study on adults with UC that fecal calprotectin <250 μg/g indicated good therapy response, while levels >250 μg/g required dose escalation [67]. They also demonstrated that infliximab trough levels of 3–7 μg/ml was indicative of good drug response, while <3 μg/ml trigger a dose escalation and >7 μg/ml a dose de-escalation. Similar results were published by Vande Casteele et al. where they found that infliximab trough level between 3 and 7 μg/ml demonstrated a better efficacy of the drug [36]. Very few studies of drug monitoring in children with UC have been published [40, 68]. Although these studies showed the potential benefit of trough levels and antidrug antibody measurement, specific cutoff levels have yet to be defined.

Infliximab and the Incidence of Surgeries in Pediatric UC

The long-term effect of infliximab and the incidence on colectomy in children with UC is not clear at this time. In adults, the ACT1 and 2 studies showed a colectomy rate of 10% in patients treated with infliximab at 54 weeks compared to 17% on the placebo group [63]. In the study performed by Hyams in the pediatric population, 72% of the patients avoided colectomy at 1 year and 61% at 2 years, and for those on continuous medication, 84% did not require surgical intervention at 1 year and 74% at 2 years [64]. Colombel et al. also demonstrated that patients being treated with infliximab and who achieved complete mucosal healing were able to achieve corticosteroid-free and colectomy-free remission at 54 weeks

[69]. Further studies need to be conducted in order to establish a better understanding of the efficacy of infliximab in reducing the rate of colectomy in children.

Side Effects and Safety Profile of Infliximab

Infusion Reactions

Infusion reaction is a side effect of infliximab therapy which may limit longer-term use of the medication for some patients. *Acute infusion reactions* may resemble anaphylaxis with urticaria, blood pressure changes, respiratory symptoms, and chest pain. While a portion of acute infusion reactions may occur in the absence of autoantibodies, prevention of autoantibodies with targeted therapeutic drug monitoring protocols, avoidance of episodic infliximab therapy, and concomitant IMM appear to have a role in prevention of some of these reactions [22, 70–73]. In pediatrics, infusion reactions have been reported in 5–16% of patients receiving infliximab, but targeted drug monitoring and early dose escalation in patients with greater disease extent or severity may have the ability to improve durability of infliximab therapy [25, 74–76]. Acute infusions reactions may be prevented in part by pretreatment with antihistamines or corticosteroids though this is controversial, and there is wide variation in this practice across centers [77, 78]. Treatment may vary based on the type of reaction and could include corticosteroids, antihistamines, or slowing of the infusion rate, and could ultimately result in change to alternative medication if reaction is severe, or consideration of a desensitization protocol.

Autoimmune phenomena may occur as an additional side effect of infliximab therapy. *Delayed reactions* may happen days after an infliximab infusion and mimic a serum sickness reaction [77]. These reactions are more typical in patients with high antibody levels or in patients who have not had infliximab exposure for an extended period of time (i.e., episodic therapy or attempted resumption of infliximab after a period of time off the drug). These reactions are thought to result from deposition of antibodies to infliximab (ATI)-induced immune complexes being deposited in the tissues and blood vessels and present with myalgia, arthralgia, and other systemic symptoms requiring treatment with corticosteroids and likely switching to alternative medication [77]. Autoantibody formation has been described in large numbers of patients with IBD and other conditions receiving infliximab therapy, with up to half of patients with IBD developing antinuclear antibodies (ANA) and about 25% developing antibodies to double-stranded DNA (anti-dsDNA) [79, 80]. Fortunately, only about 1% of patients with ANA or dsDNA develop true lupus, whether being treated for IBD or other conditions [79–81]. Development of

Coombs negative anemias, demyelinating lesions, and optic neuritis has also been described, but these are rare phenomena and typically improve with steroids or withdrawal of infliximab [81, 82].

Skin-related side effects also present a complication to infliximab therapy which may warrant discussion prior to initiating infliximab therapy. Development of new psoriasis or other skin conditions can occur in up to 30% of patients receiving infliximab [83]. In most instances, these conditions are not associated with ATI and may be treated with topical and sometimes oral therapy without necessitating discontinuation of anti-TNF. In most cases the skin-related side effects will be related to any anti-TNF, but if the condition is severe enough that discontinuation of the offending agent is being considered, a trial of alternative anti-TNF can be considered [84, 85].

Infections

Infection remains one of the more predictable risks of anti-TNF therapy. As with other IMM, infections may occur more commonly in patients receiving these medications. In the "REACH" study, which evaluated the safety of infliximab in pediatric CD, 80% of reported serious infections (pneumonia, herpes zoster, and abscess) occurred in patients receiving infliximab every 8 weeks compared to 20% occurring in patients receiving infliximab every 12 weeks [25]. As a whole, many infections were respiratory in nature, but severe infections included sepsis and fever, pneumonia, colitis, and skin infections such as MRSA adenitis or furunculosis. Infections reported have in some cases been described as "severe" but are not a common cause of mortality from infliximab use alone [86]. Ultimately, the rate of serious infections associated with both infliximab and adalimumab in pediatrics has been reported to be 352 per 10,000 patient years and is similar between both anti-TNF agents as well as the expected rate of infections for IMM which is estimated at 333 per 10,000 patient years [86]. Systemic corticosteroids pose a significantly higher risk of about 730 infections per 10,000 patient years compared to infliximab [81, 86]. Pooled analyses of adults after longer-term use of infliximab do not demonstrate a significant risk of infections or serious infections for infliximab monotherapy, and data from the adult "TREAT" registry (Crohn's Therapy, Resource, Evaluation, and Assessment Tool) suggests that active moderate-to-severe disease and the use of steroids are much more likely to be predictors of infection [87, 88]. Opportunistic infections remain a significant risk as described in the adult "TREAT" registry and may occur in 1.81 of 1000 patients, but pediatric data is limited [88, 89]. While respiratory infections remain the most commonly reported infection in pediatrics, opportunistic infections such as *Candida albicans*,

Listeria monocytogenes, herpes simplex virus (HSV), *cyto-megalovirus* (CMV), and *Epstein-Bar virus* (EBV) have been reported and are the highest risk in elderly patients rather than in young patients [88, 90]. Regional risk of opportunistic infections such as histoplasmosis may warrant screening and treatment prior to initiating therapy [91].

Rare but serious infections such as tuberculosis (TB) reactivation have been associated with anti-TNF therapy [92]. Although first described in the setting of infliximab, reactivation of TB is a concern for other anti-TNFs as well and has led to standard screening guidelines for latent TB prior to initiation of anti-TNF therapy [93, 94], with recommendations to treat in case of a positive screen prior to initiation of anti-TNF therapy [95, 96].

Vaccination

Patients with IBD should receive all routine pediatric vaccinations. While live attenuated viruses are contraindicated for patients on anti-TNF therapy, all inactivated, attenuated viruses should be offered, particularly annual influenza vaccine [93, 95]. Of particular interest are vaccinations such as hepatitis B and varicella since these infections may pose serious health risks if reactivated or contracted during anti-TNF therapy. These vaccinations should be offered if no evidence of serologic response is detected at diagnosis or prior to initiating anti-TNFs [94, 96, 97]. Hepatitis B vaccine can also be administered once infliximab has started. Varicella vaccine, however, is live and so contraindicated once a patient is on anti-TNF therapy; the clinician must weigh the risks and benefits of delaying therapy to provide vaccination for a patient without prior appropriate varicella vaccination. Response to vaccines may be suboptimal in patients on biologic therapies such as infliximab, but up to 76% may have an amnestic response to hepatitis B vaccine [98]. Protection against human papilloma virus is indicated due to increased risk of cervical dysplasia in IBD patients on immune suppression [99].

Rapid or One-Hour Infusions

Time burden and costs associated with prolonged infliximab infusions have resulted in investigation of decreasing infusion time. Most infusions are given over a period of 2–4 h, but shorter 1-h infusions appear to be safe in adults, with no increased risk of infusion reactions even for those receiving larger drug doses up to 10 mg/kg [100, 101]. These shorter infusions have been shown to correlate with improvement in overall, social, and job-related quality of life [102]. While there is a paucity of pediatric specific data, it does appear that rapid infusions are likely safe for pediatric patients if they have demonstrated tolerance of several standard infusions [100, 103].

Malignancy

Cancers such as colorectal cancer remain a risk for patients with IBD and active inflammation, but the additional risk of malignancy related to treatment remains a consideration for patients requiring immunosuppressive therapies such as biologics. One of the most significant concerns has been for hepatosplenic T-cell lymphoma; a report in 2010 by Diak et al. described 31 cases of malignancy in pediatric patients receiving infliximab therapy, of whom most patients had IBD ($n = 24$), and all of the cases of hepatosplenic T-cell lymphoma ($n = 9$) occurred in IBD patients [104]. Analysis of this report revealed that most of these patients were also on TP. A subsequent report of 36 patients with IBD and hepatosplenic T-cell lymphoma suggested that monotherapy with anti-TNF therapy was not associated with hepatosplenic T-cell lymphoma [26]. IMM had previously been described to be associated with lymphomas and EBV-driven processes in patients receiving these medications, so it appears that the TP component of therapy is likely a driver for these types of cancers and is the highest risk for older men and men less than age 30 after about 2 years of therapy [26, 105–107]. Regarding other types of cancers, Lichtenstein et al., in a long-term safety registry of Crohn disease patients (TREAT registry), reported similar crude cancer incidences between infliximab and "other treatments only" exposed patients [108].

Other forms of malignancies such as skin cancers have been described during longer-term follow-up of patients on infliximab therapy, but the highest risk seems to be from older age and longer disease duration rather than infliximab [81]. Infliximab does not appear to increase risk for nonmelanoma skin cancer after adjustment for TP therapy, but patients receiving infliximab may have an increased risk of melanoma skin cancer related to the disease itself or potentially related to anti-TNF therapy [109]. Cervical cancer remains a risk for women with IBD which may be unrelated to treatment but warrants appropriate vaccination for HPV in this high-risk population [110].

The discussion of malignancy risk for patients undergoing anti-TNF therapy represents a unique opportunity to include families in a shared decision making approach to medical treatment. There is no single consensus about approach to anti-TNF monotherapy or combination therapy for young patients, so this particular aspect of treatment may call for a more customized approach to care, discussion of medications with presumed lower risk of cancers such as methotrexate, and clear communication about differences in treatment plans.

Mortality

Mortality associated with anti-TNF use, particularly in pediatrics, is not common. Dulai et al. described seven deaths for patients on anti-TNFs, but two of these were felt to be unrelated to medication [86]. The five patient deaths on anti-TNFs totaled a rate of 5.3 per 10,000 patient years follow-up. Of the three patients who expired on infliximab therapy, the cause of death was attributed to bone marrow transplant complication, cardiac complication (in the setting of a previously described arrhythmia), or azathioprine-induced neutropenia which led to sepsis (5). Deaths due to lymphoma, particularly hepatosplenic T-cell lymphoma, have been described as well, but we now know that this may be associated with concomitant thiopurine use [81, 104].

Summary

The advent of infliximab has revolutionized the treatment of moderate-to-severe IBD in both children and adults. It has shown to be effective in inducing and maintaining remission, is steroid sparing, and restores growth, an important consideration in this particular patient group. Experience has shown us that scheduled dosing, rather than episodic, seems to be not only more efficacious but also prevents ATI formation, thereby leading to durable and sustained response. The safety profile of infliximab is overall favorable although continued vigilance remains necessary for the occurrence of infrequent but serious events, including opportunistic infection and malignancies, especially in patients with concomitant immunosuppressive treatment.

References

1. Burnham JM, Shults J, Semeao E, et al. Body-composition alterations consistent with cachexia in children and young adults with Crohn disease. Am J Clin Nutr. 2005;82:413–20.
2. Markowitz J, Hyams J, Mack D, LeLeiko N, et al. Corticosteroid therapy in the age of infliximab: acute and 1 year outcomes in newly diagnosed children diagnosed with Crohn's disease. Clin Gastroenterol Hepatol. 2006;4:1124–9.
3. Hyams JS, Markowitz J, Lerer T, Griffiths A, et al. The natural history of corticosteroid therapy for ulcerartive colitis in children. Clin Gastroenterol Hepatol. 2006;4:1118–23.
4. Munkholm P, Langholz E, Davidsen M, Binder V. Frequency of glucocorticoid resistance and dependency in Crohn disease. Gut. 1994;35:360–2.
5. Faubion Jr WA, Loftus Jr EV, Harmsen WS, et al. The natural history of corticosteroid therapy for inflammatory bowel disease: a population-based study. Gastroenterology. 2001;121:255–60.
6. Markowitz J, Grancher K, Kohn N, et al. A multicenter trial of 6-mercaptopurine and prednisone in children with newly diagnosed Crohn disease. Gastroenterology. 2000;119:895–902.
7. Sunseri W, Hyams JS, Lerer T, et al. Retrospective cohort study of methotrexate use in the treatment of pediatric Crohn's disease. Inflamm Bowel Dis. 2014;20(8):1341–5.
8. Hyams JS, Lerer T, Mack D, Bousvaros A, Griffiths A. Outcome following thiopurine use in children with ulcerative colitis: a prospective multicenter registry study. Am J Gastroenterol. 2011;106(5):981–7.
9. Borrelli O, Cordischi L, Cirulli M, et al. Polymeric diet alone versus corticosteroids in the treatment of active pediatric Crohn's disease: a randomized controlled open-label trial. Clin Gastroenterol Hepatol. 2006;4(6):744–53.
10. Griffiths AM, Ohlsson A, Sherman PM, et al. Meta-analysis of enteral nutrition as a primary treatment of active Crohn disease. Gastroenterology. 1995;108:1056–67.
11. Reinecker HC, Steffen M, Witthoeft T, et al. Enhanced secretion of tumour necrosis factor-alpha IL-6, and IL-1 beta by isolated lamina propria mononuclear cells from patients with ulcerative colitis and Crohn disease. Clin Exp Immunol. 1993;94:174–81.
12. Nicholls S, Stephens S, Braegger CP, et al. Cytokines in stools of children with inflammatory bowel disease or infective diarrhea. J Clin Pathol. 1993;46:757–60.
13. Breese E, Michie C, Nicholls S, et al. Tumor necrosis factor alpha-producing cells in the intestinal mucosa of children with inflammatory bowel disease. Gastroenterology. 1994;106:1455–66.
14. Cornillie F, Shealy D, D'Haens G, et al. Infliximab induces potent anti-inflammatory and local immunomodulatory activity but no systemic immune suppression in patients with Crohn disease. Aliment Pharmacol Ther. 2001;15:463–73.
15. Lugering A, Schmidt M, Lugering N, et al. Infliximab induces apoptosis in monocytes from patients with chronic active Crohn disease by using a caspase-dependent pathway. Gastroenterology. 2001;121:1145–57.
16. ten Hove T, van Montfrans C, Peppelenbosch MP, van Deventer SJ. Infliximab treatment induces apoptosis of lamina propria T lymphocytes in Crohn disease. Gut. 2002;50:206–11.
17. Van den Brande JM, Braat H, van den Brink GR, et al. Infliximab but not etanercept induces apoptosis in lamina propria T-lymphocytes from patients with Crohn disease. Gastroenterology. 2003;124:1774–85.
18. Shen C, Maerten P, Geboes K, et al. Infliximab induces apoptosis of monocytes and T lymphocytes in a human-mouse chimeric model. Clin Immunol. 2005;115:250–9.
19. Scallon BJ, Moore MA, Trinh H, et al. Chimeric anti-TNF-alpha monoclonal antibody cA2 binds recombinant transmembrane TNF-alpha and activates immune effector functions. Cytokine. 1995;7:251–9.
20. Abraham C, Cho JH. Inflammatory bowel disease. N Engl J Med. 2009;361:2066–78.
21. Targan SR, Hanauer SB, van Deventer SJ, et al. A short-term study of chimeric monoclonal antibody cA2 to tumor necrosis factor alpha for Crohn's disease. Crohn's Disease cA2 Study Group. N Engl J Med. 1997;337(15):1029–35.
22. Hanauer SB, Feagan BG, Lichtenstein GR, et al. ACCENT I Study Group. Maintenance infliximab for Crohn disease: the ACCENT I randomised trial. Lancet. 2002;359:1541–9.
23. Kugathasan S, Werlin SL, Martinez A, et al. Prolonged duration of response to infliximab in early but not late pediatric Crohn's disease. Am J Gastroenterol. 2000;95:3189–94.
24. Baldassano R, Braegger CP, Escher JC, et al. Infliximab (REMICADE) therapy in the treatment of pediatric Crohn's disease. Am J Gastroenterol. 2003;98:833–8.
25. Hyams J, Crandall W, Kugathasan S, et al. Induction and maintenance infliximab therapy for the treatment of moderate to severe Crohn's disease in children. Gastroenterology. 2007;132:863–73.
26. Kotlyar DS, Osterman MT, Diamond RH, et al. A systematic review of factors that contribute to hepatosplenic T-cell lymphoma in patients with inflammatory bowel disease. Clin Gastroenterol Hepatol. 2011;9:36–41. e31
27. Colombel JF, Sandborn WJ, Reinisch W, et al. Infliximab, azathioprine, or combination therapy for Crohn's disease. N Engl J Med. 2010;362:1383–95.
28. Walters TD, Kim MO, Denson LA, et al. Increased effectiveness of early therapy with anti-tumor necrosis factor-alpha vs an immu-

nomodulator in children with Crohn's disease. Gastroenterology. 2014;146:383–91.

29. Grossi V, Lerer T, Griffiths A, et al. Concomitant use of immunomodulators affects the durability of infliximab therapy in children with Crohn's disease. Clin Gastroenterol Hepatol. 2015;13:1748–56.

30. Feagan BG, McDonald JW, Panaccione R, et al. Methotrexate in combination with infliximab is no more effective than infliximab alone in patients with Crohn's disease. Gastroenterology. 2014;146:681–8. e681

31. Osterman MT, Haynes K, Delzell E, et al. Effectiveness and safety of immunomodulators with anti-tumor necrosis factor therapy in Crohn's disease. Clin Gastroenterol Hepatol. 2015;13:1293–301.

32. Zubin G, Peter L. Predicting endoscopic Crohn's disease activity before and after induction therapy in children: a comprehensive assessment of PCDAI, CRP, and fecal calprotectin. Inflamm Bowel Dis. 2015;21:1386–91.

33. Khanna R, Sattin BD, Afif W, et al. Review article: a clinician's guide for therapeutic drug monitoring of infliximab in inflammatory bowel disease. Aliment Pharmacol Ther. 2013;38:447–59.

34. Minar P, Saeed SA, Afreen M, et al. Practical use of infliximab concentration monitoring in pediatric Crohn's disease. J Pediatr Gastroenterol Nutr. 2016;62:715–22.

35. Paul S, Del Tedesco E, Marotte H, et al. Therapeutic drug monitoring of infliximab and mucosal healing in inflammatory bowel disease: a prospective study. Inflamm Bowel Dis. 2013;19:2568–76.

36. Vande Casteele N, Ferrante M, Van Assche G, et al. Trough concentrations of infliximab guide dosing for patients with inflammatory bowel disease. Gastroenterology. 2015;148:1320–9.

37. Brandse JF, van den Brink GR, Wildenberg ME, et al. Loss of infliximab into feces is associated with lack of response to therapy in patients with severe ulcerative colitis. Gastroenterology. 2015;149:350–5.

38. Afif W, Loftus Jr EV, Faubion WA, et al. Clinical utility of measuring infliximab and human anti-chimeric antibody concentrations in patients with inflammatory bowel disease. Am J Gastroenterol. 2010;105:1133–9.

39. Dubinsky MC, Lamothe S, Yang HY, et al. Pharmacogenomics and metabolite measurement for 6-mercaptopurine therapy in inflammatory bowel disease. Gastroenterology. 2000;118:705–13.

40. Singh N, Rosenthal CJ, Melmed GY, et al. Early infliximab trough levels are associated with persistent remission in pediatric patients with inflammatory bowel disease. Inflamm Bowel Dis. 2014;20:1708–13.

41. Vaughn BP, Martinez-Vazquez M, Patwardhan V, et al. Proactive therapeutic concentration monitoring of infliximab may improve outcomes for patients with inflammatory bowel disease: results from a pilot observational study. Inflamm Bowel Dis. 2014;20:1996–2003.

42. Vande Casteele N, Gils A, Singh N, et al. Antibody response to infliximab and its impact on pharmacokinetics can be transient. Am J Gastroenterol. 2013;108:962–71.

43. Ungar B, Levy I, Yavne Y, et al. Optimizing anti-TNF-α therapy: serum levels of infliximab and adalimumab are associated with mucosal healing in patients with inflmmatory bowel diseases. Clin Gastroenterol Hepatol. 2016;14:550–7.

44. Baert F, Noman M, Vermeire S, et al. Influence of immunogenicity on the long-term efficacy of infliximab in Crohn's disease. N Engl J Med. 2003;348(7):601–8.

45. Wang SL, Ohrmund L, Hauenstein S, et al. Development and validation of a homogeneous mobility shift assay for the measurement of infliximab and antibodies-to-infliximab levels in patient serum. J Immunol Methods. 2012;382(1–2):177–88.

46. Steenholdt C, Ainsworth MA, Tovey M, et al. Comparison of techniques for monitoring infliximab and antibodies against infliximab in Crohn's disease. Ther Drug Monit. 2013;35:530–8.

47. Gupta N, Cohen SA, Bostrom AG, et al. Risk factors for initial surgery in pediatric patients with Crohn's disease. Gastroenterology. 2006;130:1069–77.

48. Park KT, Sin A, Wu M, et al. Utilization trends of anti-TNF agents and health outcomes in adults and children with inflammatory bowel diseases: a single-center experience. Inflamm Bowel Dis. 2014;20:1242–9.

49. Hansen LF, Jakobsen C, Paerregaard A, et al. Surgery and postoperative recurrence in children with Crohn disease. J Pediatr Gastroenterol Nutr. 2015;60:347–51.

50. Van Assche G, Dignass A, Reinisch W, et al. The second European evidence-based consensus on the diagnosis and management of Crohn's disease: special situations. J Crohns Colitis. 2010;4:63–101.

51. Jones GR, Kennedy NA, Lees CW, et al. Systematic review: The use of thiopurines or anti-TNF in post-operative Crohn's disease maintenance–progress and prospects. Aliment Pharmacol Ther. 2014;39:1253–65.

52. Regueiro M, Schraut W, Baidoo L, et al. Infliximab prevents Crohn's disease recurrence after ileal resection. Gastroenterology. 2009;136:441–50. e441; quiz 716.

53. Kemp R, Dunn E, Schultz M. Immunomodulators in inflammatory bowel disease: an emerging role for biologic agents. BioDrugs. 2013;27:585–90.

54. Akiho H, Yokoyama A, Abe S, et al. Promising biological therapies for ulcerative colitis: a review of the literature. World J Gastrointest Pathophysiol. 2015;6:219–27.

55. Rutgeerts P, Sandborn WJ, Feagan BG, et al. Infliximab for induction and maintenance therapy for ulcerative colitis. N Engl J Med. 2005;353:2462–76.

56. Turner D, Griffiths AM. Acute severe ulcerative colitis in children: a systematic review. Inflamm Bowel Dis. 2011;17:440–9.

57. Turner D, Mack D, Leleiko N, et al. Severe pediatric ulcerative colitis: a prospective multicenter study of outcomes and predictors of response. Gastroenterology. 2010;138:2282–91.

58. Turner D, Otley AR, Mack D, et al. Development, validation, and evaluation of a pediatric ulcerative colitis activity index: a prospective multicenter study. Gastroenterology. 2007;133:423–32.

59. McGinnis JK, Murray KF. Infliximab for ulcerative colitis in children and adolescents. J Clin Gastroenterol. 2008;42:875–9.

60. Fanjiang G, Russell GH, Katz AJ. Short- and long-term response to and weaning from infliximab therapy in pediatric ulcerative colitis. J Pediatr Gastroenterol Nutr. 2007;44:312–7.

61. Russell GH, Katz AJ. Infliximab is effective in acute but not chronic childhood ulcerative colitis. J Pediatr Gastroenterol Nutr. 2004;39:166–70.

62. Kugathasan S. Infliximab outcome in children and adults with ulcerative colitis. Gastroenterology. 2002;122:a615.

63. Hyams JS, Lerer T, Griffiths A, et al. Outcome following infliximab therapy in children with ulcerative colitis. Am J Gastroenterol. 2010;105:1430–6.

64. Hyams J, Damaraju L, Blank M, et al. Induction and maintenance therapy with infliximab for children with moderate to severe ulcerative colitis. Clin Gastroenterol Hepatol. 2012;10:391–9. e1

65. Taxonera C, Barreiro-de Acosta M, Calvo M, et al. Infliximab dose escalation as an effective strategy for managing secondary loss of response in ulcerative colitis. Dig Dis Sci. 2015;60:3075–84.

66. Falaiye TO, Mitchell KR, Lu Z, et al. Outcomes following infliximab therapy for pediatric patients hospitalized with refractory colitis-predominant IBD. J Pediatr Gastroenterol Nutr. 2014;58:213–9.

67. Huang VW, Prosser C, Kroeker KI, et al. Knowledge of fecal calprotectin and infliximab trough levels alters clinical decision-making for IBD outpatients on maintenance infliximab therapy. Inflamm Bowel Dis. 2015;21:1359–67.

68. Joosse ME, Samsom JN, van der Woude CJ, Escher JC, van Gelder T. The role of therapeutic drug monitoring of anti-tumor necrosis factor alpha agents in children and adolescents with inflammatory bowel disease. Inflamm Bowel Dis. 2015;21:2214–21.

69. Colombel JF, Rutgeerts P, Reinisch W, et al. Early mucosal healing with infliximab is associated with improved long-term clinical outcomes in ulcerative colitis. Gastroenterology. 2011;141:1194–201.

70. Rutgeerts P, Feagan BG, Lichtenstein GR, et al. Comparison of scheduled and episodic treatment strategies of infliximab in Crohn's disease. Gastroenterology. 2004;126:402–13.

71. Dassopoulos T, Sultan S, Falck-Ytter YT, Inadomi JM, Hanauer SB. American Gastroenterological Association Institute technical review on the use of thiopurines, methotrexate, and anti-TNF-alpha biologic drugs for the induction and maintenance of remission in inflammatory Crohn's disease. Gastroenterology. 2013;145:1464–78. e1–5

72. Lichtenstein GR, Diamond RH, Wagner CL, et al. Clinical trial: benefits and risks of immunomodulators and maintenance infliximab for IBD-subgroup analyses across four randomized trials. Aliment Pharmacol Ther. 2009;30:210–26.

73. Baert F, Drobne D, Gils A, et al. Early trough levels and antibodies to infliximab predict safety and success of reinitiation of infliximab therapy. Clin Gastroenterol Hepatol. 2014;12:1474–81. e2; quiz e91

74. Friesen CA, Calabro C, Christenson K, et al. Safety of infliximab treatment in pediatric patients with inflammatory bowel disease. J Pediatr Gastroenterol Nutr. 2004;39:265–9.

75. Turner D. Severe acute ulcerative colitis: the pediatric perspective. Dig Dis. 2009;27:322–6.

76. Shapiro JM, Subedi S, Machan JT, et al. Durability of infliximab is associated with disease extent in children with inflammatory bowel disease. J Pediatr Gastroenterol Nutr. 2016;62:867–72.

77. Lichtenstein L, Ron Y, Kivity S, et al. Infliximab-related infusion reactions: systematic review. J Crohns Colitis. 2015;9:806–15.

78. Adler J, Sandberg KC, Shpeen BH, Eder SJ, et al. Variation in infliximab administration practices in the treatment of pediatric inflammatory bowel disease. J Pediatr Gastroenterol Nutr. 2013;57(1):35–8.

79. Vermeire S, Noman M, Van Assche G, et al. Autoimmunity associated with anti-tumor necrosis factor alpha treatment in Crohn's disease: a prospective cohort study. Gastroenterology. 2003;125:32–9.

80. Vaz JL, Fernandes V, Nogueira F, Arnobio A, Levy RA. Infliximab-induced autoantibodies: a multicenter study. Clin Rheumatol. 2016;35:325–32.

81. Fidder H, Schnitzler F, Ferrante M, et al. Long-term safety of infliximab for the treatment of inflammatory bowel disease: a single-centre cohort study. Gut. 2009;58:501–8.

82. Zabana Y, Domenech E, Manosa M, et al. Infliximab safety profile and long-term applicability in inflammatory bowel disease: 9-year experience in clinical practice. Aliment Pharmacol Ther. 2010;31:553–60.

83. Cleynen I, Van Moerkercke W, Billiet T, et al. Characteristics of skin lesions associated with anti-tumor necrosis factor therapy in patients with inflammatory bowel disease: a cohort study. Ann Intern Med. 2016;164:10–22.

84. Coutzac C, Chapuis J, Poullenot F, et al. Association between infliximab trough levels and the occurrence of paradoxical manifestations in patients with inflammatory bowel disease: a case-control study. J Crohns Colitis. 2015;9:982–7.

85. Fiorino G, Danese S, Pariente B, Allez M. Paradoxical immune-mediated inflammation in inflammatory bowel disease patients receiving anti-TNF-alpha agents. Autoimmun Rev. 2014;13:15–9.

86. Dulai PS, Thompson KD, Blunt HB, Dubinsky MC, Siegel CA. Risks of serious infection or lymphoma with anti-tumor necrosis factor therapy for pediatric inflammatory bowel disease: a systematic review. Clin Gastroenterol Hepatol. 2014;12:1443–51; quiz e88–9.

87. Lichtenstein GR, Rutgeerts P, Sandborn WJ, et al. A pooled analysis of infections, malignancy, and mortality in infliximab- and immunomodulator-treated adult patients with inflammatory bowel disease. Am J Gastroenterol. 2012;107:1051–63.

88. Lichtenstein GR, Feagan BG, Cohen RD, et al. Serious infections and mortality in association with therapies for Crohn's disease: TREAT registry. Clin Gastroenterol Hepatol. 2006;4:621–30.

89. Veereman-Wauters G, de Ridder L, Veres G, et al. Risk of infection and prevention in pediatric patients with IBD: ESPGHAN IBD Porto Group commentary. J Pediatr Gastroenterol Nutr. 2012;54:830–7.

90. Toruner M, Loftus EV, Harmsen WS, et al. Risk factors for opportunistic infections in patients with inflammatory bowel disease. Gastroenterology. 2008;134:929–36.

91. Hage CA, Bowyer S, Tarvin SE, Helper D, Kleiman MB, Wheat LJ. Recognition, diagnosis, and treatment of histoplasmosis complicating tumor necrosis factor blocker therapy. Clin Infect Dis. 2010;50:85–92.

92. Keane J, Gershon S, Wise RP, et al. Tuberculosis associated with infliximab, a tumor necrosis factor alpha-neutralizing agent. N Engl J Med. 2001;345:1098–104.

93. Singh JA, Saag KG, Bridges Jr SL, et al. 2015 American college of rheumatology guideline for the treatment of rheumatoid arthritis. Arthritis Rheumatol. 2016;68:1–26.

94. Rufo PA, Denson LA, Sylvester FA, et al. Health supervision in the management of children and adolescents with IBD: NASPGHAN recommendations. J Pediatr Gastroenterol Nutr. 2012;55:93–108.

95. Rampton DS. Preventing TB in patients with Crohn's disease needing infliximab or other anti-TNF therapy. Gut. 2005;54:1360–2.

96. Rahier JF, Magro F, Abreu C, et al. Second European evidence-based consensus on the prevention, diagnosis and management of opportunistic infections in inflammatory bowel disease. J Crohns Colitis. 2014;8:443–68.

97. Shale MJ, Seow CH, Coffin CS, Kaplan GG, Panaccione R, Ghosh S. Review article: chronic viral infection in the anti-tumour necrosis factor therapy era in inflammatory bowel disease. Aliment Pharmacol Ther. 2010;31:20–34.

98. Moses J, Alkhouri N, Shannon A, et al. Hepatitis B immunity and response to booster vaccination in children with inflammatory bowel disease treated with infliximab. Am J Gastroenterol. 2012;107:133–8.

99. Mahadevan U, Cucchiara S, Hyams JS, et al. The London position statement of the world congress of gastroenterology on biological therapy for IBD with the European Crohn's and Colitis Organisation: pregnancy and pediatrics. Am J Gastroenterol. 2011;106:214–23; quiz 24.

100. Neef HC, Riebschleger MP, Adler J. Meta-analysis: rapid infliximab infusions are safe. Aliment Pharmacol Ther. 2013;38:365–76.

101. Babouri A, Roblin X, Filippi J, Hebuterne X, Bigard MA, Peyrin-Biroulet L. Tolerability of one hour 10 mg/kg infliximab infusions in inflammatory bowel diseases: a prospective multicenter cohort study. J Crohns Colitis. 2014;8:161–5.

102. Principi M, Losurdo G, La Fortezza RF, et al. Does infliximab short infusion have a beneficial impact on the quality of life in

patients with inflammatory bowel diseases? A single centre prospective evaluation. J Gastrointest Liver Dis. 2015;24:165–70.

103. Yeckes AR, Hoffenberg EJ. Rapid infliximab infusions in pediatric inflammatory bowel disease. J Pediatr Gastroenterol Nutr. 2009;49:151–4.

104. Diak P, Siegel J, La Grenade L, Choi L, Lemery S, McMahon A. Tumor necrosis factor alpha blockers and malignancy in children forty-eight cases reported to the food and drug administration. Arthritis Rheum. 2010;62:2517–24.

105. Beaugerie L, Carrat F, Bouvier AM, et al. Excess risk of lymphoproliferative disorders (LPD) in inflammatory bowel diseases (IBD): interim results of the cesame cohort. Gastroenterology. 2008;134:A116–A7.

106. Kandiel A, Fraser AG, Korelitz BI, Brensinger C, Lewis JD. Increased risk of lymphoma among inflammatory bowel disease patients treated with azathioprine and 6-mercaptopurine. Gut. 2005;54:1121–5.

107. Deepak P, Sifuentes H, Sherid M, Stobaugh D, Sadozai Y, Ehrenpreis ED. T-cell non-Hodgkin's lymphomas reported to the FDA AERS with tumor necrosis factor-alpha (TNF-alpha) inhibitors: results of the REFURBISH study. Am J Gastroenterol. 2013;108:99–105.

108. Lichtenstein GR, Feagan BG, Cohen RD, et al. Drug thearpies and the risk of malignancy in Crohn's disease: results from the TREAT ™ registry. Am J Gastroenterol. 2014;109:212–23.

109. Long MD, Martin CF, Pipkin CA, Herfarth HH, Sandler RS, Kappelman MD. Risk of melanoma and nonmelanoma skin cancer among patients with inflammatory bowel disease. Gastroenterology. 2012;143:390.

110. Rungoe C, Simonsen J, Riis L, Frisch M, Langholz E, Jess T. Inflammatory bowel disease and cervical neoplasia: a population-based nationwide Cohort Study. Clin Gastroenterol Hepatol. 2015;13:693.

Anti-TNF Biologic Therapies Other than Infliximab

Calen A. Steiner, Emily P. Whitfield, Jeremy Adler, and Peter D.R. Higgins

Introduction

This chapter will review the use of anti-TNF targeted biologic therapies other than infliximab for the treatment of ulcerative colitis and Crohn's disease, with an emphasis on the use of these agents in pediatric patients. This review will focus on evidence of efficacy, safety, and relative efficacy in trials in children and adults with inflammatory bowel disease. When needed, data from clinical trials of these agents in children with psoriasis or rheumatologic diseases, or data from trials in adults with IBD will be included to provide additional information on the use of these agents in children.

The anti-TNF-α agents approved for use in inflammatory bowel disease other than infliximab include adalimumab, certolizumab, and golimumab.

Adalimumab in Children

After infliximab, adalimumab is perhaps the best studied anti-TNF therapeutic for inflammatory bowel disease. It is a fully human monoclonal IgG1 antibody against TNF-α that has been reported to have higher affinity for TNF-α than infliximab (Fig. 33.1a) [1]. Adalimumab is administered subcutaneously and has a half-life of 10–20 days and bioavailability

C.A. Steiner (✉)
Department of Internal Medicine, University of Michigan Health System, Ann Arbor, MI, USA

E.P. Whitfield • J. Adler, MD, MSc
Department of Pediatrics and Communicable Diseases, Pediatric Inflammatory Bowel Disease Program, C.S. Mott Children's Hospital, University of Michigan Health System, Ann Arbor, MI, USA
e-mail: ewhitfield@nwpedsgi.com; jeradler@med.umich.edu

P.D.R. Higgins
Department of Internal Medicine,
Inflammatory Bowel Disease Program, University of Michigan Health System, Ann Arbor, MI, USA
e-mail: phiggins@med.umich.edu

of 64% [2]. It reduces inflammation through a complex and incompletely understood interplay of actions including direct inhibition of the interaction of TNF-α with p55 and p75 TNF receptors on cell surfaces, down-regulation of IL-10 and IL-12, and induction of monocyte apoptosis in a caspase dependent manner [1, 3, 4].

Efficacy of adalimumab in pediatric inflammatory bowel disease (IBD) was first described in the Retrospective Evaluation of the Safety and Effect of Adalimumab Therapy (RESEAT) study, a multicenter, retrospective chart review of patients with pediatric Crohn's disease [5]. This retrospective uncontrolled chart review was conducted at 12 sites that were part of the Pediatric Inflammatory Bowel Disease Collaborative Research Group and included a total of 115 pediatric patients with moderate to severe Crohn's disease (54% female), who had received at least one dose of adalimumab. Indication for adalimumab, concomitant medications, and clinical outcomes at 3, 6, and 12 months were recorded using the physician global assessment (PGA) and pediatric Crohn's disease activity index (PCDAI) [6]. Ninety-five percent of patients had previous treatment with infliximab, and the reason for switch to adalimumab was identified as loss of response (47%), infusion reaction, anti-drug antibodies (45%), or preference for subcutaneous injection (9%). They found the most common induction dosing strategy to be induction with 160 mg followed by 80 mg (160/80 mg) (19%), 80/40 mg (44%), and 40/40 mg (15%) with 40 mg every other week for maintenance dosing in 88%. Clinical response measured by PGA at 3, 6, and 12 months was 65, 71, and 70%, respectively, with steroid-free remission in 22, 33, and 42%. Adverse events were also recorded and no malignancies, serious infections, or deaths occurred in the subjects. Based on these results, the authors concluded that adalimumab was a well-tolerated and effective therapy, with steroid-sparing effect, for moderate to severe Crohn's disease in children [5].

Efficacy was further demonstrated in the IMAgINE 1 trial, a prospective double-blind dosing study of adalimumab (ADA) for 192 pediatric patients (6–17 years old) with

© Springer International Publishing AG 2017
P. Mamula et al. (eds.), *Pediatric Inflammatory Bowel Disease*, DOI 10.1007/978-3-319-49215-5_33

Fig. 33.1 (**a**) Adalimumab and golimumab are fully human IgG1 monoclonal antibodies. (**b**) Certolizumab pegol is a human FAB region conjugated to polyethylene glycol

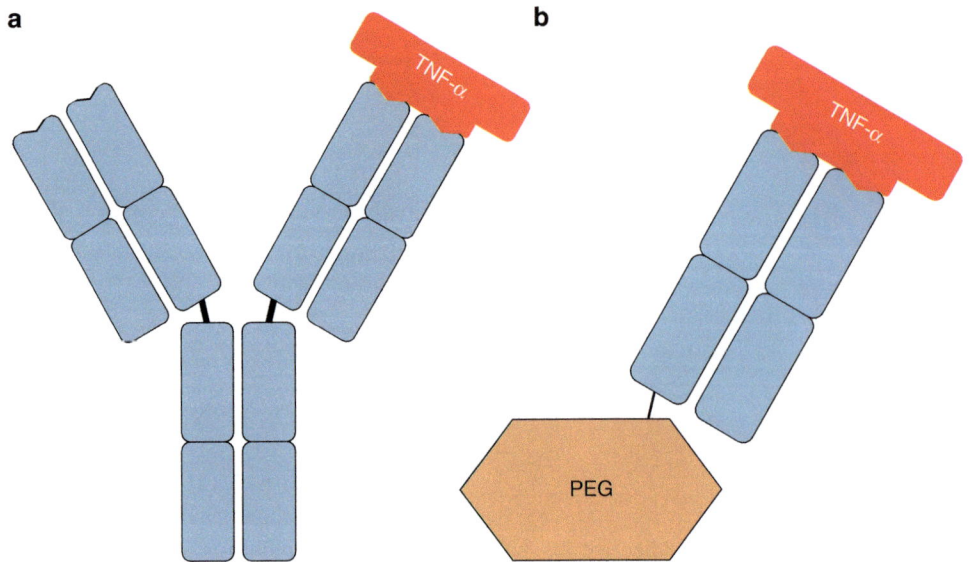

Crohn's disease who had failed conventional therapy (PCDAI >30 despite treatment with oral corticosteroid for at least 2 weeks and/or an immunomodulator for at least 8 weeks, prior to baseline). Patients previously on infliximab were permitted if they had received at least two infusions and initially responded but stopped due to infusion reaction or loss of response due to antibodies. The last dose of infliximab had to be at least 8 weeks prior to baseline. Patients were ineligible if they had received an anti-TNF other than infliximab. Patients received open-label induction therapy with adalimumab at week 0 and 2 (160 mg and 80 mg or 80 mg and 40 mg, for ≥40 kg or <40 kg, respectively), and then at week 4188, patients were randomly assigned to high-dose (40 or 20 mg every other week) or low-dose (20 or 10 mg every other week) double-blind maintenance therapy for 48 weeks, grouped according to 4-week responder status and prior exposure to infliximab.

At the 12-week study visit, patients with disease flare or non-response were switched from blinded every other week dosing to blinded weekly dosing, continuing with the same dose. After 8 more weeks, those with a disease flare or non-response could switch to open-label weekly rescue with high-dose ADA (40 or 20 mg weekly). If patients had another flare or were persistent non-responders, they could be discontinued at the investigator's discretion. One hundred and twenty-four patients completed the study. The study found that adalimumab (low dose and high dose) induced and maintained clinical response in 28–39% of patients at week 26 and 23–33% at week 52. Patients with lower CRP at baseline had higher rates of remission in both dose groups. Of note, treatment with adalimumab was associated with significant improvements in height velocity. The safety profile was found to be comparable to adult studies with infections being the most common adverse event noted, with eight serious infections [7].

The safety and efficacy of weekly dosing was described in a sub-analysis of IMAgINE 1, which analyzed the data of patients who had been escalated to weekly therapy [7]. This analysis found that escalation to weekly dosing occurred in 50.5% on low-dose and 37.6% of those on high-dose treatment, and clinical remission rates at 52 weeks were 18.8% and 31.4% for low dose and high dose, respectively. Adverse events rates were similar to those on every other week therapy [8].

A recent study evaluated the pharmacokinetics of adalimumab in children with moderate to severe Crohn's disease in a phase 3 randomized, double-blind, 52-week trial [9]. There was a 4-week open-label induction phase followed by a 48-week double-blind maintenance phase, with a standard and low-dose arm, of ADA given every other week. Trough serum adalimumab levels and antibodies were collected at baseline and then weeks 16, 26, and 52. Disease activity was analyzed at the same time points using the PCDAI. Higher body weight, higher baseline CRP, and lower baseline albumin level were associated with greater clearance of adalimumab. Additionally, an exposure (serum concentration)-efficacy relationship was observed with higher serum level associated with a higher rate of remission [9].

Adalimumab has been demonstrated to be efficacious in pediatric Crohn's disease patients after failure of infliximab therapy. Cozijnsen et al. conducted a nationwide retrospective assessment of pediatric patients in the Netherlands who were treated with adalimumab after prior treatment with infliximab [10]. Among 53 patients identified, 6% were switched to adalimumab after primary non-response to infliximab, 64% after loss of response to infliximab, 21% after allergic reaction to infliximab, and 9% after adverse reactions to infliximab. Among those started on adalimumab, dosage was based on "body weight (20–40 mg for patients <40 kg, 40–80 mg for patients >40 kg)." Seventy-four percent started with double-dosage induction sequence followed by maintenance dosing, while the remainder went straight to maintenance dosing. They found that 64% of patients reached remission within 3 months of starting adalimumab and 50% maintained remission for 2 years. Patients who had primary non-response to infliximab were more likely to fail to respond to adalimumab than those who had lost response to infliximab. Those who developed antibodies to infliximab were more likely to respond to subsequent adalimumab therapy.

The RESEAT trial found similar response rate to adalimumab after prior infliximab therapy. In that study, only six patients (5%) were treated with adalimumab as their first anti-TNF-α agent, and the authors did not comment on the efficacy of adalimumab in these small number of TNF-α-naïve patients.

Growth and Bone Health

Children who clinically respond to adalimumab therapy appear to have improved linear growth similar to that seen with infliximab. Malik et al. conducted a retrospective physician survey through the British Society of Paediatric Gastroenterology, Hepatology and Nutrition (BSPGHAN) in which they collected information on anthropometry and treatment information. Of the 70 patients included in the survey, 36 had been treated with adalimumab and had sufficient growth data at 3 points in time to assess growth. Of these patients, 34 (94%) had prior treatment with infliximab. Despite prior medical therapy, the authors demonstrated improved linear growth comparing growth 6 months prior to initiation of adalimumab to the first 6 months on adalimumab therapy. Of the 17 children who were Tanner stage 1–3 at the start of adalimumab, there was a significant increase in the height Z score after 6 months of adalimumab.

Veerappan et al. prospectively assessed markers of bone formation and resorption in children with Crohn's disease treated with adalimumab and compared their findings to those in control children without IBD. All of these children had previously been treated with immune suppressive therapy, most of whom had had prior treatment with infliximab. They found an increase in bone formation markers (osteocalcin and procollagen type 1 N-terminal propeptide) at 1 and 3 months after starting adalimumab. They also found increased osteoblast differentiation after 6 months, which the authors suggested was likely related to new bone formation.

Pain

In addition to efficacy and safety, pain with adalimumab injection is important to address, since this can impact patient adherence. Pain at the adalimumab injection site has been reported in both pediatric and adult studies. Hirai et al. conducted a survey of patient satisfaction with adalimumab self-injection [11]. They surveyed 124 patients (age 13–70 years) who were currently receiving adalimumab therapy. The majority of patients (88%) reported pain at the injection site, 28% of whom had "strong pain" at the injection site. Strategies that patients reported to help alleviate pain included "slow injection" and "warming the drug solution with their palms."

There was one report of mixing lidocaine into adalimumab prior to injection to minimize pain at the injection site. Ayala and colleagues presented findings of a study in which they recruited pediatric and adult patients treated with adalimumab who experienced pain and anxiety or were younger [12]. They added 0.2 ml of 1% lidocaine directly into the prefilled syringes of 0.8 ml adalimumab. They tested this in 15 patients who reported decreased pain at the injection site.

Adalimumab in Adults

Adalimumab has demonstrated efficacy in controlled trials in multiple disease states and received FDA approval for rheumatoid arthritis in adults in 2002, psoriatic arthritis in 2005, ankylosing spondylitis in 2006, plaque psoriasis in 2008, and juvenile idiopathic arthritis in 2008 [13–22]. Adalimumab achieved FDA approval for Crohn's disease in adults in 2007 and for ulcerative colitis in 2012. The efficacy in Crohn's disease in adults was established by four placebo-controlled trials demonstrating efficacy for induction as well as maintenance of remission [23–26]. Since these studies were published, additional randomized controlled trials have demonstrated efficacy of adalimumab in induction and maintenance of mucosal healing in adults with Crohn's disease [27] and in patients who recently underwent intestinal resection surgery [28]. Four-year maintenance data has also recently been published [29]. The efficacy of adalimumab in ulcerative colitis has been established primarily by two randomized controlled trials [30, 31], with recent 4-year maintenance data now available [32].

CLASSIC I

The CLASSIC I and CLASSIC II trials investigated the efficacy of adalimumab in patients who were anti-TNF therapy naïve with moderate to severe Crohn's disease [24, 25]. CLASSIC I first evaluated adalimumab as an induction therapy. This multicenter, randomized, double-blind, placebo-controlled trial enrolled 299 patients receiving loading doses of adalimumab in three different dose groups vs. placebo, with the primary endpoint being differences in rates of remission (defined by Crohn's Disease Activity Index [CDAI] [33] scores of < 150) at week 4 [24]. Patients were randomized to receive loading dose regimens at weeks 0 and 2 of placebo, adalimumab 40 mg/20 mg, 80 mg/ 40 mg, or 160 mg/ 80 mg. Based on pharmacokinetic data obtained in trials for rheumatoid arthritis, the investigators anticipated a target dose of 40 mg every other week for efficacy in Crohn's disease. A dose group above and below that target was selected (20 mg every other week and 40 mg weekly or 80 mg every other week), and the loading doses were selected based on early dosing pharmacokinetic data. At week 4, rates of remission were 18% in the 40 mg/20 mg group ($p = 0.36$), 24% in the 80 mg/40 mg group ($p = 0.06$), 36% in the 160 mg/80 mg group ($p = 0.001$), and 12% in the placebo group. Differences in response when compared with placebo achieved significance as early as week 1 in the 80 mg/40 mg group. This study demonstrated that induction therapy with adalimumab is more effective than placebo, with the best tested loading dose being 160 mg/80 mg at weeks 0 and 2. Additionally, adalimumab was well tolerated, with similar rates of adverse events across groups, except for injection site reactions, which occurred more frequently in the ADA groups.

CLASSIC II

The CLASSIC II trial evaluated adalimumab for maintenance therapy in moderate to severe Crohn's disease in patients who were naïve to anti-TNF therapy and then responded to ADA, for a total of 56 weeks [25]. This trial was a continuation of CLASSIC I and enrolled 276 of the 299 patients from CLASSIC I. All patients who entered CLASSIC II from CLASSIC I received 40 mg ADA at week 0 (week 4 of CLASSIC 1) and week 2. At week 4, the 55 patients who had achieved remission at weeks 0 and 4 were re-randomized to receive placebo, adalimumab 40 mg every other week, or adalimumab 40 mg weekly. The primary endpoint was again defined as a CDAI score <150. At week 56, 79% of patients in the 40 mg every other week and 83% of patients in the 40 mg weekly were in remission vs. 44% of the placebo group ($p < 0.05$). At week 4, 204 patients who had not achieved remission at week 0 and week 4 entered a separate open-label arm and received 40 mg every other week. Patients in this arm could escalate to 40 mg weekly for a flare or nonresponse. In this arm, 71 continued on 40 mg every other week, while 60 had dose escalation to 40 mg weekly. At the end of 56 weeks, 46% of patients in this arm were in remission. Additionally, 65% had a 100-point clinical response, and 72% had a 70-point clinical response. The rates of patients achieving 70-point clinical response were not significantly affected by concomitant use of immunosuppressant therapy. Thus adalimumab is more effective than placebo as maintenance therapy in adults with Crohn's disease.

CHARM

The CHARM trial was a randomized, double-blind, multicenter placebo-controlled trial that studied adalimumab for the maintenance of remission in patients who had responded to induction therapy with adalimumab [23]. This study permitted concomitant use of a stable dose of immunosuppressant therapy, 5-ASA therapy, Crohn's disease-related antibiotics, and steroids and included adults with moderate to severe Crohn's disease. This study also included patients who had previously been on a TNF antagonist, so long as it was more than 12 weeks prior to screening, and excluding those with primary non-response. Eight hundred and fifty-four patients enrolled and received open-label adalimumab loading doses of 80 mg and 40 mg at week 0 and week 2, respectively. Patients were then assessed and stratified at week 4 based on response (decrease in CDAI score of 70 or greater), and 58% of patients were randomized to placebo, adalimumab 40 mg every other week, or adalimumab 40 mg weekly up to 56 weeks. Patients who experienced a flare or nonresponse were allowed to switch to 40 mg every other week after week 12. Two primary endpoints were evaluated as percentages of the randomized responder arms achieving remission at weeks 26 and 56 (defined as CDAI score <150). At week 26 the rates of remission were 17, 40, and 47% in the placebo, adalimumab 40 mg every other week, and adalimumab 40 mg weekly groups, respectively. At week 56, these rates were 12, 36, and 41%, respectively. This demonstrated that each adalimumab group achieved significantly greater rates of remission when compared pairwise with placebo ($p < 0.001$). Differences between the two adalimumab treatment groups did not achieve significance ($P = 0.22$ at week 26 and $p = 0.34$ at week 56). Differences in the rates of remission between treatment and placebo groups were seen as early as week 6, and most patients (81%) in the treatment groups who achieved remission at week 26 remained in remission at week 56, compared to 48% in the placebo group. Adalimumab achieved superiority to placebo regardless of concomitant use of immunosuppressive therapy or prior use of TNF-antagonists. Adalimumab was also demonstrated to be steroid sparing, with both treatment groups having a greater percentage of patients achieving steroid-free remission at 26 weeks ($p < 0.001$ for each treatment group vs. placebo) and 56 weeks ($p < 0.001$ for the 40 mg every other week group vs. placebo, $p = 0.008$ for adalimumab 40 mg weekly vs. placebo). This study demonstrated that treatment with adalimumab 40 mg every other week or 40 mg weekly is an effective therapy for maintenance of remission in adults with Crohn's disease. Recently, data regarding remission rates at 4 years has been released using data from the CHARM trial and its open-label extension, ADHERE [23, 29, 34]. These studies demonstrated good durability of response, with 54% of patients who achieved remission at 1 year still in remission at 4 years [29].

GAIN

The GAIN trial was a 4-week, randomized, double-blind, placebo-controlled trial designed to ascertain adalimumab efficacy in inducing remission in Crohn's disease patients with symptoms despite infliximab therapy or an inability to take infliximab secondary to adverse events [26]. In this study 325 adults with moderate to severe Crohn's disease who were either intolerant to infliximab or had initially responded but then lost response to infliximab were randomly assigned to receive placebo or adalimumab 160 mg at week 0 and 80 mg at week 2. Patients who did not ever respond to infliximab were excluded. At week 4, 21% of adalimumab-treated patients vs. 7% of placebo-treated patients achieved remission defined as CDAI<150 ($p < 0.001$). Rates of 70-point response in adalimumab vs. placebo at weeks 1, 2, and 4 were 35% vs. 21%, 52% vs. 33%, and 52% vs. 34%, respectively, with statistically significant response seen at week 1. Total CDAI scores were also significantly lower in the adalimumab group vs. placebo at weeks 1, 2, and 4. Subgroup analysis revealed that adalimumab demonstrated efficacy regardless of concomitant immunosuppressive therapy, previous intolerance to infliximab, previous loss of response to infliximab, previous intolerance of and loss of response to infliximab, or presence of antibodies to infliximab. Based on this study, adalimumab is safe and effective for use in patients with Crohn's disease who had previously responded and discontinued infliximab due to adverse events or a loss of response, but no conclusions can be drawn about infliximab primary non-responders.

EXTEND Trial in Mucosal Healing in CD

The EXTEND trial is the first randomized, double-blind, multicenter placebo-controlled trial investigating the efficacy of adalimumab in the induction and maintenance of mucosal healing in adults with moderate to severe ileocolonic Crohn's disease [27]. One hundred and thirty-five patients received open-label adalimumab 160 mg at week 0 and 80 mg at week 2. At week 4, 129 patients who remained in the study were randomized to receive maintenance therapy with adalimumab 40 mg every other week or placebo. Patients who experienced flares or non-response could receive open-label adalimumab 40 mg every other week, with the potential to increase dosage to 40 mg weekly. Absence of mucosal ulceration at week 12 was defined as the primary endpoint. Mucosal ulceration was defined as a score of least two on the ulcerated surface subscore of the Simple Endoscopic Score for Crohn's Disease (SES-CD) [35] in at least one of five ileocolonic segments. Secondary endpoints assessed included mucosal healing at week 52, Crohn's Disease Endoscopic Index of Severity (CDEIS) [36] remission (defined as a score of 4 or less) at

week 12 and week 52, and CDAI remission (score<150) and response (100-point reduction and 70-point reduction in CDAI score) at week 12 and week 52. The primary endpoint of mucosal healing at week 12 was achieved in 27% of the continuous adalimumab group compared to 13% of the induction/placebo group ($p = 0.056$). This p-value improved to 0.046 when applying a prespecified per-protocol analysis which excluded some patients for major protocol deviations. Secondary endpoint analysis at 52 weeks revealed that 24% of the adalimumab-continuous arm and none of the induction/placebo arm achieved mucosal healing ($p < 0.001$). Similarly, all secondary endpoints achieved statistically significant superiority of continuous adalimumab compared to induction/placebo at week 52. At week 12, CDEIS remission rates and CDAI remission rates of the continuous adalimumab group achieved statistical superiority over the induction/placebo group, but not for CDEIS 75% responders nor CDAI score reductions of > 100 or >70. Ultimately this study demonstrated superiority of adalimumab maintenance therapy in mucosal healing of adults with moderate to severe Crohn's disease at 52 weeks, but not at 12 weeks post-induction. Despite the lack of statistical superiority of adalimumab on mucosal healing at week 12, this could be due to the lingering efficacy of the induction therapy that all participants received or that mucosal healing in patients with severe disease takes longer than 12 weeks. Overall this study demonstrates that adalimumab is efficacious in mucosal healing in addition to its established efficacy in clinical response and remission in Crohn's disease.

ADA in Postoperative CD

An additional randomized controlled trial (POCER) has evaluated the efficacy of adalimumab in preventing disease recurrence in patients with Crohn's disease who have undergone intestinal resection surgery [28]. This study was a randomized, prospective, open-label trial that included 51 patients with ileal or ileocolonic Crohn's disease who underwent an intestinal resection. Patients were randomized to receive adalimumab, azathioprine, or mesalamine following surgery for a period of 2 years. For the adalimumab arm, subcutaneous injections were administered as a loading dose of 160 mg/80 mg at weeks 0 and 2, respectively, followed by maintenance dosing of 40 mg every 2 weeks. The azathioprine arm received 2 mg/kg daily, while the mesalamine group received 3 g daily, divided in three doses. The primary outcome of this study was the proportion of patients with clinical and endoscopic remission at 2 years post-surgery using multiple previously developed scales, with a secondary outcome being a quality of life assessment via the previously validated IBDQ [28, 37]. After the 2-year study period, 1 of 16 patients treated with adalimumab (6.3%), 11 of 17 patients treated with azathioprine (64.7%), and 15 of 18 patients treated with mesalamine (83.3%) experienced endoscopic recurrence. These values represent an OR = 0.036 for adalimumab compared to azathioprine and OR = 0.013 for adalimumab compared to mesalamine. Perhaps due to small sample size, there was no significant difference in endoscopic recurrence between azathioprine and mesalamine, with an OR = 0.367. With regard to clinical recurrence, using the scale proposed by Hanauer et al. [38], 2 of 16 adalimumab-treated patients (12.5%) had clinical recurrence, while 11 of 17 in the azathioprine arm and 9 of 18 in the mesalamine arm had clinical recurrence for odds ratios of 0.078 and 0.143, respectively [28]. These results were also reflected by using a CDAI >200, which results in clinical recurrence of 6.3% vs. 70.6% for OR = 0.028 and 6.3% vs. 50% for an OR = 0.067. Again, there was no significant difference in azathioprine vs. mesalamine when using these scales to measure clinical recurrence. Remission, defined as CDAI score <150, occurred in 15/16 of the adalimumab group compared with 4/17 in the azathioprine group (OR = 0.021) and 6/18 in the mesalamine group (OR = 0.033), with no difference between the azathioprine and mesalamine groups. Very similar outcomes were obtained when analyzing the secondary endpoint of quality of life using the IBDQ. Thus, adalimumab was shown to be superior to azathioprine and mesalamine in the prevention of disease recurrence in adults with Crohn's disease who underwent intestinal resection.

ULTRA/UC Data

The efficacy of adalimumab in ulcerative colitis was established primarily through two different phase-three clinical trials, ULTRA-1 (Ulcerative Colitis Long-Term Remission and maintenance with Adalimumab) and ULTRA-2 [30, 31]. ULTRA-1 was a multicenter, randomized, double-blind, placebo-controlled trial that lasted 8 weeks [30]. This enrolled adult patients with moderate to severe ulcerative colitis who had been treated with immunosuppressant therapy and/or corticosteroids but still had Mayo score [39] ≥6 and endoscopic subscore ≥2. All patients were naïve to anti-TNF agents. This study initially included 186 patients randomized to receive either placebo or induction therapy with adalimumab 160 mg at week 0 and 80 mg at week 4, followed by 40 mg maintenance dosing at week 4 and week 6. The protocol was amended to include a second treatment group with a regimen of 80 mg adalimumab at week 0, followed by 40 mg at weeks 2, 4, and 6 at the behest of European regulatory authorities. Ultimately, the primary endpoint of this study was assessed in 390 patients randomized to adalimumab 160 mg/80 mg/40 mg/40 mg, 80 mg/40 mg/40 mg/40 mg, or placebo. The primary endpoint was defined as clinical remission at week 8 as defined as Mayo score ≤2 with no individual subscore >1. At week 8, 18.5% of the 160 mg/80 mg group, 10.0% of the 80 mg/40 mg group, and 9.2% of the placebo group achieved remission (p = 0.031 for 160 mg/80 mg vs. placebo, p = 0.833 for 80 mg/40 mg vs. placebo). Serious adverse events occurred in 4.0% of the adalimumab 160 mg/80 mg group, 3.8% of the adalimumab 80 mg/40 mg group, and 7.6% of the placebo group. Evaluation of the primary endpoint leads to the conclusion that adalimumab 160 mg/80 mg induction dose followed by 40 mg every other week for 2 weeks is a safe and effective induction regimen for ulcerative colitis in adults when compared to placebo. Additionally, this study leads to the conclusion that loading doses of 80 mg/40 mg are not effective for induction of remission in ulcerative colitis.

ULTRA-2 was a randomized, double-blind, multicenter, placebo-controlled trial that included 494 patients with moderate to severe ulcerative colitis that were on immunosuppressant therapy and/or oral corticosteroids [31]. This study included both patients who had prior exposure to TNF-antagonists and those who had not. Patients were randomized to receive either placebo or adalimumab 160 mg at week 0, 80 mg at week 2, followed by 40 mg every other week. Remission in this study was also defined as Mayo score ≤2 with no individual subscore >1, with primary endpoints being remission at week 8 and week 52. The rate of clinical remission at week 8 was 16.5% of the treatment group vs. 9.3% of the placebo group, p = 0.019. At 52 weeks, the rates of clinical remission were 17.3% and 8.5% in the treatment and placebo groups, respectively, p = 0.004. Secondary analysis revealed that clinical response was achieved in 50.4% of the treatment group vs. 34.6% of the placebo group at week 8 and 30.2% of the treatment group vs. 18.3% of the placebo group at week 52, for p values of $p < 0.001$ at week 8 and p = 0.002 at week 52. In patients who were anti-TNF naïve, 21.3% of the treatment group and 11% of the placebo group achieved remission at week 8 and 22% vs. 12.4% at week 52 for p values of 0.017 and 0.039, respectively. For patients who had received prior anti-TNF therapy, rates of remission at week 8 were 9.2% in the treatment group vs. 6.9% in the placebo group and 10.2% in the treatment arm vs. 3% in the placebo arm at week 52, for p values of 0.559 and 0.039, respectively. This study demonstrated that adalimumab is superior to placebo for the induction and maintenance of remission in adults with ulcerative colitis, with markedly better efficacy in patients who are anti-TNF naïve compared to those with prior anti-TNF exposure. Recently, long-term data from adalimumab-treated patients in ULTRA-1, ULTRA-2, and the open-label extension ULTRA-3 has been published [32]. This study demonstrated that 199 of 600 patients randomized to receive adalimumab in the intent-to-treat analysis of ULTRA-1 and ULTRA-2 remained on adalimumab and demonstrated a rate of remission of 24.7% by partial Mayo score at week 208.

Levels and Antibodies

Approximately 18% of adult and pediatric Crohn's disease patients who are primary responders will lose response to adalimumab, with an annual risk of over 20% per patient-year, and 37% will require dose intensification, with an annual risk of nearly 25% [40]. The importance of drug levels has been emphasized in several studies evaluating endpoints such as mucosal healing, and endoscopic and clinical indicators of disease [41–48]. Typically drug levels are evaluated with either HMSA or ELISA, which have been found to be roughly equivalent [49]. Several groups have proposed different drug level thresholds to achieve mucosal healing, with levels as low as 4.9 µg/mL (via ELISA) [44] and as high as 8.14 µg/mL (HMSA) [43] being proposed. One study proposes levels as high as 8–12 µg/mL [45]. Anti-adalimumab antibodies are thought to be primarily responsible for the observed loss of response [50, 51], with rates of anti-adalimumab antibody formation reported to range from 3% in the CLASSIC II trial [25] to as high as 21% [50]. Further, anti-adalimumab antibodies have been shown to be inversely associated with adalimumab drug levels and achievement of good clinical outcomes [42, 49]. More studies are needed to cement our understanding of the relationship between adalimumab levels, anti-adalimumab antibodies, and response, as not all studies have demonstrated such a clear relationship. One large cross-sectional study demonstrated no difference between mucosal healing rates in patients with anti-adalimumab antibodies and those without [45]. However, that comparison was made in patients who had adequate adalimumab drug levels, and the lack of separation could have been due to individuals overcoming the anti-adalimumab antibodies effect via other means. In addition to increasing drug levels, research has been done to investigate the effect of immunomodulators on the rate of formation of anti-drug antibodies [2]; however this data is limited to patients being treated with infliximab. Another proposed mechanism for loss of response is tissue inflammation itself acting to reduce levels of anti-TNF agents [47], although this is less well studied. Despite the importance of adequate drug levels in achieving remission in IBD, recent studies (TAXIT, TAILORX) using infliximab and adalimumab have demonstrated that there is no significant value in prospective drug monitoring during successful maintenance therapy and suggest that therapeutic drug monitoring should be used largely during induction or upon loss of response [52].

Certolizumab in Children

There are no completed pediatric studies of certolizumab pegol use in IBD. There was one phase 2 open-label prospective study called "The Use of Certolizumab Pegol for Treatment of Active Crohn's Disease in Children and Adolescents (NURTURE)." This study was terminated due to "higher than projected discontinuation rate during the Maintenance Phase" [53]. However some preliminary data were presented in abstract form at Digestive Disease Week 2011 [54]. This abstract presented pharmacokinetic findings in children 6–17 years of age, after 6 weeks of certolizumab therapy. Patients received an induction sequence of certolizumab subcutaneously every 2 weeks for 3 doses (weeks 0, 2, 4). The dosing was 400 mg for patients ≥40 kg and 200 mg for patients 20–40 kg. In their first 14 pediatric patients with active Crohn's disease, they found that plasma concentrations of certolizumab during the 6 weeks of induction period were similar to those observed in adult patients, though younger children (6–11 years) had slightly higher serum concentrations than older patients (12–17 years).

Despite the lack of pediatric studies of certolizumab for IBD, there are studies in juvenile idiopathic arthritis (JIA). Tzaribachev et al. reported outcomes of 22 pediatric patients with JIA who were treated with certolizumab, most of whom had previously been treated with two prior anti-TNF-α agents (5 had 1 prior and 18 had 2 prior anti-TNF-α agents) [55]. By weeks 24–36, most (68%) had no active joint inflammation. There were no serious adverse reactions, but one child developed a transient skin reaction.

Certolizumab in Adults

Certolizumab is an antibody Fab' fragment that is humanized and conjugated to polyethylene glycol (Fig. 33.1b). Certolizumab binds and inhibits TNF-α, both soluble and membrane bound. It lacks an Fc region, and as such does not fix complement nor cause cell-mediated cytotoxicity. It is administered subcutaneously, with bioavailability of approximately 80%. Certolizumab has an indication for adults with moderate to severe Crohn's disease who have not had an adequate response to conventional therapy, as well as adult indications in rheumatoid arthritis, psoriatic arthritis, and ankylosing spondylitis [33]. The efficacy of certolizumab in Crohn's disease has been assessed in multiple phase II and phase III trials including the PEGylated Antibody Fragment Evaluation in Crohn's Disease Safety and Efficacy (PRECiSE) trials [56–59], and more recently the Mucosal Healing Study in Crohn's Disease (MUSIC) trial [60, 61]. Certolizumab has also been assessed for efficacy in patients who failed infliximab after previous clinical response in the WELCOME trial [62, 63].

Initial Phase 2 Trials

Two small phase 2 studies initially assessing certolizumab demonstrated that it is well tolerated and efficacious, but these studies failed to achieve their primary endpoint [64, 65]. Both were randomized, double-blind, placebo-controlled multicenter studies. One study evaluated the safety and efficacy of certolizumab in 92 adults with Crohn's disease, who received certolizumab at doses of 1.25 mg/kg, 5 mg/kg, 10 mg/kg, or 20 mg/kg or placebo [65], which was later adjusted. The 1.25 mg/kg arm was dropped based on efficacy results in a study of rheumatoid arthritis. The primary endpoint was clinical response (CDAI score reduction of at least 100 points) or remission (CDAI score ≤ 150) at 4 weeks. While the treatment groups and placebo groups all had similar percentages of patients achieving these endpoints at week 4 (47.8–60.0%), the 10 mg/kg group did demonstrate significant separation in remission at week 2 (47.1 vs. 16.0%, p = 0.041). The second phase 2 trial included 292 patients with moderate to severe Crohn's disease randomized to 100, 200, 300, or 400 mg subcutaneous certolizumab or placebo at weeks 0, 4, and 8 [64]. This study again assessed response and remission as defined in the prior study but evaluated the endpoints at week 12. All treatment groups achieved significant separation from placebo at week 2, but this significance was not maintained. The 400 mg treatment group (roughly 6 mg/kg) maintained the highest response rate at all time points, with the most robust separation at week 10 with 52.8% vs. 30.1% for placebo (p = 0.006). However, this separation was lost in all groups at the primary endpoint analysis at week 12. It is not clear why a 700 mg (or 10 mg/kg) arm was not evaluated in phase 2.

PRECISE Trials

The PRECiSE 1 trial was the first major randomized, double-blind, placebo-controlled phase III trial evaluating the efficacy of certolizumab in adults with moderate to severe Crohn's disease [57]. This trial included 662 patients who were first stratified based on CRP ≥ 10 mg/L or CRP<10 mg/L and then randomized to receive 400 mg subcutaneous certolizumab or placebo at weeks 0, 2, and 4 followed by every 4 weeks thereafter. The primary endpoint was a decrease in CDAI score of at least 100 points at week 6, and at both week 6 and week 26, in the group with baseline CRP ≥10 mg/L. At week 6, 37% of the treatment group achieved response compared to 26% in the placebo group (p = 0.04). At both weeks 6 and 26, response was achieved in 22% of the treatment group and 12% of the placebo group (p = 0.05). These results were consistent with those in the overall population, with response rates of 35% in the treatment group vs. 27% in the placebo group at week 6 and 23% treatment vs. 16% placebo at weeks 6 and 26 (p = 0.02 in both instances). Rates of remission did not achieve statistical significance in treatment vs. placebo. The use of concomitant glucocorticoids,

previous infliximab treatment, smoking status, and immunosuppressive therapy was not associated with the magnitude of response.

PRECiSE 2 was a randomized, double-blind, placebo-controlled trial evaluating the efficacy of certolizumab for maintenance therapy in adults with moderate to severe Crohn's disease [59]. In this study 668 patients entered the open-label induction phase, in which 400 mg subcutaneous certolizumab was administered at weeks 0, 2, and 4. Of the 668 subjects entering the induction phase, 428 had a response at week 6 as defined by at least a 100-point reduction in CDAI. Those patients were then randomized to receive 400 mg certolizumab or placebo at weeks 8, 12, 16, and 20. Patients were again stratified based on CRP level as well as concurrent use of glucocorticoids and concurrent use of immunosuppressive therapy. The primary endpoint was defined as clinical response at week 26 in the CRP ≥10 mg/L group. Clinical response was achieved in this group at week 26 in 62% of the treatment arm compared to 34% of placebo (p < 0.001). When assessing the intention-to-treat population, the clinical response at 26 weeks was 63% in the treatment group vs. 36% in the placebo arm (p < 0.001). Remission (CDAI ≤150) was achieved in 48% of the treatment group vs. 29% in the placebo group (p < 0.001). Secondary analysis revealed that when the patients were stratified into those who had received prior infliximab and those who had not, both groups experienced a significant difference in response at week 26 in treatment vs. placebo.

PRECiSE 3 is an open-label extension of PRECiSE 2 in which patients who completed PRECiSE 2 were eligible to receive 400 mg certolizumab every 4 weeks long term, with data published at 54 weeks (week 80 of PRECiSE 2) [56]. This study utilized the Harvey Bradshaw Index [66] (HBI) to assess response and remission in patient groups that received uninterrupted certolizumab and interrupted certolizumab at 54 weeks (week 80 of PRECiSE 2). Of the patients responding at week 26 of PRECiSE 2, the rates of response in the continuous and interruption groups were 66.1 and 63.3%, respectively. In patients that achieved remission at week 26, rates of remission at week 80 in the continuous and interruption groups were 62.1 and 63.2%, respectively. These data suggest that certolizumab is efficacious in maintaining response and remission in certolizumab responders.

PRECiSE 4 is an open-label evaluation of patients in PRECiSE 2 who entered the randomization phase but who relapsed before week 26 [58]. In this study, patients who relapsed from the treatment group received a single extra dose of 400 mg certolizumab, and patients from the placebo group received reinduction with 400 mg certolizumab at weeks 0, 2, and 4, followed by 400 mg certolizumab every 4 weeks. This study again utilized the HBI to assess response rates. At week 4, response was attained in 63% of the continuous therapy group and 65% of the drug interruption group. At week 52, this clinical response was maintained in 55% of the continuous treatment group and 59% of the certolizumab-interrupted group. Based on this study, rescue or reinduction therapy with certolizumab in patients with an initial response may be a viable treatment option.

Certolizumab in Loss of Response to Infliximab

While the PRECiSE trials did not exclude patients on prior infliximab and were able to perform subgroup analysis on these patients, an additional randomized controlled trial has been published assessing the efficacy of certolizumab specifically in patients with Crohn's disease who experienced non-primary treatment failure on infliximab due to hypersensitivity or loss of response [63]. Five hundred and thirty-nine adults with moderate to severe Crohn's disease and secondary failure to infliximab enrolled in this 26-week trial [63]. This study also contained an open-label induction period with subsequent randomization and blinding at week 6. Patients received open-label certolizumab 400 mg subcutaneously at weeks 0, 2, and 4 and were assessed for response (CDAI reduction of ≥ 100). This was the primary endpoint and was achieved in 62.0% of patients entering the trial. Three hundred and twenty-nine patients who responded were then enrolled in the randomized, double-blind maintenance therapy portion of the trial and received certolizumab either every 4 weeks or every 2 weeks. Ultimately, response was achieved in 38.3% of patients at week 26, with no significant difference in rates of the every 4-week vs. every 2-week dosing groups. This trial was not placebo controlled but did demonstrate that good response and remission rates can be produced with certolizumab therapy in adults with Crohn's disease and prior secondary failure of infliximab.

TNF-Naïve Patients

One randomized trial evaluated the efficacy of certolizumab in adults with moderate to severe Crohn's disease but excluded patients who had received prior infliximab [67]. In this randomized, double-blind, placebo-controlled trial, 439 patients were randomized to receive either placebo or 400 mg subcutaneous certolizumab at weeks 0, 2, and 4. The primary endpoint for this trial assessed clinical remission (CDAI ≤ 150) at week 6. This study failed to achieve significance of its primary endpoint, with 32% of the treatment arm vs. 25% of the placebo arm achieving remission at week 6 ($p = 0.174$). The following subgroups did achieve significance: Men, patients ≤ 40 years old, patients with CRP ≥ 10 mg/L,

ileocolonic or colonic involvement, disease duration less than mean, CDAI ≥ 300, and patients with no prior intestinal resection. When these results are taken with the body of knowledge around TNF-α inhibitors, they seem to suggest that certolizumab is efficacious in the treatment of Crohn's disease but may be best utilized after failure of another anti-TNF such as infliximab.

MUSIC

A recent study has evaluated the efficacy of certolizumab to achieve endoscopic mucosal healing of intestinal lesions [61]. This study was open label, and patients received certolizumab 400 mg subcutaneous at weeks 0, 2, 4, and every 4 weeks thereafter up to week 52. This study demonstrated good rates of endoscopic response and remission at week 10 and week 54, with rates of endoscopic response, endoscopic remission, complete endoscopic remission, and complete mucosal healing at week 54 of 49%, 27%, 14%, and 8%, respectively. While assessment of mucosal healing is a valuable emerging measure of disease activity and subsequently efficacy, more investigation via a placebo-controlled trial would be useful.

Trough Certolizumab Levels and Anti-drug Antibodies

Antibodies to certolizumab developed in 8% of patients treated with certolizumab in the PRECiSE I trial, including 4% of patients treated with concomitant immunosuppressive therapy and 10% who were not treated with concomitant immunosuppressive therapy [57]. The importance of adequate drug levels has also been demonstrated in certolizumab through post hoc analysis of clinical trial data [60]. This study demonstrated that higher levels of certolizumab were significantly associated with response and remission at week 10 ($p = 0.0016$ and 0.0302 respectively) as well as remission ($p = 0.0206$) at week 54 of the MUSIC trial [60, 61]. Additionally, there was a significant inverse relationship between levels of certolizumab in plasma and body weight ($p = 0.0373$) and C-reactive protein ($p = 0.0014$) [60]. This publication did not speculate as to what an adequate trough level may be, but the range of plasma concentration of certolizumab at week 54 in the response and remission groups was 14.9–38.1 µg/mL [60]. It appears that certolizumab at 400 mg q4 weeks in adults (roughly 6 mg/kg) may be significantly underdosed, as the highest quartile of serum drug levels had the highest response, and no dose plateau has been reached. Given the best responses in phase 2 studies were at 10 mg/kg dosing, higher doses and higher serum trough levels may be needed to produce optimal responses to certolizumab.

Golimumab in Children

Golimumab is a fully human IgG antibody specific for TNF-α (Fig. 33.1a) that has approved indications in adults for the treatment of rheumatoid arthritis, psoriatic arthritis, ankylosing spondylitis, and ulcerative colitis. It is administered subcutaneously with bioavailability of approximately 53% [40]. Golimumab binds bioactive TNF-α, both membrane bound and soluble, and through inhibition of TNF-α reduces levels of several cytokines and inflammatory proteins such as IL-6 and C-reactive protein, with unclear contribution towards antibody, complement, and apoptotic cell lysis [68].

The Program of Ulcerative Colitis Research Study Utilizing an Investigational Treatment in Pediatrics Pharmacokinetics (PURSUIT-PEDS PK) Study Group presented abstracts at Advances in IBD in 2015 and DDW 2016 describing an open-label pharmacokinetic study of golimumab in pediatric patients with moderate to severe ulcerative colitis who had failed corticosteroids or immunomodulators but were anti-TNF-α naïve [69–71]. The induction dosing sequence was given at weeks 0, 2, and 6. Dosing was weight based and administered subcutaneously. Patients <45 kg were given 90 mg/m^2 for the initial dose, followed by 45 mg/m^2/dose thereafter, while those ≥45 kg were given 200 mg followed by 100 mg/dose. In this study, 35 patients achieved similar serum concentration to published adult data at weeks 2, 4, 6, and 14. By week 6 of induction, 60% had clinical response and 43% achieved clinical remission. By week 6, partial mucosal healing (Mayo endoscopy subscore 0 or 1) was achieved in 54% and complete healing (subscore 0) in 23%. Fifteen patients (43%) discontinued the drug prior to week 14, 12 of whom discontinued at week 6 for nonresponse. Severe adverse events were reported including exacerbation of disease (n = 10) and pancreatitis. Mild injection site reactions were reported in 6 (17%). There were no opportunistic infections. Three patients (9%) developed antibodies to golimumab by week 14.

A case series of golimumab therapy in six pediatric patients with Crohn's disease was recently published by Merras-Salmio et al. [72]. They describe six patients, all from one clinic in Helsinki, with moderate to severe Crohn's disease based on endoscopy 1–3 months prior to initiation of golimumab. All patients had previously been treated with infliximab or adalimumab, and five of the six had been initial responders to anti-TNF-α therapy. The interval between the last anti-TNF-α dose and the first golimumab dose ranged from 1 month to 4.5 years. Four of the six patients had undergone surgery (jejunal/ileal resection n = 2; colectomy n = 2). They noted that these patients were the most therapy-resistant cases of Crohn's disease in their clinic. All patients underwent the same induction with injections of 200 mg, 100 mg, and 50 mg given at 0, 2, and 6 weeks, respectively. All

patients noted a subjective benefit within a few days after the first dose, which was also objectively seen in acute phase reactants and fecal calprotectin. However, the response did not last, and all six patients required therapy escalation within 2 to 6 months of initiation of golimumab therapy. Four of the patients discontinued therapy due to lack of response within 1 year, with length of therapy ranging from 4 to 12 months. Two patients remained on golimumab with continued response at the time of the report, with total therapy time of 18–19 months. One patient was on 100 mg every 3 weeks and the other was one 50 mg every 2 weeks. All patients tolerated the injections well, and no adverse effects related to golimumab were reported [72].

There are no published studies of golimumab in JIA. However Brunner et al. presented an abstract describing a three-part double-blind placebo-controlled trial of patients treated with golimumab and concomitant methotrexate therapy, and then they were randomized to golimumab vs. placebo while continuing methotrexate [73]. They enrolled 173 patients aged 2–17 years with polyarticular JIA. After 48 weeks, they described serious adverse events (SAE) in 13% and serious infections in 3%. The most common SAE was exacerbation of JIA. The rate of serious infections with golimumab was reported to be 3.0 per 100 person-years [74].

Golimumab in Adults

The efficacy of golimumab in ulcerative colitis was established in the Program of Ulcerative Colitis Research Studies Utilizing an Investigational Treatment (PURSUIT) trials [75–77].

PURSUIT

The PURSUIT-SC and PURSUIT-IV were phase II/III randomized, double-blind, placebo-controlled, multicenter trials that assessed the efficacy of golimumab for induction therapy in patients with moderate to severe ulcerative colitis [75, 76]. The PURSUIT-IV trial study utilized intravenous golimumab in the treatment arm, while the PURSUIT-SC trial used subcutaneous golimumab. Patients enrolled in these studies had Mayo scores of 6–12, with an endoscopic subscore ≥2. Eligibility required that patients had failed therapy with one or more conventional therapies or were corticosteroid dependent and excluded patients who had previously been on anti-TNF therapy.

PURSUIT-IV, the intravenous dosing study, was ultimately assigned 291 patients randomized to receive one-time induction doses of 1 mg/kg, 2 mg/kg, or 4 mg/kg of golimumab intravenously or placebo [75]. Enrollment in the phase III portion was stopped due to lack of efficacy in the phase II portion, with 44.0% and 41.6% of the 2 mg/kg and 4 mg/kg groups, respectively, achieving clinical response compared to 30.1% for placebo at week 6 ($p = 0.081$ and 0.145, respectively). Clinical response was defined as Mayo score decrease from baseline $\geq$ 30% and $\geq$3 points, with rectal bleeding subscore of 0 or 1, or a decrease from baseline rectal bleeding score of $\geq$1.

PURSUIT-SC utilized subcutaneous dosing to evaluate 1064 adults with ulcerative colitis [76]. Enrollment criteria were the same as described above for PURSUIT-IV. Clinical response was again defined as Mayo score decrease from baseline $\geq$ 30% and $\geq$3 points, with rectal bleeding subscore of 0, or 1, or a decrease from baseline rectal bleeding score of $\geq$ 1. Remission was defined as Mayo score $\leq$ 2 with no individual subscore >1. Mucosal healing was defined as having an endoscopy subscore of 0 or 1. Initially, 169 adults were randomized to receive induction dosing at week 0 and week 2 of golimumab with doses of 100 mg/50 mg, 200 mg/100 mg, or 400 mg/200 mg, respectively, or placebo. Of these, 164 were analyzed for efficacy and the information was used for dose finding. One hundred and twenty-two additional patients were randomized using the same dosages, and data from this group were included in safety reports and analysis of pharmacokinetics. The 200 mg/100 mg and 400 mg/200 mg doses were selected based on these results for phase III development. In the phase III studies, 774 patients were randomized to receive golimumab at doses of 200 mg/100 mg or 400 mg/200 mg or placebo as induction therapy at week 0 and week 2, respectively. Seven hundred and sixty-one subjects were analyzed in the primary efficacy analysis. At week 6, the proportion of patients achieving clinical response was 51.0% for the 200 mg/100 mg group, 54.9% for the 400 mg/200 mg, and 30.3% of the placebo group ($p < 0.0001$ for both groups vs. placebo). Both treatment groups also achieved statistical significance vs. placebo for proportion of patients achieving clinical remission, mucosal healing, and IBDQ improvement from baseline. Based on this study, golimumab at induction doses of both 200 mg/100 mg and 400 mg/200 mg at week 0 and week 2 was established as efficacious therapy for adults with moderate to severe ulcerative colitis.

PURSUIT-M was a study of golimumab for maintenance therapy [77]. In this randomized, double-blind trial, the 464 patients who responded to golimumab induction from the prior PURSUIT trial were then randomized to receive placebo or golimumab at doses of 50 mg or 100 mg every 4 weeks through 52 weeks. Primary endpoint analysis was performed in 456 of the original 464 patients, with the primary endpoint being continued maintenance of clinical response (as defined in PURSUIT-SC) through week 54. This was achieved in 49.7% of the 100 mg treatment group and 47.0% of the 50 mg treatment group compared to 31.2% of the placebo group ($p < 0.001$ and $p = 0.010$, respectively).

Secondary endpoints in this trial were not unanimously significant for both treatment groups vs. placebo, but taken as a whole, this study indicates that golimumab is more effective than placebo for maintenance therapy in adults with ulcerative colitis who initially responded to induction therapy with golimumab.

Little data on the effects of golimumab drug levels on clinical or mucosal response is available, but anti-drug antibody rates are low, as 0.4% of patients assessed for antibodies were found to have antibodies to golimumab [76].

Safety Data

There are extensive safety data in adult studies and post-marketing surveillance studies of adults with IBD treated with anti-TNF therapies. One of the largest studies of adverse events associated with adalimumab therapy in adults is a long-term safety analysis by Burmester et al., which is summarized in Fig. 33.2 [78]. Adverse events with other anti-TNF therapies in adults are similar in type and in rate per patient-year. Pediatric-specific data are limited.

As the most often cited concerns regarding anti-TNF risks are cancer and infection, Dulai et al. performed a systematic review of the literature to quantify the incidence of serious infection, lymphoma, and death with anti-TNF therapy in children with Crohn's disease and ulcerative colitis [79]. They searched MEDLINE, Embase, Cochran Library, and Web of Knowledge through March 22, 2013. Any case series with less than five patients were excluded. They included 65 studies, with a total of 5528 patients and 9516 patient-years of follow-up (PYF), in their final analyses. The majority of studies reported on fewer than 100 patients and had a follow-up period shorter than 2 years. Eighty-four percent of the patients had Crohn's disease, 11% ulcerative colitis, and 5% indeterminate colitis. Ten percent of the patients with Crohn's disease were on adalimumab, the remainder of Crohn's disease, UC, and indeterminate colitis patients were on infliximab. They reported that among prospective studies, 16 of 294 patients on adalimumab developed serious infection during 545 PYF. This rate was similar to that seen in patients on infliximab. They reported 2 patients who developed lymphoma, both of whom had been on infliximab, yielding a rate of 2.1 per 10,000 PYF. They reported on seven patient deaths, two of which were believed to be unrelated to anti-TNF-α therapy. The remaining 5 yielded an absolute rate of 5.3 per 10,000 PYF. Two of the five had been on adalimumab, and both died from central-line-related sepsis while receiving parenteral nutrition.

Another systematic review of the efficacy and safety of adalimumab in pediatric Crohn's disease by Dziechciarz et al. was recently published [80]. They searched MEDLINE, EMBASE, the Cochrane Library, and abstracts from the

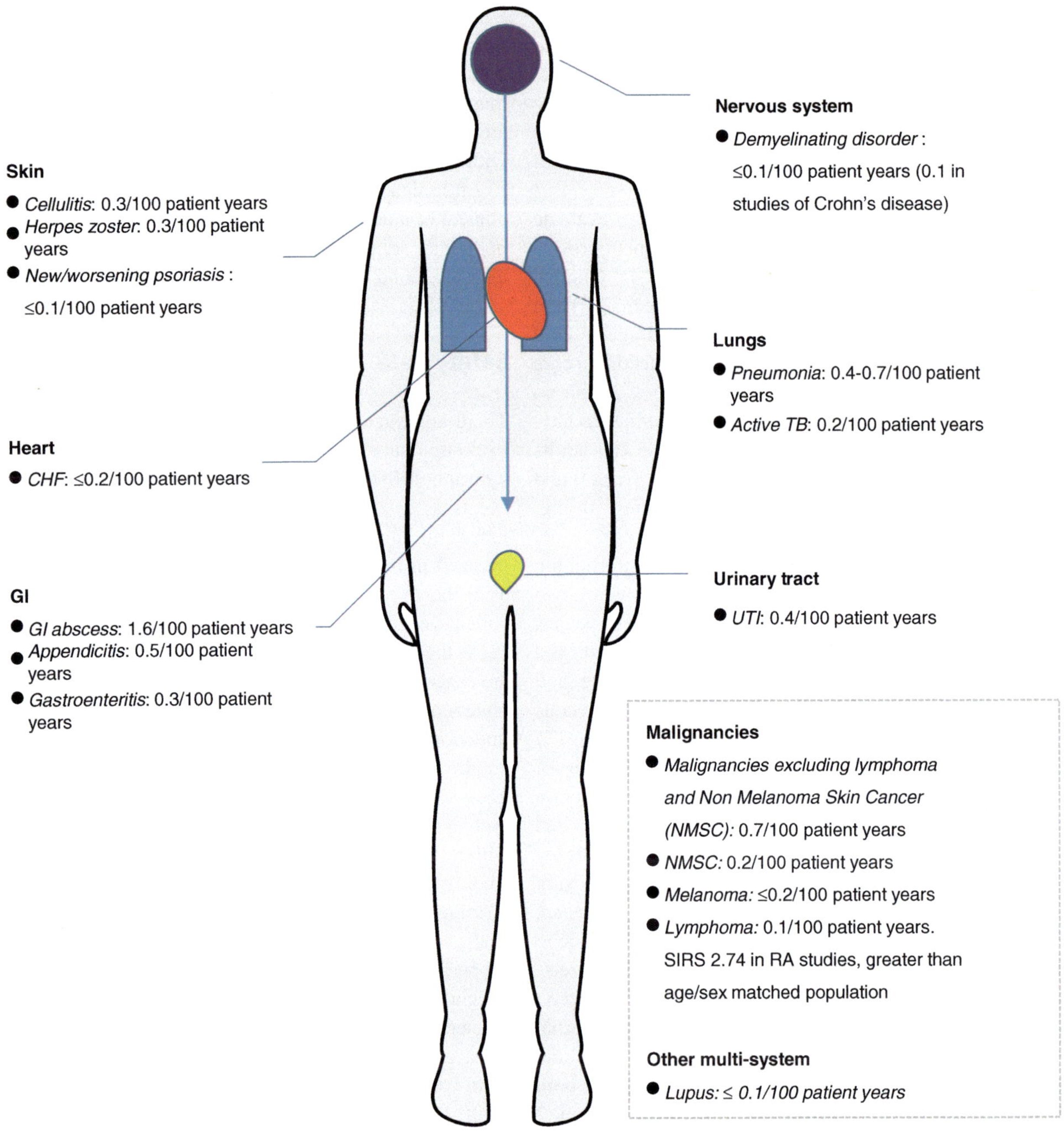

Skin

- *Cellulitis*: 0.3/100 patient years
- *Herpes zoster*: 0.3/100 patient years
- *New/worsening psoriasis* : ≤0.1/100 patient years

Heart

- *CHF*: ≤0.2/100 patient years

GI

- *GI abscess*: 1.6/100 patient years
- *Appendicitis*: 0.5/100 patient years
- *Gastroenteritis*: 0.3/100 patient years

Nervous system

- *Demyelinating disorder* : ≤0.1/100 patient years (0.1 in studies of Crohn's disease)

Lungs

- *Pneumonia*: 0.4-0.7/100 patient years
- *Active TB*: 0.2/100 patient years

Urinary tract

- *UTI*: 0.4/100 patient years

Malignancies

- *Malignancies excluding lymphoma and Non Melanoma Skin Cancer (NMSC)*: 0.7/100 patient years
- *NMSC*: 0.2/100 patient years
- *Melanoma*: ≤0.2/100 patient years
- *Lymphoma*: 0.1/100 patient years. SIRS 2.74 in RA studies, greater than age/sex matched population

Other multi-system

- *Lupus:* ≤ 0.1/100 patient years

[1] Adalimumab is the most studied of the three anti-TNFs covered in this chapter. The data shown is derived from a long term safety analysis of 23,458 patients (36,730.5 patient years) from clinical trials of adalimumab [Burmester, et. al]

[2] Adverse Event highlights [Burmester, et. al]:

- Most common serious AEs were infections
- Malignancies, excluding non-melanomatous skin cancer, were similar to that expected in the general population
- AE leading to death: ≤ 0.8/100 patient years
- Serious opportunistic infections: <0.1/100 patient years

[3] In a recent large meta-analysis, certolizumab was statistically more likely to cause a serious adverse event vs. placebo (OR 1.57), while adalumumab and golimumab were not [Singh et. al]

Fig. 33.2 Adverse events associated with anti-TNF biologics in adults based on long-term data with adalimumab and certolizumab[1–3]

main gastroenterology meetings from the past 5 years for randomized controlled trials (RCTs) or observational studies in children and adolescents with onset of Crohn's disease before the age of 18. Case series of less than five patients were not included. Eleven of the 14 articles included in the review reported on safety data, in 599 patients. Forty-nine percent of patients (n = 293/599) reported adverse effects, with infection (n = 162) and injection site reactions (n = 89) the most commonly cited. Other cited adverse events included arthralgia/myalgias (n = 7), xerosis (n = 6), abdominal pain (n = 5), headache (n = 5), nausea (n = 5), allergy (n = 4), depigmentation acne (n = 3), fever (n = 3), rash (n = 3), psoriasis (n = 2), tiredness (n = 2), tympanic membrane perforation (n = 1), dizziness (n = 1), hair loss (n = 1), dyspnea (n = 1), transient visual loss (n = 1), stomal bleeding (n = 1), itching (n = 1), and numbness (n = 1). Twelve percent (n = 69/599) reported serious adverse events, including death due to central-line sepsis (n = 2), medulloblastoma (n = 1), meningitis (n = 1), hematologic related AE (n = 24), allergic reactions (n = 10), hepatic related AE (n = 10), C. difficile infection (n = 2), perianal abscess (n = 2), anal abscess (n = 1), stomal abscess with fistula (n = 1), abdominal abscess (n = 3), colonic obstruction and abscess (n = 1), seton placement (n = 1), staphylococcus folliculitis (n = 1), scarlet fever (n = 1), disseminated histoplasmosis (n = 1), gastroenteritis (n = 1), H1N1 influenza (n = 1), viral infection (n = 1), and Yersinia infection (n = 1). One study cited a 35% (n = 64/182) withdrawal rate due to adverse events.

We found no additional studies reporting safety data for adalimumab in pediatric patients with inflammatory bowel disease that had not been included in either of these systematic reviews.

Comparative Effectiveness

Many authors have independently evaluated the efficacy of anti-TNF therapy in the treatment of inflammatory bowel disease [81–87]. In network meta-analyses (NMA) evaluating patients with Crohn's disease, infliximab, adalimumab, and certolizumab have all been found to be superior to placebo [82, 84]. These studies found trends toward superiority of infliximab relative to the other agents that did not reach significance [82, 84]. Additionally, one study found that when assessing the subcutaneous agents, adalimumab was superior to certolizumab for induction of remission [84].

Similarly, network meta-analysis of the anti-TNFs approved for ulcerative colitis have demonstrated that infliximab, adalimumab, and golimumab are all superior to placebo in measures of induction and maintenance of response and remission [81, 85, 86]. When taken as a whole, these studies also suggest that infliximab trends toward superiority to the other anti-TNF agents in the treatment of ulcerative

colitis [81, 85, 86]. Similar to the network meta-analysis of Crohn's disease, this value determination is based on trends as opposed to statistically significant findings or superiority that is only statistically significant in a subset of measures. Of note, one NMA that specifically evaluated golimumab vs. infliximab vs. adalimumab for the treatment of ulcerative colitis found that golimumab and infliximab are comparable in efficacy, with golimumab being superior to adalimumab for sustained outcomes and infliximab being superior to adalimumab in the period following induction [87].

While these data support the use of the anti-TNF biologics discussed in this chapter for Crohn's disease and ulcerative colitis, an important additional consideration is choosing an initial anti-TNF agent in the biological therapy-naïve patient. One large systematic review specifically looked at biologic-naïve patients with Crohn's disease and concluded that infliximab is numerically the most efficacious anti-TNF agent to initiate therapy in Crohn's disease [83]. In this study both infliximab and adalimumab (but not certolizumab) were more likely to induce remission than placebo, and no significant direct differentiation between agents was able to be made [83]. Similarly, a network meta-analysis comparing infliximab to adalimumab in anti-TNF-naïve patients with ulcerative colitis found that both were superior to placebo and that infliximab trended toward superiority to adalimumab for induction of remission, mucosal healing, and response at 8 weeks, but not statistically significantly different in these measures at 52 weeks [86].

References

1. Hu S, Liang S, Guo H, et al. Comparison of the inhibition mechanisms of adalimumab and infliximab in treating tumor necrosis factor alpha-associated diseases from a molecular view. J Biol Chem. 2013;288(38):27059–67.
2. Ben-Horin S, Waterman M, Kopylov U, et al. Addition of an immunomodulator to infliximab therapy eliminates antidrug antibodies in serum and restores clinical response of patients with inflammatory bowel disease. Clin Gastroenterol Hepatol. 2013;11(4):444–7.
3. Shen C, Assche GV, Colpaert S, et al. Adalimumab induces apoptosis of human monocytes: a comparative study with infliximab and etanercept. Aliment Pharmacol Ther. 2005;21(3):251–8.
4. Slevin SM, Egan LJ. New Insights into the Mechanisms of Action of Anti-tumor Necrosis Factor-Alpha Monoclonal Antibodies in Inflammatory Bowel Disease. Inflamm Bowel Dis. 2015;21(12):2909–20.
5. Rosh JR, Lerer T, Markowitz J, et al. Retrospective Evaluation of the Safety and Effect of Adalimumab Therapy (RESEAT) in pediatric Crohn's disease. Am J Gastroenterol. 2009;104(12):3042–9.
6. Turner D, Griffiths AM, Walters TD, et al. Mathematical weighting of the pediatric Crohn's disease activity index (PCDAI) and comparison with its other short versions. Inflamm Bowel Dis. 2012;18(1):55–62.
7. Hyams JS, Griffiths A, Markowitz J, et al. Safety and efficacy of adalimumab for moderate to severe Crohn's disease in children. Gastroenterology. 2012;143(2):365–74 e362.

8. Dubinsky MC, Rosh J, Faubion Jr WA, et al. Efficacy and Safety of Escalation of Adalimumab Therapy to Weekly Dosing in Pediatric Patients with Crohn's Disease. Inflamm Bowel Dis. 2016;22(4): 886–93.

9. Sharma S, Eckert D, Hyams JS, et al. Pharmacokinetics and exposure-efficacy relationship of adalimumab in pediatric patients with moderate to severe Crohn's disease: results from a randomized, multicenter, phase-3 study. Inflamm Bowel Dis. 2015;21(4): 783–92.

10. Cozijnsen M, Duif V, Kokke F, et al. Adalimumab therapy in children with Crohn disease previously treated with infliximab. J Pediatr Gastroenterol Nutr. 2015;60(2):205–10.

11. Hirai F, Watanabe K, Matsumoto T, et al. Patients' assessment of adalimumab self-injection for Crohn's disease: a multicenter questionnaire survey (The PEARL Survey). Hepatogastroenterology. 2014;61(134):1654–60.

12. Ayala RS, Groh BP, Robbins LM, Scalzi L, Bingham CA. The addition of injectable lidocaine to adalimumab results in decreased injection site pain and increased acceptance of therapy. Arthritis Rheum. 2008;58(9):S858–8..

13. den Broeder A, van de Putte L, Rau R, et al. A single dose, placebo controlled study of the fully human anti-tumor necrosis factor-alpha antibody adalimumab (D2E7) in patients with rheumatoid arthritis. J Rheumatol. 2002;29(11):2288–98.

14. Furst DE, Schiff MH, Fleischmann RM, et al. Adalimumab, a fully human anti tumor necrosis factor-alpha monoclonal antibody, and concomitant standard antirheumatic therapy for the treatment of rheumatoid arthritis: results of STAR (Safety Trial of Adalimumab in Rheumatoid Arthritis). J Rheumatol. 2003;30(12):2563–71.

15. Keystone EC, Kavanaugh AF, Sharp JT, et al. Radiographic, clinical, and functional outcomes of treatment with adalimumab (a human anti-tumor necrosis factor monoclonal antibody) in patients with active rheumatoid arthritis receiving concomitant methotrexate therapy: a randomized, placebo-controlled, 52-week trial. Arthritis Rheum. 2004;50(5):1400–11.

16. Mease PJ, Gladman DD, Ritchlin CT, et al. Adalimumab for the treatment of patients with moderately to severely active psoriatic arthritis: results of a double-blind, randomized, placebo-controlled trial. Arthritis Rheum. 2005;52(10):3279–89.

17. Rau R, Simianer S, van Riel PL, et al. Rapid alleviation of signs and symptoms of rheumatoid arthritis with intravenous or subcutaneous administration of adalimumab in combination with methotrexate. Scand J Rheumatol. 2004;33(3):145–53.

18. van de Putte LB, Atkins C, Malaise M, et al. Efficacy and safety of adalimumab as monotherapy in patients with rheumatoid arthritis for whom previous disease modifying antirheumatic drug treatment has failed. Ann Rheum Dis. 2004;63(5):508–16.

19. van de Putte LB, Rau R, Breedveld FC, et al. Efficacy and safety of the fully human anti-tumour necrosis factor alpha monoclonal antibody adalimumab (D2E7) in DMARD refractory patients with rheumatoid arthritis: a 12 week, phase II study. Ann Rheum Dis. 2003;62(12):1168–77.

20. van der Heijde D, Kivitz A, Schiff MH, et al. Efficacy and safety of adalimumab in patients with ankylosing spondylitis: results of a multicenter, randomized, double-blind, placebo-controlled trial. Arthritis Rheum. 2006;54(7):2136–46.

21. Weinblatt ME, Keystone EC, Furst DE, et al. Adalimumab, a fully human anti-tumor necrosis factor alpha monoclonal antibody, for the treatment of rheumatoid arthritis in patients taking concomitant methotrexate: the ARMADA trial. Arthritis Rheum. 2003;48(1): 35–45.

22. Weisman MH, Moreland LW, Furst DE, et al. Efficacy, pharmacokinetic, and safety assessment of adalimumab, a fully human anti-tumor necrosis factor-alpha monoclonal antibody, in adults with rheumatoid arthritis receiving concomitant methotrexate: a pilot study. Clin Ther. 2003;25(6):1700–21.

23. Colombel JF, Sandborn WJ, Rutgeerts P, et al. Adalimumab for maintenance of clinical response and remission in patients with Crohn's disease: the CHARM trial. Gastroenterology. 2007;132(1): 52–65.

24. Hanauer SB, Sandborn WJ, Rutgeerts P, et al. Human anti-tumor necrosis factor monoclonal antibody (adalimumab) in Crohn's disease: the CLASSIC-I trial. Gastroenterology. 2006;130(2):323–33. ; quiz 591

25. Sandborn WJ, Hanauer SB, Rutgeerts P, et al. Adalimumab for maintenance treatment of Crohn's disease: results of the CLASSIC II trial. Gut. 2007;56(9):1232–9.

26. Sandborn WJ, Rutgeerts P, Enns R, et al. Adalimumab induction therapy for Crohn disease previously treated with infliximab: a randomized trial. Ann Intern Med. 2007;146(12):829–38.

27. Rutgeerts P, Van Assche G, Sandborn WJ, et al. Adalimumab induces and maintains mucosal healing in patients with Crohn's disease: data from the EXTEND trial. Gastroenterology. 2012; 142(5):1102–11 e1102.

28. Savarino E, Bodini G, Dulbecco P, et al. Adalimumab is more effective than azathioprine and mesalamine at preventing postoperative recurrence of Crohn's disease: a randomized controlled trial. Am J Gastroenterol. 2013;108(11):1731–42.

29. Panaccione R, Colombel JF, Sandborn WJ, et al. Adalimumab maintains remission of Crohn's disease after up to 4 years of treatment: data from CHARM and ADHERE. Aliment Pharmacol Ther. 2013;38(10):1236–47.

30. Reinisch W, Sandborn WJ, Hommes DW, et al. Adalimumab for induction of clinical remission in moderately to severely active ulcerative colitis: results of a randomised controlled trial. Gut. 2011;60(6):780–7.

31. Sandborn WJ, van Assche G, Reinisch W, et al. Adalimumab induces and maintains clinical remission in patients with moderate-to-severe ulcerative colitis. Gastroenterology. 2012;142(2):257–65 e251–3.

32. Colombel JF, Sandborn WJ, Ghosh S, et al. Four-year maintenance treatment with adalimumab in patients with moderately to severely active ulcerative colitis: data from ULTRA 1, 2, and 3. Am J Gastroenterol. 2014;109(11):1771–80.

33. Best WR, Becktel JM, Singleton JW, Kern Jr F. Development of a Crohn's disease activity index. National Cooperative Crohn's Disease Study. Gastroenterology. 1976;70(3):439–44.

34. Panaccione R, Colombel JF, Sandborn WJ, et al. Adalimumab sustains clinical remission and overall clinical benefit after 2 years of therapy for Crohn's disease. Aliment Pharmacol Ther. 2010;31(12): 1296–309.

35. Daperno M, D'Haens G, Van Assche G, et al. Development and validation of a new, simplified endoscopic activity score for Crohn's disease: the SES-CD. Gastrointest Endosc. 2004;60(4): 505–12.

36. Mary JY, Modigliani R. Development and validation of an endoscopic index of the severity for Crohn's disease: a prospective multicentre study. Groupe d'Etudes Therapeutiques des Affections Inflammatoires du Tube Digestif (GETAID). Gut. 1989;30(7): 983–9.

37. Irvine EJ, Feagan B, Rochon J, et al. Quality of life: a valid and reliable measure of therapeutic efficacy in the treatment of inflammatory bowel disease. Canadian Crohn's Relapse Prevention Trial Study Group. Gastroenterology. 1994;106(2):287–96.

38. Hanauer SB, Korelitz BI, Rutgeerts P, et al. Postoperative maintenance of Crohn's disease remission with 6-mercaptopurine, mesalamine, or placebo: a 2-year trial. Gastroenterology. 2004;127(3): 723–9.

39. Schroeder KW, Tremaine WJ, Ilstrup DM. Coated oral 5-aminosalicylic acid therapy for mildly to moderately active ulcerative colitis. A randomized study. N Engl J Med. 1987;317(26): 1625–9.

40. Billioud V, Sandborn WJ, Peyrin-Biroulet L. Loss of response and need for adalimumab dose intensification in Crohn's disease: a systematic review. Am J Gastroenterol. 2011;106(4):674–84.

41. Bodini G, Giannini EG, Savarino EV, Savarino V. Adalimumab trough levels and response to biological treatment in patients with inflammatory bowel disease: a useful cutoff in clinical practice. Am J Gastroenterol. 2015;110(3):472–3.

42. Bodini G, Savarino V, Peyrin-Biroulet L, et al. Low serum trough levels are associated with post-surgical recurrence in Crohn's disease patients undergoing prophylaxis with adalimumab. Dig Liver Dis. 2014;46(11):1043–6.

43. Karmiris K, Paintaud G, Noman M, et al. Influence of trough serum levels and immunogenicity on long-term outcome of adalimumab therapy in Crohn's disease. Gastroenterology. 2009;137(5):1628–40.

44. Roblin X, Marotte H, Rinaudo M, et al. Association between pharmacokinetics of adalimumab and mucosal healing in patients with inflammatory bowel diseases. Clin Gastroenterol Hepatol. 2014; 12(1):80–4 e82.

45. Ungar B, Levy I, Yavne Y, et al. Optimizing anti-TNF-alpha Therapy: Serum Levels of Infliximab and Adalimumab Are Associated With Mucosal Healing in Patients With Inflammatory Bowel Diseases. Clin Gastroenterol Hepatol. 2016;14(4):550–7 e2.

46. Yarur AJ, Jain A, Hauenstein SI, et al. Higher Adalimumab Levels Are Associated With Histologic and Endoscopic Remission in Patients with Crohn's Disease and Ulcerative Colitis. Inflamm Bowel Dis. 2016;22(2):409–15.

47. Yarur AJ, Jain A, Sussman DA, et al. The association of tissue anti-TNF drug levels with serological and endoscopic disease activity in inflammatory bowel disease: the ATLAS study. Gut. 2016;65(2): 249–55.

48. Zittan E, Kabakchiev B, Milgrom R, et al. Higher Adalimumab Drug Levels are Associated with Mucosal Healing in Patients with Crohn's Disease. J Crohns Colitis. 2016;10(5):510–5.

49. Bodini G, Giannini EG, Furnari M, et al. Comparison of Two Different Techniques to Assess Adalimumab Trough Levels in Patients with Crohn's Disease. J Gastrointest Liver Dis. 2015; 24(4):451–6.

50. Frederiksen MT, Ainsworth MA, Brynskov J, Thomsen OO, Bendtzen K, Steenholdt C. Antibodies against infliximab are associated with de novo development of antibodies to adalimumab and therapeutic failure in infliximab-to-adalimumab switchers with IBD. Inflamm Bowel Dis. 2014;20(10):1714–21.

51. Roblin X, Rinaudo M, Del Tedesco E, et al. Development of an algorithm incorporating pharmacokinetics of adalimumab in inflammatory bowel diseases. Am J Gastroenterol. 2014;109(8): 1250–6.

52. Vande Casteele N, Ferrante M, Van Assche G, et al. Trough concentrations of infliximab guide dosing for patients with inflammatory bowel disease. Gastroenterology. 2015;148(7):1320–C e1323.

53. ClinicalTrials.gov. 2016; https://clinicaltrials.gov/ct2/show/NCT00 899678?term=certolizumab+NURTURE&rank=1. Accessed 7 Aug 2016.

54. Hussain SZ, Feagan BG, Samad A, Forget S, Sen DL, Lacroix BD. Use of Certolizumab Pegol in Children and Adolescents With Active Crohn's Disease: Pharmacokinetics Over 6 Weeks in the NURTURE Study. Gastroenterology. 2011;140(5):S265–5.

55. Tzaribachev N. Certolizumab pegol is effective in children with JIA not responsive to other TNF alpha antagonists. Ann Rheum Dis. 2013;71(Suppl 3):435.

56. Lichtenstein GR, Thomsen OO, Schreiber S, et al. Continuous therapy with certolizumab pegol maintains remission of patients with Crohn's disease for up to 18 months. Clin Gastroenterol Hepatol. 2010;8(7):600–9.

57. Sandborn WJ, Feagan BG, Stoinov S, et al. Certolizumab pegol for the treatment of Crohn's disease. N Engl J Med. 2007;357(3): 228–38.

58. Sandborn WJ, Schreiber S, Hanauer SB, et al. Reinduction with certolizumab pegol in patients with relapsed Crohn's disease: results from the PRECiSE 4 Study. Clin Gastroenterol Hepatol. 2010;8(8):696–702 e691.

59. Schreiber S, Khaliq-Kareemi M, Lawrance IC, et al. Maintenance therapy with certolizumab pegol for Crohn's disease. N Engl J Med. 2007;357(3):239–50.

60. Colombel JF, Sandborn WJ, Allez M, et al. Association between plasma concentrations of certolizumab pegol and endoscopic outcomes of patients with Crohn's disease. Clin Gastroenterol Hepatol. 2014;12(3):423–31 e421.

61. Hebuterne X, Lemann M, Bouhnik Y, et al. Endoscopic improvement of mucosal lesions in patients with moderate to severe ileocolonic Crohn's disease following treatment with certolizumab pegol. Gut. 2013;62(2):201–8.

62. Feagan BG, Sandborn WJ, Wolf DC, et al. Randomised clinical trial: improvement in health outcomes with certolizumab pegol in patients with active Crohn's disease with prior loss of response to infliximab. Aliment Pharmacol Ther. 2011;33(5):541–50.

63. Sandborn WJ, Abreu MT, D'Haens G, et al. Certolizumab pegol in patients with moderate to severe Crohn's disease and secondary failure to infliximab. Clin Gastroenterol Hepatol. 2010;8(8):688–95 e682.

64. Schreiber S, Rutgeerts P, Fedorak RN, et al. A randomized, placebo-controlled trial of certolizumab pegol (CDP870) for treatment of Crohn's disease. Gastroenterology. 2005;129(3):807–18.

65. Winter TA, Wright J, Ghosh S, Jahnsen J, Innes A, Round P. Intravenous CDP870, a PEGylated Fab' fragment of a humanized antitumour necrosis factor antibody, in patients with moderate-to-severe Crohn's disease: an exploratory study. Aliment Pharmacol Ther. 2004;20(11–12):1337–46.

66. Harvey RF, Bradshaw JM. A simple index of Crohn's-disease activity. Lancet. 1980;1(8167):514.

67. Sandborn WJ, Schreiber S, Feagan BG, et al. Certolizumab pegol for active Crohn's disease: a placebo-controlled, randomized trial. Clin Gastroenterol Hepatol. 2011;9(8):670–8 e673.

68. Shealy DJ, Cai A, Staquet K, et al. Characterization of golimumab, a human monoclonal antibody specific for human tumor necrosis factor alpha. MAbs. 2010;2(4):428–39.

69. Hyams J, Griffiths A, Veereman G, et al. A Multicenter Open-Label Study Assessing Pharmacokinetics, Efficacy, and Safety of Subcutaneous Golimumab in Pediatric Subjects with Moderately-Severely Active Ulcerative Colitis. Inflamm Bowel Dis. 2016; 22:S39–40.

70. Hyams JS, Griffiths AM, Veereman G, et al. A Multicenter Open-Label Study Assessing Pharmacokinetics, Efficacy, And Safety Of Subcutaneous Golimumab In Pediatric Subjects With Moderately-Severely Active Ulcerative Colitis. Gastroenterology. 2016;150(4): S-132.

71. Adedokun OJ, Chan D, Padgett L, et al. Pharmacokinetics and Exposure-Response Relationships of Golimumab in Pediatric Patients With Moderate to Severe Ulcerative Colitis: Results From a Multicenter Open Label Study. Gastroenterology. 2016;150(4): S-590.

72. Merras-Salmio L, Kolho KL. Golimumab Therapy in Six Patients with Severe Pediatric Onset Crohn's Disease. J Pediatr Gastroenterol Nutr. 2016;63(3):344–7.

73. Brunner HI, Ruperto N, Tzaribachev N, et al. A Multi-Center, Double-Blind, Randomized-Withdrawal Trial of Subcutaneous Golimumab in Pediatric Patients with Active Polyarticular Course Juvenile Idiopathic Arthritis Despite Methotrexate Therapy: Week 48 Results. Arthritis Rheumatol. 2014;66:S414–5.

74. Horneff G. Biologic-associated infections in pediatric rheumatology. Curr Rheumatol Rep. 2015;17(11):66.

75. Rutgeerts P, Feagan BG, Marano CW, et al. Randomised clinical trial: a placebo-controlled study of intravenous golimumab induc-

tion therapy for ulcerative colitis. Aliment Pharmacol Ther. 2015;42(5):504–14.

76. Sandborn WJ, Feagan BG, Marano C, et al. Subcutaneous golimumab induces clinical response and remission in patients with moderate-to-severe ulcerative colitis. Gastroenterology. 2014; 146(1):85–95. ; quiz e14–85

77. Sandborn WJ, Feagan BG, Marano C, et al. Subcutaneous golimumab maintains clinical response in patients with moderate-to-severe ulcerative colitis. Gastroenterology. 2014;146(1):96–109 e101.

78. Burmester GR, Panaccione R, Gordon KB, McIlraith MJ, Lacerda APM. Ann Rheum Dis. 2013;72(4):517–24.

79. Dulai PS, Thompson KD, Blunt HB, Dubinsky MC, Siegel CA. Risks of serious infection or lymphoma with anti-tumor necrosis factor therapy for pediatric inflammatory bowel disease: a systematic review. Clin Gastroenterol Hepatol: the official clinical practice journal of the American Gastroenterological Association. 2014; 12(9):1443–51. quiz e1488-1449

80. Dziechciarz P, Horvath A, Kierkus J. Efficacy and safety of adalimumab for pediatric Crohn's disease: a systematic review. J Crohns Colitis. 2016;10(10):1237–44.

81. Danese S, Fiorino G, Peyrin-Biroulet L, et al. Biological agents for moderately to severely active ulcerative colitis: a systematic review and network meta-analysis. Ann Intern Med. 2014;160(10):704–11.

82. Hazlewood GS, Rezaie A, Borman M, et al. Comparative effectiveness of immunosuppressants and biologics for inducing and maintaining remission in Crohn's disease: a network meta-analysis. Gastroenterology. 2015;148(2):344–54 e345. ; quiz e314-345

83. Singh S, Garg SK, Pardi DS, Wang Z, Murad MH, Loftus Jr EV. Comparative efficacy of biologic therapy in biologic-naive patients with Crohn disease: a systematic review and network meta-analysis. Mayo Clin Proc. 2014;89(12):1621–35.

84. Stidham RW, Lee TC, Higgins PD, et al. Systematic review with network meta-analysis: the efficacy of anti-TNF agents for the treatment of Crohn's disease. Aliment Pharmacol Ther. 2014; 39(12):1349–62.

85. Stidham RW, Lee TC, Higgins PD, et al. Systematic review with network meta-analysis: the efficacy of anti-tumour necrosis factor-alpha agents for the treatment of ulcerative colitis. Aliment Pharmacol Ther. 2014;39(7):660–71.

86. Thorlund K, Druyts E, Mills EJ, Fedorak RN, Marshall JK. Adalimumab versus infliximab for the treatment of moderate to severe ulcerative colitis in adult patients naive to anti-TNF therapy: an indirect treatment comparison meta-analysis. J Crohns Colitis. 2014;8(7):571–81.

87. Thorlund K, Druyts E, Toor K, Mills EJ. Comparative efficacy of golimumab, infliximab, and adalimumab for moderately to severely active ulcerative colitis: a network meta-analysis accounting for differences in trial designs. Expert Rev Gastroenterol Hepatol. 2015;9(5):693–700.

Therapeutic Drug Monitoring in Pediatric Inflammatory Bowel Disease

Namita Singh and Marla C. Dubinsky

Introduction

A key management strategy in the care of inflammatory bowel disease (IBD) patients includes maximizing the efficacy of IBD medications while minimizing their toxicity. The recognition of factors leading to a therapeutic response and remission allows for individualized dosing regimens to meet these goals. Standard dosing of immunomodulator and anti-TNF therapy is often insufficient giving inter-patient variability with regard to response and tolerability. Therapeutic drug monitoring (TDM) is a concept worth understanding in order to optimize drug efficacy with the goal of achieving a sustained and durable remission. The concept of dose optimization initially started over a decade ago with the use of thiopurines and is now utilized with antitumor necrosis factor (TNF) therapies. Given the limited number of approved medications available for young patients with IBD and the need for durable treatment strategies, TDM is an invaluable tool to guide treatment decisions. This chapter will review the historical and current utilization of TDM, as well as the accompanying challenges, in treating pediatric patients with IBD.

Thiopurine Monitoring

Thiopurine S-methyltransferase (TPMT) and thiopurine metabolite levels are measured in current clinical practice to help manage IBD patients receiving thiopurines, including 6-mercaptopurine (6-MP) and azathioprine (AZA). 6-MP

and its prodrug, AZA, undergo intestinal and hepatic metabolism by numerous enzymes including hypoxanthine phosphoribosyltransferase (HPRT), TPMT, xanthine oxidase (XO), and inosine monophosphate dehydrogenase (IMPDH), to produce the active metabolites, 6-thioguanine nucleotides (6-TGN) and 6-methylmercaptopurine ribonucleotides (6-MMP) [1] (Fig. 34.1). Through the study of these enzymes and metabolites, the mechanisms of drug efficacy and toxicity have been well described [2].

Prior to initiating a thiopurine, obtaining a TPMT level is considered a standard practice, as this determines the starting dose for an individual patient. For the majority (89%) of patients with a normal TPMT level, standard initial dosing is 2.5 mg/kg/day of AZA or 1.5 mg/kg/day of 6-MP. For the 10% of patients who are heterozygote for the TPMT gene, known as intermediate metabolizers, the clinician should prescribe half the standard dose to minimize high 6-TGN levels and the risks including leukopenia. In patients who are homozygote for the TPMT gene (1 in 300), thiopurines are contraindicated given the risk of life-threatening leukopenia [3]. TPMT-guided dosing avoids subtherapeutic use, as knowledge of TPMT activity identifies the variability in metabolism, improving clinician confidence in dosing selection.

TPMT levels drive initial dosing, yet 6-TGN and 6-MMP metabolites influence the subsequent efficacy and safety. In 1996, Cuffari et al. showed that higher 6-TGN metabolite concentrations correlate with clinical remission in pediatric Crohn's disease (CD) patients [4]. Subsequent pediatric studies demonstrated that the therapeutic response doubled in patients whose 6-TGN levels were >235 pmol/8 × 10(8) RBC (78% vs. 41%, $p < 0.001$) [5]. The odds of responding to thiopurines was five times higher in patients with 6-TGN levels >235 pmol/8 × 10(8) RBC, as compared to those below this therapeutic threshold [5]. A 6-TGN level of 235 pmol/8 × 10(8) RBC has been supported as a cut point in other pediatric and adult studies, and a meta-analysis also reported that patients with 6-TGN concentrations above this threshold had a

N. Singh, MD (✉)
Pediatric IBD Center at Cedars-Sinai Medical Center,
Los Angeles, CA, USA

David Geffen School of Medicine at UCLA,
Los Angeles, CA, USA
e-mail: Namita.Singh@cshs.org

M.C. Dubinsky, MD
Icahn School of Medicine at Mount Sinai, New York, NY, USA

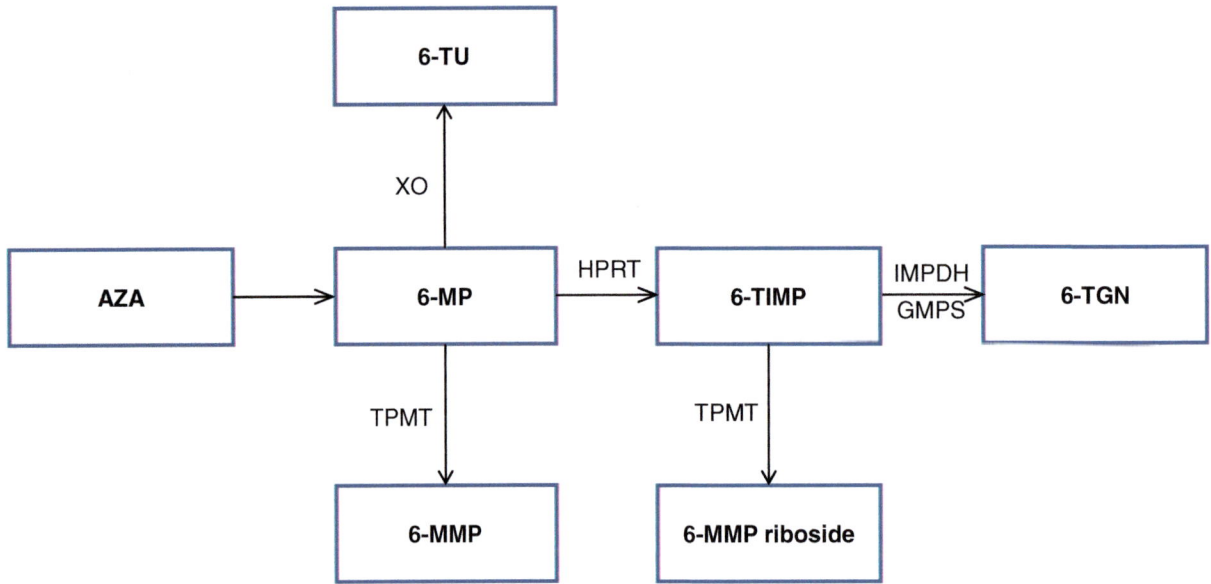

AZA, azathioprine; GMPS, guanosine monophosphate synthetase; HPRT, hypoxanthine phosphoribosyltransferase; IMPDH, inosine monophosphate dehydrogenase; 6-MMP, -methylmercaptopurine; 6-MP, 6-mercaptopurine; 6-TG, 6-thioguanine; 6-TIMP, 6-thioinosine monophosphate; TPMT, thiopurine *S*-methyltransferase; 6-TU, 6-thiouricacid; XO, xanthineoxidase

Fig. 34.1 Azathioprine/6-mercaptopurine metabolism pathways. *AZA* azathioprine, *GMPS* guanosine monophosphate synthetase, *HPRT* hypoxanthine phosphoribosyltransferase, *IMPDH* inosine monophosphate dehydrogenase, *6-MMP* 6-methylmercaptopurine, *6-MP* 6-mercaptopurine, *6-TG* 6-thioguanine, *6-TIMP* 6-thioinosine monophosphate, *TPMT* thiopurine S-methyltransferase, *6-TU* 6-thiouric acid, *XO* xanthine oxidase

threefold increased odds of being in remission than those below this threshold (62% vs. 36%; pooled odds ratio 3.3, 95% confidence interval, 1.7–6.3; $p < 0.001$) [6–9]. In a patient not clinically responding to standard thiopurine dosing, obtaining a 6-TGN and 6-MMP level could be useful to ensure therapeutic dosing. If 6-TGN levels are < 235 pmol/8 × 10(8) RBC, dose escalation is warranted; if therapeutic (235–400 pmol/8 × 10(8) RBC) levels are noted, switching to a non-thiopurine therapy might be reasonable.

Leukopenia is the most concerning toxicity associated with the use of thiopurines. This is most commonly attributable to high 6-TGN metabolite levels. Patients that are homozygous deficient for TPMT polymorphisms are most at risk of thiopurine-related myelosuppression. Colombel et al., however, reported that only one-third of myelosuppression cases were secondary to a low TPMT activity, indicating other factors contributing to leukopenia, such as effects of concomitant medications and secondary viral infections (EBV, CMV, parvovirus) [10]. It is unclear what 6-TGN level is considered "too high"; however, a level >400 pmol/8 × 10(8) RBC has been suggested as the cut point which clinicians should avoid [11].

Hepatotoxicity is another risk with thiopurine use, with some studies associating it with 6-MMP concentrations above 5700 pmol/8 × 10(8) RBC ($p < 0.05$) [5, 11]. If a patient has a therapeutic 6-TGN level with a 6-MMP level >5700 pmol/8 × 10(8) RBC and normal liver enzymes, more frequent clinical monitoring of liver enzymes is indicated, rather than a reflexive thiopurine dose decrease. If a patient, however, has both a high 6-TGN level (>400 pmol/8 × 10(8) RBC) *and* 6-MMP level (>5700 pmol/8 × 10(8) RBC), then dose de-escalation should be considered in order to minimize the risk of leukopenia and hepatotoxicity. Perhaps the most important application of high 6-MMP levels is in the patient who also has a low 6-TGN level, with subsequent dose escalation resulting in decreasing 6-TGN and increasing 6-MMP [12]. This group has been defined as being "thiopurine-resistant," or "6-MMP preferential metabolizers," and such patients would benefit from changing to another class of medication, such as methotrexate or biologic therapy. The proposed use of allopurinol in these patients to reverse the metabolism to favor more 6-TGN, and less 6-MMP may carry additional toxicity risks with relation to leukopenia but has been shown to be an effective strategy [13]. The understanding of the importance of thiopurine drug monitoring paved the way for applying the TDM concept to other IBD therapies, more specifically anti-TNF agents.

Anti-TNF Drug Concentrations

Only recently have studies examined the durability of anti-TNF agents and their pharmacokinetic (pk) profiles, despite their having being approved since 1998 in adults and 2006 in pediatric patients. Most studies have examined infliximab (IFX), with evolving literature for the other anti-TNF agents, including adalimumab, certolizumab pegol (CZP), and a paucity of data with golimumab.

Although the response to IFX induction is highly successful in 75–90% of pediatric IBD patients, maintenance of a sustained and durable remission can be more challenging [14, 15]. In the REACH trial, only 60% of pediatric CD patients who responded to induction were in remission at 1 year, and half of these patients required dose modification after losing response [14]. In a meta-analysis of adult IBD patients on IFX, 23–46% required dose escalation and 5–13% discontinued the drug at 1 year [16]. Using TDM, one can better understand the etiology of primary nonresponse and secondary loss of response, and TDM may augment clinical management by increasing the likelihood of sustained response to therapy.

In 2003, initial studies found higher serum IFX concentrations to be correlated with longer duration of response [17]. It was reported in 2006 that detectable serum IFX concentrations were associated with a higher rate of clinical remission, endoscopic improvement, and lower CRP values in CD patients [18]. Other studies also support that detectable IFX concentrations are predictive of a sustained response in CD patients [19]. In UC, the data is just as strong, with detectable IFX concentrations associated with higher remission rates, endoscopic improvement, and a significant decrease in colectomy risk (55% vs. 7%, OR 9.3; 95% CI 2.9–29.9; $p < 0.001$) [20]. In the post hoc analysis of the ACT trials, higher IFX concentrations in UC patients were associated with an increased likelihood of achieving clinical remission and mucosal healing with increasing quartiles of IFX levels [21]. Patients with drug levels in the third or fourth quartile had remission rates at week 30 closer to 60% as compared to those in the second quartile whose remission rates were 25%. Similarly, studies have found that higher adalimumab concentrations correspond to mucosal healing and clinical remission, higher CZP concentrations in CD patients are associated with endoscopic remission and response, and higher golimumab concentrations were associated with clinical remission [22–24].

The minimum anti-TNF trough concentration associated with improved outcomes remains debatable. Murthy et al. demonstrated that an IFX concentration of >2 µg/mL in UC patients was associated with a higher rate of corticosteroid-free remission, compared to a trough concentration of <2 µg/mL (69% vs. 16%; $p < 0.001$) [25]. A trough concentration >3 µg/mL during IFX maintenance therapy has been shown by Vande Casteele et al. to be independently associated with a lower CRP and has been proposed as a cutoff to improve outcomes [26]. More studies suggest that yet even higher IFX trough drug concentrations at week 14, the time of the first maintenance dose, are associated with better 1-year efficacy outcomes (≥3.5 µg/mL to >5 µg/mL) [27, 28].

Differing cutoffs have also been suggested for adalimumab concentrations. Velayos et al. found that an adalimumab concentration of >5 µg/mL was associated with decreased CRP level; Yarur et al. confirmed this association [29, 30]. Karmiris et al. suggested an even higher therapeutic threshold of >8 mg/ml [31]. For CZP, in the post hoc analysis of the WELCOME trial, evaluating induction therapy of CZP in 203 patients, remission rates were higher among patients whose CZP concentration fell within the two highest quartiles during induction at weeks 0, 2, 4, and 6 (27.5 to 33.8 µg/ml and ≥33.8 µg/ml, respectively); thus, a CZP concentration of >27.5 µg/ml has been proposed for clinical use [32]. For golimumab, patients with drug concentrations in the highest quartile with a concentration of >3.1 µg/ml had higher rates of clinical remission at 30 and 54 weeks when compared to the lower quartiles [24].

Anti-TNF Drug Antibodies and Outcomes

Despite a high primary response rate to the anti-TNF agents, two-thirds of patients losing response do so within the first year [16]. The loss of response to anti-TNF agents is most often due to an individual's unique physiologic profile driven by drug clearance – factors that influence drug clearance include a low serum albumin concentration, high baseline CRP levels, large body size, male sex, and high degree of systemic inflammation [33]. Additionally, the development of antidrug antibodies (ADAs), referred to as immunogenicity, remains a significant driver of loss of response. It should be noted that non-chimeric anti-TNF therapies have the same issues with ADA formation as chimeric anti-TNF agents [34]. The presence of ADA increases the clearance of the drug, resulting in lower drug concentrations. This, in turn, results in shorter duration of response, which has been demonstrated in multiple studies [17, 18, 22, 33, 35–38]. In a prospective study of patients receiving IFX therapy, ATI development preceded clinical loss of response in over half of patients [39]. Similar results have been reported with adalimumab, with 20% of patients developing anti-adalimumab antibodies, which predicted biochemical and clinical loss of response [40]. Another study also confirmed the association of anti-adalimumab antibodies with increased markers of inflammation and with clinical indices indicating increased disease activity [41]. Antibodies to certolizumab were also found to be associated with reduced remission rates through week 26 in the PRECISE-2 trial (71 vs 62%), with similar findings in the WELCOME trial [42, 43]. In addition to the negative effect ADAs have on efficacy, they also increase toxicity, with the example of anti-infliximab-antibodies (ATIs) being associated with infusion reactions [36]. Additionally, a recent pediatric study found that the presence of ATIs was a predictor of lower IFX concentrations and a higher risk of surgery [44].

Recent data demonstrate that ATIs may be transient. Vande Casteele et al. retrospectively found that in 28% of patients' ATIs disappeared over time, whereas they were sustained in 72% of patients [38]. It is unclear whether lower concentrations of ATI may be overcome by IFX dose escalation. However, Vande Casteele's study suggested that higher ATI concentrations of >9.1 U/ml were less likely to be overcome, with a likelihood ratio of 3.6 of failure [38], and thus such patients should be changed to another anti-TNF therapy.

The knowledge of the presence of ADA is also important in the setting of re-induction of anti-TNF therapies after a prolonged interruption or "drug holiday." Baert et al. reported that the presence of ATI 2 weeks after the first re-induction dose of IFX was associated with lower response rates and higher rates of infusion reactions [45]. The data suggest that if a patient has discontinued IFX for at least 6 months, it is important to check for the presence of ATIs prior to administering the second induction dose. It remains unclear whether, following a drug holiday, a patient should be re-induced with the standard initial induction regimen (0, 2, 6 weeks) or forego re-induction and resume with every 8-week interval.

The reported rates of ADA are entirely dependent on the specific assay used to measure ADA. Several techniques are available for measuring anti-TNF concentrations and ADA. Thus, comparison of results from different assays should be performed with caution, as there remains no standardization between different assays. Drug concentrations are generally detected sensitively between assay types, yet the detection and accurate quantification of ADAs have been more challenging. First-generation assays, such as the enzyme-linked immunosorbent assay (ELISA), have less clinical utility, given the lower sensitivity for measuring ADAs. Using the ELISA assay, serum anti-TNF drug competes with the ADA detection moiety, and thus when drug is detected in the sample, ADA is unable to be accurately measured. Radioimmune assay (RIA) is sensitive and specific for drug and ADA detection, yet disadvantages include the complexity of the test, prolonged incubation time, expense, and the handling of radioactive materials [46, 47]. The homogenous mobility shift assay (HMSA), using high-performance liquid chromatography, has the advantage of separating and quantifying the drug and antibody concentrations independently, making it feasible to detect ADAs in the presence of anti-TNF drug. ELISA and ELISA-like assays (LabCorp, Esoterix Inc) as well as HMSA assays (Prometheus labs) are currently commercially available for IFX and adalimumab.

Given the negative effects of ADA on therapeutic efficacy, durability, and association with infusion reactions, attempts should be made to reduce the likelihood of ADA formation. Various strategies have been recommended in order to do so, such as the addition of an immunomodulator and even proactive optimization of drug concentrations.

Immunomodulator Use with Anti-TNF Agents

In the ACCENT 1 trial, concomitant immunomodulator use with IFX was associated with lower rates of ATI formation [48]. In another prospective CD cohort, patients who received concomitant immunomodulator therapy had higher IFX concentrations and less likelihood of ATI formation than those not receiving a concomitant immunomodulator (43% vs. 75%; $p < 0.01$) [17]. A logistic regression analysis further demonstrated that the only significant variable predictive of IFX concentrations was the use of a concomitant immunosuppressive agent ($p < 0.001$) [17]. The SONIC trial demonstrated that combination therapy of IFX with AZA is superior to IFX monotherapy in achieving clinical remission and mucosal healing [37]. This is potentially due to less formation of antibodies and higher trough levels associated with combination therapy. Likewise, patients receiving an immunomodulator in combination with adalimumab have been noted to have higher drug concentrations than those on monotherapy [30]. Additionally, with golimumab therapy, patients receiving a concomitant immunomodulator had a lower incidence of antibody formation (1.1% vs 3.8% $p = 0.01$) [24].

Studies also suggest that addition of concomitant immunomodulator can help recapture response for patients with low anti-TNF drug concentrations. Ben Horin et al. reported in a small case series that the addition of an immunomodulator to maintenance infliximab monotherapy increased IFX concentrations and lowered antibody concentrations, improving patient outcomes by restoring clinical response [49]. Other small studies have shown that the addition of a thiopurine in patients losing response to anti-TNF monotherapy was an effective strategy to recapture response [50]. Overall, these studies suggest that concomitant immunomodulator use not only decreases immunogenicity preemptively as suggested by SONIC but may also augment recapture of response in patients with low drug concentrations.

In pediatric patients, particularly in males, the substitution of methotrexate (MTX) for thiopurines may provide a safety advantage, given the rare yet positive association between combination therapy of IFX with thiopurines and malignancy, including hepatosplenic T-cell lymphoma. The efficacy of combining an anti-TNF agent with methotrexate (MTX) has been examined as well. In the rheumatoid arthritis literature, a low dose of 7.5 mg weekly was associated with lower rates of ATI development in IFX-treated patients [51]. In a cohort of pediatric IBD patients, concomitant MTX use for at least 6 months was found to be associated with increase of IFX durability, with those on MTX with IFX for >6 months having a higher 5-year probability of remaining on IFX than those without concomitant MTX use (0.97 ± 0.03 vs. 0.41 ± 0.11, $p < 0.001$) [52]. The dose of methotrexate varied, with no clear dose threshold identified. In another pediatric study, no clinical benefit in IFX durability or efficacy was found when using very low-dose oral MTX (<10 mg/week) as concomitant therapy in pediatric IBD patients [53]. It has been proposed that a dose of at least 12.5 mg of oral MTX is needed to avoid immunogenicity. The COMMIT trial found that patients on IFX combination therapy with 25 mg of weekly subcutaneous MTX were significantly less likely to develop ATIs and had higher IFX concentrations, yet no clear benefit was found in inducing and maintaining clinical remission [54]. A German group found that concomitant use of MTX with infliximab had a positive effect in the treatment of refractory CD adult patients, using a MTX dose of 20 mg weekly, either parenterally or orally administered [55]. The ideal dose of MTX remains unclear, with suggestions of using a dose of 12.5–15 mg orally weekly.

Proactive Dose Optimization

Perhaps the most important utilization of TDM is proactively preventing the loss of response, rather than awaiting a treatment failure. This can be accomplished by dose adjusting early in the treatment course. Researchers have attempted to determine whether a drug concentration obtained early in maintenance is a predictor of a more durable response. Bortlik et al. found that, on retrospective evaluation, an IFX cut point of greater than 3 µg/mL at either the week 14 or week 22 dose was predictive of a sustained response [19]. Vande Casteele et al. described that low IFX concentrations at 14 weeks (<2.2 µg/ml) predicted IFX discontinuation due to persistent loss of response and was associated with increased incidence of ATIs [38]. In a recent post hoc analysis of ACCENT 1, patients with post-induction week 14 IFX concentrations of ≥3.5 µg/mL and a ≥60% CRP decrease were significantly associated with durable sustained response at week 54 [28]. Using a cohort of pediatric IBD patients, Singh et al. were the first to prospectively determine the optimal cut point for a week 14 IFX trough concentration in predicting 1-year durable remission. In this study, a concentration of at least 5.5 µg/mL was described as optimal ($p = 0.01$) [27]. Recently, using

a cohort of pediatric IBD patients on IFX therapy, Stein et al. found that IFX concentrations of ≥9.1 µg/mL at week 10 was found to be predictive of continuing IFX at 12 months, with a sensitivity of 80% and specificity of 60% [56].

Given the growing body of literature supporting the role of TDM, prospective trials using TDM-based dose adjustment have been performed. The TAXIT trial showed that proactive dose adjustments, maintaining a IFX concentration between 3 and 7 µg/mL, resulted in improved disease activity, even in patients who were seemingly responding favorably to therapy. Additionally, up to 30% of the TAXIT patients may be able to have their IFX dose de-escalated without clinical loss of response, again suggesting a cost-saving potential of proactive, individualized TDM [57]. Another recent study demonstrated that proactive dose adjustment using TDM, keeping IFX drug concentrations between 5 and 10 µg/mL, was associated with sustained remission as compared to those with concentrations lower than 5 µg/mL or without TDM monitoring [58].

Practical Use of TDM

TDM is integral to treating IBD patients on anti-TNF therapy. It may more readily establish the mechanism for loss of response or lack of response, and allow the clinician to appropriately tailor therapy for the individual patient. It is important that IFX and ATI be evaluated in the context of each other and thus that a drug-tolerant assay is used. Our suggested guideline for TDM in a patient on IFX therapy is outlined in Fig. 34.2.

In a patient with a therapeutic IFX concentration and no ATI present, ongoing therapy should continue if in remission; if remission is not ultimately achieved despite therapeutic IFX concentrations and lack of ATI, that patient is likely a nonresponder to the anti-TNF class of medications, and changing to another class of medications should be considered. If a patient is in deep remission and therapeutic IFX concentrations with low ATI is present (ATI <9.1 µg/mL [38]), attempt should be made to overcome the low ATI and stay on drug.

In a patient with low or undetectable IFX concentrations without ATI, optimizing IFX dose by escalating therapy is warranted and may prevent development of ATI. In a patient with low/undetectable IFX concentrations and high ATI, if that patient has prior anti-TNF response, then switching to another anti-TNF agent is indicated. However, if no response to anti-TNF therapy has been evidenced, switching out of class would best serve the patient. With low/undetectable IFX and low ATI, options would be to dose escalate and add an immunomodulator to overcome low ATI or to entirely switch out of class. With each change, if staying within class, TDM should be repeated after 2–3 infusions, once reaching a drug steady state.

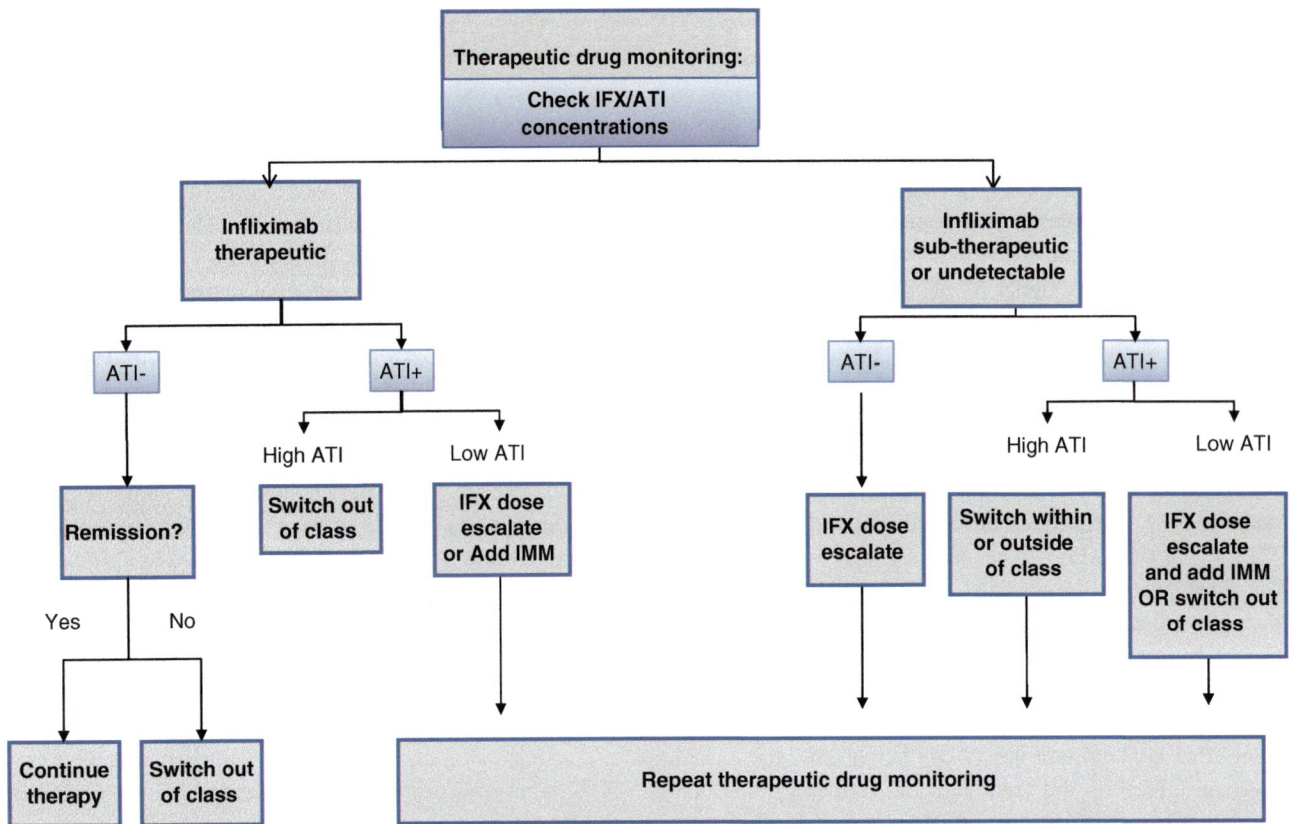

ATI anti-infliximab antibody; IFX infliximab; IMM immunomodulator

Fig. 34.2 Utilizing therapeutic drug monitoring (IFX). *ATI* anti-infliximab antibody, *IFX* infliximab, *IMM* immunomodulator

Conclusion

The body of evidence correlating serum anti-TNF drug and ADA concentrations to clinical outcomes is growing, and the value of TDM is now increasingly recognized. The use of TDM allows clinicians to gain insight into the etiology of loss of response and enables the optimization of therapy for an individual patient. With increasing prospective studies on TDM of anti-TNF therapies, new algorithms will be developed with the goal of achieving a sustained, durable remission on these therapies. Issues related to TDM, including clearance and immunogenicity, are not unique to anti-TNF therapies, and these concepts will be applicable to other biologics used in IBD patients. In this era of personalized medicine, TDM allows for optimized, individualized dosing, and improved care for IBD patients of all ages.

References

1. Lennard L. The clinical pharmacology of 6-mercaptopurine. Eur J Clin Pharmacol. 1992;43(4):329–39.
2. de Boer NK, van Bodegraven AA, Jharap B, de Graaf P, Mulder CJ. Drug Insight: pharmacology and toxicity of thiopurine therapy in patients with IBD. Nat Clin Pract Gastroenterol Hepatol. 2007;4(12):686–94.
3. Weinshilboum RM, Sladek SL. Mercaptopurine pharmacogenetics: monogenic inheritance of erythrocyte thiopurine methyltransferase activity. Am J Hum Genet. 1980;32(5):651–62.
4. Cuffari C, Theoret Y, Latour S, Seidman G. 6-Mercaptopurine metabolism in Crohn's disease: correlation with efficacy and toxicity. Gut. 1996;39(3):401–6.
5. Dubinsky MC, Lamothe S, Yang HY, et al. Pharmacogenomics and metabolite measurement for 6-mercaptopurine therapy in inflammatory bowel disease. Gastroenterology. 2000;118(4):705–13.
6. Pozler O, Chladek J, Maly J, et al. Steady-state of azathioprine during initiation treatment of pediatric inflammatory bowel disease. J Crohns Colitis. 2010;4(6):623–8.
7. Grossman AB, Noble AJ, Mamula P, Baldassano RN. Increased dosing requirements for 6-mercaptopurine and azathioprine in inflammatory bowel disease patients six years and younger. Inflamm Bowel Dis. 2008;14(6):750–5.
8. Ooi CY, Bohane TD, Lee D, Naidoo D, Day AS. Thiopurine metabolite monitoring in paediatric inflammatory bowel disease. Aliment Pharmacol Ther. 2007;25(8):941–7.
9. Osterman MT, Kundu R, Lichtenstein GR, Lewis JD. Association of 6-thioguanine nucleotide levels and inflammatory bowel disease activity: a meta-analysis. Gastroenterology. 2006;130(4):1047–53.
10. Colombel JF, Ferrari N, Debuysere H, et al. Genotypic analysis of thiopurine S-methyltransferase in patients with Crohn's disease and severe myelosuppression during azathioprine therapy. Gastroenterology. 2000;118(6):1025–30.

11. Roblin X, Peyrin-Biroulet L, Phelip JM, Nancey S, Flourie B. A 6-thioguanine nucleotide threshold level of 400 pmol/8 × 10(8) erythrocytes predicts azathioprine refractoriness in patients with inflammatory bowel disease and normal TPMT activity. Am J Gastroenterol. 2008;103(12):3115–22.

12. Dubinsky MC, Yang H, Hassard PV, et al. 6-MP metabolite profiles provide a biochemical explanation for 6-MP resistance in patients with inflammatory bowel disease. Gastroenterology. 2002;122(4):904–15.

13. Gearry RB, Day AS, Barclay ML, Leong RW, Sparrow MP. Azathioprine and allopurinol: a two-edged interaction. J Gastroenterol Hepatol. 2010;25:653–5.

14. Hyams J, Crandall W, Kugathasan S, et al. Induction and maintenance infliximab therapy for the treatment of moderate-to-severe Crohn's disease in children. Gastroenterology. 2007;132(3):863–73. quiz 1165-1166

15. Hyams J, Damaraju L, Blank M, et al. Induction and maintenance therapy with infliximab for children with moderate to severe ulcerative colitis. Clin Gastroenterol Hepatol. 2012;10(4):391–9.e391.

16. Ben-Horin S, Chowers Y. Review article: loss of response to anti-TNF treatments in Crohn's disease. Aliment Pharmacol Ther. 2011;33(9):987–95.

17. Baert F, Noman M, Vermeire S, et al. Influence of immunogenicity on the long-term efficacy of infliximab in Crohn's disease. N Engl J Med. 2003;348(7):601–8.

18. Maser EA, Villela R, Silverberg MS, Greenberg GR. Association of trough serum infliximab to clinical outcome after scheduled maintenance treatment for Crohn's disease. Clin Gastroenterol Hepatol. 2006;4(10):1248–54.

19. Bortlik M, Duricova D, Malickova K, et al. Infliximab trough levels may predict sustained response to infliximab in patients with Crohn's disease. J Crohns Colitis. 2013;7(9):736–43.

20. Seow CH, Newman A, Irwin SP, Steinhart AH, Silverberg MS, Greenberg GR. Trough serum infliximab: a predictive factor of clinical outcome for infliximab treatment in acute ulcerative colitis. Gut. 2010;59(1):49–54.

21. Reinisch W, Sandborn WJ, Rutgeerts P, et al. Long-term infliximab maintenance therapy for ulcerative colitis: the ACT-1 and -2 extension studies. Inflamm Bowel Dis. 2012;18(2):201–11.

22. Colombel JF, Sandborn WJ, Allez M, et al. Association between plasma concentrations of certolizumab pegol and endoscopic outcomes of patients with Crohn's disease. Clin Gastroenterol Hepatol. 2014;12(3):423–31.

23. Roblin X, Marotte H, Rinaudo M, et al. Association between pharmacokinetics of adalimumab and mucosal healing in patients with inflammatory bowel diseases. Clin Gastroenterol Hepatol. 2014;12(1):80–4.

24. Sandborn WJ, Feagan BG, Marano C, et al. Subcutaneous golimumab maintains clinical response in patients with moderate-to-severe ulcerative colitis. Gastroenterology. 2014;146(1):96–109.e101.

25. Murthy SKD, Seow CH, et al. Association of serum infliximab and antibodies to infliximab to long-term clinical outcome in acute ulcerative colitis. Gastroenterol Hepatol. 2012;8(8):S5. 12

26. Vande Casteele N, Khanna R, Levesque BG, et al. The relationship between infliximab concentrations, antibodies to infliximab and disease activity in Crohn's disease. Gut. 2015;64(10):1539–45.

27. Singh N, Rosenthal CJ, Melmed GY, et al. Early infliximab trough levels are associated with persistent remission in pediatric patients with inflammatory bowel disease. Inflamm Bowel Dis. 2014;20(10):1708–13.

28. Cornillie F, Hanauer SB, Diamond RH, et al. Postinduction serum infliximab trough level and decrease of C-reactive protein level are associated with durable sustained response to infliximab: a retrospective analysis of the ACCENT I trial. Gut. 2014;63(11):1721–7.

29. Velayos FSS, Lockton S, et al. Prevalence of Antibodies to Adalimumab (ATA) and Correlation Between ATA and Low Serum Drug Concentration on CRP and Clinical Symptoms in a Prospective Sample of IBD Patients. Gastroenterology. 2013;144(5):S-91.

30. Yarur AJ, Deshpande AR, Sussman DA, et al. Serum adalimumab levels and antibodies correlate with endoscopic intestinal inflammation and inflammatory markers in patients with inflammatory bowel disease. Gastroenterology. 2013;144(5):S-774.

31. Karmiris K, Paintaud G, Noman M, et al. Influence of trough serum levels and immunogenicity on long-term outcome of adalimumab therapy in Crohn's disease. Gastroenterology. 2009;137(5):1628–40.

32. Sandborn WJ, Hanauer SB, Pierre-Louis B, et al. Certolizumab pegol plasma concentration and clinical remission in Crohn's Disease. Gastroenterology. 2012;142(5):S-563.

33. Ordas I, Feagan BG, Sandborn WJ. Therapeutic drug monitoring of tumor necrosis factor antagonists in inflammatory bowel disease. Clin Gastroenterol Hepatol. 2012;10(10):1079–87.

34. Cassinotti A, Travis S. Incidence and clinical significance of immunogenicity to infliximab in Crohn's disease: a critical systematic review. Inflamm Bowel Dis. 2009;15(8):1264–75.

35. Miele E, Markowitz JE, Mamula P, Baldassano RN. Human antichimeric antibody in children and young adults with inflammatory bowel disease receiving infliximab. J Pediatr Gastroenterol Nutr. 2004;38(5):502–8.

36. Farrell RJ, Alsahli M, Jeen YT, Falchuk KR, Peppercorn MA, Michetti P. Intravenous hydrocortisone premedication reduces antibodies to infliximab in Crohn's disease: a randomized controlled trial. Gastroenterology. 2003;124(4):917–24.

37. Colombel JF, Sandborn WJ, Reinisch W, et al. Infliximab, azathioprine, or combination therapy for Crohn's disease. N Engl J Med. 2010;362(15):1383–95.

38. Vande Casteele N, Gils A, Singh S, et al. Antibody response to infliximab and its impact on pharmacokinetics can be transient. Am J Gastroenterol. 2013;108(6):962–71.

39. Ungar B, Chowers Y, Yavzori M, et al. The temporal evolution of antidrug antibodies in patients with inflammatory bowel disease treated with infliximab. Gut. 2014;63(8):1258–64.

40. Baert F, Kondragunta V, Lockton S, et al. Antibodies to adalimumab are associated with future inflammation in Crohn's patients receiving maintenance adalimumab therapy: a post hoc analysis of the Karmiris trial. Gut. 2016;65(7):1126–31.

41. Imaeda H, Takahashi K, Fujimoto T, et al. Clinical utility of newly developed immunoassays for serum concentrations of adalimumab and anti-adalimumab antibodies in patients with Crohn's disease. J Gastroenterol. 2014;49(1):100–9.

42. Sandborn WJ, Abreu MT, D'Haens G, et al. Certolizumab pegol in patients with moderate to severe Crohn's disease and secondary failure to infliximab. Clin Gastroenterol Hepatol. 2010;8(8):688–95.e682.

43. Schreiber S, Khaliq-Kareemi M, Lawrance IC, et al. Maintenance therapy with certolizumab pegol for Crohn's disease. N Engl J Med. 2007;357(3):239–50.

44. Zitomersky NL, Atkinson BJ, Fournier K, et al. Antibodies to infliximab are associated with lower infliximab levels and increased likelihood of surgery in pediatric IBD. Inflamm Bowel Dis. 2015;21(2):307–14.

45. Baert F, Drobne D, Gils A, et al. Early trough levels and antibodies to infliximab predict safety and success of re-initiation of infliximab therapy. Clin Gastroenterol Hepatol. 2014;12(9):1474–81.e2.

46. Wang SL, Ohrmund L, Hauenstein S, et al. Development and validation of a homogeneous mobility shift assay for the measurement of infliximab and antibodies-to-infliximab levels in patient serum. J Immunol Methods. 2012;382(1–2):177–88.

47. Ordas I, Mould DR, Feagan BG, Sandborn WJ. Anti-TNF monoclonal antibodies in inflammatory bowel disease: pharmacokinetics-based dosing paradigms. Clin Pharmacol Ther. 2012;91(4):635–46.

48. Hanauer SB, Feagan BG, Lichtenstein GR, et al. Maintenance infliximab for Crohn's disease: the ACCENT I randomised trial. Lancet. 2002;359(9317):1541–9.

49. Ben-Horin S, Waterman M, Kopylov U, et al. Addition of an immunomodulator to infliximab therapy eliminates antidrug antibodies in serum and restores clinical response of patients with inflammatory bowel disease. Clin Gastroenterol Hepatol. 2013;11(4):444–7.

50. Ong DE, Kamm MA, Hartono JL, Lust M. Addition of thiopurines can recapture response in patients with Crohn's disease who have lost response to anti-tumor necrosis factor monotherapy. J Gastroenterol Hepatol. 2013;28(10):1595–9.

51. Maini RN, Breedveld FC, Kalden JR, et al. Therapeutic efficacy of multiple intravenous infusions of anti-tumor necrosis factor alpha monoclonal antibody combined with low-dose weekly methotrexate in rheumatoid arthritis. Arthritis Rheum. 1998;41(9):1552–63.

52. Grossi V, Lerer T, Griffiths A, et al. Concomitant Use of Immunomodulators Affects the Durability of Infliximab Therapy in Children With Crohn's Disease. Clin Gastroenterol Hepatol. 2015;13(10):1748–56.

53. Vahabnezhad E, Rabizadeh S, Dubinsky MC. A 10-year, single tertiary care center experience on the durability of infliximab in pediatric inflammatory bowel disease. Inflamm Bowel Dis. 2014;18:18.

54. Feagan BG, McDonald JW, Panaccione R, et al. Methotrexate in combination with infliximab is no more effective than infliximab alone in patients with Crohn's disease. Gastroenterology. 2014;146(3):681–8.

55. Schroder O, Blumenstein I, Stein J. Combining infliximab with methotrexate for the induction and maintenance of remission in refractory Crohn's disease: a controlled pilot study. Eur J Gastroenterol Hepatol. 2006;18(1):11–6.

56. Stein R, Lee D, Leonard MB, et al. Serum Infliximab, Antidrug Antibodies, and Tumor Necrosis Factor Predict Sustained Response in Pediatric Crohn's Disease. Inflamm Bowel Dis. 2016;22(6):1370–7.

57. Vande Casteele N, Gils A, Ballet V, et al. Randomised Controlled Trial of Drug Level Versus Maintenance Therapy in IBD: Final Results of the TAXIT Study. United European Gastroenterol J. 2013;1:A1–A134.

58. Vaughn BP, Martinez-Vazquez M, Patwardhan VR, Moss AC, Sandborn WJ, Cheifetz AS. Proactive therapeutic concentration monitoring of infliximab may improve outcomes for patients with inflammatory bowel disease: results from a pilot observational study. Inflamm Bowel Dis. 2014;20(11):1996–2003.

New Non-anti-TNF-α Biological Therapies for the Treatment of Inflammatory Bowel Disease

Farzana Rashid and Gary R. Lichtenstein

Introduction

Blockade of the tumor necrosis factor alpha (TNF-α) pathway has been a major advancement for the treatment of inflammatory bowel disease (IBD). A substantial proportion of patients with moderate to severe Crohn's disease (CD) do not have a response to treatment with TNFα antagonists (primary nonresponse), and among patients who do have a response, it is often not sustained (secondary nonresponse) or side effects require discontinuation of medical therapy. As a consequence of this, there is an ongoing need to develop new biologics with different mechanisms of action. This chapter will discuss the major non-anti-TNF-α biological agents in the pipeline that are currently undergoing evaluation in order to effectively and safely treat patients with IBD. Figures 35.1 and 35.2 illustrate the drugs currently in the pipeline and Table 35.1 is a summary of the treatments that will be discussed in this chapter.

Cytokine Targets

IL-12/IL-23

Interleukin (IL)-12 and IL-23 have been shown to have a central role in the inflammatory pathway in Crohn's disease, psoriasis and multiple sclerosis [2]. The IL-12 family of cytokines (which includes IL-23) is involved in stimulating innate immunity and developing adaptive immunity. Interleukin-12 and interleukin-23 are key proinflammatory cytokines involved in type 1 helper T (Th1) cell response, which is characterized by a marked accumulation of macrophages making interleukin-12, the major Th1-inducing

factor, in Crohn's disease mucosa [3, 4]. Risk for developing CD and UC has been demonstrated through genome-wide association studies studying variants of the gene encoding the IL-23 receptor and the locus for the gene encoding the p40 chain [5]. It was also suggested that the production of both IL-12 and IL-23 is downregulated in patients with Crohn's disease but not with ulcerative colitis following administration of IL-12p40 monoclonal antibody [6].

IL-12 is a heterodimer of p40 and p35 subunits. IL-12 induces the differentiation of naïve CD4+ T cells into T helper 1 cells that produce interferon (IFN) gamma and mediates cellular immunity [7]. IL-23 is a heterodimer of the same p40 subunit and a p19 subunit which induces naïve CD4+ T cells into T helper 17 cells which then induce the production of proinflammatory cytokines such as IL-17, IL-6, and TNF-α [8].

Ustekinumab

Ustekinumab (originally known as CNTO 1275) is a human monoclonal antibody (IgG1) that targets the IL-12/23 shared p40 subunit. The result is the inhibition of IL-12 and IL-23 binding to their receptor on the surface of T cells, natural killer cells, and antigen-presenting cells (see Fig. 35.3).

Ustekinumab has been shown to be clinically effective in the treatment of moderate to severe CD in phase II studies. There were two groups studied with population 1 being double-blind, placebo-controlled, parallel-group, crossover at week 8 study and population 2 being an open-label study [10]. Both groups were followed up for 28 weeks. Group 1 comprised of 104 patients with moderate to severe Crohn's disease despite treatment with 5-ASA, antibiotics, corticosteroids, infliximab, and/or immunomodulators who were randomly assigned to one of four arms of treatment: subcutaneous placebo at weeks 0–3 followed by subcutaneous ustekinumab 90 mg at weeks 8–11; subcutaneous ustekinumab 90 mg at weeks 0–3 followed by subcutaneous placebo at weeks 8–11; intravenous placebo at week 0 followed by intravenous ustekinumab 4.5 mg/kg at week 8; or intravenous ustekinumab 4.5 mg/kg at week 0 followed by

F. Rashid, MD (✉)
The University of Pennsylvania, Philadelphia, PA, USA
e-mail: farzana.rashid@uphs.upenn.edu

G.R. Lichtenstein, MD, FACP, FACG, AGAF
Inflammatory Bowel Disease Center, The University of Pennsylvania, Philadelphia, PA, USA

© Springer International Publishing AG 2017
P. Mamula et al. (eds.), *Pediatric Inflammatory Bowel Disease*, DOI 10.1007/978-3-319-49215-5_35

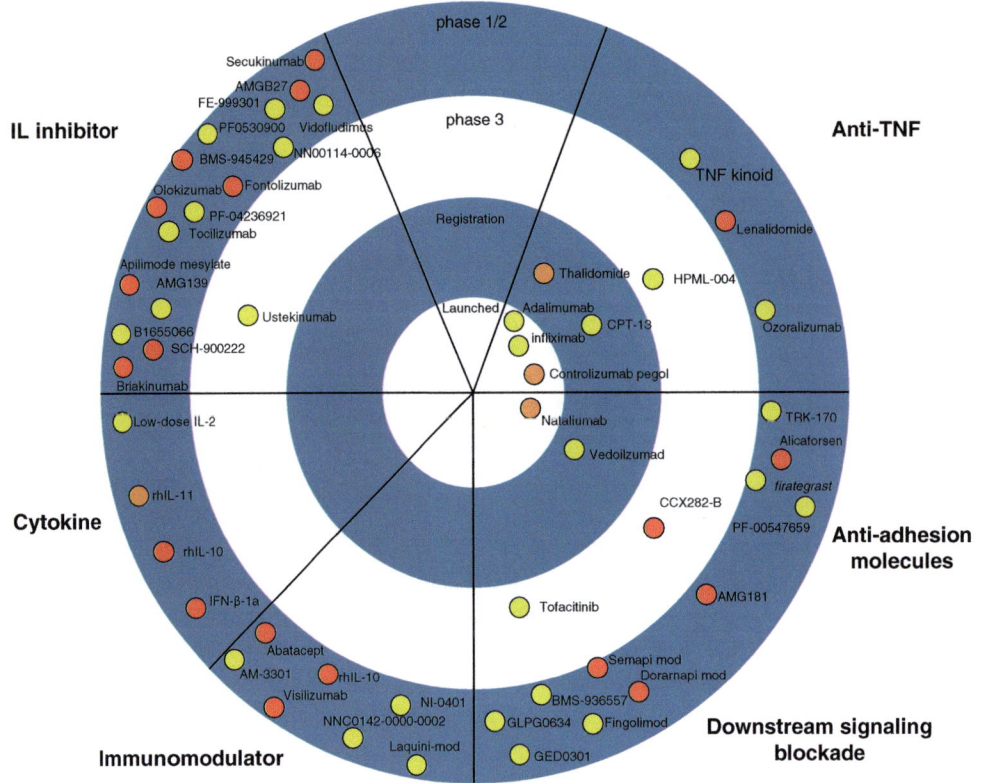

Fig. 35.1 Drugs in pipeline for CD (Amiot and Peyrin-Biroulet [1])

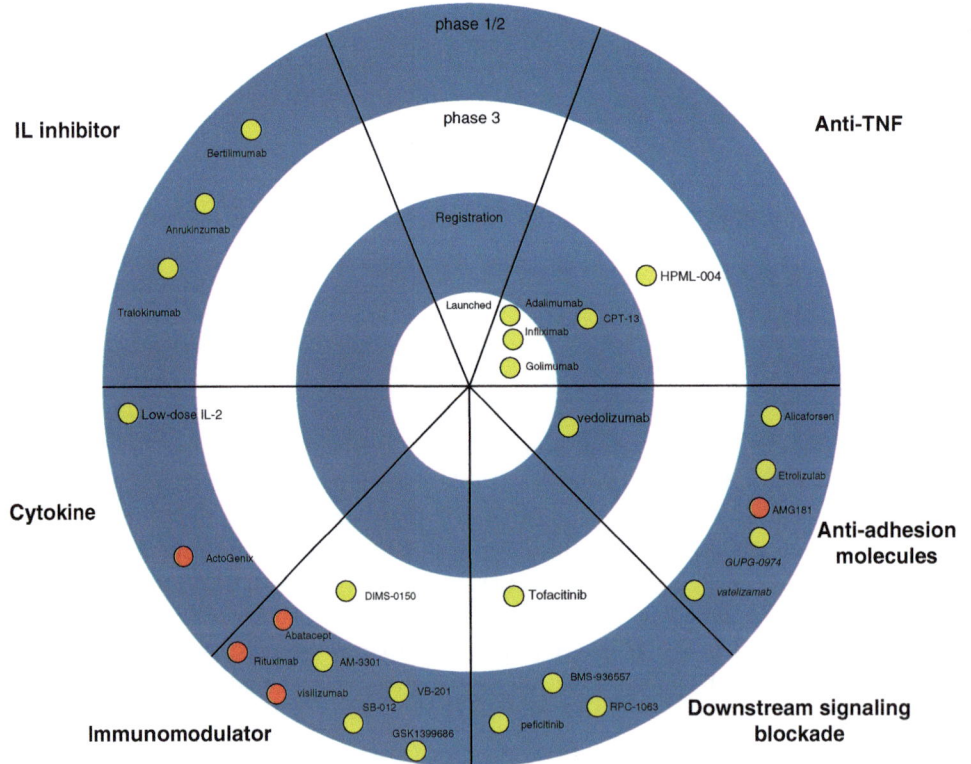

Fig. 35.2 Drugs in pipeline for UC (Amiot and Peyrin-Biroulet [1])

intravenous placebo at week 8. Group 2 consisted of 27 patients who previously failed to respond to a three-dose induction of infliximab 5 mg/kg or lost response to inflix-

imab maintenance every 8 weeks despite dose escalation to 10 mg/kg who were randomly assigned to open-label therapy with either 4 weekly subcutaneous injections ustekinumab

Table 35.1 Treatments discussed in this chapter

Target	Name	Development in IBD	Mechanism of action
Cytokines			
IL-12/IL-23	Ustekinumab MEDI 2070 (AMG 139) BI 655066 (risukizumab)	Phase III (CD, UC) Phase II (CD)	Inhibits p40 subunit Blocks binding of IL-23 to its receptor Inhibits the p19 unit
IL-6	PF-04236921	Phase II (CD)	IL-6 inhibitor
IL-13	Tralokinumab QAX576 Bertilimumab	Phase II (UC) Phase II (CD) Phase II (CD, UC)	IL-13 receptor antagonist Inhibits of IL-13 Blocks the activity of eotaxin-1
IL-17	Vidofludimus	Phase II	Inhibits IL-17 secretion
IL-21	ATR107 NNC0114-0006	Phase I Phase II (CD)	Anti-IL-21 receptor antibody IL-21 inhibitor
Signaling pathways mediated by cytokines			
JAK/STAT	Tofacitinib GLPG0634 (Filgotinib)	Phase III (UC) Phase II (CD)	Inhibits JAK1 and JAK3 JAK1 inhibitor
TGF-b	GED0301 (Mongersen)	Phase III/II (CD/UC)	SMAD7 antisense oligonucleotide
Chemokines			
IL-10 antagonist	BMS936557 (eldelumab)	Phase II (CD, UC)	CXCL-10 inhibitor
Antiadhesion molecules	Natalizumab	Approved (CD)	α4 integrin antaogmist
	Vedolizumab	Approved (CD, UC)	α4β7 integrin antagonist
	Etrolizumab	Phase III (CD, UC)	Blocks β7 subunit of α4β7 and αEβ7 integrins
	PF-00547659	Phase II (CD, UC)	MAdCAM-1 protein inhibitor
	AJM300	Phase III (UC)	α4 integrin antagonist
	Alicaforsen	Phase III (UC)	Targets intercellular adhesion molecule 1 (ICAM-1)
	AMG181 (abrilumab)	D/c'd	α4β7 integrin antagonist
	Firategrast		α4 integrin antagonist
	GLPG0974	Phase II (UC)	Against FFA2
	TRK-170	Phase II (CD)	α4β1/α4β7 integrin antagonist
Anti-inflammatory cytokine	IL-10		IL-10 replacement
T-cell stimulation and induction of apoptosis blockades	Laquinimod DIMS0150	Phase II (CD) Phase III (UC)	Modulation of immune cells Activates TLR9
Spingosine-1-phosphate receptor modulators	Fingolimod APD334 RPC1063 (ozanimod)	Phase II (UC) Phase III/II (UC/CD)	Traps lymphocytes in lymph nodes

90 mg at weeks 0–3 or single intravenous ustekinumab 4.5 mg/kg at week 0. The primary endpoint was clinical response at week 8 (a reduction of at ≥25 % and 70 points in the CDAI score from baseline). In group 1 the primary endpoint was assessed for combined subcutaneous and intravenous ustekinumab administered before crossover to placebo ($n = 51$) versus combined subcutaneous and intravenous placebo administered before crossover to ustekinumab ($n = 53$). There was no significant difference in rates of clinical response between ustekinumab and placebo at week 8 (49 % vs. 40 %, $P = 0.34$). However, superiority of ustekinumab over placebo was observed in achieving clinical response at week 4 and at week 6 (53 % vs. 30 % at both time points, $P = 0.02$). Of note, among patients in group 1 who

had prior exposure to infliximab given at submaximal infliximab doses or regimens ustekinumab was significantly superior to placebo with clinical response rates of 59 % and 26 %, respectively ($P = 0.022$). Among group 2, clinical response rates at week 8 were 43 % and 54 % for subcutaneous and intravenous route of administration of ustekinumab, respectively. It was thus concluded that ustekinumab has the potential of inducing clinical response in patients with moderate to severe active Crohn's disease with the most prominent effect at weeks 4 through 6 and in patients with prior exposure to infliximab.

Ustekinumab in CD was further studied in a phase IIb randomized, double-blind, placebo-controlled trial with an 8-week induction and 26-week maintenance evaluation

Fig. 35.3 Ustekinumab mechanism of action (Onuora [9])

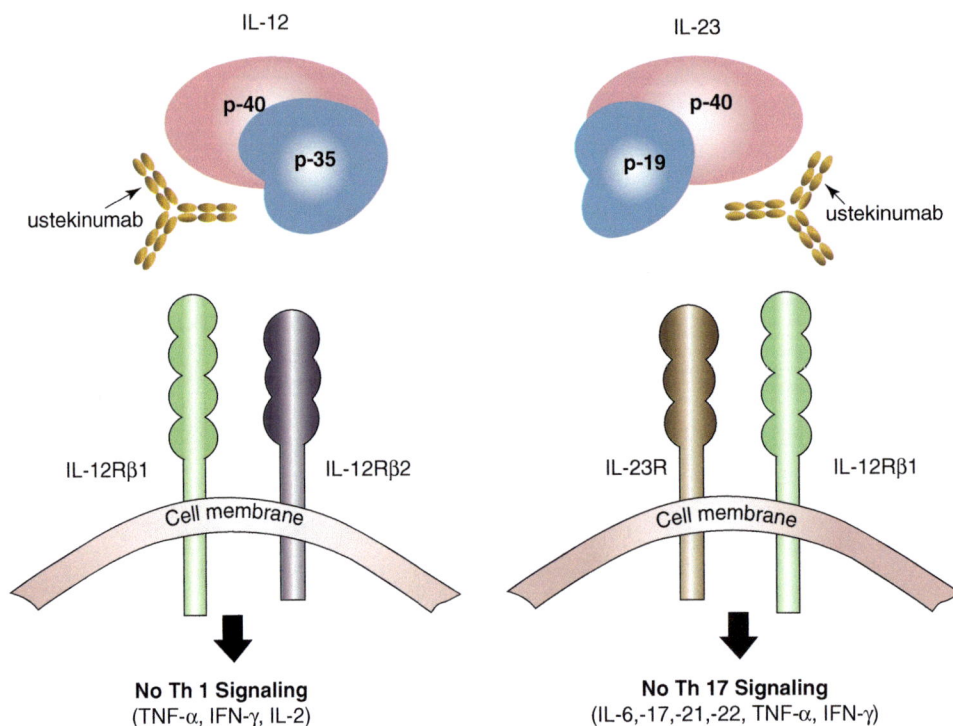

period for patients previously exposed to anti-TNF therapy who either had primary nonresponse, secondary nonresponse or intolerance to anti-TNF treatment [11]. During the induction phase, 526 patients were randomly assigned to receive a weight-based dose of intravenous (IV) ustekinumab (1, 3, or 6 mg/kg) or placebo. Responders and nonresponders were separately randomized to subcutaneous (SC) ustekinumab 90 mg or placebo at weeks 8 and 16. The primary endpoint was clinical response ($\geq$100-point decrease from baseline CDAI) at week 6. 39.7 % of patients at 6 mg/kg vs. 23.5 % of patients receiving placebo achieved clinical response at week 6 ($P = 0.005$). Clinical remission rates at week 6, however, were similar between the ustekinumab and placebo groups. Among patients with a response to ustekinumab in the induction phase, 69.4 % vs. 42.5 % and 41.7 % vs. 27.4 % of patients receiving 90 mg of ustekinumab vs. placebo in the maintenance phase continued to have a clinical response and clinical remission at week 22. In addition, 30.6 % vs. 17.8 % of patients in the ustekinumab vs. placebo group were in glucocorticoid-free remission at week 22 ($p = 0.048$). Of note, for those patients who did not achieve clinical response after induction with ustekinumab, further therapy with the drug was no different than placebo in terms of clinical response at week 22.

Mucosal healing was also evaluated in the phase IIb trial. Fifty patients were evaluated and 1 out of 9 vs. 8 out of 41 patients achieved mucosal healing in the placebo vs. ustekinumab group respectively ($P = 1.00$) [11].

Having had promising results with the phase II trials, two phase III trials are completed and a third is underway. UNITI-1 (NCT01369329) is a multicenter, double-blind, placebo-controlled study of ustekinumab for induction of remission in moderate to severe CD in patients with prior failure or intolerance to TNF antagonist therapy [12]. Patients with moderate-severely active CD (defined as a CDAI 220–450) who previously failed or were intolerant to at least 1 TNF-antagonist were randomized (1:1:1) to receive a single dose of IV placebo (PBO), ustekinumab 130 mg, or weight-based tiered ustekinumab dosing approximating 6 mg/kg (260 mg [weight $\leq$55 kg], 390 mg [weight >55 kg and $\leq$85 kg], and 520 mg [weight >85 kg]) at week 0. The primary endpoint was clinical response at week 6, defined as reduction from baseline in the CDAI score of >100 points; patients with baseline CDAI score 220–248 were considered to have had a clinical response if a CDAI score of <150 was present. At week 8, patients either transitioned to the UNITI maintenance study (see below) or were followed to week 20. Seven hundred and forty-one patients had had a history of anti-TNF therapy failure either primary nonresponse, secondary nonresponse or intolerance to at least one anti-TNF agent. Primary and secondary endpoints were met at both intravenous doses of ustekinumab. 33.7 % of the ~6 mg/kg and 34.3 % of the 130 mg ustekinumab groups versus 21.5 % in placebo ($P = 0.003$ and 0.002, respectively) achieved clinical response at week 6. 20.9 % of the ~6 mg/kg group and 15.9 % of the 130 mg ustekinumab group versus

7.3 % on placebo ($P < 0.001$, $P = 0.003$, respectively) were found to be in clinical remission (CDAI <150) at week 8. 37.8 % of the ~6 mg/kg and 33.5 % of the 130 mg ustekinumab groups, versus 20.2 % on placebo (each $P \leq 0.001$) had a clinical response at week 8. Both intravenous ustekinumab induction doses compared to placebo resulted in significant improvements in CDAI, IBDQ, CRP, fecal lactoferrin, and calprotectin. AEs, SAEs, and infections were similar in the treated and placebo groups. One opportunistic infection (*Listeria* meningitis) was reported in the ~6 mg/kg UST group; otherwise no tuberculosis, malignancies, deaths, or major adverse cardiovascular events occurred in ustekinumab treated patients through the week 20 observation.

UNITI-2 (NCT01369342) is identical in design to UNITI-1 and involves patients who have failed conventional treatment (corticosteroids, immunomodulators) or who are corticosteroid dependent without previous failure or intolerance to TNF antagonist therapy. The data were recently presented at the American College of Gastroenterology (Oct 2015 [13]). Six hundred and twenty-eight patients with moderate to severely active Crohn's disease were randomized to receive a single dose of IV placebo ($n = 210$), 130 mg of ustekinumab ($n = 209$) or weight-based tiered dosing of 6 mg/kg of ustekinumab ($n = 209$). The primary endpoint was clinical response at 6 weeks and at 8 weeks, patients either transitioned to the maintenance study or were followed through to 20 weeks. 51.7 % of patients who received 130 mg of ustekinumab and 55.5 % of patients who received 6 mg/kg of ustekinumab vs. 28 % of patients who received placebo ($P < 0.001$) achieved a clinical response at 6 weeks. 47 % of patients who received 130 mg of ustekinumab and 58 % of patients who received 6 mg/kg of ustekinumab vs. 32 % of patients who received placebo ($P < 0.001$) achieved clinical response at week 8. 31 % who received 130 mg of ustekinumab and 40 % of patients who received 6 mg/kg of ustekinumab achieved clinical remission at 8 weeks. Adverse events and serious adverse events were similar between the groups and no malignancies, deaths, opportunistic infections or tuberculosis occurred in patients treated with ustekinumab.

Patients with a clinical response to IV ustekinumab in UNITI-1 or UNITI-2 as mentioned above were eligible for enrollment in the maintenance trial, IM-UNITI (NCT01369355). This study is still ongoing [14]. Patients will be randomized to 90 mg of ustekinumab every 8 weeks, every 12 weeks, or placebo. Patients who receive placebo or ustekinumab every 12 weeks and who lose response are eligible to cross over to receive ustekinumab 90 mg every 8 weeks. The primary outcome will be clinical remission at week 44. Secondary endpoints clinical remission in patients who have previously failed TNF antagonists, clinical response, and corticosteroid-free remission at week 44. Patients who are continuing to do well at week 44 will be eligible to continue to receive ustekinumab in the long-term extension study with follow-up to 3 additional years.

Pediatric Data

Data regarding efficacy of ustekinumab in pediatric CD are lacking. However, Rinawi and colleagues attempted to induce remission with ustekinumab in a 6-year-old patient with active colonic disease, chronic arthritis, and failure to respond to all approved therapies for pediatric CD. The child received three subcutaneous doses of ustekinumab (1.3 mg/kg) at months 0, 1, and 3 which resulted in complete clinical and biochemical remission with no observed adverse events. Clinical response including resolution of diarrhea and arthritis was achieved within the first 2 months of treatment. Furthermore, 1 year after the induction, a weight gain of 3 kg and growth of 8 cm were noted and inflammatory blood markers (CRP, ESR) had normalized and albumin and hemoglobin increased. Remission was maintained with azathioprine 1 year following induction [15].

Bishop and colleagues recently described the use of ustekinumab in four adolescent patients with pediatric Crohn's disease – ages of initiation were 12, 13, 16, and 17. All patients had previously received corticosteroids, methotrexate, azathioprine/6-mercaptopurine, and both infliximab and adalimumab. Two patients showed clinical response and remained on ustekinumab, but two patients discontinued therapy due to continued symptoms and disease complications and required multiple hospitalizations [16].

Safety

In the phase II trials in Crohn's disease, there were no increase in the number of adverse or serious adverse events in patients given ustekinumab through week 8 compared with placebo [10]. There were no serious or opportunistic infections. 14 % vs. 8 % of patients in the placebo group vs. drug group reported worsening CD. Three patients (6 %) in the placebo group experienced one or more serious adverse events: small intestinal stenosis and nonsteroidal anti-inflammatory drug–induced gastrointestinal ulceration, worsening CD and erythema nodosum, worsening CD disease and small intestinal obstruction. Two patients (4 %) in the ustekinumab group experienced one or more serious adverse events: small intestinal obstruction and coronary artery disease.

In the patients in the open-label trial followed through week 28, six patients (6 %) in the population 1 group experienced one or more serious adverse events: worsening CD ($n = 2$), colonic stenosis and pneumothorax ($n = 1$), small intestinal obstruction ($n = 2$), and prostate cancer ($n = 1$).

Four patients (15 %) in the population 2 group experienced one or more serious adverse events: viral gastroenteritis ($n = 1$), nephrolithiasis ($n = 1$), worsening CD ($n = 1$), worsening CD, syncope, and disseminated histoplasmosis ($n = 1$, in a patient receiving prednisone (80 mg/day), azathioprine during the trial and with approximately 3 years prior infliximab use).

In the phase IIb trial, the overall rates of infection were also similar between the ustekinumab and placebo groups during the induction phase [11]. Serious infections were reported in five patients receiving ustekinumab 6 mg/kg (*Clostridium difficile* infection, viral gastroenteritis, urinary tract infection, anal abscess, and vaginal abscess). In one patient receiving ustekinumab 1 mg/kg, there was central catheter infection with *Staphylococcus*, and in one patient receiving placebo, there was an anal abscess. Infusion reactions were similar between the ustekinumab and the placebo groups.

In the maintenance phase, there were no deaths, major adverse cardiovascular events, tuberculosis, or other serious opportunistic infections. One patient who received 1 mg/kg ustekinumab followed by 90 mg of ustekinumab was reported to have basal-cell carcinoma. The most commonly reported adverse events in the maintenance phase, other than those related to CD, were nonserious infections (39.2 %), abdominal pain (7.2 %), nausea (6.1 %), and nasopharyngitis (6.1 %) in the ustekinumab group and these were all numerically lower than events in the placebo group, except for the rate of nasopharyngitis (3.3 %).

The long-term safety profile of ustekinumab has been evaluated in the treatment of psoriasis. Pooled safety data from four clinical trials of ustekinumab for psoriasis revealed a total of 3117 patients received at least one dose of ustekinumab, with a total of 8998 person-years of follow-up, with at least 4 years of exposure in 1482 patients [17]. At year 5, events per 100 patient years of follow-up for ustekinumab 45 mg and 90 mg were as follows: serious adverse events was 7.0 and 7.2, serious infections 0.98 and 1.19, nonmelanoma skin cancers 0.64 and 0.44, and major adverse cardiovascular events (MACE) including myocardial infarction, cerebrovascular accident or cardiovascular death 0.56 and 0.36. Adverse events or rates of overall mortality and other malignancy did not seem to increase over time compared with an age-matched and sex-matched US population.

There has been one case report of central demyelination in 63-year-old woman with CD. This patient had previous exposure to immunomodulator therapy, infliximab, adalimumab, and certolizumab and received ustekinumab through the clinical trial program and afterwards for compassionate reasons. About 1 year after first receiving ustekinumab, she developed progressive weakness and was diagnosed with primary progressive multiple sclerosis [18].

AMG139 (MEDI2070)

In contrast to IL-12 inhibition, IL-23 inhibition has been previously shown to be associated with a decreased incidence of tumor formation [19]. In addition, there have been concerns regarding the safety of ustekinumab and/or briakinumab regarding the incidence of serious infections and major adverse cardiovascular events [19]. Therefore, it is thought that IL-23-specific antagonism may provide similar or greater efficacy than blocking IL-12/23p40 and without the potential risks associated with blocking IL-12. Accordingly, a human IgG2 monoclonal antibody called AMG139 was developed to specifically bind to the IL-23 p19 unit and block binding of IL-23 specifically to its receptor. A phase I trial was just completed assessing the safety and tolerability of AMG139 following the administration of multiple intravenous (IV) or subcutaneous (SC) doses in healthy subjects and in subjects with mild to severe CD [20].

Phase IIb studies are ongoing at the writing of this chapter.

Pediatric Data

At the time of writing this chapter, there are no published data on the use of AMG139 in children or adolescents with IBD.

BI 655066

BI 655066 is a monoclonal antibody that also targets IL-23p19. It is being investigated as a subcutaneous drug in both psoriasis and Crohn's disease. A proof of concept, multicenter, randomized, double-blind, placebo-controlled, parallel-group phase II dose-ranging study of BI 655066 in patients with moderately to severely active Crohn's disease is ongoing. The primary outcome measure is clinical remission at week 12, defined as a CDAI score of <150. Secondary outcome measures include CDEIS remission, CDEIS response, mucosal healing, deep remission, and clinical response at week 12 [21]. There is another ongoing an open-label, single-group, long-term safety extension trial ongoing for subjects who responded to treatment with BI 655066 in a preceding trial [22].

Pediatric Data

At the time of writing this chapter, there are no published data on the use of BI 655066 in children or adolescents with IBD.

Safety

Selectively blocking IL-23 vs. IL-12 has been thought to be more targeted with less side effects as a result [23].

A single-rising dose, multicenter, randomized, double-blind, placebo-controlled, within-dose phase I trial was the first-in-human proof-of-concept study and in this study the clinical and biological effects of BI 655066 was evaluated in patients with moderate to severe plaque psoriasis. Patients received 0.01, 0.05, 0.25, 1, 3, or 5 mg/kg BI 655066 intravenously, 0.25 or 1 mg/kg BI 655066 subcutaneously, or matched placebo. Thirty nine patients received single-dose BI 655066 intravenously (*n* = 18) or subcutaneously (*n* = 13) or placebo (*n* = 8). BI 655066 was well tolerated. The number of adverse events were similar between the BI 655066 and placebo groups. Four serious adverse events were reported among BI 655066-treated patients and were thought not to be treatment related [24].

IL-6

Interleukin-6 (IL-6) is a cytokine with central roles in immune regulation, inflammation, hematopoiesis, and oncogenesis. It is a contributor of Th-17 differentiation [1]. Increased levels of IL-6 and soluble IL-6 receptor have been demonstrated in both serum and intestinal tissues of the patients with active Crohn's disease and with a more severe form [25].

PF-04236921
PF-04236921 is a monoclonal antibody against IL-6. A phase II placebo-controlled study has been completed to evaluate the safety and efficacy of this subcutaneously administered antibody in patients with active CD (the ANDANTE study) [26]. There were limitations of the study including early termination which led to small numbers of participants and technical problems with measurement resulting in unreliable or uninterpretable data.

Phase I/II studies are ongoing at the time of writing of the chapter.

Pediatric Data
At the time of writing this chapter, there are no published data on the use of PF-04236921 in children or adolescents with IBD.

IL-13

Interleukin-13 (IL-13) is a central cytokine in the T helper 2 immune response [27–29]. IL-13 has effects on many cell types including B cells, monocytes, macrophages, epithelial cells, smooth muscle cells and neurons and has been indicated in the pathogenesis of many disease including asthma, scleroderma in addition to IBD [30]. Its upregulation has been proposed to be a key driver of mucosal inflammation – specifically in UC.

Tralokinumab
Tralokinumab (CAT-354) is an IL-13-specific human immunoglobulin G4 monoclonal antibody that binds to and neutralizes IL-13 [31, 32]. Tralokinumab is being evaluated in phase III clinical studies in patients with asthma and in a phase II study in idiopathic pulmonary fibrosis and may be a treatment for UC.

In a phase IIa, randomized, double-blind, placebo-controlled, parallel-group, multicenter trial, 111 patients with UC (total Mayo score ≥6) were randomized to tralokinumab 300 mg subcutaneous or placebo [33]. The primary endpoint of clinical response at week 8 was 38 % (21/56) for tralokinumab vs. 33 % (18/55) for placebo (*P* = 0.406). Clinical remission rate at week 8 was 18 % (10/56) vs. 6 % (3/55) (*P* = 0.033) and mucosal healing rate was 32 % (18/56) vs. 20 % (11/55) (*P* = 0.104) for tralokinumab vs. placebo.

Pediatric Data
At the time of writing this chapter, there are no published data on the use of tralokinumab in children or adolescents with IBD.

Safety
Tralokinumab had an acceptable safety profile in the only phase IIa study to date [33]. The median duration of exposure was 84 days. The number of patients who experienced adverse events was similar in the tralokinumab and placebo groups. The most frequently reported adverse events were symptoms of UC and headache. The number of patients discontinuing treatment because of adverse events was similar in both groups and the most common adverse event leading to discontinuation was symptoms of UC.

QAX576
QAX576 is a highly potent and specific inhibitor of human IL-13 activity in cell-based in vitro assays. It has been used to treat eosinophilic esophagitis with success [34] and studied in asthma and idiopathic pulmonary fibrosis.

A phase II study to assess the safety and efficacy of intravenously administered QAX576 in patients with fistulizing Crohn's disease has been completed [35]. Another phase II study to test the safety and efficacy of the drug in the treatment of perianal fistulas has also been completed [36]. Results are not available of either of the studies.

Pediatric Data
At the time of writing this chapter, there are no published data on the use of QAX576 in children or adolescents with IBD.

Bertilimumab
Bertilimumab is a fully human, IgG4-type monoclonal antibody that blocks the activity of a protein called eotaxin-1. Eotaxin-1 plays an important role in inflammation and causes eosinophils to migrate towards sites of inflammation where

they become activated and release substances that result in tissue damage and enhance inflammation.

A randomized, double blind, placebo-controlled, parallel-group, multicenter study in adult patients with active moderate to severe UC is ongoing. Patients are currently being and eligible patients will be randomly assigned in a 2:1 ratio to one of two treatment groups, bertilimumab 10 mg/kg intravenously or matching placebo, respectively [37].

Pediatric Data
At the time of writing this chapter, there are no published data on the use of Bertilimumab in children or adolescents with IBD.

IL-17

Vidofludimus
Vidofludimus (4SC-101) is a novel oral immunomodulatory drug that inhibits dihydro-orotate dehydrogenase and lymphocyte proliferation in vitro and inhibits interleukin (IL)-17 secretion in vitro independently of effects on lymphocyte proliferation [38].

A phase IIa open-label, single-arm trial with vidofludimus (ENTRANCE trial) in inflammatory bowel disease was performed. The primary outcome was to assess remission-maintenance potential in steroid dependent IBD patients upon steroid weaning (ECCO 2011). There were 26 CD and UC patients. There was an 88.5 % response rate of both complete and partial responders in patients on vidofludimus vs. 20 % placebo. 53.9 % (14/26) patients were complete responders, 34.6 % (9/26) patients were partial responders and 11.5 % (3/26) patients were nonresponders. There was no difference in response rates between Crohn's disease (85.7 %) and ulcerative colitis (91.7 %). In addition, the average prednisolone consumption dramatically dropped during treatment with the drug. All 26 patients reached a relapse-free prednisolone dose which was significantly ($p < 0.001$) lower than their individual threshold doses at which they experienced relapses prior to entering the study. Mean prednisolone consumption was significantly lowered from 26.5 mg/day (± 8.0) at the start of treatment to 1.0 mg/day (± 2.7) at week 12.

Pediatric Data
At the time of writing this chapter, there are no published data on the use of vidofludimus in children or adolescents with IBD.

Safety
Vidofludimus was safe and well tolerated by all patients in the ENTRANCE trial. A total of 75 adverse events were reported (53 mild, 18 moderate, 4 severe) of which 19

adverse events were judged as possibly or probably drug related and included nasopharyngitis, abdominal pain, fatigue, insomnia, glucosuria, leucocyturia, microhematuria, musculoskeletal pain, myalgia, tachycardia, and dyspepsia. No drug related serious adverse events were reported.

IL-21

ATR-107
ATR-107 is a fully human anti-IL-21 receptor (IL-21R) monoclonal antibody designed to block IL-21 from binding and activating the receptor as a novel approach to treatment of systemic lupus erythematosus and other autoimmune diseases [39–41]. The ATR-107 target, IL-21R, is expressed on many lymphoid cells, including B cells, activated T cells, natural killer cells, monocytes and dendritic cells and thus ATR-107 is expected to block the effects of IL-21 activation of its receptor (enhanced proliferation of lymphoid cells, B cell differentiation to memory cells and plasma cells, and development of T helper type 17 (Th17) cells) [42, 43]. In addition, anti-inflammatory efficacy resulting from IL-21R blockade has been observed in animal models [44].

Phase I studies are ongoing at the writing of this chapter.

Pediatric Data
At the time of writing this chapter, there are no published data on the use of ATR-107 in children or adolescents with IBD.

NNC0114-0006
NNC0114-0006 is an anti-IL-21-antibody. A randomized, double-blind, placebo-controlled, parallel-group trial phase II study to assess clinical efficacy and safety of NNC0114-0006 in subjects with active Crohn's disease has been completed. Results are not yet known.

Pediatric Data
At the time of writing this chapter, there are no published data on the use of NNC0114-0006 in children or adolescents with IBD.

Blockade of the Downstream Signaling Pathways Mediated by Cytokine

JAK/STAT Pathway

Janus kinases (JAK) 1, 2 and 3 are extremely important in cytokine signaling that is involved in lymphocyte survival, proliferation, differentiation and apoptosis [45]. JAK3 is found only in hematopoietic cells and is part of the signaling pathway activated by IL-2, IL-4, IL-7, IL-9, IL-15, and IL-21 which is crucial in the activation, function and proliferation of lymphocytes [46] (see Fig. 35.4).

Tofacitinib

Tofacitinib (CP-690,550) is an oral small molecule inhibitor of JAK 1 and 3. In vitro studies have shown that it interferes with Th2 and Th17 cell differentiation and blocks the production of IL-17 and IL-22 [48].

In a phase II, double-blind, placebo-controlled trial, the efficacy of tofacitinib in 194 adults with moderately to severely active ulcerative colitis was evaluated [49]. Patients were randomly assigned to receive tofacitinib at a dose of 0.5 mg, 3 mg, 10 mg, or 15 mg or placebo twice daily for 8 weeks. The primary outcome was a clinical response at 8 weeks and occurred in 32 %, 48 %, 61 %, and 78 % of patients receiving tofacitinib at a dose of 0.5 mg ($P = 0.39$), 3 mg ($P = 0.55$), 10 mg ($P = 0.10$), and 15 mg ($P < 0.001$), respectively – compared with 42 % of patients receiving placebo. Clinical remission (Mayo score ≤ 2 with no subscore >1) at 8 weeks occurred in 13 %, 33 %, 48 %, and 41 % of patients receiving tofacitinib at a dose of 0.5 mg ($P = 0.76$), 3 mg ($P = 0.01$), 10 mg ($P < 0.001$), and 15 mg ($P < 0.001$), respectively, as compared with 10 % of patients receiving placebo. Treatment with the drug resulted in reduced C-reactive protein and fecal calprotectin levels.

Tofacitinib was also evaluated in patients with moderate to severe active CD. Patients were randomized to receive tofacitinib twice daily for 4 weeks at doses of 1 mg, 5 mg, 15 mg, or placebo [50]. The primary endpoint was not met in this phase II trial in CD patients receiving tofacitinib, but the placebo response rate was high. Although no significant clinical differences were observed between actively treated patients and placebo, a reduction in CRP and fecal calprotectin levels among patients given 15 mg tofacitinib twice daily indicated its biologic activity. The primary endpoint was clinical response at week 4 and the rates were as follows: 36 % ($P = 0.467$), 58 % ($P = 0.466$), and 46 % ($P \geq 0.999$) in those patients given 1, 5, or 15 mg tofacitinib twice daily versus 47 % given placebo. A secondary endpoint was clinical remission at week 4 and this was seen in 31 % ($P = 0.417$), 24 % ($P = 0.776$), and 14 % ($P = 0.540$) of patients given 1, 5, and 15 mg tofacitinib, versus 21 % of patients given placebo. As the clinical response was not significant, the trial was negative. However, the placebo response and remission rates were unexpectedly high and in addition, the reduction in fecal calprotectin and C-reactive protein levels among patients receiving 15 mg tofacitinib twice daily suggested biologic activity of the drug. A repeat phase II trial with stricter inclusion criteria defining active Crohn's disease is ongoing [51].

There is currently an ongoing multicenter, randomized, double-blind, placebo-controlled, parallel-group study eval-

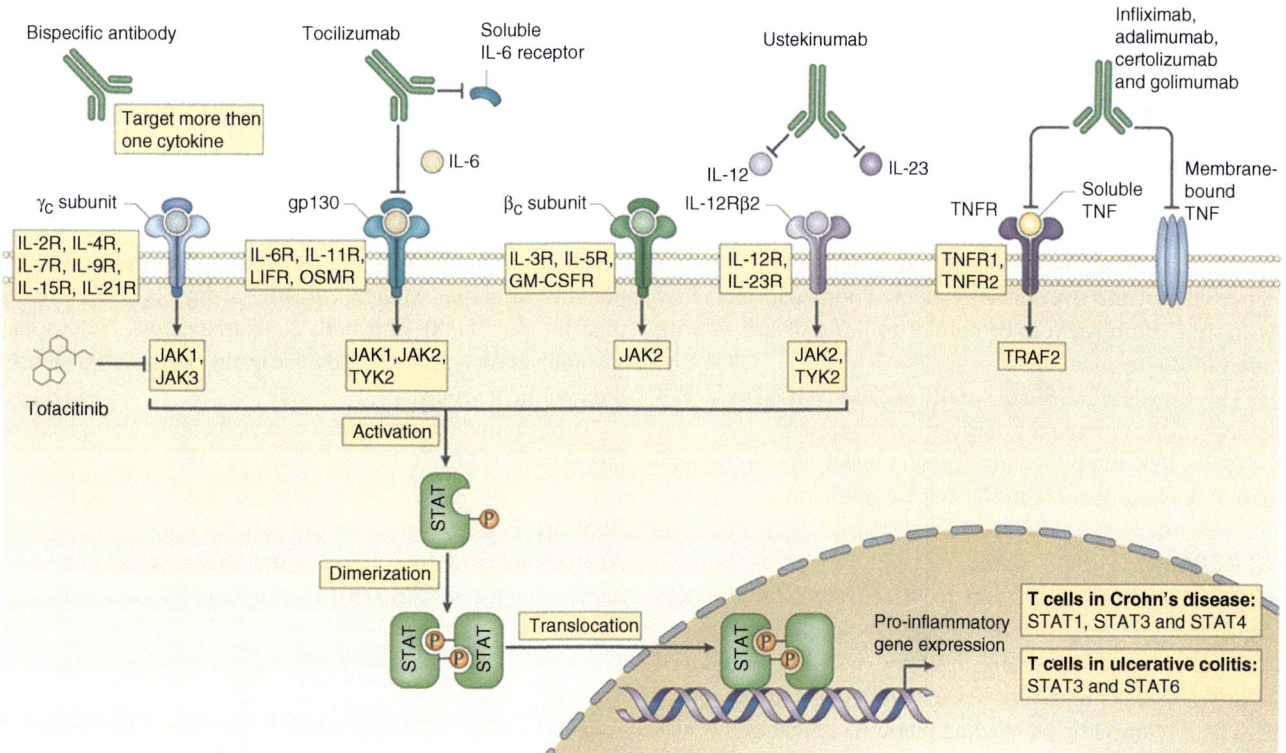

Fig. 35.4 JAK pathway inhibitors (Neurath [47])

uating tofacitinib as a maintenance therapy in patients with ulcerative colitis. Patients will either be given placebo orally twice daily, tofacitinib 5 mg orally twice daily or tofacitinib 10 mg orally twice daily. The primary endpoint is the proportion of subjects in remission at week 52. Secondary outcomes that will be measured is the proportion of patients with mucosal healing at week 52 and number of patients in sustained steroid free remission [52].

Pediatric Data
At the time of writing this chapter, there are no published data on the use of tofacitinib in children or adolescents with IBD.

Safety
Tofacitinib has generally been well tolerated in clinical trials. The most commonly reported adverse events related to infection reported by Sandborn and colleagues were influenza and nasopharyngitis [49, 50]. Two patients receiving the 10 mg dose twice daily had serious adverse events from infection (postoperative abscess, anal abscess). Of significance but uncertain long term consequence, a dose-dependent increase in low-density and high-density lipoprotein cholesterol was seen after 8 weeks of treatment which were reversible after discontinuing the study drugs [49, 50]. It is not clear what the long-term effects of this is. Three patients treated with tofacitinib (one at dose of 10 mg twice daily and two at dose of 15 mg twice daily) had an absolute neutrophil count of less than 1500 (with none being <1000) [53, 54]. Tofacitinib is a true immunosuppressant and there is a concern for increased risk of infections and lymphoma with using this drug compared to other biologics. However, this drug can be used as monotherapy which makes it a very appealing option. Herpes zoster infections have been observed quite frequently and in rheumatoid arthritis, several cases of lymphoma were reported, but the overall risks of infections and mortality with tofacitinib seem to be similar to those observed with other biologic agents [51].

This drug is administered orally and can be used as monotherapy, which makes it a very appealing option.

Other JAK inhibitors are currently under clinical investigation in phase II for both CD and UC [51].

GLPG0634
GLPG0634, has been shown to selectively inhibit JAK1-dependent signaling in cellular and whole blood assays as well as showed remarkable efficacy in collagen induced arthritis disease models for RA in both mouse and rat [55].

There is currently an ongoing phase II clinical trial evaluating the efficacy, safety and tolerability and pharmacokinetics of GLP0634 on Crohn's disease during a 20-week period of time [56].

Pediatric Data
At the time of writing this chapter, there are no published data on the use of GLPG0634 in children or adolescents with IBD.

TGF-B

One mechanism by which Crohn's disease develops involves transforming growth factor (TGF)-b which is a suppressive cytokine [57, 58]. SMAD7 is an endogenous inhibitor of the immunosuppressive cytokine transforming growth factor-β1. In Crohn's disease, TGF-b1 activity is inhibited by high Smad7, an intracellular protein that binds to the TGF-b1 receptor and prevents TGF-b1-driven signaling [59, 60]. Studies in mice have consistently shown that the induction of experimental CD-like colitis is associated with enhanced expression of Smad7 and reduced TGF-b1 activity [59]. The inhibition of Smad7 in CD mucosal cells with a specific antisense oligonucleotide has been demonstrated to restore TGF-b1 activity which therefore down-regulates the production of inflammatory cytokines [61].

GED0301 (Mongersen)
GED0301 is an antisense oligonucleotide targeting SMAD7 and is an oral gastro-resistant compound with a pH-dependent, delayed-release of the oligonucleotide in the terminal ileum and right colon.

A phase I clinical trial was performed which showed that GED0301 in active, steroid dependent/resistant CD patients resulted in a clinical benefit in all patients [62, 63].

In a placebo-controlled phase II study in patients with active CD [64], patients were randomized to receive induction treatment with different doses of GED0301 (Mongersen) or placebo for 2 weeks. The primary endpoint was clinical remission and this was seen in 55.0, 65.1, and 9.5 % of patients receiving Mongersen 40 mg/day, 160 mg/day, or placebo ($p < 0.0001$, for both comparisons) at 15 days and maintained for ≥2 weeks. Adverse events were similar across the treatment groups.

This promising molecule is now being investigated in larger trials [51].

Pediatric Data
At the time of writing this chapter, there are no published data on the use of GED0301 in children or adolescents with IBD.

Safety
A phase I clinical trial using GED0301 in active, steroid dependent/resistant CD patients was safe and well tolerated [62]. Adverse events were similar across the treatment groups in a phase II clinical trial [64].

Targeting Chemokines

Chemokines are cytokine proteins expressed in lymphoid and nonlymphoid tissue, thought to be involved in leukocyte trafficking. Their effects are mediated by g-protein coupled transmembrane receptors, which are classified by cysteine residues. Persistent, aberrant leukocyte chemotaxis to inflamed mucosa is thought to play a role in the pathogenesis of inflammatory bowel disease. Increased expression of several chemokines has been reported in patients with ulcerative colitis and Crohn's disease.

IP-10 Antagonists

Interferon-γ-inducible protein-10 (IP-10 or CXCL10) is a chemokine that plays an important role in the migration of cells into sites of inflammation by influencing activation and migration of activated T-cells, monocytes, eosinophils, natural killer, epithelial and endothelial cells [65, 66].

The receptor for CXCL-10 is CXCR3 but IL-10 also seems to modulate cellular function independently of CXCR3 [65]. CXCL10 has been found to be expressed in higher levels in the colonic tissue and plasma of patients with UC [67, 68]. In animal models of UC, blocking CXCL10 has been shown to modify disease progression [53, 66, 69–71].

BMS936557 (MDX-1100, Eldelumab)

BMS-936557 (Eldelumab) is a fully human, monoclonal antibody to CXCL10. A phase I, open-label, dose-escalation study of MDX-1100 was been performed in patients with UC using MDX-1100 [54]. The primary objective of this was to evaluate the safety of single doses of the drug in patients with ulcerative colitis having exacerbation on stable doses of standard therapy. Patients were off anti-TNF therapy for at least 8 weeks prior to the study. Cohorts of patients were given a single infusion of the drug at doses of 0.3, 1.0, 3.0, or 10 mg/kg and were followed for at least 70 days post infusion. A clinical response was defined as UCDAI decrease by ≥3 points at day 29 compared to baseline. Patients who responded were allowed to receive up to three additional infusions at the time of relapse. Peripheral blood mononuclear cells and colon biopsy specimens were studied for expression of CXCL10 and CXCL10-induced proteins. Three patients in the 1.0 mg/kg and two patients in the 3.0 mg/kg cohorts had clinical responses; however, one patient in the 1.0 mg/kg cohort also was started on concomitant immunomodulator therapy 2 months prior to MDX-1100 administration. Two of three responding patients who relapsed after 50, 85, and 93 days, respectively who had then been given additional MDX-1100 doses responded to retreatment. One patient in the 3.0 mg/kg cohort was admitted to the hospital for anemia and worsening UC requiring a colectomy but otherwise the drug was well tolerated.

Mayer, and colleagues in 2014 published data from an 8-week phase II, double-blind, multicenter, randomized study in patients with active ulcerative colitis [65]. Patients with moderately to severely active UC were given either BMS-936557 (10 mg/kg) or placebo intravenously every other week. The primary endpoint was the rate of clinical response at day 57 and secondary endpoints were clinical remission and mucosal healing rates. Fifty-five patients received the drug and 54 patients received placebo. Primary and secondary endpoints were not met. However, what was found was that with higher steady-state trough levels of BMS-936557 (108–235 µg/ml), there was an increased clinical response (87.5 % vs. 37 % $p < 0.001$) and histological improvement (73 % vs. 41 % $P = 0.004$) compared to placebo. Infections occurred in 12.7 % of BMS-936557 treated patients and 5.8 % placebo-treated patients. Two patients (or 3.6 %) discontinued due to adverse events.

In a phase IIb study of patients with ulcerative colitis [65, 72] patients ($n = 121$) with CDAI ≥220 and ≤450 were randomly assigned 1:1:1 to placebo or intravenous eldelumab 10 or 20 mg/kg given on days 1 and 8 and then every other week. Endoscopy videos were collected for all patients at baseline. Patients with a score of 2–3 on the ulcerated surface subscore of the Simplified Endoscopic Score for Crohn's Disease (SES-CD) in at least 1 of 5 segments had a follow up endoscopy at 11 weeks. A central reader read endoscopies in a blinded fashion. Trial endpoints included week 11 clinical response which was defined as a reduction in CDAI 100 points from baseline or an absolute CDAI score <150, clinical remission which was defined as CDAI <150 and endoscopic improvement. There was a trend towards efficacy as remission and response rates at week 11 for the 10 mg/kg dose, 20 mg/kg and placebo groups were 22.5 and 47.5 %, 29.3 and 41.5 %, vs. 20 and 35 % and were higher in anti-TNF-naive patients versus those patients who experienced anti-TNF failures. Both drug groups achieved a greater reduction from baseline in mean endoscopy scores compared to placebo and were similar in the eldelumab-treated groups across the anti-TNF-naive and anti-TNF failure subgroups [73].

Pediatric Data

At the time of writing this chapter, there are no published data on the use of BMS936557 in children or adolescents with IBD.

Safety

Serious adverse events were more common in the eldelumab groups (7.5 and 9.8 %) compared with placebo (5 %) in a phase IIb study of patients with ulcerative colitis [65, 73, 72].

Antiadhesion Molecules

Natalizumab

Natalizumab is a humanized IgG$_4$ monoclonal antibody against the adhesion molecule α4 integrin, which is involved in migration of leukocytes across the endothelium, and is upregulated in sites of inflamed endothelium. It is administered intravenously every 4 weeks. The efficacy of natalizumab for the treatment of multiple sclerosis has been demonstrated in controlled trials [74, 75, 76]. In November 2004 natalizumab was approved by the Food and Drug Administration (FDA) for the treatment of multiple sclerosis with subsequent withdrawal from the market in February 2005, and then reintroduction with certain restrictions for the treatment of multiple sclerosis in September 2006.

Six randomized, double-blind, placebo-controlled trials assessed the efficacy of in patients with Crohn's disease, whereas only one uncontrolled pilot study has been conducted in patients with ulcerative colitis.

An initial phase IIa trial comprised of 30 patients with active Crohn's disease who received randomly allocated single infusion of either natalizumab 3 mg/kg or placebo and had CDAI evaluated 2 weeks after infusion [77]. There was a significant decrease in baseline CDAI score in patients treated with natalizumab at week 2 (mean drop 45 points, $P = 0.02$), while no significant decrease was observed in placebo arm (mean drop 11 points, $P = 0.2$). It demonstrated a higher rate of clinical remission at week 2 in patients given natalizumab 3 mg/kg compared to placebo (39 % vs. 8 %, $P = 0.1$) [74]. There was no significant difference between natalizumab and placebo in achieving remission at week 2 (39 % vs. 8 %, $P = 0.1$). This pilot trial did not show any significant superiority of natalizumab over placebo in treating patients with Crohn's disease.

The second trial compared natalizumab (single infusion of 3 mg/kg, two infusions of 3 mg/kg or two infusions of 6 mg/kg) versus placebo in 248 patients with moderate to severe Crohn's disease [78]. The primary endpoint (remission, CDAI < 150 points at week 6) rates were 29 % for single infusion of natalizumab ($P = 0.757$), 44 % for two infusions of natalizumab 3 mg/kg ($P = 0.030$) and 31 % for two infusions of natalizumab 6 mg/kg ($P = 0.533$) versus 27 % in placebo arm. Only two doses of natalizumab 3 mg/kg had statistically significant superiority over placebo in achieving clinical remission.

Three Phase III trials have been conducted in Crohn's disease. In Efficacy of Natalizumab as Active Crohn Therapy (ENACT-1), 905 patients with moderate to severe Crohn's disease were randomly assigned to receive induction therapy at weeks 0, 4, and 8 with either natalizumab 300 mg or placebo [79]. The primary endpoint in the induction trial was clinical response defined as at least 70-point decrease in

baseline CDAI score at week 10 and it was achieved in 56 % and 49 % of natalizumab and placebo recipients, respectively ($P = 0.05$) [79]. In ENACT-2, 339 patients who had a response to natalizumab in induction ENACT-1 trial at both week 10 and 12 were randomly reassigned to receive 300 mg of natalizumab or placebo every 4 weeks from week 12 through week 56 [79]. The primary endpoint in ENACT-2 trial was a sustained response through week 36. Patients with at least 70-point increase in CDAI score after week 12 with an absolute CDAI score of at least 220 or needed therapeutic intervention after week 12 were considered losing response. Rates of sustained response at week 36 were 61 % in patients receiving maintenance treatment with natalizumab and 28 % in those receiving placebo maintenance ($P < 0.001$). It was demonstrated that maintenance treatment with natalizumab is significantly superior to placebo in patients who responded to induction treatment. Concomitant immunosuppressants did not improve the rates of clinical remission or response [80]. Patients who maintained remission on natalizumab over 12 months in the ENACT-2 trial were enrolled into a subsequent phase III, open-label, 2-year open-label extension trial designed to assess long-term efficacy and safety of natalizumab [81]. This open-label trial comprised of 146 patients who received 12 natalizumab infusions over 12 months. The proportion of patients who maintained remission after 6 (week 24) and 12 (week 48) additional infusions of natalizumab was 89 % and 84 %, respectively. This open-label extension trial supported data from ENACT-2 trial that natalizumab maintains remission over additional 12 months in patients with sustained remission on natalizumab in the preceding 12 months.

In the ENCORE trial, 509 patients with moderate to severe Crohn's disease with elevated C-reactive protein concentrations at baseline were randomized to receive natalizumab 300 mg or placebo at weeks 0, 4, and 8 [82]. Natalizumab was significantly superior over placebo in inducing remission at week 8 that was sustained through week 12 (primary endpoint defined as at least 70-point decrease in CDAI score) with respective proportions of patients of 48 % vs. 32 % ($P < 0.001$). In addition natalizumab was also significantly superior over placebo in achieving additional efficacy endpoint, namely clinical remission at week 8 sustained through week 12 CDAI <150 that was observed in 26 % of natalizumab-treated patients and 16 % of placebo recipients ($P = 0.002$).

Finally, Sands et al. performed a placebo-controlled trial in which 79 patients with active Crohn's disease during ongoing treatment with infliximab 5 mg/kg every 8 weeks for at least 10 weeks before initiation of randomization were randomly assigned to receive three intravenous infusions of either natalizumab 300 mg or placebo every 4 weeks while continuing their initial infliximab regimen during duration of the trial [83]. At week 6 patients treated with natalizumab plus infliximab experienced mean decrease in their CDAI score of 37.7 points, while those treated with placebo plus infliximab experienced small increase in CDAI score of a mean of 3.5 points ($P = 0.084$). A trend towards greater efficacy of combined treatment with natalizumab and infliximab over infliximab alone was shown in patients with active Crohn's disease not responding to infliximab therapy.

Gordon et al. published results of one small open-label study of 10 patients with active ulcerative colitis who were treated with a single infusion of natalizumab 3 mg/kg [84]. All patients had their disease activity evaluated using Powell-Tuck score 2 weeks after infusion. Treatment with natalizumab resulted in significant decrease in median disease activity score from 10 at baseline to 6 at 2 weeks postinfusion ($P = 0.004$). It was suggested that future randomized, placebo-controlled trials are warranted to further assess the efficacy of natalizumab in ulcerative colitis.

Pediatric Data

There was only one open-label study conducted in 38 pediatric patients (ages 12–17 years) with active Crohn's disease that assessed the efficacy of natalizumab in a pediatric population [84]. Among 38 enrolled patients 31 of them received three intravenous infusions of natalizumab 3 mg/kg at weeks 0, 4, and 8. Disease activity was measured using Pediatric Crohn's disease Activity Index (PCDAI) at baseline and then every 2 weeks through week 12. There was a significant decrease observed in PCDAI score from baseline at every time point ($P < 0.001$) with the greatest decrease observed at week 10 with 55 % of patients achieving clinical response (>15-point decrease from baseline) and 29 % of patients achieving clinical remission (PCDAI <10). These promising findings however need to be validated in large randomized controlled trials.

Safety

In one study in patients with Crohn's disease, 7 % of patients given one or two induction doses of natalizumab (at weeks 0 and 4) had formed anti-natalizumab antibodies at 12 weeks [78]. Patients in the ENACT-2 trial who received concomitant immunosuppressants did not develop persistent anti-natalizumab antibodies, compared to 7.5 % of patients who received natalizumab alone [79]. In patients with multiple sclerosis, the rate of formation of anti-natalizumab antibodies was 9 %, with persistence in 6 % (antibodies detected ≥ 2 more than 42 days apart) [85].

The largest ENACT-1 ($n = 905$) and ENACT-2 ($n = 339$) trials of natalizumab observed that serious adverse events occurred in similar proportion of patients in both trials (7 % in natalizumab and placebo arms in induction ENACT-1 trial and 8 % in natalizumab arm and 10 % in placebo arm in maintenance trial) [81]. However, one patient died (three doses of natalizumab combined with azathioprine during ENACT-1, placebo with azathioprine during ENACT-2 and

-5 doses of natalizumab alone after completion of ENACT-2 trial) from progressive multifocal leukoencephalopathy, associated with the JC virus was observed [85]. The other large induction trial ENCORE on 509 patients Adverse events observed similar proportion of adverse events between natalizumab (85 %) and placebo (82 %) arms without any deaths [82]. The most common adverse events that were observed in at least 10 % among either treatment arms were headache, nausea, abdominal pain, nasopharyngitis, dizziness, fatigue, and exacerbation of Crohn's disease. There was a significant greater proportion of patients in natalizumab group versus placebo that experienced nasopharyngitis (11 % vs. 6 %, $p < 0.05$), headache (29 % vs. 21 %, $p < 0.05$) and hypersensitivity reaction (4 % vs. 0.8 %, $p < 0.05$). On the other hand, exacerbation of Crohn's disease was observed in greater proportion of placebo treated patients when compared to natalizumab (13 % vs. 7 %, $P < 0.05$). Antibodies to natalizumab were detected in 9.5 of 241 tested patients treated with natalizumab and in 0.8 % of 236 tested placebo recipients ($P < 0.05$).

A placebo-controlled trial by Sands et al. assessed primarily safety of concurrent therapy with natalizumab in 79 patients with Crohn's disease already receiving infliximab [83]. The observed incidence of adverse events was similar in the treatment groups (natalizumab plus infliximab vs. infliximab plus placebo). The most frequent adverse events in both groups were headache, Crohn's disease exacerbation, nausea, and nasopharyngitis. No one experienced a hypersensitivity-like reaction to natalizumab, whilst 4 patients (5 %) experienced such reactions to infliximab. The development of antibodies to natalizumab was reported in 4%of patients whereas antibodies to infliximab were detected in 14 % of patients.

Data from pediatric open-label study showed that the most common adverse events were headache (26 %), pyrexia (21 %) and exacerbation of Crohn's disease (24 %) [86]. Anti-natalizumab antibodies were detected in 8 % of patients.

Clinical trials and marketing of natalizumab were suspended in February 2005 after two patients with multiple sclerosis treated with natalizumab and interferon beta-1A developed progressive multifocal leukoencephalopathy (PML) from reactivation of the latent human Jacob Creutzfeldt polyoma virus [87, 88]. A third patient treated with natalizumab and prior exposure to azathioprine was reclassified from malignant astrocytoma to PML [89]. An independent adjudication committee performed a safety evaluation in all patients who had recently been treated with natalizumab in clinical trials [90]. Evaluation consisted of a referral to a neurologist, brain magnetic resonance imaging, and polymerase chain reaction analysis of cerebral spinal fluid and serum for JC virus. Of 3826 initial patients enrolled in clinical trials of natalizumab, safety evaluation included 87 % (1275), 91 % (2248), and 92 % (296) of patients with Crohn's disease, multiple sclerosis, and rheumatoid arthritis patients. No additional cases of PML were identified [90]. The median duration of treatment for all patients was 17.9 months, while that of patients with Crohn's disease was 7 months. The absolute risk of developing PML during treatment with natalizumab was 1:1000 (0.1 %) with 95 % confidence intervals of 1:200–1:2800 [91]. The FDA reapproved natalizumab for multiple sclerosis in September 2006, with the requirement of mandatory participation in a risk management and registry program called the TOUCH program [85].

Vedolizumab (MLN-002, MLN-02, Entyvio®)

Vedolizumab (also known as MLN-002 and MLN-02) is a recombinant IgG1 humanized monoclonal antibody against the adhesion molecule $\alpha 4\beta 7$ integrin and is the first gut-selective humanized monoclonal antibody. In contrast to natalizumab, vedolizumab specifically targets $\alpha 4\beta 7$ integrins that are exclusively present on gut homing T cells and as a result the interaction between $\alpha 4\beta 7$ and antimucosal vascular addressin cell adhesion molecule (MAdCAM)-1 is blocked.

GEMINI I was a double-blind, phase III trial in patients with moderate to severe UC [92]. Patients were randomized to receive vedolizumab (300 mg intravenously) or placebo on day 1 and day 15. The primary endpoint of the induction trial was clinical response at week 6 and this was achieved in 47 % vs. 26 % of patients receiving vedolizumab and placebo, respectively ($P < 0.0001$). Clinical remission at week 6 was seen in 17 % versus 5 % on vedolizumab vs. placebo ($P = 0.0009$) and mucosal healing was seen in 41 and 25 % in the vedolizumab versus placebo groups ($P = 0.0012$). Patients who achieved a clinical response after induction therapy were randomized to receive placebo or further intravenous vedolizumab at 300 mg at 4- or 8-week dosing intervals up to 46 weeks. Clinical remission rates at week 52 were 42 and 45 % in the vedolizumab 8- and 4-weekly groups, respectively, versus 16 % in the placebo arm; $P < 0.0001$. Mucosal healing rates were also significantly higher in the vedolizumab group – 52 and 56 % in the vedolizumab 8- and 4-weekly group versus 20 % in the placebo group; $P < 0.0001$. The overall clinical efficacy was higher with vedolizumab in those patients naive to anti-TNF-naïve compared to those who had a prior failure or intolerance to anti-TNF therapy.

GEMINI II was a clinical trial evaluating vedolizumab in patients with moderate to severe CD [93]. Week 6 clinical remission rates were 13.3 vs. 9.7 % ($P = 0.157$) and 22.7 vs. 10.6 % ($P = 0.005$) in patients who had failed anti-TNF therapy vs. those who were naive to anti-TNF therapy compared to placebo. Week 10 clinical remission rates were 21.7 versus 11 % ($P = 0.0008$) and 24.7 versus 15.4 % ($P = 0.044$) in patients who had failed anti-TNF therapy and anti-TNF naive patients compared to placebo, respectively. Week 52 clinical remission rates were 52 and 27 % in vedolizumab vs.

placebo groups naive to anti-TNF but in those patients who had failed anti-TNF therapy, the clinical response rate was lower (28 versus 13 % in the vedolizumab and placebo groups, respectively).

GEMINI III is a placebo-controlled phase III induction trial evaluating the efficacy and safety of vedolizumab in CD patients who had failed anti-TNF therapy [94]. At week 6, clinical remission rates were not found to be superior in vedolizumab vs. placebo groups (15.2 and 12.1 % ($P = 0.433$)). However, at week 10 the therapeutic efficacy of vedolizumab was detected and vedolizumab was statistically superior to placebo for inducing clinical remission at week 10 (26.6 % versus 12.1 % in the vedolizumab vs. placebo groups, respectively ($P = 0.001$).

Overall, the results with vedolizumab seem to be somewhat better in UC compared to CD and the 6-week time point in CD was thought to have been set too early to appreciate optimal efficacy given the mode of action of this agent. In the open-label long-term extension study (GEMINI LTS) there was a suggestion that certain patients benefited from an increase in vedolizumab dosing frequency from every 8 weeks to every 4 weeks.

This drug was approved in 2014 by the FDA and EMA for both UC and CD, refractory to standard therapy and/or anti-TNF agents. It has the potential to become the first line biologic agent in UC given its higher efficacy in TNF-naïve patients.

Pediatric Data

Data on efficacy and safety of vedolizumab are currently not available in literature. However, Zoet and colleagues described an adolescent boy with ulcerative colitis who was started on monotherapy with vedolizumab at the age of 16 after having failed prior treatments including anti-TNF therapy. Before initiation of therapy, endoscopy showed severe ulcerative. After the first two doses of vedolizumab, the patient dramatically improved clinically. At 8 weeks post induction of the drug, endoscopic assessment demonstrated complete mucosal healing and the PUCAI score had improved to 5. At 4 months post induction, no side effects of vedolizumab were seen [95].

Safety

Patients with UC (GEMINI I) and CD (GEMINI II) who completed 52 weeks of vedolizumab treatment were enrolled in GEMINI LTS for an additional 52 weeks. The 2-year efficacy data of vedolizumab in CD and in UC was presented [96] and this showed the safety of vedolizumab in the GEMINI program. To date, there have been no cases of PML. Furthermore, Milch and colleagues conducted a study to determine whether vedolizumab alters T cell subpopulations in cerebrospinal fluid and no significant changes in T cell populations were observed [97]. Also, the incidence of systemic and gastrointestinal infections was similar among patients on vedolizumab or placebo [98].

Only 4 % of patients in the pooled UC and CD patients from GEMINI I and II tested positive for anti-vedolizumab antibodies during maintenance treatment with vedolizumab. Similar rates of antidrug antibodies were observed in the vedolizumab monotherapy and combination (3 % vs. 4 %). Antivedolizumab antibodies might have clinical implications, but further studies are needed to clarify their importance [51].

Furthermore, safety data (May 2009–June 2013) from six trials of vedolizumab were integrated and treatment with vedolizumab for up to 5 years demonstrated a favorable safety profile. In total, 2830 patients had 4811 person-years of vedolizumab. No increased risk of any infection or serious infection was associated with vedolizumab exposure. No cases of progressive multifocal leucoencephalopathy were observed. Infusion-related reactions as defined by the investigator were reported for ≤5 % of patients in each study. Eighteen vedolizumab-exposed patients (<1 %) were diagnosed with a malignancy [99].

Etrolizumab (rhuMAb β7)

Etrolizumab is a humanized monoclonal antibody that selectively targets the β7 subunit of α4β7 and αEβ7 integrins and as a result blocks leucocyte migration.

In a placebo-controlled, randomized phase II trial, patients with moderate to severe UC received subcutaneous etrolizumab (100 mg at weeks 0, 4, and 8, with placebo at week 2 or 420 mg at week 0 and 300 mg etrolizumab at weeks 2, 4, and 8) or placebo [100]. At week 10, etrolizumab was found to be more effective in achieving clinical remission (primary endpoint) as compared to placebo – 21 and 10 % of patients in the 100- or 300 mg etrolizumab group, respectively, and in 0 % of patients receiving placebo; the low placebo rate was thought to be a result of very careful patient selection. This study also revealed the potential role of αE as a biomarker to identify patients that are most likely to benefit from etrolizumab treatment as patients who had a clinical benefit in UC had increased αE expression levels in the inflamed colon.

Phase III studies are now underway in UC and CD.

Pediatric Data
At the time of writing this chapter, there are no published data on the use of etrolizumab in children or adolescents with IBD.

PF-00547659

PF-00547659 is a fully human monoclonal antibody that binds specifically to human MAdCAM-1. Functional assays have shown the drug to block the adhesion of a4b7 integrin expressing cells to MAdCAM-1 [101].

In a randomized, placebo-controlled trial evaluating the safety and efficacy of PF-00547659 in patients with active UC, 80 patients received a single or three doses of PF-00547659 (0.03–10 mg/kg, intravenously or subcutaneously administered) or placebo at 4-week dosing intervals [102]. No statistical differences were found between patients given the drug compared to placebo although some benefits were seen in the actively treated group in terms of clinical and endoscopic improvements. Clinical response at week 4 was seen in 32 and 52 % of patients on placebo or PF-0054659 (all doses) ($P = 0.102$) and clinical response at week 12 was 21 versus 42 % in the placebo and PF-00547659 groups, respectively ($P = 0.156$). Adverse events were similar between the PF-00547659 versus placebo groups with the most common adverse event being abdominal pain [73, 103].

Larger clinical trials evaluating efficacy of PF-00547659 in UC and CD were completed in 2015. The TURANDOT study was a phase II trial evaluating the safety and efficacy of PF-00547659 in patients with UC [104]. Three hundred and fifty-seven adults with UC (with disease extending more than 15 cm beyond the rectum and with a total Mayo Score at least 6 and endoscopic subscore of at least 2) who had failed at least one prior therapy were randomized to receive 7.5, 22.5, 75, or 225 mg of PF-00547659 or placebo every 4 weeks for three doses. Clinical remission at week 12 was the primary endpoint defined as total Mayo score 2 or less with no subscore more than 1. Clinical response (Mayo score decrease 3 and 30 % decrease from baseline) at week 12 and mucosal healing (Mayo endoscopy subscore 1) were secondary endpoints. Clinical remission at week 12 was significantly greater in the 7.5, 22.5, and 75 mg dose groups compared with placebo. Clinical response was greater for the 22.5 and 225 mg groups and mucosal healing was significantly greater in the 22.5 and 75 mg dose groups compared with placebo. Greater differences compared with placebo were observed in anti-TNF naive patients (43 % of patients had not had prior anti-TNF therapy). The 22.5 mg dose was the most effective dose for all endpoints – clinical remission: 16.7 % vs. 2.7 % clinical remission rates, 54.2 % vs. 28.8 % clinical response rates and 27.8 % versus 8.2 % mucosal healing in drug vs. placebo groups (all $P < 0.05$). Overall and serious adverse event rates were similar between all groups.

OPERA is a randomized, multicenter double-blind, placebo-controlled study evaluating the safety and efficacy of PF-00547659 in patients with Crohn's disease [105]. Two hundred and sixty seven adults with moderate to severe Crohn's disease (CDAI 220–450), who had failed or did not tolerate other therapy (anti-TNF and/or immunosuppressant drugs), had C-reactive protein (CRP) more than 3.0 mg/l and ulcers on colonoscopy were randomized to placebo or PF-00547659 at the dose of 22.5 mg, 75 mg, or 225 mg. The primary endpoint was CDAI-70 response at week 8 or 12.

Secondary endpoints included clinical remission and CDAI-100 response. The frequency and level of b7 expression on peripheral CD4þ central memory T cells, CRP and soluble MAdCAM-1 levels were also evaluated. The CDAI-70 response was not significantly different between any of PF-00547659 doses and placebo but in patients who had a baseline CRP level more than 18 remission at week 12 was higher in the drug groups compared to placebo (37 %, 24 and 39 % with increasing doses vs. 14 % placebo). At week 2, soluble MAdCAM-1 decreased significantly in a dose-dependent manner and remained low during the study in patients who received drug. Circulating b7 CD4þ central memory T-lymphocytes had increased in a dose-dependent manner at weeks 8 and 12 in patients treated with PF-00547659. PF-00547659 was well tolerated with the most common adverse events related to the underlying disease.

Pediatric Data

At the time of writing this chapter, there are no published data on the use of PF-00547659 in children or adolescents with IBD.

AJM300

AJM300 is an orally active small molecule with antagonistic properties to α4-integrin. The only trial published in an abstract from a randomized trial involving 71 patients with active Crohn's disease. This study compared oral treatment with either AJM300 (40 mg tid, 120 mg tid, or 240 mg tid) to placebo for 8 weeks [106]. The primary endpoint was the decrease of CDAI score from baseline to final evaluation at week 4 or later, while the secondary efficacy endpoint was clinical response (≥70 point decrease in CDAI). There was no significant difference in clinical response was observed between active treatment and placebo arms. Among patients with high CDAI at baseline a significant decrease from baseline CDAI score (mean decrease 41.5 points, $P = 0.0485$) was observed in those treated with AJM300 at the dose of 120 mg tid and mean 41.6 point decrease from baseline CDAI in those treated with AJM300 at the dose of 240 mg tid (p-value not reported). In addition, patients treated with AJM at the dose of 240 mg tid had significant twofold decrease in C-reactive protein from baseline over 8 weeks ($P = 0.0220$). The investigators suggested that AJM300 at dose 120 mg tid and 240 mg tid showed clinical efficacy in treating patients with active Crohn's disease [106].

Pediatric Data

At the time of writing this chapter there are no published data on the use of AJM300 in children or adolescents with IBD.

Safety

AJM300 was tolerated well with incidence of adverse events that was not dose-dependent (0.0 %, 23.5 %, and 22.2 % for AJM300 40 mg, 120 mg and 240 mg treated patients, respectively, vs. 16.7 % for placebo-treated patients, p-value not reported) [106].

Alicaforsen

Alicaforsen (ISIS 2302) is a 20 base phosphorothioate oligodeoxy-nucleotide that hybridizes to a sequence in the 3′ untranslated region of intercellular adhesion molecule 1 (ICAM-1) mRNA [107]. The translated oligonucleotide-RNA serves as a substrate for the nuclease RNase-H, an ubiquitous intracellular endoribonuclease that recognizes DNA:RNA heteroduplexes as substrate for selective RNA hydrolysis. This results in reduction of ICAM-1 RNA expression and protein levels. Intravenous, subcutaneous, and rectal enema formulations have been studied in patients with Crohn's disease or ulcerative colitis.

There have been three randomized, placebo-controlled trials that assessed the efficacy of alicaforsen administered intravenously [108, 109, 110] and one randomized, placebo-controlled trial that evaluated the efficacy of this agent administered subcutaneously [111] in patients with active Crohn's disease.

A phase IIA, double-blind, randomized, placebo-controlled trial of 20 patients with active Crohn's disease suggested the efficacy of intravenously administered alicaforsen [109]. Patients were randomly assigned to be treated with 13 infusions of either alicaforsen (0.5, 1, or 2 mg/kg, $n = 15$) or placebo ($n = 5$) over the period of 26 days with subsequent 6-month follow-up [111]. The rates of clinical remission (CDAI < 150) at the end of treatment were 47 % and 20 % in active drug and placebo arms, respectively (p-value not reported) [111]. ISIS 2302 showed corticosteroid sparing effect with significantly lower dose of corticosteroids over time when compared to placebo ($p = 0.0001$). Data from subsequent dose ranging pharmacokinetic trial of high-dose alicaforsen administered intravenously at the dose of 300 or 350 mg three times a week for 4 weeks in 22 patients with active Crohn's disease demonstrated that 41 % of patients achieved clinical remission indicating that this agent might be efficacious in treating Crohn's disease. Unfortunately, large randomized, placebo-controlled trials with intravenous alicaforsen did not support these preliminary findings.

In the subsequent large clinical trial that comprised of 299 patients with active steroid dependent (prednisone 10–40 mg) Crohn's disease patients were randomly assigned to intravenous treatment three times a week with either ISIS 2302 (2 mg/kg) or placebo for 2 or 4 weeks and the regimen was then repeated after 1 month without treatment [108]. The corticosteroid-free remission (CDAI < 150) at week 14 (primary endpoint) was comparable between combined ISIS 2302 and placebo arms (20.2 % vs. 18.8 %, p-value not reported). On the other hand, a significantly greater proportion of patients receiving ISIS 2302 than placebo had successful corticosteroids withdrawal at week 14 (78 % vs. 64 %; P = 0.032). According to pharmacodynamic analysis statistically significant results for clinical remission, improvement in CDAI and quality of life based on IBD questionnaire were observed in the highest area under the curve subgroup of ISIS 2302 arm when compared to placebo. Finally, data from two double-masked, placebo-controlled trials of patients with Crohn's disease who received intravenous treatment with either alicaforsen (n = 221) or placebo (n = 110) three times a week for 4 weeks did not show any benefit of alicaforsen over placebo in achieving clinical remission at week 12 with respective remission rates of 33.9 % and 34.5 % (P = 0.89) [110]. Subcutaneous administration of alicaforsen also did not demonstrate any superiority over placebo in achieving clinical remission in patients with Crohn's disease. Schreiber et al. randomized 75 patients with corticosteroid-refractory Crohn's disease to subcutaneous treatment with either ISIS 2302 or placebo [111]. The primary endpoint, corticosteroid-free remission at week 14 (CDAI < 150) was observed in 3.3 % of ISIS-2302-treated and 0 % of placebo treated patients. On the other hand, there was a trend towards efficacy of ISIS 2302 in achieving one of the secondary endpoints, namely corticosteroid-free remission at week 26 (13.3 % vs. 6.7 %, p-value not reported). Similarly, a greater proportion of patients receiving active drug when compared to placebo achieved a corticosteroid dose <10 mg/day at week 14 (48.3 % vs. 33.3 %) and week 26 (55.0 % vs. 40.0 %) and a prednisone equivalent dose of 0 mg at week 26 [23.3 % vs. 6.7 %, respectively].

There have been three randomized, placebo-controlled trials assessing the efficacy of alicaforsen enemas in patients with active left-side ulcerative colitis [91, 103, 112].

Van Deventer et al. performed a randomized, placebo-controlled trial of alicaforsen enema in 40 patients with mild to moderately active distal ulcerative colitis who received 60 mL of alicaforsen enema (0.1, 0.5, 2, or 4 mg/mL) or placebo once daily for 28 consecutive days. There was observed a significant dose-dependent reduction in disease activity index in patients treated with active drug than placebo at day 29 that was observed for alicaforsen given at the highest dose 4 mg/mL (70 % vs. 28 %, P = 0.004). After 3 months alicaforsen 2 mg/mL and 4 mg/mL caused significant reduction in disease activity index when compared to placebo by 72 % and 68 %, respectively (vs. 11.5 % for placebo, P = 0.016 and 0.021, respectively). In the subsequent phase II dose ranging, double-blind, placebo-controlled study of alicaforsen enema (120 mg daily for 10 days, then

every other day; 240 mg every other day; 240 mg daily for 10 days, then every other day; 240 mg daily) given daily for 6 weeks in 112 patients presenting with acute exacerbation of mild to moderate left-sided ulcerative colitis there was no significant difference observed between active drug and placebo in reduction of disease activity index at week 6 [91]. However, a greater proportion of patients receiving alicaforsen 240 mg daily had prolonged clinical improvement at week 18 (51 % vs. 18 %) and week 30 (50 % vs. 11 %) when compared to placebo. Finally, Miner et al. compared two dose formulations of alicaforsen enema (120 mg or 240 mg) with 4 g mesalamine enema given for 6 weeks in 159 patients with mild to moderate left-sided ulcerative colitis [103]. There was no difference observed between treatment arms in reduction of disease activity index at week 6 with reduction in mean disease activity index when compared to baseline of 50 % for the mesalamine arm and 40 % and 41 % for the 120 and 240 mg alicaforsen groups (P = 0.27 and 0.32, respectively). However, higher dose of alicaforsen enema was significantly more efficacious than mesalamine in achieving clinical remission at week 18 (20 % vs. 6 %, P = 0.03) [103].

An open-label study of alicaforsen enema given at daily dose of 240 mg for 6 weeks to 15 patients with active ulcerative colitis showed a 46 % reduction in mean disease activity index and 33 % rate of complete mucosal healing at the end of treatment [113]. In addition, alicaforsen concentrations were greater in mucosal colonic tissue biopsies than those observed in plasma suggesting that alicaforsen enemas allow for achieving high local concentrations with little systemic exposure. Another open-label study of 12 patients with chronic pouchitis following an ileal pouch-anal anastomosis for ulcerative colitis showed that alicaforsen enemas given at dose of 240 mg daily for 6 weeks resulted in significant reduction in the mean pouchitis disease activity index from baseline value of 11.42 points to 6.83 points at 6 weeks (P = 0.001) [114].

Pediatric Data

At the time of writing this chapter there are no published data on the use of alicaforsen in children or adolescents with IBD.

Safety

Data from large trial of 331 patients treated with intravenous alicaforsen or placebo showed that the only adverse events that occurred in greater proportion of patients treated with alicaforsen were symptoms related to infusion reactions such as fever (22.6 % vs. 14.7 %, p-not significant), chills (14 % vs. 1.8 %, P = 0.0005), and myalgia (5.4 % vs. 0.92 %) [110]. Data from the second largest trial of 299 patients with Crohn's disease receiving alicaforsen or placebo intravenously showed that the only adverse events that occurred in significantly greater proportion of patients treated with active drug than placebo were infusion reactions described as transient facial flushing or a feeling of warmth during infusion (11.6 % vs. 4 %, $P = 0.03$) [108]. There was a significantly greater average transient aPTT increase without bleeding sequelae (8.66 s vs. 0.8 s, $P +0.0001$) after alicaforsen than placebo infusion [108]. Safety analysis of alicaforsen administered subcutaneously in the largest trial of 75 patients determined that injection site reactions, headache, pain, fever, rash, arthritis, asthenia, and flu-like symptoms injection site reactions occurred in greater proportion of patients treated with active drug than placebo with injection site reactions demonstrating the largest difference (23.3 % vs. 0 %, p-value not reported) [111].

Gastrointestinal complaints were associated with the alicaforsen enemas in a dose-dependent fashion. Community-acquired pneumonia and sinusitis were also reported and were associated with the study drug [91, 103, 112, 113, 114].

AMG181

AMG181 is a human monoclonal IgG2 antibody that specifically binds to a4b7 heterodimers.

A phase I first inhuman randomized, double-blind, placebo-controlled study conducted in healthy subjects and subjects with UC evaluating the pharmacokinetics and pharmacodynamics, safety, tolerability, and effects of subcutaneous or intravenous AMG181 was performed [115]. Sixty-eight healthy male subjects received a single dose of AMG181 or placebo at 0.7, 2.1, 7, 21, 70 mg SC (or IV), 210 mg SC (or IV), 420 mg IV or placebo. Four patients with UC received 210 mg AMG181 or placebo SC (3:1). Among the findings, AMG181-treated UC subjects were in remission with mucosal healing at weeks 6, 12, and/or 28 and the placebo-treated UC subject experienced a colitis flare at week 6. No treatment-related serious adverse events were observed.

AMG181 is currently being tested in subjects with UC or CD in phase II clinical trials.

Pediatric Data

At the time of writing this chapter, there are no published data on the use of AMG181 in children or adolescents with IBD.

Firategrast (SB 683699)

Firategrast is an orally bioavailable small molecule α4-integrin antagonist [116].

A phase II studies evaluating the effectiveness and safety of the 683,699 in treating subjects with moderately to severely active CD has been completed. Results are not available [117].

Pediatric Data

At the time of writing this chapter, there are no published data on the use of Firategrast in children or adolescents with IBD.

GLPG0974

Free fatty acids (FFA) act as inflammatory signaling molecules through receptors such as FFA2, which is activated by short chain fatty acids (SCFA). Through FFA2, SCFAs induce neutrophil activation and migration. In IBD patients, FFA2 expression is up-regulated in the colon.

GLPG0974 is a potent and selective antagonist of FFA2, inhibiting SCFA-induced neutrophil migration and activation in vitro.

In a 4-week, first-in-UC study with GLPG0974 in patients with mild to moderate UC, GLPG0974 was well tolerated and safe. Biomarkers (MPO and FC) indicate that GLPG0974 reduces neutrophil activation and influx, suggesting a role for FFA2 in neutrophil migration in UC. The reduction in neutrophil influx is not sufficient to induce a measurable clinical difference between GLPG0974 treated patients and placebo within 4 weeks [118].

Phase II studies are ongoing.

Pediatric Data

At the time of writing this chapter, there are no published data on the use of GLPG0974 in children or adolescents with IBD.

TRK-170

TRK-170 is a novel orally active alpha4beta1/alpha4beta7 integrin antagonist. A study evaluated the effect of TRK-170, as compared to an anti-alpha4 antibody and prednisolone, on 2, 4, 6-trinitrobenzene sulfonic acid (TNBS)-induced colitis. Oral administration of TRK-170 significantly inhibited the increase of macroscopic damage scores. TRK-170 also reduced the elevation of myeloperoxidase activity in colons, and the increase in colon weight. Efficacy of TRK-170 is almost comparable to the anti-alpha4 antibody and prednisolone at this dosage and dose regimen. Detailed mechanisms of action of TRK-170, such as potential effects on immune cells, are being characterized. These results indicate that TRK-170 is expected to provide an attractive approach for the future therapy of IBD. Because TRK-170 is orally active unlike anti-alpha4 antibody, TRK-170 may be more beneficial than the antibody [119].

Phase II clinical studies are ongoing.

Pediatric Data

At the time of writing this chapter, there are no published data on the use of TRK-170 in children or adolescents with IBD.

Administration of Anti-inflammatory Cytokine

Interleukin-10 (IL-10)

Interleukin-10 is secreted by T helper cells, B cells, monocytes, macrophages, dendritic cells and keratinocytes. It suppresses inflammation by reducing HLA class I expression decreasing secretion of IL-2 and diminishing production of IL-1α, Il-1β, IL-6, IL-8, and TNF-α. The recombinant human rHuIL-10 may be administered subcutaneously, intravenously, or orally via a genetically modified *Lactococcus lactis* (LL-Thy12) in which the thymidylate synthase gene is replaced with a synthetic sequence encoding mature human interleukin-10.

Interleukin-10 has shown efficacy in treatment of chronic hepatitis C [120] , and modest improvement in skin but not arthritic manifestations of psoriasis in a Phase II trial [121]. Open-label and Phase I trials in patients with rheumatoid arthritis failed to show clinical efficacy or decrease in inflammation from synovial biopsies [122, 123].

Several placebo-controlled trials assessed the efficacy of either intravenously or subcutaneously administered rhu-IL-10 in the treatment of patients with active Crohn's disease. A randomized, double-blind, placebo-controlled phase IIa trial by Van Deventer et al. suggested that intravenous bolus of recombinant human IL-10 once daily for 7 consecutive days (rhu-IL-10) might be efficacious for the treatment of active Crohn's disease [124]. Among 46 patients with active steroid-resistant Crohn's disease who were treated with rhu-IL-10 (0.5, 1, 5, 10, or 25 µg/kg) or placebo 50 % treated with active drug and 23 who received placebo achieved a complete remission (decrease in baseline CDAI <150 and >100-point decrease in CDAI when compared to baseline) at any time during 3-week follow-up (*p*-value not reported). The second randomized, placebo-controlled trial of subcutaneous rhuIL-10 (1, 5, 10, or 20 µ/kg) given for 28 consecutive days with subsequent 20-week follow-up in 95 patients with active Crohn's disease observed that only rhu-IL-10 administered at dose 5 µg/kg showed benefit over placebo with 23.5 % (CI, 6.8–49.9 %) and 0 % (CI, 0–14.8 %) rates of complete remission (CDAI <150 and at ≥100 point decrease in CDAI from baseline with improvement or resolution in on endoscopy) measured on day 29 [125].

A double-blind, placebo-controlled phase III trial of 329 patients with chronic, active and refractory to corticosteroids Crohn's disease randomly allocated patients to receive subcutaneous injections with either rhu_IL-10 (1, 4, 8, or 20 µ/kg) or placebo daily for 28 days [126].

There was no significant difference between any of rhu-IL-10 dose and placebo in inducing primary endpoint, clinical remission (CDAI ≤ 150 with concomitant decrease in CDAI ≥ 100 points from baseline) with rates of 18 % for dose 1 µg/kg (*P* = 0.79 vs. placebo), 20 % for dose 4 µg/kg (*P* = 0.76), 20 % for dose 8 µg/kg (*P* = 0.76), 28 % for dose 20 µg/kg (*P* = 0.17) when compared to 18 % for placebo-treated patients [126]. There was a significant superiority in achieving clinical improvement (decrease in CDAI ≥100 points when compared to baseline) in patients who received rhu-IL-10 at the dose 8 µg/kg when compared to placebo (46 % vs. 27 %, *P* = 0.034).

A subsequent randomized, double-blind, placebo-controlled phase III trial (published only in an abstract form) assessed the efficacy of rhu-IL-10 in 373 patients with corticosteroid-dependent Crohn's disease who received once daily subcutaneously for 2 weeks then 3 times per week for 26 weeks either rhu-IL-10 (4 µg/kg or 8 µg/kg) or placebo [127]. Rhu-IL-10 4 µg/kg or 8 µg/kg was not statistically significant more efficacious than placebo in achieving the ability to discontinue corticosteroids by 16 weeks and to maintain clinical remission (CDAI<150) by week 28 with respective rates of 25 %, 32 %, and 29 % (*p*-value not reported). It was suggested that IL-10 at the highest dose 20 µg/kg may increase the production of IFN-γ and neopterin and thus increasing proinflammatory cytokines such as TNF-α, IL-1β and increasing nitric oxide production [128]. Colombel et al. analyzed 65 patients with Crohn's disease after curative ileal or ileocolonic resection and primary anastomosis who were randomized within 2 weeks after surgery to subcutaneous injections of either rhu-IL-10 4 µg/kg once daily, rhu-IL-10 8 µg/kg twice weekly or placebo and were followed-up for 12 weeks [129].

Of 65 patients 58 underwent endoscopy at the end of follow-up that showed that 46 % of patients treated with active drug and 52 % of placebo recipients had recurrent lesions (*p* not significant) [129]. Successful treatment of a murine model of colitis with *L. lactis* secreting interleukin-10 has been reported [130]. Methods for biological containment and formulation for delivery to the human intestine have been developed [131–133]. A pilot Phase Ia study has demonstrated the potential of a genetically modified *L. lactis* (LL-Thy12) given orally at the dose of 10 capsules with 1 × 10^{10} colony-forming units (CFU) of LLThy12 twice daily for 7 days to 10 patients with active Crohn's disease [134]. In LL-Thy12 the thymidylate synthase gene has been replaced with a synthetic sequence encoding mature human interleukin-10 [133]. Clinical benefit was observed in 8 of 10 patients with 5 patients achieving complete remission (CDAI <150) and 3 patients experiencing clinical response (decrease in CDAI >70) [134]. Future clinical trials are needed to validate these preliminary findings.

Pediatric Data
At the time of writing this chapter there is no published data on the use of rhu-IL-10 in children or adolescents with IBD.

Safety
The only clinical trial that assessed safety of intravenously administered rhu-IL-10 observed similar proportion of adverse events between active drug and placebo arms. [124] The only exception was the abdominal pain that was reported in 9 % of patients receiving rhu-IL-10 and 31 % of placebo recipients. Data from 329 patients with Crohn's disease who were treated with either rhu-IL-10 ($n = 262$) or placebo ($n = 66$) provided the largest population of patients that was assessed for safety of rhu-IL-10 and showed that both active drug and placebo arms had comparable proportion of adverse events (95 % vs. 94 %) [126]. The only events that occurred in greater proportion of patients treated with rhu-IL-10 than placebo were headache ($P = 0.02$), fever ($P = 0.02$), back pain ($P = 0.01$), decrease in hemoglobin concentration ($P = 0.0007$), dizziness ($P = 0.005$), and thrombocytopenia ($P = 0.0006$) [126]. Severe adverse events were observed in 28 % 17 % of patients treated with rhu-IL-10 and placebo, respectively ($P = 0.057$). A dose-dependent decrease in hemoglobin of unknown mechanism occurred in 33 % of patients treated with rhuIL-10 at the dose of 20 μg/kg when compared to 8 % of placebo patients ($P = 0.0003$). Thrombocytopenia of unknown mechanism was also observed in greater proportion of patients receiving rhuIL-10 at the dose 8 μg/kg (6, $P = 0.04$) and rhuIL-10 at the dose 20 μg/kg (27 %, $P < 0.0001$) when compared to 0 % among placebo recipients. All hematologic abnormalities were reversible upon cessation of study medication.

Reversible anemia and thrombocytopenia are common, as are mild to moderate headaches, fever, back pain, diarrhea, arthralgias, and dizziness. Antibodies to IL-10 have not been detected [129, 126].

Blockade of T Cell Stimulation and Induction of Apoptosis

Laquinimod

Laquinimod is an oral agent that produces anti-inflammatory effects by modulating immune cells with result of reduced synthesis of several cytokines. Laquinimod has been used in multiple sclerosis with success and seems to be a safe medication [135] and is being evaluated in Crohn's disease.

A phase IIa trial was performed using different doses of laquinimod (0.5, 1, 1.5, or 2 mg/day) for 8 weeks in patients with active Crohn's disease [136]. Clinical remission rates at week 8 were as follows: 48.3, 26.7, 13.8, and 17.2 % of patients receiving 0.5, 1, 1.5, and 2 mg laquinimod versus 15.9 % placebo. Overall, induction treatment with laquinimod was tolerated and the most common adverse effects were headache, abdominal pain, nausea, vomiting, and musculoskeletal pain. This may be an effective treatment of Crohn's disease and further studies are needed.

Pediatric Data
At the time of writing this chapter, there are no published data on the use of laquinimod in children or adolescents with IBD.

DIMS0150

DNA based immunomodulatory sequence (DIMS0150) is a single stranded partially modified synthetic oligonucleotide of 19 bases in length and activates the Toll-Like Receptor 9 (TLR9) present in immune cells such as T and B cells, macrophages and plasmacytoid dendritic cells (pDCs) that are found in abundance on mucosal surfaces such as the colonic mucosa. Activation of TLR9 by DIMS0150 results in the local production of potent anti-inflammatory cytokines such as IL-10 and type I interferons from human peripheral blood mononuclear cells (PBMCs) that have also interestingly been shown to increase steroid sensitivity in steroid resistant UC patients and human monocytes [137]. Administration of DIMS0150 in the form of an enema in steroid-refractory subjects with UC allows the drug to come into direct contact with a large number of target cells harboring the TLR9 receptor and has been shown to be beneficial in steroid refractory patients with UC. These cells when activated release steroid sensitizing cytokines which induce a local and peripheral steroid-sensitizing effect [138].

In a study where a single dose of DIMS0150 was given to steroid unresponsive IBD patients on concomitant steroid therapies, single doses of 3 and 30 mg were effective in inducing a clinical response [139]. Five of seven patients (70 %) that received active treatment had a clinical response 1 week after therapy and after more than 8 years, two remained in glucocorticoid free remission.

In a phase II study, 151 patients with mild or moderately active UC were given DIMS0150 as a single rectal dose at one of four dose levels (0.3, 3, 30, and 100 mg) with the hopes of inducing clinical remission. No significant benefit was demonstrated at any dose level.

Another phase IIa proof of concept study was conducted in steroid dependent or steroid resistant UC patients on concomitant steroid therapies evaluating DIMS0150 at a single dose level of 30 mg [140]. Thirty-four patients were randomized to receive a single rectal administration of placebo or 30 mg of DIMS0150. Blood derived PBMCs were obtained before dosing and assayed to evaluate for a steroid enhancing effect in the presence of DIMS0150 and the established steroid sensitivity marker IL-6 [140] was also used to determine the steroid sensitivity status of the subjects. The study showed that glucocorticoid refractory UC patients most likely to benefit from DIMS0150 treatment.

In an uncontrolled, prospective treatment series, eight patients with chronic active severe UC on concomitant glucocorticoid therapy were given DIMS0150 [138]. Seven patients received a single topical dose of 30 mg and one special case received three doses (given in 4 week intervals). Evaluation of drug efficacy was determined by measuring colitis activity index, endoscopic improvement and histologic disease activity at week 12 with a follow up period of 2 years. In addition, glucocorticoid sensitivity was assayed by measurement of IL-6. All patients showed a rapid reduction in their colitis activity index within 1 week after administration of DIMS0150. At week 4, clinical response was 71 % and clinical remission was in 43 %. By week 12, clinical response was 82 % and clinical remission was 71 %. In the 2-year posttreatment period, all but one of the treated patients avoided colectomy. In addition, treatment with DIMS0150 restored glucocorticoid sensitivity.

DIMS0150 is currently in phase III trials.

Pediatric Data
At the time of writing this chapter, there are no published data on the use of DIMS0150 in children or adolescents with IBD.

Sphingosine-1-Phosphate Receptor Modulators

Sphingolipids are ubiquitous building blocks of eukaryotic cell membranes. S1P (sphingosine-1-phosphate) is a bioactive sphingolipid and its concentration gradient (between tissues and blood) regulates lymphocyte recirculation [141]. In order for lymphocytes to leave lymph nodes, the S1P receptors on the surface of the lymphocyte must bind to S1P and S1P modulators cause the S1P receptors on the surface of lymphocytes to be internalized and degraded preventing lymphocytes from leaving the lymph nodes. As a result lymphocytes are trapped in lymph nodes resulting in a reduction of the peripheral lymphocyte count and circulating effector T cells making fewer immune cells available in the circulating blood to effect tissue damage.

Fingolimod (FTY720, Gilenya™)

FTY720, the prototype drug, is a small-molecule agonist of S1P receptors 1,3,4,5 and is approved by the FDA as the first oral drug for the treatment of MS [142]. Its therapeutic effect is through a poorly understood mechanism independent of leukocyte integrin pathways. It has been found that S1P1 modulation was the driving force behind FTY720's efficacy and that the FTY720-mediated sequestration of circulating lymphocytes or immune modulation correlated with positive therapeutic outcomes [141].

Newer compounds are seemingly more promising for example in the treatment of IBD with a higher selectivity window for S1P1 over S1P3, while still having S1P5 activity as they are structured to have shorter half-lives and a shorter duration of lymphopenia, in contrast to the long-lasting actions of FTY20 [142].

Pediatric Data
At the time of writing this chapter, there are no published data on the use of Fingolimod in children or adolescents with IBD.

APD334

APD334, an orally available S1P$_1$ receptor modulator, discovered by Arena, has therapeutic potential in autoimmune diseases such as ulcerative colitis.

Phase II trial currently underway in UC [143].

Pediatric Data
At the time of writing this chapter, there are no published data on the use of APD334 in children or adolescents with IBD.

RPC1063 (Ozanimod)

RPC1063 is an oral selective agonist for S1P receptors 1 and 5 and has been shown in phase II studies to be effective for the treatment of both multiple sclerosis and ulcerative colitis [144].

The UC TOUCHSTONE phase II study evaluated the safety and efficacy of 0.5 and 1 mg RPC1063 compared to placebo and after the 8 week induction period, there was a continuing maintenance period for responders [145]. One hundred and ninety-seven patients with moderate to severe ulcerative colitis (Mayo score of 6–12 with an endoscopic subscore 2). The primary endpoint of clinical remission (Mayo score 2, no subscore >1) at week 8 was 16.4 % for high dose ($P = 0.048$ versus placebo), 13.8 % for low dose ($P = 0.14$), and 6.2 % for placebo. Secondary endpoints included the proportion of patients exhibiting clinical response (reduction in Mayo score of 3 and 30 % with a decrease in the rectal bleeding score of 1 or a rectal bleeding score 1), proportion of patients with mucosal improvement (endoscopy score 1), and a change in Mayo score. Ninety five percent of patients completed the induction portion of the study. Clinical response was 56.7 % for high dose ($P = 0.01$), 53.8 % for low dose ($P = 0.06$), and 36.9 % for placebo. Mucosal improvement was 34.3 % for high dose ($P = 0.002$), 27.7 % for low dose ($P = 0.03$), and 12.3 % for placebo. The improvement in Mayo score from baseline was 3.3 points for high dose ($P = 0.003$), 2.6 points for low dose ($P = 0.098$), and 1.9 for placebo. The adverse event profiles were comparable between groups (about 31 % of experiencing a treatment emergent event across all groups) and the most common in the treatment event was worsening of ulcerative colitis and anemia/decreased hemoglobin. Modest effects on heart rate occurred with no notable cardiac, pulmonary, ophthalmologic, or malignancy observed and transient transaminase (ALT 3×) occurred in three patients and decreased with continued treatment.

A phase III trial in ulcerative colitis and a phase II trial in Crohn's disease are being planned.

Pediatric Data

At the time of writing this chapter, there are no published data on the use of RPC1063 in children or adolescents with IBD.

Summary

Blockade of the TNF-a pathway has provided significant strides in the treatment of IBD. However, still a substantial proportion of patients with inflammatory bowel disease specifically moderate to severe Crohn's disease do not have a response to treatment with TNF antagonists and are primary or secondary nonresponders or they develop side effects or intolerances leading to discontinuation of medical therapy. As discussed in this chapter, several new biologic treatments utilizing different mechanisms of action to treat IBD are currently in the pipeline and these therapies are to date are proving to be promising new treatments for IBD.

References

1. Amiot A, Peyrin-Biroulet L. Current, new and future biological agents on the horizon for the treatment of inflammatory bowel diseases. Ther Adv Gastroenterol. 2015;8(2):66–82.
2. Toussirot E. The IL23/Th17 pathway as a therapeutic target in chronic inflammatory diseases. Inflamm Allergy Drug Targets. 2012;11:159–68.
3. Peluso I, Pallone F, Monteleone G. Interleukin-12 and Th1 immune response in Crohn's disease: pathogenetic relevance and therapeutic implication. World J Gastroenterol. 2006;12:5606–10.
4. Neurath MF. IL-23: a master regulator in Crohn's disease. Nat Med. 2007;13:26–8.
5. Niederreiter L, Adolph TE, Kaser A. Anti-IL-12/23 in Crohn's disease: bench and bedside. Curr Drug Targets. 2013;14(12):1379–84.
6. Fuss IJ, Becker C, Yang Z, Groden C, Hornung RL, Heller F, Neurath MF, Strober W, Mannon PJ. Both IL-12p70 and IL-23 are synthesized during active Crohn's disease and are down-regulated by treatment with anti-IL-12 p40 monoclonal antibody. Inflamm Bowel Dis. 2006;12:9–15.
7. Parrello T, Monteleone G, Cucchiara S, et al. Up-regulation of the IL-12 receptor beta 2 chain in Crohn's disease. J Immunol. 2000;165:7234–9.
8. Iwakura Y, Ishigame H. The IL-23/IL-17 axis in inflammation. J Clin Invest. 2006;116:1218–22.
9. Onuora S. Ustekinumab after anti-TNF failure: a step closer to the PSUMMIT of psoriatic arthritis therapy? Nat Rev Rheumatol. 2014;10:125.
10. Sandborn WJ, Feagan BG, Fedorak RN, Scherl E, Fleisher MR, Katz S, Johanns J, Blank M, Rutgeerts P. A randomized trial of Ustekinumab, a human interleukin-12/23 monoclonal antibody, in patients with moderate-to-severe Crohn's disease. Gastroenterology. 2008;135:1130–41.
11. Sandborn WJ, Gasink C, Gao LL, et al. Ustekinumab induction and maintenance therapy in refractory Crohn's disease. N Engl J Med. 2012;367:1519–28.
12. Sandborn W, et al. A multicenter, double-blind, placebo-controlled phase3 study of ustekinumab, a human IL-12/23P40 mAB, in moderate-service Crohn's disease refractory to anti-TFNα: UNITI-1. Inflamm Bowel Dis. 2016;22 Suppl 1:S1.
13. ACG October 2015. http://www.healio.com/gastroenterology/inflammatory-bowel-disease/news/online/%7B3319d496-e8ac-41db-8729-1e14070f0af8%7D/uniti-2-trial-stelara-effective-for-treating-crohns-disease.
14. A study to evaluate the safety and efficacy of ustekinumab maintenance therapy in patients with moderately to severely active Crohn's disease (IM-UNITI). Available at: http://clinicaltrials.gov/show/NCT01369355. http://clinicaltrials.gov/show/NCT01369355. Accessed Jan 2016.
15. Rinawi F, et al. Ustekinumab for resistant pediatric Crohn's disease. J Pediatr Gastroenterol Nutr. 2014. [Epub ahead of print].
16. Bishop C, et al. Ustekinumab in pediatric Crohn's disease patients: case review. J Pediatr Gastroenterol Nutr. 2016;63(3): 348–51.
17. Papp KA, Griffiths CE, Gordon K, et al. Long-term safety of ustekinumab in patients with moderate-to-severe psoriasis: final results from 5 years of follow-up. Br J Dermatol. 2013;168:844–54. Leung, Y, Panaccione R. Update on Ustekinumab for the treatment of Crohn's disease. Gastroenterol Clin N Am. 43(2014):619–30.
18. Badat Y, Meissner WG, Laharie D. Demyelination in a patient receiving ustekinumab for refractory Crohn's disease. J Crohns Colitis. 2014;8:1138–9.
19. Kock K, et al. Preclinical development of AMG 139, a human antibody specifically targeting IL-23. Br J Pharmacol. 2015;172:159–72.
20. Multiple ascending doses of AMG 139 in healthy and Crohn's disease subjects, www.clinicaltrials.gov/ct2/show/NCT01258205?term=AMG139&rank=1.
21. A phase II, multicenter, randomized, double-blind, multiple dose, placebo-controlled, parallel-group study to evaluate the efficacy, pharmacokinetics, and safety of BI 655066, an IL-23 p19 antagonist monoclonal antibody, in patients with moderately to severely active Crohn's disease, who are naïve to, or were previously treated with anti-TNF therapy. https://clinicaltrials.gov/ct2/show/NCT02031276. Accessed Jan 2016.

22. A long term extension trial of BI 655066 in patients with moderately to severely active Crohn's disease. https://clinicaltrials.gov/ct2/show/NCT02513459. Accessed Jan 2016.

23. BI 655066 dose ranging in psoriasis, active comparator ustekinumab. https://www.clinicaltrials.gov/ct2/show/NCT02054481?term=BI+655066&rank=3.

24. Krueger JG, et al. Anti-IL-23A mAb BI 655066 for treatment of moderate-to-severe psoriasis: safety, efficacy, pharmacokinetics, and biomarker results of a single-rising-dose, randomized, double-blind, placebo-controlled trial. J Allergy Clin Immunol. 2015;136(1):116–24.e7

25. Ito H. IL-6 and Crohns disease. Curr Drug Targets Inflamm Allergy. 2003;2(2):125–30.

26. A study to assess the efficacy and safety of PF-04236921 in subjects with Crohn's disease who failed anti-TNF therapy (ANDANTE). https://www.clinicaltrials.gov/ct2/show/NCT01287897?term=PF-04236921&rank=3.

27. Fuss IJ, Strober W. The role of IL-13 and NK T cells in experimental and human ulcerative colitis. Mucosal Immunol. 2008;1(Suppl 1):S31–3.

28. Heller F, Florian P, Bojarski C, et al. Interleukin-13 is the key effector Th2 cytokine in ulcerative colitis that affects epithelial tight junctions, apoptosis, and cell restitution. Gastroenterology. 2005;129:550–64.

29. Fuss IJ, Heller F, Boirivant M, et al. Nonclassical CD1d-restricted NK T cells that produce IL-13 characterize an atypical Th2 response in ulcerative colitis. J Clin Invest. 2004;113:1490–7.

30. Hua F, et al. A pharmacokinetic comparison of anrukinzumaban anti- IL-13 monoclonal antibody, among healthy volunteers, asthma and ulcerative colitis patients. Br J Clin Pharmacol. 2015;80(1):101–9.

31. May RD, Monk PD, Cohen ES, et al. Preclinical development of CAT-354, an IL-13 neutralizing antibody, for the treatment of severe uncontrolled asthma. Br J Pharmacol. 2012;166:177–93.

32. Oh CK, Faggioni R, Jin F, et al. An open-label, single-dose bioavailability study of the pharmacokinetics of CAT-354 after subcutaneous and intravenous administration in healthy males. Br J Clin Pharmacol. 2010;69:645–55.

33. Danese S, et al. Tralokinumab for moderate-to-severe UC: a randomised, double-blind, placebo-controlled, phase IIa study. Gut. 2015;64:243–9.

34. Rothenberg ME, et al. Intravenous anti–IL-13 mAb QAX576 for the treatment of eosinophilic esophagitis. J Allergy Clin Immunol. 2015;135(2):500–7.

35. A multi-center, randomized, double-blind, active controlled study to assess the efficacy, safety and tolerability of the anti-IL13 monoclonal antibody QAX576 in the treatment of perianal fistulas in patients suffering from Crohn's disease. https://clinicaltrials.gov/ct2/show/NCT01355614?term=QAX576&rank=9.

36. A study to assess efficacy, safety and tolerability of the Anti-IL-13 monoclonal antibody QAX576 in the treatment of perinanal fistulas in patients suffering from Crohn's disease. https://clinicaltrials.gov/ct2/show/NCT01316601?term=QAX576&rank=15.

37. A randomized, double-blind, placebo-controlled, parallel group, multi-center study designed to evaluate the safety, efficacy, pharmacokinetic and pharmacodynamic profile of bertilimumab in patients with active moderate to severe ulcerative colitis. clinicaltrials.gov/ct2/show/NCT01671956?term=Bertilimumab&rank=1. Accessed Jan 2016.

38. Fitzpatrick LR. Vidofludimus inhibits colonic interleukin-17 and improves hapten-induced colitis in rats by a unique dual mode of action. J Pharmacol Exp Ther. 2012;342(3):850–60.

39. Xue L, et al. Contribution of enhanced engagement of antigen presentation machinery to the clinical immunogenicity of a human interleukin (IL)-21 receptor-blocking therapeutic antibody. Clin Exp Immunol. 2016;183:102–13.

40. Hua F, et al. Anti-IL21 receptor monoclonal antibody (ATR-107): safety, pharmacokinetics, and pharmacodynamic evaluation in healthy volunteers: a phase I, first-in-human study. J Clin Pharmacol. 2014;54(1):14–22.

41. Vugmeyster Y, Guay H, Szklut P, et al. In vitro potency, pharmacokinetic profiles, and pharmacological activity of optimized anti-IL-21R antibodies in a mouse model of lupus. MAbs. 2010;2:335–46.

42. Vallieres F, Girard D. IL-21 enhances phagocytosis in mononuclear phagocyte cells: identification of spleen tyrosine kinase as a novel molecular target of IL-21. J Immunol. 2013;190:2904–12.

43. Spolski R, Leonard WJ. Interleukin-21: a double-edged sword with therapeutic potential. Nat Rev Drug Discov. 2014;13:379–95.

44. Young DA, Hegen M, Ma HL, et al. Blockade of the interleukin-21/interleukin-21 receptor pathway ameliorates disease in animal models of rheumatoid arthritis. Arthritis Rheum. 2007;56:1152–63.

45. Rietdijk ST, D'Haens GR. Recent developments in the treatment of inflammatory bowel disease. J Dig Dis. 2013;14(6):282–7.

46. Ghoreschi K, Laurence A, O'Shea J. Janus kinases in immune cell signaling. Immunol Rev. 2009;228:273–87.

47. Neurath M. Cytokines in inflammatory bowel disease. Nat Rev Immunol. 2014;14:329–34.

48. Ghoreschi K, Jesson MI, Lee JL, et al. Modulation of innate and adaptive immune responses by tofacitinib (CP-690,550). J Immunol. 2011;186:4234–43.

49. Sandborn WJ, Ghosh S, Panes J, Vranic I, Su C, Rousell S, Niezychowski W, Study A3921063 Investigators. Tofacitinib, an oral Janus kinase inhibitor, in active ulcerative colitis. N Engl J Med. 2012;367(7):616–24.

50. Sandborn WJ, Ghosh S, Panes J, Vranic I, Wang W, Niezychowski W. A phase 2 study of tofacitinib, an oral Janus kinase inhibitor, in patients with Crohn's disease. Clin Gastroenterol Hepatol. 2014;12:1485–93.

51. Lowenberg M, D'Haens G. Next-generation therapeutics for IBD. Curr Gastroenterol Rep. 2015;17:21.

52. A study of oral CP-690,550 as a maintenance therapy for ulcerative colitis (OCTAVE). ClinicalTrials.gov Identifier: NCT01458574. Last accessed Jan 2016.

53. Hyun JG, Lee G, Brown JB, et al. Anti-interferon-inducible chemokine, CXCL10, reduces colitis by impairing T helper-1 induction and recruitment in mice. Inflamm Bowel Dis. 2005;11:799–805.

54. Hardi R, Mayer L, Targan SR, et al. A phase 1 open-label, single-dose, dose-escalation study of MDX-1100, a high-affinity, neutralizing, fully human Igg1 (kappa) anti-CXCL10 (Ip10) monoclonal antibody, in ulcerative colitis. Gastroenterology. 2008;134:A-99–100.

55. Van Rompaey L, et al. Preclinical characterization of GLPG0634, a selective inhibitor of JAK1, for the treatment of inflammatory diseases. J Immunol. 2013;191:3568–77.

56. Efficacy and safety of GLPG0634 in subjects with active Crohn's disease. https://clinicaltrials.gov/ct2/show/NCT02048618?term=GLPG0634&rank=2.

57. Wahl SM. Transforming growth factor beta: the good, the bad, and the ugly. J Exp Med. 1994;180:1587–90.

58. Letterio JJ, Roberts AB. Regulation of immune responses by TGF-beta. Annu Rev Immunol. 1998;16:137–61.

59. Monteleone G, Kumberova A, Croft NM, Mc Kenzie C, Steer HW, Mac Donald TT. Blocking Smad7 restores TGF-beta1 signaling in chronic inflammatory bowel disease. J Clin Invest. 2001;108:601–9.

60. Monteleone G, Boirivant M, Pallone F, Mac Donald TT. TGF-beta1 and Smad7 in the regulation of IBD. Mucosal Immunol. 2008;1(Suppl 1):S50–3.

61. Boirivant M, Pallone F, Di Giacinto C, et al. Inhibition of Smad7 with a specific antisense oligonucleotide facilitates TGF-beta1-mediated suppression of colitis. Gastroenterology. 2006;131:1786–98.

62. Monteleone G, Fantini MC, Onali S, et al. Phase I clinical trial of Smad7 knockdown using antisense oligonucleotide in patients with active Crohn's disease. Mol Ther. 2012;20:870–6.

63. Zorzi F, et al. A phase 1 open-label trial shows that smad7 anti-sense oligonucleotide (GED0301) does not increase the risk of small bowel strictures in Crohn's disease. Aliment Pharmacol Ther. 2012;36:850–7.

64. Monteleone G et al. Abstract presentation UEGW 2014, OP203. Vienna.

65. Mayer L, Sandborn WJ, Stepanov Y, Geboes K, Hardi R, Yellin M, Tao X, Xu LA, Salter-Cid L, Gujrathi S, Aranda R, Luo AY. Anti-IP-10 antibody (BMS-936557) for ulcerative colitis: a phase II randomised study. Gut. 2014;63(3):442–50.

66. Kuhne M, Preston B, Wallace S, Chen S, Vasudevan G, Witte A, Cardarelli P. MDX-1100, a fully human anti-CXCL10 (IP-10) antibody, is a high affinity, neutralizing antibody that has entered phase I clinical trials for the treatment of Ulcerative Colitis (UC). J Immunol. 2007;178:S241.

67. Uguccioni M, Gionchetti P, Robbiani DF, et al. Increased expression of IP-10, IL-8,MCP-1, and MCP-3 in ulcerative colitis. Am J Pathol. 1999;155:331–6.

68. Witte A, Kuhne MR, Preston BT, et al. W1170 CXCL10 expression and biological activities in inflammatory bowel disease. Gastroenterology. 2008;134:A-648.

69. Soejima K, BJ R. A functional IFN – inducible protein-10/CXCL10-specific receptor expressed by epithelial and endothelial cells that is neither CXCR3 nor glycosaminoglycan. J Immunol. 2001;167:6576–82.

70. Sasaki S, Yoneyama H, Suzuki K, et al. Blockade of CXCL10 protects mice from acute colitis and enhances crypt cell survival. Eur J Immunol. 2002;32:3197–205.

71. Singh UP, Singh S, Taub DD, et al. Inhibition of IFN-gamma-inducible protein-10 abrogates colitis in IL-10−/− mice. J Immunol. 2003;171:1401–6.

72. Sandborn WJ, Rutgeerts PJ, Colombel J-F, et al. 827 phase IIA, randomized, placebo-controlled evaluation of the efficacy and safety of induction therapy with eldelumab (anti-IP-10 antibody; BMS-936557) in patients with active Crohn's disease. Gastroenterology. 2015;148:S-162–3.

73. Rivera-Nieves J. Strategies that target leukocyte traffic in inflammatory bowel diseases: recent developments. Curr Opin Gastroenterol. 2015;31:441–8.

74. Rudick RA, Stuart WH, Calabresi PA, Confavreux C, Galetta SL, Radue EW, Lublin FD, Weinstock-Guttman B, Wynn DR, Lynn F, Panzara MA, Sandrock AW, Investigators S. Natalizumab plus interferon beta-1a for relapsing multiple sclerosis. N Engl J Med. 2006;354:911–23.

75. Miller DH, Khan OA, Sheremata WA, Blumhardt LD, Rice GP, Libonati MA, Willmer-Hulme AJ, Dalton CM, Miszkiel KA, O'Connor PW, International Natalizumab Multiple Sclerosis Trial Group. A controlled trial of natalizumab for relapsing multiple sclerosis [see comment]. N Engl J Med. 2003;348:15–23.

76. Polman CH, O'Connor PW, Havrdova E, Hutchinson M, Kappos L, Miller DH, Phillips JT, Lublin FD, Giovannoni G, Wajgt A, Toal M, Lynn F, Panzara MA, Sandrock AW, Investigators A. A randomized, placebo-controlled trial of natalizumab for relapsing multiple sclerosis. N Engl J Med. 2006;354:899–910.

77. Gordon FH, Lai CW, Hamilton MI, Allison MC, Srivastava ED, Fouweather MG, Donoghue S, Greenlees C, Subhani J, AmLot PL, Pounder RE. A randomized placebo-controlled trial of a humanized monoclonal antibody to alpha4 integrin in active Crohn's disease. Gastroenterology. 2001;121:268–74.

78. Ghosh S, Goldin E, Gordon FH, Malchow HA, Rask-Madsen J, Rutgeerts P, Vyhnalek P, Zadorova Z, Palmer T, Donoghue S. Natalizumab for active Crohn's disease. N Engl J Med. 2003;348:24–32.

79. Sandborn WJ, Colombel JF, Enns R, Feagan BG, Hanauer SB, Lawrance IC, Panaccione R, Sanders M, Schreiber S, Targan S, van Deventer S, Goldblum R, Despain D, Hogge GS, Rutgeerts P. Natalizumab induction and maintenance therapy for Crohn's disease. N Engl J Med. 2005;353:1912–25.

80. Sandborn W, Colombel J, Enns R, Feagan B, Hanauer S, Lawrance I, Panaccione R, Rutgeerts P, Schreiber S, Targan S, van Deventer S. Maintenance therapy with natalizumab does not require use of concomitant iImmunosuppressants for sustained efficacy in patients with active Crohn's disease: results from the ENACT-2 study. Gastroenterology. 2006;130:A-482 Abstract 1137.

81. Panaccione R, Colombel J, Enns R, Feagan B, Hanauer S, Lawrance I, Rutgeerts P, Sandborn W, Schreiber S, Targan S, van Deventer S. Natalizumab maintains remission in patients with moderately to severely active Crohn's disease for up to 2-years: results from an open-label extension study. Gastroenterology. 2006;130:A-111 Abstract 768.

82. Targan SR, Feagan BG, Fedorak RN, Lashner BA, Panaccione R, Present DH, Spehlmann ME, Rutgeerts PJ, Tulassay Z, Volfova M, Wolf DC, Hernandez C, Bornstein J, Sandborn WJ. Natalizumab for the treatment of active Crohn's disease: results of the ENCORE Trial. Gastroenterology. 2007;132:1672–83.

83. Sands BE, Kozarek R, Spainhour J, Barish CF, Becker S, Goldberg L, Katz S, Goldblum R, Harrigan R, Hilton D, Hanauer SB. Safety and tolerability of concurrent natalizumab treatment for patients with Crohn's disease not in remission whil receiving infliximab. Inflamm Bowel Dis. 2007;13:2–11.

84. Gordon FH, Hamilton MI, Donoghue S, Greenlees C, Palmer T, Rowley-Jones D, Dhillon AP, AmLot PL, Pounder RE. A pilot study of treatment of active ulcerative colitis with natalizumab, a humanized monoclonal antibody to alpha-4 integrin. Aliment Pharmacol Ther. 2002;16:699–705.

85. Prescribing information for Tysabri (natalizumab). 2007. http://www.accessdata.fda.gov/drugsatfda_docs/label/2012/125104s0576lbl.pdf; https://www.biogen.com.au/content/dam/corporate/en_AU/pdfs/products/TYSABRI/bdptysab11116.pdf.

86. Hyams JS, Wilson DC, Thomas A, Heuschkel R, Mitton S, Mitchell B, Daniels R, Libonati MA, Zanker S, Kugathasan S, International Natalizumab CD305 Trial Group. Natalizumab therapy for moderate to severe Crohn's disease in adolescents. J Pediatr Gastroenterol Nutr. 2007;44:185–91.

87. Kleinschmidt-DeMasters BK, Tyler KL. Progressive multifocal leukoencephalopathy complicating treatment with natalizumab and interferon beta-1a for multiple sclerosis. [see comment]. N Engl J Med. 2005;353:369–74.

88. Langer-Gould A, Atlas SW, Green AJ, Bollen AW, Pelletier D. Progressive multifocal leukoencephalopathy in a patient treated with natalizumab. [see comment]. N Engl J Med. 2005;353:375–81.

89. Van Assche G, Van Ranst M, Sciot R, Dubois B, Vermeire S, Noman M, Verbeeck J, Geboes K, Robberecht W, Rutgeerts P. Progressive multifocal leukoencephalopathy after natalizumab therapy for Crohn's disease. [see comment]. N Engl J Med. 2005;353:362–8.

90. Yousry TA, Major EO, Rysckewitsch C, Fahle G, Fischer S, Hou J, Curfman B, Miszkiel K, Mueller-Lenke N, Sanchez E, Barkhof F, Radue EW, Jager HR, Clifford DB. Evaluation of patients treated with natalizumab for progressive multifocal leukoencephaolopathy. N Engl J Med. 2006;354:924–33.

91. Van Deventer SJH, Wedel MK, Baker BF, Xia S, Chuang E, Miner PB. A phase II dose ranging, double-blind, placebo-controlled study of alicaforsen enema in subjects with acute exacerbation of mild to moderate left-sided ulcerative colitis. Aliment Pharmacol Ther. 2006;23:1415–25.

92. Feagan BG, Rutgeerts P, Sands BE, Hanauer S, Colombel JF, Sandborn WJ, et al. Vedolizumab as induction and maintenance therapy for ulcerative colitis. N Engl J Med. 2013;369:699–710.

93. Sandborn WJ, Feagan BG, Rutgeerts P, Hanauer S, Colombel JF, Sands BE, et al. Vedolizumab as induction and maintenance therapy for Crohn's disease. N Engl J Med. 2013;369:711–21.

94. Sands BE, Feagan BG, Rutgeerts P, Colombel JF, Sandborn WJ, et al. Effects of vedolizumab induction therapy for patients with Crohn's disease in whom tumor necrosis factor antagonist treatment failed. Gastroenterology. 2014;147:618–27.

95. Zoet ID, et al. Successful vedolizumab therapy in a sixteen-year-old boy with refractory ulcerative colitis. J Crohns Colitis. 2015;10(3):373–4.

96. Poster presentation UEGW 2014, P1059, Hanauer S et al., poster presentation UEGW 2014, P1667, Feagan B et al.

97. Milch C, Wyant T, Xu J, Parikh A, Kent W, Fox I, et al. Vedolizumab, a monoclonal antibody to the gut homing alpha-4beta7 integrin, does not affect cerebrospinal fluid T-lymphocyte immunophenotype. J Neuroimmunol. 2013;264:123–6.

98. Lowenberg M, D'Haens G. Novel targets for inflammatory bowel disease therapeutics. Curr Gastroenterol Rep. 2013;15:311.

99. Colombel J-F, et al. The safety of vedolizumab for ulcerative colitis and Crohn's disease. Gut. 2016;0:1–13.

100. Vermeire S, O'Byrne S, Keir M, Williams M, Lu TT, Mansfield JC, et al. Etrolizumab as induction therapy for ulcerative colitis: a randomised, controlled, phase 2 trial. Lancet. 2014;384:309–18.

101. Pullen N, Molloy E, Carter D, et al. Pharmacological characterization of PF-00547659, an antihuman MAdCAM monoclonal antibody. Br J Pharmacol. 2009;157:281–93.

102. Vermeire S, Ghosh S, Panes J, Dahlerup JF, Luegering A, Sirotiakova J, et al. The mucosal addressin cell adhesion molecule antibody PF-00547,659 in ulcerative colitis: a randomised study. Gut. 2011;60:1068–75.

103. Miner PB, Wedel MK, Xia S, Baker BF. Safety and efficacy of two dose formulations of alicaforsen enema compared with mesalazine enema for treatment of mild to moderate left-sided ulcerative colitis: a randomized, double-blind, active-controlled trial. Aliment Pharmacol Ther. 2006;23:1403–13.

104. Reinisch W, Sandborn W, Danese S, et al. 901a A randomized, multicenter double-blind, placebo-controlled study of the safety and efficacy of anti-MAdCAM Antibody PF-00547659 (PF) in patients with moderate to severe ulcerative colitis: results of the TURANDOT study. Gastroenterology. 2015;148:S-1193.

105. Sandborn W, Lee SD, Tarabar D, et al. 825 anti-MAdCAM-1 antibody (PF-00547659) for active refractory Crohn's disease: results of the OPERA study. Gastroenterology. 2015;148:S-162.

106. Takazoe M, Watanabe M, Kawaguchi T, Matsumoto T, Oshitani N, Hiwatashi N, Hibi T. Oral alpha-4 integrin inhibitor (AJM300) in patients with active Crohn disease – a randomized, double-blind, placebo-controlled trial. Gastroenterology. 2009;136:A-181.

107. Shanahan Jr WR. ISIS 2302, an antisense inhibitor of intercellular adhesion molecule 1. Expert Opin Investig Drugs. 1999;8:1417–29.

108. Yacyshyn BR, Chey WY, Goff J, Salzberg B, Baerg R, Buchman AL, Tami J, Yu R, Gibiansky E, Shanahan WR. Double blind, placebo controlled trial of the remission inducing and steroid sparing properties of an ICAM-1 antisense oligodeoxynucleotide, alicaforsen (ISIS 2302), in active steroid dependent Crohn's disease. Gut. 2002;51:30–6.

109. Yacyshyn BR, Bowen-Yacyshyn MB, Jewell L, Tami JA, Bennett CF, Kisner DL, Shanahan Jr WR. A placebo-controlled trial of ICAM-1 antisense oligonucleotide in the treatment of Crohn's disease. Gastroenterology. 1998;114:1133–42.

110. Yacyshyn B, Chey WY, Wedel MK, Yu RZ, Paul D, Chuang E. A randomized, double-masked, placebo-controlled study of alicaforsen, an antisense inhibitor of intercellular adhesion molecule 1, for the treatment of subjects with active Crohn's disease. Clin Gastroenterol Hepatol. 2007;5:215–20.

111. Schreiber S, Nikolaus S, Malchow H, Kruis W, Lochs H, Raedler A, Hahn EG, Krummenerl T, Steinmann G. Absence of efficacy of

112. van Deventer SJ, Tami JA, Wedel MK. A randomised, controlled, double blind, escalating dose study of alicaforsen enema in active ulcerative colitis. Gut. 2004;53:1646–51.

113. Miner Jr PB, Geary RS, Matson J, Chuang E, Xia S, Baker BF, Wedel MK. Bioavailability and therapeutic activity of alicaforsen (ISIS 2302) administered as a rectal retention enema to subjects with active ulcerative colitis. Aliment Pharmacol Ther. 2006;23:1427–34.

114. Miner P, Wedel M, Bane B, Bradley J. An enema formulation of alicaforsen, an antisense inhibitor of intercellular adhesion molecule-1, in the treatment of chronic, unremitting pouchitis. Aliment Pharmacol Ther. 2004;19:281–6.

115. Pan WJ, et al. Clinical pharmacology of AMG 181, a gut-specific human anti-α4β7 monoclonal antibody, for treating inflammatory bowel diseases. Br J Clin Pharmacol. 2014;78(6):1315–33.

116. Prat A, Stuve O. Firategrast: natalizumab in a pill? Lancet Neurol. 2012;11(2):120–1.

117. A randomized, double-blind, placebo-controlled, parallel-group study to investigate the efficacy and safety of nine-weeks administration of three doses of SB-683699 in subjects with moderately to severely active Crohn's disease. Clinicaltrials.gov. NCT00101946.

118. Digital Oral Presentation, ECCO 2015.

119. Koga Y, Kainoh M. PP-065-15 effect of an orally active small molecule alpha4beta1/alpha4beta7 integrin antagonist, TRK-170, on experimental colitis in mice. International Immunology Meeting Abstracts. Kobe. 2010.

120. Nelson DR, Tu Z, Soldevila-Pico C, Abdelmalek M, Zhu H, Xu YL, Cabrera R, Liu C, Davis GL. Long-term interleukin 10 therapy in chronic hepatitis C patients has a proviral and anti-inflammatory effect. Hepatology. 2003;38:859–68.

121. McInnes IB, Illei GG, Danning CL, Yarboro CH, Crane M, Kuroiwa T, Schlimgen R, Lee E, Foster B, Flemming D, Prussin C, Fleisher TA, Boumpas DT. IL-10 improves skin disease and modulates endothelial activation and leukocyte effector function in patients with psoriatic arthritis. J Immunol. 2001;167:4075–82.

122. Maini R, Paulus HE, Breedveld FC. rHuIL-10 in subjects with active rheumatoid arthritis (RA): a phase I and cytokine response study. Arthritis Rheum. 1997;1997:S224.

123. Smeets TJ, Kraan MC, Versendaal J, Breedveld FC, Tak PP. Analysis of serial synovial biopsies in patients with rheumatoid arthritis: description of a control group without clinical improvement after treatment with interleukin 10 or placebo. J Rheumatol. 1999;26:2089–93.

124. van Deventer SJ, Elson CO, Fedorak RN. Multiple doses of intravenous interleukin 10 in steroid-refractory Crohn's disease. Crohn's disease Study Group. Gastroenterology. 1997;113:383–9.

125. Fedorak RN, Gangl A, Elson CO, Rutgeerts P, Schreiber S, Wild G, Hanauer SB, Kilian A, Cohard M, LeBeaut A, Feagan B. Recombinant human interleukin 10 in the treatment of patients with mild to moderately active Crohn's disease. The Interleukin 10 Inflammatory Bowel Disease Cooperative Study Group. Gastroenterology. 2000;119:1473–82.

126. Schreiber S, Fedorak RN, Nielsen OH, Wild G, Williams CN, Nikolaus S, Jacyna M, Lashner BA, Gangl A, Rutgeerts P, Isaacs K, van Deventer SJ, Koningsberger JC, Cohard M, LeBeaut A, Hanauer SB. Safety and efficacy of recombinant human interleukin 10 in chronic active Crohn's disease. Crohn's disease IL-10 Cooperative Study Group. Gastroenterology. 2000;119:1461–72.

127. Fedorak R, Nielsen O, Williams N, Malchow H, Forbes A, Stein B, Wild G, Lashner B, Renner E, Buchman A, Hardi R, The Interleukin-10 Study Group. Human recombinant interleukin-10 is safe and well tolerated but does not induce remission in steroid dependent Crohn's disease. Gastroenterology. 2001;120:A-127.

128. Tilg H, van Montfrans C, van den Ende A, Kaser A, van Deventer SJ, Schreiber S, Gregor M, Ludwiczek O, Rutgeerts P, Gasche C, Koningsberger JC, Abreu L, Kuhn I, Cohard M, LeBeaut A, Grint

P, Weiss G. Treatment of Crohn's disease with recombinant human interleukin 10 induces the proinflammatory cytokine interferon gamma. [see comment]. Gut. 2002;50:191–5.

129. Colombel JF, Rutgeerts P, Malchow H, Jacyna M, Nielsen OH, Rask-Madsen J, Van Deventer S, Ferguson A, Desreumaux P, Forbes A, Geboes K, Melani L, Cohard M. Interleukin 10 (Tenovil) in the prevention of postoperative recurrence of Crohn's disease. Gut. 2001;49:42–6.

130. Steidler L, Hans W, Schotte L, Neirynck S, Obermeier F, Falk W, Fiers W, Remaut E. Treatment of murine colitis by Lactococcus lactis secreting interleukin- 10. Science. 2000;289:1352–5.

131. Steidler L, Neirynck S, Huyghebaert N, Snoeck V, Vermeire A, Goddeeris B, Cox E, Remon JP, Remaut E. Biological containment of genetically modified Lactococcus lactis for intestinal delivery of human interleukin 10. Nat Biotechnol. 2003;21:785–9.

132. Huyghebaert N, Vermeire A, Neirynck S, Steidler L, Remaut E, Remon JP. Evaluation of extrusion/spheronisation, layering and compaction for the preparation of an oral, multi-particulate formulation of viable, hIL-10 producing Lactococcus lactis. Eur J Pharm Biopharm. 2005;59:9–15.

133. Huyghebaert N, Vermeire A, Neirynck S, Steidler L, Remaut E, Remon JP. Development of an enteric-coated formulation containing freeze-dried, viable recombinant Lactococcus lactis for the ileal mucosal delivery of human interleukin-10. Eur J Pharm Biopharm. 2005;60:349–59.

134. Braat H, Rottiers P, Hommes DW, Huyghebaert N, Remaut E, Remon JP, van Deventer SJ, Neirynck S, Peppelenbosch MP, Steidler L. A phase I trial with transgenic bacteria expressing interleukin-10 in Crohn's disease. Clin Gastroenterol Hepatol. 2006;4:754–9.

135. Comi G, Jeffery D, Kappos L, Montalban X, Boyko A, Rocca MA, et al. Placebo-controlled trial of oral laquinimod for multiple sclerosis. N Engl J Med. 2012;366:1000–9.

136. D'Haens G, Sandborn WJ, Colombel JF, Rutgeerts P, Brown K, Barkay H, Sakov A, Haviv A, Feagan BG. A phase II study of laquinimod in Crohn's disease. Gut. 2015;64(8):1227–35. doi:10.1136/gutjnl-2014-307118. Epub 2014 Oct 3.

137. Creed TJ, Lee RW, Newcomb PV, di Mambro AJ, Raju M, Dayan CM. The effects of cytokines on suppression of lymphocyte proliferation by dexamethasone. J Immunol. 2009;183:164–71.

138. Musch E, et al. Topical treatment with the toll-like receptor agonist DIMS0150 has potential for lasting relief of symptoms in patients with chronic active ulcerative colitis by restoring glucocorticoid sensitivity. Inflamm Bowel Dis. 2013;19: 283–92.

139. Lofberg R, Neurath M, Ost A, Pettersson S. Topical NFκB p65 antisense oligonucleotide in patients with active distal colonic IBD: a randomized, controlled, pilot trial. Gastroenterology. 2001;122(Suppl 41):503A.

140. Kuznetsov NV, et al. Biomarkers can predict potential clinical responders to DIMS0150 a toll-like receptor 9 agonist in ulcerative colitis patients. BMC Gastroenterol. 2014;14:79.

141. Gonzalez-Cabrera PJ. S1P signaling: new therapies and opportunities. F1000Prime Rep. 2014;6:109.

142. Masopust D, Choo D, Vezys V, et al. Dynamic T cell migration program provides resident memory within intestinal epithelium. J Exp Med. 2010;207:553–64.

143. Safety and efficacy of APD334 in patients with ulcerative colitis (clinical trials.gov NCT02447302).

144. Sandborn W. New targets for small molecules in inflammatory bowel disease. Gastroenterol Hepatol. 2015;11(5):338–40.

145. Sandborn W, Feagan BG, Wolf DC, et al. 445 the TOUCHSTONE study: a randomized, double-blind, placebo-controlled induction trial of an oral S1P receptor modulator (RPC1063) in moderate to severe ulcerative colitis. Gastroenterology. 2015; 148:S-93.

Medical Treatment of Perianal Crohn's Disease Fistulae

Mark T. Osterman and Gary R. Lichtenstein

Background

Classification

Perianal fistulae historically have been classified in a variety of ways. The most clinical useful way to classify fistulae was recently proposed by the American Gastroenterological Association in a position statement and technical review on perianal CD [1–4]. They stratify perianal fistulae into two groups: simple and complex. Simple fistulae are low, that is, below the dentate line, and have a superficial, low intersphincteric, or low trans-sphincteric origin. These fistulae also have a single external opening, have no associated pain or fluctuation to suggest an abscess, and have no evidence of a rectovaginal fistula or anorectal stricture. Complex fistulae, on the other hand, are high in origin (high intersphincteric, high trans-sphincteric, or suprasphincteric), may have multiple external openings, may have associated pain or fluctuation to suggest an abscess, and may have evidence of a rectovaginal fistula or anorectal stricture. The distinction between the two types of perianal fistula is clinically important, not only because the management varies, but also because several studies have demonstrated higher rates of healing with simple fistulae [5–8].

Pathogenesis

The transmural nature of the inflammation that typifies CD predisposes patients to fistula formation. Although the pathogenesis of perianal fistulae is not known precisely, two mechanisms seem plausible [9]. Perianal fistulae may develop locally as deeppenetrating ulcers in the anus or rectum, which then extend over time as feces is forced into the ulcers during defecation [10]. Alternatively, these fistulae may develop after anal gland infections or abscesses [11]. Since some of the anal glands penetrate into the intersphincteric space, infection in this space can readily extend to the external anal sphincter or skin.

Natural History

The reported incidence of fistulae in patients with CD ranges from 17% to 43% in referral-center-based case series [12–21]. Population-based studies have also examined the natural history of CD fistulae [22, 23]. A study by Hellers et al. included 826 patients diagnosed with CD in Stockholm County, Sweden, from 1955 to 1974, and observed a 23% cumulative incidence of perianal fistulae [22]. The authors noticed that the frequency of perianal fistulae increased as the inflammatory disease became more distal, with a 12% incidence in ileal disease, 15% in ileocolonic disease, 41% in colonic without rectal disease, and 92% in colonic with rectal disease. A later study by Schwartz et al. examined 176 patients diagnosed with CD in Olmsted County, Minnesota, from 1970 to 1993 and found a cumulative incidence of at least one fistula (at any site) of 21% at 1 year, 26% at 5 years, 33% at 10 years, and 50% at 20 years [23]. The corresponding cumulative incidences of at least one perianal fistula were 12% at 1 year, 15% at 5 years, 21% at 10 years, and 26% at 20 years. Taken collectively, fistulae were located as follows: 54% perianal, 24% enteroenteric, 9% rectovaginal, 6% enterocutaneous, 3% enterovesical, and 3% entero-intra-abdominal. Interestingly, 45% of patients developed a perianal fistula before or at the time of diagnosis

M.T. Osterman, MD, MSCE (✉)
Division of Gastroenterology, Department of Medicine,
Penn Presbyterian Medical Center, University of Pennsylvania
School of Medicine, 218 Wright Saunders Building,
51 N. 39th Street, Philadelphia, PA 19104, USA
e-mail: mark.osterman@uphs.upenn.edu

G.R. Lichtenstein, MD
Division of Gastroenterology, Department of Medicine,
Hospital of the University of Pennsylvania,
University of Pennsylvania School of Medicine,
3400 Spruce Street, Philadelphia,
PA 19104, USA

© Springer International Publishing AG 2017
P. Mamula et al. (eds.), *Pediatric Inflammatory Bowel Disease*, DOI 10.1007/978-3-319-49215-5_36

of CD, an observation first noted by Gray et al. in 1965 [24] and also seen in the study by Hellers et al. [22]. This observation highlights the frequent difficulties encountered in attempting to diagnose CD in patients with isolated perianal disease.

In pediatrics, the presence of fistulas in the first year of life should prompt concern for underlying immunodeficiency or monogenic defect. These patients should undergo an immunological evaluation.

The clinical course of perianal fistulae depends somewhat on their complexity. Simple fistulae may heal spontaneously in up to 50% of cases [16, 25], whereas complex fistulae rarely heal spontaneously [26]. A number of studies have demonstrated that simple perianal fistulae tend to heal more completely and recur less than complex fistulae [6, 8, 25, 27, 28].

Diagnosis

Since healing rates seem to decrease when fistulae transform from simple to complex, it is tantamount to recognize and treat perianal CD fistulae as soon as symptoms manifest themselves. Thus, fistula location and extent must be accurately ascertained prior to commencing therapy. Unfortunately, digital rectal examination alone is not sufficient in this capacity, with accuracy as low as 62% [29]. Fortunately, a variety of other modalities exist, including fistulography, pelvic CT, pelvic magnetic resonance imaging (MRI), anorectal endoscopic ultrasound (EUS), and examination under anesthesia (EUA). Fistulography, which may cause significant patient discomfort and more importantly may disseminate septic fistula content, has a reported diagnostic accuracy of 16–50%, which is too low to be clinically useful [30–34]. Similarly, CT, with its limited diagnostic accuracy of 24–60%, is also not particularly useful [35–41]. Pelvic MRI, on the contrary, represents a vast improvement with a reported diagnostic accuracy of 76–100% and is often used to delineate anorectal and pelvic anatomy [42–50]. Anorectal EUS is also a clinically useful diagnostic modality with diagnostic accuracy ranging from 56% to 100% [41, 49, 51–56]. Of note, both pelvic MRI and anorectal EUS have been found to change surgical management in 10–15% of cases [44–50, 56]. EUA performed by an experienced colorectal surgeon has long been considered the gold standard for diagnosis of perianal fistulae in CD. However, this view has recently been challenged by Schwartz et al. who compared EUA, MRI, and EUS in a prospective blinded study of 34 patients with suspected CD perianal fistulae [49]. In this study, a consensus gold standard was determined for each patient. The authors observed a diagnostic accuracy exceeding 85% for all three modalities, specifically 91% for EUA and EUS and 87% for MRI. Of note, when any two of the tests were combined, diagnostic accuracy increased to 100%.

Medical Treatment

5-Aminosalicylic Acid Derivatives

5-Aminosalicylic acid derivatives have not been shown to be efficacious in inducing remission in luminal CD and also have never been studied for the treatment of CD fistulae in controlled trials. Thus, they cannot be recommended for the treatment of fistulizing CD.

Corticosteroids

There are no controlled studies evaluating the use of steroids in the management of CD fistulae. Unfortunately, neither the National Cooperative Crohn's Disease trial nor the European Cooperative Crohn's Disease trial provided data on response in the subgroup of patients with fistulae. However, two large uncontrolled studies have shown that corticosteroid use may actually be detrimental to patients with fistulizing CD, as it was associated with higher rates of surgical intervention [57, 58]. A retrospective case–control study of 432 patients with CD studied risk of intra-abdominal or pelvic abscess with systemic corticosteroid use during the previous 3 months [59]. The authors found a significant ninefold increased risk of intra-abdominal or pelvic abscess in patients with perforating CD who had received systemic corticosteroids during the prior 3 months (adjusted OR = 9.03, 95% CI = 2.40–33.98). In patients with relapsed active disease, they also reported a significant ninefold increased risk of abscess in patients receiving systemic steroids in the 3 months prior to presentation (unadjusted OR = 9.31, 95% CI = 1.03–83.91). For these reasons, corticosteroids should not be avoided whenever possible in patients with fistulizing CD.

Antibiotics

Although antibiotics are the most commonly used medication for the treatment of fistulae in CD, there are limited controlled data indicating that these agents are effective in this regard. The use of antibiotics in fistulizing CD is largely based upon a number of uncontrolled case series, each with a small number of patients [60–69]. Metronidazole, the most commonly used antibiotic, was first discovered in 1975 to have possible efficacy by Ursing and Kamme, who reported perianal fistula closure in three patients [60]. Bernstein et al. treated 21 consecutive patients with perianal CD fistulae with metronidazole at a dose of 20 mg/kg/day and observed clinical improvement in all patients, fistula closure in 83%, and complete healing in 56% [61]. These responses typically occurred within 6–8 weeks of commencement of therapy. The same group published a follow-up study, comprised of

17 of the 21 original patients and 9 additional consecutive patients, and found that dosage reduction was associated with relapse in all patients [63]. However, rapid healing was noted in all patients upon readministration of metronidazole. Thus, while efficacious in the induction of improvement, metronidazole is limited in that maintenance therapy is often required. Three other small, uncontrolled studies have also observed efficacy with metronidazole in fistulizing CD with fistula closure rates of 40–50%, but a high rate of relapse after cessation of therapy was seen in one of these studies [62, 64, 65]. The typical dose of metronidazole in the treatment of fistulizing CD ranges from 750 to 1500 mg/day. Adverse events associated with metronidazole are quite common, often leading to intolerance and discontinuation of the drug, and include a distal sensory neuropathy with paresthesias, nausea, dyspepsia, fatigue, glossitis, metallic taste, and a disulfiram-like reaction to alcohol ingestion [70].

Given that adverse events are commonly problematic with metronidazole, ciprofloxacin began to be used in the late 1980s and early 1990s to treat CD fistulae [66–69]. The first report of ciprofloxacin use in this setting was by Turunen et al. who studied eight patients with severe perianal disease and one patient with enterocutaneous fistula refractory to metronidazole [66]. In this study, in which patients were given 1000–1500 mg/day of ciprofloxacin for 3–12 months, the authors found that all patients demonstrated initial improvement, but 50% continued to have persistent drainage, which required surgical intervention in several patients. As with metronidazole, relapses were common upon cessation of therapy, but improvement was seen upon reinstitution of therapy in most cases. A subsequent study, published only in abstract form by Wolf et al., noted improvement in four out of five patients with severe perianal disease within 5 weeks of treatment [67]. Combination therapy with ciprofloxacin and metronidazole has been examined by Solomon et al. in a retrospective study of 14 patients [68]. They observed improvement in nine patients and fistula closure in three patients within 12 weeks, but like previous antibiotic studies, they also reported that relapse was the norm following discontinuation of therapy. The typical dose of ciprofloxacin in the treatment of fistulizing CD ranges from 1000 to 1500 mg/day. Adverse events with ciprofloxacin are uncommon and include headache, nausea, diarrhea, rash, and spontaneous tendon rupture [71, 72].

The only randomized controlled trial of antibiotic use for fistulizing CD, sponsored by the Crohn's and Colitis Foundations of America and Canada, compared ciprofloxacin, metronidazole, and placebo given for 10 weeks [73]. In this study, remission was defined as closure of all fistulae, and response was defined as closure of at least 50% of all fistulae that were draining at baseline. The authors planned to recruit 168 patients in total (56 for each treatment arm), but only 25 patients were able to be recruited, and the study was terminated early due to low enrollment. Among the 25 patients who completed the study, remission and response rates for the ciprofloxacin ($n = 10$), metronidazole ($n = 7$), and placebo ($n = 8$) groups were 30% and 40%, 0% and 14%, and 13% and 13%, respectively.

Azathioprine/6-Mercaptopurine

No controlled trials examining fistula healing with azathioprine or 6-mercaptopurine (6MP) as a primary endpoint have ever been published. In the very first publication documenting use of azathioprine in CD, Brooke et al. reported that all six patients with fistulizing disease who had received azathioprine demonstrated marked clinical improvement in their fistulae [74]. Since then, five randomized controlled trials, which investigated healing of fistulae as a secondary endpoint, have been published (Table 36.1) [75–79]. The studies used improvement or complete healing of fistulae as the outcome measure. With the exception of the trial by Present et al., the studies had very few patients with fistulizing disease. The studies were quite heterogeneous with respect to duration of therapy; there was also some variability in medication used and dosage. Three of the five trials observed higher rates of fistula improvement with azathioprine or 6MP [76, 77, 79]. Of note, the study by Present et al. observed a 31% rate of complete closure of the fistulae in the group receiving 6MP versus 6% for the placebo group [79]. A meta-analysis of these five trials reported an overall response rate (defined as improvement or complete healing) in 54% of patients treated with azathioprine or 6MP compared to 21% in patients treated with placebo [80]. The corresponding pooled odds ratio for fistula healing with azathioprine or 6MP was 4.44 (95% CI = 1.50–13.20). When interpreting the results of this meta-analysis, it is important to keep in mind that the majority of the fistulous cases (46/70, or 66%) were derived from a single study conducted at a single center [79]. Moreover, as mentioned previously, fistula healing was not a primary endpoint for any of the individual trials.

In addition, two uncontrolled case series, one in adults and one in children, have been published [81, 82]. The adult series, by Korelitz et al., treated 34 patients with 6MP at a dose of 1.5 mg/kg/day with various types of fistulae, including perianal (18 patients), abdominal wall (8 patients), enteroenteric (7 patients), rectovaginal (6 patients), and vulvar (2 patients) [81]. Complete fistula closure was achieved in 39% of patients, with an additional 26% showing improvement. This study also underscored the importance of maintenance therapy. Fistulae remained closed for 1–5 years in 46% of patients (6/13) who remained on 6MP, and relapses tended to occur within 2 weeks to 9 months after discontinuation of the drug. Healing was once again achieved upon readministration of 6MP. Furthermore, the authors noted that

Table 36.1 Randomized controlled trials for treatment of fistulizing Crohn's disease with azathioprine or 6-mercaptopurine

Author, year	N	Drug, dose	Rx time	Response drug	Response placebo	p-value
Willoughby et al., 1971 [75]	3	AZA, 2 mg/kg/day	24 weeks	0/2 (0%)	0/1 (0%)	NR
Rhodes et al., 1971 [76]	6	AZA, 2 mg/kg/day	2 months	2/4 (50%)	0/2 (0%)	NR
Klein et al., 1974 [77]	10	AZA, 3 mg/kg/day	4 months	4/5 (80%)	2/5 (40%)	NR
Rosenberg et al., 1975 [78]	5	AZA, 2 mg/kg/day	26 weeks	0/4 (0%)	1/1 (100%)	NR
Present et al., 1980 [79]	46	6MP, 1.5 mg/kg/day	1 year	16/29 (55%)	4/17 (24%)	NR

Fistula outcome not a primary endpoint

Abbreviations: *N* number of patients, *Rx* treatment, *AZA* azathioprine, *NR* not reported, *6MP* 6-mercaptopurine

although all types of fistulae responded to 6MP, abdominal wall and enteroenteric fistulae responded particularly well.

The combination of azathioprine and antibiotics has also been investigated. Dejaco et al. published a prospective, open-label study evaluating the use of an 8-week course of ciprofloxacin and/or metronidazole as a bridge to azathioprine in the treatment of 52 patients with perianal fistulae [83]. In this trial, 17 patients had been taking azathioprine prior to the start of the study, and another 14 patients were initiated on azathioprine after the 8-week course of antibiotics. At week 8, 50% of patients had improved and 25% had achieved complete healing. At week 20, improvement was seen overall in 35% of patients, with complete healing in 18%. Patients who received azathioprine were significantly more likely to achieve response at week 20 than those who did not receive azathioprine (48% vs. 15%, p = 0.03). Thus, more evidence is provided that maintenance therapy is critical to continued fistula healing.

The cost–utility of the combination of metronidazole and 6MP with or without infliximab has been studied by Arseneau et al., who designed a 1-year Markov model for therapy of perianal CD fistulae [84]. They observed that all treatment strategies had similar effectiveness, but strategies involving infliximab were much more expensive. Their conclusion, therefore, was that the incremental benefit of infliximab may not justify the higher cost over a 1-year period. Metronidazole combined with 6MP appears to have the highest initial cost–utility in the treatment of fistulizing perianal Crohn's disease.

Typical doses of azathioprine and 6MP used in clinical trials were 1–1.5 mg/kg/day and 2–3 mg/kg/day, respectively. Currently, there is some debate as to whether dosing according to the level of the active metabolites, the 6-thioguanine nucleotides, should be employed routinely. A meta-analysis has demonstrated that higher 6-thioguanine nucleotide levels (especially >230–260 pmol/10^8 red blood cells) were associated with clinical remission [85]. Adverse events are common with azathioprine and 6MP, occurring in 9–15% of patients, and include allergic reactions, bone marrow suppression (especially leukopenia), pancreatitis, infection, hepatotoxicity, non-Hodgkin's lymphoma, and other gastrointestinal side effects (nausea, vomiting, and abdominal pain) [80, 86, 87].

Methotrexate

Methotrexate has been shown to be effective in the induction and maintenance of remission of CD in several controlled trials. Unfortunately, these studies did not address fistulizing disease. To date, only two retrospective case series have been published which examined the use of methotrexate for CD [88, 89]. The first, by Vandeputte et al., analyzed 20 patients, 8 of whom had fistulae, refractory to azathioprine and requiring continuous corticosteroid treatment [88]. The authors reported improvement in 70% of patients overall with parental methotrexate within 12 weeks but did not specify the outcome of the patients with fistulae. The other series, by Mahadevan et al., included 37 courses of intramuscular and/or oral methotrexate given to 33 patients, 16 of whom had fistulae and were intolerant or refractory to 6MP [89]. Complete fistula closure was achieved in 25%, with another 31% showing improvement. Similar to other medications, fistulae often recurred when the dose of intramuscular methotrexate was decreased or when the route of administration was changed to oral. Thus, methotrexate may represent a reasonable alternative to patients who fail or cannot tolerate azathioprine or 6MP, and long-term maintenance therapy is likely necessary; however, prospective randomized placebo-controlled trials are still needed to evaluate formally the efficacy of methotrexate for fistulizing CD. The initial dose of methotrexate suggested is 25 mg intramuscularly every week. Concurrent administration of folate is advocated to lessen nausea. Adverse events are common and include hepatic fibrosis, bone marrow suppression, pneumonitis and pulmonary fibrosis, nausea, and teratogenicity [90, 91].

Cyclosporine A

There are no controlled trials documenting the efficacy of cyclosporine for the treatment of fistulizing CD. Ten case series, with a total of 64 patients, assessing cyclosporine in Crohn's fistula have been published [92–101]. The largest series, by Present and Lichtiger, looked at 16 patients with various types of CD fistulae (perianal, rectovaginal, and enterocutaneous) treated with intravenous cyclosporine at a dose of 4 mg/kg/day and observed improvement in 88% with complete fistula closure in 44% [96]. The mean time to response was rather short at just over 7 days. The authors noted that 36% of patients relapsed when converted to oral cyclosporine. Taken collectively, the 10 case series showed an initial response rate of fistulizing CD to intravenous cyclosporine of 83% at doses of 2.5–5 mg/kg/day (mostly 4 mg/kg/day). The overall rate of fistula recurrence after discontinuing oral cyclosporine was 62%, however, and thus, most authorities will use cyclosporine as a bridge to other maintenance therapies, such as azathioprine or 6MP [9, 26, 102]. The recommended initiation intravenous dose of cyclosporine is 4 mg/kg/day for 1 week, followed by oral formulation, typically 6–8 mg/kg/day, all dosed by levels. Adverse events are common and include paresthesias, hirsutism, hypertension, tremor, renal insufficiency, headache, opportunistic infections, gingival hyperplasia, seizures, and hepatotoxicity [90, 103].

Tacrolimus

Several uncontrolled case series, with a total of 16 patients with CD fistulae, have suggested that tacrolimus may have efficacy in the management of fistulizing disease [104–107]. The only controlled trial of tacrolimus for fistulizing CD is a randomized, double-blind, placebo-controlled study of 48 patients with perianal or enterocutaneous fistulae by Sandborn et al. [108]. In this study, patients received oral tacrolimus at 0.2 mg/kg/day or placebo for 10 weeks. The primary endpoint, fistula improvement (defined as closure of >50% of draining fistulae and maintenance of closure for at least 4 weeks), occurred in 43% of patients receiving tacrolimus, compared to 8% of patients on placebo ($p = 0.004$). There was no difference in the secondary endpoint, fistula remission (defined as closure of all fistulae and maintenance of that closure for at least 4 weeks), between the two groups (10% of tacrolimus-treated patients vs. 8% of placebo-treated patients). Of note, 38% of patients treated with tacrolimus developed increases in serum creatinine to >1.5 mg/dL, necessitating dose reduction. Gonzalez-Lama et al. conducted a small, uncontrolled, prospective, open-label study of long-term oral tacrolimus at a dose of 0.1 mg/kg/day in 10 patients with Crohn's fistulae refractory to all conventional therapy, including infliximab [109]. Patients in the study had perianal, enterocutaneous, and rectovaginal fistulae. The authors found that after 6–24 months of follow-up, 50% of patients achieved complete response and an additional 40% showed improvement. Importantly, no relapses and no cases of nephrotoxicity occurred throughout the follow-up period. In addition to nephrotoxicity, other adverse events associated with tacrolimus include headache, insomnia, paresthesias, tremor, and leg cramps [108].

Infliximab

Given that inflammation in CD is associated with high levels of tissue tumor necrosis factor-α (TNF-α) expression, therapies directed against this cytokine have become a recent focus of interest. Infliximab, a chimeric (75% human, 25% murine) IgG1 monoclonal antibody directed against TNF-α, is the prototype anti-TNF-α agent, and has now become the cornerstone in medical therapy of fistulizing CD. Several uncontrolled studies have shown efficacy of infliximab in this regard [110–112]. Infliximab has also been shown to be efficacious in the treatment of CD in two multicenter randomized, double-blind, placebo-controlled trials [113, 114], and thus has the most robust data of any medication for the treatment of CD fistulae. The first, by Present et al., randomized 94 patients with draining abdominal (10% of patients) or perianal (90% of patients) fistulae to placebo, infliximab at a dose of 5 mg/kg, or infliximab at 10 mg/kg, administered intravenously at weeks 0, 2, and 6 [113]. The primary endpoint was a reduction in the number of draining fistulae by >50%, which was maintained for at least 4 weeks, and a secondary endpoint was closure of all fistulae. The authors found that the primary endpoint was achieved in 68% of patients who received infliximab at 5 mg/kg and 56% of patients who received infliximab at 10 mg/kg, compared to 26% of patients who received placebo ($p = 0.002$ and $p = 0.02$, respectively). Closure of all fistulae was achieved in 55% of patients who received infliximab at 5 mg/kg and 38% of patients who received infliximab at 10 mg/kg, compared to only 13% of patients who received placebo ($p = 0.001$ and $p = 0.04$, respectively). The median time to response was 14 days for infliximab-treated patients versus 42 days for patients assigned to placebo, and the majority of infliximab-treated patients achieved fistula closure prior to the third infusion. Eleven percent of infliximab-treated patients developed a perianal abscess, possibly resulting from premature closure of the cutaneous end before the closure of the rest of the fistula tract. However, the overall rates of infection did not differ between the infliximab and placebo groups.

In the study by Present et al., the median duration of response was 3 months, suggesting that, similar to the treatment of CD fistula with other medications, maintenance therapy may be required. In addition, since the treatment of luminal CD with infliximab often necessitates maintenance therapy, it should not come as a surprise that maintenance infliximab may be of benefit in the management of fistulizing CD. The other multicenter, randomized, double-blind, placebo-controlled trial of infliximab for CD fistula, the ACCENT II trial (*A C*rohn's Disease *C*linical Trial *E*valuating Infliximab in a *N*ew Long-Term *T*reatment Regimen in Patients with Fistulizing Crohn's Disease) reported by Sands et al., followed 282 patients with draining perianal, abdominal, and rectovaginal fistulae [114]. All patients were induced with infliximab at 5 mg/kg at weeks 0, 2, and 6, and response, defined as a reduction in the number of draining fistulae by >50% for at least 4 weeks, was achieved in 195 patients (69%), similar to the induction response rate reported by Present et al. At week 14, these 195 responders were then randomly assigned to receive infusions of either infliximab 5 mg/kg or placebo every 8 weeks until week 54. The primary endpoint was time to loss of response. The authors observed a median time to loss of response of 40 weeks in infliximab-maintained patients versus 14 weeks in placebo-assigned patients ($p = 0.001$). Overall, 42% of patients in the infliximab group had a loss of response, compared to 62% in the placebo group. At week 54, 46% of patients treated with infliximab still had a response, versus 23% of patients treated with placebo ($p = 0.001$). In addition, at week 54, 36% of patients in the infliximab group had a complete absence of draining fistulae, compared to 19% in the placebo group ($p = 0.009$). Sands et al. performed a post-hoc analysis of the ACCENT II data looking at the efficacy of infliximab induction and maintenance in the subset of women with rectovaginal fistulae [115]. Twenty-five of the original 138 women had a total of 27 draining rectovaginal fistulae at baseline. At week 14, 64% of these 25 women had responded and were then randomized to receive infliximab or placebo maintenance therapy. The authors reported a median time to loss of response of 46 weeks for the infliximab group versus 33 weeks in the placebo group.

The social impact of infliximab in patients with active fistulizing CD has also been investigated in two recent studies. Cadahia et al. were interested in the effect of infliximab induction treatment on health-related quality of life, and thus, they conducted a prospective observational study of 25 patients who received three-dose induction infliximab therapy for single or multiple draining abdominal or perianal fistulae [116]. The authors found that health-related quality of life, as measured by the SF-36, demonstrated significant improvement in the physical domain after 4 and 10 weeks. In addition, a significant increase in IBDQ score was seen after 4 weeks. More recently, Lichtenstein et al. evaluated the impact of infliximab maintenance therapy on the number of hospitalizations, surgeries, and procedures in patients with fistulizing CD [117]. Using data from the ACCENT II trial, they revealed that compared to patients who received placebo, patients who received maintenance infliximab had significantly fewer number of mean hospitalization days (0.5 vs. 2.5 days), hospitalizations (0.11 vs. 0.31), total surgeries and procedures (65 vs. 126), inpatient surgeries and procedures (7 vs. 41), and major surgeries (2 vs. 11).

Mechanistically, infliximab's effects on mucosal cytokine profiles may predict which patients with fistulizing CD will relapse. Agnholt et al. recently collected tissue samples for cytokine analysis from 26 patients with CD fistulae [118]. They observed that fistula healing was associated with decreased production of TNF-α, interferon-γ, and interleukin-10, while relapse was associated with increased production of interferon-γ.

Despite all of its reported success, the use of infliximab may not obviate the need for surgical management of CD fistulae in many cases. Poritz et al. retrospectively examined surgical rates in patients treated with infliximab for fistulizing CD at a single institution [119]. Among the 26 patients with various types of fistulae, 46% experienced a partial response to infliximab, and an additional 23% had fistula closure. However, 54% of patients overall still required surgery after infliximab therapy, and another 23% continued to open fistulous drainage but refused surgery. Of note, none of the patients with either enterocutaneous or peristomal fistulae were healed with infliximab treatment.

The effectiveness of infliximab in combination with other medical therapies for fistulizing CD has also been investigated in several studies [120–122]. West et al. conducted a double-blind, placebo-controlled trial of ciprofloxacin overlapping with infliximab in patients with perianal CD fistulae [120]. In this study, 24 patients were randomized to receive either ciprofloxacin at 1000 mg/day or placebo for 12 weeks in addition to infliximab at 5 mg/kg at weeks 6, 8, and 12. Patients were followed for 18 weeks, and the primary endpoint was reduction in the number of draining fistulae by >50%. The authors reported that 73% of the ciprofloxacin-treated patients responded, compared to 39% in the placebo group. One caveat is that the response rate to infliximab alone was much less than in other infliximab studies, in which at least 60% of patients responded. Infliximab has also been evaluated in combination with immunomodulator therapy. Ochsenkühn et al. performed an uncontrolled pilot study of long-term azathioprine (at 2–2.5 mg/kg/day) or 6MP (at 1 mg/kg/day) in combination with induction infliximab in 16 patients [121]. They found that 75% of patients achieved complete fistula closure, which persisted for more than 6 months (median time of 10 months). As seen previously, the median time to fistula closure was 14 days. A similar uncontrolled pilot study by Schröder et al. followed 12 consecutive patients with CD fistulae intolerant or resistant to azathioprine [122]. Patients were treated with induction infliximab and long-term methotrexate at 20 mg/week (intravenously for 6 weeks, followed by oral thereafter). The authors observed that 33% of patients experienced complete fistula closure for at least 6 months (median 13 months), and 25% had a partial response. While providing a suggestion of efficacy of combination therapy for the treatment of fistulizing CD, controlled trials have yet to be performed.

The combination of infliximab with surgical intervention (i.e., seton placement) in the treatment of CD perianal fistulae has been assessed in several studies [6, 7, 123–125]. Three single-center retrospective case series, from Calgary, Leeds, and Oxford, each of which included 21 patients, have documented favorable rates of fistula healing with seton placement followed by induction and maintenance infliximab, with complete and partial healing rates of 67% and 19%, 47% and 53%, and 21% and 42%, respectively [7, 123, 124]. Two studies were able to compare the outcomes of patients treated with infliximab and seton placement to those treated with infliximab and/or seton placement alone [6, 125]. The first, by Regueiro and Mardini, retrospectively analyzed 32 consecutive patients with perianal CD fistulae, all of whom had received at least three induction doses of infliximab and some of whom had additionally undergone an EUA with seton placement prior to infliximab treatment [6]. Response was defined as complete closure and cessation of drainage from the fistula. They found that compared to patients treated with infliximab alone ($n = 23$), patients who had a preinfusional EUA with seton placement ($n = 9$) had a significantly higher rate of initial response (100% vs. 83%, $p = 0.014$), lower rate of recurrence (44% vs. 79%, $p = 0.001$), and longer time to recurrence (13.5 months vs. 3.6 months, $p = 0.0001$). The second, by Scaudione et al., prospectively subdivided 35 consecutive patients with complex perianal fistulae into three groups: infliximab with seton placement ($n = 14$), infliximab alone ($n = 11$), and seton placement alone ($n = 10$) [125]. The authors reported that patients in the combination group had a nonsignificantly higher rate of complete response, defined as closure of all draining fistulae and cessation of drainage for 3 months, of 79% vs. 64% and 70%, respectively, and a significantly longer time to recurrence of 10.1 months vs. 2.6 and 3.6 months, respectively ($p < 0.02$).

The combination of infliximab with immunomodulators and seton placement has also been investigated more recently. A prospective open-label study of 34 patients from three hospitals in France, by Roumeguere et al., had patients undergo seton placement 3 months prior to the start of medical therapy, followed by initiation of methotrexate 25 mg/week, followed by induction infliximab, after which patients were maintained on methotrexate alone [126]. At 14 weeks, 74% of patients had a complete response and another 11% had a partial response. Of patients with initial response, 90% had

maintained at least a partial response after 56 weeks. A prospective study of 41 patients from St. Mark's Hospital in London, by Tozer et al., assessed long-term fistula response and remission rates after treatment with infliximab (or adalimumab in nine patients who lost response to infliximab) combined with thiopurines, in which 73% of patients had seton placement which was removed after 2–6 weeks [127]. They reported rates of fistula response and remission at 2 years of 35% and 29%, respectively, and at 3 years of 37% and 21%, respectively. A large retrospective study from two referral centers in France, by Bouguen et al., assessed long-term rates of initial and sustained fistula closure in 156 patients treated with infliximab and immunomodulators (in 58%) and seton placement (in 62%) [128]. They observed rates of initial fistula closure of 59%, 73%, and 88% at 3, 5, and 10 years, respectively, and rates of sustained fistula closure of 22%, 43%, and 57% at 3, 5, and 10 years, respectively. Interestingly, the use of infliximab for more than 118 weeks and the use of combination therapy were associated with significantly higher rates of initial fistula closure.

Adverse events with infliximab treatment are common and include infusion reactions, delayed-type hypersensitivity reactions, formation of human antichimeric antibodies, formation of antinuclear and anti-double-stranded DNA antibodies, and drug-induced lupus-like reactions [129–131]. In addition, infectious complications seem to be increased, but serious infections, such as pneumonia, sepsis, tuberculosis, and opportunistic infections, including listeriosis, aspergillosis, histoplasmosis, coccidiomycosis, and *Pneumocystis carinii* pneumonia, occur only rarely [132–136]. Finally, there have been isolated case reports of hepatic necrosis and non-Hodgkin's lymphoma in patients treated with infliximab, although it has not been determined whether these events were the direct consequence of infliximab therapy.

Adalimumab and Certolizumab Pegol

Like infliximab, the other commonly used anti-TNF-α medications for CD treatment, adalimumab and certolizumab pegol, have shown efficacy in the treatment of fistulizing disease. However, although data in patients with fistulae for both adalimumab and certolizumab pegol were obtained from randomized placebo-controlled studies, fistula healing was not a primary endpoint in these studies. Adalimumab, a fully human IgG1 monoclonal antibody, was found to be efficacious for maintenance of remission in the Crohn's Trial of the Fully *H*uman Antibody *A*dalimumab for *R*emission *M*aintenance (CHARM), in which 854 patients received open-label induction treatment with subcutaneous adalimumab 80 mg at week 0 and 40 mg at week 2, followed by randomized maintenance treatment with adalimumab 40 mg every week or every other week or placebo up to week

56, with a co-primary endpoint of clinical remission at weeks 26 and 56 [137]. In this study, 117 patients had draining fistulae, and 113 of these had perianal fistulae. A subgroup analysis of these patients, in which complete fistula healing was defined as the absence of draining fistulae at the last two consecutive post-baseline evaluations, reported complete fistula healing rates of 30% for the combined adalimumab groups versus 13% for the placebo group at week 26 (*p* < 0.05), and 33% for the combined adalimumab groups versus 13% for the placebo group at week 56 (*p* < 0.05) [138]. The authors also observed that these rates of fistula healing were largely maintained for up to 2 years of follow-up in a long-term extension study of CHARM called ADHERE [139].

Certolizumab pegol, a pegylated humanized Fab fragment of an anti-TNF-α monoclonal antibody, was shown to have efficacy in the maintenance of remission in active Crohn's disease in the Pegylated Antibody Fragment Evaluation in Crohn's Disease: Safety and Efficacy 2 (PRECISE 2) randomized placebo-controlled trial, in which 668 patients received open-label induction treatment with subcutaneous certolizumab pegol 400 mg at weeks 0, 2, and 4, followed by randomized maintenance treatment with certolizumab pegol 400 mg or placebo every 4 weeks through week 24 and followed to week 26 [140]. In this study, 58 patients had draining fistulae, and 55 of these had perianal fistulae. A subgroup analysis of these patients, in which complete and partial fistula closure were defined as closure of 100% and at least 50%, respectively, of all draining fistulae at two consecutive post-baseline evaluations at least 3 weeks apart, reported complete fistula healing rates of 36% for the certolizumab pegol group versus 17% for the placebo group (*p* = 0.038), and partial fistula healing rates of 54% for the certolizumab pegol group versus 43% for the placebo group (*p* = NS) at week 26 [141].

Adverse events associated with adalimumab and certolizumab pegol are similar to those seen with infliximab.

Other Anti-TNF-α Agents

Other anti-TNF-α medications, including CDP571 and thalidomide, have also been preliminarily investigated for the treatment of fistulizing CD; of note, golimumab has not been studied for the treatment of CD fistulae. CDP571, a humanized (95% human, 5% murine) IgG4 monoclonal antibody, has been assessed for efficacy in the treatment of CD fistulae in two multicenter, randomized, double-blind, placebo-controlled trials [142, 143]. The first study, by Feagan et al., published only in abstract form, treated 71 patients with steroid-dependent CD with intravenous CDP571 at 20 mg/kg or placebo at week 0, followed by a second infusion of CDP571 at 10 mg/kg or placebo at week 8 [142]. At week 16, among the subgroup of patients with draining perianal fistulae, fistula closure was achieved in 25% of patients who

received CDP571, compared to none in the placebo group. The other study, by Sandborn et al., followed 169 patients for 24 weeks, during which patients received an initial infusion of CDP571 at either 10 or 20 mg/kg or placebo, followed by CDP571 at 10 mg/kg or placebo every 8–12 weeks [143]. This study included 37 patients with open perianal or enterocutaneous fistulae and reported that 50% of patients treated with CDP571 achieved fistula closure versus 15% of patients who received placebo. Adverse events due to CDP571 include infusion reactions, formation of anti-idiotype antibodies, development of new antinuclear or anti-double-stranded DNA antibodies, insomnia, pruritus, and rash [142, 143].

Thalidomide has also been preliminarily evaluated in the treatment of fistulizing CD in two open-label pilot studies [144, 145]. The first study, by Ehrenpreis et al., enrolled 22 patients with refractory CD to receive oral thalidomide at 200 or 300 mg/day for 12 weeks [144]. At week 4, of the 13 patients with fistulae, 9 patients (69%) responded, 3 patients (23%) achieved remission, and 2 patients (15%) had closure of all fistulae. Nine patients with fistulizing disease completed the 12 weeks of treatment. Of these nine patients, all (69%) were responders, six patients (46%) achieved remission, and five patients (38%) had complete closure of all fistulae. The other pilot study, by Vasiliauskas et al., treated 12 patients with steroid-dependent CD with 50 or 100 mg/day of thalidomide for 12 weeks [145]. Of the six patients with active perianal fistulae at the time of entry into the study, five (83%) had improvement in symptoms after 4 weeks. Four of these six patients with fistulizing disease completed 12 weeks of treatment. Fistula closure was achieved in one patient (17%) at week 12, with improvement in another two patients (33%). Adverse events are common with thalidomide therapy and include severe somnolence, peripheral neuropathy, teratogenicity, peripheral edema, constipation, seborrheic dermatitis, hypertension, muscle spasm, and diffuse rash [144, 145].

Vedolizumab

Anti-integrin therapy has been used more recently in the treatment of CD as a way to target reduction of lymphocyte trafficking to the gut. The α4β7 integrin, a cell-surface glycoprotein expressed on lymphocytes, helps to regulate lymphocyte migration into inflamed intestinal tissue via interaction with mucosal addressin-cell adhesion molecule 1 (MAdCAM-1) on intestinal blood vessels [146]. Natalizumab, which is not gut-specific as it binds both α4β7 and α4β1 integrins (the latter which are located in the central nervous system), was shown to be effective for the treatment of CD in a large randomized controlled trial, but patients with draining fistulae were exluded [147]. However, the use of natalizumab is associated with an increased risk of progressive multifocal leukoencephalopathy [148], and thus vedolizumab was developed as a purely gut-selective blocker of α4β7. Vedolizumab was shown to be efficacious for the treatment of moderate-to-severe active Crohn's disease in the GEMINI 2 double-blind randomized placebo-controlled trial [149]. Although fistula treatment was not the primary endpoint in this trial, 57 patients had actively draining fistulae at baseline. Treatment with vedolizumab 300 mg every 8 weeks was associated with a significantly higher rate of fistula closure than treatment with placebo after 52 weeks (41% vs. 18%, $p = 0.03$).

Other Therapies

A variety of other therapies for fistulizing CD have been suggested to be of possible benefit in uncontrolled case series or anecdotally. These include elemental diets, bowel rest with total parental nutrition, mycophenolate mofetil, granulocyte-colony stimulating factor, hyperbaric oxygen, and coagulation factor XIII [150–170]. However, controlled trials are required before any of these modalities

can be recommended for routine use. Other novel therapies are also currently under investigation (refer to www.clinicaltrials.gov).

Conclusion

The treatment of perianal fistulizing CD has evolved greatly in the last 15 years, due largely to improvements in medical therapy. Tables 36.2 and 36.3 summarize all published controlled and uncontrolled trials of immunomodulator and anti-TNF-α therapy for the treatment of CD. The advent of immunomodulators and anti-TNF-α agents has transformed the treatment of CD from almost exclusively surgical to placing a much larger emphasis on medical therapy, either as initial therapy alone, with surgery reserved for refractory cases, or in combination with surgery from the start. For this reason, gastroenterologists and surgeons must work in concert in order to provide the best care for each patient. Proper fistula management also relies heavily on accurate diagnosis, especially defining the anatomy of the fistula, ascertaining whether abscess formation is present, and determining the location and extent of intestinal inflammation.

Table 36.2 Controlled trials for treatment of fistulizing Crohn's disease with immunomodulators or anti-TNF-α agents

Author, Year	N	(Drug), dose	Rx time	Response drug	Response placebo	p-value
Immunomodulators						
Azathioprine/6MP[a]						
Willoughby et al., 1971 [75]	3	AZA, 2 mg/kg/day	24 wk	0/2 (0%)	0/1 (0%)	NR
Rhodes et al., 1971 [76]	6	AZA, 2 mg/kg/day	2 mo	2/4 (50%)	0/2 (0%)	NR
Klein et al., 1974 [77]	10	AZA, 3 mg/kg/day	4 mo	4/5 (80%)	2/5 (40%)	NR
Rosenberg et al., 1975 [78]	5	AZA, 2 mg/kg/day	26 wk	0/4 (0%)	1/1 (100%)	NR
Present et al., 1980 [79]	46	6MP, 1.5 mg/kg/day	1 yr	16/29 (55%)	4/17 (24%)	NR
Total	70			22/44 (50%)	7/26 (27%)	
Tacrolimus						
Sandborn et al., 2003 [108]	48	0.2 mg/kg/day	10 wk	9/21 (43%)	2/25 (8%)	0.004
Anti-TNF-α agents						
Infliximab						
Present et al., 1999 [113]	94	5 mg/kg 10 mg/kg	14 wk	21/31 (68%) 18/32 (56%)	8/31 (26%)	0.002 0.02
Sands et al., 2004 [114]	195	5 mg/kg	54 wk	42/91 (46%)	23/98 (23%)	0.001
Total	289			81/154 (53%)	31/129 (24%)	
Adalimumab[a]						
Colombel et al., 2009 [138]	117	40 mg EOW or Qwk	56 wk	6/47 (13%)	23/70 (33%)	<0.05
Certolizumab Pegola						
Schreiber et al., 2011 [141]	58	400 mg Q4 wk	26 wk	10/28 (36%)	5/30 (17%)	0.038
CDP571[a]						
Sandborn et al., 2001 [143]	37	CDP571, 10 or 20 mg/kg	24 wk	12/24 (50%)	2/13 (15%)	0.074
Vedolizumab						
Sandborn et al. 2013 [149]	57	300 mg Q8 wk 300 mg Q4 wk	52 wk	7/17 (41%) 5/22 (23%)	2/18 (11%)	0.03 0.32

Abbreviations: *N* number of patients, *Rx* treatment, *AZA* azathioprine, *d* day, *wk* week(s), *NR* not reported, *mo* month(s); 6MP, 6-mercaptopurine, *yr* year(s), *EOW* every other week, *Q* every
[a]Fistula outcome not a primary endpoint

Table 36.3 Uncontrolled trials for treatment of fistulizing Crohn's disease with immunomodulators or anti-TNF-α agents

Author, year	N	Drug, dose	Initial response	Sustained response
Immunomodulators				
Methotrexate				
Mahadevan et al., 2003 [89]	16	Methotrexate, 25 mg/week im	9/16 (56%)	3/16 (19%)
Cyclosporine A				
Fukushima et al., 1989 [92]	1	Cyclosporine A, 8 mg/kg/day po	1/1 (100%)	1/1 (100%)
Lichtiger, 1990 [93]	10	Cyclosporine A, 4 mg/kg/day iv	6/10 (60%)	NR
Markowitz et al., 1990 [94]	1	Cyclosporine A, 4 mg/kg/day iv	0/1 (0%)	0/1 (0%)
Hanauer et al., 1993 [95]	5	Cyclosporine A, 4 mg/kg/day iv	5/5 (100%)	2/5 (40%)
Present et al., 1994 [96]	16	Cyclosporine A, 4 mg/kg/day iv	14/16 (88%)	9/16 (56%)
Abreu-Martin et al., 1996 [97]	2	Cyclosporine A, 2.5 mg/kg/day iv	2/2 (100%)	1/2 (50%)
O'Neill et al., 1997 [98]	8	Cyclosporine A, 4 mg/kg/day iv	7/8 (88%)	0/8 (0%)
Hinterleitner et al., 1997 [99]	7	Cyclosporine A, 5 mg/kg/day iv	9/9 (100%)	4/9 (44%)
Egan et al., 1998 [100]	9	Cyclosporine A, 4 mg/kg/day iv	7/9 (78%)	2/8 (25%)
Gurudu et al., 1999 [101]	3	Cyclosporine A, 4 mg/kg/day iv	2/3 (67%)	NR
Total	64		53/64 (83%)	19/50 (38%
Anti-TNF-α agents				
Thalidomide				
Ehrenpreis et al., 1999 [144]	13	Thalidomide, 200 or 300 mg/day	9/13 (69%)	NR
Vasiliauskas et al., 1999 [145]	6	Thalidomide, 50 or 100 mg/day	1/6 (17%)	NR
Total	19		10/19 (53%)	NR

Abbreviations: *N* number of patients, *NR* not reported, *im* intramuscular, *po* oral, *iv* intravenous

References

1. Crohn BB, Ginzburg L, Oppenheimer GD. Regional ileitis: a pathologic and clinical entity. JAMA. 1932;99:1323–9.
2. Bissell AD. Localized chronic ulcerative colitis. Ann Surg. 1934;99:957–66.
3. American Gastroenterological Association. American Gastroenterological Association medical position statement: perianal Crohn's disease. Gastroenterology. 2003;125:1503–7.
4. American Gastroenterological Association. AGA technical review on perianal Crohn's disease. Gastroenterology. 2003;125:1508–30.
5. Scott HJ, Northover JM. Evaluation of surgery for perianal Crohn's fistulas. Dis Colon Rectum. 1996;39:1039–43.
6. Regueiro M, Mardini H. Treatment of perianal fistulizing Crohn's disease with infliximab alone or as an adjunct to exam under anesthesia with seton placement. Inflamm Bowel Dis. 2003;9:98–103.
7. Topstad DR, Panaccione R, Heine JA, Johnson DR, MacLean AR, Buie WD. Combined seton placement, infliximab infusion, and maintenance immunosuppressives improve healing rates in fistulizing anorectal Crohn's disease: a single center experience. Dis Colon Rectum. 2003;46:577–83.
8. Bell SJ, Williams AB, Wiesel P, Wilkinson K, Cohen RC, Kamm MA. The clinical course of fistulating Crohn's disease. Aliment Pharmacol Ther. 2003;17:1145–51.
9. Schwartz DA, Herdman CR. Review article: the medical treatment of Crohn's perianal fistulas. Aliment Pharmacol Ther. 2004;19:953–67.
10. Hughes L. Surgical pathology and management of anorectal Crohn's disease. J R Soc Med. 1978;71:644–51.
11. Parks A. The pathogenesis and treatment of fistula-in-ano. Br Med J. 1961;1:463–9.
12. Fielding JF. Perianal lesions in Crohn's disease. J R Coll Surg Edinb. 1972;17:32–7.

13. Greenstein AJ, Kark AE, Drelling DA. Crohn's disease of the colon I. Fistula in Crohn's disease colon, classification presenting features and management in 63 patients. Am J Gastroenterol. 1974;62:419–29.
14. Farmer R, Hawk W, Turnbull RJ. Clinical patterns in Crohn's disease. A statistical study of 615 cases. Gastroenterology. 1975;68:627–35.
15. Rankin GB, Watts HD, Melnyk CS, Kelley Jr ML. National Cooperative Crohn's Disease Study: extraintestinal manifestations and perianal complications. Gastroenterology. 1979;77:914–20.
16. Buchmann P, Keighly MR, Allan RN, Thompson H, Alexander-Williams J. Natural history of perianal Crohn's disease. Ten year follow-up: a plea for conservatism. Am J Surg. 1980;140:642–4.
17. Williams DR, Coller JA, Corman ML, Nugent FW, Veidenheimer MC. Anal complications in Crohn's disease. Dis Colon Rectum 1981;24:22–4.
18. Marks CG, Ritchie JK, Lockhart-Mummery HE. Anal fistulas in Crohn's disease. Br J Surg. 1981;68:525–7.
19. Hobbiss JH, Schofield PF. Management of perianal Crohn's disease. J R Soc Med. 1982;75:414–7.
20. Van Dongen LM, Lubbers E. Perianal fistulas in patients with Crohn's disease. Arch Surg. 1986;121:1187–90.
21. Goebell H. Perianal complications in Crohn's disease. Neth J Med. 1990;37:S47–51.
22. Hellers G, Bergstrand O, Ewerth S, Homstrom B. Occurrence and outcome after primary treatment of anal fistulae in Crohn's disease. Gut. 1980;21:525–7.
23. Schwartz DA, Loftus EV, Tremaine WJ, Pananccione R, Harmsen WS, Zinsmeister AR, Sandborn WJ. The natural history of fistulizing Crohn's disease in Olmstead County, Minnesota. Gastroenterology. 2002;122:875–80.
24. Gray BK, Lockhart-Mummery HE, Morson BC. Crohn's disease of the anal region. Gut. 1965;6:515–24.

25. Halme L, Sainio AP. Factors related to frequency, type, and outcome of anal fistulas in Crohn's disease. Dis Colon Rectum. 1995;38:55–9.
26. Judge TA, Lichtenstein GR. Treatment of fistulizing Crohn's disease. Gastroenterol Clin N Am. 2004;33:421–54.
27. Bayer I, Gordon PH. Selected operative management of fistula-in-ano in Crohn's disease. Dis Colon Rectum. 1994;37:760–5.
28. Makowiec F, Jehle EC, Becker HD, Starlinger M. Perianal abscess in Crohn's disease. Dis Colon Rectum. 1997;40:443–50.
29. Van Beers B, Grandin C, Kartheuser A. MRI of complicated anal fistulae: comparison with digital examination. J Comput Assist Tomogr. 1994;18:87–90.
30. Fazio VW, Wilk P, Turnbull Jr RB, Jagelman DG. The dilemma of Crohn's disease: ileosigmoidal fistula complicating Crohn's disease. Dis Colon Rectum. 1977;20:381–6.
31. Kuijpers HC, Schulpen T. Fistulography for fistula-in-ano. Is it useful? Dis Colon Rectum. 1985;28:103–4.
32. Glass RE, Ritchie JK, Lennard-Jones JE, Hawley PR, Todd IP. Internal fistulas in Crohn's disease. Dis Colon Rectum. 1985;28:557–61.
33. Pomerri F, Pittarello F, Dodi G, Pianon P, Muzzio PC. Radiologic diagnosis of anal fistulae with radio-opaque markers. Radiol Med. 1988;75:632–7.
34. Weisman RI, Orsay CP, Pearl RK, Abcarian H. The role of fistulography in fistula-in-ano. Report of five cases. Dis Colon Rectum. 1991;34:181–4.
35. Berliner L, Redmond P, Purow E, Megna D, Scottile V. Computed tomography in Crohn's disease. Am J Gastroenterol. 1982;77:584–53.
36. Goldberg HI, Gore RM, Margulis AR, Moss AA, Baker EL. Computed tomography in the evaluation of Crohn's disease. Am J Roentgenol. 1983;140:277–82.
37. Kerber GW, Greenberg M, Rubin JM. Computed tomography evaluation of local and extraintestinal complications of Crohn's disease. Gastrointest Radiol. 1984;9:143–8.
38. Fishman EK, Wolf EJ, Jones B, Bayless TM, Siegelman SS. CT evaluation of Crohn's disease: effect on patient management. Am J Roentgenol. 1987;148:537–40.
39. Yousem DM, Fishman EK, Jones B. Crohn's disease: perirectal and perianal findings at CT. Radiology. 1988;167:331–4.
40. Van Outryve MJ, Pelckmans PA, Michielsen PP, Van Maercke YM. Value of tranrectal ultrasonography in Crohn's disease. Gastroenterology. 1991;101:1171–7.
41. Schratter-Sehn AU, Lochs H, Vogelsang H, Schurawitzki H, Herold C, Schratter M. Endoscopic ultrasonography versus computed tomography in the differential diagnosis of perianorectal complications in Crohn's disease. Endoscopy. 1993;25:582–6.
42. Koelbel G, Schmiedl U, Majer MC, Weber P, Jenss H, Kueper K, Hess CF. Diagnosis of fistulae and sinus tracts in patients with Crohn's disease: value of MR imaging. Am J Roentgenol. 1989;152:999–1003.
43. Skalej M, Makowiec F, Weinlich M, Jenss H, Laniado M, Starlinger M. Magnetic resonance imaging in perianal Crohn's disease. Dtsch Med Wochenschr. 1993;118:1791–6.
44. Lunniss PJ, Barker PG, Sultan AH, Armstrong P, Reznek RH, Bartram CI, Cottam KS, Phillips RK. Magnetic resonance imaging of fistula-in-ano. Dis Colon Rectum. 1994;37:708–18.
45. Barker PG, Lunniss PJ, Armstrong P, Reznek RH, Cottam KS, Phillips RK. Magnetic resonance imaging of fistula-in-ano: technique, interpretation, and accuracy. Clin Radiol. 1994;49:7–13.
46. Haggert PJ, Moore NR, Shearman JD, Travis SP, Jewell DP, Mortensen NJ. Pelvic and perianal complications of Crohn's disease: assessment using magnetic resonance imaging. Gut. 1995;36:407–10.
47. DeSouza NM, Hall AS, Puni R, Gilderdale DJ, Young IR, Kmiot WA. High resolution magnetic resonance imaging of the anal sphincter using a dedicated endoanal coil. Comparison of magnetic resonance imaging with surgical finding. Dis Colon Rectum. 1996;39:926–34.
48. Spencer JA, Chapple K, Wilson D, Ward J, Windsor AC, Ambrose NS. Outcome after surgery for perianal fistula: predictive value of MR imaging. Am J Roentgenol. 1998;171:403–6.
49. Schwartz DA, Wiersema MJ, Dudiak KM, Fletcher JG, Clain JE, Tremaine WJ, Zinsmeister AR, Norton ID, Boardman LA, Devine RM, Wolff BG, Young-Fadok TM, Diehl NN, Pemberton JH, Sandborn WJ. A comparison of endoscopic ultrasound, magnetic resonance imaging, and exam under anesthesia for evaluation of Crohn's perianal fistulas. Gastroenterology. 2001;121:1064–72.
50. Beets-Tan RG, Beets GL, van der Hoop AG, Kessels AG, Vliegen RF, Baeten CG, van Engelshoven JM. Preoperative MR imaging of anal fistulas: does it really help the surgeon? Radiology. 2001;218:75–84.
51. Tio TL, Mulder CJ, Wijers OB, Sars PR, Tytgat GN. Endosonography of peri-anal and per-colorectal fistula and/or abscess in Crohn's disease. Gastrointest Endosc. 1990;36:331–6.
52. Wijers O, Tio T, Tytgat G. Endosonography (transrectal and transvaginal) in the assessment of perianorectal fistulas and abscesses: experience with 127 cases. In: Demling L, Fruhmorgan P, editors. Non-neoplastic diseases of the anorectum. London: Kluwer; 1992. p. 65–78.
53. Solomon MJ. Fistulae and abscesses in symptomatic perianal Crohn's disease. Int J Color Dis. 1996;11:222–6.
54. Orsoni P, Barthet M, Portier F, Panuel M, Desjeux A, Grimaud JC. Prospective comparison of endosonography, magnetic resonance imaging and surgical findings in anorectal fistula and abscess complicating Crohn's disease. Br J Surg. 1999;86:360–4.
55. Stewart LK, McGee J, Wilson SR. Transperineal and transvaginal sonography of perianal inflammatory bowel disease. Am J Roentgenol. 2001;177:627–32.
56. Sloots CE, Felt-Bersma RJ, Poen AC, Cuesta MA, Meuwissen SG. Assessment and classification of fistula-in-ano in patients with Crohn's disease by hydrogen peroxide enhanced transanal ultrasound. Int J Color Dis. 2001;16:292–7.
57. Sparberg M, Kirsner JB. Long-term corticosteroid therapy for regional enteritis: an analysis of 58 courses in 54 patients. Am J Dig Dis. 1966;11:865–80.
58. Jones JH, Lennard-Jones JF. Corticosteroids and corticotropin in the treatment of Crohn's disease. Gut. 1966;7:181–7.
59. Agrawal A, Durrani S, Leiper K, Ellis A, Morris AI, Rhodes JM. Effect of systemic corticosteroid therapy on risk for intra-abdominal or pelvic abscess in non-operated Crohn's disease. Clin Gastroenterol Hepatol. 2005;3:1215–20.
60. Ursing B, Kamme C. Metronidazole for Crohn's disease. Lancet. 1975;1:775–7.
61. Bernstein LH, Frank MS, Brandt LJ, Boley SJ. Healing of perianal Crohn's disease with metronidazole. Gastroenterology. 1980;79:357–65.
62. Schneider MU, Strobel S, Riemann JF, Demling L. Treatment of Crohn's disease with metronidazole. Dtsch Med Wochenschr. 1981;106:1126–9.
63. Brandt LJ, Bernstein LH, Boley SJ, Frank MS. Metronidazole therapy for perianal Crohn's disease: a follow-up study. Gastroenterology. 1982;83:383–7.
64. Jakobovits J, Schuster MM. Metronidazole therapy for Crohn's disease and associated fistulae. Am J Gastroenterol. 1984;79:533–40.
65. Schneider MU, Laudage G, Guggenmoos-Holzmann I, Riemann JF. Metronidazole in the treatment of Crohn's disease. Results of a controlled randomized prospective study. Dtsch Med Wochenschr. 1985;110:1724–30.
66. Turunen U, Farkkila M, Seppala K. Long-term treatment of perianal or fistulous Crohn's disease with ciprofloxacin. Scand J Gastroenterol Suppl. 1989;24:144.

67. Wolf JL. Ciprofloxacin may be useful in Crohn's disease (abstr). Gastroenterology. 1990;98:A212.

68. Solomon MJ, McLeod RS, O'Connor BI, Steinhart AH, Greenberg GR, Cohen Z. Combination ciprofloxacin and metronidazole in severe perianal Crohn's disease. Can J Gastroenterol. 1993;7:571–3.

69. Turunen U, Farkkila M, Valtonen V. Long-term outcome of ciprofloxacin treatment in severe perianal or fistulous Crohn's disease (abstr). Gastroenterology. 1993;104:A793.

70. Freeman CD, Klutman NE, Lamp KC. Metronidazole. A therapeutic review and update. Drugs. 1997;54:679–708.

71. Davis R, Markham A, Balfour JA. Ciprofloxacin. An updated review of its pharmacology, therapeutic efficacy and tolerability. Drugs. 1996;51:1019–74.

72. Casparian JM, Luchi M, Moffat RE, Hinthorn D. Quinolones and tendon ruptures. South Med J. 2000;93:488–91.

73. Thia KT, Mahadevan U, Feagan BG, Wong C, Cockeram A, Bitton A, Bernstein CN, Sandborn WJ. Ciprofloxacin or metronidazole for the treatment of perianal fistulas in patients with Crohn's disease: a randomized, double-blind, placebo-controlled pilot study. Inflamm Bowel Dis. 2009;15:17–24.

74. Brooke BN, Hoffman DC, Swarbrick ET. Azathioprine for Crohn's disease. Lancet. 1969;2:612–4.

75. Willoughby JM, Beckett J, Kumar PJ, Dawson AM. Controlled trial of azathioprine in Crohn's disease. Lancet. 1971;2:944–7.

76. Rhodes J, Bainton D, Beck P, Campbell H. Controlled trial of azathioprine in Crohn's disease. Lancet. 1971;2:1273–6.

77. Klein M, Binder HJ, Mitchell M, Aaronson R, Spiro H. Treatment of Crohn's disease with azathioprine: a controlled evaluation. Gastroenterology. 1974;66:916–22.

78. Rosenberg JL, Levin B, Wall AJ, Kirsner JB. A controlled trial of azathioprine in Crohn's disease. Am J Digest Dis. 1975;20:721–6.

79. Present DH, Korelitz BI, Wisch N, Glass JL, Sachar DB, Pasternack BS. Treatment of Crohn's disease with mercaptopurine. A long-term, randomized, double-blind study. N Engl J Med. 1980;302:981–7.

80. Pearson D, May G, Fick G, Sutherland L. Azathioprine and 6-mercaptopurine in Crohn's disease: a meta analysis. Ann Intern Med. 1995;123:132–42.

81. Korelitz BI, Present DH. Favorable effect of mercaptopurine on fistulae of Crohn's disease. Digest Dis Sci. 1985;30:58–64.

82. Jeshion WC, Larsen KL, Jawad AF, Piccoli DA, Verma R, Maller ES, Baldassano RN. Azathioprine and 6-mercaptopurine for the treatment of perianal Crohn's disease in children. J Clin Gastroenterol. 2000;30:294–8.

83. Dejaco C, Harrer M, Waldhoer T, Miehsler W, Vogelsang H, Reinisch W. Antibiotics and azathioprine for the treatment of perianal fistulas in Crohn's disease. Aliment Pharmacol Ther. 2003;18:1113–20.

84. Arseneau KO, Cohn SM, Cominelli F, Connors Jr AF. Cost-utility of initial medical management for Crohn's disease perianal fistulae. Gastroenterology. 2001;120:1640–56.

85. Osterman MT, Kundu R, Lichtenstein GR, Lewis JD. Association of 6-thioguanine nucleotide levels and inflammatory bowel disease activity: a meta-analysis. Gastroenterology. 2006;130: 1047–53.

86. Present DH, Meltzer SJ, Krumholz MP, Wolke A, Korelitz BI. 6-Mercaptopurine in the management of inflammatory bowel disease: short- and long-term toxicity. Ann Intern Med. 1989;111: 641–9.

87. Dayharsh GA, Loftus Jr EV, Sandborn WJ, Tremaine WJ, Zinsmeister AR, Witzig TE, Macon WR, Burgart LJ. Epstein-Barr virus-positive lymphoma in patients with inflammatory bowel disease treated with azathioprine or 6-mercaptopurine. Gastroenterology. 2002;122:72–7.

88. Vandeputte L, D'Haens G, Beart F, Rutgeerts P. Methotrexate in refractory Crohn's disease. Inflamm Bowel Dis. 1999;5:11–5.

89. Mahadevan U, Marion JF, Present DH. Fistula response to methotrexate in Crohn's disease: a case series. Aliment Pharmacol Ther. 2003;18:1003–8.

90. Sandborn WJ. A review of immune modifier therapy for inflammatory bowel disease: azathioprine, 6-mercaptopurine, cyclosporine, and methotrexate. Am J Gastroenterol. 1996;91:423–33.

91. Lemann M, Zenjari T, Bouhnik Y, Cosnes J, Mesnard B, Rambaud JC. Methotrexate in Crohn's disease: long-term efficacy and toxicity. Am J Gastroenterol. 2000;95:1730–4.

92. Fukushima T, Sugita A, Masuzawa S, Yamazaki Y, Tsuchiya S. Effects of cyclosporine A on active Crohn's disease. Gastroenterol Jpn. 1989;24:12–5.

93. Lichtiger S. Cyclosporin therapy in inflammatory bowel disease: open-label experience. Mt Sinai J Med. 1990;57:315–9.

94. Markowitz J, Rosa J, Grancher K, Aiges H, Daum F. Long-term 6-mercaptopurine treatment in adolescents with Crohn's disease. Gastroenterology. 1990;99:1347–51.

95. Hanauer SB, Smith MB. Rapid closure of Crohn's disease fistulas with continuous intravenous cyclosporin A. Am J Gastroenterol. 1993;88:646–9.

96. Present DH, Lichtiger S. Efficacy of cyclosporine in treatment of fistula of Crohn's disease. Dig Dis Sci. 1994;39:374–80.

97. Abreu-Martin J, Vasilauskas E, Gaiennie J, Voigt B, Targan SR. Continuous infusion cyclosporine is effective for acute severe Crohn's disease...but for how long (abstr)? Gastroenterology. 1996;110:A851.

98. O'Neill J, Pathmakanthan S, Goh J, Costello S, MacMathuna P, O'Connell R, Crowe J, Lennon J. Cyclopsorine A induces remission in fistulous Crohn's disease but relapses occur upon cessation of treatment (abstr). Gastroenterology. 1997;112:A1056.

99. Hinterleitner TA, Petritsch W, Aichbichler B, Fickert P, Ranner G, Krejs GJ. Combination of cyclosporine, azathioprine and prednisone for perianal fistulas in Crohn's disease. Z Gastroenterol. 1997;35:603–8.

100. Egan LJ, Sandborn WJ, Tremaine WJ. Clinical outcome following treatment of refractory inflammatory and fistulizing Crohn's disease with intravenous cyclosporine. Am J Gastroenterol. 1998;93: 442–8.

101. Gurudu SR, Griffel LH, Gialanella RJ, Das KM. Cyclosporine therapy in inflammatory bowel disease: short- and long-term results. J Clin Gastroenterol. 1999;29:151–4.

102. Present DH. Crohn's fistula: current concepts in management. Gastroenterology. 2003;124:1629–35.

103. Sandborn WJ. A critical review of cyclosporine therapy in inflammatory bowel disease. Inflamm Bowel Dis. 1995;1:48–63.

104. Sandborn WJ. Preliminary report on the use of oral tacrolimus (FK506) in the treatment of complicated proximal small bowel and fistulizing Crohn's disease. Am J Gastroenterol. 1997; 92:876–9.

105. Fellerman K, Ludwig D, Stahl M, David-Walek T, Stange EF. Steroid-unresponsive acute attacks of inflammatory bowel disease: immunomodulation by tacrolimus (FK506). Am J Gastroenterol. 1998;93:1860–6.

106. Lowry PW, Weaver AL, Tremaine WJ, Sandborn WJ. Combination therapy with oral tacrolimus (FK506) and azathioprine or 6-mercaptopurine for treatment-refractory Crohn's disease perianal fistulae. Inflamm Bowel Dis. 1999;5:239–45.

107. Ierardi E, Principi M, Rendina M, Francavilla R, Ingrosso M, Pisani A, Amoruso A, Panella C, Francavilla A. Oral tacrolimus (FK506) in Crohn's disease complicated by fistulae of the perineum. J Clin Gastroenterol. 2000;125(30):200–2.

108. Sandborn WJ, Present DH, Isaacs KL, Wolf DC, Greenberg E, Hanauer SB, Feagan BG, Mayer L, Johnson T, Galanko J, Martin C, Sandler RS. Tacrolimus for the treatment of fistulas in patients with Crohn's disease: a randomized, placebo-controlled trial. Gastroenterology. 2003;125:380–8.

109. Gonzalez-Lama Y, Abreu L, Vera MI, Pastrana M, Tabernero S, Revilla J, Duran JG, Escartin P. Long-term oral tacrolimus therapy in refractory to infliximab fistulizing Crohn's disease: a pilot study. Inflamm Bowel Dis. 2005;11:8–15.
110. Cohen RD, Tsang JF, Hanauer SB. Infliximab in Crohn's disease: first anniversary clinical experience. Am J Gastroenterol. 2000;95:3469–77.
111. Farrell RJ, Shah SA, Lodhavia PJ, Alsahli M, Falchuk KR, Michetti P, Peppercorn MA. Clinical experience with infliximab therapy in 100 patients with Crohn's disease. Am J Gastroenterol. 2000;95:3490–7.
112. Ricart E, Panaccione R, Loftus EV, Tremaine WJ, Sandborn WJ. Infliximab for Crohn's disease in clinical practice at the Mayo Clinic: the first 100 patients. Am J Gastroenterol. 2001;96:722–9.
113. Present DH, Rutgeerts P, Targan S, Hanauer SB, Mayer L, van Hogezand RA, Podolsky DK, Sands BE, Braakman T, DeWoody KL, Schaible TF, van Deventer SJH. Infliximab for the treatment of fistulas in patients with Crohn's disease. N Engl J Med. 1999;340:1398–405.
114. Sands BE, Anderson FH, Bernstein CN, Chey WY, Feagan BG, Fedorak RN, Kamm MA, Korzenik JR, Lashner BA, Onken JE, Rachmilewitz D, Rutgeerts P, Wild G, Wolf DC, Marsters PA, Travers SB, Blank MA, van Deventer SJ. Infliximab maintenance therapy for fistulizing Crohn's disease. N Engl J Med. 2004;350:876–85.
115. Sands BE, Blank MA, Patel K, van Deventer SJ. Long-term treatment of rectovaginal fistulas in Crohn's disease: response to infliximab in the ACCENT II study. Clin Gastroenterol Hepatol. 2004;2:912–20.
116. Cadahia V, Garcia-Carbonero A, Vivas S, Fuentes D, Nino P, Rebollo P, Rodrigo L. Infliximab improves quality of life in the short-term in patients with fistulizing Crohn's disease in clinical practice. Rev Esp Enferm Dig. 2004;96:369–74.
117. Lichtenstein GR, Yan S, Bala M, Blank M, Sands BE. Infliximab maintenance treatment reduces hospitalization, surgeries, and procedures in fistulizing Crohn's disease. Gastroenterology. 2005;128:862–9.
118. Agnholt J, Dahlerup JF, Buntzen S, Tøttrup A, Lyhne Nielsen S, Lundorf E. Response, relapse and mucosal immune regulation after infliximab treatment in fistulating Crohn's disease. Aliment Pharmacol Ther. 2003;17:703–10.
119. Poritz LS, Rowe WA, Koltun WA. Remicade does not abolish the need for surgery in fistulizing Crohn's disease. Dis Colon Rectum. 2002;45:771–5.
120. West RL, van der Woude CJ, Hansen BE, Felt-Bersma RJF, van Tilburg AJP, Drapers JAG, Kuipers EJ. Clinical and endosonographic effect of ciprofloxacin on the treatment of perianal fistulae in Crohn's disease with infliximab: a double-blind placebo-controlled study. Aliment Pharmacol Ther. 2004;20:1329–36.
121. Ochsenkühn T, Göke B, Sackmann M. Combining infliximab with 6-mercaptopurine/azathioprine for fistula therapy in Crohn's disease. Am J Gastroenterol. 2002;97:2022–5.
122. Schröder O, Blumenstein I, Schulte-Buckholt A, Stein J. Combining infliximab and methotrexate in fistulizing Crohn's disease resistant or intolerant to azathioprine. Aliment Pharmacol Ther. 2004;19:295–301.
123. Talbot C, Sagar PM, Johnston MJ, Finan PJ, Burke D. Infliximab in the surgical management of complex fistulating anal Crohn's disease. Color Dis. 2005;7:164–8.
124. Hyder SA, Travis SL, Jewell DP, Mortensen NJM, George BD. Fistulating anal Crohn's disease: results of combined surgical and infliximab treatment. Dis Colon Rectum. 2006;49:1837–41.
125. Scaudione G, Di Stazio C, Limongelli P, Guadagni I, Pellino G, Riegler G, Coscione P, Selvaggi F. Treatment of complex perianal fistulas in Cohn disease: infliximab, surgery, or combined approach. Can J Surg. 2010;5:299–304.
126. Roumeguere P, Bouchard D, Pigot F, et al. Combined approach with infliximab, surgery, and methotrexate in severe fistulizing anoperineal Crohn's disease: results from a prospective study. Inflamm Bowel Dis. 2011;17:69–76.
127. Tozer P, Ng SC, Siddiqui MR, et al. Long-term MRI-guided combined anti-TNF-α and thiopurine therapy for Crohn's perianal fistulas. Inflamm Bowel Dis. 2012;18:1825–34.
128. Bouguen G, Siproudhis L, Gizard E, et al. Long-term outcome of perianal fistulizing Crohn's disease treated with infliximab. Clin Gastroenterol Hepatol. 2013;11:975–81.
129. Sandborn WJ, Hanauer SB. Antitumor necrosis factor therapy for inflammatory bowel disease: a review of agents, pharmacology, clinical results, and safety. Inflamm Bowel Dis. 1999;5:119–33.
130. Schaible TF. Long-term safety of infliximab. Can J Gastroenterol. 2000;14:29C–32C.
131. Remicade (infliximab) for IV injection. Package Insert, 2002.
132. Keane J, Gershon S, Wise RP, Mirabile-Levens E, Kasznica J, Schwieterman WD, Siegel JN, Braun MM. Tuberculosis associated with infliximab, a tumor necrosis factor alpha-neutralizing agent. N Engl J Med. 2001;345:1098–104.
133. Morelli J, Wilson FA. Does administration of infliximab increase susceptibility to listeriosis? Am J Gastroenterol. 2000;95:841–2.
134. Kamath BM, Mamula P, Baldassano RN, Markowitz JE. Listeria meningitis after treatment with infliximab. J Pediatr Gastroenterol Nutr. 2002;34:410–2.
135. Warris A, Bjorneklett A, Gaustad P. Invasive pulmonary aspergillosis associated with infliximab therapy. N Engl J Med. 2001;344:1099–100.
136. Nakelchik M, Mangino JE. Reactivation of histoplasmosis after treatment with infliximab. Am J Med. 2002;112:78.
137. Colombel JF, Sandborn WJ, Rutgeerts P, Enns R, Hanauer SB, Panaccione R, Schreiber S, Byczkowski D, Li J, Kent JD, Pollack PF. Adalimumab for maintenance of clinical response and remission in patients with Crohn's disease: the CHARM trial. Gastroenterology. 2007;132:52–65.
138. Colombel JF, Scwartz DA, Sandborn WJ, Kamm MA, D'Haens G, Rutgeerts P, Enns R, Panccione R, Schreiber S, Li J, Kent JD, Lomax KG, Pollack PF. Adalimumab for the treatment of fistulas in patients with Crohn's disease. Gut. 2009;940:8.
139. Panaccione R, Colombel JF, Sandborn WJ, et al. Adalimumab sustains clinical remission and overall clinical benefit after 2 years of therapy for Crohn's disease. Aliment Pharmacol Ther. 2010;31:1296–309.
140. Schreiber S, Khaliq-Kareemi M, Lawrance IC, Thomson OØ, Hanauer SB, McColm J, Bloomfield R, Sandborn WJ, PRECiSE 2 Study Investigators. Maintenance therapy with certolizumab pegol for Crohn's disease. N Engl J Med. 2007;357:239–50.
141. Schreiber S, Lawance IC, Thomson OØ, Hanauer SB, Bloomfield R, Sandborn WJ. Randomised clinical trial: certolizumab pegol for fistulas in Crohn's disease – subgroup results from a placebo-controlled trial. Aliment Pharmacol Ther. 2011;33:185–93.
142. Feagan BG, Sandborn WJ, Baker JP, Cominelli F, Sutherland LR, Elson CD, Salzberg B, Archambault A, Bernstein CN, Lichtenstein GR, Heath PK, Hanauer SB. A randomized, double-blind, placebo-controlled multicenter trial of the engineered human antibody to TNF (CDP571) for steroid sparing and maintenance of remission in patients with steroid-dependent Crohn's disease (abstr). Gastroenterology. 2000;118:A655.
143. Sandborn WJ, Feagan BG, Hanauer SB, Present DH, Sutherland LR, Kamm MA, Wolf DC, Baker JP, Hawkey C, Archambault A, Bernstein CN, Novak C, Heath PK, Targan SR. An engineered human antibody to TNF (CDP571) for active Crohn's disease: a randomized double-blind placebo-controlled trial. Gastroenterology. 2001;120:1330–8.
144. Ehrenpreis ED, Kane SV, Cohen LB, Cohen RD, Hanauer SB. Thalidomide therapy for patients with refractory Crohn's disease: an open-label trial. Gastroenterology. 1999;117:1271–7.

145. Vasilauskas EA, Kam LY, Abreu-Martin MT, Hassard PV, Papadakis KA, Yang H, Zeldis JB, Targan SR. An open-label pilot study of low-dose thalidomide in chronically active, steroid-dependent Crohn's disease. Gastroenterology. 1999;117:1278–87.

146. Erle DJ, Briskin MJ, Butcher EC, et al. Expression and function of the MAdCAM-1 receptor, integrin α4β7, on human leukocytes. J Immunol. 1994;153:517–28.

147. Sandborn WJ, Colombel JF, Enns R, et al. Natalizumab induction and maintenance therapy for Crohn's disease. N Engl J Med. 2005;353:1912–25.

148. Van Assche G, Van Ranst M, Sciot R, et al. Progressive multifocal leukoencephalopathy after natalizumab therapy for Crohn's disease. N Engl J Med. 2005;353:362–8.

149. Sandborn WJ, Feagan BG, Rutgeerts P, et al. Vedolizumab as induction and maintenance therapy for Crohn's disease. N Engl J Med. 2013;369:711–21.

150. Voitk AJ, Echave V, Brown RA, Gurd FN. Use of elemental during the adaptive stage of short gut syndrome. Gastroenterology. 1973;65:419–26.

151. Segal AW, Levi AJ, Loewi G. Levamisole in the treatment of Crohn's disease. Lancet. 1977;2:382–5.

152. Axelsson C, Jarnum S. Assessment of the therapeutic value of an elemental diet in chronic inflammatory bowel disease. Scand J Gastroenterol. 1977;12:89–95.

153. Russell RI, Hall MJ. Elemental diet therapy in the management of complicated Crohn's disease. Scott Med J. 1979;24:291–5.

154. Calam J, Crooks PE, Walker RJ. Elemental diets in the management of Crohn's perianal fistulae. J Parenter Enter Nutr. 1980;4:4–8.

155. Teahon K, Bjarnason I, Pearson M, Levi AJ. Ten years' experience with an elemental diet in the management of Crohn's disease. Gut. 1990;31:1133–7.

156. Jones VA. Comparison of total parenteral nutrition and elemental diet in induction of remission of Crohn's disease. Dig Dis Sci. 1987;32:100S–7S.

157. Fukuda Y, Kosaka T, Okui M, Hirakawa H, Shimoyama T. Efficacy of nutritional therapy for active Crohn's disease. J Gastroenterol. 1995;30:83–7.

158. Harford FJ, Fazio VW. Total parenteral nutrition as primary therapy for inflammatory bowel disease of the bowel. Dis Colon Rectum. 1978;21:555–7.

159. Milewski PJ, Irving MH. Parenteral nutrition in Crohn's disease. Dis Colon Rectum. 1980;23:395–400.

160. Greenberg GR, Fleming CR, Jeejeebhoy KN, Rosenberg IH, Sales D, Tremaine WJ. Controlled trial of bowel rest and nutritional support in the management of Crohn's disease. Gut. 1988;29:1309–15.

161. Fickert P, Hinterleitner TA, Wenzl HH, Aichbichler BW, Petritsch W. Mycopheylate mofetil in patients with Crohn's disease. Am J Gastroenterol. 1998;93:2529–32.

162. Vaughan D, Drumm B. Treatment of fistulas with granulocyte colony-stimulating factor in a patient with Crohn's disease. N Engl J Med. 1999;340:239–40.

163. Korzenik J, Dieckgraefe B. Immunostimulation in Crohn's disease: results of a pilot study of G-CSF (R-Methug-CSF) in mucosal and fistulizing Crohn's disease (abstr). Gastroenterology. 2000;118:A874.

164. Dieckgraefe BK, Korzenik JR. Treatment of active Crohn's disease with recombinant human granulocyte-macrophage colony-stimulating factor. Lancet. 2002;360:1478–80.

165. Brady III CE, Cooley BJ, Davis JC. Healing of severe perianal and cutaneous Crohn's disease with hyperbaric oxygen. Gastroenterology. 1989;97:756–60.

166. Nelson Jr EW, Bright DE, Villar LF. Closure of refractory perianal Crohn's lesion. Integration of hyperbaric oxygen into case management. Dig Dis Sci. 1990;35:1561–6.

167. Brady III CE. Hyperbaric oxygen and perianal Crohn's disease: a follow-up. Gastroenterology. 1993;105:1264.

168. Lavy A, Weisz G, Adir Y, Ramon Y, Melamed Y, Eidelman S. Hyperbaric oxygen for perianal Crohn's disease. J Clin Gastroenterol. 1994;19:202–5.

169. Colombel JF, Mathieu D, Bouault JM, Lesage X, Zavadil P, Quandalle P, Cortot A. Hyperbaric oxygen in severe perianal Crohn's disease. Dis Colon Rectum. 1995;38:609–14.

170. Oshitani N, Nakamura S, Matsumoto T, Kobayashi K, Kitano A. Treatment of Crohn's disease fistulas with coagulation factor XIII. Lancet. 1996;347:119–20.

Treatment of Acute Severe Ulcerative Colitis

37

Jess L. Kaplan and Harland S. Winter

Case

A 13-year-old boy was previously well until he acutely developed nonbloody diarrhea while on a skiing vacation. The following day he continued to have nausea, vomiting, and diarrhea, and started a clear liquid diet. On day 3 of this acute illness, he continued to pass 6–8 liquid stools daily and began to notice red blood in the stool. He was treated in the local emergency room with intravenous fluids and discharged. Stool cultures for enteric pathogens, including *Escherichia coli* 0157, ova, and parasites and *Clostridium difficile*, were all negative. His white blood cell count (WBC) was 15,900, hemoglobin 130 g/L, and hematocrit 37%. Liver function tests, amylase, and lipase were all normal. C-reactive protein (CRP) was elevated at 25 mg/dL.

On day 6 of the illness, he noted increased bloody diarrhea and was admitted to the local hospital. Despite being kept nil per os (NPO), he continued to pass 3–4 loose, grossly bloody stools daily. On the seventh day of the illness, he became febrile to 39 °C and continued to pass 5–6 bloody stools daily. His albumin was decreased at 2.2 g/dL. He was transferred to a tertiary care facility.

On transfer, his vital signs were stable and he was afebrile. His weight was 46 kg. He appeared pale but was resting comfortably. He had no oral ulcers. His chest and cardiac examinations were normal. His abdomen was soft with diffuse but mild tenderness without guarding or rebound tenderness. He had no organomegaly. Upon admission, an upper endoscopy was normal, but the ileocolonoscopy revealed

pancolitis (Fig. 37.1) with a normal-appearing terminal ileum, consistent with ulcerative colitis. His PUCAI score was 65. He was made NPO, given intravenous fluids at 1.5 times maintenance, and started on intravenous methylprednisolone sodium succinate 20 mg every 12 h. Repeat stool analysis was negative for enteric pathogens. Biopsies of the colon showed moderate-to-severe chronic pancolitis without evidence of granulomas, and biopsies of the terminal ileum were normal. Electrolytes were monitored daily and corrected as necessary; hematocrit was maintained over 30% with packed red blood cell transfusions; albumin was replaced with salt-poor albumin (1 g/kg) when below 3.0 g/dL. After 3 days of intravenous corticosteroids, his PUCAI was 55, and methylprednisolone was increased to 30 mg intravenously every 12 h. Because of ongoing diarrhea and bleeding, a peripherally inserted central catheter (PICC) was placed for nutritional support and total parenteral nutrition was started. His PUCAI score on day 5 of intravenous corticosteroids was 60. Options for rescue therapy were discussed with the patient and family, and the pediatric surgery team was consulted. On hospital day 6, he was given 5 mg/kg of infliximab intravenously. Over the next 2 days, stool output decreased; he was restarted on oral feedings and was discharged on day 10. He returned in 2 weeks for his second infliximab infusion, passing formed stools without visible blood, and a prednisone taper was started.

He continued to do well, and maintenance infliximab therapy was continued after induction therapy was complete. Approximately 7 months later, hematochezia and abdominal cramping returned 6 weeks following an infliximab dose. The infliximab trough concentration was 9 µg/mL, and the presence of anti-infliximab antibodies could not be determined. Stool cultures were negative for enteric pathogens, and *Clostridium difficile* testing was also negative. Oral prednisone was started, but symptoms did not improve. He was passing 10–12 grossly bloody liquid stools daily, with three nocturnal stools with peridefecatory cramping and fecal urgency. He was admitted to the hospital, made NPO, and started on intravenous methylprednisolone sodium suc-

J.L. Kaplan, MD (✉)
Harvard Medical School, Pediatric Gastroenterology, MassGeneral Hospital for Children, Boston, MA, USA
e-mail: jlkaplan@mgh.harvard.edu

H.S. Winter, MD (✉)
Harvard Medical School, Pediatric IBD Program, MassGeneral Hospital for Children, Boston, MA, USA
e-mail: hwinter@mgh.harvard.edu

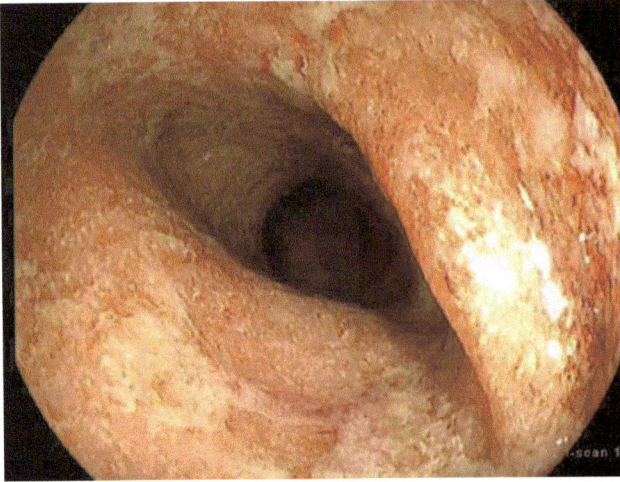

Fig. 37.1 Sigmoid colon: Diffuse inflammation with loss of vascular pattern and ulceration, typical of the pattern seen in ulcerative colitis

cinate 20 mg every 12 h. On day 3, his PUCAI score was 60. A sigmoidoscopy was performed that revealed severe proctitis. Rectal biopsy showed severely active chronic colitis without evidence of granulomas, and immunohistochemistry for cytomegalovirus (CMV) was negative. A 5 mg/kg dose of infliximab was given (6.5 weeks following the previous dose) without clinical improvement. He developed fever to 38.5 °C, and intravenous ampicillin, gentamicin, and metronidazole were given. Total parenteral nutrition was started on day 4. On day 6 of intravenous steroids, his stool output was >2 L, and he required a blood transfusion for symptomatic anemia. His C-reactive protein was 10 times the upper limit of normal. On day 9 of the hospitalization, he underwent a total abdominal colectomy and ileostomy. He was discharged 6 days later and subsequently returned for completion of the colectomy, creation of a J-pouch with ileostomy reversal, and ileal pouch anal anastomosis (IPAA).

Introduction

The clinical course of ulcerative colitis (UC) in children is unpredictable. Compared to patients with adult-onset disease, children with UC have more extensive disease and often a more severe course, manifest by higher rates of corticosteroid use and dependency and shorter time to surgery [1, 2].

Severe exacerbations of UC are common in both children and adults, and cause significant morbidity. These exacerbations can occur both at disease onset and as relapse in patients with established disease.

In 2008, the European Crohn's and Colitis Organization (ECCO) defined acute severe colitis (ASC) in adults as an exacerbation with more than six bloody stools per day with at least one of the following: tachycardia (>90 b/min), temperature >37.8 °C, anemia (hemoglobin <10.5 g/dL), or an erythrocyte sedimentation rate (ESR) >30 mm/h [3]. In children, ASC is generally defined by a Pediatric Ulcerative Colitis Activity Index (PUCAI) score ≥65 [4], a cutoff that has been validated in independent cohorts and has predictive value with regard to response to intravenous corticosteroid (IVCS) therapy [5, 6] (see Chap. 46, Appendix C-3 for more details regarding PUCAI scoring). In adults, fulminant colitis has been defined by >10 stools per day with continuous bleeding, abdominal tenderness and distension, systemic toxic symptoms such as fever and anorexia, and blood transfusion requirement; this can progress to toxic megacolon with severe colonic distension (>6 cm), hypotension, altered mental status, and high mortality [7]. While colonic dilation is a hallmark of current or impending toxic megacolon (TMC), precise criteria for TMC in children have not been established. One study showed that in children ≥10 years of age, a transverse colon diameter ≥5.6 cm was suggestive of TMC [8], while in children younger than 10 years of age, a diameter >4 cm is concerning for toxic megacolon [9].

The frequency of ASC in children with UC is not fully known, but it is suggested that rates are as or even higher than the rates in adults. For example, over a 3-year period, in the greater Toronto area, it was estimated that 28% of all children with UC developed a severe exacerbation requiring hospitalization for intravenous corticosteroids before the age of 15 [10]. The remainder of this chapter addresses the management and ASC in children.

Initial Management

ASC is a serious and potentially life-threatening exacerbation of pediatric UC. As such, care for patients with ASC should be in the hospital setting so that frequent monitoring of clinical status, disease progression, and potential complications can take place. The goals of management are medical stabilization, treating exacerbating factors such as certain infections, and implementing a stepwise active treatment approach typically beginning with intravenous corticosteroids (IVCS) in order to control gastrointestinal hemorrhage while avoiding/limiting complications from the disease and/ or therapy. Response to therapy should be frequently reassessed by a multidisciplinary team of providers, including, in many cases, surgeons with experience in IBD, in order to help guide plans for subsequent treatment.

The initial management of ASC includes a complete history and physical examination, beginning with assessment of vital signs and general appearance which may reveal signs of systemic toxicity such as hypotension, fever, significant tachycardia, or altered mental status. Abdominal tenderness should be assessed, keeping in mind that tenderness and even colonic perforation and peritoneal signs may be masked in patients on high-dose corticosteroids. The absence of bowel sounds is an ominous prognostic indicator. Frequent reassessment is necessary as progression to fulminant disease may be rapid. A PUCAI score should be calculated at the onset of symptoms and then daily during the exacerbation until improvement and disposition. A PUCAI score over 65 correlates with severe disease. This validated scoring system not only gives the provider an idea of the general well-being of the child, but also predicts response to IVCS and helps guide the timing of subsequent "rescue" therapy [6].

Hospitalized patients with ASC should have intravenous access and be fluid-resuscitated to assure adequate hydration. Laboratory studies including a complete blood count, serum electrolytes, albumin, ESR, and CRP should be obtained and repeated frequently. Despite the lack of randomized controlled clinical trials to provide evidence-based guidance for optimal therapy, expert opinion suggests that mucosal healing is best achieved by keeping the hematocrit over 30%, the albumin over 3 g/dL, and the electrolytes in the normal range. Although not evidence-based, in theory, avoiding anemia and hypoalbuminemia may enhance delivery of oxygen to the intestinal tissues and improve mucosal blood flow. Normal electrolytes decrease the likelihood of stasis related to poor motility. Measurement of fecal calprotectin or lactoferrin may be useful to establish a baseline so that repeated assessment can help define response to medical therapy.

Patients with IBD are at higher risk for being diagnosed with *Clostridium difficile* infection (CDI). In one single-center study, 18.4% of children with UC had a positive polymerase chain reaction (PCR) for the toxin B gene of *C. difficile* [11]. The percentages may be even higher in hospitalized children with IBD [12]. CDI is implicated in disease exacerbation and increases the risk for complications such as colectomy in adults with UC [13, 14]. Although there is not yet direct evidence that treating CDI in children with ASC improves outcomes, testing for and treatment of CDI is current standard practice and was recommended in the joint ECCO/European Society for Pediatric Gastroenterology, Hepatology, and Nutrition (ESPGHAN) ASC guidelines [9]. Stools should be screened for both toxins A and B. Stool should also be cultured for other potentially treatable bacterial pathogens.

Plain films of the abdomen are recommended as part of the initial evaluation of severe colitis if there are any signs of systemic toxicity that may suggest fulminant disease or TMC [9]. However, since examination findings can be masked by corticosteroid, our practice is to obtain a KUB on every hospitalized patient with ASC at baseline. As previously mentioned, transverse colon dilation $\geq$ 56 mm and $\geq$ 40 mm is suggestive of TMC in children $\geq$10 and <10 years of age, respectively. Colonic dilation has also been shown to predict response to IVCS therapy in this setting [15].

Although children with ASC may not wish to eat or drink due to their physical symptoms, unless surgery is imminent, they should be allowed to do so, since available evidence from the adult literature shows that while bowel rest may decrease stool frequency and volume, it does not improve outcomes and may worsen nutritional status [16]. If a regular diet cannot be tolerated by the third or fourth day, then enteral or parenteral nutrition should be considered, as a further malnourished state may prevent healing and clinical improvement. The risks of parenteral nutrition, including complications from central venous catheters (e.g., infection, thrombus) and electrolyte abnormalities, need to be balanced with potential benefit. There is no evidence to support any particular oral diet or diet restrictions in ASC.

Unlike in Crohn's disease, antibiotics are generally not indicated in ulcerative colitis, unless there is evidence for toxicity or infection. Since bowel perforations may be silent in patients on high doses of corticosteroids, any clinical sign of infection should be investigated and treated. In well-controlled trials in adults with ASC, intravenous (IV) antibiotics including ciprofloxacin [17] and metronidazole [18] have not been shown to improve ASC outcomes when used as adjunctive therapy to corticosteroids. No large or controlled pediatric studies directly address the efficacy of antibiotics in ASC; however, the recommendations are to treat with IV antibiotics if infection is suspected or while awaiting confirmatory testing [9]. ASC patients with fulminant disease or suspicion or diagnosis of TMC should be treated with IV antibiotics. The antibiotics agent(s) used should target enteric bacteria, including anaerobes.

Adults who are hospitalized with ASC are routinely treated with anticoagulants for venous thromboembolism (VTE) prophylaxis. Hospitalized children with IBD are also at increased risk for VTE [19]. The prothrombotic tendency in IBD is thought to be attributable to many different factors including an increase in procoagulants, decrease in anticoagulants, thrombocytosis, as well as endothelial and immunologic factors [20]. VTE is more common in children with active IBD than in those who have quiescent disease [21]. This risk may be augmented by relative immobility of sick, hospitalized IBD patients. In one study, risk factors for VTE in hospitalized children with IBD included older age, central venous catheters, parenteral nutrition, and the presence of a hypercoagulable condition [19]. Children with colonic IBD appear to be at higher risk for VTE [22]. Despite this, the overall incidence of VTE in hospitalized children remains low (11.8/1000 hospitalizations) [19], and there have been no pediatric studies assessing the benefits and risks of prophylactic anticoagulation in ASC or in IBD in general. As such, the routine use of anticoagulation in children with ASC is not currently recommended [9]. However, noninvasive methods of VTE prophylaxis like frequent mobilization, adequate hydration, and pneumatic/mechanical devices are advised, as they are of low risk, even if not well supported by current evidence. It is reasonable to consider anticoagulation in patients with other risk factors for VTE, including known hereditary causes of thrombophilia, smoking, and the use of oral contraceptives. When used, anticoagulation does not seem to worsen bleeding during IBD flares.

Intravenous corticosteroids (IVCS) are the recommended first-line treatment for ASC in children. IVCS have been used for acute exacerbations of UC for more than 60 years and have been shown to reduce mortality in adults [23]. There are no randomized trials evaluating the comparative efficacy of various CS doses in children. The current recommendations for CS dosing are for 1–1.5 mg/kg/day of methylprednisolone up to 40–60 mg/day [9]. The daily dose is often divided over two daily doses. Doses above 60 mg/day have not been found to be more effective in adults with ASC [24]. More recently, a prospective pediatric cohort study which followed 283 children with ASC for 1 year concluded that an IVCS dose of 2 mg/kg/day was not more effective than doses of 1–1.25 mg/kg/day in preventing the need for salvage therapy during the hospitalization or by 1 year, although day 5 PUCAI scores were improved in the high-dose CS group before sensitivity analysis [25]. In this study, IVCS dosing was at the discretion of the provider (not randomized), but propensity matching was performed to limit bias. Interestingly, glucocorticoid bioactivity in serum did not predict response to IVCS in a study of children with ASC [26].

Not all children with ASC improve with IVCS. A systematic review found a 34% (range 9–47%) IVCS failure rate in a pooled analysis of five studies of children with ASC [27]. In the one prospective study included in the analysis, 37 of 128 children (29%) failed to respond to IVCS and required second-line treatment [6]. Multiple predictors for poor response to IVCS in children have been identified. A multicenter prospective study that followed 128 children with ASC found response to IVCS less likely in older patients and in patients with established disease [6]. The same study showed that after multivariate analysis, additional day 3 and day 5 predictors of IVCS failure included high stool frequency and large amount of blood in the stool. A high CRP at day 5 also predicted CS failure. The PUCAI score outperformed other clinical indices in predicting IVCS failure at both days 3 and 5. A PUCAI score >45 on day 3 predicted CS failure with a sensitivity of 92% and negative predictive value (NPV) of 94%, indicating a high likelihood of response if the PUCAI score is ≤45. On day 5, a PUCAI score of >70 had a specificity and positive predictive value (PPV) of 100% for CS failure, while a score of >65 has specificity and PPV of 96% and 82%, respectively. The addition of fecal calprotectin or CRP to the model did not improve the accuracy of the PUCAI score. The findings from this study and others have formed the basis of recommendations for disease monitoring and for the timing

of second-line/rescue therapy in children with ASC. Additional predictors of poor response to IVCS have also been identified. A prior single-center study found that a high number of nocturnal stools and high CRP were predictive of CS failure at days 3 and 5 [10]. The presence of megacolon, defined as a transverse colon diameter >40 mm and >60 mm in children <12 and >12 years of age, respectively, and ulceration on abdominal X-ray may also predict IVCS failure [15]. A separate study showed that day 3 interleukin (IL)-6 levels predicted IVCS failure, although this did not hold true after multivariate analysis [28]. Finally, there is limited evidence that IVCS nonresponders have decreased fecal microbial richness/diversity compared to responders, though this is not yet clinically applicable [29].

Monitoring Response to Corticosteroids

In general, monitoring for response to initial therapy begins with careful and frequent reassessment of vital signs, stool frequency, volume, blood loss, and abdominal pain as well as of changes in the abdominal examination. The validation of the PUCAI score in predicting IVCS failure has led to a suggested algorithm and the following recommendations for disease monitoring and for the timing of second-line, also referred to as "rescue" or "salvage", therapy [9]. A PUCAI score >45 on day 3 of IVCS should initiate preparation for second-line therapy, including discussion of potential risks and benefits with patients and families and inclusion of a surgeon with experience in IBD. A PUCAI score >65 on day 5 should prompt initiation of second-line therapy. Patients with PUCAI scores between 35 and 65 on day 5 can continue IVCS for an additional 2–5 days, at which point further recommendations are based on PUCAI score at that time. Patients who improve on IVCS and have a PUCAI score <35 on day 5 are unlikely to require rescue therapy before discharge [9]. Thiopurines can be considered in IVCS responders, particularly in those who were previously naive, but therapeutic benefit is often delayed for 2–3 months; so, they have little role in the acute setting.

There is no current evidence to support the value of repeat colonoscopic evaluation in ASC patients who are improving on IVCS in the clinical setting. However, repeat sigmoidoscopy is suggested if the day 3 PUCAI score is >45 in order to search for evidence of Crohn's disease such as granulomas and to exclude cytomegalovirus (CMV) colitis, which can complicate ASC and may alter therapy. While the prevalence of CMV colitis in children with ASC is not known, it is relatively common in adults with UC, particularly in those with steroid refractory disease [30]. Mucosal biopsies should be obtained and evaluated for signs of CMV disease (deep ulcerations and viral inclusions) as well as immunohistochemistry [9]. CMV colitis should prompt an infectious disease consultation, and antiviral treatment should be considered [31].

Medical Rescue Therapy

Patients with ASC with poor response to IVCS require rescue therapy. About one-third of children with ASC require rescue therapy before discharge from the hospital. In adults, the earlier use of rescue therapy appears to decrease mortality [24], and extending IVCS without rescue treatment beyond 14 days is unlikely to provide benefit and may increase the risk for complications, including, but not limited to, opportunistic infections, metabolic and electrolyte abnormalities, osteopenia/porosis, and psychiatric disturbance. The goals of rescue therapy are to improve symptoms and allow for eventual discontinuation of CS. Current rescue therapy options for children with ASC include infliximab, calcineurin inhibitors (cyclosporine and tacrolimus), and colectomy. Although the data supporting these rescue therapies are primarily in CS refractory patients, these treatments are also used without IVCS in patients with contraindications or prior lack of response to CS.

Infliximab (IFX) is a monoclonal antibody against TNF-α that can induce and maintain remission in pediatric UC [32]. Pooled data from six pediatric case series ($n = 126$) of ASC patients treated with IFX showed a 75% (67–83%, 95% CI) response rate by the time of hospital discharge and a 64% colectomy-free rate during follow-up which ranged from a few months to a few years [27]. In one prospective study, 76% (25/33) of children with ASC refractory to IVCS had short-term response to IFX [6]. The remaining 24% underwent colectomy. At 1 year, 55% had sustained response to IFX and 45% had CS-free sustained response, while an additional 28% required colectomy by 1 year. In a more recent retrospective study from a single center in Italy, 80% of ASC patients had short-term response to IFX, but 50% of these patients went on to colectomy by 24 months [33]. Predictors of IFX failure may include shorter disease duration and more active disease at the time of admission and day 3 of IVCS [6]. IFX is typically dosed at 5 mg/kg at baseline and then repeated at 2 and 6 weeks following the initial dose. The pharmacokinetics of IFX in children with moderate-to-severe UC appears to be similar to that in adults [34]. However, many pediatric centers use higher doses (10 mg/kg) and/or shorter dosing intervals of IFX in ASC. While there is currently a lack of direct evidence to support this practice, some have suggested that IFX clearance may be higher in patients with acute severe disease leading to a requirement for higher dosing [35]. A recent retrospective study of children with IBD (CD and UC) showed that patients with a larger colonic inflammatory burden were more likely to require IFX dose escalation by 12 months than patients with limited or moderate disease and that 43% of patients who started at 5 mg/kg dosing did not improve with dose escalation [36]. Although this study was not limited to ASC patients, it does provide some indirect evidence that children with more extensive disease may benefit from higher IFX doses at the start of treatment. ECCO/ESPGHAN guidelines recommend IFX as the preferred rescue therapy in patients with previous thiopurine failure as IFX can also be effective as a maintenance agent in UC [9]. Prior to starting IFX, tuberculosis and Hepatitis B status should be documented.

Cyclosporine (CsA) is a calcineurin inhibitor that has been shown to be effective at inducing remission in adults with ASC [37, 38]. Support for the use of CsA in children with ASC comes from eight retrospective case series ($n = 94$) [27]. Pooled short-term response rates were 81% (76–86%, 95% CI), but long-term colectomy-free rates dropped to 39% (29–49%, 95% CI) in patients treated with CsA. There is heterogeneity in the eight studies with regard to CsA dose, route of administration, and duration of follow-up, which makes interpretation difficult. CsA is generally used for 3–6 months as a bridge to a maintenance therapy, often thiopurine treatment, which can take 2–3 months to become effective. CsA has not been studied as a long-term maintenance agent in UC. More prolonged use of CsA is limited by serious potential side effects such as hypertension, electrolyte disturbance, and renal and neurologic toxicity. Dosing is generally started intravenously, and then transitioned to oral dosing (4–8 mg/kg/day) once response is achieved [9]. Trough levels should be monitored frequently with preferred levels starting in the range of 150–300 ng/mL. Clinical response is generally seen in 5–7 days. Adult guidelines suggest that *Pneumocystis jiroveci* prophylaxis should be routinely given to patients treated with CsA, who are also treated with other immunosuppressive agents [39].

Tacrolimus, another calcineurin inhibitor, also appears effective as short-term rescue therapy for children with CS-resistant ASC. Retrospective studies report short-term response rates between 50% and 89% with long-term colectomy-free rates ranging from 0% to 40% [40–42]. The largest of these studies reported a 40% colectomy-free rate at 26 months, with most patients having been bridged to either thiopurines or IFX [40]. Hypertension (52%), tremor (46%), and hyperglycemia (35%) were common side effects of tacrolimus treatment. Initial dosing is typically 0.1 mg/kg/dose twice daily (0.2 mg/kg/day), and the dose adjusted to reach levels of 10–15 ng/mL during induction and 5–10 ng/mL during maintenance therapy [40]. Tacrolimus may have more reliable oral absorption and may be better tolerated than CsA. Otherwise, time to response and side effects are similar to those of CsA, as is the need for *P. jiroveci* prophylaxis when used with other immunosuppressive agents.

There are no pediatric studies that directly compare the efficacy of medical rescue options in ASC. A prospective, multicenter, randomized open-label trial in adults with ASC refractory to IVCS found no difference in the efficacy of CsA and IFX [43]. A recent meta-analysis confirmed that these two treatments were equally successful in randomized trials but concluded that IFX appeared slightly more effective than CsA in nonrandomized trials [44]. Adverse events, postoperative complications, and mortality were similar with both treatments. Two small retrospective studies have compared tacrolimus and IFX rescue in adults with ACS [45, 46]. Neither study showed a difference in short-term efficacy, but the larger of the two studies showed that IFX was more effective than a tacrolimus bridge to thiopurine strategy in the longer term [46].

There is limited evidence from retrospective adult studies that a second medical rescue therapy (IFX following calcineurin inhibitor or vice versa) can prevent colectomy in ~30–70% of ASC patients following failure of a first rescue agent [47–49]. However, due to the high risk for serious toxicity with this approach, the use of a second rescue agent is not currently recommended for children with ASC until additional data on efficacy and safety can be obtained [9].

Surgery

The indications for surgical treatment in ASC are perforation, toxic megacolon, massive hemorrhage, or failure to respond to maximal medical management. However, in rare circumstances in which there are contraindications to medical rescue therapy, surgery may be considered first. The details of surgical options for UC are detailed in Chap. 42. The current surgical standard of care for UC is a restorative proctocolectomy consisting of a total colectomy, rectal mucosectomy with ileal pouch anal anastomosis (IPAA). This procedure can be done in one, two, or three steps. The first step in a three-step procedure includes a subtotal colectomy with ileostomy and Hartmann's pouch creation. This is followed by completion of the colectomy, rectal mucosectomy, and restorative IPAA with diverting ileostomy (step 2), and finally by ileostomy takedown reversal (step 3). In a typical two-step procedure, bowel continuity is immediately restored when the ileal pouch is formed (step 2), without a diverting ileostomy. Alternatively, the abdominal colectomy and mucosectomy may be performed with IPAA and diverting ileostomy in step 1 followed by ileostomy takedown (step 2). At some centers, abdominal colectomy and mucosectomy with IPAA may be done as a single operation [50]. The decision on which operation(s) to select is highly dependent on the experience and expertise of the surgical team.

High-dose corticosteroids have been shown to increase short-term complications such as postoperative infection [51]. Additionally, adult studies show a lower risk of IPAA leak in patients with a temporary protective ileostomy [52]. For these reasons, it is recommended that a three-step procedure be

considered in more complicated patients including those requiring emergent surgery, for those treated with high-dose corticosteroids, or those with significant malnutrition [9]. In a retrospective pediatric study, preoperative exposure to calcineurin inhibitors or thiopurines within 30 days of surgery or to IFX within 90 days of surgery was not associated with an increase of postoperative complications [53]. Whenever possible, efforts should be made to maximize nutritional status before surgery. Postoperative risks as well as typical outcomes should be discussed with patients and families to help form realistic goals. Additional issues that need to be discussed include the risk for pouchitis and potential issues with future fertility in female patients [54]. Patients also need to be aware that the risk for an eventual diagnosis of Crohn's disease following restorative proctocolectomy for UC is 5–10% [55]. In addition to medical and surgical management, stress management and support for the patient and family are essential components to the multidisciplinary approach needed to optimally care for children with ASC.

Future Directions/Conclusions

Recommendations for the management of ASC in children are somewhat limited by the lack of data from pediatric studies. Important questions remain unanswered, and the rarity of ASC in children makes prospective interventional trials challenging to complete. Large, multicenter collaborative studies may be best positioned to answer some of these questions. Specific gaps in knowledge include longer-term outcomes of children with ASC, the most effective dosing regimens for rescue medications like IFX and calcineurin inhibitors, and the role of CMV in pediatric ASC. There needs to be improved understanding of predictors of response to first-line rescue therapy which can help personalize care going forward. The role for established UC treatments like adalimumab and vedolizumab in ASC need to be elucidated. Additionally, newer therapies, such as combination antibiotics, that have showed some promise in small, open-label trials [56], should be evaluated in larger, controlled studies. Acute severe colitis is a serious complication in children with UC. Despite recent improvements in medical treatment, many patients continue to require surgical intervention before discharge, and still more within the following 12 months.

References

1. Van Limbergen J, Russell RK, Drummond HE, Aldhous MC, Round NK, Nimmo ER, et al. Definition of phenotypic characteristics of childhood-onset inflammatory bowel disease. Gastroenterology. 2008;135(4):1114–22.
2. Jakobsen C, Bartek Jr J, Wewer V, Vind I, Munkholm P, Groen R, et al. Differences in phenotype and disease course in adult and

paediatric inflammatory bowel disease – a population-based study. Aliment Pharmacol Ther. 2011;34(10):1217–24.

3. Travis SP, Stange EF, Lémann M, Oresland T, Bemelman WA, Chowers Y, et al.; European Crohn's and Colitis Organisation (ECCO). European evidence-based Consensus on the management of ulcerative colitis: current management. J Crohns Colitis. 2008;2(1):24–62.

4. Turner D, Otley AR, Mack D, Hyams J, de Bruijne J, Uusoue K, et al. Development, validation, and evaluation of a pediatric ulcerative colitis activity index: a prospective multicenter study. Gastroenterology. 2007;133(2):423–32.

5. Turner D, Hyams J, Markowitz J, Lerer T, Mack DR, Evans J, et al.; Pediatric IBD Collaborative Research Group. Appraisal of the pediatric ulcerative colitis activity index (PUCAI). Inflamm Bowel Dis. 2009;15(8):1218–23.

6. Turner D, Mack D, Leleiko N, Walters TD, Uusoue K, Leach ST, et al. Severe pediatric ulcerative colitis: a prospective multicenter study of outcomes and predictors of response. Gastroenterology. 2010;138(7):2282–91.

7. Travis SP, Farrant JM, Ricketts C, Nolan DJ, Mortensen NM, et al. Predicting outcome in severe ulcerative colitis. Gut. 1996;38(6): 905–10.

8. Benchimol EI, Turner D, Mann EH, Thomas KE, Gomes T, McLernon RA, et al. Toxic megacolon in children with inflammatory bowel disease: clinical and radiographic characteristics. Am J Gastroenterol. 2008;103(6):1524–31.

9. Turner D, Travis SP, Griffiths AM, Ruemmele FM, Levine A, Benchimol EI, et al.; European Crohn's and Colitis Organization; Porto IBD Working Group, European Society of Pediatric Gastroenterology, Hepatology, and Nutrition. Consensus for managing acute severe ulcerative colitis in children: a systematic review and joint statement from ECCO, ESPGHAN, and the Porto IBD Working Group of ESPGHAN. Am J Gastroenterol. 2011; 106(4):574–88.

10. Turner D, Walsh CM, Benchimol EI, Mann EH, Thomas KE, Chow C, et al. Severe paediatric ulcerative colitis: incidence, outcomes and optimal timing for second-line therapy. Gut. 2008;57(3):331–8.

11. Lamousé-Smith ES, Weber S, Rossi RF, Neinstedt LJ, Mosammaparast N, Sandora TJ, et al. Polymerase chain reaction test for Clostridium difficile toxin B gene reveals similar prevalence rates in children with and without inflammatory bowel disease. J Pediatr Gastroenterol Nutr. 2013;57(3):293–7.

12. Pascarella F, Martinelli M, Miele E, Del Pezzo M, Roscetto E, Staiano A. Impact of Clostridium difficile infection on pediatric inflammatory bowel disease. J Pediatr. 2009;154(6):854–8.

13. Ananthakrishnan AN, McGinley EL, Binion DG. Excess hospitalisation burden associated with Clostridium difficile in patients with inflammatory bowel disease. Gut. 2008;57(2):205–10.

14. Negrón ME, Rezaie A, Barkema HW, Rioux K, De Buck J, Checkley S, et al. Ulcerative colitis patients with clostridium difficile are at increased risk of death, colectomy, and postoperative complications: a population-based inception cohort study. Am J Gastroenterol. 2016;111(5):691–704.

15. Livshits A, Fisher D, Hadas I, Bdolah-Abram T, Mack D, Hyams J, et al. Abdominal X-ray in pediatric acute severe colitis and radiographic predictors of response to intravenous steroids. J Pediatr Gastroenterol Nutr. 2016;62(2):259–63.

16. McIntyre PB, Powell-Tuck J, Wood SR, Lennard-Jones JE, Lerebours E, Hecketsweiler P, et al. Controlled trial of bowel rest in the treatment of severe acute colitis. Gut. 1986;27(5):481–5.

17. Mantzaris GJ, Petraki K, Archavlis E, Amberiadis P, Kourtessas D, Christidou A, et al. A prospective randomized controlled trial of intravenous ciprofloxacin as an adjunct to corticosteroids in acute, severe ulcerative colitis. Scand J Gastroenterol. 2001;36(9):971–4.

18. Chapman RW, Selby WS, Jewell DP. Controlled trial of intravenous metronidazole as an adjunct to corticosteroids in severe ulcerative colitis. Gut. 1986;27(10):1210–2.

19. Nylund CM, Goudie A, Garza JM, Crouch G, Denson LA. Venous thrombotic events in hospitalized children and adolescents with inflammatory bowel disease. J Pediatr Gastroenterol Nutr. 2013;56(5):485–91.

20. Zitomersky NL, Verhave M, Trenor 3rd CC. Thrombosis and inflammatory bowel disease: a call for improved awareness and prevention. Inflamm Bowel Dis. 2011;17(1):458–70.

21. Lazzerini M, Bramuzzo M, Maschio M, Martelossi S, Ventura A. Thromboembolism in pediatric inflammatory bowel disease: systematic review. Inflamm Bowel Dis. 2011;17(10):2174–83.

22. Zitomersky NL, Levine AE, Atkinson BJ, Harney KM, Verhave M, Bousvaros A, et al. Risk factors, morbidity, and treatment of thrombosis in children and young adults with active inflammatory bowel disease. J Pediatr Gastroenterol Nutr. 2013;57(3):343–7.

23. Truelove SC, Witts LJ. Cortisone in ulcerative colitis; final report on a therapeutic trial. Br Med J. 1955;2(4947):1041–8.

24. Turner D, Walsh CM, Steinhart AH, Griffiths AM. Response to corticosteroids in severe ulcerative colitis: a systematic review of the literature and a meta-regression. Clin Gastroenterol Hepatol. 2007;5(1):103–10.

25. Choshen S, Finnamore H, Auth MK, Bdolah-Abram T, Shteyer E, Mack D, et al. Corticosteroid dosing in pediatric acute severe ulcerative colitis: a propensity score analysis. J Pediatr Gastroenterol Nutr. 2016;63:58–64.

26. Turner D, Kolho KL, Mack DR, Raivio T, Leleiko N, Crandall W, et al. Glucocorticoid bioactivity does not predict response to steroid therapy in severe pediatric ulcerative colitis. Inflamm Bowel Dis. 2010;16(3):469–73.

27. Turner D, Griffiths AM. Acute severe ulcerative colitis in children: a systematic review. Inflamm Bowel Dis. 2011;17(1):440–9.

28. Wine E, Mack DR, Hyams J, Otley AR, Markowitz J, Crandall WV, et al. Interleukin-6 is associated with steroid resistance and reflects disease activity in severe pediatric ulcerative colitis. J Crohns Colitis. 2013;7(11):916–22.

29. Michail S, Durbin M, Turner D, Griffiths AM, Mack DR, Hyams J, et al. Alterations in the gut microbiome of children with severe ulcerative colitis. Inflamm Bowel Dis. 2012; 18(10):1799–808.

30. Ayre K, Warren BF, Jeffery K, Travis SP. The role of CMV in steroid-resistant ulcerative colitis: a systematic review. J Crohns Colitis. 2009;3(3):141–8.

31. Rahier JF, Magro F, Abreu C, Armuzzi A, Ben-Horin S, Chowers Y, et al.; European Crohn's and Colitis Organisation (ECCO). Second European evidence-based consensus on the prevention, diagnosis and management of opportunistic infections in inflammatory bowel disease. J Crohns Colitis. 2014;8(6):443–68.

32. Hyams J, Damaraju L, Blank M, Johanns J, Guzzo C, Winter HS, et al.; T72 Study Group. Induction and maintenance therapy with infliximab for children with moderate to severe ulcerative colitis. Clin Gastroenterol Hepatol. 2012;10(4):391–9.

33. Aloi M, D'Arcangelo G, Capponi M, Nuti F, Vassallo F, Civitelli F, et al. Managing paediatric acute severe ulcerative colitis according to the 2011 ECCO-ESPGHAN guidelines: efficacy of infliximab as a rescue therapy. Dig Liver Dis. 2015;47(6):455–9.

34. Adedokun OJ, Xu Z, Padgett L, Blank M, Johanns J, Griffiths A, et al. Pharmacokinetics of infliximab in children with moderate-to-severe ulcerative colitis: results from a randomized, multicenter, open-label, phase 3 study. Inflamm Bowel Dis. 2013;19(13): 2753–62.

35. Rosen MJ, Minar P, Vinks AA. Review article: applying pharmacokinetics to optimise dosing of anti-TNF biologics in acute severe ulcerative colitis. Aliment Pharmacol Ther. 2015;41(11):1094–103.

36. Shapiro JM, Subedi S, Machan JT, Cerezo CS, Ross AM, Shalon LB, et al. Durability of infliximab is associated with disease extent in children with inflammatory bowel disease. J Pediatr Gastroenterol Nutr. 2016;62(6):867–72.

37. Lichtiger S, Present DH, Kornbluth A, Gelernt I, Bauer J, Galler G, et al. Cyclosporine in severe ulcerative colitis refractory to steroid therapy. N Engl J Med. 1994;330(26):1841–5.

38. Shibolet O, Regushevskaya E, Brezis M, Soares-Weiser K. Cyclosporine A for induction of remission in severe ulcerative colitis. Cochrane Database Syst Rev. 2005;1:CD004277.

39. Okafor PN, Nunes DP, Farraye FA. Pneumocystis jiroveci pneumonia in inflammatory bowel disease: when should prophylaxis be considered? Inflamm Bowel Dis. 2013;19(8):1764–71.

40. Watson S, Pensabene L, Mitchell P, Bousvaros A. Outcomes and adverse events in children and young adults undergoing tacrolimus therapy for steroid-refractory colitis. Inflamm Bowel Dis. 2011; 17(1):22–9.

41. Ziring DA, Wu SS, Mow WS, Martín MG, Mehra M, Ament ME. Oral tacrolimus for steroid-dependent and steroid-resistant ulcerative colitis in children. J Pediatr Gastroenterol Nutr. 2007;45(3):306–11.

42. Navas-López VM, Blasco Alonso J, Serrano Nieto MJ, Girón Fernández-Crehuet F, Argos Rodriguez MD, Sierra SC. Oral tacrolimus for pediatric steroid-resistant ulcerative colitis. J Crohns Colitis. 2014;8(1):64–9.

43. Laharie D, Bourreille A, Branche J, Allez M, Bouhnik Y, Filippi J, et al.; Groupe d'Etudes Thérapeutiques des Affections Inflammatoires Digestives. Ciclosporin versus infliximab in patients with severe ulcerative colitis refractory to intravenous steroids: a parallel, open-label randomised controlled trial. Lancet. 2012;380(9857):1909–15.

44. Narula N, Marshall JK, Colombel JF, Leontiadis GI, Williams JG, Muqtadir Z, et al. Systematic review and meta-analysis: infliximab or cyclosporine as rescue therapy in patients with severe ulcerative colitis refractory to steroids. Am J Gastroenterol. 2016;111(4):477–91.

45. Minami N, Yoshino T, Matsuura M, Koshikawa Y, Yamada S, Toyonaga T, et al. Tacrolimus or infliximab for severe ulcerative colitis: short-term and long-term data from a retrospective observational study. BMJ Open Gastroenterol. 2015;2(1):e000021.

46. Endo K, Onodera M, Shiga H, Kuroha M, Kimura T, Hiramoto K, et al. A comparison of short- and long-term therapeutic outcomes of infliximab- versus tacrolimus-based strategies for steroid-refractory ulcerative colitis. Gastroenterol Res Pract. 2016;2016:3162595.

47. Maser EA, Deconda D, Lichtiger S, Ullman T, Present DH, Kornbluth A. Cyclosporine and infliximab as rescue therapy for each other in patients with steroid-refractory ulcerative colitis. Clin Gastroenterol Hepatol. 2008;6(10):1112–6.

48. Leblanc S, Allez M, Seksik P, Flourié B, Peeters H, Dupas JL, et al.; GETAID. Successive treatment with cyclosporine and infliximab in steroid-refractory ulcerative colitis. Am J Gastroenterol. 2011; 106(4):771–7.

49. Narula N, Fine M, Colombel JF, Marshall JK, Reinisch W. Systematic review: sequential rescue therapy in severe ulcerative colitis: do the benefits outweigh the risks? Inflamm Bowel Dis. 2015;21(7):1683–94.

50. Ryan DP, Doody DP. Restorative proctocolectomy with and without protective ileostomy in a pediatric population. J Pediatr Surg. 2011;46(1):200–3.

51. Ferrante M, D'Hoore A, Vermeire S, Declerck S, Noman M, Van Assche G, et al. Corticosteroids but not infliximab increase short-term postoperative infectious complications in patients with ulcerative colitis. Inflamm Bowel Dis. 2009;15(7):1062–70.

52. Weston-Petrides GK, Lovegrove RE, Tilney HS, Heriot AG, Nicholls RJ, Mortensen NJ, et al. Comparison of outcomes after restorative proctocolectomy with or without defunctioning ileostomy. Arch Surg. 2008;143(4):406–12.

53. Schaufler C, Lerer T, Campbell B, Weiss R, Cohen J, Sayej W, et al. Preoperative immunosuppression is not associated with increased postoperative complications following colectomy in children with colitis. J Pediatr Gastroenterol Nutr. 2012; 55(4):421–4.

54. Rajaratnam SG, Eglinton TW, Hider P, Fearnhead NS. Impact of ileal pouch-anal anastomosis on female fertility: meta-analysis and systematic review. Int J Color Dis. 2011;26(11):1365–74.

55. Melmed GY, Fleshner PR, Bardakcioglu O, Ippoliti A, Vasiliauskas EA, Papadakis KA, et al. Family history and serology predict Crohn's disease after ileal pouch-anal anastomosis for ulcerative colitis. Dis Colon Rectum. 2008;51(1):100–8.

56. Turner D, Levine A, Kolho KL, Shaoul R, Ledder O. Combination of oral antibiotics may be effective in severe pediatric ulcerative colitis: a preliminary report. J Crohns Colitis. 2014;8(11): 1464–70.

Dietary Therapies for Inflammatory Bowel Disease

38

Ronen Stein and Robert N. Baldassano

Abbreviations

CD	Crohn's disease
CDED	Crohn's disease exclusion diet
DHA	Docosahexaenoic acid
EEN	Exclusive enteral nutrition
FODMAP	Fermentable oligosaccharides, disaccharides, monosaccharides, and polyols
IBD	Inflammatory bowel disease
IBD-AID	Inflammatory bowel disease anti-inflammatory diet
n-3	Omega-3
n-6	Omega-6
PEN	Partial enteral nutrition
PUFA	Polyunsaturated fatty acids
SCD	Specific carbohydrate diet
UC	Ulcerative colitis

Introduction

The inflammatory bowel diseases (IBD), Crohn's disease (CD) and ulcerative colitis (UC), are chronic, relapsing, and remitting inflammatory conditions of the gastrointestinal tract. They are complex disorders with genetics, environmental influences, and the immune system all involved in disease development and progression [1]. To date, over 200 genetic polymorphisms have been associated with the development of IBD [2]. However, data from twin studies have demonstrated that genetics alone cannot entirely explain the etiology of IBD as the concordance rates for CD and UC among monozygotic twins are only 45% and 15%, respectively [3]. This indicates that environmental factors play a large role in the development of IBD. The current understanding of the etiology of IBD is that in a genetically susceptible host, environmental factors may trigger dysregulation of the innate and adaptive immune response and lead to chronic inflammation in the gastrointestinal tract [4].

The two largest environmental exposures for the gastrointestinal tract are the microbiota and dietary intake, although cigarette smoking, antibiotics, nonsteroidal anti-inflammatory drugs, and infectious agents are among the other environmental exposures associated with IBD [5]. As mentioned in Chap. 4, there is strong evidence from multiple studies that the gut microbiota is involved in the pathogenesis of IBD, as many of the genetic polymorphisms associated with IBD regulate the body's interactions with microbes [6]. As we will describe later in the chapter, there have been multiple studies showing that dietary intake itself plays an important role in the composition and function of the gut microbiota. Therefore, diet is likely involved in the pathogenesis of IBD and may be a potential therapeutic target.

In this chapter we will summarize epidemiological data supporting the role of diet in IBD, show that the composition of the gut microbiota is heavily influenced by diet, and describe the relationship between macronutrients, food additives, oral supplements, and IBD. We will also review the literature on a number of structured diets proposed to treat IBD.

R. Stein, MD (✉) • R.N. Baldassano, MD (✉)
Department of Pediatrics, The Children's Hospital of Philadelphia, Philadelphia, PA, USA

Perelman School of Medicine at the University of Pennsylvania, Philadelphia, PA, USA

Division of Gastroenterology, Hepatology, and Nutrition, The Children's Hospital of Philadelphia, 3401 Civic Center Blvd, Philadelphia, PA 19104, USA
e-mail: Baldassano@email.chop.edu

© Springer International Publishing AG 2017
P. Mamula et al. (eds.), *Pediatric Inflammatory Bowel Disease*, DOI 10.1007/978-3-319-49215-5_38

Diet and Worldwide Trends in IBD

The incidence and prevalence of IBD varies by region, with the highest rates in developed nations, particularly in North America and Northern Europe. The overall global incidence of IBD is rapidly increasing worldwide, not only in westernized societies, but also in developing countries with historically low rates [7, 8]. The influences of globalization and industrialization in countries such as China, India, Japan, and South Korea have resulted in increased urbanization, improved sanitation, increased antibiotic use, sedentary lifestyles, and refrigeration [9, 10]. However, this has also resulted in adaptation of a westernized diet, which has been shown to be associated with development of CD in a newly industrialized population [11].

Population migration studies also suggest that westernization may be a risk factor for the development of IBD. Children who immigrate to western countries from developing nations have a higher risk of IBD than their counterparts from their country of origin but a lower risk than children in their new country [12, 13]. The younger the child is at the time of immigration, the higher the risk of IBD [12]. However, second-generation immigrants have an even higher risk of developing IBD and in fact assume the same incidence of IBD as their peers in their new country [12, 9]. This may indicate that environmental exposures, such as a westernized diet, particularly early in life, impact the development of IBD.

Diet and the Gut Microbiota

Multiple studies have shown that the composition of the gut microbiota differs between healthy controls and individuals with IBD [14–17]. There is decreased microbial diversity in IBD with an increased proportion of bacteria in the phyla *Actinobacteria* and *Proteobacteria*, including *Escherichia coli*, and a decrease in *Firmicutes*, specifically in the group *Clostridia* [18, 19]. This dysbiosis, or alteration in the balance between commensal and pathogenic microorganisms, has been hypothesized to be involved in the pathogenesis of IBD. *Clostridia*, including *Faecalibacterium prausnitzii*, produce butyrate, a short-chain fatty acid that is an important energy source associated with colonic epithelial health. Conversely, adherent invasive *E. coli*, which are able to cross across ileal epithelium and can be found within granulomas in CD patients, may be linked to development of IBD [20].

Dietary patterns can alter the composition of the gut microbiota starting at infancy. The composition of the gut microbiota differs between breastfed and formula-fed infants. The intestinal tract of formula-fed infants is colonized with increased numbers of *E. coli*, whereas in breast-fed infants, *Bifidobacterium* species predominate and account for approximately 75% of microorganisms in the intestinal tract [21]. The human milk oligosaccharides contained in breast milk are felt to selectively promote growth of *Bifidobacterium* species [22], which may have anti-inflammatory properties [23]. A decrease in *Bifidobacterium* species has been found among CD patients [15]. The effect of breastfeeding on *Bifidobacterium* species may help explain why breastfeeding has been shown to have a protective effect against development of pediatric CD [24].

Long-term dietary patterns also affect the microbiome. Individuals on a westernized diet, high in animal fat and low in fiber, have high levels of *Bacteroides* species, whereas in those on a high-carbohydrate, low-fat diet, *Prevotella* species predominate [25]. Likewise, another study compared the microbiome of healthy children from a village in rural Africa on a low-fat, high-fiber diet to counterparts in Europe on a westernized diet. The African children had a high proportion of *Prevotella* species compared to the European children [26].

Mounting evidence shows that the composition of the gut microbiota is heavily influenced by diet. However, in addition to changing the makeup of the microbiome, animal models have shown that dietary intake can also affect its function [27]. A diet high in milk fat was found to induce colitis in IL-10 knockout mice by facilitating the growth of *Bilophila wadsworthia*. Sulfur is an important nutrient necessary for *B. wadsworthia* to thrive. Milk fat was found to stimulate secretion of sulfur-containing taurine-conjugated bile acids thereby creating an environment that preferentially promoted the growth of *B. wadsworthia*. Increased populations of *B. wadsworthia* were associated with greater inflammatory cytokine burden and development of colitis in IL-10 knockout mice. *B. wadsworthia* may also have exerted its effect by production of hydrogen sulfide leading to disruption of the intestinal epithelial barrier [28]. This indicates that by affecting the composition and function of the microbiome, dietary intake can stimulate immune responses in genetically susceptible hosts, leading to the development of chronic inflammation [29].

Dietary Components and IBD

The typical westernized diet contains high amounts of saturated fats, refined sugars, red meat, and processed foods with limited fresh fruits, vegetables, and fiber [30]. Many studies have investigated the dietary risk factors associated with new-onset IBD and have identified many components of a westernized diet as being risk factors [31]. In particular, a diet high in animal fats, omega-6 (n-6) fatty acids, and refined sugars has been associated with an increased risk of IBD. Conversely, high vegetable intake has been associated

Table 38.1 Dietary components and IBD

Dietary component	Dietary sources	Association with IBD
Saturated fat	Animal fat, milk fat	Increased risk of CD with high intake of saturated fat [32] Milk fat induces colitis in IL-10 knockout mice [28]
Omega-3-polyunsaturated fatty acid (n-3 PUFA)	Fish, flaxseed	Decreased risk of CD and UC with high intake of n-3 PUFA [33] Decreased risk of CD and UC with high docosahexaenoic acid intake [34, 35] Supplementation with n-3 PUFA not shown to have benefit as maintenance therapy in UC or CD ([36, 37])
Omega-6-polyunsaturated fatty acid (n-6 PUFA)	Avocado, egg, nuts, poultry, red meat, vegetable oils	Increased risk of CD and UC with high intake of n-6 PUFA [32] High ratio of n-6 PUFA to n-3 PUFA associated with increased risk of CD [33]
Simple carbohydrates	Candy, refined sugars, sweetened drinks	Increased risk of CD and UC with high intake of simple carbohydrates [32]
Complex carbohydrates/fiber	Fruits, legumes, vegetables, whole grains	High fiber, fruit, and vegetable intake associated with decreased CD risk [33] and high vegetable intake associated with lower UC risk [32]
Maltodextrin	Artificial sweeteners, breakfast cereals (selected), candy, infant formulas, processed snack foods	Maltodextrin promotes adhesion of adherent invasive *E. coli* based on in vitro studies [38]
Emulsifiers (e.g., carboxymethylcellulose, polysorbate-80)	Bread, coffee creamers, dressings, ice cream, margarine, mayonnaise, processed cheeses, sauces	Positive correlation between emulsifier intake and CD incidence [39] Emulsifiers induce mild colitis in wild-type mice and severe colitis in IL-10 knockout mice [40]
Curcumin	Turmeric, oral supplementation	Supplementation with pure curcumin was superior to placebo for induction of remission [41] and maintenance of remission [42] in UC
Iron	Heme iron (fish, red meat, poultry), non-heme iron (fortified cereals, fruits, vegetables), oral supplementation	Increased risk of CD and UC with high meat intake [32] Increased risk of UC flares with red meat consumption [43] Oral iron supplementation worsens colitis by generating oxidative stress in animal models [44]

with a decreased UC risk, and a diet high in fruits and fiber has been associated with a decreased CD risk [32]. Below, we review the literature on the relationship between different dietary components and IBD based on in vitro studies, animal models, and epidemiological data (summarized in Table 38.1).

Fat

High total fat intake, a component of the westernized diet, is associated with the development of IBD [32]. Even among healthy subjects, a high-fat diet has been shown to increase markers of systemic inflammation [45]. A study of dietary intake among the Japanese population annually from 1966 to 1985 found that total fat intake was strongly correlated with development of CD [11].

Although increased total fat intake is associated with IBD, the specific type of fat consumed may be a more important risk factor. Fatty acids are comprised of saturated fats, polyunsaturated fatty acids (PUFA), and monounsaturated fats [31]. Products with animal and milk fat contain a high proportion of saturated fat [28]. Multiple studies have found high intake of saturated fat to be a risk factor for development of IBD [32]. Likewise, in animal models, milk fat has

been shown to induce colitis in susceptible hosts [28]. Moreover, among subjects with known UC, studies have found increased red meat consumption to be a risk factor for disease flares [43].

Increased intake of PUFA has also been linked to IBD [32]. PUFA are comprised of n-6 and omega-3 (n-3), and it is the relative ratio of these fatty acids that is important [33]. The westernized diet contains a high ratio of n-6 to n-3 PUFA, which has been shown to be a risk factor for IBD [30]. In animal and in vitro models, n-3 PUFA has been found to have anti-inflammatory properties, including inhibition of macrophage TNFα production, while n-6 PUFA is broken down into byproducts that are pro-inflammatory [46, 47]. Foods higher in n-3 PUFA include fish and flaxseed [48]. Vegetable oils, poultry, and red meats are high in n-6 PUFA [30]. Among the n-3 PUFAs, docosahexaenoic acid (DHA) may have the strongest anti-inflammatory effects, as several studies have found an inverse association between DHA intake and risk of developing UC and CD, although no association was found with eicosapentaenoic acid, another n-3 PUFA [34, 35]. Despite these promising epidemiological results, systematic reviews of n-3 PUFA supplementation have not shown any benefit as maintenance therapy for patients already diagnosed with UC and CD [36, 37].

Carbohydrates

Carbohydrates are comprised of monosaccharides, disaccharides, oligosaccharides, and polysaccharides. Monosaccharides (e.g., glucose and fructose) and disaccharides (e.g., lactose and sucrose) are also called simple carbohydrates, whereas oligosaccharides and polysaccharides are complex carbohydrates [31]. Processed simple sugars are known as refined sugars. There is no association between total carbohydrate intake and risk of developing IBD. However, studies have found increased consumption of simple carbohydrates to be associated with a higher risk of both CD and UC [32].

Dietary fibers are nondigestible oligosaccharides and polysaccharides and are comprised of insoluble and soluble fiber. Insoluble fibers pass through the gastrointestinal tract mostly undigested, adding bulk and reducing transit time for stool. Cellulose is an important insoluble fiber found in fruits, vegetables, flaxseed, and quinoa. Soluble fibers, such as inulin and pectin, are found in grains and nuts. They are digested via fermentation by the gut microbiota producing short-chain fatty acids, such as acetate, butyrate, and propionate [48]. Not only is butyrate a critical energy source for colonocytes, but it is also felt to help maintain gastrointestinal homeostasis [31, 48]. In vitro studies have shown that fiber can enhance epithelial barrier function [49]. Additionally, multiple epidemiological studies have associated increased fiber intake with a decreased risk of developing CD and UC [32, 33].

A low-residue, low-fiber diet has been the historical dietary recommendation for patients with active IBD including those without stricturing disease [48]. However, there has been no proven benefit to this dietary therapy in non-stricturing disease. A study comparing a low-residue diet to an unlimited diet among CD patients with a non-stricturing disease phenotype showed no difference in symptoms, hospitalizations, or complications, including need for surgery [50]. Additionally, a semi-vegetarian diet, high in fiber, has been shown to improve clinical outcomes in a small cohort of adult CD patients [51].

Food Additives

Maltodextrin is a polysaccharide food additive commonly found in infant formula, breakfast cereals, candy, artificial sweeteners, and processed snack foods [52]. In animal studies, maltodextrin has been found to interfere with the integrity of the gastrointestinal epithelial barrier [53]. Adherent invasive E. coli exposed to maltodextrin have enhanced biofilm formation and improved adhesion to intestinal epithelial cells. Additionally, in vitro, maltodextrin promotes adhesion of adherent invasive E. coli [38]. There is no literature on the effects of maltodextrin in patients with IBD.

Emulsifiers are common food additives that have both hydrophilic and lipophilic properties, which allow for the mixture of otherwise immiscible substances. Common emulsifiers include carboxymethylcellulose, carrageenan, and polysorbate-80 [31, 40]. Emulsifiers are found in processed foods, including store-bought bread, processed cheeses, ice cream, dressings, margarine, mayonnaise, sauces, and coffee creamers [54–59]. In vitro studies have shown that carrageenan decreases gastrointestinal epithelial integrity [60]. Increased intake of emulsifiers has been positively correlated with CD incidence [39]. Recently, consumption of carboxymethylcellulose and polysorbate-80 in wild-type and IL-10 knockout mice was studied over 12 weeks [40]. Emulsifier consumption resulted in low-grade chronic colitis in wild-type mice and severe colitis in IL-10 knockout mice. Intestinal permeability increased as a result of emulsifier intake with bacterial-epithelial distance inversely correlated with severity of inflammation. This suggests that emulsifier exposure is associated with translocation of bacteria, confirming the findings of a previous in vitro study [49]. The importance of host-microbiota interactions were further supported by the observation that colitis did not occur in germ-free mice exposed to emulsifiers. However, when the microbiota from emulsifier-exposed mice was transferred to emulsifier-naïve mice, inflammation resulted [40]. Human intervention studies investigating emulsifier consumption and IBD are needed to better understand the association between emulsifiers and IBD.

Oral Supplements

Curcumin

Curcumin is the major pigment found in turmeric and has historically been used in traditional Chinese medicine to treat a variety of inflammatory conditions [41]. In vitro studies have shown curcumin to have antioxidant and anti-inflammatory properties, while in mice, curcumin has been found to improve colitis via downregulation of TNFα and nuclear transcription factor kappa B [61]. A pilot study of five patients with ulcerative proctitis and five patients with CD who received an oral pure curcumin preparation for 2–3 months found improvement in inflammatory markers and disease activity scores [62]. A multicenter, double-blind placebo trial of 82 subjects with quiescent UC on mesalamine or sulfasalazine therapy showed that curcumin was superior to placebo for maintenance of remission [42]. Recently, another multicenter, double-blind, clinical trial of 50 patients with active mild-to-moderate UC found that the addition of a 95% pure curcumin preparation to mesalamine therapy was superior to combination therapy with placebo in inducing clinical and endoscopic remission [41]. After 1 month of therapy, 14/26 (53.8%) subjects receiving curcumin were in clinical remission compared to none in the placebo group. Likewise, 8/22 (36.3%) subjects who underwent endoscopic evaluation were found to be in endoscopic remission compared to 0/16 subjects receiving placebo. Despite these promising results, the quantity of curcumin used in these studies was much higher than the amount that can be consumed exclusively through diet. Larger clinical trials are needed to confirm these findings in UC and to investigate whether curcumin has a therapeutic role in CD.

Iron

Iron deficiency anemia is a common complication of IBD, and oral iron supplementation is often used for treatment [63]. Iron is a catalyst for reactions that generate reactive oxygen species. In animal models of IBD, oral iron supplementation has been shown to worsen colitis by generating oxidative stress [44]. It is unclear if oral iron can generate oxidative stress and worsen disease activity in IBD patients, as there is conflicting evidence in the literature. A small study of ten CD patients receiving 1 week of ferrous fumarate supplementation showed a rise in oxidative stress and disease activity scores [64]. However, another study of 33 IBD patients supplemented with ferrous sulfate for 4 weeks did not show an increase in reactive oxygen species. Clinical disease activity scores worsened for the UC subjects, but there was no difference in rectosigmoid endoscopic activity or laboratory parameters [65]. As the adverse effects of oral iron supplementation include gastrointestinal symptoms such as abdominal pain, it is unclear if the increases in clinical disease activity scores truly reflect inflammatory activity.

In terms of dietary sources of iron, heme iron, which is found in red meat, has been found to worsen colitis in animal models [66]. Studies have also found increased red meat consumption to be a risk factor for disease flares in UC [43]. There are no published studies on the effects of non-heme iron sources, such as those found in fruits, vegetables, or iron-fortified cereals, on disease activity in IBD.

Structured Diets

A number of structured diets have been proposed for the treatment of IBD (Tables 38.2 and 38.3). These diets are based on exclusion of dietary components felt to be pro-inflammatory. However, with the exception of enteral nutrition therapy, there is currently a lack of robust data to support the efficacy of any structured diet in IBD. This partially reflects the challenges of performing prospective trials of dietary therapies. Because patients in diet trials are often on concurrent medical therapies, the efficacy of the dietary intervention is more difficult to interpret. Accurately assessing dietary intake and adherence is another challenge of diet studies. Moreover, as opposed to scientifically rigorous pharmaceutical trials, clinical trials involving dietary interventions cannot be double-blinded or have a placebo arm [9]. Whereas many study drugs are only available by enrolling in

Table 38.2 Supporting evidence for proposed IBD structured diets

Diet	Description	Supporting evidence
Exclusive enteral nutrition (EEN)	Polymeric, semi-elemental, or elemental formula taken as the sole source of nutrition	Multiple prospective studies support the use of EEN for induction of remission, mucosal healing, and growth impairment in pediatric CD
Partial enteral nutrition (PEN)	Same as EEN except formula is the nonexclusive source of nutrition	Retrospective and prospective studies support the use of PEN for induction of remission and maintenance therapy in pediatric CD
Specific carbohydrate diet	Consumption of monosaccharides is allowed, but disaccharides, oligosaccharides, and polysaccharides are eliminated	Limited evidence. Small retrospective study demonstrated improved clinical disease activity scores. Small prospective study showed improvement in mucosal healing
IBD anti-inflammatory diet	Multiple-phase diet derived from the SCD. Certain carbohydrates and fats are restricted and intake of pre- and probiotics is encouraged	Limited evidence. Small retrospective case series of adult IBD subjects demonstrated improvement in disease activity scores
Crohn's disease exclusion diet	Structured diet that reduces or eliminates exposure to animal fats, dairy products, gluten, and processed foods	Limited evidence. Retrospective study demonstrated improvement in disease activity and mucosal healing in adult and pediatric CD
Semi-vegetarian diet	Diet containing fruits, vegetables, dairy, and eggs with limited fish and meat	Limited evidence. Prospective study showed improvement in symptom-based remission compared to free diet
Low-FODMAP diet	Diet low in fermentable oligosaccharides, disaccharides, monosaccharides, and polyols	No published data on the effect of the diet on disease activity in IBD
Gluten-free diet	Gluten (found in rice, barley, and wheat) is completely excluded	No published data on the effect of the diet on disease activity in IBD
Paleolithic diet	Exclusion diet allowing foods presumed to be available in prehistoric times, including most fruits, vegetables, and game meat	No published scientific literature

Table 38.3 Allowed and restricted foods in proposed IBD structured diets

Structured diet	Allowed foods	Restricted foods
Specific carbohydrate diet[1, 2]	Fresh or frozen meat, poultry, fish, eggs Most fruits (fresh or dried), vegetables (fresh or frozen), and certain legumes Certain cheeses (cheddar, Colby, Swiss, farmers); fully fermented yogurt Oats, flax; nut and legume flours Honey Unsweetened fruit juices	Processed or smoked meats/fish Canned fruits and vegetables, potatoes, chickpeas, soybeans Most forms of dairy Wheat, barley, rye, corn, rice Refined sugars Maple syrup, mayonnaise
IBD anti-inflammatory diet[3]	Lean meat, poultry, fish, omega-3 eggs Most fruits, vegetables, and legumes Certain cheeses (aged, cheddar, farmers), fresh-cultured yogurt, kefir Oats, flax, nuts; legume and nut flours Honey, maple syrup, mayonnaise Unsweetened fruit juices	Non-lean cuts of meat Fruits with seeds and vegetables with stems (depending on diet phase) Most forms of dairy Wheat, barley, rye, corn, rice Hydrogenated oils Refined sugars
Crohn's disease exclusion diet[4]	Fresh fish and chicken breast; eggs; limited fresh beef Select fruits and vegetables White rice; rice noodles Honey; sugar for cooking Freshly squeezed orange juice	Processed or smoked meats/fish Canned fruits and vegetables, soy Dairy products Wheat, cereals, breads, baked goods Refined sugars Packaged snacks
Low-FODMAP diet[5]	Meat, poultry, fish, eggs Low-FODMAP fruits (e.g., banana, orange, strawberry) and vegetables (carrot, celery, potato) Lactose-free dairy, hard cheeses Rice, quinoa, corn, peanut Maple syrup	High-FODMAP fruits (e.g., apple, pear, watermelon), vegetables (e.g., asparagus, cauliflower, garlic, onion), and legumes (e.g., beans, chickpeas, lentils) Most forms of dairy Wheat, barley, rye High-fructose corn syrup, honey

[1]Cohen et al. [67]
[2]Obih et al. (2015)
[3]Oldenzki et al. (2014)
[4]Sigall-Boneh et al. [68]
[5]Gibson and Shepherd [69]

a clinical trial, structured diets are often well known and can be followed outside the confines of a clinical trial, rendering recruitment difficult.

Exclusive Enteral Nutrition

Exclusive enteral nutrition (EEN) has been extensively studied in pediatric IBD and has been shown to be an effective treatment modality for induction of remission [70–72]. Formula is the sole source of nutrition in EEN, and the duration of treatment can range from 3 to 12 weeks. The formula can be taken orally or through a nasogastric tube with equal efficacy; with nasogastric tube feedings, the formula can be administered while asleep [73]. Additionally, there is no difference in efficacy between polymeric, semi-elemental, or elemental formulas. Polymeric formulas may be more palatable and increase compliance with oral EEN [71, 73]. Although early studies had indicated that response to EEN was strongest among CD patients with small bowel disease, more recent studies have not shown any difference in efficacy based on disease location in CD [74].

Meta-analyses have shown that 73% of pediatric CD patients treated with EEN achieve clinical remission [71]. In

children with CD, EEN is as effective as corticosteroids for induction therapy [75]. Additionally, EEN has been found to be significantly better than corticosteroids at achieving mucosal healing [76]. Whereas corticosteroids are known to impair growth, EEN has been shown to improve growth among children with IBD [77]. Based on these data, the latest pediatric CD treatment guidelines by the European Society of Pediatric Gastroenterology, Hepatology and Nutrition recommend EEN as first-line therapy for the induction of remission in children with active luminal CD [71].

Partial Enteral Nutrition

Although EEN is an effective therapy for induction of remission in pediatric IBD, it may be too restrictive for many children, as it requires avoidance of all foods. Even among children who do elect to use EEN for induction, it may not be a feasible long-term treatment modality for maintenance therapy. Partial enteral nutrition (PEN) refers to the nonexclusive use of formula for the treatment of IBD with typically at least 50% of calories from formula. Studies have shown that PEN may also be effective for induction of remission among children with CD [78, 79]. The use of a diet providing 80–90% of caloric needs from formula, with the remainder of calories coming from a free diet, was found to induce remission in 65% of children with CD [78].

In pediatric CD, PEN has also been shown to be an effective maintenance therapy. Children who received PEN that provided 50–60% of caloric needs for 4–5 nights per week were less likely to relapse compared to those on a free diet over a 1-year follow-up period after induction of remission [80]. PEN is also effective as maintenance therapy in adult CD. Patients with CD who received 50% of calories through formula and the remainder of calories via table foods were more likely than those on a free diet to be in clinical and endoscopic remission after 1–2 years [81, 82]. Among adult CD patients, PEN has been found to be as effective as 6-mercaptopurine in maintaining long-term remission [83].

Head-to-head comparisons of PEN and EEN have found EEN to be a more efficacious treatment for pediatric CD [79, 84]. A recent study compared children with active CD receiving either infliximab, EEN, or PEN (80% of caloric feeds from formula) and found that infliximab and EEN were superior to PEN in terms of mucosal healing [79]. The PEN and EEN groups were similar in the amount of calories received from formula. However, the amount of table food consumed was significantly higher among the PEN group. This suggests that the mechanism of action of EEN may result from the elimination of table food rather than from any intrinsic therapeutic properties from the formula.

Specific Carbohydrate Diet

The specific carbohydrate diet (SCD) was developed in the 1920s as a treatment for celiac disease and proposed as a treatment for IBD in the 1990s. The diet allows for consumption of monosaccharides, but not disaccharides, oligosaccharides, or polysaccharides, which are felt to be poorly absorbed and felt to influence the composition of the microbiota [30]. Fruits, fresh meat and fish, eggs, fully fermented yogurt, and most vegetables are allowed, although potatoes, corn, and some legumes are not. Grains, including wheat, barley, and rice, as well as most forms of dairy are excluded. Processed foods and refined sugars are also eliminated. Nut flours can be used as substitutes to make baked goods. Because the diet is restrictive and weight loss is common, close follow-up with a dietician is likely warranted [85].

There have been several small studies investigating the use of the SCD in pediatric IBD. A retrospective study of 20 CD and 6 UC subjects on the SCD demonstrated improved clinical disease activity scores and serum inflammatory markers on the diet but noted that weight loss occurred in nine subjects (35%) [85]. A prospective study of ten pediatric subjects with active CD starting the SCD showed improvement in disease activity scores after 12 weeks of therapy. Video capsule endoscopy demonstrated mucosal healing in 4/10 (40%) subjects. Seven subjects were followed to 52 weeks with mucosal healing seen in 2/7 (29%) subjects [67]. Larger cohort prospective studies, with a control group, are needed to further study the efficacy of the SCD in pediatric IBD.

IBD Anti-inflammatory Diet

The IBD anti-inflammatory diet (IBD-AID) is a structured diet derived from the SCD [86]. There are four phases to the diet based on disease activity. The diet restricts certain carbohydrates, including lactose and refined sugars. Most grains, with the exception of oats, are also eliminated. The diet encourages consumption of foods that are prebiotics and probiotics, including fermented foods and those high in soluble fiber. Allowed foods are high in n-3 PUFA and low in saturated fats. In conjunction with a dietician, food intolerances and nutritional deficiencies are identified. Food textures are modified based on clinical disease activity.

There has only been a single retrospective case series reporting experience with the IBD-AID among 27 adult participants with IBD [86]. Self-reported symptoms improved in 24/27 (89%) of subjects. More extensive chart reviews, including disease activity scores, were reported for only 11 subjects (8 CD and 3 UC) among whom all reported improved symptoms and were able to de-escalate medication therapies. All 11 subjects were in clinical remission as defined by the Harvey Bradshaw Index and the Modified Truelove and Witts Severity Index for the CD and UC subjects, respectively. Large, randomized, clinical trials with assessment of disease activity and mucosal healing are needed to define the therapeutic role of the IBD-AID.

Crohn's Disease Exclusion Diet

The Crohn's disease exclusion diet (CDED) is a structured diet that reduces or eliminates exposure to animal fats, dairy products, gluten, many packaged products, canned goods, and products containing emulsifiers. There has been one published study with a small cohort of 47 children and young adults with active CD who followed this diet [68]. Most subjects also received PEN and consumed 50% of calories from formula. Subjects were allowed to be on concomitant immunomodulator therapy, as the primary endpoint was at 6 weeks, prior to the expected full onset of action of such medications. At 6 weeks, clinical remission was achieved in 70% of patients with significant improvements in inflammatory markers and serum albumin. Among the seven subjects who consumed all calories from table food and did not receive

PEN, six were in clinical remission at 6 weeks, suggesting that the exclusion diet without PEN may also be efficacious. Fifteen subjects in clinical remission practicing the diet for at least 6 months were assessed for mucosal healing, with 73% found to have evidence of healing based on endoscopy or the combination of imaging and fecal calprotectin. Despite these encouraging results, randomized studies with a larger cohort are needed to evaluate the efficacy of the CDED for both induction and maintenance therapy in pediatric CD.

Semi-Vegetarian Diet

There has been one published study on the use of a semi-vegetarian diet for maintenance of remission among 22 adults with CD [51]. This cohort was instructed to consume a diet containing brown rice, vegetables, fruits, yogurt, eggs, and milk. Fish was limited to once a week and meat to once every 2 weeks. During the study period, subjects were treated with either mesalamine or sulfasalazine. The cohort was followed for 2 years with 16 subjects remaining on the diet and six subjects consuming an omnivorous diet. Of the subjects on the semi-vegetarian diet, 15/16 (94%) were in remission compared to 2/6 (33%) subjects on free diet. This study is limited by the small sample size and the definition of remission as based on clinical symptoms rather than biochemical or endoscopic parameters. Additionally, all patients were offered this diet, with the treatment group including those who were compliant while the control group was comprised of those who were noncompliant. A study with a larger cohort using established clinical endpoints is needed to assess the efficacy of this dietary intervention.

Low-FODMAP Diet

A diet low in fermentable oligosaccharides, disaccharides, monosaccharides, and polyols (FODMAP) has been shown to reduce clinical symptoms in irritable bowel syndrome [87], but the data are limited in IBD. FODMAPs contain food products that are poorly absorbed by the human body, which leads to an influx of luminal water via osmosis. Additionally, FODMAPs are easily fermentable by the gastrointestinal microbiota into hydrogen byproducts. Together, luminal water and hydrogen production lead to luminal distention and clinical discomfort in patients with functional gastrointestinal disorders [69]. Functional abdominal pain is common in childhood with 13% of pediatric CD patients in remission meeting criteria [88]. Therefore, it is possible that a low-FODMAP diet may have some benefit among IBD patients with overlap functional gastrointestinal disorders. Moreover, since the prevalence of lactose malabsorption is high among patients with small bowel CD [48], a diet low in

lactose, such as the low-FODMAP diet, may improve clinical symptoms.

Two small studies have investigated the use of a low-FODMAP diet in IBD. A cohort of eight UC patients who had undergone colectomy and started on a low-FODMAP diet was retrospectively found to have decreased stool frequency on the diet. However, a prospective arm of five subjects did not show a dietary effect [89]. A retrospective study of 52 CD and 20 UC patients started on a low-FOMAP diet demonstrated improvement in overall gastrointestinal symptoms in 56% and 55% of CD and UC patients, respectively. Patient-reported improvements in abdominal pain, diarrhea, and bloating were most common [90]. However, the study had no control group, and disease activity was not objectively measured. Therefore, it is unclear if the improved symptoms were related to a placebo effect, an underlying functional gastrointestinal disorder, or improvement in IBD clinical activity. As such, there is currently no data to support the use of a low-FODMAP diet for induction of remission or maintenance therapy in IBD.

Gluten-Free Diet

Adherence to a gluten-free diet is common among IBD patients with a recent cross-sectional questionnaire study finding that approximately 19% of patients had previously followed the diet. Approximately two-thirds of patients on a gluten-free diet reported improvement in gastrointestinal symptoms [91]. Self-reported non-celiac gluten sensitivity has been shown to be common in IBD and possibly associated with active disease activity in CD [92]. Gliadin has been shown to increase intestinal permeability even among individuals without celiac disease [93], suggesting that gluten restriction could be a logical dietary target in IBD. Currently, there is no evidence to support the use of a gluten-free diet for induction of remission or maintenance therapy in IBD. Prospective studies are needed to study the effect of a gluten-free diet on clinical disease activity and mucosal healing in IBD.

The Paleolithic Diet

The theory behind the Paleolithic diet is that the increased prevalence of diseases like IBD is due to a change in the human diet from foods obtained by hunting and gathering to agricultural-based foods. Therefore, the diet excludes farm-based foods, such as grains, legumes, and meats from domesticated animals, and allows fruits, most vegetables, and game meat [30, 48]. Although the Paleolithic diet has been promoted in the lay literature, there have been no published studies regarding its use in IBD.

Conclusion

The westernized diet, consisting of high amounts of animal fat, refined sugars, and processed foods with limited amounts of fresh fruits, vegetables, and fiber, has been associated with the rise in worldwide IBD. Patients and families with IBD commonly seek dietary guidance from their medical providers. Unfortunately, there is currently no strong evidence to support the use of any structured diet, with the exception of enteral nutrition, for the treatment of pediatric IBD. Until a structured diet is developed that is proven to induce and/or maintain remission in IBD, clinicians can use data from epidemiological, microbiome, and animal-model studies to provide general dietary guidelines to their patients. Pending additional data, a recommendation of a well-balanced diet high in fresh fruits, fresh vegetables, and whole grains with limited processed foods, red meat, and saturated fat may be warranted for pediatric IBD patients.

References

1. Loddo I, Romano C. Inflammatory bowel disease: genetics, epigenetics, and pathogenesis. Front Immunol. 2015;6:551.
2. Bianco AM, Girardelli M, Tommasini A. Genetics of inflammatory bowel disease from multifactorial to monogenic forms. World J Gastroenterol. 2015;21(43):12296–310.
3. Halme L, Paavola-Sakki P, Turunen U, Lappalainen M, Farkkila M, Kontula K. Family and twin studies in inflammatory bowel disease. World J Gastroenterol. 2006;12(23):3668–72.
4. Rosen MJ, Dhawan A, Saeed SA. Inflammatory bowel disease in children and adolescents. JAMA Pediatr. 2015;169(11):1053–60.
5. Dutta AK, Chacko A. Influence of environmental factors on the onset and course of inflammatory bowel disease. World J Gastroenterol. 2016;22(3):1088–100.
6. Kostic AD, Xavier RJ, Gevers D. The microbiome in inflammatory bowel disease: current status and the future ahead. Gastroenterology. 2014;146(6):1489–99.
7. Benchimol EI, Fortinsky KJ, Gozdyra P, Van den Heuvel M, Van Limbergen J, Griffiths AM. Epidemiology of pediatric inflammatory bowel disease: a systematic review of international trends. Inflamm Bowel Dis. 2011;17(1):423–39.
8. Cosnes J, Gower-Rousseau C, Seksik P, Cortot A. Epidemiology and natural history of inflammatory bowel diseases. Gastroenterology. 2011;140(6):1785–94.
9. Lee D, Albenberg L, Compher C, Baldassano R, Piccoli D, Lewis JD, et al. Diet in the pathogenesis and treatment of inflammatory bowel diseases. Gastroenterology. 2015a;148(6):1087–106.
10. Prideaux L, Kamm MA, De Cruz PP, Chan FK, Ng SC. Inflammatory bowel disease in Asia: a systematic review. J Gastroenterol Hepatol. 2012;27(8):1266–80.
11. Shoda R, Matsueda K, Yamato S, Umeda N. Epidemiologic analysis of Crohn disease in Japan: increased dietary intake of n-6 polyunsaturated fatty acids and animal protein relates to the increased incidence of Crohn disease in Japan. Am J Clin Nutr. 1996;63(5):741–5.
12. Benchimol EI, Mack DR, Guttmann A, Nguyen GC, To T, Mojaverian N, et al. Inflammatory bowel disease in immigrants to Canada and their children: a population-based cohort study. Am J Gastroenterol. 2015;110(4):553–63.
13. Li X, Sundquist J, Hemminki K, Sundquist K. Risk of inflammatory bowel disease in first- and second-generation immigrants in Sweden: a nationwide follow-up study. Inflamm Bowel Dis. 2011;17(8):1784–91.
14. Fujimoto T, Imaeda H, Takahashi K, Kasumi E, Bamba S, Fujiyama Y, et al. Decreased abundance of Faecalibacterium prausnitzii in the gut microbiota of Crohn's disease. J Gastroenterol Hepatol. 2013;28(4):613–9.
15. Joossens M, Huys G, Cnockaert M, De Preter V, Verbeke K, Rutgeerts P, et al. Dysbiosis of the faecal microbiota in patients with Crohn's disease and their unaffected relatives. Gut. 2011;60(5):631–7.
16. Machiels K, Joossens M, Sabino J, De Preter V, Arijs I, Eeckhaut V, et al. A decrease of the butyrate-producing species Roseburia hominis and Faecalibacterium prausnitzii defines dysbiosis in patients with ulcerative colitis. Gut. 2014;63(8):1275–83.
17. Sartor RB. Microbial influences in inflammatory bowel diseases. Gastroenterology. 2008;134(2):577–94.
18. Kaakoush NO, Day AS, Huinao KD, Leach ST, Lemberg DA, Dowd SE, et al. Microbial dysbiosis in pediatric patients with Crohn's disease. J Clin Microbiol. 2012;50(10):3258–66.
19. Vidal R, Ginard D, Khorrami S, Mora-Ruiz M, Munoz R, Hermoso M, et al. Crohn associated microbial communities associated to colonic mucosal biopsies in patients of the western Mediterranean. Syst Appl Microbiol. 2015;38(6):442–52.
20. Tawfik A, Flanagan PK, Campbell BJ. Escherichia coli-host macrophage interactions in the pathogenesis of inflammatory bowel disease. World J Gastroenterol. 2014;20(27):8751–63.
21. Saavedra JM, Dattilo AM. Early development of intestinal microbiota: implications for future health. Gastroenterol Clin North Am. 2012;41(4):717–31.
22. LoCascio RG, Desai P, Sela DA, Weimer B, Mills DA. Broad conservation of milk utilization genes in Bifidobacterium longum subsp. infantis as revealed by comparative genomic hybridization. Appl Environ Microbiol. 2010;76(22):7373–81.
23. Imaoka A, Shima T, Kato K, Mizuno S, Uehara T, Matsumoto S, et al. Anti-inflammatory activity of probiotic Bifidobacterium: enhancement of IL-10 production in peripheral blood mononuclear cells from ulcerative colitis patients and inhibition of IL-8 secretion in HT-29 cells. World J Gastroenterol. 2008;14(16):2511–6.
24. Barclay AR, Russell RK, Wilson ML, Gilmour WH, Satsangi J, Wilson DC. Systematic review: the role of breastfeeding in the development of pediatric inflammatory bowel disease. J Pediatr. 2009;155(3):421–6.
25. Wu GD, Chen J, Hoffmann C, Bittinger K, Chen YY, Keilbaugh SA, et al. Linking long-term dietary patterns with gut microbial enterotypes. Science. 2011;334(6052):105–8.
26. De Filippo C, Cavalieri D, Di Paola M, Ramazzotti M, Poullet JB, Massart S, et al. Impact of diet in shaping gut microbiota revealed by a comparative study in children from Europe and rural Africa. Proc Natl Acad Sci U S A. 2010;107(33):14691–6.
27. Holmes E, Li JV, Marchesi JR, Nicholson JK. Gut microbiota composition and activity in relation to host metabolic phenotype and disease risk. Cell Metab. 2012;16(5):559–64.
28. Devkota S, Wang Y, Musch MW, Leone V, Fehlner-Peach H, Nadimpalli A, et al. Dietary-fat-induced taurocholic acid promotes pathobiont expansion and colitis in Il10−/− mice. Nature. 2012;487(7405):104–8.
29. Sartor RB. Gut microbiota: diet promotes dysbiosis and colitis in susceptible hosts. Nat Rev Gastroenterol Hepatol. 2012;9(10):561–2.
30. Knight-Sepulveda K, Kais S, Santaolalla R, Abreu M. Diet and inflammatory bowel disease. Gastroenterol Hepatol. 2015;11(8):511–20.

31. Dixon LJ, Kabi A, Nickerson KP, McDonald C. Combinatorial effects of diet and genetics on inflammatory bowel disease pathogenesis. Inflamm Bowel Dis. 2015;21(4):912–22.

32. Hou JK, Abraham B, El-Serag H. Dietary intake and risk of developing inflammatory bowel disease: a systematic review of the literature. Am J Gastroenterol. 2011;106(4):563–73.

33. Amre DK, D'Souza S, Morgan K, Seidman G, Lambrette P, Grimard G, et al. Imbalances in dietary consumption of fatty acids, vegetables, and fruits are associated with risk for Crohn's disease in children. Am J Gastroenterol. 2007;102(9):2016–25.

34. Chan SS, Luben R, Olsen A, Tjonneland A, Kaaks R, Lindgren S, et al. Association between high dietary intake of the n-3 polyunsaturated fatty acid docosahexaenoic acid and reduced risk of Crohn's disease. Aliment Pharmacol Ther. 2014;39(8):834–42.

35. John S, Luben R, Shrestha SS, Welch A, Khaw KT, Hart AR. Dietary n-3 polyunsaturated fatty acids and the aetiology of ulcerative colitis: a UK prospective cohort study. Eur J Gastroenterol Hepatol. 2010;22(5):602–6.

36. Lev-Tzion R, Griffiths AM, Leder O, Turner D. Omega 3 fatty acids (fish oil) for maintenance of remission in Crohn's disease. Cochrane Database Syst Rev. 2014;(2):CD006320.

37. Turner D, Shah PS, Steinhart AH, Zlotkin S, Griffiths AM. Maintenance of remission in inflammatory bowel disease using omega-3 fatty acids (fish oil): a systematic review and meta-analyses. Inflamm Bowel Dis. 2011;17(1):336–45.

38. Nickerson KP, McDonald C. Crohn's disease-associated adherent-invasive Escherichia coli adhesion is enhanced by exposure to the ubiquitous dietary polysaccharide maltodextrin. PLoS One. 2012;7(12):e52132.

39. Roberts CL, Rushworth SL, Richman E, Rhodes JM. Hypothesis: Increased consumption of emulsifiers as an explanation for the rising incidence of Crohn's disease. J Crohns Colitis. 2013;7(4):338–41.

40. Chassaing B, Koren O, Goodrich JK, Poole AC, Srinivasan S, Ley RE, et al. Dietary emulsifiers impact the mouse gut microbiota promoting colitis and metabolic syndrome. Nature. 2015;519(7541):92–6.

41. Lang A, Salomon N, Wu JC, Kopylov U, Lahat A, Har-Noy O, et al. Curcumin in combination with mesalamine induces remission in patients with mild-to-moderate ulcerative colitis in a randomized controlled trial. Clin Gastroenterol Hepatol. 2015;13(8):1444–9.e1.

42. Hanai H, Iida T, Takeuchi K, Watanabe F, Maruyama Y, Andoh A, et al. Curcumin maintenance therapy for ulcerative colitis: randomized, multicenter, double-blind, placebo-controlled trial. Clin Gastroenterol Hepatol. 2006;4(12):1502–6.

43. Jowett SL, Seal CJ, Pearce MS, Phillips E, Gregory W, Barton JR, et al. Influence of dietary factors on the clinical course of ulcerative colitis: a prospective cohort study. Gut. 2004;53(10):1479–84.

44. Carrier J, Aghdassi E, Platt I, Cullen J, Allard JP. Effect of oral iron supplementation on oxidative stress and colonic inflammation in rats with induced colitis. Aliment Pharmacol Ther. 2001;15(12):1989–99.

45. Pendyala S, Walker JM, Holt PR. A high-fat diet is associated with endotoxemia that originates from the gut. Gastroenterology. 2012;142(5):1100–1101.e2.

46. Costea I, Mack DR, Lemaitre RN, Israel D, Marcil V, Ahmad A, et al. Interactions between the dietary polyunsaturated fatty acid ratio and genetic factors determine susceptibility to pediatric Crohn's disease. Gastroenterology. 2014;146(4):929–31.

47. Novak TE, Babcock TA, Jho DH, Helton WS, Espat NJ. NF-kappa B inhibition by omega −3 fatty acids modulates LPS-stimulated macrophage TNF-alpha transcription. Am J Physiol Lung Cell Mol Physiol. 2003;284(1):L84–9.

48. Shah ND, Parian AM, Mullin GE, Limketkai BN. Oral diets and nutrition support for inflammatory bowel disease: what is the evidence? Nutr Clin Pract. 2015;30(4):462–73.

49. Roberts CL, Keita AV, Duncan SH, O'Kennedy N, Soderholm JD, Rhodes JM, et al. Translocation of Crohn's disease Escherichia coli across M-cells: contrasting effects of soluble plant fibres and emulsifiers. Gut. 2010;59(10):1331–9.

50. Levenstein S, Prantera C, Luzi C, D'Ubaldi A. Low residue or normal diet in Crohn's disease: a prospective controlled study in Italian patients. Gut. 1985;26(10):989–93.

51. Chiba M, Abe T, Tsuda H, Sugawara T, Tsuda S, Tozawa H, et al. Lifestyle-related disease in Crohn's disease: relapse prevention by a semi-vegetarian diet. World J Gastroenterol. 2010;16(20): 2484–95.

52. Pfeffer-Gik T, Levine A. Dietary clues to the pathogenesis of Crohn's disease. Dig Dis. 2014;32(4):389–94.

53. Nickerson KP, Homer CR, Kessler SP, Dixon LJ, Kabi A, Gordon IO, et al. The dietary polysaccharide maltodextrin promotes Salmonella survival and mucosal colonization in mice. PLoS One. 2014;9(7):e101789.

54. Ahmad A, Arshad N, Ahmed Z, Bhatti MS, Zahoor T, Anjum N, et al. Perspective of surface active agents in baking industry: an overview. Crit Rev Food Sci Nutr. 2014;54(2):208–24.

55. Charles M, Rosselin V, Beck L, Sauvageot F, Guichard E. Flavor release from salad dressings: sensory and physicochemical approaches in relation with the structure. J Agric Food Chem. 2000;48(5):1810–6.

56. Lal SN, O'Connor CJ, Eyres L. Application of emulsifiers/stabilizers in dairy products of high rheology. Adv Colloid Interface Sci. 2006;123–126:433–7.

57. Ogawa A, Cho H. Role of food emulsifiers in milk coffee beverages. J Colloid Interface Sci. 2015;449:198–204.

58. Ogutcu M, Temizkan R, Arifoglu N, Yilmaz E. Structure and stability of fish oil organogels prepared with sunflower wax and monoglyceride. J Oleo Sci. 2015;64(7):713–20.

59. Rahmati K, Mazaheri Tehrani M, Daneshvar K. Soy milk as an emulsifier in mayonnaise: physico-chemical, stability and sensory evaluation. J Food Sci Technol. 2014;51(11):3341–7.

60. Choi HJ, Kim J, Park SH, Do KH, Yang H, Moon Y. Proinflammatory NF-kappaB and early growth response gene 1 regulate epithelial barrier disruption by food additive carrageenan in human intestinal epithelial cells. Toxicol Lett. 2012;211(3): 289–95.

61. Aggarwal BB, Gupta SC, Sung B. Curcumin: an orally bioavailable blocker of TNF and other pro-inflammatory biomarkers. Br J Pharmacol. 2013;169(8):1672–92.

62. Holt PR, Katz S, Kirshoff R. Curcumin therapy in inflammatory bowel disease: a pilot study. Dig Dis Sci. 2005;50(11):2191–3.

63. Koutroubakis IE, Ramos-Rivers C, Regueiro M, Koutroumpakis E, Click B, Schoen RE, et al. Persistent or recurrent anemia is associated with severe and disabling inflammatory bowel disease. Clin Gastroenterol Hepatol. 2015;13(10):1760–6.

64. Erichsen K, Hausken T, Ulvik RJ, Svardal A, Berstad A, Berge RK. Ferrous fumarate deteriorated plasma antioxidant status in patients with Crohn disease. Scand J Gastroenterol. 2003;38(5):543–8.

65. de Silva AD, Tsironi E, Feakins RM, Rampton DS. Efficacy and tolerability of oral iron therapy in inflammatory bowel disease: a prospective, comparative trial. Aliment Pharmacol Ther. 2005;22(11–12):1097–105.

66. Le Leu RK, Young GP, Hu Y, Winter J, Conlon MA. Dietary red meat aggravates dextran sulfate sodium-induced colitis in mice whereas resistant starch attenuates inflammation. Dig Dis Sci. 2013;58(12):3475–82.

67. Cohen SA, Gold BD, Oliva S, Lewis J, Stallworth A, Koch B, et al. Clinical and mucosal improvement with specific carbohydrate diet in pediatric Crohn disease. J Pediatr Gastroenterol Nutr. 2014;59(4): 516–21.

68. Sigall-Boneh R, Pfeffer-Gik T, Segal I, Zangen T, Boaz M, Levine A. Partial enteral nutrition with a Crohn's disease exclusion diet

is effective for induction of remission in children and young adults with Crohn's disease. Inflamm Bowel Dis. 2014;20(8): 1353–60.

69. Gibson PR, Shepherd SJ. Evidence-based dietary management of functional gastrointestinal symptoms: the FODMAP approach. J Gastroenterol Hepatol. 2010;25(2):252–8.

70. Grover Z, Muir R, Lewindon P. Exclusive enteral nutrition induces early clinical, mucosal and transmural remission in paediatric Crohn's disease. J Gastroenterol. 2014;49(4):638–45.

71. Ruemmele FM, Veres G, Kolho KL, Griffiths A, Levine A, Escher JC, et al. Consensus guidelines of ECCO/ESPGHAN on the medical management of pediatric Crohn's disease. J Crohns Colitis. 2014;8(10):1179–207.

72. Soo J, Malik BA, Turner JM, Persad R, Wine E, Siminoski K, et al. Use of exclusive enteral nutrition is just as effective as corticosteroids in newly diagnosed pediatric Crohn's disease. Dig Dis Sci. 2013;58(12):3584–91.

73. Critch J, Day AS, Otley A, King-Moore C, Teitelbaum JE, Shashidhar H, et al. Use of enteral nutrition for the control of intestinal inflammation in pediatric Crohn disease. J Pediatr Gastroenterol Nutr. 2012;54(2):298–305.

74. Buchanan E, Gaunt WW, Cardigan T, Garrick V, McGrogan P, Russell RK. The use of exclusive enteral nutrition for induction of remission in children with Crohn's disease demonstrates that disease phenotype does not influence clinical remission. Aliment Pharmacol Ther. 2009;30(5):501–7.

75. Dziechciarz P, Horvath A, Shamir R, Szajewska H. Meta-analysis: enteral nutrition in active Crohn's disease in children. Aliment Pharmacol Ther. 2007;26(6):795–806.

76. Borrelli O, Cordischi L, Cirulli M, Paganelli M, Labalestra V, Uccini S, et al. Polymeric diet alone versus corticosteroids in the treatment of active pediatric Crohn's disease: a randomized controlled open-label trial. Clin Gastroenterol Hepatol. 2006;4(6): 744–53.

77. Grover Z, Lewindon P. Two-year outcomes after exclusive enteral nutrition induction are superior to corticosteroids in pediatric Crohn's disease treated early with thiopurines. Dig Dis Sci. 2015;60(10):3069–74.

78. Gupta K, Noble A, Kachelries KE, Albenberg L, Kelsen JR, Grossman AB, et al. A novel enteral nutrition protocol for the treatment of pediatric Crohn's disease. Inflamm Bowel Dis. 2013;19(7): 1374–8.

79. Lee D, Baldassano RN, Otley AR, Albenberg L, Griffiths AM, Compher C, et al. Comparative effectiveness of nutritional and biological therapy in North American children with active Crohn's disease. Inflamm Bowel Dis. 2015b;21(8):1786–93.

80. Wilschanski M, Sherman P, Pencharz P, Davis L, Corey M, Griffiths A. Supplementary enteral nutrition maintains remission in paediatric Crohn's disease. Gut. 1996;38(4):543–8.

81. Takagi S, Utsunomiya K, Kuriyama S, Yokoyama H, Takahashi S, Iwabuchi M, et al. Effectiveness of an 'half elemental diet' as maintenance therapy for Crohn's disease: a randomized-controlled trial. Aliment Pharmacol Ther. 2006;24(9):1333–40.

82. Yamamoto T, Nakahigashi M, Saniabadi AR, Iwata T, Maruyama Y, Umegae S, et al. Impacts of long-term enteral nutrition on clinical and endoscopic disease activities and mucosal cytokines during remission in patients with Crohn's disease: a prospective study. Inflamm Bowel Dis. 2007;13(12):1493–501.

83. Hanai H, Iida T, Takeuchi K, Arai H, Arai O, Abe J, et al. Nutritional therapy versus 6-mercaptopurine as maintenance therapy in patients with Crohn's disease. Dig Liver Dis. 2012;44(8):649–54.

84. Johnson T, Macdonald S, Hill SM, Thomas A, Murphy MS. Treatment of active Crohn's disease in children using partial enteral nutrition with liquid formula: a randomised controlled trial. Gut. 2006;55(3):356–61.

85. Obih C, Wahbeh G, Lee D, Braly K, Giefer M, Shaffer ML, et al. Specific carbohydrate diet for pediatric inflammatory bowel disease in clinical practice within an academic IBD center. Nutrition. 2016;32(4):418–25.

86. Olendzki BC, Silverstein TD, Persuitte GM, Ma Y, Baldwin KR, Cave D. An anti-inflammatory diet as treatment for inflammatory bowel disease: a case series report. Nutr J. 2014;13:5. doi:10.1186/1475-2891-13-5.

87. Halmos EP, Power VA, Shepherd SJ, Gibson PR, Muir JG. A diet low in FODMAPs reduces symptoms of irritable bowel syndrome. Gastroenterology. 2014;146(1):67–75.e5.

88. Zimmerman LA, Srinath AI, Goyal A, Bousvaros A, Ducharme P, Szigethy E, et al. The overlap of functional abdominal pain in pediatric Crohn's disease. Inflamm Bowel Dis. 2013;19(4): 826–31.

89. Croagh C, Shepherd SJ, Berryman M, Muir JG, Gibson PR. Pilot study on the effect of reducing dietary FODMAP intake on bowel function in patients without a colon. Inflamm Bowel Dis. 2007;13(12):1522–8.

90. Gearry RB, Irving PM, Barrett JS, Nathan DM, Shepherd SJ, Gibson PR. Reduction of dietary poorly absorbed short-chain carbohydrates (FODMAPs) improves abdominal symptoms in patients with inflammatory bowel disease-a pilot study. J Crohns Colitis. 2009;3(1):8–14.

91. Herfarth HH, Martin CF, Sandler RS, Kappelman MD, Long MD. Prevalence of a gluten-free diet and improvement of clinical symptoms in patients with inflammatory bowel diseases. Inflamm Bowel Dis. 2014;20(7):1194–7.

92. Aziz I, Branchi F, Pearson K, Priest J, Sanders DS. A study evaluating the bidirectional relationship between inflammatory bowel disease and self-reported non-celiac gluten sensitivity. Inflamm Bowel Dis. 2015;21(4):847–53.

93. Hollon J, Puppa EL, Greenwald B, Goldberg E, Guerrerio A, Fasano A. Effect of gliadin on permeability of intestinal biopsy explants from celiac disease patients and patients with non-celiac gluten sensitivity. Nutrients. 2015;7(3):1565–76.

Jennifer Panganiban, Jessi Erlichman, and Maria Mascarenhas

Introduction

Complementary and alternative medicine (CAM) is an umbrella term encompassing a broad range of modalities, healing philosophies, and approaches. CAM is often classified into one of the five domains: (1) whole medical systems, (2) mind-body medicine, (3) biologically based practices, (4) manipulative and body-based practices, and (5) energy medicine. Whole medical systems represent the theories and practices of traditional Chinese medicine, Ayurvedic medicine and homeopathy, for example. Mind-body interventions involve modalities such as prayer and meditation and are meant to facilitate the connection between the mind and body. Herbal products, dietary supplements, and diets comprise the category of biologically based therapies. Body-based practices employ human touch to manipulate the physical body, such as massage or craniosacral therapy. Finally, the domain of energy therapies harnesses the body's energy fields to promote health and healing. Examples include tai chi and reiki. These classification entities encompass a wide range of diverse therapies and may have disparate, but interrelated, therapeutic targets.

Recently, in the United States, the National Center for Complementary and Integrative Health has moved toward a two-subgroup classification system: mind and body practices or natural products. Furthermore, the identification that most Americans use nonmainstream practices in conjunction with, not as an alternative to, conventional treatments has lead the development of the term integrative medicine or health.

J. Panganiban, MD (✉)
Division of Gastroenterology, Hepatology and Nutrition,
The Children's Hospital of Philadelphia,
Perelman School of Medicine, University of Pennsylvania,
Philadelphia, PA, USA
e-mail: panganibaj@email.chop.edu

J. Erlichman, MPH • M. Mascarenhas, MBBS
The Children's Hospital of Philadelphia, Division of
Gastroenterology, Hepatology and Nutrition,
Philadelphia, PA, USA

Integrative health (IH) refers to the incorporation and integration of complementary approaches into mainstream healthcare practices.

Use of CAM or IH practices is common. National survey data in the United States suggest 33.2% of adults and 11.6% of children used complementary health approaches in 2012. The rates of IH use in chronic disease populations frequently exceed those in the general population. Prevalence of CAM use in pediatric chronic disease populations also exceeds that of general pediatric population [1]. In this chapter we explore the interest, utilization, and efficacy of a subset of IH modalities for the adjuvant treatment of IBD in pediatrics.

Integrative Health Use in IBD

Multiple studies confirm CAM use is common among children with IBD, with prevalence estimates ranging between 6.7 and 72% [2]. Pediatric prevalence rates are compatible with or exceed CAM use in adult IBD [2–6]. Surveys also suggest that high proportions of IBD patients who do not use CAM would consider using it in the future [7]. These surveys indicate that biologically based therapies are the most common IH domain utilized in pediatric IBD populations [5, 6, 8]. The use of CAM in conjunction with prescribed medications is also common. In a study by Wong et al., 43.6% of all patients with IBD used both prescription medications and IH therapies in the treatment of their disease [5].

Across surveys, however, prevalence of IH and predictors of use vary and are inconsistent. Variation in prevalence rates may be attributed to methodologic differences in survey instruments and sampling approaches, regional and geographic differences, and ethnic, cultural, and other demographic influences [9]. The high degree of variability in use estimates may also be due to how IH is defined. For example, in surveys where prayer, specifically for health reasons, is included as a mind-body modality, 62% of US adults used CAM in the past 12 months. Whereas when prayer was excluded, utilization estimates decreased to 36% [10].

There are myriad factors associated with the use of IH in pediatric IBD populations. These factors can be categorized into sociodemographic characteristics or disease-related characteristics. Parents' use of CAM, parental education level, parental age, and age of child may predict CAM use in children with IBD [5, 8, 11, 12]. Disease-related attributes associated with CAM use may include dissatisfaction with traditional treatment, low self-reported health-related quality of life (HRQOL), desire to have more control over child's condition, symptom management, and to avoid side effects of medicine, extent of out-of-pocket expenditures on prescription medication, and CD vs. UC [6, 8, 12].

However, disease-related characteristics do not consistently predict IH use. In part, this may be due to how disease severity or activity is defined across studies. In several studies, low HRQOL, increased school absences, greater out-of-pocket spending, and frequency of use of certain conventionally prescribed medications were associated with pediatric CAM use [6, 8, 11]. Yet in other studies, school absences, hospital admissions, and prescription medication were not associated or predictive of CAM use [8, 13–17].

Irrespective of whether the child used any IH modalities, parental attitudes toward use at time of IBD diagnosis or as an adjuvant treatment with child's current medical regimen is high, suggesting parental receptivity toward CAM utilization [12]. CAM may confer a sense of control over the child's disease as the parent voluntarily chooses which modalities to use, whereas the clinician prescribes a treatment. Interestingly, when parents perceive conventional medical treatment as effective or if they worry about CAM interactions, they are unlikely to recommend CAM for their child [18].

IH Modality Use in Pediatric IBD

There is an emerging body of literature focused on use of mind-body therapies to mitigate psychosocial stress and improve HRQOL among IBD patients. Considering that stressful event experiences are perceived as possible triggers for relapse and increased disease activity, the application of mind-body CAM to enhance stress coping skills may enhance durability of remission [19, 20]. Mind-body CAM includes modalities such as meditation, yoga, and deep breathing, for example, and may be a useful adjuvant treatment for pediatric IBD patients. These modalities are relatively inexpensive, safe, easily integrated, and readily accessible and available. Furthermore, the known association between stress and physical symptom exacerbation and the prevalence of comorbid affective disorders in patients with GI conditions suggest that mind-body IH may be effective in symptom amelioration [21]. Future studies exploring this interaction are warranted. The

remainder of this chapter will focus on the available literature as it pertains to the safety and efficacy of a number of biologically based modalities frequently used in IBD.

Biologically Based Therapies for the Treatment of IBD

The specific role of CAM in the treatment of IBD has not yet been established. CAM products that have been evaluated in clinical studies for the treatment of IBD include biologically based therapies (herbs, dietary supplements, and specialized diets) and mind-body medicine. The use of herbal remedies or nutritional supplements in pediatric IBD has been reported to be high as ~20% and ~36%, respectively. Although research has explored many of these products, scientific evidence regarding their efficacy or safety has not been adequate. The most common biologically based therapies in the treatment of IBD are those stated below (Table 39.1):

Herbal Therapies

Aloe Vera

Aloe Vera (Xanthorrhoeaceae) is a stemless, drought-resisting succulent plant of the lily family. It is indigenous to hot countries and has been shown to have anti-inflammatory and antioxidant properties. *Aloe vera* gel is the mucilaginous aqueous extract of the leaf pulp of Aloe barbadensis and can act as a barrier such as in colitis. *Aloe vera* contains an abundance of phytochemical substances such as mannans and anthraquinone. Its immunomodulating activity is thought to work through the induction of maturation of dendritic cells and in vitro inhibition of prostaglandin E2 and IL-8. Topical administration of aloe gel is considered safe but if taken orally has been found to cause abdominal cramps, diarrhea, and dehydration. This has also been linked to thyroid dysfunction, acute hepatitis, and perioperative bleeding.

Aloe vera gel has been used in the treatment of mild-to-moderate ulcerative colitis. A randomized double-blind controlled trial from the United Kingdom showed that aloe vera gel, when administered to patients with moderately active ulcerative colitis for 4 weeks, was superior to placebo. The primary outcome measures were clinical remission (Simple Clinical Colitis Activity Index < 2), sigmoidoscopic remission (Baron score < 1), and histological remission (Saverymuttu score < 1). Aloe vera gel taken for 4 weeks appeared to be safe, produced a clinical response ($p < 0.05$), reduction in median SSCAI ($p<0.01$), and reduction in histological disease activity ($p < 0.03$) in comparison to placebo. [22].

Table 39.1 Biologically based therapies in the treatment of inflammatory bowel disease

Biologically based therapy	Year	Indication	Subjects	Comparator	Duration	Response on CAM (%)	Response on comparator (%)	Author, Ref
I. Herbal therapies:								
Aloe vera	2004	UC	44	Placebo	4 weeks	30	7	Langmead, [22]
Triticum aestivum	2002	UC	23	Placebo	4 weeks	91	42	Ben-Arye, [23]
Andrographis paniculata (HMPL-004)	2011	UC	120	Mesalamine	8 weeks	76	82	Tang, [24]
	2013	UC	224	Placebo	8 weeks	60	40	Sandborn, [25]
Jian Pi Ling tablet	1994	UC	153	Sulfasalazine (S) Placebo (P)	90 days	53	28 (S) 19 (P)	Chen, [26]
Yukui tang tablets	1999	UC	118	Prednisolone, neomycin, vitamin B	40 days	33	17	Chen, [27]
Cannabis (THC)	2013	CD	21	Placebo	8 weeks	90	40	Naftali, [48]
II. Non herbal therapies:								
Plantago ovata seeds	1999	UC	105	Mesalamine	12 months	60	65	Fernandez-Bernares, [44]
NAG (Pediatric Pilot)	2000	UC + CD	12	None	Not specified	Oral: 8/12 Rectal 2/9	–	Salvatore, [45]
Curcumin	2006	UC	89	Placebo	6 months	95	79	Hanai, [31]
	2015	UC	50	Placebo	4 weeks	65	12.5	Lang, [32]
Open label	2005	CD	5	None	3 months	80	–	Holt, [33]
Pediatric	2013	CD + UC	11	None	9 weeks	–	–	Suskind, [34]
Boswellia serrata (BS)	2001	UC	30	Sulfasalazine	6 weeks	70	40	Gupta, [35]
BS Extract H15	2001	CD	102	Mesalamine	8 weeks	36	31	Gerhardt, [36]
BS Boswelan-PS0201Bo	2010	CD	108	Placebo	52 weeks	60	55	Holtmeier, [37]
Artemisia absinthium	2007	CD	40	Placebo	10 weeks	65	0	Omer, [38]
	2010	CD	20	Placebo	6 weeks	80	20	Krebs, [39]
Tripterygium wilfordii	2007	CD	20	Placebo	12 weeks	–	–	Ren, [40]
	2009	Post op CD	45	Mesalamine	6 months 12 months	82 (6 months) 68 (12 months)	78 (6 months) 61 (12 months)	Tao, [41]
	2009	Post op CD	39	Sulfasalazine	52 weeks	94	75	Liao, [42]
III. Rectal enema therapies:								
Kui Jie Qing enemas	1997	UC	106	Sulfasalazine, prednisolone (oral and enema)	20 days	72	9	Wang, [49]
Xilei-san enema	2013	UC	35	Dexamethasone enema	8 weeks	–	–	Zhang, [50]
Xilei-san suppository	2013	UC	30	Placebo suppository	2 weeks	46	0	Fukunaga, [51]
Bovine colostrum enema	2002	UC	14	Placebo (albumin)	4 weeks	88	0	Khan, [52]

Triticum aestivium

Triticum aestivum (Poaceae) or better known as wheat grass is prepared by sprouting wheat seeds in water for 7–10 days before harvesting the leaves. It has antioxidant properties and a natural source of vitamins and minerals. It contains agropyrene that has antibiotic activity and apigenin, which has anti-inflammatory properties by inhibiting adhesion of leucocytes to endothelial cells. It is relatively safe but can cause nausea, anorexia, and constipation.

Wheat grass has shown significant benefit as single or adjuvant treatment for active distal ulcerative colitis. In a randomized, double-blind, multicenter study from Israel, 23 patients with active distal UC were given either daily wheat grass juice or placebo for 4 weeks. Patients were found to have clinical improvement (reduction in rectal bleeding, abdominal pain, physical global assessment score) in 10/11 patients on wheat grass (91%) vs. 5/12 on placebo (42%). Gross improvement was also seen on sigmoidoscopy in 78% or 7/9 patients on wheat grass vs. 30% or 3/10 on placebo [23].

Andrographis paniculata

Andrographis paniculata (Acanthaceae) is a bitter-tasting annual plant in Asia. This has been marketed in China as Kan Jang, Kold Kare, KalmCold, and Paractin. *Andrographis* has been found to have antibacterial, antioxidant, anti-inflammatory, anticancer, and immune-stimulating properties. Its active constituents are diterpenoid lactones known as andrographolides. Its anti-inflammatory activity works by inhibiting nitric oxide production, cyclooxygenase-2 expression, and TNF-alpha, IL-1b, and NF-kB. Side effects include headache, fatigue, hypersensitivity, lymphadenopathy, nausea, diarrhea, altered taste, transaminitis, and acute kidney injury. *Andrographis* extract may inhibit 1A2, 2C9, and 3A4 and induce CYP1A1. These two properties can affect the intracellular concentration of drugs metabolized by these enzymes.

Andrographis has been found to be an efficacious alternative to mesalamine in the treatment of active UC. A randomized double-blind multicenter 8-week parallel-group study showed that *Andrographis paniculata* (HMPL-004) was as effective as mesalamine (response 76% vs. 82%; remission 21% vs. 16%) in the treatment of mild-to-moderate ulcerative colitis, but there was no difference in endoscopic remission rates at 8 weeks between the two groups, 28% vs. 24% [24]. This was followed up by a larger randomized, double-blind controlled trial in 224 adults with mild-to-moderate ulcerative colitis. HMPL-004 given at a higher dose (1800 mg daily) was associated with a greater clinical response than placebo (60% vs. 40%; $P = 0.018$) although remission rates at 8 weeks were not different between both groups, 38% vs. 34%; $P = 0.101$ [25].

Jian Pi Ling

Jian Pi Ling (JPL) tablet and *Yukui tang* tablets are herbal therapies that have been studied in China in the treatment for ulcerative colitis [26, 27, 28, 29]. In a randomized controlled trial, 153 patients with UC were randomly assigned to three groups: group I, Jian Pi Ling (JPL) tablet with retention enema of *Radix Sophorae Flavescentis* and Flos Sophora decoction; group II, sulfasalazine and retention enema of dexamethasone; and group III, placebo and retention enema of decoction. Remission rates at 3 months in group 1 were significantly higher (53%) than those in the other two groups (28 and 19%, respectively) [26, 27]. Another study evaluated 118 patients with active UC who were treated with oral Yukui tang tablets and herbal decoction enemas, in addition to oral prednisolone 15 mg daily, neomycin, and vitamin B for 40 days. Eighty-six control patients who received only low-dose prednisolone, neomycin, and vitamin B were used for comparison. The remission rates and response rates were 33 and 51%, respectively, in the active group, compared with 17 and 43%, in the control group [26, 27].

Oenothera biennis

Oenothera biennis also known as evening primrose oil, night willow herb, fever plant, and king's cure-all. Evening primrose oil is rich in omega-6 gamma-linolenic acid (GLA), which can be converted directly to the prostaglandin precursor dihomo-GLA (DGLA). It has been demonstrated to have anti-inflammatory activity and inhibits platelet aggregation. Administration of the oil may benefit individuals unable to metabolize cis-linolenic acid to GLA, producing subsequent intermediates of metabolic significance including prostaglandins. Side effects include abdominal pain, indigestion, nausea, softening of stools, and headaches. This may cause increased bleeding when taken with anticoagulants or anti-platelet medication. Although there are no interactions reported with antihypertensive medications, evening primrose oil was identified to increase both systolic and diastolic blood pressures, with a clinically meaningful difference for systolic blood pressure in a large population-based study.

Primrose oil has been used in the treatment of ulcerative colitis. In a placebo-controlled study, 43 patients with stable ulcerative colitis were randomized to receive MaxEPA (*Oenothera biennis*) ($n = 16$), super evening primrose oil ($n = 19$), or olive oil as placebo ($n = 8$) for 6 months, in addition to their normal treatment. Evening primrose oil significantly improved stool consistency, and the difference was maintained even after treatment was discontinued. There was no difference in stool frequency, rectal bleeding, disease relapse, sigmoidoscopic appearance, or histology in the three treatment groups [30].

Curcumin

Curcumin is the active yellow pigment of the spice turmeric. It is an herb belonging to the ginger family native to India and Southeast Asia. Curcumin is commonly used in Indian traditional cuisine and medicine. It has been found to have anti-inflammatory, antioxidant, and antitumor effects. Curcumin is thought to cause the suppression of the nuclear factor kappa-light chain enhancer of activated B cells (NF-KB).

Furthermore, curcumin activity includes suppression of inter-leukin-1 (IL-1) and tumor necrosis factor alpha (TNF α), two main cytokines that play important roles in the regulation of inflammatory responses. Side effects include dyspepsia, diarrhea, distension, GERD, gassiness, nausea, and vomiting. It also has been found to interact with anticoagulants, hypoglycemic medications, and iron and can increase sulfasalazine levels. Thus, this must be discontinued at least 2 weeks prior to any surgery.

Curcumin has been used in the treatment of both ulcerative colitis and Crohn's disease. A 2012 Cochrane review found curcumin is safe and an effective therapy for maintenance of remission in quiescent UC when given as adjunctive therapy along with mesalamine or sulfasalazine. A multicenter randomized double-blind Japanese study evaluated 89 patients who were randomized to receive either curcumin (1 g twice daily) or placebo, in addition to sulfasalazine or mesalamine, for 6 months. Relapse rate was significantly lower in the curcumin group, 4.7% compared to placebo 20.5%, $p = 0.04$ [31]. This was reinforced by a multicenter double-blind randomized control trial, which evaluated 50 patients with active mild-moderate UC on 5-ASA, who did not respond to 2 weeks of max 5-ASA oral and topical therapy. Patients were randomly assigned to curcumin 3 g/d ($n = 26$) or placebo ($n = 24$) × 4 weeks. Clinical response (reduction of ≥3 points in SCCAI) was achieved by 17 patients (65.3%) in the curcumin group vs. three patients (12.5%) in the placebo group ($P < 0.001$). Endoscopic remission (partial Mayo score ≤1) was observed in 8 of the 22 patients evaluated in the curcumin group (38%), compared with 0 of 16 patients evaluated in the placebo group $p = 0.04$ [32]. Curcumin has been also evaluated in Crohn's disease. A pilot study of five patients demonstrated that 360 mg of curcumin TID could cause a mean reduction in CDAI of 55 points, ESR reduction of 10 mm/hr, and CRP reduction of 0.1 mg/dl [33]. A pediatric tolerability study was performed in 11 patients with mild UC or CD. Three patients had a decrease in their PUCAI or PCDAI scores and none had a relapse or worsening of symptoms [34].

Boswellia

Boswellia (Burseraceae) also known as Indian frankincense is a tree prevalent in India, the Middle East, and North Africa. The gummy exudate or the resin obtained by peeling away the bark is commonly known as "frankincense" or "olibanum." Boswellic acids act as an anti-inflammatory by noncompetitive inhibition of 5-lipoxygenase and decrease in pro-inflammatory makers such as TNF α. Side effects include gastric irritation and nausea. It has been shown to interact with cytochrome P450 substrates and immunosuppressants.

Boswellia has been used in the treatment of ulcerative colitis and Crohn's disease. Two studies had compared the efficacy of herbal therapy to mesalamine. In the first study,

30 patients with chronic active UC were randomized to gum resin of *Boswellia serrata* (900 mg daily in three doses; $n = 20$) or sulfasalazine (3 g daily in three doses; $n = 10$) for 6 weeks. Fourteen of 20 patients treated with *Boswellia* gum resin and 4 of 10 treated with sulfasalazine achieved remission. Eighteen of 20 patients treated with *Boswellia* gum resin and 6 of 10 patients on sulfasalazine showed an improvement in one of more of the parameters including stool properties, histopathology, and scanning electron microscopy [35].

In a randomized, double-blind, non-inferiority, parallel-group control trial done in Germany, 102 patients with Crohn's disease were randomized. Forty-four patients were treated with *Boswellia* extract (H15) and thirty-nine with mesalamine. CDAI decreased by 90 in the *Boswellia* group and 53 in mesalamine group [36]. A subsequent double-blind, placebo-controlled, randomized, parallel study from 22 centers in Germany evaluated the long-term efficacy and safety of *Boswellia serrata* extract (Boswelan, PS0201Bo) in maintaining remission in 108 patients with Crohn's disease. At 52 weeks, there was no significant difference in the proportion of patients in clinical remission between those who were actively treated or on the placebo group (59.9% vs. 55.3%). The mean time to relapse was also not different between the two groups [37].

Artemisia absinthium

Artemisia absinthium (Asteraceae) is commonly known as wormwood or sweet sagewort and has been used in traditional Chinese medicine. Dihydroartemisinin (DHA) is a semisynthetic derivative of artemisinin and has been found to have anti-inflammatory properties. It is believed to attenuate COX-2 production via downregulation of serine/threonine kinase (AKT) and mitogen-activated protein kinase (MAPK) pathways and decrease TNF α. Side effects include hepatitis and patients with a history of ulcers should not take *Artemisia*. *Artemisia* can also induce seizures resulting from decreased efficacy of antiseizure medications. Extracts from *Artemisia* induce CYP2B6 and CYP3A4 and may affect the serum concentration of drugs metabolized by these enzymes.

Wormwood has been used in the treatment of Crohn's disease. A double-blind study carried out at five sites in Germany evaluated 40 patients suffering from Crohn's disease receiving a stable daily dose of steroids at an equivalent of 40 mg or less of prednisone for at least 3 weeks. They were randomized to receive either an herbal blend containing wormwood herb (3 × 500 mg/day) or placebo for 10 weeks. There was a steady improvement in CD symptoms in 18 patients (90%) who received wormwood in spite of tapering of steroids as shown by Crohn's Disease Activity Index (CDAI) questionnaire, Inflammatory Bowel Disease Questionnaire (IBDQ), Hamilton Depression Scale (HAMD), and Visual Analogue Scale (VA-Scale). After

8 weeks of treatment with wormwood, there was almost complete remission of symptoms in 13 (65%) patients in this group as compared to none in the placebo group. This remission persisted till the end of the observation period that was week 20, and the addition of steroids was not necessary. This study strongly suggest that wormwood has a steroid-sparing effect with improvement of mood and quality of life based on HAMD scale, which is not achieved by other standard medications [38].

In a separate controlled trial, 20 patients with active CD were given either dried powdered wormwood or placebo, in addition to their existing CD therapy. At 6 weeks, 8 of 10 patients (80%) on wormwood and 2 of 10 patients (20%) on placebo achieved clinical remission defined as a Crohn's disease activity index (CDAI) below 170 or a reduction in CDAI by 70 points. Six of ten patients on woodworm had a clinical response compared to none on placebo [39].

Tripterygium wilfordii Hook F (TWHF)

Tripterygium wilfordii Hook F (TWHF) or known by its mandarin name "léi gōng téng" sometimes called thunder god vine is a vine used in traditional Chinese medicine that has both immunomodulatory and anti-inflammatory activities. It is a dipterpene tripoxide from an extract obtained from *Tripterygium wilfordii*. Side effects include amenorrhea and nonspecific gastrointestinal symptoms. *Tripterygium* is used in the treatment and in the prevention of postoperative recurrence of Crohn's disease. A study evaluated 20 adult patients with active Crohn's disease who were treated with *Tripterygium* pills for 12 weeks. CDAI scores dropped during the first 8 weeks, and endoscopic improvements were observed at week 12. Furthermore, a significant decrease in serum levels of C-reactive protein and pro-inflammatory cytokines were reported [40].

Two placebo-controlled studies assessed the role of *Tripterygium wilfordii* (GTW) in preventing postoperative recurrence of CD. Forty-five patients with CD were randomly assigned to receive GTW or mesalamine after their operation. No clinical recurrence occurred in both groups at 3 months. There were no significant differences in clinical relapse at 6 months (18% vs. 22%) or 12 months (32% vs. 39%) between the GTW and mesalamine groups. Endoscopic recurrence at 12 months was also similar in the two groups, 46% vs. 61% [41]. This was followed by a subsequent study, which randomized 39 CD patients to GTW ($n = 21$) or sulfasalazine ($n = 18$) 2 weeks after resection for Crohn's disease. Clinical recurrence was reported in 6% on GTW and 25% on sulfasalazine, and endoscopic recurrence was reported in 22% on GTW and 56% on sulfasalazine. GTW appeared to be as effective, if not more effective, than mesalamine in preventing recurrence of postoperative Crohn's disease [42].

Belladonna

Belladonna (Tincture of belladonna) *Atropa belladonna* or *Atropa bella-donna*, commonly known as belladonna or deadly nightshade, is a perennial herbaceous plant in the tomato family Solanaceae. This is native to Europe, North Africa, Western Asia, and some parts of Canada and the United States. The active agents in belladonna include atropine, hyoscine, and hyoscyamine that have anticholinergic properties. Side effects include dilated pupils, sensitivity to light, blurred vision, tachycardia, loss of balance, staggering, headache, rash, flushing, severely dry mouth, urinary retention, constipation, confusion, hallucinations, delirium, and convulsions. This has been for its anticholinergic properties and symptomatic treatment of pain in inflammatory bowel disease. Its side effect is suppression of gastrointestinal motility and thus can precipitate toxic megacolon. Thus, use is not recommended.

Cannabis

Cannabis is a genus of flowering plant that includes three species *sativa*, *indica*, and *ruderalis*. The plant is indigenous to Central Asia and the Indian subcontinent. D9-tetrahydrocannabinol (THC) and cannabidiol (CBD) seem to be the most active cannabinoids. Two cannabinoid receptors in the gut have been identified, cannabinoid receptor CB1 and CB2. They act mainly through cannabinoid receptor 2 which causes downregulation of cytokines, specifically tumor necrosis factor (TNF)-α and interleukin-1. They also act by suppressing cell-mediated immunity and enhancing humoral immunity. Cannabinoid exposure antagonizes release of prostaglandins, histamine, and matrix-active proteases from mast cells. Side effects can include dry mouth, drowsiness, palpitations, paranoia, anxiety, memory loss [43], altered state of consciousness, distorted perceptions of time and space, bloodshot eyes, dilated pupils, increased appetite, and impaired coordination and concentration.

Cannabinoids have been used within gastroenterology to treat anorexia, emesis, abdominal pain, gastroenteritis, diarrhea, intestinal inflammation, and diabetic gastroparesis [44]. Endogenous endocannabinoids have been discovered which may modulate intestinal inflammation [45], and animal models suggest cannabis play a role in the treatment of colitis [46]. THC has been used in the symptomatic relief in inflammatory bowel disease in adults. A retrospective study found that 21 out of 30 CD patients had clinical improvement ($p < 0.001$) based upon Harvey-Bradshaw Index and a decreased need for escalation of therapy and surgery after cannabis treatment [47]. A double-blinded prospective study evaluated 21 with Crohn's Disease Activity Index (CDAI) scores greater than 200 who did not respond to therapy with steroids, immunomodulators, or antitumor necrosis factor-α agents. Patients were randomized to receive cigarettes containing 115 mg of D9 tetrahydrocannabinol (THC) or placebo containing cannabis flowers from which the THC had been extracted twice daily for 8 weeks. Complete remission (CDAI score, <150) was achieved by 5 of 11 subjects in the cannabis group and 1 of 10 in the placebo group (p 0.43), and a clinical response (decrease in CDAI score of >100) was observed 90% in the cannabis group and 40% in the placebo group (p = 0.028). THC-rich cannabis produced significant clinical, steroid-free benefits with active Crohn's disease, compared with placebo, without side effects [48]. There have been no studies in children, not has mucosal healing been assessed with this treatment to date.

Non-herbal Therapies

Fatty Acids

Fish Oil (Omega-3 FFA)

Fish oil (omega-3 FFA) is a type of polyunsaturated fatty acid (PUFA) derived mainly from fish oil. It has been found to have anti-inflammatory and immunomodulatory properties. They suppress mediators of immune function by reducing cytokine production (IL-1, IL-2, IL-6 TNF α), suppressing T and B cell proliferation and decreasing antibody production. Omega-3 fatty acids may also reduce inflammation in patients with ulcerative colitis by reducing rectal dialysate leukotriene $\beta 4$. This is generally safe but side effects include fishy aftertaste, nausea, diarrhea, and heartburn. Fish oil can have additive anticoagulant/antiplatelet effects and interact with NSAIDS. This may also potentiate some of the adverse effects of glucocorticoids.

It has been used in the treatment of both ulcerative colitis and Crohn's disease. Despite its generally accepted use, results in clinical studies have been inconsistent. A 2014 Cochrane review of 6 studies with 1039 patients demonstrated marginal benefit of therapy for maintenance of remission. The overall quality of evidence was very low, and the two best quality studies showed no benefit. In two systematic reviews, omega-3 fatty acids are not effective for the maintenance of remission in Crohn's disease [49].

Blond Psyllium

Blond psyllium comes from the husk surrounding the seeds of an herb called *Plantago ovata* (Plantaginaceae). When exposed to water, psyllium swells and forms a gel-like mass called mucilage. The colonic fermentation of psyllium in the gastrointestinal tract produces butyrate. Butyrate has an anti-inflammatory effect and inhibits cytokine production. Side effects include transient flatulence, abdominal pain, diarrhea, constipation, dyspepsia, and nausea. Contraindications for its use in IBD include fecal impaction, GI tract narrowing,

obstruction, swallowing disorders, and treatment within 2 weeks of surgery.

Blond psyllium has been used to prevent relapse and improve associated ulcerative colitis symptoms. Blond psyllium has been used as a butyrate enema and is effective for the treatment of diversion colitis. In an open-label, parallel-group, multicenter, randomized clinical trial, 105 patients with UC in remission were randomized into groups to receive *Plantago ovata* seeds (10 g twice daily), mesalamine (500 mg three times daily), and *Plantago ovata* seeds plus mesalamine at the same doses. Primary outcome was maintenance of remission for 1 year. Relapse rate at 12 months were similar in the three groups, psyllium 40% vs. mesalamine 35% vs. combination 30%. There was a significant increase in fecal butyrate with psyllium. Side effects were mild and included constipation and/or flatulence [50].

N-Acetyl Glucosamine (NAG)

N-acetyl glucosamine (NAG) is a chemical that comes from the outer shells of shellfish. It is an amino sugar form of glucosamine. NAG is thought to restore the gastrointestinal protective glycoprotein layer that is broken down with mucosal inflammation. It has been shown to block adherence of *Candida* to gastrointestinal mucosa and stimulates growth of beneficial *Bifidobacteria*. Side effects include gastrointestinal upset and it is not advised in patients with shellfish allergy. It may interact with acetaminophen, hypoglycemic medication, and warfarin and is contraindicated in asthmatics.

NAG has been used in the treatment of both ulcerative colitis and Crohn's disease. A pediatric pilot study evaluated 12 children with severe treatment-resistant bowel disease (10 CD, 2 UC). Seven of the twelve patients had symptomatic strictures. Patients were given 3–6 grams of NAG orally as adjunctive therapy. Similar doses were given rectally as monotherapy to 9 children with distal UC or proctitis resistant to steroids and antibiotics. Eight of the twelve children who were given oral treatment improved but four required resection. Two of the nine children given rectal therapy achieved remission and three improved, and there was no effect seen in the remaining two patients. Histological improvement was seen in all nine cases biopsied [51].

Chitosan

Chitosan is the N-deacetylated form of chitin extracted from shells of crustaceans and has a structure similar to cellulose. It is a water-insoluble dietary fiber that helps improve bowel habits and prevents colon cancer. Evidence suggests positively charged chitosan polymers bind to negatively charged bile acids in the intestines. This is generally safe but side effects include gastrointestinal upset, nausea, flatulence, increased stool bulk, constipation, and shellfish allergy. It has also been shown to reduce absorption of calcium, magnesium, selenium, fat-soluble vitamins, and warfarin. This has been studied in the treatment of Crohn's disease. A pilot trial of 11 patients with Crohn's was given chitosan and ascorbic acid mixture (1.05 g/d) for 8 weeks. Patients continued their regular therapy. They found that bowel movements slightly increased but nutritional, inflammatory markers, and CDAI did not change. There have been no studies in children. Based on data, this is not recommended in the treatment of IBD [52].

Bromelain

Bromelain (*Ananas comosus*) is a proteolytic enzyme derived from pineapple stem. It can decrease expression of mRNAs encoding pro-inflammatory cytokines by human leukocytes in vitro. It has also been shown to decrease secretion of granulocyte-macrophage colony-stimulating factor, IFN-gamma, and TNF-α in ulcerative colitis and Crohn's disease colon biopsies in vitro [53]. Side effects include mild nausea and vomiting, diarrhea, and excessive menstrual bleeding, and it has been seen to interact with anticoagulants, sedatives, and antibiotics. It has been used in refractory ulcerative colitis. There has been a case report of two patients who entered and remained in clinical and endoscopic remission after self-treatment [54].

Rutin

Rutin is a flavonoid with antioxidant properties. It is found in buckwheat, Japanese pagoda tree, eucalyptus, lime tree flowers, elder flowers, hawthorn leaves, St John's wort, *Ginkgo biloba*, and apples. It is safe in small amounts such as present in fruits and vegetables. Side effects include headache, flushing, rashes, and gastrointestinal disturbance. This has shown some benefit in improving inflammatory bowel disease in rats, yet there are no human studies.

Probiotics and Dietary Therapy

Probiotics and Dietary Therapy have shown marked promise in the treatment of inflammatory bowel disease. This will be discussed separately in their own chapters.

Rectal Enema Therapies

Kui Jie Qing (KJQ)

Kui jie qing (KJQ) is a traditional Chinese remedy that has been used as an enema in the treatment of active ulcerative colitis. A randomized controlled trial from China evaluated 95 patients with active UC who were treated with Kui jie qing enemas four times a day. This form of treatment was compared with conventional anti-IBD drugs, including sulfasalazine (1.5 g 3 times daily), oral prednisolone (30 mg once daily), and prednisone enemas (20 mg 4 times daily). After 20 days of treatment, authors reported a 95% effective-

ness rate for KJQ and 62% for conventional drugs, based on the comparison of cure and improvement between the groups. Effective "cure" was shown in 72% of KJQ-treated patients but only in 9% of controls although the definition of "cure" or "improvement" in this study was not clear [55].

Xilei-San

Xilei-san is used in traditional Chinese herbal medicine for its anti-inflammatory properties. This has been used in the treatment of ulcerative proctitis. In an 8-week double-blind randomized study, Xilei-san enema was compared with dexamethasone enemas in 35 subjects with mild-to-moderate active ulcerative proctitis. Subjects were followed up for 12 weeks. Both treatments showed significant improvement in clinical, endoscopic, and histological score compared to baseline [56].

In another randomized control trial, Xilei-san was used to induce remission in 30 patients with intractable ulcerative proctitis. Subjects were treated with topical mesalamine or corticosteroids for 4 weeks and then randomized into Xilei-san suppositories or placebo for 2 weeks. In the Xilei-san-treated group, significantly more patients achieved remission (clinical disease index ≤ 4) compared with placebo ($P < 0.04$). Histologic improvements, as well as relapse rate at 180 days, were significantly lower in Xilei-san-treated group compared with placebo [57].

Bovine Colostrum

Bovine colostrum is cow's milk secreted during the first few days following calving. It is rich in immunoglobulins, growth factors, and cytokines and confers immune protection to the newborn calf from opportunistic infections. Bovine colostrum is postulated to enhance the immune response. Although the high concentration of immunoglobulins may account for bovine colostrum's effects, the exact mechanism is not known. This may not be used in patients who have cow's milk allergy. Bovine colostrum has been used as an enema in the treatment of ulcerative proctitis. Fourteen patients with mild-to-moderate active UC were treated with bovine colostrum enemas or placebo containing albumin solution twice daily for 4 weeks in addition to mesalamine. Only the colostrum group showed a mean reduction in symptom score in 7 out of 8 patients and an improvement in the histological score in 5/8 patients vs. 2/6 in the placebo group [58].

Conclusion

Conventional treatment for IBD focuses on induction or maintenance of remission and symptom management primarily through medication administration. No therapy is curative. The physical and psychological effects of this chronic disease have an enduring impact on HRQOL and may be refractory to treatment. Conventional treatment may have untoward health effects. Parents and patients may seek opportunities to gain a sense of control over the child's disease and therefore may seek out CAM.

Clinicians ought to appreciate the prevalence of CAM utilization in the pediatric IBD population, parent's receptivity toward these modalities as adjuvant therapies, and the reticence to disclose utilization. Concurrent use of biologically based CAM, such as herbals and supplements, and prescription medication is common and may cause untoward drug interactions. While the survey literature on IBD CAM prevalence rates is robust, there is a dearth of high-quality studies assessing safety and efficacy of these modalities. Randomized controlled trials are infrequently employed. The methodologic quality of small pilot studies limits extrapolation of study conclusions. Evidence to support the use of biologically based therapies is still lacking. Stronger randomized control trials are needed in pediatrics to support their use.

Pediatric gastroenterologists should routinely inquire about CAM use and maintain open, nonjudgmental channels of communication about modality use. The maintenance of a cursory level of understanding and awareness of CAM modalities, including knowledge of efficacy, interactions, and contraindications, is essential to ensure patient safety.

References

1. Birdee GS, Phillips RS, Davis RB, Gardiner P. Factors associated with pediatric use of complementary and alternative medicine. Pediatrics. 2010;125:249–56.
2. Hilsden RJ, Verhoef MJ, Rasmussen H, Porcino A, DeBruyn JCC. Use of complementary and alternative medicine by patients with inflammatory bowel disease. Inflamm Bowel Dis. 2011;17:655–62.
3. Rawsthorne P et al. An international survey of the use and attitudes regarding alternative medicine by patients with inflammatory bowel disease. Am J Gastroenterol. 1999;94:1298–303.
4. Hung A, Kang N, Bollom A, Wolf JL, Lembo A. Complementary and alternative medicine use is prevalent among patients with gastrointestinal diseases. Dig Dis Sci. 2015;60:1883–8.
5. Wong AP et al. Use of complementary medicine in pediatric patients with inflammatory bowel disease: results from a multicenter survey. J Pediatr Gastroenterol Nutr. 2009;48:55–60.
6. Markowitz JE et al. Patterns of complementary and alternative medicine use in a population of pediatric patients with inflammatory bowel disease. Inflamm Bowel Dis. 2004;10:599–605.
7. Langhorst J et al. Patterns of complementary and alternative medicine (CAM) use in patients with inflammatory bowel disease: perceived stress is a potential indicator for CAM use. Complement Ther Med. 2007;15:30–7.
8. Heuschkel R et al. Complementary medicine use in children and young adults with inflammatory bowel disease. Am J Gastroenterol. 2002;97:382–8.
9. Surette S, Vanderjagt L, Vohra S. Surveys of complementary and alternative medicine usage: A scoping study of the paediatric literature. Complement Ther Med. 2013;21:S48–53.
10. Barnes PM, Powell-Griner E, McFann K, Nahin RL. Complementary and alternative medicine use among adults: United States (Number 343). Advance Data from Vital and Health Statistics. 2004;343:1–19.
11. Gerasimidis K, McGrogan P, Hassan K, Edwards CA. Dietary modifications, nutritional supplements and alternative medicine in paediatric patients with inflammatory bowel disease. Aliment Pharmacol Ther. 2008;27:155–65.
12. Ceballos C et al. Complementary and alternative medicine use at a single pediatric inflammatory bowel disease center. Gastroenterol Nurs. 2014;37:265–71.
13. Day AS, Whitten KE, Bohane TD. Use of complementary and alternative medicines by children and adolescents with inflammatory bowel disease. J Paediatr Child Health. 2004;40:681–4.
14. Nousiainen P, Merras-Salmio L, Aalto K, Kolho K. Complementary and alternative medicine use in adolescents with inflammatory bowel disease and juvenile idiopathic arthritis. BMC Complement Altern Med. 2014;14:124.
15. Hilsden RJ, Meddings JB, Verhoef MJ. Complementary and alternative medicine use by patients with inflammatory bowel disease: An Internet survey. Can J Gastroenterol. 1999;13:327–32.
16. Hilsden RJ, Scott CM, Verhoef MJ. Complementary medicine use by patients with inflammatory bowel disease. Am J Gastroenterol. 1998;93:697–701.
17. Cotton S et al. Mind-body complementary alternative medicine use and quality of life in adolescents with inflammatory bowel disease. Inflamm Bowel Dis. 2010;16:501–6.
18. Otley AR, Verhoef MJ, Best A, Hilsden RJ. Prevalence and determinants of use of complementary and alternative medicine in a Canadian pediatric inflammatory bowel disease (IBD) population. Gastroenterology. 2001;120:A213
19. Levenstein S et al. Stress and exacerbation in ulcerative colitis: a prospective study of patients enrolled in remission. Am J Gastroenterol. 2000;95:1213–20.
20. Farhadi A et al. Heightened responses to stressors in patients with inflammatory bowel disease. Am J Gastroenterol. 2005;100:1796–804.
21. Anton PA. Stress and mind-body impact on the course of inflammatory bowel diseases. Semin Gastrointest Dis. 1999;10:14–9.
22. Langmead L et al. Randomized, double-blind, placebo-controlled trial of oral aloe vera gel for active ulcerative colitis. Aliment Pharmacol Ther. 2004;19:739–47.
23. Ben-Arye E et al. Wheat grass juice in the treatment of active distal ulcerative colitis: a randomized double-blind placebo-controlled trial. Scand J Gastroenterol. 2002;37:444–9.
24. Tang T et al. Randomised clinical trial: herbal extract HMPL-004 in active ulcerative colitis - a double-blind comparison with sustained release mesalazine. Aliment Pharmacol Ther. 2011;33:194–202.
25. Sandborn WJ et al. Andrographis paniculata extract (HMPL-004) for active ulcerative colitis. Am J Gastroenterol. 2013;108:90–8.
26. Chen ZS, Nie ZW, Sun QL. Clinical study in treating intractable ulcerative colitis with traditional Chinese medicine. Zhongguo Zhong Xi Yi Jie He Za Zhi. 1994;14:400–2.
27. Chen Q, Zhang H. Clinical study on 118 cases of ulcerative colitis treated by integration of traditional Chinese and Western medicine. J Tradit Chin Med. 1999;19:163–5.
28. Ng SC et al. Systematic review: the efficacy of herbal therapy in inflammatory bowel disease. Aliment Pharmacol Ther. 2013;38:854–63.
29. Triantafyllidi A, Xanthos T, Papalois A, Triantafillidis J. Herbal and Plant therapy in patients with inflammatory bowel disease. Ann Gastroenterol. 2015;28:210–20.
30. Greenfield SM et al. A randomized controlled study of evening primrose oil and fish oil in ulcerative colitis. Aliment Pharmacol Ther. 1993;7:159–66.

31. Hanai H et al. Curcumin maintenance therapy for ulcerative colitis: randomized, multicenter, double-blind, placebo-controlled trial. Clin Gastroenterol Hepatol Off Clin Pract J Am Gastroenterol Assoc. 2006;4:1502–6.

32. Lang A et al. Curcumin in combination with 5-aminosalycilate induces remission in patients with mild to moderate ulcerative colitis in a randomized controlled trial. Clin Gastroenterol Hepatol. 2015;1–7. doi:10.1016/j.cgh.2015.02.019.

33. Holt PR, Katz S, Kirshoff R. Curcumin therapy in inflammatory bowel disease: A pilot study. Dig Dis Sci. 2005;50:2191–3.

34. Suskind DL et al. Tolerability of curcumin in pediatric inflammatory bowel disease: a forced-dose titration study. J Pediatr Gastroenterol Nutr. 2013;56:277–9.

35. Gupta I et al. Effects of gum resin of Boswellia serrata in patients with chronic colitis. Planta Med. 2001;67:391–5.

36. Gerhardt H, Seifert F, Buvari P, Vogelsang H, Repges R. Therapy of active Crohn disease with Boswellia serrata extract H 15. Z Gastroenterol. 2001;39:11–7.

37. Holtmeier W et al. Randomized, placebo-controlled, double-blind trial of Boswellia serrata in maintaining remission of Crohn's disease. Inflamm Bowel Dis. 2011;17:573–82.

38. Omer B, Krebs S, Omer H, Noor TO. Steroid-sparing effect of wormwood (Artemisia absinthium) in Crohn's disease: a double-blind placebo-controlled study. Phytomedicine. 2007;14:87–95.

39. Krebs S, Omer TN, Omer B. Wormwood (Artemisia absinthium) suppresses tumour necrosis factor alpha and accelerates healing in patients with Crohn's disease - a controlled clinical trial. Phytomedicine. 2010;17:305–9.

40. Ren J, Tao Q, Wang X, Wang Z, Li J. Efficacy of T2 in active Crohn's disease: a prospective study report. Dig Dis Sci. 2007;52:1790–7.

41. Tao Q et al. Maintenance effect of polyglycosides of Tripterygium wilfordii on remission in postoperative Crohn disease. Zhonghua Wei Chang Wai Ke Za Zhi. 2009;12:491–3.

42. Liao N et al. Efficacy of polyglycosides of Tripterygium wilfordii in preventing postoperative recurrence of Crohn disease. Zhonghua Wei Chang Wai Ke Za Zhi. 2009;12:167–9.

43. Lal S et al. Cannabis use amongst patients with inflammatory bowel disease. Eur J Gastroenterol Hepatol. 2011;23:891–6.

44. Izzo AA, Camilleri M. Emerging role of cannabinoids in gastrointestinal and liver diseases: basic and clinical aspects. Gut. 2008;57:1140–55.

45. Izzo AA, Sharkey KA. Cannabinoids and the gut: New developments and emerging concepts. Pharmacol Ther. 2010;126:21–38.

46. Borrelli F et al. Beneficial effect of the non-psychotropic plant cannabinoid cannabigerol on experimental inflammatory bowel disease. Biochem Pharmacol. 2013;85:1306–16.

47. Naftali T et al. Treatment of Crohn's disease with cannabis: an observational study. Isr Med Assoc J. 2011;13:455–8.

48. Naftali T et al. Cannabis induces a clinical response in patients with Crohn's disease: a prospective placebo-controlled study. Clin Gastroenterol Hepatol. 2013;11:1276–1280.e1.

49. Feagan BG et al. Omega-3 free fatty acids for the maintenance of remission in Crohn disease: the EPIC Randomized Controlled Trials. JAMA. 2008;299:1690–7.

50. Fernández-Bañares F et al. Randomized clinical trial of Plantago ovata seeds (Dietary fiber) as compared with mesalamine in maintaining remission in ulcerative colitis. Am J Gastroenterol. 1999;94:427–33.

51. Salvatore S et al. A pilot study of N-acetyl glucosamine, a nutritional substrate for glycosaminoglycan synthesis, in paediatric chronic inflammatory bowel disease. Aliment Pharmacol Ther. 2000;14:1567–79.

52. Tsujikawa T et al. Supplement of a chitosan and ascorbic acid mixture for Crohn's disease: a pilot study. Nutrition. 2003;19:137–9.

53. Onken JE, Greer PK, Calingaert B, Hale LP. Bromelain treatment decreases secretion of pro-inflammatory cytokines and chemokines by colon biopsies in vitro. Clin Immunol. 2008;126:345–52.

54. Kane S, Goldberg M. Use of bromelain for mild ulcerative colitis. Ann Intern Med. 2000;132:680.

55. Wang B, Ren S, Fend W, Zhong Z, Qin C. Kui jie qing in the treatment of chronic non-specific ulcerative colitis. J Tradit Chin Med. 1997;17:10–3.

56. Zhang F, Li Y, Xu F, Chu Y, Zhao W. Comparison of Xilei-san, a Chinese herbal medicine, and dexamethasone in mild/moderate ulcerative proctitis: a double-blind randomized clinical trial. J Altern Complement Med. 2013;19:838–42.

57. Fukunaga K et al. Placebo controlled evaluation of Xilei San, a herbal preparation in patients with intractable ulcerative proctitis. J Gastroenterol Hepatol. 2012;27:1808–15.

58. Khan Z et al. Use of the 'nutriceutical', bovine colostrum, for the treatment of distal colitis: results from an initial study. Aliment Pharmacol Ther. 2002;16:1917–22.

Management of Intra-abdominal Complications of Inflammatory Bowel Disease

Elizabeth C. Maxwell, Peter Mattei,
and Andrew B. Grossman

Introduction

While the initial phenotype of Crohn disease (CD) is most commonly inflammatory in pediatric patients, the pathogenesis is characterized by transmural inflammation, which can lead to complications such as fistulae, bowel perforation, and intra-abdominal and pelvic abscesses. This chapter will describe the evaluation for patients with suspected intra-abdominal complications of CD and considerations for management, with a focus on intra-abdominal and pelvic abscess resulting from internal penetrating disease. In particular, medical and surgical options for treatment will be compared. Surgical emergencies and elective procedures in CD for the indications of perforation, obstruction, and stricture are discussed in more detail in Chap. 41. The approach for managing penetrating perianal disease is covered in Chap. 36. Surgical treatment of ulcerative colitis (UC) is the focus of Chap. 42, but the complication of toxic megacolon will also be described here.

Intra-abdominal and Pelvic Abscess

It is estimated that 10–28% of patients with CD will develop intra-abdominal or pelvic abscess, and in some patients, abscess is part of the initial disease presentation [1]. Once recognized, the key principles of treatment are source control of the infection and, if possible, drainage. Traditionally, intra-abdominal and pelvic abscesses were treated with surgical drainage, often involving bowel resection and creation of an ostomy (either temporary or permanent) in an acutely ill patient [1]. More recent evidence has shown that antibiotics and percutaneous drainage, if feasible, may have a more favorable outcome compared to surgery as initial therapy, though this issue continues to be debated. Other treatment considerations include the role of disease-specific medical therapies to control underlying inflammatory disease in the setting of active infection and how to best optimize nutritional status in these patients.

Pathogenesis

Abscesses tend to form in dependent areas including the paracolic gutters, pelvis, subdiaphragmatic region, and in-between loops of bowel [1]. Figure 40.1 illustrates the progression from mucosal ulceration to penetrating disease with abscess formation. Alternatively, abscesses can also be formed via hematologic seeding from a remote section of diseased bowel or from contamination at the time of bowel surgery [1]. Approximately half of CD-related abscesses are spontaneous and half result after bowel surgery [1]. Culture from pelvic and intra-abdominal abscesses may not always be obtained, but one report found that at least 80% of abscesses are comprised of mixed bacterial pathogens [1]. They may also be sterile and may contain fungal organisms, particularly in the case of immunosuppressed patients and in the setting of chronic abscess [1].

Evaluation

The most common presenting symptoms and signs in patients with internal penetrating disease include abdominal pain (84%), fever (49%), nausea and vomiting (41%), diarrhea (25%), and presence of a fistula (14%) [2]. There may also be features of partial bowel obstruction, including a colicky nature of the pain, vomiting, abdominal distention, and/or

E.C. Maxwell, MD (✉) • A.B. Grossman, MD
Division of Gastroenterology, Hepatology, and Nutrition,
The Children's Hospital of Philadelphia, 3401 Civic Center
Boulevard, Philadelphia, PA 19104, USA
e-mail: maxwelle@email.chop.edu

P. Mattei, MD
Division of General, Thoracic and Fetal Surgery,
The Children's Hospital of Phladelphia, 3401 Civic
Center Boulevard, Philadelphia, PA, USA

© Springer International Publishing AG 2017
P. Mamula et al. (eds.), *Pediatric Inflammatory Bowel Disease*, DOI 10.1007/978-3-319-49215-5_40

Fig. 40.1 Proposed mechanism of pathogenesis of internal penetrating Crohn disease (Adapted from Pfefferkorn et al. [2])

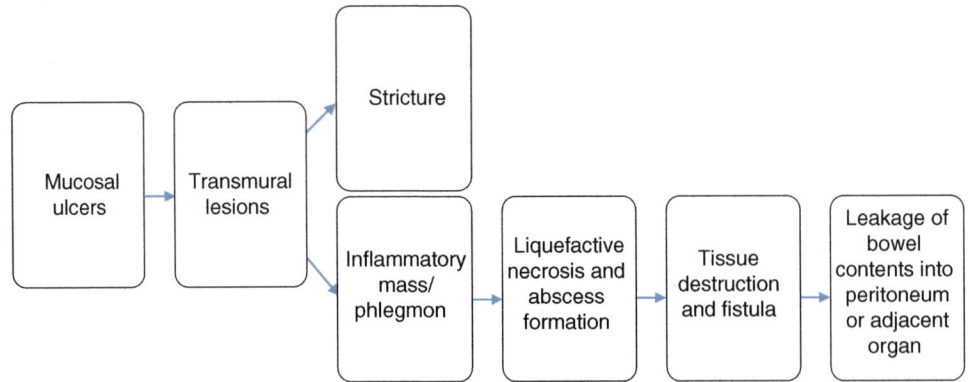

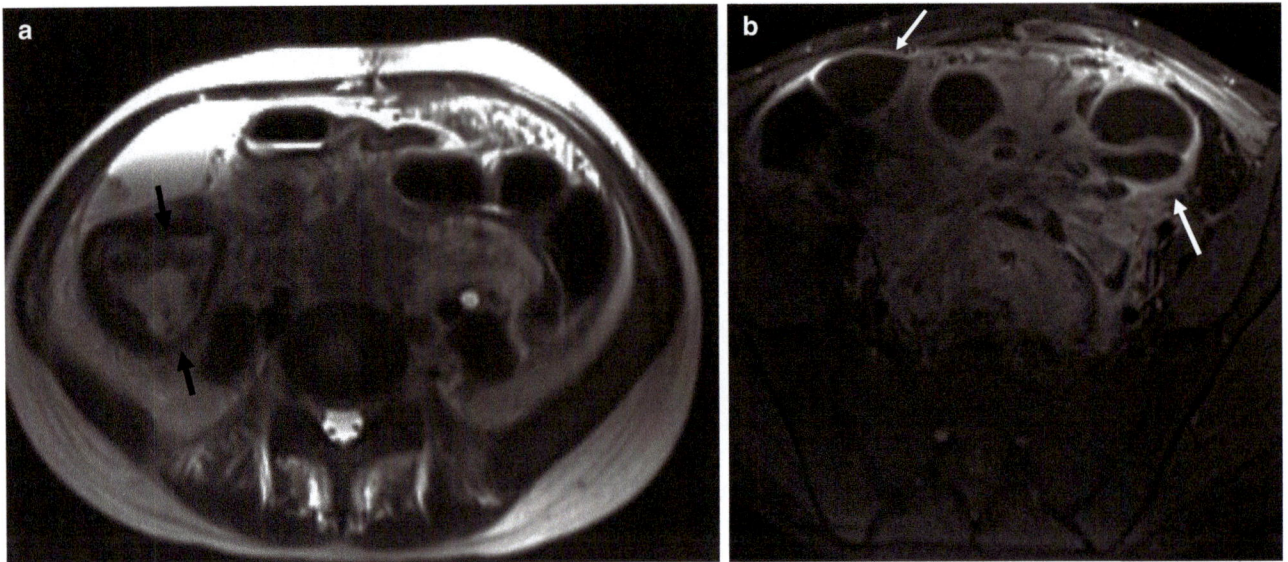

Fig. 40.2 15-year-old female with history of Crohn disease initially worked up at an outside hospital presenting with prolonged IBD flare and significant weight loss. (**a**) Axial T2-weighted HASTE sequence from an MR enterography shows marked thickening of the cecum in the right upper quadrant (*arrows*). (**b**) Axial post-contrast T1-weighted image shows marked enhancement and thickening of other segments of the colon in the right and left abdomen (*arrows*) (Images courtesy of Sudha Anupindi MD, The Children's Hospital of Philadelphia)

intermittent constipation [3]. Additional symptoms may be present depending on the nature and location of the abscess. The right lower quadrant is the most common location of abscess, followed by the pelvis [4]. If an abscess is adjacent to the bladder, a patient may have urinary symptoms, while local irritation of the psoas muscle from an abscess in the distal ileal region can present as refusal to walk or bear weight [2].

Physical examination may demonstrate localized tenderness and an abdominal mass may be palpable. Peritoneal signs such as rebound tenderness and involuntary guarding may also be present. Abscess in the right lower quadrant secondary to ileal disease can be difficult to distinguish from acute appendicitis on physical examination. Pelvic abscess may be palpable as a tender bulge on rectal exam. In a patient with known CD, development of intra-abdominal abscess may also be coupled with other signs of active disease, such as poor growth or weight loss, extraintestinal manifestations including oral ulcers or arthritis, or perianal findings such as tags or fistulae [2].

Laboratory evaluation will not be specific for an intra-abdominal process, but there may be abnormalities in complete blood count (leukocytosis, anemia, thrombocytosis), complete metabolic panel (electrolyte disturbances, hypoalbuminemia), and elevation of C-reactive protein and/or erythrocyte sedimentation rate. It can be useful to compare these values to previous results to establish a trend or deterioration from a patient's baseline. In patients with abdominal pain and vomiting, liver and pancreatic enzymes should be investigated, and urinalysis and urine culture should be obtained in any patient with urinary symptoms. Blood cultures should be obtained in any febrile and acutely ill-appearing patient [2].

Cross-sectional imaging is a key component in the evaluation of patients with a suspected intra-abdominal complication of CD [2]. Magnetic resonance enterography (MRE) is often considered the optimal imaging modality in pediatrics because it is radiation-sparing (Fig. 40.2). However, in the acutely ill child, standard computed

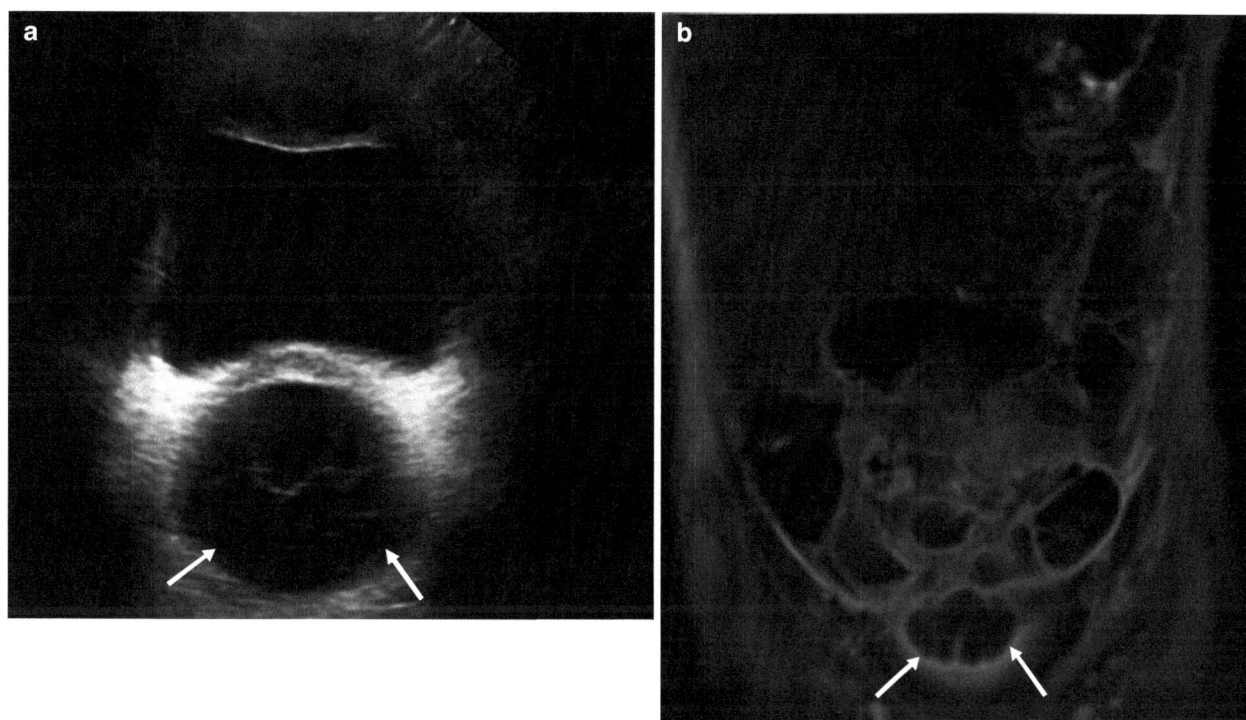

Fig. 40.3 15-year-old female with history of Crohn disease presenting with prolonged symptoms and significant weight loss. (**a**) Transverse ultrasound image shows a complex collection (*arrows*) representing an abscess in the pelvis behind the bladder. (**b**) The same abscess is seen on the correlative coronal post-contrast T1-weighted image from an MR enterography (*arrows*) (Images courtesy of Sudha Anupindi MD, The Children's Hospital of Philadelphia)

tomography (CT) may be the most readily available option [5]. Cross-sectional imaging is able to demonstrate bowel wall thickening, bowel dilation, and mesenteric fat proliferation. Both CT and MR can detect presence of fistulae, particularly if utilizing oral contrast and performing full MRE or CT enterography (CTE) [2]. Bowel ultrasound (US), which is also radiation-sparing, can be useful in certain clinical scenarios as well, particularly serial monitoring for improvement or disease progression as well as detection of phlegmon or intra-abdominal abscess if performed and interpreted by an experienced team (Fig. 40.3) [5]. The administration of enteral contrast may improve the quality of bowel US [6]. US can be limited by bowel gas, which is not an issue with CT or MR [2]. Lastly, magnetic resonance imaging (MRI) of the pelvis is usually the modality of choice to evaluate complicated perianal disease [7]. One challenge is successfully being able to distinguish a phlegmon, which is an inflammatory mass, from a pus-filled abscess cavity, particularly in cases of extensive bowel inflammation. CT, MR, and ultrasound may allow for this differentiation using presence of gas, fluid, and/or color Doppler signals, though without these clear features, discerning abscess and phlegmon can be difficult in practice [8]. This can be a clinically critical delineation, as phlegmons cannot usually be drained, while drainage is a mainstay of abscess treatment, as described later in this chapter.

The role of endoscopy in the evaluation of intra-abdominal abscess has not been well defined in the literature. In general, endoscopy can be useful to better define overall disease activity and assess for infectious complications of disease or immunosuppression, such as cytomegalovirus, and may provide guidance for overall disease management, particularly when surgery is being considered [2]. However, there is concern regarding higher rate of complication of endoscopic assessment in the setting of an active abscess secondary to penetrating disease. Optimal timing of endoscopy following treatment of intra-abdominal abscess is also debated, with most sources citing a window of 4–6 weeks after therapy as the ideal interval [1].

Antimicrobial Therapy

Antimicrobial coverage is indicated in all cases of intra-abdominal and pelvic abscess and is aimed at enteric gram-negative aerobic and facultative bacilli, enteric gram-positive *streptococci*, and obligate anaerobic bacilli [1]. Coverage should also target nosocomial pathogens, as many patients with CD and abscess will have had multiple exposures to the healthcare system [2]. Initial broad-spectrum options include a carbapenem, a B-lactam/B-lactamase inhibitor combination, or an advanced-generation cephalosporin, plus metronidazole [2]. Narrowing of coverage may be possible if abscess material is obtained for culture and sensitivity. Consulting with an infectious disease specialist can provide additional guidance related to local resistance patterns and other special considerations such as recent antibiotic exposure [2].

Route of administration of antimicrobials has not been directly compared in the literature, but the decision regarding parenteral versus oral antibiotics is usually determined based on the clinical course and severity [1]. Duration of therapy depends primarily on the ability to successfully drain the collection. Antibiotics are usually continued for 3–7 days after successful drainage [9]. Longer courses are required if the abscess cannot be drained adequately [1].

Some adult studies have shown that antibiotics alone, without percutaneous or operative drainage, can be successful in the treatment of CD-related intra-abdominal abscesses. Cases that may be more likely to respond to medical management alone include abscesses of small size (<3 cm), absence of associated fistula(e), and patients who are immunomodulator-naïve [10–13]. Despite these described associations in several studies, there are not clear indications for which patients will respond to this approach [1]. The recurrence rate after medical treatment for intra-abdominal abscess in CD ranges from 37 to 50% [1].

Percutaneous Interventional Drainage

Percutaneous abscess drainage is performed by positioning a catheter or drain into the abscess cavity guided by imaging techniques such as ultrasound or CT scan [10]. In the past, this technique was avoided because of the perceived risk of creating a post-drainage enterocutaneous fistula, but more recent studies have shown favorable results in certain clinical scenarios [2], particularly since the advent of biologic therapies to treat CD [1]. It is done in conjunction with antibiotics and can either serve as definitive therapy or as an intended bridge therapy prior to a surgical procedure [10]. There are also cases of failure of percutaneous drainage to fully treat the abscess where eventual surgery is required [10].

Factors related to success of percutaneous drainage have been described to include abscess size, number, etiology, location, presence of fistula, and proximity to vital structures (10), though studies have shown mixed results when analyzing these variables. In general, a unilocular, well-defined cavity, >2–3 centimeters in size, without direct contact with major vessels or organs, is most likely to be successfully drained [14]. The expectation is that clinical improvement should be seen within 3–5 days after drain placement, with decreasing volumes of drainage [10]. When drainage decreases to <10 mL/day (5 mL/day in neonates), and the patient is clinically improved, the drain can be removed [2, 15]. If clinical improvement is not seen, reimaging is indicated to reassess if abscess has been drained adequately. If it has not, repositioning of the drain or plan for surgical intervention usually follows [10].

Persistent drainage raises the concern for fistula formation, in which case an abscessogram can be performed using injected contrast [2]. Studies examining continued treatment with the percutaneous drain combined with medical therapy, bowel rest, and parenteral nutrition have reported varying success in addressing these fistulae [16–18].

Rypens and colleagues published a retrospective series of 14 pediatric patients with CD and intra-abdominal or pelvic abscess who underwent percutaneous abscess drainage as an initial intervention. All but two patients eventually had the affected bowel segment resected, though the authors indicated definitive surgical management was the preferred therapy at their institution; thus, percutaneous drainage had not been intended to be definitive therapy. They concluded that, following the percutaneous drainage, the patients had improved clinical status prior to surgery, which was thought to contribute to a less invasive and technically easier surgical procedure [19]. Other studies, which were not designed to examine this exact question, have shown reduced postoperative complications in patients who have percutaneous drainage preoperatively [20–22].

Percutaneous drainage is a relatively safe procedure [14]. Complications have been reported in approximately 5–11% of cases and include sepsis, small bowel fistulae, colon perforation, and death [14, 19]. Minor complications such as bacteremia or infection at the catheter site have been reported in about 3% of cases [14].

Surgical Intervention

Traditionally, surgical drainage had been the primary treatment option for intra-abdominal abscesses in CD [10]. Surgical drainage of intra-abdominal or pelvic abscess involves exploration of the region, evacuation of all abscess contents, irrigation and debridement of the abscess cavity, and commonly resection of the affected bowel [1]. Importantly, surgical resection of diseased bowel is not considered curative in Crohn disease as postoperative recurrence of disease, particularly at the surgical anastomosis, is common. Surgical drainage can be associated with significant morbidity, particularly as it is performed in ill patients. Potential complications include wound infections, small bowel fistulae, and anastomotic leakage [10]. Often ostomy creation is indicated or cannot be avoided [10].

As will be discussed in more detail in the following section, surgical intervention may be necessary when medical and percutaneous drainage measures are unsuccessful in achieving abscess resolution and, in some cases, may be the primary intervention selected along with antimicrobial therapy and CD-specific treatment, based on a variety of factors [2]. General principles of surgical management include preservation of intestinal length and resection with macroscopically disease-free margins [2]. Laparoscopy has become the preferred approach over time due to the benefits of shorter postoperative recovery time, decreased wound-related complications, formation of fewer intra-abdominal adhesions, and better cosmesis when compared to an open approach [23]. Laparotomy, however, is still considered a safe and reasonable approach in patients who cannot tolerate or have too many adhesions from prior surgery to allow the insufflation of the abdomen with carbon dioxide needed for laparoscopy [2]. Diverting ileostomy or colostomy may be necessary when there is significant intra-abdominal soilage, inflammatory thickening of the intestinal wall, and intraoperative instability precluding safe additional operating time to construct an anastomosis [2]. Ostomy creation may be temporary.

Complication rates vary in the literature but have been reported to be as high as 25% [24] and may be influenced by several factors, including preoperative percutaneous drainage, discussed in more detail in the next section. Otherwise, weight loss, number of structures involved in the inflammatory mass, peritonitis and free air, smoking, and previous intestinal surgery have also been associated with postoperative complications [25]. Nutritional status and decreasing steroid dose may reduce surgical complication rates [2] and are discussed in more detail in later sections of this chapter.

Percutaneous Versus Surgical Drainage

Several studies have retrospectively analyzed outcomes of percutaneous drainage compared to surgical drainage of intra-abdominal abscesses in CD [10]. Consistent conclusions are difficult to draw, however, given the mostly retrospective nature, mixed results, and small sample sizes. The decision regarding initial intervention therefore continues to be a challenging one, and treatment strategy for each individual patient continues to be based on patient factors and experience and practice patterns of the treating physicians and institutions.

To address the question of efficacy, the most recent and comprehensive assessment of prior retrospective studies is a meta-analysis by He and colleagues published in 2015. The authors compared clinical outcomes between percutaneous drainage (with or without further elective surgery) and initial surgery in adult patients with CD-related intra-abdominal abscesses [26]. Nine studies involving a total of 513 patients were included. In five studies, percutaneous drainage was used as a definitive therapy and compared to initial surgical management; four of the studies compared surgical outcomes in those patients who first underwent preoperative percutaneous drainage and those who did not. When initial percutaneous drainage was compared to surgery, there were no significant differences between groups regarding patient sex, previous abdominal surgery, abscess location, single or multiple abscesses, abscess size, perioperative immunomodulator or steroid use, or length of follow-up period.

While several previous studies have indicated success with percutaneous drainage as definitive management of intra-abdominal abscesses [27–30], this larger meta-analysis found that over one third of patients treated by percutaneous drainage as the intended definitive therapy did ultimately require surgery [26]. Even when eventual surgery is needed, several studies suggest preoperative percutaneous drainage is beneficial, contributing to less surgical technical difficulty and decreased risk of ostomy creation [1, 19]. Given the multitude of factors contributing to success and risk in both options, there may still be a subset of less ill patients with intra-abdominal abscess who will do quite well with percutaneous drainage. In fact, there were 12 patients identified in one study who successfully underwent percutaneous drainage procedures on an outpatient basis and received oral antibiotics at home [31].

Regarding safety, several studies have reported increased complication rates in patients undergoing surgical drainage compared to percutaneous drainage, specifically longer lengths of stay in the hospital [31] and increased need for ostomy creation [26, 32]. Another study noted fewer postoperative complications in patients who first underwent percutaneous abscess drainage, including anastomotic leaks, postoperative abscess formation, intestinal fistula, leaks of intestinal stumps, and leaks of sutured secondary internal fistulae, though these trends (25% vs. 11% complication rates) did not reach statistical significance [25]. Again, there are potential biases in these analyses as more severe illness and disability may be present in the patients who were treated primarily surgically [31]. In the large recent meta-analysis by He and colleagues, initial surgery was associated with significantly higher overall complication rate compared to initial percutaneous drainage. However, there was no difference in rates of specific complications such as enterocutaneous fistula, wound infection, anastomotic leak, postoperative abscess, and recurrent abscess [26]. There may be some advantages to preoperative percutaneous drainage to decrease overall complications, but data regarding this question was mixed. Four studies showed a decrease in complications when percutaneous drainage was used prior to surgery but three showed comparable complication rates [26].

To date, randomized controlled trials comparing the two approaches are lacking [1, 10]. Several consensus guidelines including the North American Society for Pediatric Gastroenterology, Hepatology, and Nutrition (NASPGHAN) [2] and the American College of Radiology [12, 13] have recommended percutaneous drainage as an initial step, provided it is technically feasible [10]. When abscesses are not amenable to percutaneous drainage because of size or location, or persist despite percutaneous drainage and antimicrobial therapy, surgical drainage is warranted [10].

Treatment of Phlegmon

A phlegmon is an ill-defined inflammatory mass that can form as a result of a sealed-off perforation. Phlegmons in CD typically involve the mesentery and adjacent loops of bowel. Though it is known that penetrating disease affects 40% of CD patients within the first 5 years of diagnosis, there are no specific data related to prevalence of phlegmons [33]. One review of about 350 adult patients with CD who had median duration of disease of about 10 years reported penetrating disease in 20% and phlegmon in 3.4% using CTE [34]. Treatment has traditionally included antibiotics, bowel rest, drainage of an associated abscess collection if present, and eventually surgical resection of the mass. CD-specific medications may also play an important therapeutic role as described in the next section [33]. In the future, radiologic terminology may be moving away from the term "phlegmon" to more illustrative descriptions of findings, such as "inflammatory mass with or without abscess."

Crohn Disease-Specific Therapy

In addition to antimicrobials and drainage of abscess, CD-specific therapy should also be considered as part of the management plan. Aminosalicylates have not been shown to be effective in the treatment of internal penetrating CD, but may be continued if already a component of a patient's maintenance regimen [2]. Corticosteroids should be avoided in the presence of known fistulizing disease because of increased risk of abscess formation [35]. If a patient is already on steroids at the time an abscess is diagnosed, there does not seem to be additional morbidity associated with continuing the steroids if the abscess is otherwise being addressed [1]. Weaning steroids to a lower dose may reduce risk of perioperative complications when surgical intervention is required [24, 36], with some recommending reduction to less than 20 mg daily [2, 20].

There are no randomized prospective clinical trials examining efficacy and safety of biologic agents (infliximab, adalimumab) or immunomodulators (6-mercaptopurine, azathioprine, methotrexate) in the setting of acute abscess in CD. Post hoc analysis of the ACCENT II study explored whether fistula-related abscess formation was impacted by exposure to infliximab; no increased formation of abscess was found in the group treated with infliximab compared to placebo [37]. Nguyen and colleagues examined the role of initiation of anti-TNFα therapy after initial management of intra-abdominal abscess in 95 adult patients, 55 of whom underwent image-guided percutaneous drainage and 40 of whom had laparotomy [31]. In the patients who underwent laparotomy as initial treatment of abscess, 30% were not on any therapy for CD at the time. After treatment for the abscess, treatment with an anti-TNFα agent either alone or in combination with a thiopurine was protective against abscess recurrence compared to no therapy. There is also data in adults to suggest that 30% of fistulas are partially or completely closed on immunomodulator therapy (azathioprine, 6-mercaptopurine, methotrexate), but require ongoing treatment to maintain closure [35, 38]. Taken together, expert opinion based on this adult data indicates that immunomodulators and/or biologic agents can be given soon after drainage of the abscess and are beneficial [1].

Cullen et al. retrospectively described initiation of anti-TNFα therapy following antibiotics in 13 adult patients with CD and abdominal phlegmon [33]. Abscess was detected by imaging in 12 patients initially, but had resolved or was drained prior to initiation of anti-TNFα in all but 5 patients who had small undrainable collections. At a mean of 2.3 years of follow-up, no patients developed infection or new abscess. Two patients eventually had surgery after failure of anti-TNFα therapy, and 10 of the 11 patients who remained on anti-TNFα therapy were asymptomatic at the conclusion of the study. Although this was a small study in adult patients, the results suggest that initiation of anti-TNFα therapy after antibiotics in patients with intestinal phlegmon can be safe and successful [33].

Nutritional Considerations

Nutritional support and rehabilitation are important in all patients with CD, particularly those with complications of the disease and when surgery is being considered. Nutritional status is one of the few modifiable risk factors related to surgical outcomes and should be optimized whenever possible before proceeding to surgery [2]. Historical and daily weights should be obtained and compared and serum albumin and prealbumin monitored. Bowel rest and support with total parental nutrition may be considered until drainage of the abscess can be achieved. Once the abscess is drained without evidence of reaccumulation, enteral feeds can be initiated and are usually tolerated [2]. Presence of an actively flowing fistula may be another indication to select bowel rest over enteral feedings [2]. Some studies, however, have shown a benefit to nutritional rehabilitation with enteral feedings in the setting of internal penetrating disease [21], and exclusive enteral nutrition is a proven therapy to induce remission in CD [39].

Summary

Internal penetrating disease represents a complicated type of CD and leads to several possible complications, including fistulae, phlegmon, and abscess. There are many factors that determine the optimal management approach in each individual patient, including overall clinical status and risk for deterioration, severity of underlying disease, nutritional status, and features of the collection including size and location. Source control of infection using antimicrobial agents and drainage of abscess when possible are the mainstays of therapy. CD-specific therapy and nutritional optimization are also important aspects of management in these patients.

Other Complications from Internal Penetrating CD

Perforation

Spontaneous free perforation of the small intestine in CD is rare, with a quoted prevalence of 1–3% in adult patients with Crohn disease over their disease course [40]. One series of 1000 consecutive adult patients found 15 cases of perforation over the course of 20 years. Spontaneous free perforation was the presenting feature leading to CD diagnosis in 9 of those 15 patients (60%) [41]. An older case series in 1415 adult patients with CD over 23 years found a similar incidence of spontaneous free perforation in 21 (1.5%) patients; this series included ten patients with small bowel perforation, ten with colonic perforation, and one with perforation in both small bowel and colon [42]. There are no large series of pediatric patients with CD and spontaneous intestinal perforation but it has been described in case reports [43]. Perforation is managed operatively, which is urgent in the setting of peritonitis to prevent sepsis. Typically the diseased area of bowel is resected, and primary anastomosis is attempted if deemed safe or a diverting ostomy, which is often temporary, is performed [41].

Small Bowel Obstruction

Fibrostenotic CD usually presents with obstructive symptoms. The most common location for a stricture is the ileocecal region. Obstructive symptoms related to narrowing and stricture formation may be aggravated by superimposed edema from active inflammation [44]. Therefore, a trial of medical management with corticosteroids may be attempted to evaluate whether the obstruction can be relieved without surgery [45]. It was previously thought that preexisting bowel stenosis was a contraindication for therapy with anti-TNFα agents, but further study has demonstrated that some patients with mixed strictures (both fibrotic and inflammatory components) can benefit from infliximab therapy [46–48].

If medical management is unsuccessful, balloon dilation, stricturoplasty, or surgical resection is considered [44]. One large meta-analysis of 13 studies of endoscopic balloon dilation of mostly postsurgical strictures reported a technical success rate of 86% [49]. In that study, long-term clinical efficacy was 58%, with mean follow-up of 33 months and major complication rate of 2%. Short strictures of ≤4 cm were most likely to avoid need for surgery. Stricturoplasty is a surgical intervention which increases bowel diameter without any resection. It is technically feasible for short strictures [44]. Compared to resection, results are comparable when analyzing resolution of obstructive symptoms, reoperation rate, and time to recurrence of symptoms [50]. Stricturoplasty may be performed in conjunction with a bowel resection [50]. Limited resection for stenotic CD is effective in relieving obstruction, but multiple respective bowel surgeries are avoided if possible, to reduce the risk of short bowel syndrome [44].

Toxic Megacolon

Toxic megacolon is a serious complication of inflammatory bowel disease (IBD) and is a syndrome of systemic toxicity and colonic dilation (>6 cm) in the setting of active colitis with high morbidity and mortality. Toxic megacolon is most often seen in IBD patients with UC, though it has been described in Crohn's colitis, as well as other non-IBD entities such as Hirschsprung disease and *Clostridium difficile* infection [51]. Toxic megacolon in pediatric IBD is rare, but the true incidence is not known. A small case-control study of ten pediatric IBD patients with toxic megacolon identified diagnostic features of fever, tachycardia, dehydration, and electrolyte abnormalities to be significantly more common in patients with toxic megacolon compared with hospitalized age-matched controls with UC. Also, a mean luminal transverse colon diameter of ≥56 mm was highly suggestive of toxic megacolon in children. Altered mental status and hypovolemic shock have been described more commonly in adults with toxic megacolon than in pediatric cases [52]. New narcotic requirement in a patient admitted with acute severe colitis can be a red flag sign of evolving toxic megacolon. This and other suggestive symptoms should prompt evaluation of toxic megacolon with an abdominal X-ray (Fig. 40.4).

The goal of treatment of toxic megacolon is to reduce colitis and likelihood of colonic perforation [51]. Immediate surgical consultation should be initiated at the time toxic megacolon is suspected. Medical therapy includes complete bowel rest and NG tube and/or rectal tube for decompression. Patients are frequently monitored in the ICU setting for serial exams, and should have laboratory studies (complete blood count, electrolytes) and abdominal radiographs reviewed every 12 hours, initially. IV corticosteroids can be used to reduce inflammation, and broad-spectrum antibiotics are recommended to decrease risk of septic complications. Anticholinergic and narcotic medications should be

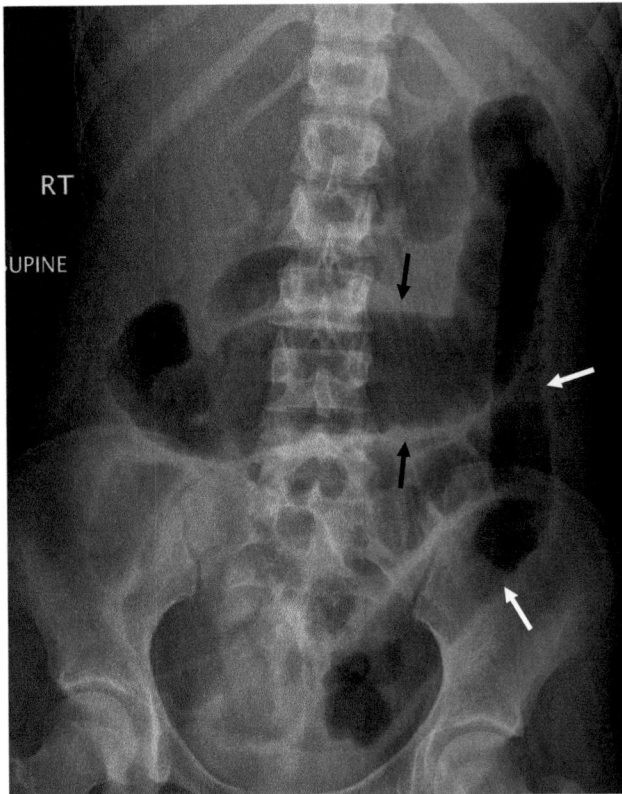

Fig. 40.4 15-year-old female with ulcerative colitis: Supine radiograph of the abdomen shows dilated featureless, ahaustral transverse, and left colon to sigmoid with thumb printing (*white arrows*) indicative of submucosal edema or hemorrhage. In addition the transverse colon is disproportionately dilated suggestive of toxic megacolon (*black arrows*) (Images courtesy of Sudha Anupindi MD, The Children's Hospital of Philadelphia)

discontinued. Resolution of toxic appearance, decreased fluid and transfusion requirement, improvement in colonic dilation and abdominal distention, and improved laboratory derangements are signs that toxic megacolon is resolving. Absolute indications for surgery are free perforation, massive hemorrhage, increasing transfusion requirements, progression of colonic dilation, and/or worsening toxicity. Subtotal colectomy with end ileostomy is the surgical procedure of choice in urgent or emergent situations [51]. There is a paucity of data regarding outcome of toxic megacolon for pediatric inflammatory bowel disease; seven of ten patients in the aforementioned case series underwent colectomy [52].

References

1. Feagins LA, Holubar SD, Kane SV, Spechler SJ. Current strategies in the management of intra-abdominal abscesses in Crohn's disease. Clin Gastroenterol Hepatol. 2011;9(10):842–50.
2. Pfefferkorn MD, Marshalleck FE, Saeed SA, Splawski JB, Linden BC, Weston BF. NASPGHAN clinical report on the evaluation and treatment of pediatric patients with internal penetrating Crohn disease: intraabdominal abscess with and without fistula. J Pediatr Gastroenterol Nutr. 2013;57(3):394–400.
3. Jawhari A, Kamm MA, Ong C, Forbes A, Bartram CI, Hawley PR. Intra-abdominal and pelvic abscess in Crohn's disease: results of noninvasive and surgical management. Br J Surg. 1998;85(3):367–71.
4. Ayuk P, Williams N, Scott NA, Nicholson DA, Irving MH. Management of intra-abdominal abscesses in Crohn's disease. Ann R Coll Surg Engl. 1996;78(1):5–10.
5. Anupindi SA, Grossman AB, Nimkin K, Mamula P, Gee MS. Imaging in the evaluation of the young patient with inflammatory bowel disease: what the gastroenterologist needs to know. J Pediatr Gastroenterol Nutr. 2014;59(4):429–39.
6. Pallotta N, Civitelli F, Di Nardo G, Vincoli G, Aloi M, Viola F, et al. Small intestine contrast ultrasonography in pediatric Crohn's disease. J Pediatr. 2013;163(3):778–84. e1
7. Maltz R, Podberesky DJ, Saeed SA. Imaging modalities in pediatric inflammatory bowel disease. Curr Opin Pediatr. 2014;26(5):590–6.
8. Ripolles T, Martinez-Perez MJ, Paredes JM, Vizuete J, Garcia-Martinez E, Jimenez-Restrepo DH. Contrast-enhanced ultrasound in the differentiation between phlegmon and abscess in Crohn's disease and other abdominal conditions. Eur J Radiol. 2013;82(10):e525–31.
9. Solomkin JS, Mazuski JE, Bradley JS, Rodvold KA, Goldstein EJ, Baron EJ, et al. Diagnosis and management of complicated intra-abdominal infection in adults and children: guidelines by the Surgical Infection Society and the Infectious Diseases Society of America. Clin Infect Dis. 2010;50(2):133–64.
10. de Groof EJ, Carbonnel F, Buskens CJ, Bemelman WA. Abdominal abscess in Crohn's disease: multidisciplinary management. Dig Dis. 2014;32(Suppl 1):103–9.
11. Bermejo F, Garrido E, Chaparro M, Gordillo J, Manosa M, Algaba A, et al. Efficacy of different therapeutic options for spontaneous abdominal abscesses in Crohn's disease: are antibiotics enough? Inflamm Bowel Dis. 2012;18(8):1509–14.
12. Lorenz JM, Funaki BS, Ray Jr CE, Brown DB, Gemery JM, Greene FL, et al. ACR Appropriateness Criteria on percutaneous catheter drainage of infected fluid collections. J Am Coll Radiol. 2009;6(12):837–43.
13. Kumar RR, Kim JT, Haukoos JS, Macias LH, Dixon MR, Stamos MJ, et al. Factors affecting the successful management of intra-abdominal abscesses with antibiotics and the need for percutaneous drainage. Dis Colon Rectum. 2006;49(2):183–9.
14. Golfieri R, Cappelli A. Computed tomography-guided percutaneous abscess drainage in coloproctology: review of the literature. Tech Coloproctol. 2007;11(3):197–208.
15. Hogan MJ, Hoffer FA. Biopsy and drainage techniques in children. Tech Vasc Interv Radiol. 2010;13(4):206–13.
16. Gervais DA, Hahn PF, O'Neill MJ, Mueller PR. Percutaneous abscess drainage in Crohn disease: technical success and short- and long-term outcomes during 14 years. Radiology. 2002;222(3):645–51.
17. Schuster MR, Crummy AB, Wojtowycz MM, McDermott JC. Abdominal abscesses associated with enteric fistulas: percutaneous management. J Vasc Interv Radiol. 1992;3(2):359–63.
18. LaBerge JM, Kerlan Jr RK, Gordon RL, Ring EJ. Nonoperative treatment of enteric fistulas: results in 53 patients. J Vasc Interv Radiol. 1992;3(2):353–7.
19. Rypens F, Dubois J, Garel L, Deslandres C, Saint-Vil D. Percutaneous drainage of abdominal abscesses in pediatric Crohn's disease. AJR Am J Roentgenol. 2007;188(2):579–85.
20. Alves A, Panis Y, Bouhnik Y, Pocard M, Vicaut E, Valleur P. Risk factors for intra-abdominal septic complications after a first ileocecal resection for Crohn's disease: a multivariate analysis in 161 consecutive patients. Dis Colon Rectum. 2007;50(3):331–6.

21. Smedh K, Andersson M, Johansson H, Hagberg T. Preoperative management is more important than choice of sutured or stapled anastomosis in Crohn's disease. Eur J Surg. 2002;168(3):154–7.

22. Goyer P, Alves A, Bretagnol F, Bouhnik Y, Valleur P, Panis Y. Impact of complex Crohn's disease on the outcome of laparoscopic ileocecal resection: a comparative clinical study in 124 patients. Dis Colon Rectum. 2009;52(2):205–10.

23. Laituri CA, Fraser JD, Garey CL, Aguayo P, Sharp SW, Ostlie DJ, et al. Laparoscopic ileocecectomy in pediatric patients with Crohn's disease. J Laparoendosc Adv Surg Tech A. 2011;21(2):193–5.

24. Yamamoto T, Bain IM, Mylonakis E, Allan RN, Keighley MR. Stapled functional end-to-end anastomosis versus sutured end-to-end anastomosis after ileocolonic resection in Crohn disease. Scand J Gastroenterol. 1999;34(7):708–13.

25. Iesalnieks I, Kilger A, Glass H, Obermeier F, Agha A, Schlitt HJ. Perforating Crohn's ileitis: delay of surgery is associated with inferior postoperative outcome. Inflamm Bowel Dis. 2010;16(12): 2125–30.

26. He X, Lin X, Lian L, Huang J, Yao Q, Chen Z, et al. Preoperative Percutaneous Drainage of Spontaneous Intra-Abdominal Abscess in Patients With Crohn's Disease: A Meta-Analysis. J Clin Gastroenterol. 2015;49(9):e82–90.

27. Casola G. vanSonnenberg E, Neff CC, Saba RM, Withers C, Emarine CW. Abscesses in Crohn disease: percutaneous drainage. Radiology. 1987;163(1):19–22.

28. Sahai A, Belair M, Gianfelice D, Cote S, Gratton J, Lahaie R. Percutaneous drainage of intra-abdominal abscesses in Crohn's disease: short and long-term outcome. Am J Gastroenterol. 1997;92(2): 275–8.

29. Golfieri R, Cappelli A, Giampalma E, Rizzello F, Gionchetti P, Laureti S, et al. CT-guided percutaneous pelvic abscess drainage in Crohn's disease. Tech Coloproctol. 2006;10(2):99–105.

30. Gutierrez A, Lee H, Sands BE. Outcome of surgical versus percutaneous drainage of abdominal and pelvic abscesses in Crohn's disease. Am J Gastroenterol. 2006;101(10):2283–9.

31. Nguyen DL, Sandborn WJ, Loftus Jr EV, Larson DW, Fletcher JG, Becker B, et al. Similar outcomes of surgical and medical treatment of intra-abdominal abscesses in patients with Crohn's disease. Clin Gastroenterol Hepatol. 2012;10(4):400–4.

32. Xie Y, Zhu W, Li N, Li J. The outcome of initial percutaneous drainage versus surgical drainage for intra-abdominal abscesses in Crohn's disease. Int J Colorectal Dis. 2012;27(2):199–206.

33. Cullen G, Vaughn B, Ahmed A, Peppercorn MA, Smith MP, Moss AC, et al. Abdominal phlegmons in Crohn's disease: outcomes following antitumor necrosis factor therapy. Inflamm Bowel Dis. 2012;18(4):691–6.

34. Bruining DH, Siddiki HA, Fletcher JG, Tremaine WJ, Sandborn WJ, Loftus Jr EV. Prevalence of penetrating disease and extraintestinal manifestations of Crohn's disease detected with CT enterography. Inflamm Bowel Dis. 2008;14(12):1701–6.

35. Present DH. Crohn's fistula: current concepts in management. Gastroenterology. 2003;124(6):1629–35.

36. Aberra FN, Lewis JD, Hass D, Rombeau JL, Osborne B, Lichtenstein GR. Corticosteroids and immunomodulators: postoperative infectious complication risk in inflammatory bowel disease patients. Gastroenterology. 2003;125(2):320–7.

37. Sands BE, Blank MA, Diamond RH, Barrett JP, Van Deventer SJ. Maintenance infliximab does not result in increased abscess development in fistulizing Crohn's disease: results from the ACCENT II study. Aliment Pharmacol Ther. 2006;23(8):1127–36.

38. Mahadevan U, Marion JF, Present DH. Fistula response to methotrexate in Crohn's disease: a case series. Aliment Pharmacol Ther. 2003;18(10):1003–8.

39. Griffiths AM. Enteral nutrition in the management of Crohn's disease. JPEN J Parenter Enteral Nutr. 2005;29(4 Suppl):S108–12. discussion S12-7, S84-8

40. Werbin N, Haddad R, Greenberg R, Karin E, Skornick Y. Free perforation in Crohn's disease. Isr Med Assoc J. 2003;5(3):175–7.

41. Freeman HJ, James D, Mahoney CJ. Spontaneous peritonitis from perforation of the colon in collagenous colitis. Can J Gastroenterol. 2001;15(4):265–7.

42. Greenstein AJ, Sachar DB, Mann D, Lachman P, Heimann T, Aufses Jr AH. Spontaneous free perforation and perforated abscess in 30 patients with Crohn's disease. Ann Surg. 1987;205(1):72–6.

43. Kambouri K, Gardikis S, Agelidou M, Vaos G. Local peritonitis as the first manifestation of Crohn's disease in a child. J Indian Assoc Pediatr Surg. 2014;19(2):100–2.

44. Schoepfer AM, Safroneeva E, Vavricka SR, Peyrin-Biroulet L, Mottet C. Treatment of fibrostenotic and fistulizing Crohn's disease. Digestion. 2012;86(Suppl 1):23–7.

45. Sandborn WJ, Feagan BG, Hanauer SB, Lochs H, Lofberg R, Modigliani R, et al. A review of activity indices and efficacy endpoints for clinical trials of medical therapy in adults with Crohn's disease. Gastroenterology. 2002;122(2):512–30.

46. Pelletier AL, Kalisazan B, Wienckiewicz J, Bouarioua N, Soule JC. Infliximab treatment for symptomatic Crohn's disease strictures. Aliment Pharmacol Ther. 2009;29(3):279–85.

47. Louis E, Boverie J, Dewit O, Baert F, De Vos M, D'Haens G, et al. Treatment of small bowel subocclusive Crohn's disease with infliximab: an open pilot study. Acta Gastroenterol Belg. 2007;70(1):15–9.

48. Holtmann M, Wanitschke R, Helisch A, Bartenstein P, Galle PR, Neurath M. Anti-TNF antibodies in the treatment of inflammatory intestinal stenoses in Crohn's disease. Z Gastroenterol. 2003;41(1): 11–7.

49. Hassan C, Zullo A, De Francesco V, Ierardi E, Giustini M, Pitidis A, et al. Systematic review: Endoscopic dilatation in Crohn's disease. Aliment Pharmacol Ther. 2007;26(11–12):1457–64.

50. Dietz DW, Laureti S, Strong SA, Hull TL, Church J, Remzi FH, et al. Safety and longterm efficacy of strictureplasty in 314 patients with obstructing small bowel Crohn's disease. J Am Coll Surg. 2001;192(3):330–7. discussion 7-8.

51. Gan SI, Beck PL. A new look at toxic megacolon: an update and review of incidence, etiology, pathogenesis, and management. Am J Gastroenterol. 2003;98(11):2363–71.

52. Benchimol EI, Turner D, Mann EH, Thomas KE, Gomes T, McLernon RA, et al. Toxic megacolon in children with inflammatory bowel disease: clinical and radiographic characteristics. Am J Gastroenterol. 2008;103(6):1524–31.

Surgical Management of Crohn Disease in Children

Daniel von Allmen

Introduction

Surgery plays an important role in the treatment of Crohn disease. Crohn disease has a major impact on quality of life in the pediatric population [1], and, unfortunately, despite the dramatic improvements in medical therapies, 70–80% of patients who carry the diagnosis of Crohn disease undergo some type of surgical procedure at some point during the course of their disease [2–4]. The indications for surgery have evolved over time with a trend toward less invasive procedures [5] and fewer emergency surgery operations because of an acute complication of the disease. However, the basic role of surgery has not changed. Crohn disease cannot be cured in the operating room so the procedures are primarily employed to treat complications of the disease including obstruction, perforation, and medically refractory disease. Surgery is unavoidable in some cases and the preferred treatment option in many others.

As with many diseases in children, studies specific to the pediatric population are not always available making it necessary to extrapolate the results of adult series when considering treatment options for younger patients. Although some differences between the patient populations exist, the philosophy remains the same. Surgical intervention is an integral part of the management of patients with Crohn disease but should be invoked judiciously to avoid the potential for long-term consequences of multiple bowel resections, and procedures should always be carried out with the long-term potential for short bowel syndrome in mind.

D. von Allmen, MD
Division of Pediatric General and Thoracic Surgery,
Cincinnati Children's Hospital Medical Center, 3333 Burnet
Avenue, ML 2023, Cincinnati, OH 45229, USA
e-mail: Daniel.vonallmen@cchmc.org

History of Surgical Therapy

When Crohn disease was first described in the early 1930s, the disease was thought to be isolated to the terminal ileum [6], and surgical therapy typically involved resection of the terminal ileum with an ileocolic anastomosis. In this era, before the development of antibiotics and sophisticated electrolyte replacement and nutritional support, the mortality for this operation was 25% [7]. In an effort to improve the surgical outcomes and reduce mortality, many surgeons moved to a two-stage approach in which the diseased segment of bowel was bypassed with an ileocolostomy leaving the diseased segment of terminal ileum as a blind pouch emptying into the cecum. Months later the patient was returned to the operating room for resection of the diseased segment. Although this approach required a second trip to the operating room to resect the bypassed segment, surgical mortality was substantially reduced. As experience with this approach increased, it became clear that the bypassed segment often improved and ceased causing problems. Many surgeons subsequently abandoned resection of the diseased segment altogether resulting in a dramatic improvement in surgical mortality. In one study mortality in 145 patients was 16% for one-stage operations, 12% for two-stage operations, and 0% in ileotransverse colostomy with exclusion [8]. Unfortunately, it became apparent that there were long-term consequences to bypassing the diseased segment and right side of the colon and leaving it in situ. Function of normal colonic tissue was sacrificed and increased risks of malignant changes in the small bowel were reported [9].

Fortunately, with improvements in perioperative surgical care, the risk of a primary definitive procedure has been reduced to the point where it has once again become the operation of first choice and is associated with extremely low mortality rates.

Operative Indications

The indications for surgical intervention in Crohn disease are varied and often patient specific, especially in children. However, the principles regarding surgical intervention are similar regardless of the age of the patient. The goal of an operation for Crohn disease is to control one of the many mechanical complications resulting from the inflammatory process in the intestine, and there are many clinical situations that warrant consideration of a surgical procedure during the course of a child's disease (Table 41.1). The timing, indications, and operative procedure performed vary considerably based on the segment of intestine involved and the specific complication being addressed. The distribution of disease in the pediatric patients has been examined in a large cohort of European children. In that study combined ileocolonic disease was found in 53% of patients followed by isolated colonic disease in 27% and limited cecal disease in 16% (Fig. 41.1) [10].

Isolated Crohn disease of the foregut is relatively rare [11] and rarely requires surgical intervention. In contrast, terminal ileal and colonic disease account for the vast major-

ity of surgical interventions in the pediatric patient. Some require urgent operation, while most are more elective in nature. The most common complications leading to a surgical intervention are obstruction, abscesses, fistulas, and failure or intolerance of pharmacological treatment [12–14].

The indications for surgery have evolved somewhat as medical treatments have improved. A study examining surgical indications in the period from 1970 to 1990 compared to the period from 1991 to 1997 revealed that active disease as an indication for surgery decreased from 64 to 25% of cases, while chronic stricture increased from 9 to 50% of cases. In addition, the time from diagnosis to initial operation increased from 3.5 to 11.5 years [15] suggesting that medical therapy has been successful in altering the course of disease but not necessarily preventing ultimate progression in many cases. Fortunately, the shift to less emergent operation likely reduces the morbidity associated with a surgical intervention.

Absolute indications for surgery are rare, and many patients present with multiple relative indications rather than an acute precipitating event. In a large cohort of adults with Crohn disease, the decision to proceed with surgery was distributed as follows: failure of medical management in 220, obstruction in 94, intestinal fistula in 68, mass in 56, abdominal abscess in 33, hemorrhage in 7, and peritonitis in 9 [16].

As our understanding of inflammatory bowel disease has increased, it has become clear that there are different variants of Crohn disease, and some phenotypes are more likely to require operative intervention. The age at diagnosis has an impact on disease characteristics and propensity to progress with younger patients having more extensive and more

Table 41.1 Surgical complications of Crohn disease

Obstruction	Bleeding
Perforation	Fistula
Phlegmon	Abscess
Drug allergies	Drug resistance
Perineal disease	Urologic complications
Progression	Growth failure

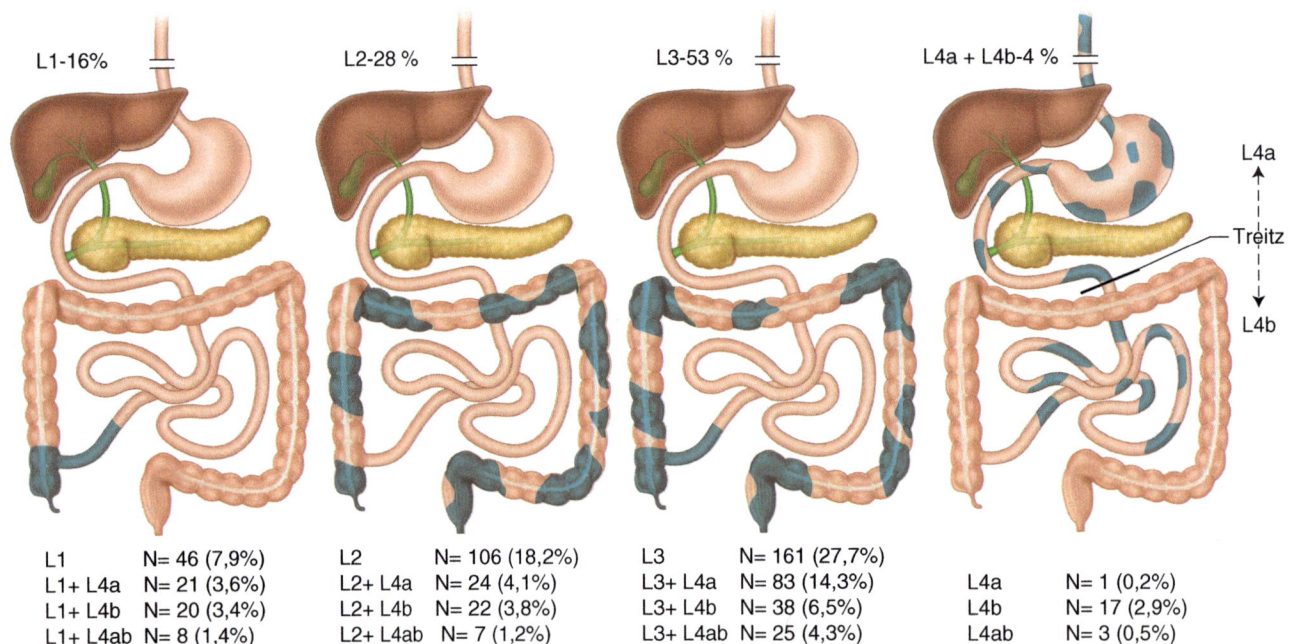

L1	N= 46 (7,9%)	L2	N= 106 (18,2%)	L3	N= 161 (27,7%)		
L1+ L4a	N= 21 (3,6%)	L2+ L4a	N= 24 (4,1%)	L3+ L4a	N= 83 (14,3%)	L4a	N= 1 (0,2%)
L1+ L4b	N= 20 (3,4%)	L2+ L4b	N= 22 (3,8%)	L3+ L4b	N= 38 (6,5%)	L4b	N= 17 (2,9%)
L1+ L4ab	N= 8 (1,4%)	L2+ L4ab	N= 7 (1,2%)	L3+ L4ab	N= 25 (4,3%)	L4ab	N= 3 (0,5%)

Fig. 41.1 Distribution of pediatric Crohn disease (de Bie et al. [10])

aggressive disease than adult-onset patients [17]. The complex associations of genetic and epigenetic alterations with specific phenotypes are beyond the scope of this chapter, but our ability to predict patterns of disease and response to therapy continues to improve. As our understanding of the relationship between genotype and phenotype grows in the future, it may be possible to target specific patient populations for specific types of surgical intervention based on response rates and specific disease characteristics.

The indications for surgical intervention in the pediatric population differ from those in adults in many cases. Mechanical complication of obstruction and perforation is the same, but the impact of medical therapy on growth and development is unique to the pediatric population [18]. In as many as 50% of pediatric patients, the indication for surgery may be failure of medical therapy with growth retardation rather than obstruction or other mechanical complicationsl [19]. In one study of children who had received extensive medical and/or nutritional treatment before surgery, 26 patients underwent intestinal resections. The indication for surgery was chronic intestinal obstruction in 13 cases and chronic intestinal disability leading to growth failure in 13 cases [20]. Furthermore, the timing of surgery for growth issues is critical in the adolescent. Surgical intervention must occur well before epiphyseal plates close to allow sufficient time for subsequent catch-up growth following the operation [21]. Surgical therapy is associated with significant catch-up growth in 6 months following operation in patients with treatment-resistant disease [22].

Fortunately, surgical treatments have evolved along with medical therapy, and current surgical procedures are safer and less invasive than at any time in the past. Surgery has progressed from a treatment of last resort for life-threatening complications to therapy for use in conjunction with medical interventions to maximize the patient's quality of life. While the specter of short bowel syndrome must be kept in mind, elective procedures to treat the complications of Crohn disease can be accomplished safely and effectively [23]. While medical therapy may one day render surgical therapy unnecessary, at present, the surgeon remains an integral part of the treatment team for patients with any inflammatory bowel disease and Crohn disease in particular.

Surgical Emergencies

Patients who develop either perforation with diffuse peritonitis or obstruction that is unresponsive to medical management are rare but may require an urgent operation. The operative goal in this situation is to control sepsis and decompress the intestine with as little risk to the patient as possible. In cases of perforation where the process is localized, percutaneous drainage and antibiotics may convert an acute situation into a more controllable elective intervention. When laparotomy is undertaken in the acute setting, the peritoneal cavity may be very hostile with inflammatory adhesions, fistulas, friable bowel, and diffuse peritonitis making extensive dissections and primary bowel anastomosis ill advised. Rather than proceed with extensive surgery, often the most prudent approach is to divert the fecal steam with a proximal ostomy [24]. Resection of the involved intestinal segment may be considered when technically possible, but proximal diversion without addressing the actual diseased bowel may be the safest option in severe cases.

Proximal diversion with an ileostomy is not without risk. Ileostomies are associated with significant complications at the ileostomy site in addition to the accompanying challenging body image and social stigmata in teenagers [25]. The risk of a diverting ostomy becoming permanent is significant. In a recent pediatric series from the Cincinnati Children's Hospital Colorectal Center, 11 pediatric patients underwent diversion and 8 (73%) had the ostomies reversed. However, three patients required re-diversion leaving only 45% of the original group without a permanent diversion (unpublished data presented at the 2012 meeting of the American Pediatric Surgery Association).

Once the intra-abdominal sepsis is controlled and the inflammatory adhesions are allowed to resolve for 6–8 weeks following emergent ileostomy, a more definitive procedure with ostomy closure can be considered. Although no one, especially teenagers and their parents, wants an ileostomy, attempting an extensive dissection or bowel anastomosis in the face of severe inflammation can result in life-threatening complications and potential loss of large segments of small bowel.

A complete bowel obstruction without accompanying sepsis that does not respond to medical therapy may also require an acute surgical intervention [26]. In a stable patient, aggressive medical management should be attempted to resolve the obstruction before committing to taking a patient to the operating room. This is especially true in cases involving difficult to treat intestinal segments like the duodenum where avoiding any surgical intervention is desirable if possible [27]. If the obstruction fails to resolve or evidence of bowel compromise is present, operation must be undertaken without the ability to prepare the bowel for primary anastomosis. At surgery the bowel is often inflamed and friable, and although a definitive resection with reanastomosis may be possible, the patient and family must be prepared for a diverting ileostomy to avoid the risks of breakdown of an attempted primary bowel anastomosis.

Patients that have had multiple previous abdominal operations may be particularly challenging because of preexisting adhesions and scar tissue. Studies suggest that as many as half of the patients undergoing reoperative surgery will require ileostomy formation [28]. In many pediatric patients, this is less of an issue because often patients are making their first trip to the operating room, but one should never hesitate to perform a temporary bowel diversion when primary anastomosis may be unsafe.

Elective Surgery

The indication for surgical intervention is more commonly not emergent, and the timing of the intervention requires the careful consideration of the surgeon, the gastroenterologist, and the family. The typical indications for surgery include failure of medical management, stricturing disease with near obstructing lesions, fistulas, and complications related to the side effects of medical therapy.

The preoperative evaluation usually includes both endoscopic and imaging studies. Traditional imaging involves contrast enemas and/or upper gastrointestinal series with small bowel follow-through. More recently, magnetic resonance enterography has been utilized to provide a more complete assessment of the entire gastrointestinal tract [29]. Some recent evidence suggests that CT enterography may provide superior imaging [30] but the differences are not dramatic, and the experience of the radiologist is probably more important when deciding between the two studies. Whichever method is chosen, enterography offers the advantage of cross-sectional imaging of the entire bowel wall rather than being limited to assessing luminal disease. This allows for more accurate surgical planning and facilitates discussions with the patient and family regarding the operative approach.

Efforts should be made to control intra-abdominal sepsis through drainage of abscess and treatment with antibiotics prior to surgery along with supporting the nutritional status of the patient. Percutaneous abscess drainage with prompt resumption of immunotherapy has been associated with avoidance of bowel resection in the pediatric Crohn disease population [31].

Methods to reduce the risk of surgical site infections (SSI) including anastomotic leaks, intra-abdominal sepsis, and wound infections have been extensively studied and remain controversial. The use of intravenous antibiotics, enteral antibiotics, and mechanical bowel preparation has all been advocated for colorectal procedures. As with many pediatric surgical procedures, most of the data comes from the adult surgical literature. The evidence pertaining to the prevention of SSI has recently been evaluated and reported by the Outcomes Committee of the American Pediatric Surgical Association [32].

The presence of a stricture alone is not an indication for operation. Areas of diseased bowel that do not present a mechanical impediment to the flow of the intestinal contents do not require intervention. However, significant chronic obstruction is suggested by dilation of bowel loops proximal to the diseased area (Fig. 41.2). These changes signify a

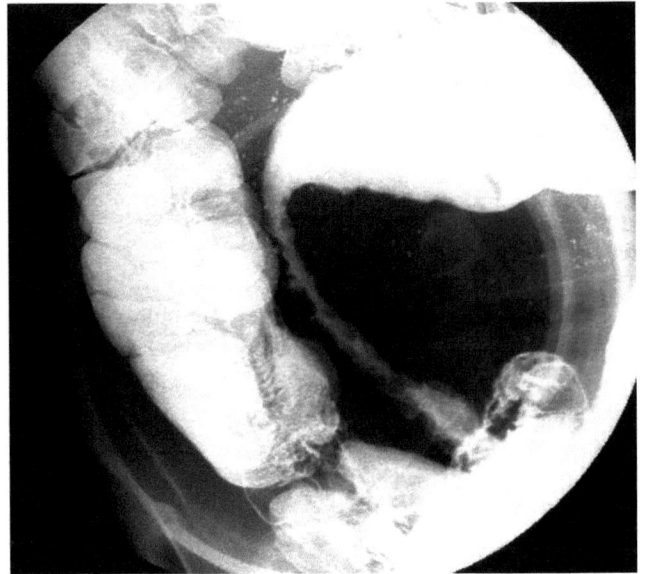

Fig. 41.2 Barium contrast study demonstrating a segmental distal ileal stricture

possible impending complete obstruction, and elective resection prior to that allows the opportunity for bowel preparation and resection with primary anastomosis rather than a two-stage procedure requiring temporary diversion with subsequent ileostomy closure. Entero-entero fistulas, chronic phlegmon, and enterocutaneous fistulas are other mechanical indications for operative intervention which can be dealt with after careful radiographic studies to delineate the anatomy and preoperative patient preparation.

Fistulas to the urinary tract with recurrent urinary tract infections may not constitute an urgent indication for operation, but continued soiling of the urinary tract could result in progressive renal dysfunction arguing for earlier rather than later intervention in these situations. Although some patients will respond to medical therapy, vast majority of patients will require surgical intervention [33–36]. Enterovesical fistulas are treated with takedown of the fistula and closure of the bladder, while ureteral fistulas may require resection with reanastomosis or reimplantation of the ureter.

Finally, progression of the disease with persistent symptoms despite maximal medical therapy may also be the impetus for considering the surgical option. Regardless of the indication, the philosophy of therapy remains the same. The surgical procedure must be tailored to the individual patient with an eye toward preserving all possible small bowel length while providing the most effective palliation of the presenting complication of the Crohn disease. Surgical intervention in patients with progressive or chronic symptoms related to stricturing or fistulizing disease in the abdomen is effective in relieving symptoms and can minimize absence from school and improve overall well-being when compared to nonoperative therapy [37].

Surgical Therapy

The procedure performed at the time of operation depends on the clinical situation and extent of the disease. As mentioned previously, in a patient that is acutely ill with sepsis or complete obstruction, simple diversion may be the most appropriate response. However, in most patients a more definitive procedure is performed. In pediatric patients with stricturing disease, the terminal ileum is the most common site involved. Often the disease extends up to include the ileocecal valve, and the most common approach is bowel resection extending from the proximal extent of the disease in the ileum to the ascending colon, which is usually uninvolved. Bowel continuity is restored with a primary anastomosis.

In an effort to preserve as much bowel length as possible, only gross disease is resected since recurrent disease may require additional surgery, and bowel length may be shorter than normal in patients with Crohn disease leaving less margin for resection before developing issues with poor absorption [38]. The actual technical aspects of the procedure vary somewhat by surgeon and are largely a matter of training and experience. Bowel resection is carried out in the standard fashion with no need to obtain clear margins or mesenteric lymph nodes as might be required for a cancer operation. The only technical aspect of the procedure that may impact outcome is the manner in which the bowel is anastomosed.

There are a number of techniques for reanastomosing bowel with the most surgeons performing either a hand-sewn end-to-end anastomosis or a side-to-side, functional end-to-end stapled anastomosis. There is some evidence to suggest that a stapled anastomosis may reduce the time to recurrence in patients with Crohn disease [39–47]. The reason for this is unclear and may have to do with the diameter of the resulting anastomosis or the nonreactive nature of the staples. Alternatively, it may have more to do with the anatomic orientation of the anastomosis rather than the manner in which the bowel is re-approximated [48]. The other reported benefit of a stapled anastomosis stems from data to suggest that anastomotic leaks and intra-abdominal abscesses are less common with the stapled anastomosis in some series but not in others [43, 49–52].

Complications following bowel resection and anastomosis in patients with Crohn disease are common and are most often infectious in nature. Wound infections are most common and occur in as many as 20% of patients, while more serious intra-abdominal infections related to anastomotic leak occur in 3–10% [43, 53]. Wound complications are treated with local care, while anastomotic complications may require reoperation with revision or temporary diversion with an ostomy.

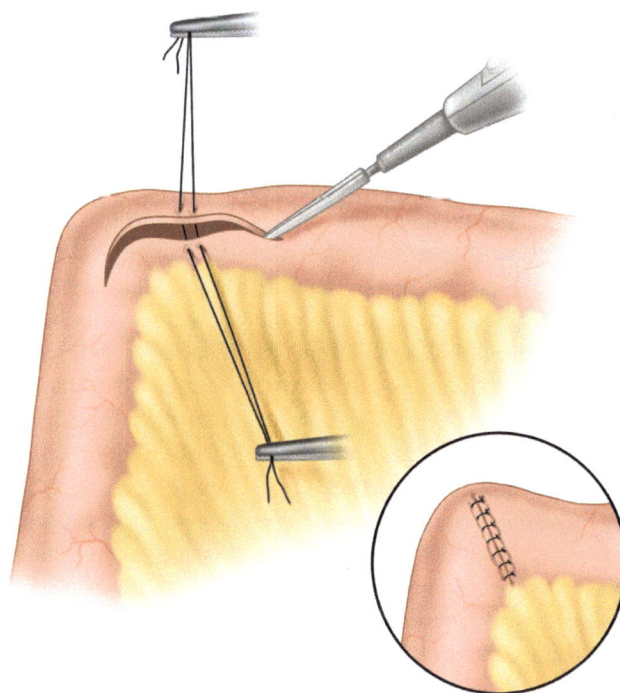

Fig. 41.3 Heineke-Mikulicz enteroplasty

Stricturoplasty

Diffuse small bowel disease with skip lesions or strictures that do not involve the ileocecal valve allows for some additional options in surgical treatment. Short segments are often resected with primary anastomosis when it represents the only area of disease. However, multiple short segments or longer segments up to 20 cm in length may be amenable to stricturoplasty rather than resection in an effort to preserve bowel length.

The technique entails a longitudinal enterotomy through the strictured segment with closure in a transverse fashion to relieve the obstruction (Heineke-Mikulicz stricturoplasty) (Fig. 41.3). While it seems somewhat counterintuitive to leave the diseased bowel in situ, the results following this operation are quite good even when applied to multiple strictures in the same patient [54]. Surprisingly, the rate at which recurrent disease occurs at the stricturoplasty site is low [55], and the technique has been used for many years with results from long-term follow-up studies supporting its use [56]. Recurrence rates following stricturoplasty are on the order of 15% at 2 years and 20% at 5 years [57].

There are a number of technical modifications of this technique that allow for longer segments to be preserved while relieving obstruction [58–62]. In a study of 102 patients undergoing a nonconventional stricturoplasty for a longer segment of the intestine, there were 48 ileoileal side-to-side isoperistaltic stricturoplasties, 41 widening ileocolic stricturoplasties, and 32 ileocolic side-to-side isoperistaltic stricturoplasties, which were associated with Heineke-Mikulicz stricturoplasties in 80 procedures or with short segmental bowel resections or both in 47 procedures. The postoperative complication rate was 5.7% which is consistent with the complication rate from the more common Heineke-Mikulicz stricturoplasty. The 10-year clinical recurrence rate was 43%, and the recurrence rate at the previously affected site was only 0.8% [60]. In another study long-segment stricturoplasty (>20 cm) was reported to have recurrence rates that are not significantly different than that for shorter-segment disease. Recurrence rates were 20–35% at 3 years, 50% at 5 years, and 60% at 10 years with no difference in complications between the groups [59].

In some very difficult situations such as long duodenal strictures, other modifications of the stricturoplasty technique can be applied. In one such case, a jejunal patch was used to successfully relieve the obstruction and avoid intestinal bypass in a patient with a difficult duodenal stricture [63].

Laparoscopy

The most recent advances in surgical treatment of intra-abdominal complications of Crohn disease have been the application of minimally invasive surgical techniques. As with many of the other conditions to which laparoscopic techniques have been applied, multiple studies have demonstrated a decrease in hospital length of stay, more rapid return to work, less postoperative narcotic use, and improved cosmetic results. Similarly, multiple studies of laparoscopic techniques applied to surgery for Crohn disease in children and adults have also suggested shorter hospital stays, decreased need for parenteral narcotics, and faster return to a regular diet [64–73]. However, a recent Cochrane analysis has shown no difference in length of stay or duration of ileus [74], and the morbidity of the laparoscopic approach is equivalent to open surgery [75]. Thus, although the benefits of the laparoscopic approach may be limited to improved cosmesis at the expense of longer operating time, there is a trend toward increased use of minimally invasive techniques, and the outcomes are at least equivalent to open surgery.

The techniques employed often use laparoscopic exploration of the abdomen with mobilization of the diseased bowel segment. Various sealer/cutting devices facilitate taking the mesentery of involved segments without additional blood loss and stapling devices allow for dividing the bowel at the margins of disease. Anastomosis may be carried out extracorporeally after the diseased segment is delivered from the abdomen through a small incision or intracorporeally using the laparoscopic stapling devices. These techniques can also be incorporated into the single-site surgical approach to achieve "scarless" operations [76] although the benefit is purely cosmetic and the outcomes have not been tested. Use of the surgical robot has also been reported with the possible benefit of reducing conversions to an open operation but no difference in other surgical morbidities [77].

Although complicated disease involving fistulas or phlegmon was considered a relative contraindication to the laparoscopic approach, many cases are now handled by experienced surgeons without an increase in complication rate [78–83]. One potential benefit of the laparoscopic approach is a reduction in postoperative adhesion formation. This carries added importance in the Crohn populations where disease recurrence is more the rule than the exception and reoperation is often necessary. Reduced adhesions facilitate subsequent operations [84] and theoretically lower the risk of injury to the bowel and ureters. Approaching recurrent disease laparoscopically is also feasible without an increased complication rate [85, 86].

In the long run, patients' quality of life does not appear to be impacted by the technique used at the time of surgery [86, 87]. However, the advantage of the minimally invasive approach likely extends beyond quality of life measurements. Reduced intra-abdominal adhesion formation, possible faster resumption of full enteral nutrition, and perhaps less psychological trauma related to body image issues are all of particular significance to the pediatric patient population.

Colonic Disease

Crohn colitis requires a different approach than for small bowel disease. Colonic disease is traditionally regarded as being more aggressive, and the colon is not necessary for the nutritional function of the intestinal tract, so some advocate subtotal colectomy rather than segmental resections when colonic involvement requires surgical intervention. However, segmental resection offers the opportunity to preserve colonic function and avoid or delay the potential for permanent ileostomy and has become the more common approach [15]. Fewer symptoms, fewer loose stools, and better anorectal function have been reported following segmental resection, and the re-resection rate did not differ from patients undergoing subtotal colectomy [88, 89]. Conversely, patients with pancolitis or severe distal colonic disease have been reported to have longer disease-free intervals [90] and wean from chronic medications more often when treated with subtotal colectomy or proctocolectomy when compared to those undergoing segmental resection. However, these patients also had a higher incidence of permanent diverting ileostomy [91, 92] suggesting that segmental resection for pediatric patients with colonic Crohn disease is preferable when possible. Laparoscopic techniques are possible and show similar advantages of those described in small bowel resection [93].

Perineal Disease

Approximately one third of patients with Crohn disease will develop perineal or rectal manifestations of the disease [94]. Patients presenting with perineal disease tend to have more aggressive disease with higher rates of both perineal and intra-abdominal operations [95].

Fistulizing perineal disease is an area in which surgical intervention has classically been avoided given the risk of nonhealing wounds and incontinence. More recently, however, the use of early surgical evaluation has been found to provide important information to help guide the medical management. While fistulotomy and incision and drainage of local abscesses were fraught with long-term complications in the past, the use of new biologic agents such as infliximab has rendered early surgical intervention not only safe but necessary for rapid control of the disease.

Medical therapy for perineal disease has been greatly improved with the advent of biologic agents yet more than half ultimately require surgical procedures [96]. Two controlled trials support the efficacy of infliximab in achieving closure of perineal fistulas [97], and the combination of infliximab and surgical treatment of fistulizing perineal disease can result in marked improvement of perineal disease which is superior to infliximab alone [98–100]. Conversely, infliximab treatment does not prevent the need for surgery for fistulizing Crohn disease [101].

Treatment algorithms in pediatric inflammatory bowel disease centers have evolved to include an aggressive surgical approach early. Examination under anesthesia is particularly useful in the pediatric population. Comprehensive rectal examination is often difficult in the clinic setting in younger patients that are unable to cooperate fully with the exam. General anesthesia in the operating room provides the ideal environment to carefully evaluate the extent of disease with delineation of fistula tracts, abscesses, and rectal strictures. A complete assessment of the extent of the disease is important to help guide medical therapy.

Once the extent of disease is determined, therapeutic measures can be performed during the same anesthetic. If fistulae-in-ano are present, they can be probed to ascertain the anatomy. Superficial tracts are treated with fistulotomy, while for more complex tracts a non-cutting seton placement is placed.

Initial surgical treatment may improve the response to subsequent pharmacologic therapy. Local infection can be controlled, strictures dilated, and complex fistulas delineated and controlled with seton placement. Following initiation of

treatment with infliximab, the seton is removed to allow the fistula tract to close. Abscesses are drained and strictures can be sized and dilated.

Unfortunately, long-term control of perianal disease remains a challenge, and diverting colostomy may be necessary to gain control of the problem in pediatric patients. In adults, as many as 20% of patients with severe perianal disease proceed to proctocolectomy with permanent ileostomy [94].

Rectal Strictures

Low rectal and anal strictures caused by chronic fibrosis from chronic inflammation can be successfully treated with transanal dilations [97]. Younger pediatric patients may require dilations under anesthesia on a regular basis, while older patients will tolerate dilations in the office or at home. Incontinence can result from overdilation of rectal strictures or operative damage to the muscles during fistulotomy, but it is often difficult to separate the impact of the dilations relative to the underlying disease process. Tight irregular strictures longer than 3–4 cm without a clear lumen are a relative contraindication to dilation because perforation of the rectum is possible, particularly in small pediatric patients. Initial dilation in the operating room guided by fluoroscopy may reduce the risk of subsequent outpatient dilations. Treatment with dilations may be needed for many months, and ultimately the result is dependent on systemic control of the disease process. Strictures that do not respond to chronic dilations may eventually require a diverting colostomy. The combination of anal stricture and colonic Crohn disease ultimately leads to fecal diversion in more than 50% of patients [102].

Impact of Medical Therapy

Many of the drugs used to treat Crohn disease have the potential to increase complications following surgical procedures. Steroids significantly impair wound healing, impact growth, and increase infectious complications. Risks of abdominal wound infection, abdominal wound dehiscence, and anastomotic dehiscence are all potentially increased in the presence of steroids. While the risks of operating on Crohn patients being treated concurrently with steroids are likely increased, the data in the literature to support that fear is circumstantial. Studies have demonstrated an apparent increased risk of early complications in patients with ulcerative colitis undergoing definitive surgery while on chronic steroids, while complications were not increased in patients weaned off steroids prior to surgery [103]. Asthma patients treated with steroids during the perioperative period failed to show an increased complication rate over controls [104] suggesting that the impact of steroids on Crohn patients may be cumulative with the other risk factors in these patients. Infliximab therapy does not appear to increase the rate of perioperative complications associated with bowel resections for Crohn disease [53, 105].

Postoperative Recurrence

Recurrence of Crohn disease following a surgical resection is common. In many cases medical therapy is discontinued following surgical treatment, but continued therapy with a number of drugs has been investigated to improve disease-free intervals. Establishing the recurrence risk for individual patients and performing endoscopic surveillance are important to help guide therapy [106]. While some studies fail to demonstrate an advantage to prophylactic therapy [107], others have proposed specific algorithms for follow-up and treatment [108, 109]. Agents including the 5-aminosalicylate formulations, antibiotics, steroids, and azathioprine have been examined. None of these therapies have convincingly been shown to prevent recurrent lesions [110]. Infliximab has been reported effective in a prospective randomized trial where remission was maintained in 93% of patients in the infliximab group and only 53% of patients in the control group [111]. Importantly, early postoperative treatment with infliximab does not appear to be associated with an increase in adverse events [106]. The use of infliximab to prevent recurrence in children has also been reported [112]. The antibiotics metronidazole and ornidazole have shown efficacy, but cannot be used in the long term because of side effects [113]. 6-Mercaptopurine and azathioprine may be more effective than mesalamine [97, 114, 115].

Given the risk of recurrent disease, it is important to resect only the grossly involved segment of the intestine at the time of the initial operation. Fortunately, there is some evidence to suggest that the involved segments of intestine in subsequent operations for ileal disease are shorter than those involved at initial presentation [116].

Adjuvant Procedures

Finally, there are well-documented complications of growth and development in the pediatric population [117]. Pediatric patients are at particular risk for nutritional complications because of the normal rapid growth and development in children. Delayed puberty, short stature, and bone demineralization may all be indications for supplemental nutritional support. Surgical adjuncts to care such as gastrostomy tubes and devices for chronic parenteral access may prove to be lifesaving measures for some patients. Compliance with medical regimens in the pediatric population can be challenging, and providing these types of devices early with minimal trauma may help minimize the impact of the disease on these nutritional issues. Low residue diets are frequently used in pediatric patients with progressive stricturing disease in the small bowel. The social impact of an indwelling nasogastric feeding tube may inhibit compliance in the teenage population making these children candidates for percutaneous or laparoscopically placed gastrostomy tubes. The laparoscopic approach allows direct visualization of the stomach to properly site the tube, secure the stomach to the abdominal wall, and place a primary button device without the scarring associated with the open approach.

Patients unable to tolerate adequate enteral feedings are often candidates for supplemental parenteral nutritional support. In these cases, surgically placed central venous access devices may significantly improve lifestyle by providing stable chronic venous access for infusions and blood sampling. Either cuffed catheters or part devices may be indicated.

References

1. Rabbett H, Elbadri A, Thwaites R, et al. Quality of life in children with Crohn disease. J Pediatr Gastroenterol Nutr. 1996;23(5): 528–33.
2. Hancock L, Windsor AC, Mortensen NJ. Inflammatory bowel disease: the view of the surgeon. Colorectal Dis. 2006;8 (Suppl 1):10–4.
3. Schraut WH. The surgical management of Crohn disease. Gastroenterol Clin North Am. 2002;31(1):255–63.
4. Poggioli G, Pierangeli F, Laureti S, Ugolini F. Review article: indication and type of surgery in Crohn disease. Aliment Pharmacol Ther. 2002;16(Suppl 4):59–64.
5. Leowardi C, Heuschen G, Kienle P, et al. Surgical treatment of severe inflammatory bowel diseases. Dig Dis. 2003;21(1):54–62.
6. Dolgin SE. Surgical management of upper gastrointestinal and small bowel Crohn disease. Semin Pediatr Surg. 2007;16:172–7.
7. Aufses Jr AH. The history of Crohn disease. Surg Clin North Am. 2001;81(1):1–11. vii
8. Garlock JHCB. Appraisal of results of surgery in the treatment of regional enteritis. JAMA. 1945;127:205–8.
9. Greenstein AJSD, Pucillo A, et al. Cancer in Crohn disease after divisionary surgery. A report of seven carcinomas occurring in excluded bowel. Am J Surg. 1978;135:86–90.
10. de Bie CI, Paerregaard A, Kolacek S, Ruemmele FM, Koletzko S, Fell JM, et al. Disease phenotype at diagnosis in pediatric Crohn's disease: 5-year analyses of the EUROKIDS registry. Inflamm Bowel Dis. 2013;19:378–85.
11. Griffiths AM, Alemayehu E, Sherman P. Clinical features of gastroduodenal Crohn disease in adolescents. J Pediatr Gastroenterol Nutr. 1989;86:259–62.
12. Dziki A, Galbfach P. Crohn disease – when to operate? Acta Chir Iugosl. 2004;51(2):61–8.
13. McLeod RS. Surgery for inflammatory bowel diseases. Dig Dis. 2003;21(2):168–79.
14. Veroux M, Angriman I, Ruffolo C, et al. Severe gastrointestinal bleeding in Crohn disease. Ann Ital Chir. 2003;74(2):213–5. ; discussion 6

15. Andersson P, Olaison G, Bodemar G, et al. Surgery for Crohn colitis over a twenty-eight-year period: fewer stomas and the replacement of total colectomy by segmental resection. Scand J Gastroenterol. 2002;37(1):68–73.
16. Hurst RD, Molinari M, Chung TP, et al. Prospective study of the features, indications, and surgical treatment in 513 consecutive patients affected by Crohn disease. Surgery. 1997;122(4):661–7. discussion 7–8
17. Freeman HJ. Natural history and long-term clinical course of Crohn's disease. World J Gastroenterol. 2014;20(1):31–6.
18. Rufo PA, Bousvaros A. Current therapy of inflammatory Bowel disease in children. Paediatr Drugs. 2006;8(5):279–302.
19. Patel HI, Leichtner AM, Colodny AH, Shamberger RC. Surgery for Crohn disease in infants and children. J Pediatr Surg. 1997;32(7):1063–7. discussion 7–8
20. Dokucu AI, Sarnacki S, Michel JL, et al. Indications and results of surgery in patients with Crohn disease with onset under 10 years of age: a series of 18 patients. Eur J Pediatr Surg. 2002;12(3):180–5.
21. Konno M, Kobayashi A, Tomomasa T, et al. Guidelines for the treatment of Crohn disease in children. Pediatr Int. 2006;48(3):349–52.
22. Heuschkel R, Salvestrini C, Beattie RM, Hildebrand H, Walters T, Griffiths A. Guidelines for the management of growth failure in childhood inflammatory bowel disease. Inflamm Bowel Dis. 2008;14(6):839–49.
23. Nissan A, Zamir O, Spira RM, et al. A more liberal approach to the surgical treatment of Crohn disease. Am J Surg. 1997;174(3):339–41.
24. Berg DF, Bahadursingh AM, Kaminski DL, Longo WE. Acute surgical emergencies in inflammatory bowel disease. Am J Surg. 2002;184(1):45–51.
25. Ecker KW, Gierend M, Kreissler-Haag D, Feifel G. Reoperations at the ileostomy in Crohn disease reflect inflammatory activity rather than surgical stoma complications alone. Int J Colorectal Dis. 2001;16(2):76–80.
26. Froehlich F, Juillerat P, Mottet C, et al. Obstructive fibrostenotic Crohn disease. Digestion. 2005;71(1):29–30.
27. Karaoglu AO, Yukselen V. Obstructing Crohn disease of the duodenum: is surgery always mandatory? Int J Clin Pract. 2004;58(2):221–3.
28. Heimann TM, Greenstein AJ, Lewis B, et al. Comparison of primary and reoperative surgery in patients with Crohns disease. Ann Surg. 1998;227(4):492–5.
29. Tillack C, Seiderer J, Brand S, Göke B, Reiser MF, Schaefer C, Diepolder H, Ochsenkühn T, Herrmann KA. Correlation of magnetic resonance enteroclysis (MRE) and wireless capsule endoscopy (CE) in the diagnosis of small bowel lesions in Crohn disease. Inflamm Bowel Dis. 2008;14(9):1219–28.
30. Siddiki HA, Fidler JL, Fletcher JG, Burton SS, Huprich JE, Hough DM, et al. Prospective comparison of state-of-the-art MR enterography and CT enterography in small-bowel Crohn's disease. AJR Am J Roentgenol. 2009;193(1):113–21.
31. Pugmire BS, Gee MS, Kaplan JL, Hahn PF, Doody DP, Winter HS, Gervais DA. Role of percutaneous abscess drainage in the management of young patients with Crohn disease. Pediatr Radiol. 2016;46:653–9.
32. Rangel SJ, Islam S, St Peter SD, Goldin AB, Abdullah F, Downard CD, Saito JM, Blakely ML, Puligandla PS, Dasgupta R, Austin M, Chen LE, Renaud E, Arca MJ, Calkins CM. Prevention of infectious complications after elective colorectal surgery in children: an American Pediatric Surgical Association Outcomes and Clinical Trials Committee comprehensive review. J Pediatr Surg. 2015;50:192–200.
33. Solem CA, Loftus Jr EV, Tremaine WJ, et al. Fistulas to the urinary system in Crohn disease: clinical features and outcomes. Am J Gastroenterol. 2002;97(9):2300–5.
34. Present DH. Urinary tract fistulas in Crohn disease: surgery versus medical therapy. Am J Gastroenterol. 2002;97(9):2165–7.
35. Gruner JS, Sehon JK, Johnson LW. Diagnosis and management of enterovesical fistulas in patients with Crohn disease. Am Surg. 2002;68(8):714–9.
36. Ben-Ami H, Ginesin Y, Behar DM, et al. Diagnosis and treatment of urinary tract complications in Crohn disease: an experience over 15 years. Can J Gastroenterol. 2002;16(4):225–9.
37. Akobeng AK, Suresh-Babu MV, Firth D, et al. Quality of life in children with Crohn disease: a pilot study. J Pediatr Gastroenterol Nutr. 1999;28(4):S37–9.
38. Glehen O, Lifante JC, Vignal J, et al. Small bowel length in Crohn disease. Int J Colorectal Dis. 2003;18(5):423–7.
39. Yamamoto T, Bain IM, Mylonakis E, et al. Stapled functional end-to-end anastomosis versus sutured end-to-end anastomosis after ileocolonic resection in Crohn disease. Scand J Gastroenterol. 1999;34(7):708–13.
40. Ikeuchi H, Kusunoki M, Yamamura T. Long-term results of stapled and hand-sewn anastomoses in patients with Crohn disease. Dig Surg. 2000;17(5):493–6.
41. Tersigni R, Alessandroni L, Barreca M, et al. Does stapled functional end-to-end anastomosis affect recurrence of Crohn disease after ileocolonic resection? Hepatogastroenterology. 2003;50(53):1422–5.
42. Yamamoto T. Factors affecting recurrence after surgery for Crohn disease. World J Gastroenterol. 2005;11(26):3971–9.
43. Resegotti A, Astegiano M, Farina EC, et al. Side-to-side stapled anastomosis strongly reduces anastomotic leak rates in Crohn disease surgery. Dis Colon Rectum. 2005;48(3):464–8.
44. Larson DW, Pemberton JH. Current concepts and controversies in surgery for IBD. Gastroenterology. 2004;126(6):1611–9.
45. Munoz-Juarez M, Yamamoto T, Wolff BG, Keighley MR. Wide-lumen stapled anastomosis vs. conventional end-to-end anastomosis in the treatment of Crohn disease. Dis Colon Rectum. 2001;44(1):20–5. discussion 5–6
46. Yamamoto T, Allan RN, Keighley MR. Strategy for surgical management of ileocolonic anastomotic recurrence in Crohn disease. World J Surg. 1999;23(10):1055–60. discussion 60–1
47. Cunningham MF, Docherty NG, Coffey JC, Burke JP, O'Connell PR. Postsurgical recurrence of ileal Crohn disease: an update on risk factors and intervention points to a central role for impaired host-microflora homeostasis. World J Surg. 2010;34(7):1615–26.
48. Scarpa M, Angriman I, Barollo M, et al. Role of stapled and hand-sewn anastomoses in recurrence of Crohn disease. Hepatogastroenterology. 2004;51(58):1053–7.
49. Smedh K, Andersson M, Johansson H, Hagberg T. Preoperative management is more important than choice of sutured or stapled anastomosis in Crohn disease. Eur J Surg. 2002;168(3):154–7.
50. Yamamoto T, Keighley MR. Stapled functional end-to-end anastomosis in Crohn disease. Surg Today. 1999;29(7):679–81.
51. Galandiuk S. Stapled and hand-sewn anastomoses in Crohn disease. Dig Surg. 1998;15(6):655.
52. Hashemi M, Novell JR, Lewis AA. Side-to-side stapled anastomosis may delay recurrence in Crohn disease. Dis Colon Rectum. 1998;41(10):1293–6.
53. Colombel JF, Loftus Jr EV, Tremaine WJ, et al. Early postoperative complications are not increased in patients with Crohn disease treated perioperatively with infliximab or immunosuppressive therapy. Am J Gastroenterol. 2004;99(5):878–83.
54. Dietz DW, Fazio VW, Laureti S, et al. Strictureplasty in diffuse Crohn jejunoileitis: safe and durable. Dis Colon Rectum. 2002;45(6):764–70.
55. Laurent S, Detry O, Detroz B, et al. Strictureplasty in Crohn disease: short- and long-term follow-up. Acta Chir Belg. 2002;102(4):253–5.
56. Dasari BV, Maxwell R, Gardiner KR. Assessment of complications following strictureplasty for small bowel Crohn Disease. Ir J Med Sci. 2010;179(2):201–5.

57. Hurst RD, Michelassi F. Strictureplasty for Crohn disease: techniques and long-term results. World J Surg. 1998;22(4):359–63.

58. Poggioli G, Laureti S, Pierangeli F, Ugolini F. A new model of strictureplasty for multiple and long stenoses in Crohn ileitis: side-to-side diseased to disease-free anastomosis. Dis Colon Rectum. 2003;46(1):127–30.

59. Shatari T, Clark MA, Yamamoto T, et al. Long strictureplasty is as safe and effective as short strictureplasty in small-bowel Crohn disease. Colorectal Dis. 2004;6(6):438–41.

60. Sampietro GM, Cristaldi M, Maconi G, et al. A prospective, longitudinal study of nonconventional strictureplasty in Crohn disease. J Am Coll Surg. 2004;199(1):8–20. discussion -2

61. Michelassi F, Upadhyay GA. Side-to-side isoperistaltic strictureplasty in the treatment of extensive Crohn disease. J Surg Res. 2004;117(1):71–8.

62. Tonelli F, Fedi M, Paroli GM, Fazi M. Indications and results of side-to-side isoperistaltic strictureplasty in Crohn disease. Dis Colon Rectum. 2004;47(4):494–501.

63. Eisenberger CF, Izbicki JR, Broering DC, et al. Strictureplasty with a pedunculated jejunal patch in Crohn disease of the duodenum. Am J Gastroenterol. 1998;93(2):267–9.

64. Milsom JW, Hammerhofer KA, Bohm B, et al. Prospective, randomized trial comparing laparoscopic vs. conventional surgery for refractory ileocolic Crohn disease. Dis Colon Rectum. 2001;44(1):1–8. discussion -9

65. Dutta S, Rothenberg SS, Chang J, Bealer J. Total intracorporeal laparoscopic resection of Crohn disease. J Pediatr Surg. 2003;38(5):717–9.

66. Tilney HS, Constantinides VA, Heriot AG, et al. Comparison of laparoscopic and open ileocecal resection for Crohn disease: a metaanalysis. Surg Endosc. 2006;20(7):1036–44.

67. Bonnard A, Fouquet V, Berrebi D, et al. Crohn disease in children. Preliminary experience with a laparoscopic approach. Eur J Pediatr Surg. 2006;16(2):90–3.

68. Maartense S, Dunker MS, Slors JF, et al. Laparoscopic-assisted versus open ileocolic resection for Crohn disease: a randomized trial. Ann Surg. 2006;243(2):143–9. discussion 50–3

69. Casillas S, Delaney CP. Laparoscopic surgery for inflammatory bowel disease. Dig Surg. 2005;22(3):135–42.

70. Hirayama I, Ide M, Shoji H, et al. Laparoscopic-assisted partial ileectomy for Crohn disease associated with chronic anemia due to frequent hemorrhage. Hepatogastroenterology. 2005;52(63):823–5.

71. Huilgol RL, Wright CM, Solomon MJ. Laparoscopic versus open ileocolic resection for Crohn disease. J Laparoendosc Adv Surg Tech A. 2004;14(2):61–5.

72. von Allmen D, Markowitz JE, York A, et al. Laparoscopic-assisted bowel resection offers advantages over open surgery for treatment of segmental Crohn disease in children. J Pediatr Surg. 2003;38(6):963–5.

73. Shore G, Gonzalez QH, Bondora A, Vickers SM. Laparoscopic vs conventional ileocolectomy for primary Crohn disease. Arch Surg. 2003;138(1):76–9.

74. Dasari BVM, McKay D, Gardiner K. Laparoscopic versus Open surgery for small bowel Crohn disease. Cochrane Database Syst Rev. 2011, Issue 1. Art. No.: CD006956. doi:10.1002/14651858.CD006956.pub2

75. Diamond IR, Gerstle JT, Kim PC, Langer JC. Outcomes after laparoscopic surgery in children with inflammatory bowel disease. Surg Endosc. 2010;24(11):2796–802.

76. Zaghiyan KN, Murrell Z, Fleshner PR. Scarless single-incision laparoscopic loop ileostomy: a novel technique. Dis Colon Rectum. 2011;54(12):1542–6.

77. Feinberg AE, Elnahas A, Bashir S, Cleghorn MC, Quereshy FA. Comparison of robotic and laparoscopic colorectal resections with respect to 30-day perioperative morbidity. Can J Surg. 2016;59:16615.

78. Wu JS, Birnbaum EH, Kodner IJ, et al. Laparoscopic-assisted ileocolic resections in patients with Crohn disease: are abscesses, phlegmons, or recurrent disease contraindications? Surgery. 1997;122(4):682–8. discussion 8–9

79. Milsom JW. Laparoscopic surgery in the treatment of Crohn disease. Surg Clin North Am. 2005;85(1):25–34. vii

80. Seymour NE, Kavic SM. Laparoscopic management of complex Crohn disease. JSLS. 2003;7(2):117–21.

81. Benoist S, Panis Y, Beaufour A, et al. Laparoscopic ileocecal resection in Crohn disease: a case-matched comparison with open resection. Surg Endosc. 2003;17(5):814–8.

82. Evans J, Poritz L, MacRae H. Influence of experience on laparoscopic ileocolic resection for Crohn disease. Dis Colon Rectum. 2002;45(12):1595–600.

83. Watanabe M, Ohgami M, Teramoto T, et al. Laparoscopic ileocecal resection for Crohn disease associated with intestinal stenosis and ileorectal fistula. Surg Today. 1999;29(5):446–8.

84. Cima RR, Wolff BG. Reoperative Crohn surgery: tricks of the trade. Clin Colon Rectal Surg. 2007;20(4):336–43.

85. Uchikoshi F, Ito T, Nezu R, et al. Advantages of laparoscope-assisted surgery for recurrent Crohn disease. Surg Endosc. 2004;18(11):1675–9.

86. Hasegawa H, Watanabe M, Nishibori H, et al. Laparoscopic surgery for recurrent Crohn disease. Br J Surg. 2003;90(8):970–3.

87. Thaler K, Dinnewitzer A, Oberwalder M, et al. Assessment of long-term quality of life after laparoscopic and open surgery for Crohn disease. Colorectal Dis. 2005;7(4):375–81.

88. Andersson P, Olaison G, Hallbook O, Sjodahl R. Segmental resection or subtotal colectomy in Crohn colitis? Dis Colon Rectum. 2002;45(1):47–53.

89. Martel P, Betton PO, Gallot D, Malafosse M. Crohn colitis: experience with segmental resections; results in a series of 84 patients. J Am Coll Surg. 2002;194(4):448–53.

90. Bernell O, Lapidus A, Hellers G. Recurrence after colectomy in Crohn colitis. Dis Colon Rectum. 2001;44(5):647–54. discussion 54

91. Fichera A, McCormack R, Rubin MA, et al. Long-term outcome of surgically treated Crohn colitis: a prospective study. Dis Colon Rectum. 2005;48(5):963–9.

92. Rieger N, Collopy B, Fink R, et al. Total colectomy for Crohn disease. Aust N Z J Surg. 1999;69(1):28–30.

93. Proctor ML, Langer JC, Gerstle JT, Kim PC. Is laparoscopic subtotal colectomy better than open subtotal colectomy in children? J Pediatr Surg. 2002;37(5):706–8.

94. Lewis RT, Maron DJ. Anorectal Crohn disease. Surg Clin North Am. 2010;90(1):83–97.

95. Zwintscher NP, Shah PM, Argawal A, Chesley PM, Johnson EK, Newton CR, Maykel JA, Steele SR. The impact of perianal disease in young patients with inflammatory bowel disease. Int J Colorectal Dis. 2015;30(9):1275–9.

96. Duff S, Sagar P, Rao M, Dolling S, Sprakes M, Hamlin PJ. Infliximab and surgical treatment of complex anal Crohn disease. Colorectal Dis. 2011; doi:10.1111/j.1463-1318.2011.02811.x. [Epub ahead of print]

97. Sandborn WJ, Fazio VW, Feagan BG, Hanauer SB. AGA technical review on perianal Crohn disease. Gastroenterology. 2003;125(5):1508–30.

98. Judge TA, Lichtenstein GR. Treatment of fistulizing Crohn disease. Gastroenterol Clin North Am. 2004;33(2):421–54. xi-xii

99. Regueiro M, Mardini H. Treatment of perianal fistulizing Crohn disease with infliximab alone or as an adjunct to exam under anesthesia with seton placement. Inflamm Bowel Dis. 2003;9(2):98–103.

100. Topstad DR, Panaccione R, Heine JA, et al. Combined seton placement, infliximab infusion, and maintenance immunosuppressives improve healing rate in fistulizing anorectal Crohn disease: a single center experience. Dis Colon Rectum. 2003; 46(5):577–83.

101. Poritz LS, Rowe WA, Koltun WA. Remicade does not abolish the need for surgery in fistulizing Crohn disease. Dis Colon Rectum. 2002;45(6):771 5.

102. Galandiuk S, Kimberling J, Al-Mishlab TG, Stromberg AJ. Perianal Crohn disease: predictors of need for permanent diversion. Ann Surg. 2005;241(5):796–801. discussion -2

103. Rintala RJ, Lindahl HG. Proctocolectomy and J-pouch ileo-anal anastomosis in children. J Pediatr Surg. 2002;37(1):66–70.

104. Su FW, Beckman DB, Yarnold PA, Grammer LC. Low incidence of complications in asthmatic patients treated with preoperative corticosteroids. Allergy Asthma Proc. 2004;25(5):327–33.

105. Marchal L, D'Haens G, Van Assche G, et al. The risk of postoperative complications associated with infliximab therapy for Crohn disease: a controlled cohort study. Aliment Pharmacol Ther. 2004;19(7):749–54.

106. Regueiro M, El-Hachem S, Kip KE, Schraut W, Baidoo L, Watson A, Swoger J, Schwartz M, Barrie A, Pesci M, Binion D. Postoperative infliximab is not associated with an increase in adverse events in Crohn disease. Dig Dis Sci. 2011;56(12): 3610–5.

107. Bordeianou L, Stein SL, Ho VP, Dursun A, Sands BE, Korzenik JR, Hodin RA. Immediate versus tailored prophylaxis to prevent symptomatic recurrences after surgery for ileocecal Crohn disease? Surgery. 2011;149(1):72–8.

108. Spinelli A, Sacchi M, Fiorino G, Danese S, Montorsi M. Risk of postoperative recurrence and postoperative management of Crohn disease. World J Gastroenterol. 2011;17(27):3213–9. Review

109. Schwartz DA, Maltz BE. Treatment of fistulizing inflammatory bowel disease. Gastroenterol Clin North Am. 2009;38(4):595–610. Review

110. Rutgeerts P. Review article: recurrence of Crohn disease after surgery – the need for treatment of new lesions. Aliment Pharmacol Ther. 2006;24(Suppl 3):29–32.

111. Yoshida K, Fukunaga K, Ikeuchi H, et al. Scheduled infliximab monotherapy to prevent recurrence of Crohn disease following ileocolic or ileal resection: a 3-year prospective randomized open trial. Inflamm Bowel Dis. 2011; doi:10.1002/ibd.21928. [Epub ahead of print]

112. Abbas PI, Peterson ML, Fallon SC, Lopez ME, Wesson DE, Walsh SM, Kellermayer R, Rodriguez JR. Evaluating the impact of infliximab use on surgical outcomes in pediatric Crohn's disease. J Pediatr Surg. 2016;51:786–9.

113. Lemann M. Review article: can post-operative recurrence in Crohn disease be prevented? Aliment Pharmacol Ther. 2006; 24(Suppl 3):22–8.

114. Sandborn WJ, Feagan BG. The efficacy of azathioprine and 6-mercaptopurine for the prevention of postoperative recurrence in patients with Crohn disease remains uncertain. Gastroenterology. 2004;127(3):990–3.

115. Rutgeerts P. Strategies in the prevention of post-operative recurrence in Crohn disease. Best Pract Res Clin Gastroenterol. 2003;17(1):63–73.

116. Pelletier AL, Stefanescu C, Vincent C, Etienney I, Mentré F, Soulé JC. Is the length of postoperative recurrence on the neo ileum terminal ileum predictable in Crohn disease? J Crohns Colitis. 2011;5(1):24–7.

117. Stephens M, Batres LA, Ng D, Baldassano R. Growth failure in the child with inflammatory bowel disease. Semin Gastrointest Dis. 2001;12(4):253–62.

Surgical Treatment of Ulcerative Colitis

42

Peter Mattei

Introduction

The surgical treatment of patients with ulcerative colitis (UC) nearly always culminates in the complete removal of the colon and rectum. Although not a cure in the traditional sense, this effectively removes the principal target organ of the disease and, with creation of a neorectum, allows the majority of children and young adults with medically refractory disease to achieve a very high quality of normal function, growth, and development. Colectomy, proctectomy, and ileoanal reconstruction have evolved from the earlier operations that included appendicostomy, which allowed colonic irrigation, and ileostomy, which diverted the fecal stream. These simpler operations allowed some patients relief of their symptoms, but because the diseased colon remained an ongoing source of symptoms and a significant risk of malignant degeneration, they were eventually treated with total colectomy and permanent ileostomy, the standard of care for many decades [1]. More recent advancements have included the ability to create a functional neorectum using the ileum and minimally invasive techniques that have improved recovery and cosmesis. There is increasing emphasis on achieving normal bowel function, minimizing complications, and improving overall quality of life; however, despite such dramatic technical advances, minimal postoperative complications, and overall excellent functional outcomes, the surgical therapy of UC remains less than ideal, principally due to the ongoing and poorly understood tribulations associated with undiagnosed Crohn disease, chronic pouchitis, and, in a significant minority of patients, pouch failure necessitating pouch removal and permanent ileostomy.

P. Mattei, MD
Department of Surgery, Perelman School of Medicine of the University of Pennsylvania, General, Thoracic and Fetal Surgery, The Children's Hospital of Philadelphia, 34th St. & Civic Center Blvd., Philadelphia, PA 19104, USA
e-mail: mattei@email.chop.edu

Indications for Surgical Intervention

The treatment of patients with UC is primarily medical [2, 3]. In fact, with modern drug treatment regimens, most patients with UC can remain largely free of debilitating symptoms for many years. Ultimately, however, approximately 30–40% of patients with UC will ultimately require an operation [4]. Indications for surgical intervention generally fall into one of the three categories (Table 42.1): debilitating symptoms that are refractory to medical management, a serious disease-related complication, or concern about malignant transformation. The most common indication for surgical referral in children is the persistence of bleeding, severe diarrhea, or pain despite maximal medical therapy, but patterns of disease progression are highly variable. Some patients present acutely with rapidly progressive symptoms and unless they respond to aggressive medical treatment are forced to consider having an operation within a few weeks or months of disease onset. Others have symptoms that steadily worsen, requiring more frequent blood product replacement and repeated hospitalizations, until they are no longer responsive to even the most aggressive treatment modalities. Still others, despite otherwise manageable chronic symptoms, will

Table 42.1 Indications for surgery

Urgent/emergent indications
Intractable bleeding
Unrelenting pain
Unremitting sepsis
Complications
Colonic perforation
Colonic stricture
Elective indications
Refractory to or complications of medical management
Chronic malnutrition
Poor growth
Delayed sexual maturation
Steroid dependence
Mucosal dysplasia
Malignant degeneration

© Springer International Publishing AG 2017
P. Mamula et al. (eds.), *Pediatric Inflammatory Bowel Disease*, DOI 10.1007/978-3-319-49215-5_42

be referred for surgery due to poor growth or delayed sexual maturation presumably due to persistent inflammation and chronic malnutrition. As always, the anticipated benefits and potential risks of an operation need to be weighed carefully against the expected consequences of disease progression.

Currently, a complication of UC or its treatment is an uncommon indication for operative intervention, especially in children. Colon *perforation*, though rare, is an indication for urgent laparotomy and should be suspected in patients with UC who present with peritonitis or evidence of free intraperitoneal air. The patient with intractable *bleeding* should also be considered a candidate for urgent colectomy [5]. *Toxic megacolon* includes the combination of sepsis and a massively dilated colon (≥ 6 cm in diameter) [6]. Though often critically ill, these patients can usually be successfully treated with fluid resuscitation and broad-spectrum antibiotics [7]. Indications for urgent laparotomy include perforation, uncontrolled bleeding, or intractable sepsis. Some complications of UC are due to the effects of having long-standing disease and are therefore rare in children. These include colonic stricture, debilitating extraintestinal manifestations of the disease, and malignancy.

Patients are sometimes referred to a surgeon because of complications from medical management or dependence on corticosteroids. Most of the drugs used in the treatment of UC are well tolerated, and there are few serious complications that would prompt consideration of an operation; however, patients who require long-term high-dose corticosteroid therapy can develop serious sequelae such as diabetes, hypertension, opportunistic infection, or psychiatric complications. They can also develop debilitating somatic changes, acne, obesity, growth failure, and osteopenia. Patients with incapacitating side effects of medication and

no effective alternative should be considered for operative intervention.

Although rare in children, mucosal dysplasia identified on colonic biopsy during routine surveillance is an indication for colectomy. Colonoscopic surveillance is recommended for most patients starting 5–8 years after the onset of disease [8]. As UC is being identified in younger patients, we might reasonably expect to see more adolescents with dysplasia being referred for consideration of early colectomy.

The success of currently available medicines has significantly reduced the likelihood that a child with UC will require an emergency operation. One typically begins to consider a surgical option in the patient who is corticosteroid-dependent or whose chronic symptoms are increasingly refractory to medical therapy. As always, the risks of an operation must be considered in the context of the risks of continued nonoperative management. Perhaps more important to consider is the anticipated functional result and life-style implications of undergoing proctocolectomy and pelvic reconstructive surgery.

Surgical Procedures

In the past, proctocolectomy (complete removal of the colon and rectum, Table 42.2) with permanent ileostomy was the standard operation for UC and in many ways remains the benchmark by which all other operations are compared. The operation removes the organ responsible for nearly all of the symptoms of the disease and can be performed in even the sickest patients with a low complication rate and negligible mortality. Patients are usually able to resume normal activities fairly soon after surgery and most adapt well to having

Table 42.2 Surgical options

Operation	Comments
Ileostomy	Rarely performed as an isolated procedure
Abdominal colectomy + Hartmann[a] + ileostomy[b]	Usually performed if an operation is needed urgently
Abdominal colectomy + ileorectostomy	Usually performed for indeterminate or Crohn colitis Requires lifelong surveillance of rectum
Proctocolectomy + end ileostomy	Formerly the standard of care Overall very good results Not popular because ileostomy is permanent
Proctocolectomy + Kock continent ileostomy	Rarely performed except at a few centers with experience Difficult operation with frequent complications
Proctocolectomy + ileal pouch-anal anastomosis	Current standard of care "J-pouch" is most common variation
1. Mucosal proctectomy + hand-sewn IPAA	Good function Leaves no rectal cuff Technically more difficult
2. Proctocolectomy + double-stapled IPAA	Good function Leaves short cuff of rectal mucosa Requires lifelong surveillance of rectal remnant

[a]Hartmann operation: the proximal end of the rectum is sutured or stapled closed; the anus is patent
[b]"Three-stage" approach: (I) Abdominal colectomy/ileostomy, (II) Ileoanal pouch procedure/ileostomy, (III) Ileostomy closure

an ileostomy. Nevertheless, many patients find the idea of a permanent ileostomy objectionable or even unbearable, which led surgeons to develop operations that remove the colon and rectum but allow near-normal bowel function without the use of a permanent ileostomy – the ileal pouch-anal anastomosis (IPAA). In current practice, the operation is typically performed in two or sometimes three stages, depending on the certainty of the diagnosis, the overall health of the patient, and whether the procedure is performed electively or more urgently.

Proctocolectomy with IPAA is a definitive operation for patients with UC; however, the clinical circumstances might dictate that a lesser operation be performed, at least initially. For example, a *diverting ileostomy* might be considered in a patient with severe and intractable colitis of unclear etiology. A typical scenario is that of a young child with severe colitis, whose diagnosis is uncertain (UC vs. Crohn disease) and an adequate trial of medical therapy has not been possible due to rapid progression of the disease. In these situations, it might be difficult for parents to accept the idea of taking such a seemingly dramatic and irreversible step as colectomy. Patients sometimes improve dramatically after ileostomy diversion, but subsequent clinical decision making can be difficult. Simple reversal of the ileostomy after a period of clinical remission often results in prompt recurrence of symptoms, while the true diagnosis remains elusive. In these patients, one should anticipate that another surgical procedure will eventually need to be performed, usually involving colectomy. If the diagnosis of UC is confirmed, the recommended operation is proctocolectomy with IPAA. The diagnosis of Crohn disease, on the other hand, could be an indication for partial colectomy and a restorative operation in which the rectum and part of the colon are preserved (ileocolostomy or ileorectostomy).

Most patients with UC who require an urgent operation are offered *abdominal (subtotal) colectomy*, in which the surgeon removes the colon, creates an ileostomy, and closes the intra-abdominal end of the rectum (Hartmann procedure). The rectum is preserved so that a restorative procedure can be performed on an elective basis after the patient has stabilized and can be prepared properly for such a delicate and demanding operation. Urgent colectomy is traditionally performed through a long midline incision but at some centers is routinely done laparoscopically. The principal risks are surgical site infection and bleeding, though the majority of children do well and recover very quickly. The advantages of a laparoscopic approach include smaller incisions, a shorter recovery time, a more rapid return to normal activities, and less scarring [9–11]. Regardless of the technique, the goal of this urgent operation is to remove most of the diseased colon as quickly and as safely as possible and to allow the patient to return to a state of good health until a more definitive restorative operation can be performed electively 2–3 months later. It also provides a

surgical specimen that can be examined histologically when the true diagnosis remains uncertain.

Despite the fact that the rectum is not removed, patients usually do quite well after abdominal colectomy. After approximately 6 weeks, plans can be made for restorative proctectomy and construction of an ileal reservoir. In the past, some patients were given the option of *ileorectostomy*, in which the rectum is preserved and an anastomosis is created between the ileum and the rectum. This preserves relatively normal rectal sensory and motor function but also retains the rectal mucosa, placing the patient at risk for persistent proctitis and eventual carcinoma. These patients require frequent and meticulous endoscopic surveillance for dysplasia for the rest of their lives. Because of concerns about the risk of cancer and the burden of a lifetime of surveillance, ileorectostomy is no longer considered a suitable option for the definitive treatment of UC in children. However, due to a higher risk of infectious complications and fistulizing perianal disease after ileal reconstruction of the rectum, it is considered a reasonable consideration for children with Crohn disease or indeterminate colitis.

Currently, the most popular restorative operation for children with UC is *ileal pouch-anal anastomosis* (IPAA): the colon and rectum are removed, the ileum is brought down through the pelvic floor musculature, and an anastomosis is created between the ileum and the anus. This creates an ileal reservoir that is intended to function as a replacement for the rectum. The ileum may be unmodified (*straight pull-through*) or can be fashioned to create a more capacious reservoir, the *ileal pouch*. The most commonly used pouch configuration is the *J-pouch*, in which the ileum is folded back on itself for a distance of approximately 8–12 cm and the common wall is obliterated using a surgical stapling device (Fig. 42.1). Other options include the *S-pouch*, in which the ileum is folded twice to create a reservoir that is three times the diameter of the ileum, and the *W-pouch*, in which the ileum is folded yet again, resulting in an even larger reservoir. In general, the larger the pouch, the sooner the patient achieves a pattern of relatively normal bowel habits, but the higher the degree of stasis and bacterial overgrowth, factors that many believe increase the likelihood of pouch inflammation and infection. Given its relative ease of construction and proven track record of excellent functional results, most surgeons currently prefer the J-pouch.

There are two accepted methods of creating the ileoanal anastomosis, both of which produce excellent results. Although the decision is based on the preference of the operating surgeon, it is an important consideration, especially in children. One involves *mucosal proctectomy with a true ileoanal anastomosis*; the other is *total proctectomy with double-stapled anastomosis*, in which case the anastomosis is made between the pouch and the rectum 1–2 cm above the start of the anal mucosa (Fig. 42.2). Mucosal

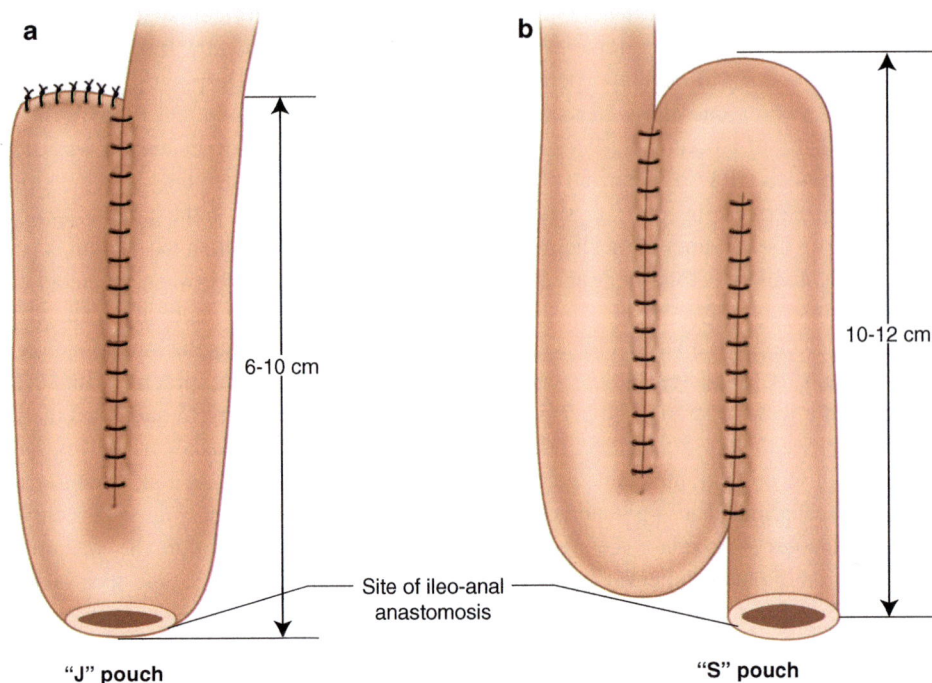

Fig. 42.1 The two most commonly used ileal pouch configurations. (**a**) J-pouch. (**b**) S-pouch. The walls of the jejunal limbs that are brought together are opened using a surgical stapling device so as to create a single lumen that is larger than that of the ileum itself. The ileoanal anastomosis is created by suturing or stapling the lower end of the pouch to the anus

proctectomy involves dissecting along a submucosal plane and removal of the rectal mucosa all the way down to the anal transition zone, with circumferential preservation of a short portion of the muscular wall of the rectum. This was originally designed as a way to remove the mucosa and submucosa, which is where the inflammation in patients with UC is found, while preserving the presumed motor and sensory function of the rectal musculature. The submucosal dissection can be arduous and rather difficult, especially in patients with severe or long-standing rectal inflammation. The ileoanal anastomosis was traditionally created using a hand-sewn technique through the anus, which is laborious but effective. Recently, a new technique has been developed that allows the creation of a circular stapled anastomosis of the pouch to the anal mucosa without having to leave a remnant of diseased rectum [12].

The classic double-stapled approach involves removing the entire thickness of the rectum, which is transected using a linear stapling device somewhere above the anal transition zone. An ileorectal anastomosis is then created using an end-to-end circular stapling device, creating a circular anastomosis. The advantages of this approach include an easier plane of dissection, a less anal sphincter dilatation (placing anastomosis stitches by hand transanally requires more anal stretching than simply inserting a stapling device), and a shorter operating time. The functional results also appear to be the same or better than those achieved using the rectal muscle-sparing hand-sewn technique. An important distinction, however, is that the traditional double-stapled technique necessitates the retention of a short segment of rectal mucosa, usually approximately 1–2 cm in length, which is at risk for ongoing inflammation and malignant degeneration [13, 14]

(Fig. 42.2). Although it is recommended that *all* patients be followed indefinitely regardless of the surgical technique used, those with retained rectal mucosa require more diligent surveillance, including frequent routine biopsies, for their entire lives, which is probably why it is the less attractive alternative for younger people [15].

At the time of ileoanal reconstruction, surgeons have traditionally also performed a temporary ileostomy, which is supposed to decrease the risk of anastomotic leak, pelvic abscess, and other postoperative septic complications. These complications have been associated with poor pouch function and a significantly diminished long-term quality of life [16, 17]. Although pelvic sepsis is relatively uncommon even without diversion, some surgeons prefer to minimize the risk as much as possible by performing a temporary ileostomy. Others feel that the risk of a severe complication is low enough that protective ileostomy can be avoided in certain patients [18, 19]; however, this remains somewhat controversial. The ileostomy can usually be reversed 6–8 weeks after surgery, usually after a water-soluble contrast enema confirms good healing, a normal pouch configuration, and good evacuation (Fig. 42.3). For most patients, this will be the second or third stage of the operation, depending on whether a subtotal colectomy was done at the first stage.

A procedure that is rarely performed anymore but deserves mention is the *Kock pouch* (or *continent ileostomy*) operation [20, 21]. The colon and rectum are completely removed, and the ileum is used to create a reservoir that resides within the abdomen. The end of the ileum is brought out through a small abdominal incision in the manner of an ileostomy, but a small intussusception is created just proximal to the outlet, essentially creating a valve that prevents the leakage of stool.

Fig. 42.2 Two commonly used methods for creation of the ileal pouch-anal anastomosis: (**a**) *Double-stapled anastomosis*, so-called because the rectum is first divided and stapled transversely, and then an anastomosis is created between the pouch and the rectum with a specialized stapling device that creates a circular staple line between two hollow viscera (**b**) *Mucosectomy with hand-sewn anastomosis*, in which the mucosa is stripped from the distal rectum, preserving a short segment of rectal musculature, and the anastomosis is performed by hand. Note that with the double-stapled technique, it is unavoidable that a short (1–2 cm) segment of rectal mucosa remains, while after mucosectomy the mucosa is excised all the way down to the anal transition zone. The J-pouch or S-pouch can be used with either method

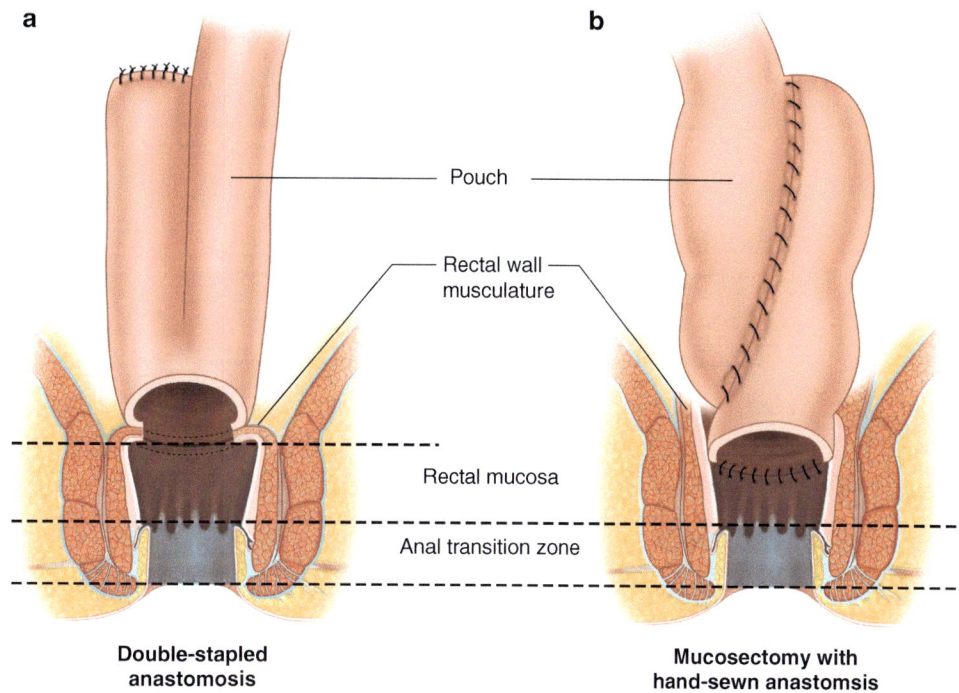

a

b

Pouch

Rectal wall musculature

Rectal mucosa

Anal transition zone

Double-stapled anastomosis

Mucosectomy with hand-sewn anastomsis

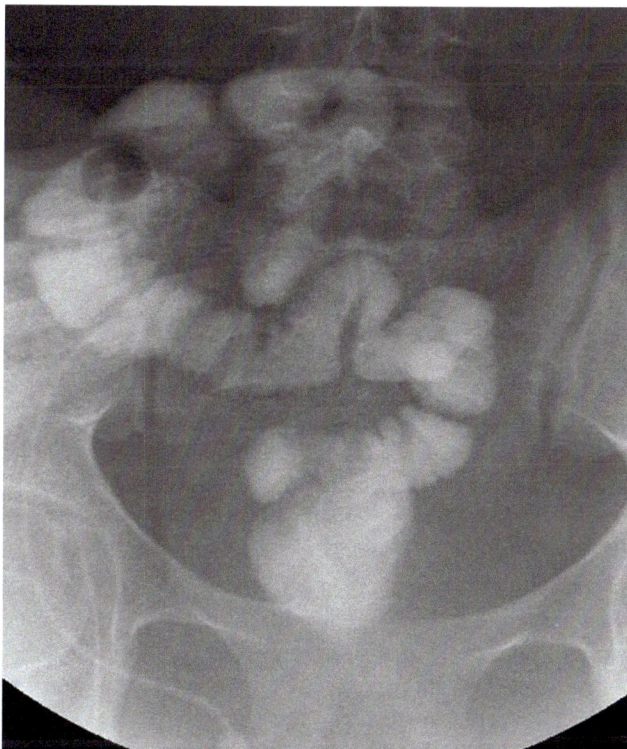

Fig. 42.3 Contrast study performed through mucous fistula of loop ileostomy. The pouch is situated low in the pelvis, is reasonably capacious without evidence of stricture, and is not twisted or volvulized. Functionally, it is important to note that the patient sensed the presence of contrast, was able to hold it for the duration of the study, and at the conclusion of the study was able to evacuate completely and voluntarily

The patient does not wear a standard ileostomy appliance and instead uses a plastic tube to evacuate the pouch several times daily as needed. The concept is certainly appealing; however, the long-term results of the Kock pouch have been somewhat disappointing and the complication rate has been unacceptably high in most centers. The procedure has for the most part been abandoned, except at a small number of institutions worldwide.

Surgical Decision Making

Recent worldwide experience has confirmed that children with UC whose disease is refractory to medical management are best served by the combination of colectomy, proctectomy, and ileal pouch-anal anastomosis, with or without a temporary protective ileostomy [22, 23]. Though classically considered a three-stage operation, and still perhaps best conceptualized as a three-stage operation, there is sometimes pressure, mostly from patients and their parents, to combine all three stages in a single operation, namely, colectomy, proctectomy, and IPAA without a temporary protective ileostomy (Fig. 42.4). There are reports in adults and in children that a one-stage approach is generally safe and appears to produce similar long-term results and functional outcomes as the two- or three-stage approaches [24, 25]. These studies are certainly promising and somewhat compelling; however, it must be noted that a true side-by-side comparison or

"Classic" 3-Stage Operation:

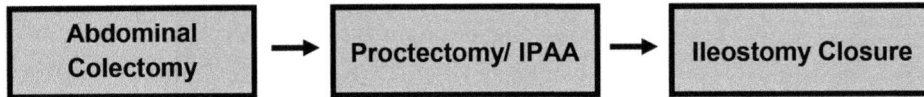

Abdominal Colectomy → Proctectomy/ IPAA → Ileostomy Closure

Traditional 2-Stage Operation:

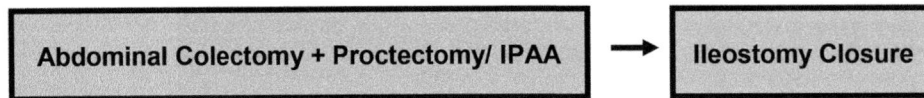

Abdominal Colectomy + Proctectomy/ IPAA → Ileostomy Closure

Contemporary 2-Stage Operation:

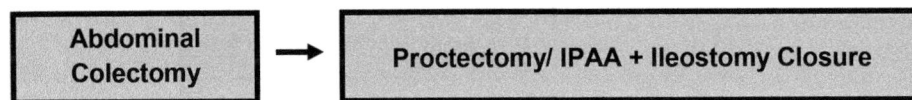

Abdominal Colectomy → Proctectomy/ IPAA + Ileostomy Closure

One-Stage Operation:

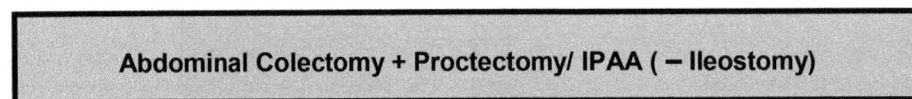

Abdominal Colectomy + Proctectomy/ IPAA (− Ileostomy)

Fig. 42.4 Each box represents a single operation, sometimes comprised of more than one operative procedure. Each *arrow* represents a typical wait time between operations of at least 6 weeks, depending on the clinical status of the patient. Patients who are healthy, with good nutrition, and on low-dose or no corticosteroids might be considered for a one-stage operation; however, currently these patients are rarely considered candidates for surgery. The more typical pediatric patient being considered for surgical intervention has at least one significant risk factor, making a two-stage operation a safer option. Functional results and patient satisfaction might be better with the contemporary two-stage operation than with the traditional two-stage operation, in which the colectomy, proctectomy/IPAA, and ileostomy are performed at the first operation. The three-stage approach is still sometimes indicated, especially in patients who are chronically ill or have anatomic features that place the pouch at significant risk of ischemia or undue tension

randomized trial has not been, and probably never will be, done. This means that there is likely some selection bias on the part of surgeons who must decide whether they feel comfortable proceeding with a single-stage procedure or not. The decision is complex and involves consideration of several factors: (1) the overall health status of the patient, especially nutrition and corticosteroid dependence; (2) whether the operation is being performed electively or emergently; (3) confidence in the diagnosis (UC or Crohn disease); (4) intraoperative factors such as the length and difficulty of the operation, blood loss, degree of soiling of the pelvis with rectal contents, blood supply of the ileal pouch, and degree of tension at the anastomosis; and (5) recent administration of biological agents such as infliximab – some [26, 27] but not all [28, 29] studies suggest an increased risk of surgical complications for up to 8 weeks. There is also the overriding concern, based on the early published series of the results of IPAA, that pouch complications such as leak and pelvic sepsis diminish pouch function for the life of the patient, [16, 17] which in children could reasonably be expected to be more than 50 years after the operation. Therefore, because most pediatric surgeons would consider long-term functional results more important than the short-term inconvenience of multiple operations or time with an ileostomy, they are more likely to prefer to err on the side of caution. Nevertheless, the progressive pediatric surgeon should evaluate the published data objectively, consider the individual risk factors and overall status of the patient on a case-by-case basis, and discuss all options with patients and their families in a frank but compassionate manner.

Patients with UC who are nutritionally robust and whose symptoms are relatively well controlled tend to be considered responsive to medical management and therefore are not considered candidates for surgical intervention. As a result, those patients who are considered for surgery tend to be acutely ill (bleeding, pain, intractable diarrhea) or severely chronically unwell (malnutrition, corticosteroid dependency, growth failure). These patients are perhaps best served by abdominal colectomy, preferably performed laparoscopically, and temporary end ileostomy. The vast majority feel better immediately, wean off corticosteroids (and all medications) rapidly, gain weight nicely, and are pleased to have had the operation. In patients for whom the diagnosis remains uncertain, this also provides a large specimen (the colon) to examine carefully for signs of Crohn disease without having "burned a bridge" by removing the rectum. (Interestingly, very few patients have symptoms due to inflammation in the diverted rectum even off all systemic medications.) On the other hand, under these same circumstances, there are some surgeons who would consider going ahead with proctectomy and IPAA and perhaps even consider avoiding the ileostomy. Provided that parents understand the risks of short-term complications are *probably* higher and that long-term pouch function *could* be affected, this might be a reasonable approach in select cases.

In some cases a compromise in the form of a two-stage approach is a reasonable option. The traditional two-stage approach is to combine the colectomy and proctectomy/IPAA but to perform a temporary protective ileostomy. (This is also the fallback position when one believes a one-stage procedure is feasible going in but then encounters technical difficulties or is unhappy with the viability or tension of the pouch during the operation.) Then again, some surgeons have found that if they perform abdominal colectomy up front and allow the patient to become healthy and come off all medications, the proctectomy/IPAA becomes technically much easier, and they are therefore more likely to forego the ileostomy. Other advantages of performing the ileostomy after the first operation include better patient acceptance of an ileostomy at a time when they are ill but are expected to begin to feel better (they often associate their improved sense of well-being with the ileostomy rather than with the colectomy); the diverted rectum is "cleaner" and often less inflamed at the time of proctectomy, and it avoids having to create a mid-ileal anastomosis at the time of the ultimate ileostomy closure – the ileostomy placed after colectomy is an "end" ileostomy, which ultimately becomes part of the pouch, while the ileostomy placed after proctectomy/IPAA is a "loop" ileostomy, closure of which entails a bowel anastomosis and potentially the increased risk of subsequent stricture or adhesive bowel obstruction.

Finally, though it might be considered "old-fashioned" and it certainly should no longer be considered the standard approach in children with UC, it is reasonable to recommend a three-stage operation when appropriate [30]. The chronically ill patient who has intraoperative complications or a pouch that is under significant tension is probably not best served by a heroic attempt at a one-stage operation. As always, surgical decision making for patients with UC demands careful consideration of the overall balance of potential risks and anticipated benefits. The opinions of patients and their parents should also be considered whenever possible.

Preparation for Surgery

Patients who need an urgent operation are prepared for surgery in the usual fashion, with intravenous fluid resuscitation and broad-spectrum prophylactic antibiotics. Patients who are anemic may require a blood transfusion, depending on the surgical and anesthetic standards of the institution. Typically 1–2 units of packed red blood cells are made available for possible use during or after the operation. For patients receiving corticosteroids, it is still standard practice at some institutions to administer a "stress dose" of corticosteroids. Lastly, if time allows, the patient should be evaluated by an enterostomal therapist so that an optimal ileostomy site can be identified and marked.

Patients who are being prepared for an elective procedure should have a formal nutritional assessment. Moderate to severe malnutrition prolongs healing and increases the risk of complications after major surgery. Enteral or parenteral nutritional supplementation is sometimes necessary, even if this means delaying the operation for several weeks. Given that chronic, high-dose corticosteroid therapy can also adversely affect wound healing and increase the risks of an operation, attempts should be made to gradually decrease the dose for patients who are scheduled for surgery, preferably down to 15–20 mg of prednisone daily. Although gradually falling out of favor for most colorectal operations, some surgeons still believe that a mechanical bowel preparation decreases the risk of septic complications after major colorectal surgery. A typical regimen includes a clear liquid diet for 24–48 h and the administration of an osmotic laxative such as polyethylene glycol or magnesium citrate solution. Antibiotics are given intravenously immediately before incision, but oral antibiotics are also sometimes used. There are recent data that suggest bowel preparation does not improve the outcome for most kinds of elective colorectal surgery [31, 32], but the potential benefit in patients who undergo proctectomy and ileoanal reconstruction is not well known.

Outcomes of Surgery

The technical results of the operations described for children with UC are generally quite good. Infectious complications and bleeding are uncommon and usually easily managed without sequelae. Even after the most complicated operations, most children recover nicely and are able to tolerate a regular diet within a few days of surgery. The short-term results for patients who undergo a minimally invasive procedure might be slightly better, with the added benefit of improved cosmesis [9–11]. Regardless of the technique, the overall risk of serious complications or death is very low.

Functional Results

The functional results of IPAA are generally very good, though there is a great deal of variation between patients and in the same patient over time. The ultimate goal of surgical intervention is for the patient to enjoy a normal lifestyle; however, there are inherent limitations in duplicating normal rectal function with a surgical construct [33]. The ideal functional result of IPAA includes (1) fecal continence day and night, (2) four or fewer stools throughout the daytime, (3) no more than one stool at night, (4) the ability to postpone evacuation for 30 min, and (5) the ability to distinguish between flatus and stool.

The J-pouch IPAA is still the most popular operation for children and adolescents with UC who need surgical intervention, and several large studies have confirmed that the majority of patients have good functional results [25, 34–38]. In most large series, patients report an average stool frequency of three per day and once or none at night. Fewer than 5% have soiling or staining, most of which occurs only at night. Approximately 90% of patients can delay defecation for at least 30 min, and most report being able to pass flatus without accidents. Many patients are able to participate in a wide variety of normal activities including athletics [36]. Studies using patient questionnaires document a very good quality of life for the majority of patients after IPAA with 90–95% of patients reported to be satisfied or very satisfied with the results of their operation [39, 40].

Because the anal dilatation required during completion of the mucosectomy and creation of the ileoanal anastomosis might result in injury to the anal sphincter, some studies have assessed anorectal function after IPAA using rectal manometry [41, 42], though few have included children [43]. Most studies confirm that although there is often a decrease in resting sphincter pressure and maximum squeeze pressure after IPAA relative to preoperative controls, these values gradually return to normal when patients are followed for more than a year. Furthermore, although the rectal inhibitory reflex is often noted to be absent, nearly all patients regain normal rectal sensation for the presence of stool.

Most large series of patients who undergo IPAA report good results regardless of pouch anatomy or method of pelvic dissection. Some surgeons continue to advocate the use of a straight ileoanal anastomosis [44, 45]. The purported benefits of avoiding a pouch include its relative ease of construction, the creation of less tension on the small bowel mesentery, and decreased stasis, which is thought to increase the risk of pouchitis. Nevertheless, the disadvantages of the procedure, including increased frequency and urgency of defecation, are felt by most surgeons to outweigh its potential advantages. A number of patients with a straight pull-through ask to be converted to a J-pouch because of the unacceptably high frequency of stooling [35]. When compared with colectomy and either Brooke or Kock ileostomy, most studies report improved functional results and quality of life in patients who have undergone colectomy with IPAA [46, 47]. However, at least one group has suggested that it is the colectomy that is responsible for most of the improvement in the quality of life for patients with UC and that restoration of normal defecation actually contributes very little [39].

When mucosal proctectomy with hand-sewn anastomosis is compared to extra-rectal proctectomy and double-stapled anastomosis, the functional results and quality of life parameters appear to be identical [15, 48–50], although the relative simplicity of the double-stapled technique may result in improved results in centers where few such procedures are performed [51]. Patients who require a revision of their pouch also tend to do better than expected [52], although it is certainly preferable for any complex reconstructive procedure to function well after the first attempt. All in all, careful analysis of the collective experience with the IPAA operation over the past two decades confirms that it is a good operation, with excellent functional results and improved quality of life for the majority of patients with UC who need surgery.

Complications

As with any complex reconstructive operation, the complication rate for IPAA is not insignificant, occurring in as many as half of all patients [16, 36, 37, 53]. Complications that occur in the immediate postoperative period – surgical site infection, postoperative ileus, and excessive ileostomy output – are usually easily managed. More serious complications such as small bowel obstruction due to adhesions, parastomal hernia, and pelvic abscess may require operative intervention.

A rare but serious complication of ileal pouch-anal anastomosis is partial or complete anastomotic disruption. This usually manifests as pelvic sepsis, often with an organizing abscess, or with a clinical picture of a perforated viscus, including peritonitis, shoulder pain, free intraperitoneal air on imaging, and occasionally frank sepsis. Partial disruptions typically take the form of a tiny leak and can sometimes be managed conservatively with fluid resuscitation, antibiotics, and percutaneous drainage of the abscess. However, patients who are clinically ill, have frank peritonitis, or show signs of more than just a small leak should undergo ileostomy diversion. The experienced surgeon will resist the strong urge to perform a repair, which, under these conditions, is futile and dangerous. Much has been made in the past about the subsequent poor function of a pouch construction that has been complicated by pelvic sepsis, which was typically used to caution surgeons to be more conservative and always create a protective ileostomy. However, although anastomotic stricture is certainly more common, it can usually be treated with anal dilation. If patients who are well-nourished and off corticosteroids are provided a well-vascularized and tension-free pouch, the risk of significant disruption is minimal and does not justify subjecting every patient to diversion.

Long-term complications are often more significant as they can interfere with the function of the pouch and may result in less than satisfactory function [54, 55]. Approximately 10–15% of patients develop a *stricture* at the ileoanal anastomosis, which increases the risk of pouch stasis and pouchitis. Symptomatic strictures usually respond to periodic anal dilatation and rarely require surgical revision or ileostomy. When an ileoanal stricture is associated with a *perirectal abscess* or *anal fistula*, the diagnosis of Crohn disease must be considered. Prolapse, stenosis, or retraction of the ileostomy may occur, but because the ileostomy is generally temporary, these complications can often be managed by early closure.

Pouchitis

Perhaps the most significant potential complication after IPAA is acute or chronic *pouchitis*. The patient with acute pouchitis typically presents with increased stool frequency, urgency, or pain and sometimes by bloody stools, tenesmus, abdominal distension, or fever. The diagnosis is usually made on clinical grounds, though endoscopic examination of the mucosa may reveal mucosal edema, ulceration, or friable granulation tissue [56]. Biopsies often reveal an acute inflammatory process, with polymorphonuclear leukocyte infiltration, crypt abscesses, or ulceration depending on the severity of the disease. The true incidence and relative severity of pouchitis has been difficult to evaluate consistently between series, perhaps because of the variable presentation and somewhat subjective manner in which the diagnosis is made. Some have therefore proposed the use of a pouchitis disease activity index score so that therapeutic trials from different institutions can be more easily assessed and compared [54, 57, 58] (Table 42.3).

Of patients who have had an IPAA for UC, perhaps as many as 40% will have at least one bout of pouchitis. Interestingly, the disease almost never occurs in patients who have had an IPAA for familial adenomatous polyposis. At the opposite extreme, it affects as many as 80% of patients with UC who have primary sclerosing cholangitis. Most patients with acute pouchitis respond promptly to a short course of

Table 42.3 Pouchitis disease activity index [57, 58]

Criteria	Score
Clinical	
Stool frequency	
Usual postoperative stool frequency	0
1–2 stools/day > postoperative usual	1
3 or more stools/day > postoperative usual	2
Rectal bleeding	
None or rare	0
Present daily	1
Fecal urgency or abdominal cramps	
None	0
Occasional	1
Usual	2
Fever (temperature >37.8 ° C)	
Absent	0
Present	1
Endoscopic inflammation	
Edema	1
Granularity	1
Friability	1
Loss of vascular pattern	1
Mucous exudates	1
Ulceration	1
Acute histologic inflammation	
Polymorphonuclear leukocyte infiltration	
Mild	1
Moderate + crypt abscess	2
Severe + crypt abscess	3
Ulceration per low-power field (mean)	
<25%	1
25–50%	2
>50%	3

A total score of 7 is considered consistent with a diagnosis of pouchitis. A modified pouchitis disease activity index (mPDAI) has been proposed [58] in which the histology component is excluded, thus avoiding the risk and cost of biopsies. Using the mPDAI, a score of 5 is considered diagnostic of pouchitis

oral metronidazole and/or ciprofloxacin. Chronic or relapsing acute pouchitis is less common but can be debilitating. Some have suggested that it represents a form of "recurrent" UC and clinically may behave as such. Approximately 5–10% of patients eventually require permanent ileostomy or removal of the pouch because of intractable pouchitis [55]. The treatment of severe chronic pouchitis is often similar to that of UC or Crohn colitis, including anti-inflammatory enemas, chronic antibiotic therapy, or infliximab [59].

The cause of pouchitis is unknown, though the fact that it occurs almost exclusively in patients with UC would suggest a specific underlying predisposition. A small but significant percentage of patients with severe pouchitis will eventually be identified as having Crohn disease. Regardless of the etiology, stasis appears to be an important factor that increases the risk of pouchitis. This is supported by the observation that pouchitis is less common after straight ileoanal pull-through. Pouchitis is also more common in the presence of an ileoanal stricture or an excessively dilated pouch. Some patients will respond to serial anal dilatations or daily rectal intubation or saline irrigation; however, surgical revision of the pouch needs to be considered in these situations. Some have found that bulking agents in the form of dietary fiber supplements reduce the incidence of pouchitis [60], perhaps by promoting more complete evacuation of the pouch. Probiotics may decrease the risk of pouchitis; however, thus far the results of clinical trials have been mixed [61–63].

As many as 13% of children who undergo IPAA will eventually be found to have Crohn disease, developing complications after IPAA including pouchitis, sinus tracts, fistulae, and pelvic abscess [64]. Although some respond well to standard medical therapy, many will eventually require removal of the pouch and permanent ileostomy. Similarly, many consider indeterminate colitis a contraindication to IPAA, though there are some who advocate the use of pelvic pouch procedures in this subgroup of patients, citing an acceptable complication rate [65]. Interestingly, the presence of terminal ileitis ("backwash" ileitis) at operation does not appear to increase the risk of complications, pouchitis, or pouch failure [64]. Patients who develop severe or recurrent pouchitis, anal fistula, or pelvic sepsis after IPAA should be evaluated for Crohn disease with small intestinal imaging, upper and lower endoscopy with biopsies, and serologic analysis for markers of Crohn disease.

Carcinoma

Long-term complications of UC include colorectal carcinoma. Patients with UC are recommended to have yearly colonoscopy with frequent biopsies starting several years after onset of symptoms, and cancer is an indication for colectomy in patients with UC [66]. Patients with high-grade dysplasia are at high risk for carcinoma and are also recommended to undergo colectomy. Those with low-grade dysplasia are observed more closely with colonoscopy every 6 months, though there are proponents of colectomy for these patients as well [67, 68]. Although malignancy is rarely an issue in children, there are several important considerations for the pediatric gastroenterologist. First, as the incidence of UC is increasing [69] and increasingly affecting younger patients, it is more likely that patients will need to begin surveillance in adolescence. Secondly, patients who undergo IPAA using a double-stapled technique invariably have a 1–2 cm cuff of native rectal mucosa distal to the ileal pouch anastomosis, which necessitates lifelong surveillance because of the risk of dysplasia or cancer within the remnant. Because of the obvious long-term implications, this is an important technical detail that should be passed along to the patient. Lastly, there are occasional reports of cancer developing within the ileal pouch itself or at the ileoanal anastomosis [70, 71], suggesting that the risk of carcinoma can never be completely eliminated in patients with UC. Patients should therefore undergo periodic endoscopic evaluation of the pouch with biopsies, although the frequency of these assessments has not been standardized [72].

Current Trends and Future Considerations

Patients with UC who have undergone IPAA surgery as children are now able to be evaluated as adults. Several series have reported a significant incidence of infertility in women who have undergone ileoanal pouch procedures [73–77], with some series suggesting that the risk is double of what is expected for women matched for age and severity of disease who are treated medically. Although fertility can be a difficult factor to assess accurately, especially in a select subgroup of chronically ill individuals, a preponderance of data appears to support this link. The risk of infertility is considerably higher for women with UC who undergo IPAA compared to those with familial polyposis and to those who have had an ileorectostomy. The risk is also significantly higher for those who require an intraoperative blood transfusion. The cause of infertility in these cases is unclear. It is thought that the degree of pelvic surgical dissection might generate adhesions, which are known to have a negative impact on fertility. This has led some groups to adopt empirically the use of enzymatic adhesion barriers during IPAA surgery, although there are no data to support that its use reduces infertility [76, 78, 79]. Nevertheless, it is an issue that should be discussed with any young woman with UC who is considering surgical intervention, as they may choose to delay the operation until after they have children.

Outcomes research generally supports the view that the functional results are better and the complication rate is lower for complex operations performed at high-volume centers. The IPAA procedure is a technically demanding operation with many pitfalls and potential complications. Although there are no large series in which a direct comparison has been done specifically for IPAA in patients with UC, there appears to be a correlation between the experience of the surgeon and favorable outcomes in a variety of complex colorectal procedures [80–82]. In addition, several studies report a significant learning curve for surgeons who perform ileoanal pouch procedures [83–85]. This suggests that the results of IPAA procedures that are done by experienced surgeons and at high-volume centers are likely to be better overall.

Minimally invasive surgery offers potential advantages such as less scarring, less pain, more rapid postoperative recovery, and improved cosmesis [86] (Fig. 42.5). Many surgeons advo-

a

b

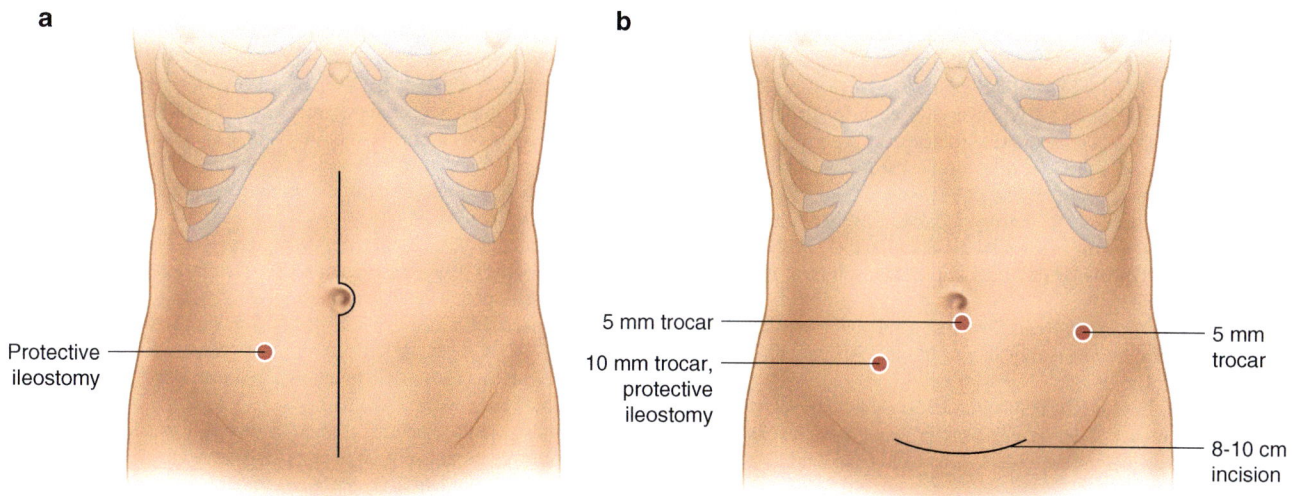

Protective ileostomy

5 mm trocar

10 mm trocar, protective ileostomy

5 mm trocar

8-10 cm incision

Fig. 42.5 Comparison of (**a**) the long midline incision used for the standard open colectomy and ileal pouch-anal anastomosis operation and (**b**) the smaller incisions used during laparoscopic colectomy and ileal pouch-anal anastomosis operation. The right lower quadrant laparoscopic incision is used for creation of an ileostomy. The low transverse incision is a Pfannenstiel incision, also referred to as a "bikini-line" incision, and is used for the creation of the ileoanal pouch after the colon is removed laparoscopically. It can also be used to allow insertion of the surgeon's hand to facilitate the laparoscopic portion of the operation ("hand-assisted" laparoscopy). The primary advantage of the minimally invasive approach is improved cosmesis; other purported advantages include shorter hospital stay and faster recovery

cate the use of a laparoscopic-assisted approach, [10, 11] in which the colectomy is performed laparoscopically, while the more delicate pelvic dissection is done through an open incision but one that is much smaller than usual. Although the initial results with this approach have been encouraging, it is too soon to know if the long-term functional results will be the same compared to the more standard open approach. As the technology continues to improve, minimally invasive approaches to complex colorectal surgery in children, including robotic techniques, will eventually become the standard of care for children with UC who need surgery.

Summary

The goals of surgical intervention for UC are to remove the affected organ, to restore normal function, and to minimize morbidity. The surgical treatment of children and adolescents with UC has improved dramatically over the past few decades, mostly because of technical refinements of the ileal pouch-anal anastomosis procedure. Ileal pouch-anal anastomosis has become the standard of care for patients with UC who require surgical intervention. The majority of patients who undergo IPAA can expect to enjoy an essentially normal lifestyle, although the operation is technically demanding and can be associated with significant morbidity. Surgeons continue to strive to develop restorative operations that more closely duplicate normal anatomy and function with fewer potentially debilitating side effects.

References

1. Onaitis MW, Mantyh C. Ileal pouch-anal anastomosis for ulcerative colitis and familial adenomatous polyposis: historical development and current status. Ann Surg. 2003;238(6 Suppl):S42–8.
2. Fell JM. Update of the management of inflammatory bowel disease. Arch Dis Child. 2012;97(1):78–83.
3. Blonski W, Buchner AM, Lichtenstein GR. Inflammatory bowel disease therapy: current state-of-the-art. Curr Opin Gastroenterol. 2011;27(4):346–57.
4. Hancock L, Windsor AC, Mortensen NJ. Inflammatory bowel disease: the view of the surgeon. Color Dis. 2006;8(Suppl.1):10–4.
5. Tsujikawa T, Andoh A, Sakaki M, et al. Operative indications for patients with refractory or severe ulcerative colitis. Hepato-Gastroenterology. 2005;52(65):1470–3.
6. Ausch C, Madoff RD, Gnant M, et al. Aetiology and surgical management of toxic megacolon. Color Dis. 2005;8(3):195–201.
7. Autenrieth DM, Baumgart DC. Toxic megacolon. Inflamm Bowel Dis. 2012;18(3):584–91.
8. Itzkowitz SH, Harpaz N. Diagnosis and management of dysplasia in patients with inflammatory bowel diseases. Gastroenterology. 2004;126(6):1634–48.
9. Diamond IR, Gerstle JT, Kim PC, Langer JC. Outcomes after laparoscopic surgery in children with inflammatory bowel disease. Surg Endosc. 2010;24(11):2796–802.
10. Holder-Murray J, Marsicovetere P, Holubar SD. Minimally invasive surgery for inflammatory bowel disease. Inflamm Bowel Dis. 2015;21(6):1443–58.
11. Kienle P, Weitz J, Benner A, et al. Laparoscopically assisted colectomy and ileoanal pouch procedure with and without protective ileostomy. Surg Endosc. 2003;17(5):716–20.
12. Geiger JD, Teitelbaum DH, Hirschl RB, Coran AG. A new operative technique for restorative proctocolectomy: the endorectal pull-through combined with a double-stapled ileo-anal anastomosis. Surgery. 2003;134(3):492–5.

13. M'Koma AE, Moses HL, Adunyah SE. Inflammatory bowel disease-associated colorectal cancer: proctocolectomy and mucosectomy do not necessarily eliminate pouch-related cancer incidences. Int J Color Dis. 2011;26(5):533–52.

14. O'Riordain MG, Fazio VW, Lavery IC, et al. Incidence and natural history of dysplasia of the anal transitional zone after ileal pouch-anal anastomosis: results of a five-year to ten-year follow-up. Dis Colon Rectum. 2000;43(12):1660–5.

15. Davis C, Alexander F, Lavery I, Fazio VW. Results of mucosal proctectomy versus extrarectal dissection for ulcerative colitis and familial polyposis in children and young adults. J Pediatr Surg. 1994;29(2):305–9.

16. Fazio VW, Kiran RP, Remzi FH, et al. Ileal pouch anal anastomosis: analysis of outcome and quality of life in 3707 patients. Ann Surg. 2013;257(4):679–85.

17. Farouk R, Dozois RR, Pemberton JH, Larson D. Incidence and subsequent impact of pelvic abscess after ileal pouch-anal anastomosis for chronic ulcerative colitis. Dis Colon Rectum. 1998;41(10):1239–43.

18. Sugerman HJ, Sugerman EL, Meador JG, et al. Ileal pouch anal anastomosis without ileal diversion. Ann Surg. 2000;232(4):530–41.

19. Kim NK, Park JS, Park JK, et al. Restorative proctocolectomy: operative safety and functional outcomes. Yonsei Med J. 2000;41(5):634–41.

20. Telander RL, Smith SL, Marcinek HM, et al. Surgical treatment of ulcerative colitis in children. Surgery. 1981;90(4):787–94.

21. Castillo E, Thomassie LM, Whitlow CB, et al. Continent ileostomy: current experience. Dis Colon Rectum. 2005;48(6):1263–8.

22. Lillehei CW et al. Restorative proctocolectomy and ileal pouch-anal anastomosis in children. Dis Colon Rectum. 2009;52(9):1645–9.

23. Patton D, Gupta N, Wojcicki JM, Garnett EA, Nobuhara K, Heyman MB. Postoperative outcome of colectomy for pediatric patients with ulcerative colitis. J Pediatr Gastroenterol Nutr. 2010;51(2):151–4.

24. Weston-Petrides GK, Lovegrove RE, Tilney HS, Heriot AG, Nicholls RJ, Mortensen NJ, Fazio VW, Tekkis PP. Comparison of outcomes after restorative proctocolectomy with or without defunctioning ileostomy. Arch Surg. 2008;143(4):406–12.

25. Gray BW, Drongowski RA, Hirschl RB, Geiger JD. Restorative proctocolectomy without diverting ileostomy in children with ulcerative colitis. J Pediatr Surg. 2012;47(1):204–8.

26. Mor IJ, Vogel JD, da Luz MA, Shen B, Hammel J, Remzi FH. Infliximab in ulcerative colitis is associated with an increased risk of postoperative complications after restorative proctocolectomy. Dis Colon Rectum. 2008;51(8):1202–7.

27. Kennedy R, Potter DD, Moir C, Zarroug AE, Faubion W, Tung J. Pediatric chronic ulcerative colitis: does infliximab increase post-ileal pouch anal anastomosis complications? J Pediatr Surg. 2012;47(1):199–203.

28. Gainsbury ML, Chu DI, Howard LA, Coukos JA, Farraye FA, Stucchi AF, Becker JM. Preoperative infliximab is not associated with an increased risk of short-term postoperative complications after restorative proctocolectomy and ileal pouch-anal anastomosis. J Gastrointest Surg. 2011;15(3):397–403.

29. Coquet-Reinier B, Berdah SV, Grimaud JC, Birnbaum D, Cougard PA, Barthet M, Desjeux A, Moutardier V, Brunet C. Preoperative infliximab treatment and postoperative complications after laparoscopic restorative proctocolectomy with ileal pouch-anal anastomosis: a case-matched study. Surg Endosc. 2010;24(8):1866–71.

30. Bikhchandani J, Polites SF, Wagie AE, Habermann EB, Cima RR. National trends of 3- versus 2-stage restorative proctocolectomy for chronic ulcerative colitis. Dis Colon Rectum. 2015;58(2):199–204.

31. Güenaga KF, Matos D, Wille-Jørgensen P. Mechanical bowel preparation for elective colorectal surgery. Cochrane Database Syst Rev. 2011;9:CD001544.

32. Van't Sant HP, Weidema WF, Hop WC, Oostvogel HJ, Contant CM. The influence of mechanical bowel preparation in elective lower colorectal surgery. Ann Surg. 2010;251(1):59–63.

33. Thompson-Fawcett MW, Jewell DP, Mortensen NJ. Ileoanal reservoir dysfunction: a problem-solving approach. Br J Surg. 1997;84(10):1351–9.

34. van Balkom KA, Beld MP, Visschers RG, van Gemert WG, Breukink SO. Long-term results after restorative proctocolectomy with ileal pouch-anal anastomosis at a young age. Dis Colon Rectum. 2012;55(9):939–47.

35. Stavlo PL, Libsch KD, Rodeberg DA, Moir CR. Pediatric ileal pouch-anal anastomosis: functional outcomes and quality of life. J Pediatr Surg. 2003;38(6):935–9.

36. Fonkalsrud EW, Thakur A, Beanes S. Ileoanal pouch procedures in children. J Pediatr Surg. 2001;36(11):1689–92.

37. Rintala RJ, Lindahl HG. Proctocolectomy and J-pouch ileo-anal anastomosis in children. J Pediatr Surg. 2002;37(1):66–70.

38. Wewer V, Hesselfeldt P, Qvist N, et al. J-pouch ileoanal anastomosis in children and adolescents with ulcerative colitis: functional outcome, satisfaction and impact on social life. J Pediatr Gastroenterol Nutr. 2005;40(2):189–93.

39. Weinryb RM, Gustavsson JP, Liljeqvist L, et al. A prospective study of the quality of life after pelvic pouch operation. J Am Coll Surg. 1995;180(5):589–95.

40. Shamberger RC, Masek BJ, Leichtner AM, et al. Quality-of-life assessment after ileoanal pull-through for ulcerative colitis and familial adenomatous polyposis. J Pediatr Surg. 1999;34(1):163–6.

41. Luukkonen P. Manometric follow-up of anal sphincter function after an ileo-anal pouch procedure. Int J Color Dis. 1988;3(1):43–6.

42. Becker JM, McGrath KM, Meagher MP, et al. Late functional adaptation after colectomy, mucosal proctectomy, and ileal pouch-anal anastomosis. Surgery. 1991;110(4):718–24. discussion 725.

43. Shamberger RC, Lillehei CW, Nurko S, Winter HS. Anorectal function in children after ileoanal pull-through. J Pediatr Surg. 1994;29(2):329–32. discussion 332–3.

44. Shilyansky J, Lelli JL, Drongowski RA, Coran AG. Efficacy of the straight endorectal pull-through in the management of familial adenomatous polyposis – a 16-year experience. J Pediatr Surg. 1997;32(8):1139–43.

45. Coran AG. A personal experience with 100 consecutive total colectomies and straight ileoanal endorectal pull-throughs for benign disease of the colon and rectum in children and adults. Ann Surg. 1990;212(3):242–7. discussion 247–8.

46. Orkin BA, Telander RL, Wolff BG, et al. The surgical management of children with ulcerative colitis. The old vs. the new. Dis Colon Rectum. 1990;33(11):947–55.

47. Kohler LW, Pemberton JH, Zinsmeister AR, Kelly KA. Quality of life after proctocolectomy. A comparison of Brooke ileostomy, Kock pouch, and ileal pouch-anal anastomosis. Gastroenterology. 1991;101(3):679–84.

48. Michelassi F, Lee J, Rubin M, et al. Long-term functional results after ileal pouch anal restorative proctocolectomy for ulcerative colitis: a prospective observational study. Ann Surg. 2003;238(3):433–41. discussion 442–5.

49. Scotte M, Del Gallo G, Steinmetz L, et al. Ileoanal anastomosis for ulcerative colitis: results of an evolutionary surgical procedure. Hepato-Gastroenterology. 1998;45(24):2123–6.

50. Choen S, Tsunoda A, Nicholls RJ. Prospective randomized trial comparing anal function after hand sewn ileoanal anastomosis with mucosectomy versus stapled ileoanal anastomosis without mucosectomy in restorative proctocolectomy. Br J Surg. 1991;78(4):430–4.

51. Kayaalp C, Nessar G, Akoglu M, Atalay F. Elimination of mucosectomy during restorative proctocolectomy in patients with ulcerative colitis may provide better results in low-volume centers. Am J Surg. 2003;185(3):268–72.

52. Baixauli J, Delaney CP, Wu JS, et al. Functional outcome and quality of life after repeat ileal pouch-anal anastomosis for complications of ileoanal surgery. Dis Colon Rectum. 2004;47(1): 2–11.

53. Bach SP, Mortensen N. Revolution and evolution: 30 years of ileoanal pouch surgery. Inflamm Bowel Dis. 2006;12(2):131–45.

54. Heuschen UA, Autschbach F, Allemeyer EH, et al. Long-term follow-up after ileoanal pouch procedure: algorithm for diagnosis, classification, and management of pouchitis. Dis Colon Rectum. 2001;44(4):487–99.

55. Prudhomme M, Dehni N, Dozois RR, et al. Causes and outcomes of pouch excision after restorative proctocolectomy. Br J Surg. 2006;93(1):82–6.

56. Shen B, Fazio VW, Remzi FH, Lashner BA. Clinical approach to diseases of ileal pouch-anal anastomosis. Am J Gastroenterol. 2005;100(12):2796–807.

57. Sandborn WJ, Tremaine WJ, Batts KP, et al. Pouchitis after ileal pouch-anal anastomosis: a pouchitis disease activity index. Mayo Clin Proc. 1994;69(5):409–15.

58. Shen B, Achkar JP, Connor JT, et al. Modified pouchitis disease activity index: a simplified approach to the diagnosis of pouchitis. Dis Colon Rectum. 2003;46(6):748–53.

59. Kooros K, Katz AJ. Infliximab therapy in pediatric Crohn pouchitis. Inflamm Bowel Dis. 2004;10(4):417–20.

60. Welters CF, Heineman E, Thunnissen FB, et al. Effect of dietary inulin supplementation on inflammation of pouch mucosa in patients with an ileal pouch-anal anastomosis. Dis Colon Rectum. 2002;45(5):621–7.

61. Shen B, Brzezinski A, Fazio VW, et al. Maintenance therapy with a probiotic in antibiotic-dependent pouchitis: experience in clinical practice. Aliment Pharmacol Ther. 2005;22(8):721–8.

62. Meier R, Steuerwald M. Place of probiotics. Curr Opin Crit Care. 2005;11(4):318–25.

63. Holubar SD, Cima RR, Sandborn WJ, Pardi DS. Treatment and prevention of pouchitis after ileal pouch-anal anastomosis for chronic ulcerative colitis. Cochrane Database Syst Rev. 2010;16(6): CD001176.

64. Mortellaro VE, Green J, Islam S, Bass JA, Fike FB, St Peter SD. Occurrence of Crohn's disease in children after total colectomy for ulcerative colitis. J Surg Res. 2011;170(1):38–40.

65. Wolff BG. Is ileoanal the proper operation for indeterminate colitis: the case for. Inflamm Bowel Dis. 2002;8(5):362–5.

66. Bernstein CN. Ulcerative colitis with low-grade dysplasia. Gastroenterology. 2004;127(3):950–6.

67. Ullman TA. Making the grade: should patients with UC and low-grade dysplasia graduate to surgery or be held back? Inflamm Bowel Dis. 2002;8(6):430–1.

68. Ullman T, Odze R, Farraye FA. Diagnosis and management of dysplasia in patients with ulcerative colitis and Crohn's disease of the colon. Inflamm Bowel Dis. 2009;15(4):630–8.

69. Ekbom A. The epidemiology of IBD: a lot of data but little knowledge. How shall we proceed? Inflamm Bowel Dis. 2004;10(Suppl 1):S32–4.

70. Branco BC, Sachar DB, Heimann TM, Sarpel U, Harpaz N, Greenstein AJ. Adenocarcinoma following ileal pouch-anal anastomosis for ulcerative colitis: review of 26 cases. Inflamm Bowel Dis. 2009;15(2):295–9.

71. Borjesson L, Willen R, Haboubi N, et al. The risk of dysplasia and cancer in the ileal pouch mucosa after restorative proctocolectomy for ulcerative proctocolitis is low: a long-term term follow-up study. Color Dis. 2004;6(6):494–8.

72. Liu ZX, Kiran RP, Bennett AE, Ni RZ, Shen B. Diagnosis and management of dysplasia and cancer of the ileal pouch in patients with underlying inflammatory bowel disease. Cancer. 2011; 117(14):3081–92.

73. Olsen KO, Joelsson M, Laurberg S, Oresland T. Fertility after ileal pouch-anal anastomosis in women with ulcerative colitis. Br J Surg. 1999;86(4):493–5.

74. Olsen KO, Juul S, Bulow S, et al. Female fecundity before and after operation for familial adenomatous polyposis. Br J Surg. 2003; 90(2):227–31.

75. Rajaratnam SG, Eglinton TW, Hider P, Fearnhead NS. Impact of ileal pouch-anal anastomosis on female fertility: meta-analysis and systematic review. Int J Color Dis. 2011;26(11):1365–74.

76. Gorgun E, Remzi FH, Goldberg JM, et al. Fertility is reduced after restorative proctocolectomy with ileal pouch anal anastomosis: a study of 300 patients. Surgery. 2004;136(4):795–803.

77. Wax JR, Pinette MG, Cartin A, Blackstone J. Female reproductive health after ileal pouch anal anastomosis for ulcerative colitis. Obstet Gynecol Surv. 2003;58(4):270–4.

78. Practice Committee of American Society for Reproductive Medicine in collaboration with Society of Reproductive Surgeons. Pathogenesis, consequences, and control of peritoneal adhesions in gynecologic surgery. Fertil Steril. 2008;90(5 Suppl):S144–9.

79. Ahmad G, O'Flynn H, Hindocha A, Watson A. Barrier agents for adhesion prevention after gynaecological surgery. Cochrane Database Syst Rev. 2015;4:CD000475.

80. Kapiteijn E, van de Velde CJ. Developments and quality assurance in rectal cancer surgery. Eur J Cancer. 2002;38(7):919–36.

81. Prystowsky JB, Bordage G, Feinglass JM. Patient outcomes for segmental colon resection according to surgeon's training, certification, and experience. Surgery. 2002;132(4):663–70. discussion 670–2.

82. McGrath DR, Leong DC, Gibberd R, et al. Surgeon and hospital volume and the management of colorectal cancer patients in Australia. ANZ J Surg. 2005;75(10):901–10.

83. Tekkis PP, Senagore AJ, Delaney CP, Fazio VW. Evaluation of the learning curve in laparoscopic colorectal surgery: comparison of right-sided and left-sided resections. Ann Surg. 2005;242(1): 83–91.

84. Tekkis PP, Fazio VW, Lavery IC, et al. Evaluation of the learning curve in ileal pouch-anal anastomosis surgery. Ann Surg. 2005;241(2):262–8.

85. Pellino G, Selvaggi F. Outcomes of salvage surgery for ileal pouch complications and dysfunctions. the experience of a referral centre and review of literature. J Crohns Colitis. 2015;9(7):548–57.

86. Linden BC, Bairdain S, Zurakowski D, Shamberger RC, Lillehei CW. Comparison of laparoscopic-assisted and open total proctocolectomy and ileal pouch anal anastomosis in children and adolescents. J Pediatr Surg. 2013;48(7):1546–50.

Postoperative Surveillance and Management of Crohn's Disease

43

Arthur M. Barrie III and Miguel Regueiro

Risk and Diagnosis of Postoperative Crohn's Disease

Early and more frequent use of immunomodulators and antitumor necrosis factor (TNF) therapies have reduced but not spared Crohn's disease (CD) patients the risk for needing an intestinal resection. Recent biologic era population studies have found that the rate or probability of a first major bowel surgery in CD is still 20–30% [1, 2]. Pediatric CD progresses slower to surgery than adult onset disease, as the reported 5-year cumulative risk for bowel surgery for pediatric CD patients is less than that for adult patients, but still significant at 13.8–17% [3, 4, 5].

Unfortunately, CD is rarely curable by surgery, and postoperative recurrence (POR) of CD is inevitable for a vast majority of patients. In the prebiologic era, natural history studies found that 70–90% of CD patients developed endoscopic evidence of POR within 1 year of their surgery, and that 30–60% of postoperative (POCD) patients became symptomatic from recurrent disease within 3–5 years of their surgery [6, 7, 8] (Fig. 43.1). Consequently, 50% of POCD patients in the prebiologic era required repeat surgery within 5 years of their first surgery. Clinical recurrence rates for postoperative pediatric CD are equally high and identical to adult rates, reported to be 60–78% at 5 years [9, 10].

Postoperative Crohn's disease recurrence is often clinically silent. Rutgeerts and colleagues found in their initial seminal study of the natural history of postoperative recurrent CD that 72% of examined patients (21 out of 29) had recurrent endoscopic CD within 1 year of curative resection and that a remarkable number of these patients were asymptomatic [11]. In a subsequent prospective cohort of 8-year follow-up study of 89 patients after resection, Rutgeerts

et al. found that only 20 and 34% of patients were symptomatic 1 and 3 years after surgery, respectively, despite endoscopic disease found in 73 and 85% of these patients [7]. Regueiro and colleagues observed similar findings in their postoperative randomized placebo-controlled infliximab (IFX) trial, as they determined the kappa coefficient of agreement between the patients' endoscopic scores, and their clinical Crohn's Disease Activity Index (CDAI) scores was only 0.12 [12].

The degree of endoscopic disease severity at 1 year, as judged by the now classified Rutgeerts score (Table 43.1), directly correlated with the progression to symptomatic recurrence and was the most statistically significant variable in predicting outcome [7]. For example, only 8.6% of patients with no or only mild endoscopic disease at 1 year, as defined by Rutgeerts score i0 or i1, had clinical symptoms at 8 years, while 100% of patients with severe endoscopic disease, as defined by Rutgeerts score i4, had symptomatic recurrence by 4 years. Although the Rutgeerts score has not been validated as a measure of treatment response, most studies now define endoscopic postoperative remission as i0 or i1, and recurrence as i2, i3, or i4.

Since symptom assessment is an unreliable and delayed measure of POR, ileocolonoscopy utilizing the Rutgeerts scoring system is the current gold standard test for POR assessment and is recommended to be performed 6 months to 1 year after surgery. The Rutgeerts scoring system defines severity of disease on a 0–4 scale based on the extent of aphthous ulcerations in the neoterminal ileum (Table 43.1) [7]. Complete endoscopic remission with no lesions is classified as i0, while mild disease consisting of five or fewer aphthous ulcers is classified as i1. Moderate disease defined by more than five aphthous lesions with normal mucosa between the lesions, or skip areas of larger lesions or lesions confined to the ileocolonic anastomosis is classified as i2. Diffuse aphthous ileitis with diffusely inflamed mucosa is classified as i3, and the most severe disease characterized by diffuse inflammation with already larger ulcers, nodules, and/or narrowing is classified as i4 disease.

A.M. Barrie III, MD, PhD • M. Regueiro, MD (✉)
Division of Gastroenterology, Hepatology, and Nutrition,
University of Pittsburgh Medical Center, 200 Lothrop Street,
C-Wing, Mezzanine, Pittsburgh, PA 15213, USA
e-mail: amb145@pitt.edu; mdr7@pitt.edu

© Springer International Publishing AG 2017
P. Mamula et al. (eds.), *Pediatric Inflammatory Bowel Disease*, DOI 10.1007/978-3-319-49215-5_43

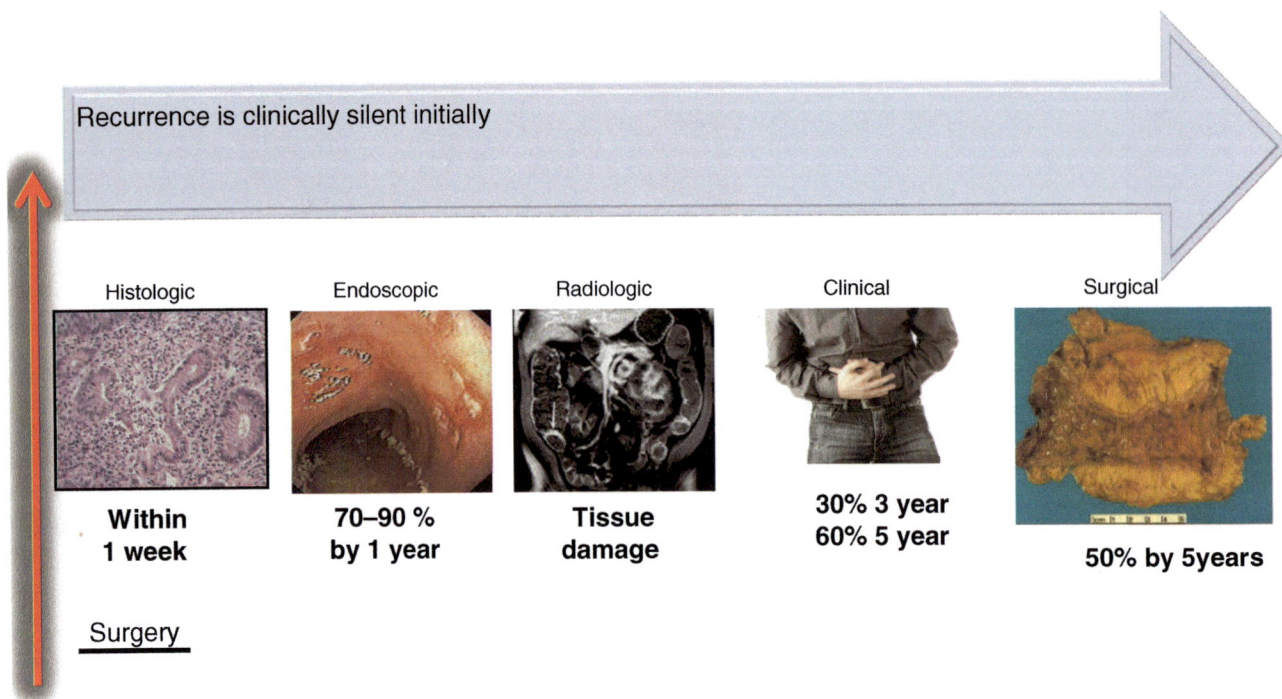

Fig. 43.1 The natural course of postoperative Crohn's disease

Table 43.1 Rutgeerts postoperative Crohn's disease endoscopic scoring system

Endoscopic score	Endoscopic findings
i0	No lesions
i1	≤5 aphthous lesions
i2	>5 aphthous lesions with normal mucosa between the lesions, or skip areas of larger lesions or lesions confined to the ileocolonic anastomosis (i.e., <1 cm in length)
i3	Diffuse aphthous ileitis with diffusely inflamed mucosa
i4	Diffuse inflammation with already larger ulcers, nodules, and/or narrowing

Though ileocolonoscopy is sensitive at detecting POR, the invasive nature of the test is associated with patient discomfort, high cost, and procedural risk. Fecal calprotectin (fCal), produced by gut leukocytes and epithelial cells at sites of mucosal injury including in Crohn's disease, is being investigated as a potential noninvasive marker of POR. Lasson et al. reported that there was no significant difference in fCal levels between POCD patients with endoscopic recurrence versus patients in endoscopic remission at 1 year after surgery, in a small study of 30 patients [13]. In contrast, Boschetti and colleagues recently published the results of their larger study of 86 asymptomatic POCD patients within 18 months after surgery in which they found that patients with endoscopic recurrence (i2-4) have significantly higher levels of fecal

calprotectin than patients in endoscopic remission (i0-1) (mean ± s.e.m.: 473 ± 78 µg/g vs. 115 ± 18 µg/g; $P < 0.0001$), and that fCal levels strongly correlate with Rutgeerts scores ($r = 0.65$, $P < 0.0001$) [14]. The authors also found that high-sensitivity C-reactive protein was elevated in patients with POR, but to a lesser degree than fCal, and concluded that fCal was a superior noninvasive marker of POR. Given the limited studies to date and their discordant findings, further research is required to determine whether the measurement of fCal is a valid assessment for POR.

Noninvasive radiographic studies such as small intestine contrast ultrasonography (SICUS) have also been investigated to evaluate POR. Calabrese et al. reported that SICUS utilizing oral contrast detected POR, defined by increased bowel wall thickness (BWT) ((>3 mm) for at least 4 cm at the perianastomotic area), in 62 out of 67 patients with endoscopic recurrent disease (i1-4) (92.5% sensitivity), and that BWT strongly correlated with the Rutgeerts score ($r = 0.67$, $P < 0.0001$) [15]. Paredes and colleagues had similar findings in their study of contrast-enhanced US utilizing IV contrast in which they found that BWT > 5 mm or contrast enhancement >46% on US had a sensitivity, specificity, and accuracy of 98, 100, and 98.3% for the diagnosis of endoscopic recurrence (i1-4) [16]. Despite these positive findings, the use of SICUS in clinical practice in the United States is currently limited as it requires experienced radiologists with advanced training.

Given the natural predisposition for POR, preventive therapy has received considerable attention, particularly for high-risk patients who have had penetrating or perforating disease, and/or multiple prior CD-related bowel surgeries, and/or cigarette smoking after surgery [17]. Identified risk factors for POR in pediatric CD patients include colonic Crohn's disease, high preoperative Pediatric Crohn Disease Activity Index (PCDAI), and immunomodulator therapy before surgery [9]. It is the authors' opinion that patients with a short (<10 years) disease duration before needing surgery and who have a long (>10 cm) stricture with active inflammation are at moderate risk for POR. Patients with long-standing (10 years or more) CD who undergo surgery for the first time for only a short noninflammatory stricture are at low risk for POR.

Nonbiologic Treatment Options for Postoperative Crohn's Disease

Standard medical therapies including antibiotics, aminosalicylates, and immunomodulators have been shown to moderately reduce the risk of clinical and endoscopic disease recurrence [18] (Table 43.2). Mesalamine is a safe but minimally effective drug to prevent POR. A Cochrane analysis by Doherty et al. found that mesalamine does reduce clinical recurrence (RR 0.76; 95% CI 0.62–0.94) and severe endoscopic recurrence (RR 0.50; 95% CI 0.29–0.84) compared to placebo, but with a number needed to treat (NNT) of 12 and 8, respectively [19]. A subsequent systemic review and meta-analysis by Ford et al. concluded that mesalamine is of only modest benefit in preventing POR compared to placebo and should only be considered if immunosuppressive therapy is not warranted or is contraindicated [20].

In the aforementioned Cochrane analysis, azathioprine (AZA)/6-mercaptopurine (6-MP) was found to significantly reduce clinical recurrence (RR 0.59; 95% CI 0.38–0.92, NNT = 7) and severe endoscopic recurrence (RR 0.64; 95 CI 0.44–0.92, NNT = 4) compared to placebo and was found to be superior to mesalamine [19]. Similar findings were reported by Peyrin-Biroulet et al. in a concurrent meta-analysis of four controlled trials, in which AZA/6-MP was determined to be more effective than placebo for preventing clinical recurrence at 1 year (mean difference, 95% CI: 8, 1–15%, $P = 0.021$, NNT = 13) and 2 years (mean difference, 95% CI: 13%, 2–24%, $P = 0.018$, NNT = 8)

after surgery, and endoscopic recurrence (i2-4) (mean difference, 95% CI: 23%, 9–37%, $P = 0.0016$, NNT = 4) at 1 year after surgery [21].

Metronidazole (20 mg/kg) may significantly reduce the incidence of severe (i3-4) endoscopic recurrent disease compared to placebo-treated patients at 3 months after surgery (3 of 23; 13% vs. 12 of 28; 43%; $P = 0.02$), and clinical recurrence at 1 year (1 of 23; 4% vs. 7 of 28; 25%; $P = 0.044$) [22]. Combining metronidazole with AZA may improve outcomes further. POCD patients treated with metronidazole for 3 months and AZA (100–150 mg qd dependent on body mass) for 12 months had significantly less endoscopic recurrent disease (i2-4) at 1 year after surgery than patients treated with metronidazole alone at 1 year after surgery (14 of 32; 43.7% vs. 20 of 29; 69.0%; $P = .048$) [23]. The limitation of metronidazole is that patients often do not tolerate high doses, and long-term prevention of recurrence is lost when the antibiotic is stopped.

Anti-TNFs for Prevention of Postoperative Crohn's Disease

Growing evidence demonstrates that anti-TNF therapy is the most effective treatment to prevent POR and may have the potential to change the natural course of Crohn's disease after surgery. Since Sorrentino and colleagues first reported the successful use of prophylactic IFX in a Crohn's colitis patient after a partial colonic resection [24], multiple small randomized and prospective open-label trials have found that IFX and adalimumab (ADA) are superior to placebo, mesalamine, and AZA at preventing POR (Table 43.3). Regueiro and colleagues performed the first randomized placebo-controlled trial examining the ability of IFX (5 mg/kg every 8 weeks) to prevent endoscopic recurrence of Crohn's disease at 1 year after ileal resection [25]. In a relatively small study of patients with ileal or ileocolonic disease at moderate to high risk for disease recurrence, the rate of endoscopic recurrence (i2-4) was significantly lower in IFX-treated patients (9.1%, $n = 11$) compared to the placebo group (84.6%, $n = 13$) ($P = 0.0006$). Several other small randomized studies verified that infliximab prevents POR [26, 27]. The protective effects of IFX appear to be a class effect of TNF inhibitors, as ADA has also been found to prevent POR

Table 43.2 Summary of postoperative Crohn's disease randomized controlled trials

Postop prevention RCTs	Clinical recurrence (%)	Endoscopic recurrence (%)
Placebo	25–77	53–79
5-ASA	24–58	63–66
Budesonide	19–32	52–57
Nitroimidazole	7–8	52–54
AZA/6-MP	34–50	42–44

Table 43.3 Postoperative Crohn's prevention trials investigating the rates of endoscopic recurrence with anti-TNF therapy versus control

	Anti-TNF (%)	Control (%)
Sorrentino (MTX/IFX vs. 5-ASA 2 year)	0	100 (5-ASA)
Regueiro (IFX vs. PBO RCT 1 year)	9	85 (PBO)
Yoshida (IFX vs. PBO Open 1 year)	21	81 (5-ASA)
Armuzzi (IFX vs. AZA Open 1 year)	9	40 (AZA)
Fernandez-Blanco (ADA)	10	N/A
Papamichael (ADA 6 m)	0	N/A
Savarino (ADA 3 year)	0	N/A
Aguas (ADA 1 year)	21	N/A
De Cruz (ADA vs. AZA 6mos)	6	38 (AZA)
Savarino (ADA vs. AZA vs. 5-ASA 2 years)	6	65 (AZA), 83 (5-ASA)

Abbreviations: *MTX* methotrexate, *PBO* placebo, *5-ASA* aminosalicylates

in several small open-label and randomized studies [28, 29, 30]. Overall, anti-TNF therapy is the most effective treatment to prevent POR as verified by recent systematic review and network meta-analysis examining the comparative efficacy of all drugs studied to prevent POR [31]. Accordingly, the authors recommend anti-TNF therapy as first-line prophylactic therapy for patients at high risk for POR or for patients who have tried and failed or are intolerant of AZA/6-MP.

Treating Postoperative Crohn's Disease: Waiting for Endoscopic Recurrence

Postoperative natural history studies have taught us that most *but not all* patients will develop recurrent disease. Thus, initiating anti-TNF therapy in all postoperative Crohn's disease patients would certainly mean overtreating a subset. Relevant to this concern, it is not known whether prophylactic anti-TNF therapy is more effective than waiting to treat recurrent disease. Yamamoto et al. investigated the impact of IFX therapy on Crohn's patients in clinical remission but who had endoscopic recurrent disease 6 months after ileocolonic resection despite prophylactic mesalamine therapy (3 gm/day) [32]. Eight such patients were started on IFX (5 mg/kg every 8 weeks), another eight were started on AZA (50 mg/day), and the remainder was maintained only on mesalamine. They found that infliximab induced complete endoscopic remission in 38%, 6 months after starting treatment, compared to only 13% of AZA-treated patients and 0% of mesalamine-treated patients ($P = 0.10$). Sorrentino and colleagues found similar results when they treated patients with endoscopic disease 6 months after surgery with either IFX (5 mg/kg every 8 weeks) or mesalamine (2.4 gm/day) [33]. Fifty-four percent of the infliximab-treated patients ($n = 13$) were in endoscopic remission 1 year after starting treatment compared to 0% of mesalamine-treated patients ($n = 11$)

($P = 0.01$). Adalimumab appears to be equally effective in treating early recurrent disease, as Papamichael et al. showed in their study that ADA promoted endoscopic healing in 60% of treated patients ($n = 15$) who had endoscopic disease 6 months after surgery [28]. Overall, these studies suggest that anti-TNF therapy may be effective at treating early recurrent disease in certain patients.

Safety of Postoperative Anti-TNFs

The risks versus benefits of continuing prophylactic anti-TNF therapy in patients in long-term remission have also been called into question, considering the cost of treatment and potential for rare, but serious, side effects. Long-term safety data for IFX in the treatment of Crohn's disease demonstrates that IFX therapy is associated with a moderate risk for infection, but does not increase the risk of mortality or malignancy [34, 35]. The same study found that severe Crohn's disease and prednisone and narcotic use are associated with a higher risk of infection than IFX therapy, and thus one could argue that the benefits of IFX to prevent severe recurrent disease outweighs the infection risk. In the initial postoperative IFX study, there was no increased risk of adverse events in IFX-treated patients compared to placebo, including postoperative complications up to 1 year after surgery [36, 12]. Preventive anti-TNF therapy has been found to be relatively safe in other postoperative studies, including the study of ADA by Savarino and colleagues who reported that ADA-treated patients had fewer adverse events than the azathioprine-treated and mesalamine-treated patients over a 2-year follow-up period [29].

In contrast, the risks of stopping postoperative anti-TNF therapy appear to be higher than continuing treatment, as Regueiro and colleagues found that patients in remission who stop IFX are at high risk for recurrent disease. After completion of the 1-year study, patients were permitted to discontinue (or start) IFX and were then followed for an additional 5 years [37]. Eight of the original 11 IFX-treated patients chose to stop therapy, and all eight developed endoscopic recurrent disease, and five subsequently required repeat surgery. The three other original IFX-treated patients continued their treatment, and none required repeat surgery during the study period. Twelve of the original 13 placebo patients had recurrence and chose to start IFX; seven of these patients achieved endoscopic remission and required no repeat surgery during the study period. Overall, Regueiro et al. found that patients who were treated with IFX for at least 60% of the 5-year study period had a significantly lower risk for repeat surgery, irrespective of their original treatment assignment (20.0% vs. 64.3%, $P = 0.047$). Sorrentino and colleagues found a similar high risk of recurrence, as they reported that 83% of patients ($n = 12$), who were previously in remission for 3 years after surgery on IFX, developed endoscopic recurrent disease 16 weeks after stopping treatment [24].

PREVENT and POCER Studies

The efficacy of prophylactic anti-TNF therapy to prevent endoscopic POR has been supported by the PREVENT study, the largest randomized placebo-controlled POR-preventive treatment trial to date [38]. The PREVENT study was a multicenter trial that enrolled 297 CD patients who had undergone ileocolonic resection and were at increased risk for POR. One hundred forty-seven patients were randomized to receive IFX (5 mg/kg every 8 weeks), and 150 patients were randomized to receive placebo treatment for a 200-week treatment period. The primary endpoint was clinical recurrence prior to or at week 76 defined by Crohn's disease activity index (CDAI) score and endoscopic recurrence (i2-4), or the development of a fistula or abscess. The secondary endpoint was endoscopic recurrence alone (i2-4) prior to or at week 76. The study reported that the proportion of subjects with clinical recurrence was numerically lower in the IFX group compared with the placebo group, but the difference was not statistically significant (12.9% vs. 20.4%, $P = 0.097$) (Fig. 43.2). However, IFX treatment significantly reduced endoscopic recurrence compared to placebo treatment (22.4% vs. 51.3%, $P < 0.001$) (Fig. 43.3). Of patients who had a score of i0, there were more receiving IFX than placebo (83.1% vs. 28.4%). Of patients who had more aggressive recurrence, i3 or i4, there were fewer receiving IFX than placebo (16.9% vs. 71.6%).

The timing of the first colonoscopy after surgery to detect endoscopic recurrence and prevent progression was recently assessed in the POCER study [39]. The primary endpoint was endoscopic recurrence at 18 months. In the

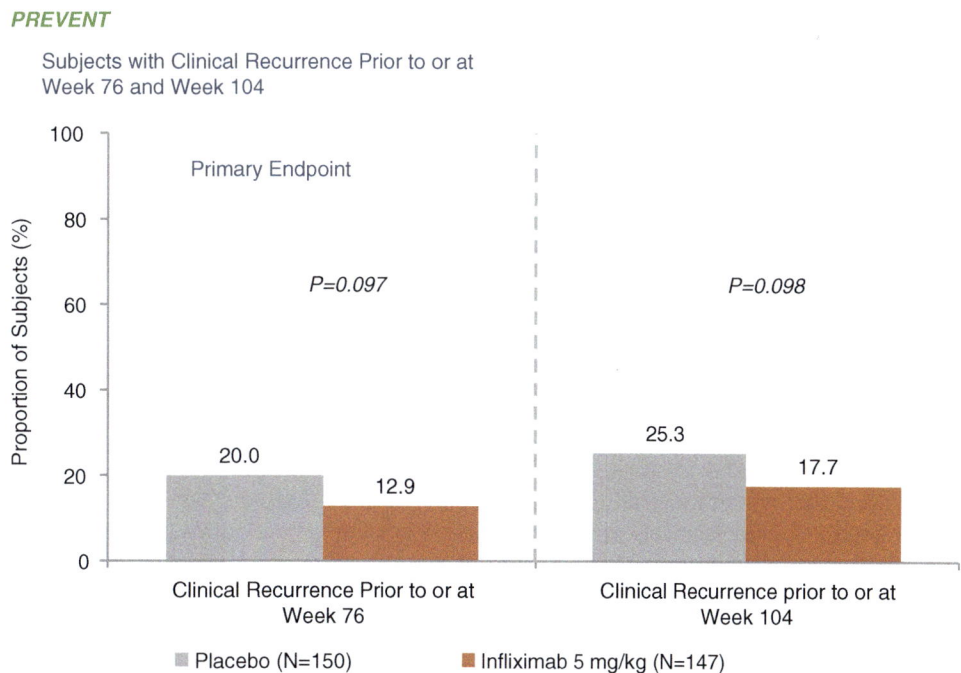

Fig. 43.2 Clinical recurrence reduced in infliximab-treated patients in the PREVENT study

P-values based on the Cochran-Mantel-Haenszel chi-square test stratified by the number of risk factors for recurrence of active CD (1 or >1) and baseline use (yes/no) of an immunosuppressive (i.e., AZA, 6-MP, or MTX).

Fig. 43.3 Endoscopic recurrence significantly reduced in infliximab-treated patients in the PREVENT study

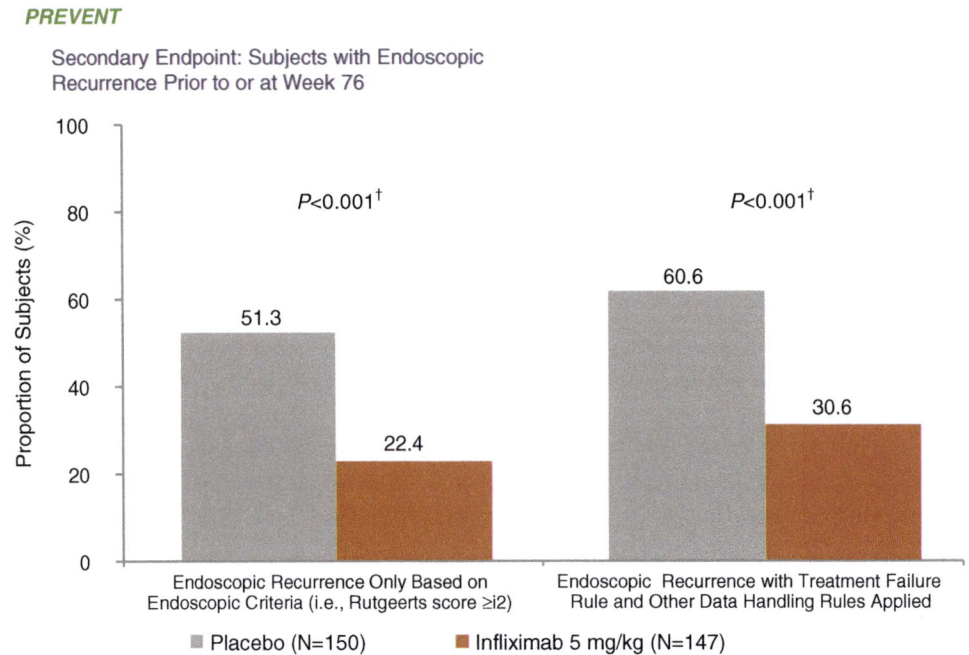

PREVENT

Secondary Endpoint: Subjects with Endoscopic Recurrence Prior to or at Week 76

† Nominal p-values based on the Cochran-Mantel-Haenszel chi-square test stratified by the number of risk factors for recurrence of active CD (1 or >1) and baseline use (yes/no) of an immunosuppressive (i.e., AZA, 6-MP, or MTX).

trial, 174 postoperative patients were randomly assigned in a 2:1 ratio to either a standard care or active care arm. The active care arm had patients undergo a colonoscopy at 6 months, and if there was active Crohn's disease ($\geq$ i2), they had a step up in their therapy, for example, starting AZA/6-MP if previously on no medication or adding ADA to AZA/6-MP. The standard care arm did not undergo a 6-month colonoscopy and only had the 18-month colonoscopy. Both study arms were given metronidazole 400 mg twice a day for 3 months. If patients were intolerant, the dose was reduced to 200 mg twice daily, or was stopped altogether. If they were of high risk (smokers or recurrent surgery or penetrating disease) but medication-naive, patients were given AZA 2 mg/kg or 6-MP 1.5 mg/kg once daily, beginning within 1 month after surgery. Patients intolerant to this regimen were administered ADA 160 mg/80 mg induction followed by 40 mg every other week. Patients without any risk factors for postoperative recurrence, that is, nonsmokers, first surgery, and absence of penetrating disease, received no additional treatment beyond 3 months of metronidazole. The 18-month primary endpoint of endoscopic recurrence was significantly lower in the active care arm compared with the standard care arm (49% vs. 67%, $p = 0.03$). Although not an endpoint of the study, it was interesting that the 6-month postoperative endoscopic recurrence rates for patients receiving AZA/6-MP and ADA were consistent to what has been previously reported (45% vs. 21%).

Strategies for Postoperative Crohn's Disease Management

The questions that remain in the practical management of postoperative Crohn's disease are: (1) which patients should receive immediate postoperative therapy, and (2) which patients would it be reasonable to wait to treat endoscopic recurrence? There are two emerging strategies to postoperative Crohn's disease management. One strategy would be to stratify postoperative treatment based on risk and treat only those patients at high risk for recurrence with AZA/6-MP, or an anti-TNF if intolerant of thiopurines (Fig. 43.4). All patients would then undergo a colonoscopy at 6 months from surgery. If the colonoscopy revealed active Crohn's disease ($\geq$ i2), untreated patients would be started on thiopurine therapy, and thiopurine-treated patients would be started on anti-TNF therapy. A second strategy, which is the authors' practice, is to start prophylactic treatment for high-risk and moderate-risk patients (Fig. 43.5). Those at low risk for recurrence would not be given postoperative medication.

Fig. 43.4 Proposed watchful waiting treatment algorithm for the management of postoperative Crohn's disease. Low risk of postop recurrence defined by long-standing Crohn's disease, first surgery, and short stricture. Moderate risk defined by less than 10 year history of Crohn's disease, long stricture, and/or inflammatory disease. High risk defined by cigarette smoking, penetrating disease, and/or two or more surgeries

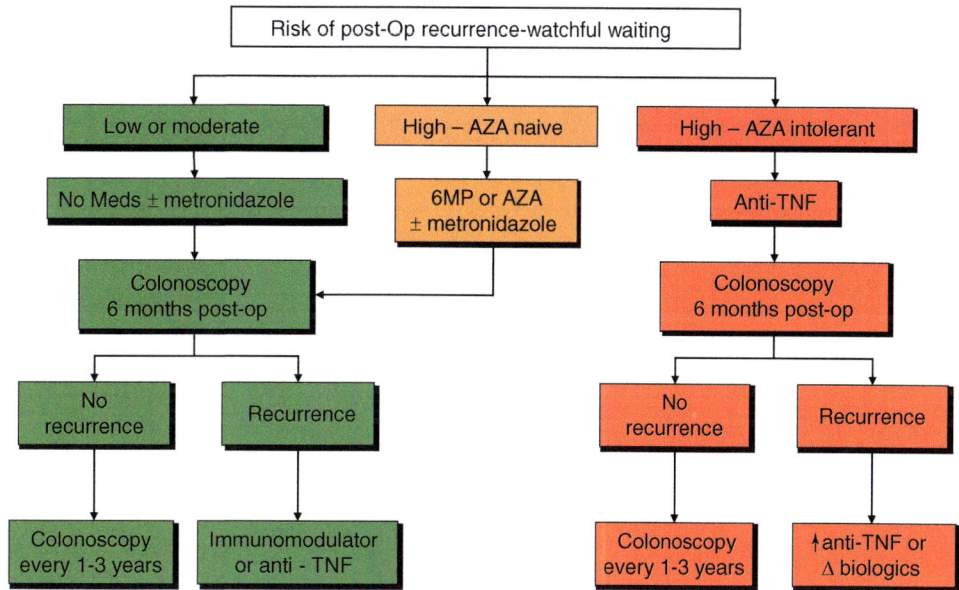

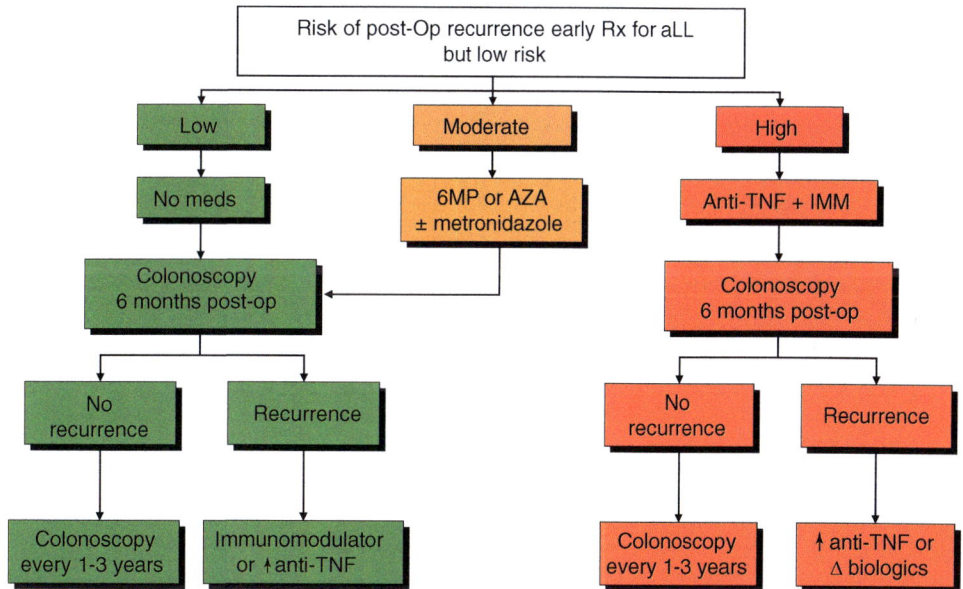

Fig. 43.5 Proposed early treatment algorithm for the management of postoperative Crohn's disease. Low risk of postop recurrence defined by long-standing Crohn's disease, first surgery, and short stricture. Moderate risk defined by less than 10 year history of Crohn's disease, long stricture, and/or inflammatory disease. High risk defined by cigarette smoking, penetrating disease, and/or two or more surgeries

Those at moderate risk for recurrence would receive AZA/6-MP after surgery. Those at high risk would receive AZA/6-MP in combination with an anti-TNF agent. All patients would then undergo a colonoscopy at 6 months from surgery with treatment escalated based on endoscopic recurrence.

Financial Disclosures Dr. Barrie – none

Dr. Regueiro – Abbvie, Janssen, UCB, Shire, Takeda

References

1. Rungoe C, Langholz E, Andersson M, Basit S, Nielsen NM, Wohlfahrt J, Jess T. Changes in medical treatment and surgery rates in inflammatory bowel disease: a nationwide cohort study 1979–2011. Gut. 2014;63(10):1607–16.
2. Vester-Andersen MK, Prosberg MV, Jess T, Andersson M, Bengtsson BG, Blixt T, Munkholm P, Bendtsen F, Vind I. Disease course and surgery rates in inflammatory bowel disease: a population-based, 7-year follow-up study in the era of immunomodulating therapy. Am J Gastroenterol. 2014;109(5):705–14.

3. Gupta N, Cohen SA, Bostrom AG, Kirschner BS, Baldassano RN, Winter HS, Ferry GD, Smith T, Abramson O, Gold BD, Heyman MB. Risk factors for initial surgery in pediatric patients with Crohn's disease. Gastroenterology. 2006;130(4):1069–77.

4. Schaefer ME, Machan JT, Kawatu D, Langton CR, Markowitz J, Crandall W, Mack DR, Evans JS, Pfefferkorn MD, Griffiths AM, Otley AR, Bousvaros A, Kugathasan S, Rosh JR, Keljo DJ, Carvalho RS, Tomer G, Mamula P, Kay MH, Kerzner B, Oliva-Hemker M, Kappelman MD, Saeed SA, Hyams JS, Leleiko NS. Factors that determine risk for surgery in pediatric patients with Crohn's disease. Clin Gastroenterol Hepatol. 2010;8(9):789–94.

5. Van Limbergen J, Russell RK, Drummond HE, Aldhous MC, Round NK, Nimmo ER, Smith L, Gillett PM, McGrogan P, Weaver LT, Bisset WM, Mahdi G, Arnott ID, Satsangi J, Wilson DC. Definition of phenotypic characteristics of childhood-onset inflammatory bowel disease. Gastroenterology. 2008;135(4):1114–22.

6. Olaison G, Smedh K, Sjodahl R. Natural course of Crohn's disease after ileocolic resection: endoscopically visualised ileal ulcers preceding symptoms. Gut. 1992;33(3):331–5.

7. Rutgeerts P, Geboes K, Vantrappen G, Beyls J, Kerremans R, Hiele M. Predictability of the postoperative course of Crohn's disease. Gastroenterology. 1990;99(4):956–63.

8. Sachar DB. The problem of postoperative recurrence of Crohn's disease. Med Clin North Am. 1990;74(1):183–8.

9. Baldassano RN, Han PD, Jeshion WC, Berlin JA, Piccoli DA, Lautenbach E, Mick R, Lichtenstein GR. Pediatric Crohn's disease: risk factors for postoperative recurrence. Am J Gastroenterol. 2001;96(7):2169–76.

10. Bobanga ID, Bai S, Swanson MA, Champagne BJ, Reynolds HJ, Delaney CP, Barksdale Jr EM, Stein SL. Factors influencing disease recurrence after ileocolic resection in adult and pediatric onset Crohn's disease. Am J Surg. 2014;208(4):591–6.

11. Rutgeerts P, Geboes K, Vantrappen G, Kerremans R, Coenegrachts JL, Coremans G. Natural history of recurrent Crohn's disease at the ileocolonic anastomosis after curative surgery. Gut. 1984;25(6):665–72.

12. Regueiro M, Kip KE, Schraut W, Baidoo L, Sepulveda AR, Pesci M, El-Hachem S, Harrison J, Binion D. Crohn's disease activity index does not correlate with endoscopic recurrence one year after ileocolonic resection. Inflamm Bowel Dis. 2011;17(1):118–26.

13. Lasson A, Strid H, Ohman L, Isaksson S, Olsson M, Rydstrom B, Ung KA, Stotzer PO. Fecal calprotectin one year after ileocaecal resection for Crohn's disease–a comparison with findings at ileocolonoscopy. J Crohns Colitis. 2014;8(8):789–95.

14. Boschetti G, Laidet M, Moussata D, Stefanescu C, Roblin X, Phelip G, Cotte E, Passot G, Francois Y, Drai J, Del Tedesco E, Bouhnik Y, Flourie B, Nancey S. Levels of fecal calprotectin are associated with the severity of postoperative endoscopic recurrence in asymptomatic patients with Crohn's disease. Am J Gastroenterol. 2015;110(6):865–72.

15. Calabrese E, Petruzziello C, Onali S, Condino G, Zorzi F, Pallone F, Biancone L. Severity of postoperative recurrence in Crohn's disease: correlation between endoscopic and sonographic findings. Inflamm Bowel Dis. 2009;15(11):1635–42.

16. Paredes JM, Ripolles T, Cortes X, Moreno N, Martinez MJ, Bustamante-Balen M, Delgado F, Moreno-Osset E. Contrast-enhanced ultrasonography: usefulness in the assessment of postoperative recurrence of Crohn's disease. J Crohns Colitis. 2013;7(3):192–201.

17. Schwartz M, Regueiro M. Prevention and treatment of postoperative Crohn's disease recurrence: an update for a new decade. Curr Gastroenterol Rep. 2011;13(1):95–100.

18. Regueiro M. Management and prevention of postoperative Crohn's disease. Inflamm Bowel Dis. 2009;15(10):1583–90.

19. Doherty G, Bennett G, Patil S, Cheifetz A, Moss AC. Interventions for prevention of post-operative recurrence of Crohn's disease. Cochrane Database Syst Rev. 2009;4:CD006873.

20. Ford AC, Khan KJ, Talley NJ, Moayyedi P. 5-aminosalicylates prevent relapse of Crohn's disease after surgically induced remission: systematic review and meta-analysis. Am J Gastroenterol. 2011;106(3):413–20.

21. Peyrin-Biroulet L, Deltenre P, Ardizzone S, D'Haens G, Hanauer SB, Herfarth H, Lemann M, Colombel JF. Azathioprine and 6-mercaptopurine for the prevention of postoperative recurrence in Crohn's disease: a meta-analysis. Am J Gastroenterol. 2009; 104(8):2089–96.

22. Rutgeerts P, Hiele M, Geboes K, Peeters M, Penninckx F, Aerts R, Kerremans R. Controlled trial of metronidazole treatment for prevention of Crohn's recurrence after ileal resection. Gastroenterology. 1995;108(6):1617–21.

23. D'Haens GR, Vermeire S, Van Assche G, Noman M, Aerden I, Van Olmen G, Rutgeerts P. Therapy of metronidazole with azathioprine to prevent postoperative recurrence of Crohn's disease: a controlled randomized trial. Gastroenterology. 2008;135(4):1123–9.

24. Sorrentino D, Paviotti A, Terrosu G, Avellini C, Geraci M, Zarifi D. Low-dose maintenance therapy with infliximab prevents postsurgical recurrence of Crohn's disease. Clin Gastroenterol Hepatol. 2010;8(7):591–599.e591. ; quiz e578–99

25. Regueiro M, Schraut W, Baidoo L, Kip KE, Sepulveda AR, Pesci M, Harrison J, Plevy SE. Infliximab prevents Crohn's disease recurrence after ileal resection. Gastroenterology. 2009;136(2):441–450. e441.; quiz 716

26. Armuzzi A, Felice C, Papa A, Marzo M, Pugliese D, Andrisani G, Federico F, De Vitis I, Rapaccini GL, Guidi L. Prevention of postoperative recurrence with azathioprine or infliximab in patients with Crohn's disease: an open-label pilot study. J Crohns Colitis. 2013;7(12):e623–9.

27. Yoshida K, Fukunaga K, Ikeuchi H, Kamikozuru K, Hida N, Ohda Y, Yokoyama Y, Iimuro M, Takeda N, Kato K, Kikuyama R, Nagase K, Hori K, Nakamura S, Miwa H, Matsumoto T. Scheduled infliximab monotherapy to prevent recurrence of Crohn's disease following ileocolic or ileal resection: a 3-year prospective randomized open trial. Inflamm Bowel Dis. 2012;18(9):1617–23.

28. Papamichael K, Archavlis E, Lariou C, Mantzaris GJ. Adalimumab for the prevention and/or treatment of post-operative recurrence of Crohn's disease: a prospective, two-year, single center, pilot study. J Crohns Colitis. 2012;6(9):924–31.

29. Savarino E, Bodini G, Dulbecco P, Assandri L, Bruzzone L, Mazza F, Frigo AC, Fazio V, Marabotto E, Savarino V. Adalimumab is more effective than azathioprine and mesalamine at preventing postoperative recurrence of Crohn's disease: a randomized controlled trial. Am J Gastroenterol. 2013;108(11):1731–42.

30. Savarino E, Dulbecco P, Bodini G, Assandri L, Savarino V. Prevention of postoperative recurrence of Crohn's disease by Adalimumab: a case series. Eur J Gastroenterol Hepatol. 2012; 24(4):468–70.

31. Singh S, Garg SK, Pardi DS, Wang Z, Murad MH, Loftus Jr EV. Comparative efficacy of pharmacologic interventions in preventing relapse of Crohn's disease after surgery: a systematic review and network meta-analysis. Gastroenterology. 2015;148(1):64–76.e62.; quiz e14

32. Yamamoto T, Umegae S, Matsumoto K. Impact of infliximab therapy after early endoscopic recurrence following ileocolonic resection of Crohn's disease: a prospective pilot study. Inflamm Bowel Dis. 2009;15(10):1460–6.

33. Sorrentino D, Terrosu G, Paviotti A, Geraci M, Avellini C, Zoli G, Fries W, Danese S, Occhipinti P, Croatto T, Zarifi D. Early diagnosis and treatment of postoperative endoscopic recurrence of Crohn's disease: partial benefit by infliximab–a pilot study. Dig Dis Sci. 2012;57(5):1341–8.

34. Lichtenstein GR, Feagan BG, Cohen RD, Salzberg BA, Diamond RH, Langholff W, Londhe A, Sandborn WJ. Drug therapies and the risk of malignancy in Crohn's disease: results from the TREAT Registry. Am J Gastroenterol. 2014;109(2):212–23.

35. Lichtenstein GR, Feagan BG, Cohen RD, Salzberg BA, Diamond RH, Price S, Langholff W, Londhe A, Sandborn WJ. Serious infection and mortality in patients with Crohn's disease: more than 5 years of follow-up in the TREAT registry. Am J Gastroenterol. 2012;107(9):1409–22.

36. Regueiro M, El-Hachem S, Kip KE, Schraut W, Baidoo L, Watson A, Swoger J, Schwartz M, Barrie A, Pesci M, Binion D. Postoperative infliximab is not associated with an increase in adverse events in Crohn's disease. Dig Dis Sci. 2011;56(12):3610–5.

37. Regueiro M, Kip KE, Baidoo L, Swoger JM, Schraut W. Postoperative therapy with infliximab prevents long-term Crohn's disease recurrence. Clin Gastroenterol Hepatol. 2014;12(9):1494–502. e1491

38. Regueiro M, Feagan BG, Zou B, Johanns J, Blank MA, Chevrier M, Plevy S, Popp J, Cornillie FJ, Lukas M, Danese S, Gionchetti P, Hanauer SB, Reinisch W, Sandborn WJ, Sorrentino D, Rutgeerts P; PREVENT Study Group. Infliximab Reduces Endoscopic, but Not Clinical, Recurrence of Crohn's Disease After Ileocolonic Resection. Gastroenterology. 2016;150(7):1568–78.

39. De Cruz P, Kamm MA, Hamilton AL, Ritchie KJ, Krejany EO, Gorelik A, Liew D, Prideaux L, Lawrance IC, Andrews JM, Bampton PA, Gibson PR, Sparrow M, Leong RW, Florin TH, Gearry RB, Radford-Smith G, Macrae FA, Debinski H, Selby W, Kronborg I, Johnston MJ, Woods R, Elliott PR, Bell SJ, Brown SJ, Connell WR, Desmond PV. Crohn's disease management after intestinal resection: a randomised trial. Lancet. 2015;385(9976):1406–17.

Pouchitis After Ileal Pouch-Anal Anastomosis

44

Jacob Kurowski, Marsha Kay, and Robert Wyllie

Introduction

Proctocolectomy with ileal pouch-anal anastomosis (IPAA) has emerged as the surgical procedure of choice for patients diagnosed with ulcerative colitis (UC) and familial adenomatous polyposis (FAP) syndrome since its introduction in the 1980s. In pediatric patients diagnosed with UC, specific indications for proctocolectomy include severe disease refractory to medications, toxic megacolon, perforation, and intractable bleeding. In addition, findings consistent with dysplasia or malignancy on biopsy specimens are strong indications to proceed with IPAA [1]. The latter two entities, however, are rare in pediatric patients. Patients with indeterminate colitis who undergo IPAA represent a special population. These patients have a complication rate similar to that of UC, unless the diagnosis of Crohn's disease (CD) is ultimately made [2].

Initially, restorative proctocolectomy was performed using straight ileoanal anastomosis (IAA) without construction of a pouch. The results of multiple subsequent studies have shown the superiority of IPAA in comparison to the straight ileoanal anastomosis [3, 4]. In the pediatric population, Telander et al. compared 121 children and young adults with either the straight IAA or the J-pouch procedure. They found the J-pouch to be superior in relation to stool frequency and nighttime stool patterns [3]. The IPAA procedure involves total abdominal colectomy with the upper internal anal sphincter and rectal muscular columnar cuff left intact. A pouch reservoir is then created utilizing the ileum, and an anastomotic connection is made to the anus. J-type, S-type, and W-type pouch reservoirs have been fashioned, but the most common and successful procedure involves using the

J-pouch (Fig. 44.1). Temporary loop ileostomies are performed at the time of the procedure to facilitate healing of the anastomotic connection and are closed at a later date, typically 2–3 months. Contraindications to IPAA include a preoperative diagnosis of pelvic floor dysfunction and decreased anal sphincter muscle tone. Crohn's disease is a relative but not absolute contraindication, and a pouch procedure can be necessary if control of colonic disease is unable to be obtained, recognizing the potential long-term complications discussed later in the chapter [5].

Long-term results are excellent with minimal mortality related to the procedure. The majority of patients are satisfied with the IPAA procedure. Maintenance of bowel continence with a satisfactory functional outcome ranks high with these patients. However, there can be significant morbidity related to IPAA. Long-term complications include pouchitis, pouch dysfunction, stenosis, and fistulae.

Definition and Incidence

Pouchitis is defined as inflammation of the ileal reservoir in patients status post proctocolectomy with IPAA. Pouchitis is the most common long-term complication of IPAA and is a significant cause of morbidity related to the procedure. Pouchitis was first described in the literature by Kock et al. in 1977. His group described the condition as inflammation in the ileal reservoir constructed after proctocolectomy [6]. Since the initial description, multiple investigators have attempted to characterize pouchitis and delineate the underlying pathophysiology which may be multifactorial. The diagnosis of pouchitis is based on clinical symptoms, endoscopic findings, and histologic findings (Fig. 44.1).

The frequency of pouchitis reported by different groups has varied significantly. However, it is well established that the incidence of pouchitis is higher for UC patients as compared to FAP patients. Lifetime incidence of pouchitis

J. Kurowski, MD • M. Kay, MD • R. Wyllie, MD (✉)
Cleveland Clinic Foundation, Department of Pediatric Gastroenterology, Hepatology and Nutrition, Cleveland, OH, USA
e-mail: wyllier@ccf.org

© Springer International Publishing AG 2017
P. Mamula et al. (eds.), *Pediatric Inflammatory Bowel Disease*, DOI 10.1007/978-3-319-49215-5_44

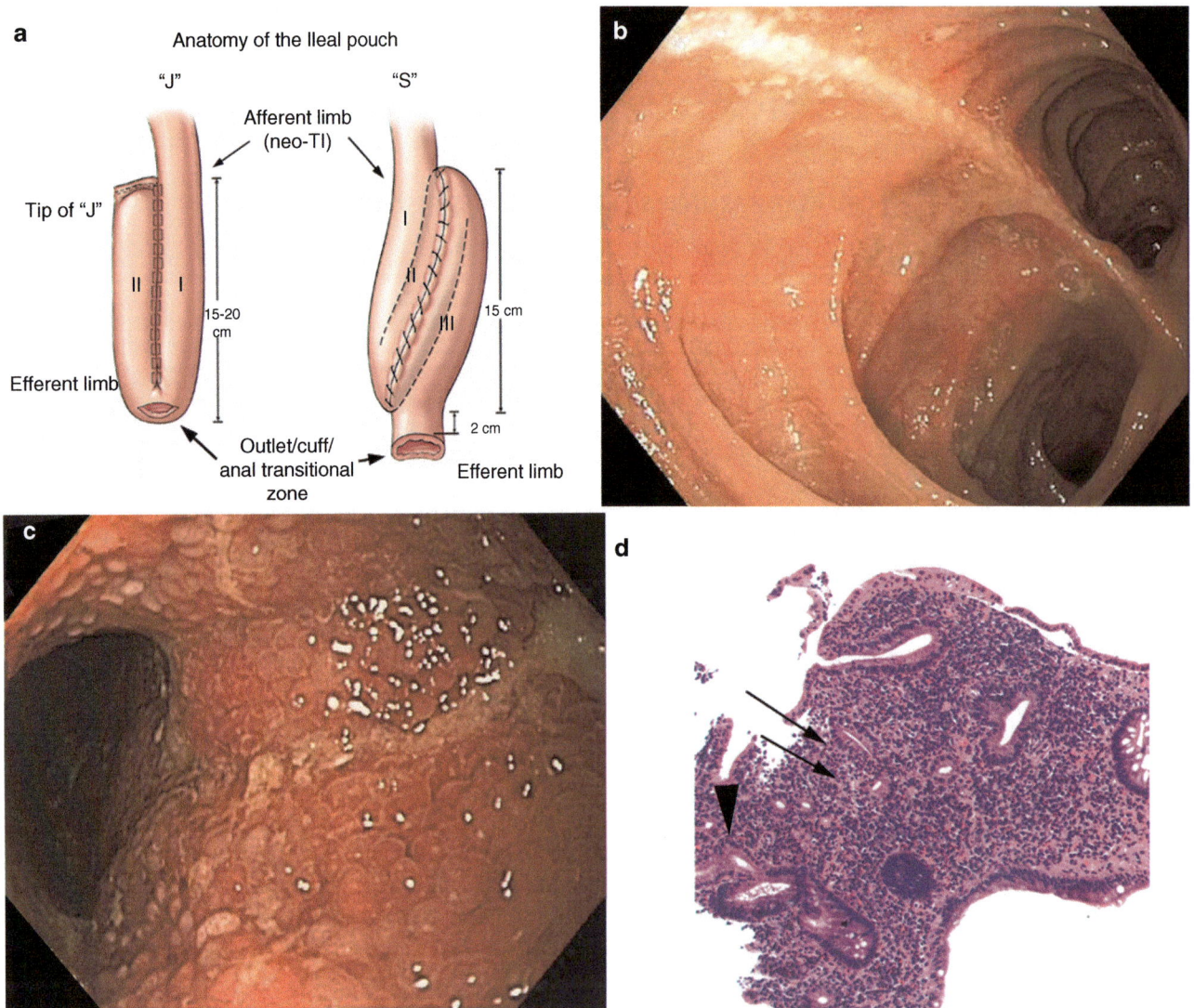

Fig. 44.1 (**a**) Schematic drawing of constructed "J"-pouch (*left*) and "S"-pouch (*right*). (**b**) Normal-appearing J-pouch with efferent (*top*) and afferent (*bottom*) giving "owl's eye" appearance. (**c**) Inflamed pouch with diffuse erythema, edema, cobblestoning, and ulceration. (**d**) Low-power magnification demonstrates distortion of villous architecture, expansion of lamina propria, and pyloric gland metaplasia (*arrows*). There is abundant active, neutrophil-mediated epithelial injury (*arrow head*) (hematoxylin and eosin stain, ×20) (Drawing and pictures courtesy of Bo Shen, MD. Pathology courtesy of Thomas Plesec, MD.)

in patients with UC varies between 15 and 53% [5, 7–10]. In comparison, the incidence of pouchitis in FAP patients ranges between 3 and 14% [11]. The overall incidence reported for pouchitis is related to the duration of clinical follow-up and the clinical definition used for the diagnosis of pouchitis [12]. In adult patients, Simchuk et al. reported that the incidence of pouchitis was 25% for patients followed for less than 6 months, 37% for patients followed for 1 year, and 50% for patients followed for 3 years [13].

In pediatric patients, Ozdemir et al. reviewed the outcomes of 433 pediatric patients after IPAA (83.4% with inflammatory bowel disease (IBD), 15.7% with FAP) and found an incidence of pouchitis of 31.9% with a mean follow-up of 9 years. The occurrence of pouchitis was not associated with specific pouch type in this mixed surgical group (J- vs. S-pouch) [14]. Shannon et al. reported a 45% incidence of pouchitis at a mean of 20-year postprocedure in a recent study of pediatric patients who had IPAA at the Cleveland Clinic between 1982 and 1997 for UC alone [15]. This cohort was originally reported on in 1996 and subsequently in 1999 by Sarigol et al. with shorter-term rates of pouchitis of 13% at 1.9 years and 45% at 5 years [16, 17]. Durno et al. reported a 44% incidence of at least one episode of pouchitis in pediatric patients with a J-pouch for UC in Toronto, Canada [18].

Etiology and Pathogenesis

Although there has been much interest in defining and classifying pouchitis, the etiology of pouchitis remains unknown. There are a number of proposed factors that may play a role in the pathogenesis. It is most likely that the development of pouchitis is multifactorial with several physiological and immunological factors contributing in a susceptible host. The frequency of pouchitis may vary based on the center, surgical experience, and follow-up medical care. Table 44.1 lists the proposed etiological factors that contribute to the development of pouchitis [19].

Immune Dysregulation

One of the most pursued areas of inflammatory bowel disease research is the influence of variations of gene loci on the development of IBD. As cytokines play a major role in the inflammatory pathway that lead to disease manifestations, many studies have focused on the role of cytokines such as interleukin (IL)-1 alpha, beta, and receptor antagonist (RA) in the etiology of IBD. IL-1 alpha and beta are proinflammatory cytokines, whereas IL-1RA is the natural inhibitor of these cytokines. Genetic polymorphisms that lead to a reduction in the ratio of IL-1 alpha and beta to IL-1RA will potentially lead to increased and/or chronic inflammation [20].

It is also possible that an imbalance in the ratio of IL-1 alpha and beta to IL-1RA may influence the initiation of inflammation leading to pouchitis in patients status post IPAA. In 2001, Carter et al. reported that patients that developed pouchitis had a higher IL-1RN*2 carrier rate as compared to patients that did not have the particular allele, 72% versus 45%, respectively [7]. IL-1RN*2 represents a polymorphism in the IL-1 gene cluster that has been associated with a change in the ratio of IL-1 alpha and beta to IL-1RA and the development of UC. This finding suggests patients with UC that carry this allele may have an increased tendency of developing pouchitis after IPAA.

Table 44.1 Proposed etiological factors of pouchitis

Immune dysregulation
Bacterial overgrowth and dysbiosis
Fecal stasis
Malnutrition
Mucosal ischemia (tension, torsion, or vascular)
Crohn's disease, undiagnosed
Colonic metaplasia associated with ulceration
Extraintestinal manifestations, including primary sclerosing cholangitis
Smoking
pANCA status

Adapted from Macafee et al. [19]

More recent studies have identified other genetic polymorphisms and cell membrane receptors that are associated with pouchitis. The NOD2/CARD15 mutations have been shown to be associated with the development of pouchitis and, in some instances, a more severe manifestation of the disease [21–23]. These mutations are associated with several markers of disease severity in pediatric CD [24]. It is therefore highly probable that these patients may actually have CD involving the pouch.

Intestinal epithelial expression of the innate Toll-like receptors (TLRs) 2, 4, and 5 is activated by bacterial peptidoglycan, lipopolysaccharides, and flagellin and leads to a complex downstream cascade of inflammatory signaling mediated by NF-κB. These TLRs have shown to be upregulated in patients with pouchitis [25]. Lammers et al. showed that patients who possess Toll-like receptor (TLR) 9-1237C and CD14-260 T alleles have a higher risk of developing chronic or relapsing pouchitis [26]. Alterations in tight junction claudin-1 and claudin-2 expression in biopsies of patients with pouchitis also indicate increased barrier dysfunction as a result of the inflammation [27].

A novel concept of immunoglobulin G4 (IgG4)-associated pouchitis has been described [28, 29]. Seril et al. demonstrated a high prevalence of IgG4-expressing plasma cells in the pouch of patients with chronic antibiotic-refractory pouchitis (CARP). Patients with CARP were also more likely to have autoimmune thyroid disease, primary sclerosing cholangitis (PSC), and serum microsomal antibodies suggestive of an autoimmune-mediated pouchitis [30]. Future studies are needed to further investigate the role of IgG4 in the etiology, pathogenesis, and prognosis of patients with pouchitis.

Fecal Stasis and Dysbiosis

The favorable response of the majority of acute episodes of pouchitis to antibiotic therapy and more recently to administration of probiotics suggests that bacterial populations are important etiological factors in the development of pouchitis. Pouchitis also rarely occurs until after takedown of the ileostomy with resultant resumption of fecal flow to the neoileum pouch. However, to date, no single microbial factor has been identified as the causative factor. Fecal stasis in the pouch may also be a contributing factor. A study of rats who received IPAA after colectomy had longer fecal retention and higher rates of inflammation in the pouch compared to rats who underwent straight ileorectal anastomosis [31]. As in patients with IBD prior to IPAA, 16 S ribosomal RNA sequencing has demonstrated altered microbial diversity in patients with pouchitis at multiple taxonomic levels with an increase in Fusobacteria and Enterobacteriaceae and a decrease in Bacteroidetes [32–34].

Other studies have looked at the role of serological markers, such as antibodies to bacteria fragments, in the pathogenesis of inflammatory bowel disease and also pouchitis. Serological markers such as anti-*Saccharomyces cerevisiae* antibodies (ASCA) have been found to be associated with postoperative fistula formation after restorative proctocolectomy (RPC) [35]. Antibodies to OmpC, an outer membrane porin from *E. coli* and I2 (antigen to *Pseudomonas fluorescens*), were found to be predictive of postoperative continuous inflammation of the pouch [36]. In 2001, Fleshner et al. studied the relationship between pouchitis and serum perinuclear antineutrophil cytoplasmic antibody (pANCA) in a prospective study. They did not find an overall significant difference in the occurrence of pouchitis in the pANCA-positive versus pANCA-negative groups. They did, however, demonstrate a significant relationship between the development of chronic pouchitis in patients with a high level of pANCA (>100 EU/ml) as compared to patients with a medium level (40–100 EU/ml), low level (<40 EU/ml), or undetectable level of pANCA [10]. A more recent study investigating the impact of preoperative pANCA and anti-CBir1 flagellin on the development of acute or chronic pouchitis showed that both pANCA and anti-CBir1 expression are associated with pouchitis after IPAA. Anti-CBir1 increases the incidence of acute pouchitis only in patients who have low-level pANCA expression and increases the incidence of chronic pouchitis in patients who have high-level pANCA expression [37]. These findings are suggestive of a pathogenic immune response to bacterial antigens.

Infection with *Clostridium difficile* has been increasingly recognized as a problematic cause of diarrhea in IBD patients with both pre- and postcolectomy with IPAA. *C. difficile* as a cause of pathogen-associated pouchitis is diagnosed in up to 10% of adults with increased risk in patients with recent hospitalization, receiving antibiotics, and males [38, 39]. When possible, PCR testing for *C. difficile* toxin B is more sensitive than enzyme immunoassay though neither is specific, and clinical context needs to be considered for patients who may be colonized [40]. Evaluation with either endoscopy or fecal calprotectin helps to establish inflammation in the setting of symptoms in patients positive for *C. difficile*. As many of the patients have already been on metronidazole, consider vancomycin as the first-line treatment. Recurrent or persistent *C. difficile* may also require fecal microbial transplant to eradicate [41].

Mucosal Ischemia

During pouchoscopy, if the pattern of inflammation is isolated to specific limb or wall of the pouch, ischemia should be considered as an etiology of the pouchitis. Ischemia can arise from tension on the pouch when it is pulled into the pelvis during surgery, either from torsion of the pouch when attached to the cuff or by leaving a long cuff resulting in a mobile base for the pouch to rotate on. Ischemia can also occur from decreased tissue perfusion as a vasculitic component of the underlying disease [42]. Ischemic pouchitis can be evaluated under fluoroscopy and by a surgeon for tension-induced ischemia which may require revision. If there is no evidence of tension on the pouch, a more global ischemic process may be the cause. Ischemia has been proposed as a contributing factor in intestinal inflammation after the observation that IBD patients improved after treatment with hyperbaric oxygen therapy (HBOT). A 1994 study demonstrated improvement in 8 of 10 patients with perianal CD, 5 of which had complete resolution [43]. A follow-up study showed decreased levels of IL-1, IL-6, and TNF-α in these patients after HBOT [44]. A 2014 review by Dulai et al. evaluated 17 studies in which HBOT was administered for either UC or CD (including perianal disease) with varying protocols of which 86% responded ($n = 613$, 8924 treatments). The most common complication from treatment was middle ear barotrauma and tympanic membrane perforation (1.5% patients, 0.1% of all treatments) [45]. A recent case report of a patient with chronic antibiotic refractory pouchitis had significant improvement in symptoms after treatment with HBOT [46]. More studies including randomized controlled trials should be completed to further evaluate such a therapeutic endeavor.

Crohn's Disease

Undiagnosed CD can present clinically as chronic pouchitis following IPAA. In adults, a 2008 study by Melmed et al. reported 16/238 (7%) patients who underwent IPAA for UC or IBD-U were later diagnosed as having CD with significant risk factors of family history of CD and/or presence of serum ASCA-IgA. Four of these patients (25%) failed medical management and had a diverting ileostomy [47]. A 2012 study by Coukos et al. also demonstrated association of ASCA-IgA, ASCA-IgG, and anti-CBir1 flagellin in the development of CD of the pouch or fistula in patients with UC after IPAA [48]. In pediatrics, Wewer et al. reported approximately a 6% detection rate for CD in 30 patients aged 7–17 years status post IPAA with a median follow-up of 3.7 years [4]. Ozdemir et al. reviewed the outcomes of 361 pediatric patients who underwent IPAA over a 27-year period and found 18 patients (5%) to be later diagnosed with CD [14]. In a more recent 2016 single-center study follow-up of 74 pediatric patients (15–30 years later) after IPAA, Shannon et al. reported 28% were ultimately diagnosed as having CD, of which 40% required take down of the pouch for pouch failure [15]. The most common manifestations of CD noted for patients status post IPAA are fistulizing disease of the pouch and prepouch ileitis.

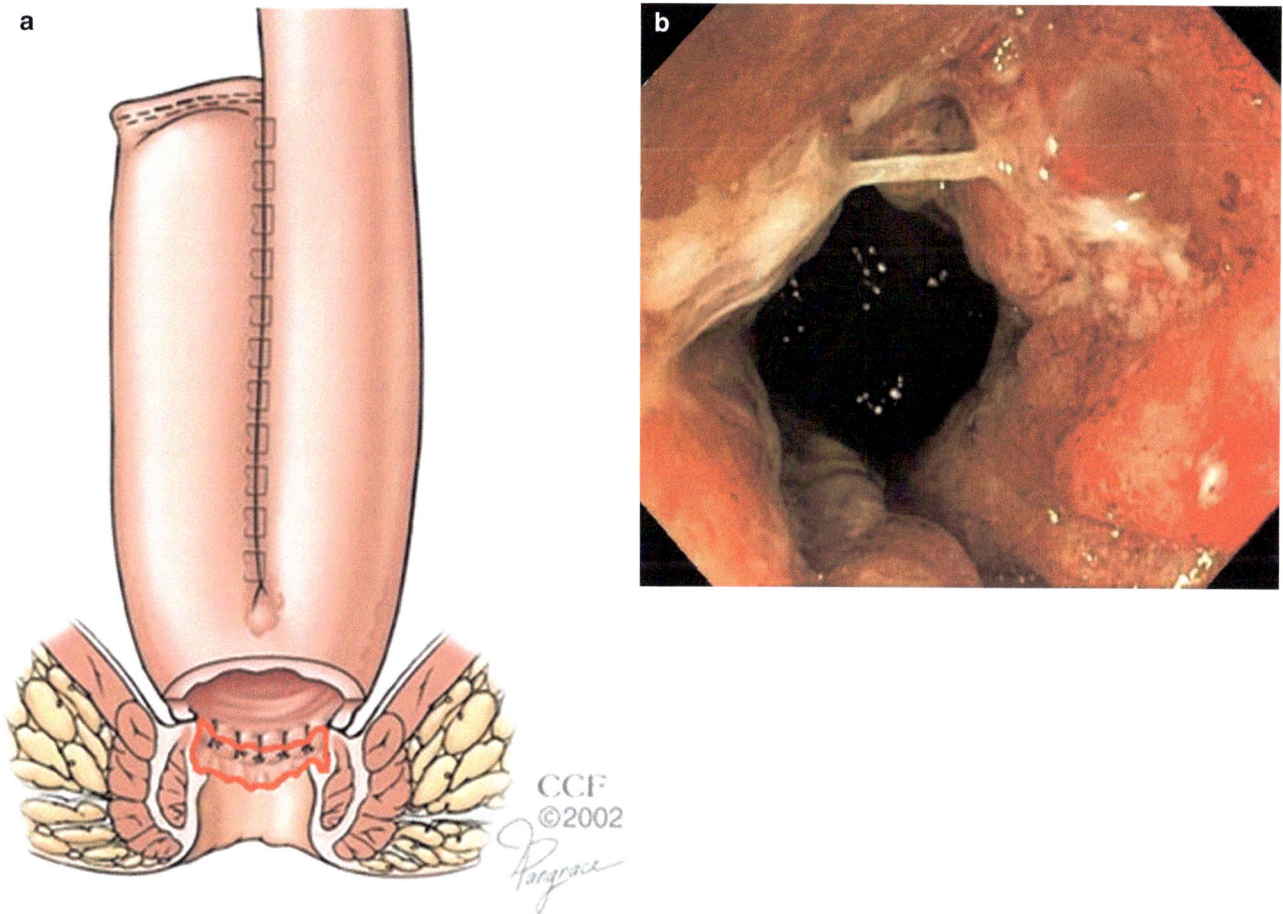

Fig. 44.2 (**a**) Schematic drawing of constructed "J"-pouch with cuff outlined in red. (**b**) Inflamed cuff or "cuffitis" at the distal end of J-pouch

Extraintestinal Manifestations

The presence of extraintestinal manifestations related to inflammatory bowel disease has been studied as possible predictors of the development and severity of pouchitis. Lohmuller et al. looked at extraintestinal manifestations such as erythema nodosum, arthritis, and uveitis to determine a relationship. Their group found that pouchitis occurred in 39% of patients with preoperative extraintestinal manifestations as compared to 26% of UC patients with no preoperative extraintestinal manifestations ($p < 0.001$). They also found an increased risk of pouchitis if postoperative extraintestinal manifestations were diagnosed [8].

Multiple groups have specifically analyzed the relationship between primary sclerosing cholangitis (PSC) and the development of pouchitis. Penna et al. found that pouchitis occurred in 63% of the patients with PSC, while pouchitis only occurred in 32% of the patients without this particular extraintestinal manifestation ($p < 0.001$). This group also reported an increased frequency of chronic pouchitis in patients with PSC versus patients without this disease, 60% and 15%, respectively ($p < 0.001$) [9]. In 2005, a study by Gorgun et al. refuted this claim. This group reported a higher

overall mortality for patients with PSC status post IPAA; however, they did not find a statistically significant relationship between chronic pouchitis and UC in patients with preoperative PSC [49]. A review of the available literature by Rahman et al. concluded that pouchitis appears to be more common in the subset of patients that have both UC and PSC [50]. Shen et al. also demonstrated that concurrent PSC appears to be associated with a significant pre-pouch ileitis on endoscopy and histology in patients with IPAA [51].

Cuffitis

After IPAA a region of colonic columnar mucosa remains unless a mucosectomy is performed [52]. It has been shown that patients have markedly better pouch function when mucosectomy is not performed, and this is the preferred treatment modality in the absence of dysplasia. As a result, a "cuff" remains above the anal transitional zone (Fig. 44.2). The length of the cuff is dependent on the type of IPAA performed. After a stapled IPAA, the preferred method by adult colorectal surgeons, a region of 1.5–2 cm of diseased mucosa, remains. A hand-sewn IPAA has traditionally been performed by pediatric surgeons and leaves a variably smaller cuff region. Neither method is superior to the other as far as complication rate, but the stapled IPAA may offer improved nocturnal continence with higher resting and squeeze pressures of the pouch demonstrated by anorectal manometry [53].

As expected, remaining diseased columnar mucosa can develop inflammation, a term coined "cuffitis." Patient symptoms include anal pain or discomfort, bleeding, discharge, or diarrhea and endoscopic features typical of colitis in the cuff region (erythema, friability, ulceration). Thompson-Fawcett et al. biopsied the cuff of 113 patients after stapled IPAA and found 13% had evidence of acute inflammation, most of which was mild and 9% were symptomatic [54]. Wu et al. followed 120 patients with cuffitis (12.9%) from their registry of 931 pouch patients over a median of 4 years and found no difference in the demographics, risk factors, and extent or severity of disease compared to controls without cuffitis. Of these patients, 33% responded to topical 5-ASA/steroid therapy, 18% relapsed after initial response to 5-ASA/steroid therapy, and 48% did not respond to topical therapy and required immunotherapy. Sixteen patients (13%) with cuffitis ultimately had failure of the pouch due to CD of the pouch, refractory cuffitis, or surgical complications (fistula, sinus) requiring diversion or pouch reconstruction [55]. As a small segment of colonic mucosa remains in situ, the risk for dysplasia remains equally present in the cuff as in the pouch [56].

Smoking

It has previously been established that cigarette smoking is associated with a reduction in the risk of developing UC. In 1996, Merrett et al. also described a link between smoking and a reduction in the incidence of pouchitis in patients after IPAA. Their study documented that 18/72 (25%) nonsmokers were diagnosed with pouchitis, while 1/17 smokers (5%) were diagnosed with pouchitis. The reason for these findings is unclear, but may be related to the effect of smoking on gut mucosal permeability [57]. Fleshner et al. performed a multivariate analysis of clinical factors associated with pouchitis after IPAA. He showed that smoking and the use of steroids prior to colectomy were associated with acute pouchitis, while smoking in of itself appeared to protect against the development of chronic pouchitis [58].

Diagnosis

The first episode of pouchitis occurs most often in the first 6 months after closure of the loop ileostomy; however, it can occur any time after IPAA is performed [11]. To accurately make a diagnosis, a combination of clinical symptoms, endoscopic appearance, and histologic findings is typically uti-

lized. In practice, a presumptive diagnosis of pouchitis is often made on clinical symptoms alone. However, endoscopic and histologic inflammation may not correspond to the degree of symptoms, for example, in irritable pouch syndrome. Pouchoscopy still remains the main tool for establishing a diagnosis and also for evaluating other differential diagnoses in suspected cases of pouchitis [59].

The clinical presentation of pouchitis typically includes a combination of increased stool frequency, abdominal cramping, hematochezia, bowel incontinence, and/or low-grade fever. Endoscopic findings involve assessing the severity of inflammation of the pouch mucosa. Signs of inflammation include erythema, edema, granularity, mucosal ulceration, and friability. The afferent and efferent limp of the pouch are most often affected and should routinely be biopsied (Fig. 44.1). In addition, if inflammation of the neoterminal ileum is visualized, this finding is suggestive of CD. Cheifetz et al. suggest that the presence of a single aphthous lesion in the terminal ileum does not confirm the diagnosis; rather the presence of serpiginous ulcers are more suggestive [60]. Histology of the pouch is graded on an ABC scale. Type A mucosa is described as normal mucosa or mild villous atrophy with no or minimal inflammation. Type B mucosa is described as transient atrophy with temporary moderate to severe inflammation followed by normalization of the architecture. Type C mucosa is described as persistent atrophy with permanent subtotal or total villous atrophy developing from the early functioning period accompanied by severe pouchitis and thus requires follow-up pouchoscopy to diagnose [61]. Type B and C mucosa are most often found in pouchitis. When a diagnosis of pouchitis is made, evidence of acute and/or chronic inflammation is typically present on biopsy samples. Chronic lymphocytic infiltrate, crypt hyperplasia, crypt abscesses, pyloric gland metaplasia, and fibromuscular obliteration of the lamina propria are specific findings that aid in the diagnosis [62].

Histologic evaluation is also invaluable in identifying some of the other secondary causes of pouchitis such as pathogens like cytomegalovirus (CMV) or Candida, ischemia, mucosal prolapse, granulomas, and dysplasia [63]. Other laboratory tests such as stool studies for *Clostridium difficile* infection may be important especially in patients with chronic antibiotic refractory pouchitis [63]. Inflammatory markers in the serum may be useful noninvasive adjuncts in the evaluation of patients with suspected pouchitis. Studies evaluating the erythrocyte sedimentation rate (ESR) as a marker of pouchitis have shown that despite its role as a nonspecific marker of inflammation, it does correlate with the pouchitis disease activity index (PDAI) and episodes of pouchitis [64, 65]. Elevation of the serum C-reactive protein is a nonspecific marker of inflammation, but this was also found to correlate with the PDAI score and the presence of endoscopic inflammation in the pouch and

Table 44.2 Pouchitis disease activity index (PDAI)

Clinical criteria	Score
Stool frequency	
Usual postoperative stool frequency	0
1–2 stools/day > postoperative usual	1
3 or more stools/day > postoperative usual	2
Rectal bleeding	
None or rare	0
Present daily	1
Fecal urgency or abdominal cramping	
None	0
Occasional	1
Usual	2
Fever (>100.5 °F)	
Absent	0
Present	1
Endoscopic criteria	
Edema	1
Granularity	1
Friability	1
Loss of vascular pattern	1
Mucus exudates	1
Ulceration	1
Acute histologic pattern	
Polymorphonuclear infiltration	
Mild	1
Moderate with crypt abscesses	2
Severe with crypt abscesses	3
Ulceration per low-power field (mean)	
<25%	1
25–50%	2
>50%	3

Adapted from Sandborn et al. [11]
Pouchitis defined as a total PDAI score of 7 or above

Table 44.3 Moskowitz criteria

Acute changes	Score
Acute inflammatory cell infiltrate	
Mild and patchy infiltrate in the surface of the epithelium	1
Moderate with crypt abscesses	2
Severe with crypt abscesses	3
Ulceration per low power field	
<25%	1
≥25–≤50%	2
>50%	3
Total possible	6
Chronic changes	
Chronic inflammatory cell infiltration	
Mild	1
Moderate	2
Severe	3
Villous atrophy	
Partial	1
Subtotal	2
Total	3
Total possible	6

Adapted from Moskowitz et al. [69]

Classification

The classification of pouchitis can be made based upon several different factors (Table 44.4). Severity varies from remission to severely active. Duration varies from acute (less than 4 weeks) to chronic (more than 4 weeks or more than three episodes of pouchitis in a 12-month period). Frequency varies from infrequent to continuous. Pouchitis can also be graded according to response to therapy. Response to therapy is described as antibiotic responsive, antibiotic dependent, or antibiotic resistant (refractory) [5, 73]. In addition, it must be considered that not all patients status post IPAA with symptoms of diarrhea and abdominal pain will truly have pouchitis. Other disease entities that may present similarly to pouchitis include irritable pouch syndrome, cuffitis, stenosis of the pouch, CD, celiac disease, and infectious bowel disease (most often secondary to *Clostridium difficile* or Cytomegalovirus).

Treatment

There are currently less than 20 randomized controlled trials that address the treatment or prophylaxis of pouchitis. None of these trials have been performed in pediatric patients. Therefore, the majority of treatment regimens for pouchitis are based on empiric data alone. Treatment approaches include both primary prophylaxis and treatment following development of symptoms.

afferent limb [59, 64]. Fecal inflammatory markers usually are reflective of the presence of intestinal inflammation. The fecal pyruvate kinase, calprotectin, and lactoferrin levels have been found to correlate with pouchitis and PDAI scores in a number of studies [66–68]. These fecal markers could serve as potential adjunctive tests in the initial evaluation of patients with pouchitis, but their role in the overall management of these patients still needs to be clearly elucidated.

Several scales for grading pouchitis have been developed over the last two decades. The most commonly used and referenced scales include the pouchitis disease activity index (PDAI) (Table 44.2), Moskowitz criteria (Table 44.3), and the Heidelberg Pouchitis Activity Score [11, 69, 70]. Another well-validated scoring system is the Cleveland Global Quality of Life (CGQL) which has patients score their current quality of life, quality of health, and energy level on a 0–10 scale (0:worst; 10:best). The total of the three items is then divided by 30 to determine their CGQL [71].

Table 44.4 Classification of pouchitis

Classification	Description
Severity	Remission
	Mildly active
	Moderately active
	Severely active
Duration	Acute (less than 4 weeks)
	Chronic (more than 4 weeks)
Frequency	Infrequent (1–2 episodes)
	Relapsing (more than 3 episodes)
	Continuous
Response to therapy	Antibiotic responsive
	Antibiotic dependent
	Antibiotic refractory

Adapted from Wu and Shen [92]

Prophylaxis

The use of probiotics is proposed to increase the normal, healthy flora of the colon such that concentrations of unhealthy microflora are reduced and the incidence and severity of pouchitis are decreased. VSL#3® (Sigma-Tau, Gaithersburg, MD) contains four strains of *Lactobacillus*, three strains of *Bifidobacterium*, and *Streptococcus thermophilus*. One week after ileostomy closure, a randomized controlled trial demonstrated 10% (2/20) of patients treated with one packet of VSL#3® (900 billion bacteria) developed acute pouchitis within 12 months versus 40% (8/20) of patients who received placebo [74]. The first episode of pouchitis has also shown to be delayed in patients given *Lactobacillus rhamnosus* GG following IPAA [75]. There is an ever-growing number of probiotics now on the market, while there is a paucity of randomized controlled trials to evaluate primary prophylaxis of pouchitis or if one particular brand of probiotics is more effective than another.

Acute Pouchitis

Acute episodes of pouchitis respond to antibiotic therapy 95% of the time. The first-line antibiotics of choice for acute pouchitis are a 14-day course of metronidazole (15–20 mg/kg/day) or ciprofloxacin (20–30 mg/kg/day). Fluoroquinolones have been associated with arthropathy and tendon rupture in all ages and should be considered when prescribing to children. In the past metronidazole alone was considered to be first-line therapy. The first controlled studies with this drug were published by Madden et al. in 1994. They performed a double-blind, crossover trail comparing metronidazole with placebo. They reported that patients with pouchitis treated with metronidazole had statistically significant improvement in their stool frequency as compared with placebo [76]. Later

studies showed the efficacy of ciprofloxacin. In an unblinded randomized controlled trial by Shen et al., it was reported that both ciprofloxacin and metronidazole significantly improved PDAI scores. In addition, the ciprofloxacin group experienced significantly larger reductions in PDAI scores and decreased side effects as compared with metronidazole [77]. Both metronidazole and ciprofloxacin are now considered first-line therapy for acute pouchitis (Fig. 44.3).

Chronic Pouchitis

The medical treatment of chronic pouchitis is less clear. Other antibiotic combinations such as tinidazole and rifaximin have been used in the treatment of chronic pouchitis. Rifaximin, an inhibitor of bacterial DNA-dependent RNA polymerase, has been used as monotherapy in a pilot study by Isaacs et al. This study showed clinical remission occurred more frequently in patients on rifaximin compared to the placebo but the difference was not significant [78]. Shen et al. conducted an open-label trial using rifaximin as a maintenance agent for adult patients with antibiotic-dependent pouchitis. These patients demonstrated a favorable response to therapy [79]. Larger trials with long-term follow-up of patients are needed to fully understand the benefits that may accrue from the use of rifaximin in the treatment of patients with pouchitis.

Tinidazole, a nitroimidazole derivative, has been used in combination with ciprofloxacin in the treatment of chronic antibiotic-refractory pouchitis (CARP). This combination led to a significant reduction in the PDAI scores and also improvement in quality of life scores after 4 weeks of therapy [80]. In 2004, a study evaluating the effectiveness of combination therapy of rifaximin and ciprofloxacin was published in patients with CARP. Eight patients with chronic pouchitis refractory to ciprofloxacin alone were treated with rifaximin and ciprofloxacin for 2 weeks. Eighty-eight percent (7/8) of the patients responded to therapy, and five went into remission for at least 6 months [81]. Additional medications that have been used in the treatment of CARP include 5-ASA products (i.e., oral mesalamine, rectal mesalamine suppositories and enemas), topical and oral steroids (i.e., prednisone or budesonide enemas), bismuth-containing products, and anti-TNF therapy.

In their randomized controlled trial published in 2000, Gionchetti et al. showed that treatment with VSL#3® for 9 months following antibiotic treatment compared with antibiotic treatment alone was statistically significant in maintaining remission from pouchitis [82]. In 2005, a double-blind placebo-controlled trial examined the expression of proinflammatory cytokines in patients diagnosed with pouchitis who were treated with VSL#3®. The results revealed that the expression of mRNA for the proinflammatory cytokines IL-1 beta, IL-8, and IFN-gamma in patients treated with VSL#3®

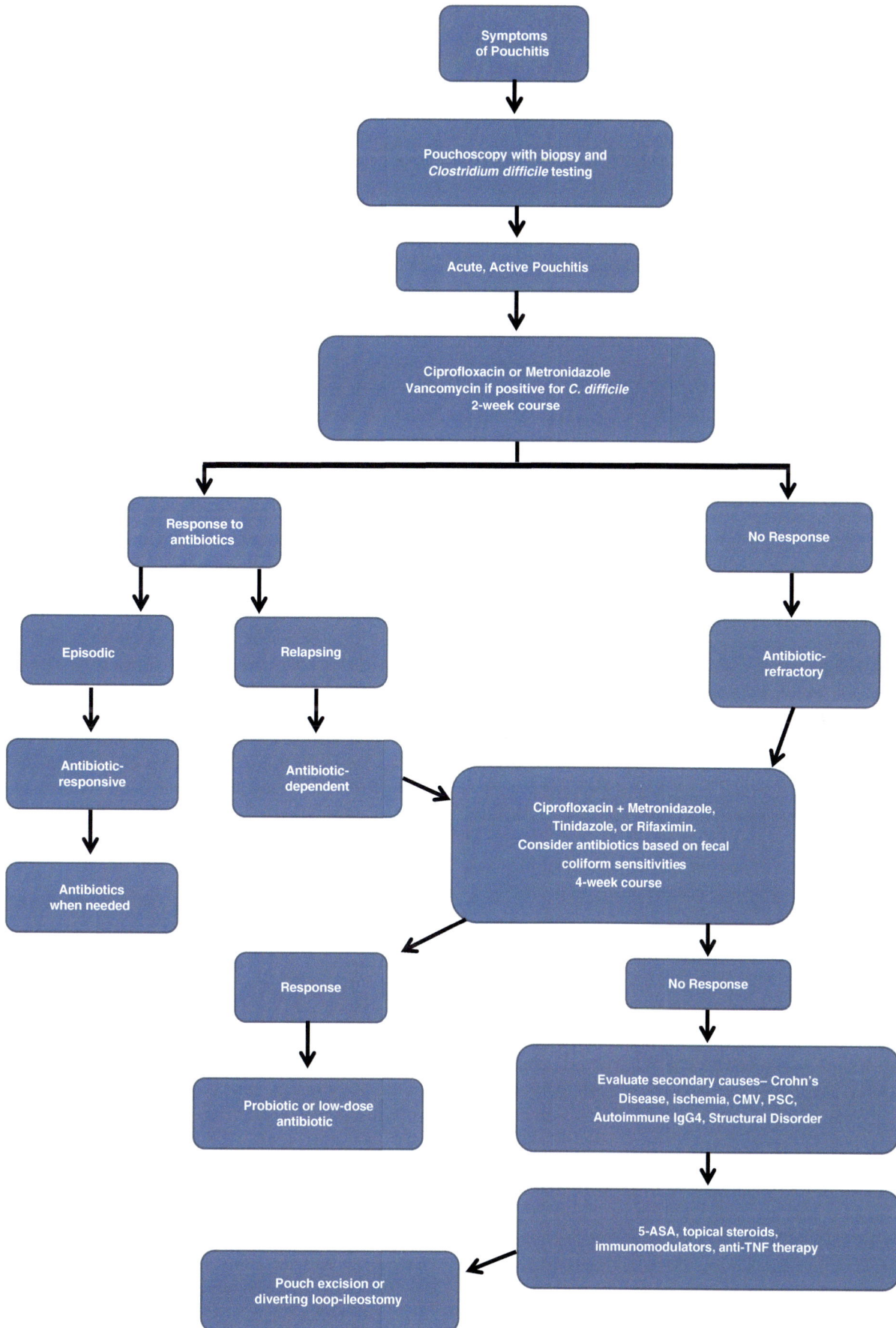

Fig. 44.3 Treatment algorithm for the management of pouchitis (Adapted from Shen [5])

was significantly decreased as compared with placebo. The levels of all of these cytokines were decreased at least two-fold [83]. A pooled meta-analysis of randomized, placebo-controlled trials on the use of probiotics showed that probiotics were beneficial in the management of pouchitis, though each study evaluated patients in different stages of disease [84].

For patients status post IPAA who are subsequently diagnosed with CD or CARP, infliximab therapy is an option that has been utilized as part of the treatment regimen. In the adult population, Columbel et al. reported in their 2003 case series that 85% percent of the patients (22/26) with CD after IPAA experienced clinical response to infliximab. Of these responders, 62% (16/26) had a complete response [85]. There is one case series in the pediatric literature supporting these findings. In this case series, four patients with CD diagnosed after IPAA were studied. The Pediatric Crohn's Disease Activity Index improved from 32.5–42.5 to 0–10 for these patients after infliximab infusions were initiated [86]. Multiple studies have since found benefit to the use of anti-TNF therapy in patients with CARP, which one could argue is on the spectrum with CD of the pouch [87–89].

The medical treatment algorithm for acute and chronic pouchitis is shown in Fig. 44.3. The antibiotic treatment of the first acute episode of pouchitis should be either metronidazole three times per day for 14 days or ciprofloxacin twice per day for 14 days. If a patient is diagnosed with antibiotic-dependent or antibiotic refractory pouchitis, alternative therapies include prolonged antibiotic therapy or combination of various antibiotic therapies with the option of additional therapy with probiotics such as VSL#3®. Failure of response to these therapeutic options should warrant the consideration of other secondary causes of pouchitis such as *Clostridium difficile* and other pathogens in the stool. The addition of anti-inflammatory or immunosuppressive therapy to the treatment regimen should be considered at this point.

Surgical

Pouch failure is an unfortunate consequence that results from a number of complications with the most common being pouch dysfunction, pouch fistulae, refractory pouchitis, pelvic sepsis, anastomotic leak, pouch prolapse, stricture, and development of CD. In adults, pouch failure occurs more commonly in CD than UC (13.3% vs. 5.1%) [73]. In pediatrics, with a mixed series of indications for IPAA over a 27-year period and mean follow-up of 9 years, 9% (39/433) had pouch failure requiring small bowel diversion or excision of the pouch, of which four were for pouchitis and three for CD [14]. Pouch failure can result in excision of the pouch, diversion with a proximal loop ileostomy, or an unreversed diverting ileostomy from primary colectomy.

Outcome

One of the most concerning potential complications of long-term inflammation of the surgically created pouch is dysplasia and progression to malignancy. Overall, the incidence of dysplasia in the pouch is more common for patients with FAP than with UC. For patients with FAP, dysplasia is more often related to the development of adenomas in the pouch. For patients with IBD, the development of dysplasia is related to chronic inflammation. A 2015 meta-analysis reported a pooled prevalence of dysplasia in the pouch of 0.6% and 3.0% at 5 and 20 years, respectively, in adults with IBD [90].

To date, no evidence of dysplasia has been noted in the biopsy specimens of pediatric patients within 5 years after the pouch has been created. Ten percent of the patients followed did have severe inflammation and villous atrophy noted in biopsy specimens which is concerning for possible neoplasia in the future [17]. No long-term studies have been performed to delineate the overall risk of malignancy in this patient population. Gullberg et al. compared the risk of dysplasia in patients status post IPAA with type A histology of the pouch (normal mucosa or mild villous atrophy) compared with type C histology of the pouch (persistent atrophy with severe inflammation). They determined that 5/7 patients with type C mucosa developed dysplasia while no patients with type A mucosa developed dysplasia [91]. These findings are consistent with other research and confirm that patients with type C mucosa are a higher risk of dysplasia and possibly malignant lesions in the pouch. Fifteen cases of adenocarcinoma in the pelvic pouches of adult patients have been described in the literature. Eight of these cases occurred with UC patients and seven occurred with FAP patients [1]. There are currently no consensus guidelines for endoscopic surveillance for dysplasia in place for adults or pediatric patients who are status post IPAA.

Summary

Ileal pouch-anal anastomosis is the surgical procedure of choice for pediatric patients with ulcerative colitis or FAP. The procedure is generally well tolerated; however, pouchitis is the most frequent cause of morbidity. The majority of patients will experience isolated acute episodes of pouchitis. However, up to 41% of adults with IPAA will ultimately be diagnosed with chronic pouchitis [72]. Pouchoscopy remains the main tool for establishing the diagnosis of pouchitis; however, other emerging noninvasive tests may serve as useful adjuncts in the diagnostic process. Therapeutic guidelines are generally empirically derived. Most patients do respond to antibiotic treatment with cipro-floxacin or metronidazole. Others may be treated with a combination of probiotics, antibiotics, anti-inflammatory medications, and/or immunosuppressive medications. Takedown of the pouch is uncommon and occurs only in a small minority of patients. There is however an increased incidence in the development of CD in pediatric patients with longer-term follow-up, but change in diagnosis to CD does not inevitably result in pouch failure. Dysplasia and malignancy are concerns for patients with chronic pouchitis and severe inflammatory changes. To date, dysplasia and malignancy of the pouch have not been diagnosed in pediatric-aged patients although they may be at a higher risk for these complications in their lifetime due to the long duration of the disease and other yet undetermined factors.

References

1. Duff SE, O'Dwyer ST, Hulten L, Willen R, Haboubi NY. Dysplasia in the ileoanal pouch. Colorectal Dis. 2002;4(6):420–9.
2. Pishori T, Dinnewitzer A, Zmora O, et al. Outcome of patients with indeterminate colitis undergoing a double-stapled ileal pouch-anal anastomosis. Dis Colon Rectum. 2004;47(5):717–21.
3. Telander RL, Spencer M, Perrault J, Telander D, Zinsmeister AR. Long-term follow-up of the ileoanal anastomosis in children and young adults. Surgery. 1990;108(4):717–23; discussion 723–5.
4. Wewer V, Hesselfeldt P, Qvist N, Husby S, Paerregaard A. J-pouch ileoanal anastomosis in children and adolescents with ulcerative colitis: functional outcome, satisfaction and impact on social life. J Pediatr Gastroenterol Nutr. 2005;40(2):189–93.
5. Shen B. Acute and chronic pouchitis–pathogenesis, diagnosis and treatment. Nat Rev Gastroenterol Hepatol. 2012;9(6):323–33.
6. Kock NG, Darle N, Hulten L, Kewenter J, Myrvold H, Philipson B. Ileostomy. Curr Probl Surg. 1977;14(8):1–52.
7. Carter MJ, Di Giovine FS, Cox A, et al. The interleukin 1 receptor antagonist gene allele 2 as a predictor of pouchitis following colectomy and IPAA in ulcerative colitis. Gastroenterology. 2001;121(4):805–11.
8. Lohmuller JL, Pemberton JH, Dozois RR, Ilstrup D, van Heerden J. Pouchitis and extraintestinal manifestations of inflammatory bowel disease after ileal pouch-anal anastomosis. Ann Surg. 1990;211(5):622–7; discussion 627–9.
9. Penna C, Dozois R, Tremaine W, et al. Pouchitis after ileal pouch-anal anastomosis for ulcerative colitis occurs with increased frequency in patients with associated primary sclerosing cholangitis. Gut. 1996;38(2):234–9.
10. Fleshner PR, Vasiliauskas EA, Kam LY, et al. High level perinuclear antineutrophil cytoplasmic antibody (pANCA) in ulcerative colitis patients before colectomy predicts the development of chronic pouchitis after ileal pouch-anal anastomosis. Gut. 2001;49(5):671–7.
11. Mahadevan U, Sandborn WJ. Diagnosis and management of pouchitis. Gastroenterology. 2003;124(6):1636–50.
12. Stocchi L, Pemberton JH. Pouch and pouchitis. Gastroenterol Clin North Am. 2001;30(1):223–41.
13. Simchuk EJ, Thirlby RC. Risk factors and true incidence of pouchitis in patients after ileal pouch-anal anastomoses. World J Surg. 2000;24(7):851–6.
14. Ozdemir Y, Kiran RP, Erem HH, et al. Functional outcomes and complications after restorative proctocolectomy and ileal pouch anal anastomosis in the pediatric population. J Am Coll Surg. 2014;218(3):328–35.
15. Shannon A, Eng K, Kay M, et al. Long-term follow up of ileal pouch anal anastomosis in a large cohort of pediatric and young adult patients with ulcerative colitis. J Pediatr Surg. 2016;51(7):1181–6.
16. Sarigol S, Caulfield M, Wyllie R, et al. Ileal pouch-anal anastomosis in children with ulcerative colitis. Inflamm Bowel Dis. 1996;2(2):82–7.
17. Sarigol S, Wyllie R, Gramlich T, et al. Incidence of dysplasia in pelvic pouches in pediatric patients after ileal pouch-anal anastomosis for ulcerative colitis. J Pediatr Gastroenterol Nutr. 1999;28(4):429–34.
18. Durno C, Sherman P, Harris K, et al. Outcome after ileoanal anastomosis in pediatric patients with ulcerative colitis. J Pediatr Gastroenterol Nutr. 1998;27(5):501–7.
19. Macafee DA, Abercrombie JF, Maxwell-Armstrong C. Pouchitis. Colorectal Dis. 2004;6(3):142–52.
20. Casini-Raggi V, Kam L, Chong YJ, Fiocchi C, Pizarro TT, Cominelli F. Mucosal imbalance of IL-1 and IL-1 receptor antagonist in inflammatory bowel disease. A novel mechanism of chronic intestinal inflammation. J Immunol. 1995;154(5):2434–40.
21. Meier CB, Hegazi RA, Aisenberg J, et al. Innate immune receptor genetic polymorphisms in pouchitis: is CARD15 a susceptibility factor? Inflamm Bowel Dis. 2005;11(11):965–71.
22. Sehgal R, Berg A, Hegarty JP, et al. NOD2/CARD15 mutations correlate with severe pouchitis after ileal pouch-anal anastomosis. Dis Colon Rectum. 2010;53(11):1487–1494.
23. Tyler AD, Milgrom R, Stempak JM, et al. The NOD2insC polymorphism is associated with worse outcome following ileal pouch-anal anastomosis for ulcerative colitis. Gut. 2013;62(10):1433–9.
24. Russell RK, Drummond HE, Nimmo EE, et al. Genotype-phenotype analysis in childhood-onset crohn's disease: NOD2/CARD15 variants consistently predict phenotypic characteristics of severe disease. Inflamm Bowel Dis. 2005;11(11):955–64.
25. Heuschen G, Leowardi C, Hinz U, et al. Differential expression of toll-like receptor 3 and 5 in ileal pouch mucosa of ulcerative colitis patients. Int J Colorectal Dis. 2007;22(3):293–301.
26. Lammers KM, Ouburg S, Morre SA, et al. Combined carriership of TLR9-1237C and CD14-260 T alleles enhances the risk of developing chronic relapsing pouchitis. World J Gastroenterol. 2005;11(46):7323–9.
27. Amasheh S, Dullat S, Fromm M, Schulzke JD, Buhr HJ, Kroesen AJ. Inflamed pouch mucosa possesses altered tight junctions indicating recurrence of inflammatory bowel disease. Int J Colorectal Dis. 2009;24(10):1149–56.
28. Navaneethan U, Venkatesh PG, Kapoor S, Kiran RP, Remzi FH, Shen B. Elevated serum IgG4 is associated with chronic antibiotic-refractory pouchitis. J Gastrointest Surg. 2011;15(9):1556–61.
29. Shen B, Bennett AE, Navaneethan U. IgG4-associated pouchitis. Inflamm Bowel Dis. 2011;17(5):1247–8.
30. Seril DN, Yao Q, Lashner BA, Shen B. Autoimmune features are associated with chronic antibiotic-refractory pouchitis. Inflamm Bowel Dis. 2015;21(1):110–20.
31. Stucchi AF, Shebani KO, Reed KL, et al. Stasis predisposes ileal pouch inflammation in a rat model of ileal pouch-anal anastomosis. J Surg Res. 2010;164(1):75–83.
32. Komanduri S, Gillevet PM, Sikaroodi M, Mutlu E, Keshavarzian A. Dysbiosis in pouchitis: evidence of unique microfloral patterns in pouch inflammation. Clin Gastroenterol Hepatol. 2007;5(3):352–60.
33. Morgan XC, Kabakchiev B, Waldron L, et al. Associations between host gene expression, the mucosal microbiome, and clinical outcome in the pelvic pouch of patients with inflammatory bowel disease. Genome Biol. 2015;16:67–015-0637-x.
34. Tyler AD, Knox N, Kabakchiev B, et al. Characterization of the gut-associated microbiome in inflammatory pouch complications following ileal pouch-anal anastomosis. PLoS One. 2013;8(9):e66934.

35. Dendrinos KG, Becker JM, Stucchi AF, Saubermann LJ, LaMorte W, Farraye FA. Anti-saccharomyces cerevisiae antibodies are associated with the development of postoperative fistulas following ileal pouch-anal anastomosis. J Gastrointest Surg. 2006;10(7):1060–4.

36. Hui T, Landers C, Vasiliauskas E, et al. Serologic responses in indeterminate colitis patients before ileal pouch-anal anastomosis may determine those at risk for continuous pouch inflammation. Dis Colon Rectum. 2005;48(6):1254–62.

37. Fleshner P, Ippoliti A, Dubinsky M, et al. Both preoperative perinuclear antineutrophil cytoplasmic antibody and anti-CBir1 expression in ulcerative colitis patients influence pouchitis development after ileal pouch-anal anastomosis. Clin Gastroenterol Hepatol. 2008;6(5):561–8.

38. Li Y, Qian J, Queener E, Shen B. Risk factors and outcome of PCR-detected clostridium difficile infection in ileal pouch patients. Inflamm Bowel Dis. 2013;19(2):397–403.

39. Shen BO, Jiang ZD, Fazio VW, et al. Clostridium difficile infection in patients with ileal pouch-anal anastomosis. Clin Gastroenterol Hepatol. 2008;6(7):782–8.

40. Kvach EJ, Ferguson D, Riska PF, Landry ML. Comparison of BD GeneOhm cdiff real-time PCR assay with a two-step algorithm and a toxin A/B enzyme-linked immunosorbent assay for diagnosis of toxigenic clostridium difficile infection. J Clin Microbiol. 2010;48(1):109–14.

41. Seril DN, Shen B. Clostridium difficile infection in patients with ileal pouches. Am J Gastroenterol. 2014;109(7):941–7.

42. Wu XR, Kirat HT, Xhaja X, Hammel JP, Kiran RP, Church JM. The impact of mesenteric tension on pouch outcome and quality of life in patients undergoing restorative proctocolectomy. Colorectal Dis. 2014;16(12):986–94.

43. Lavy A, Weisz G, Adir Y, Ramon Y, Melamed Y, Eidelman S. Hyperbaric oxygen for perianal crohn's disease. J Clin Gastroenterol. 1994;19(3):202–5.

44. Weisz G, Lavy A, Adir Y, et al. Modification of in vivo and in vitro TNF-alpha, IL-1, and IL-6 secretion by circulating monocytes during hyperbaric oxygen treatment in patients with perianal crohn's disease. J Clin Immunol. 1997;17(2):154–9.

45. Dulai PS, Gleeson MW, Taylor D, Holubar SD, Buckey JC, Siegel CA. Systematic review: the safety and efficacy of hyperbaric oxygen therapy for inflammatory bowel disease. Aliment Pharmacol Ther. 2014;39(11):1266–75.

46. Nyabanga CT, Kulkarni G, Shen B. Hyperbaric oxygen therapy for chronic antibiotic-refractory ischemic pouchitis. Gastroenterol Rep (Oxf). 2015. pii: gov038:1–2. PMID:26319238. doi:10.1093/gastro/gov038.

47. Melmed GY, Fleshner PR, Bardakcioglu O, et al. Family history and serology predict crohn's disease after ileal pouch-anal anastomosis for ulcerative colitis. Dis Colon Rectum. 2008;51(1):100–8.

48. Coukos JA, Howard LA, Weinberg JM, Becker JM, Stucchi AF, Farraye FA. ASCA IgG and CBir antibodies are associated with the development of crohn's disease and fistulae following ileal pouch-anal anastomosis. Dig Dis Sci. 2012;57(6):1544–53.

49. Gorgun E, Remzi FH, Manilich E, Preen M, Shen B, Fazio VW. Surgical outcome in patients with primary sclerosing cholangitis undergoing ileal pouch-anal anastomosis: a case-control study. Surgery. 2005;138(4):631–7. discussion 637-9

50. Rahman M, Desmond P, Mortensen N, Chapman RW. The clinical impact of primary sclerosing cholangitis in patients with an ileal pouch-anal anastomosis for ulcerative colitis. Int J Colorectal Dis. 2011;26(5):553–9.

51. Shen B, Bennett AE, Navaneethan U, et al. Primary sclerosing cholangitis is associated with endoscopic and histologic inflammation of the distal afferent limb in patients with ileal pouch-anal anastomosis. Inflamm Bowel Dis. 2011;17(9):1890–900.

52. Chambers WM, McC Mortensen NJ. Should ileal pouch-anal anastomosis include mucosectomy? Colorectal Dis. 2007;9(5):384–92.

53. Lovegrove RE, Constantinides VA, Heriot AG, et al. A comparison of hand-sewn versus stapled ileal pouch anal anastomosis (IPAA) following proctocolectomy: a meta-analysis of 4183 patients. Ann Surg. 2006;244(1):18–26.

54. Thompson-Fawcett MW, Mortensen NJ, Warren BF. "Cuffitis" and inflammatory changes in the columnar cuff, anal transitional zone, and ileal reservoir after stapled pouch-anal anastomosis. Dis Colon Rectum. 1999;42(3):348–55.

55. Wu B, Lian L, Li Y, et al. Clinical course of cuffitis in ulcerative colitis patients with restorative proctocolectomy and ileal pouch-anal anastomoses. Inflamm Bowel Dis. 2013;19(2):404–10.

56. Scarpa M, van Koperen PJ, Ubbink DT, Hommes DW, Ten Kate FJ, Bemelman WA. Systematic review of dysplasia after restorative proctocolectomy for ulcerative colitis. Br J Surg. 2007;94(5):534–45.

57. Merrett MN, Mortensen N, Kettlewell M, Jewell DO. Smoking may prevent pouchitis in patients with restorative proctocolectomy for ulcerative colitis. Gut. 1996;38(3):362–4.

58. Fleshner P, Ippoliti A, Dubinsky M, et al. A prospective multivariate analysis of clinical factors associated with pouchitis after ileal pouch-anal anastomosis. Clin Gastroenterol Hepatol. 2007;5(8):952–8. quiz 887

59. Navaneethan U, Shen B. Diagnosis and management of pouchitis and ileoanal pouch dysfunction. Curr Gastroenterol Rep. 2010;12(6):485–94.

60. Cheifetz A, Itzkowitz S. The diagnosis and treatment of pouchitis in inflammatory bowel disease. J Clin Gastroenterol. 2004;38(5 Suppl 1):S44–50.

61. Veress B, Reinholt FP, Lindquist K, Lofberg R, Liljeqvist L. Long-term histomorphological surveillance of the pelvic ileal pouch: dysplasia develops in a subgroup of patients. Gastroenterology. 1995;109(4):1090–7.

62. Nicholls RJ, Banerjee AK. Pouchitis: risk factors, etiology, and treatment. World J Surg. 1998;22(4):347–51.

63. Navaneethan U, Shen B. Secondary pouchitis: those with identifiable etiopathogenetic or triggering factors. Am J Gastroenterol. 2010;105(1):51–64.

64. M'Koma AE. Serum biochemical evaluation of patients with functional pouches ten to 20 years after restorative proctocolectomy. Int J Colorectal Dis. 2006;21(7):711–20.

65. Lu H, Lian L, Navaneethan U, Shen B. Clinical utility of C-reactive protein in patients with ileal pouch anal anastomosis. Inflamm Bowel Dis. 2010;16(10):1678–84.

66. Walkowiak J, Banasiewicz T, Krokowicz P, Hansdorfer-Korzon R, Drews M, Herzig KH. Fecal pyruvate kinase (M2-PK): a new predictor for inflammation and severity of pouchitis. Scand J Gastroenterol. 2005;40(12):1493–4.

67. Johnson MW, Maestranzi S, Duffy AM, et al. Faecal calprotectin: a noninvasive diagnostic tool and marker of severity in pouchitis. Eur J Gastroenterol Hepatol. 2008;20(3):174–9.

68. Parsi MA, Shen B, Achkar JP, et al. Fecal lactoferrin for diagnosis of symptomatic patients with ileal pouch-anal anastomosis. Gastroenterology. 2004;126(5):1280–6.

69. Moskowitz RL, Shepherd NA, Nicholls RJ. An assessment of inflammation in the reservoir after restorative proctocolectomy with ileo-anal ileal reservoir. Int J Colorectal Dis. 1986;1(3):167–74.

70. Heuschen UA, Autschbach F, Allemeyer EH, et al. Long-term follow-up after ileoanal pouch procedure: algorithm for diagnosis, classification, and management of pouchitis. Dis Colon Rectum. 2001;44(4):487–99.

71. Fazio VW, O'Riordain MG, Lavery IC, et al. Long-term functional outcome and quality of life after stapled restorative proctocolectomy. Ann Surg 1999;230(4):575–84; discussion 584–6.

72. Ferrante M, Declerck S, De Hertogh G, et al. Outcome after proctocolectomy with ileal pouch-anal anastomosis for ulcerative colitis. Inflamm Bowel Dis. 2008;14(1):20–8.

73. Fazio VW, Kiran RP, Remzi FH, et al. Ileal pouch anal anastomosis: analysis of outcome and quality of life in 3707 patients. Ann Surg. 2013;257(4):679–85.
74. Gionchetti P, Rizzello F, Helwig U, et al. Prophylaxis of pouchitis onset with probiotic therapy: a double-blind, placebo-controlled trial. Gastroenterology. 2003;124(5).1202–9.
75. Gosselink MP, Schouten WR, van Lieshout LM, Hop WC, Laman JD, Ruseler-van Embden JG. Delay of the first onset of pouchitis by oral intake of the probiotic strain lactobacillus rhamnosus GG. Dis Colon Rectum. 2004;47(6):876–84.
76. Madden MV, McIntyre AS, Nicholls RJ. Double-blind crossover trial of metronidazole versus placebo in chronic unremitting pouchitis. Dig Dis Sci. 1994;39(6):1193–6.
77. Shen B, Achkar JP, Lashner BA, et al. A randomized clinical trial of ciprofloxacin and metronidazole to treat acute pouchitis. Inflamm Bowel Dis. 2001;7(4):301–5.
78. Isaacs KL, Sandler RS, Abreu M, et al. Rifaximin for the treatment of active pouchitis: a randomized, double-blind, placebo-controlled pilot study. Inflamm Bowel Dis. 2007;13(10):1250–5.
79. Shen B, Remzi FH, Lopez AR, Queener E. Rifaximin for maintenance therapy in antibiotic-dependent pouchitis. BMC Gastroenterol. 2008;8:26-230X-8-26.
80. Shen B, Fazio VW, Remzi FH, et al. Combined ciprofloxacin and tinidazole therapy in the treatment of chronic refractory pouchitis. Dis Colon Rectum. 2007;50(4):498–508.
81. Abdelrazeq AS, Kelly SM, Lund JN, Leveson SH. Rifaximin-ciprofloxacin combination therapy is effective in chronic active refractory pouchitis. Colorectal Dis. 2005;7(2):182–6.
82. Gionchetti P, Rizzello F, Venturi A, et al. Oral bacteriotherapy as maintenance treatment in patients with chronic pouchitis: a double-blind, placebo-controlled trial. Gastroenterology. 2000;119(2):305–9.
83. Lammers KM, Vergopoulos A, Babel N, et al. Probiotic therapy in the prevention of pouchitis onset: decreased interleukin-1beta, interleukin-8, and interferon-gamma gene expression. Inflamm Bowel Dis. 2005;11(5):447–54.
84. Elahi B, Nikfar S, Derakhshani S, Vafaie M, Abdollahi M. On the benefit of probiotics in the management of pouchitis in patients underwent ileal pouch anal anastomosis: a meta-analysis of controlled clinical trials. Dig Dis Sci. 2008;53(5):1278–84.
85. Colombel JF, Ricart E, Loftus Jr EV, et al. Management of crohn's disease of the ileoanal pouch with infliximab. Am J Gastroenterol. 2003;98(10):2239–44.
86. Kooros K, Katz AJ. Infliximab therapy in pediatric crohn's pouchitis. Inflamm Bowel Dis. 2004;10(4):417–20.
87. Viazis N, Giakoumis M, Koukouratos T, et al. One-year infliximab administration for the treatment of chronic refractory pouchitis. Ann Gastroenterol. 2011;24(4):290–3.
88. Barreiro-de Acosta M, Garcia-Bosch O, Souto R, et al. Efficacy of infliximab rescue therapy in patients with chronic refractory pouchitis: a multicenter study. Inflamm Bowel Dis. 2012;18(5):812–7.
89. Kelly OB, Rosenberg M, Tyler AD, et al. Infliximab to treat refractory inflammation after pelvic pouch surgery for ulcerative colitis. J Crohns Colitis. 2016;10(4):410–7.
90. Derikx LA, Nissen LH, Smits LJ, Shen B, Hoentjen F. Risk of neoplasia after colectomy in patients with inflammatory bowel disease: a systematic review and meta-analysis. Clin Gastroenterol Hepatol. 2016;14(6):798–806.e20.
91. Gullberg K, Stahlberg D, Liljeqvist L, et al. Neoplastic transformation of the pelvic pouch mucosa in patients with ulcerative colitis. Gastroenterology. 1997;112(5):1487–92.
92. Wu H, Shen B. Pouchitis and pouch dysfunction. Gastroenterol Clin North Am. 2009;38(4):651–68.

Enteral Feeding Devices and Ostomies

45

Judith J. Stellar

Gastrostomy

Children and adolescents with inflammatory bowel disease (IBD) often suffer the consequences of malnutrition and growth failure. Enteral nutrition as a therapy has been discussed in Chap. 27. Enteral access either via nasogastric tube (NGT) feedings or direct enteral access via a gastrostomy tube (G-tube) is an option for children with inflammatory bowel disease. Once it is clear that a patient requires supplemental calories to support growth and development, a trial of feedings via NGT is often done prior to more invasive percutaneous feeding tube placement. The trial of NGT feedings demonstrates the ability to tolerate supplemental enteral formula, and allows the patient and family to become familiar with the feeding delivery system—particularly the feeding bag setup and the pump. It is essential that families are educated regarding NGT placement, feeding administration, and maintenance of the tube and equipment.

Younger children may pose difficulty in keeping the NGT in place. There are products such as the AMT Bridle®, which help prevent the patient from pulling out the tube. Older children and adolescents may choose to place the NGT in the evening and remove it in the morning so as not to have to go to school or other activities with the tube visible. For many patients and families, nasogastric tube feeding is cosmetically unappealing and difficult to maintain on a long-term basis. Eventually, this approach not only becomes burdensome, but it also causes daily discomfort. In these instances, if the supplemental feedings appear to be needed on a long-term basis, it becomes necessary to consider percutaneous gastrostomy tube (G-tube) placement.

Gastrostomy tube feeding is appealing for a number of reasons but particularly because the tube does not require daily or frequent insertions and it is not visible to the outside world. The indications for placement are to provide long-term nutrition to patients who cannot orally ingest sufficient calories for appropriate weight gain and growth and for disease treatment. There are a variety of methods for G-tube placement including open surgical, laparoscopic, percutaneous endoscopic gastrostomy (PEG), or percutaneous radiologic gastrostomy (PRG). Nonsurgical placement of a gastrostomy tube was first described 35 years ago [1, 2], and since that time the technique has been refined. Prior to endoscopic or radiologic gastrostomy tube placement, an upper gastrointestinal series should be considered in order to assure that the anatomy of the gastrointestinal tract is normal, as well as upper endoscopy to assess for the presence and severity of stomach inflammation which might interfere with the tube site healing. A percutaneously placed tube, either endoscopic or radiologic, is most likely going to be a tube that extends off the abdomen and is approximately 25–30 cm long and consists of an internal bumper and an external crossbar or securing disc (Fig. 45.1). An exception is the one-step button (Bard®) which is designed to be placed as an intitial PEG/PRG tube. Most centers would recommend waiting 12 weeks before changing an initial PEG or PRG tube to a low-profile device in order to maximize healing of the track and decrease risk of gastric dehiscence.

When a G-tube is placed surgically, the type of initial tube can vary from a standard mushroom-type tube such as the Malecot or Pezzer, a standard balloon tube such as Kimberly Clark, or a low-profile balloon tube such as AMT or MIC-KEY. The choice is often based on surgeon's preference while accounting for any clinical benefits of one type of tube or another for a particular patient. An initial surgically placed G-tube could be changed within 4–6 weeks. Regardless of the method of G-tube placement, the timing, method, and personnel involved in initial tube change vary from institution to institution. Commonly, an initial PEG- or PRG-placed tube remains in place for 12 weeks; then, it is replaced with a low-profile device or standard replacement tube under fluoroscopic guidance. Thereafter, the tube can be changed by nursing staff or parents who have been thoroughly educated on the G-tube change procedure.

It is essential that families are well educated regarding the care and maintenance of enteral feeding devices and, as mentioned, it is preferable that the success of enteral nutrition via

J.J. Stellar, MSN, CRNP, PPCNP-BC, CWOCN
Department of Nursing and General Surgery, The Children's Hospital of Philadelphia, 34th Street and Civic Ctr. Blvd., Philadelphia, PA 19104, USA
e-mail: stellar@email.chop.edu

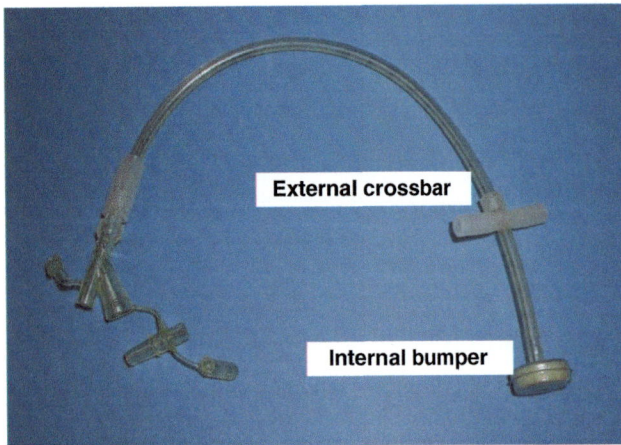

Fig. 45.1 Typical initial PEG/PRG tube with internal "bumper" and external "crossbar"

nasogastric tube has been previously documented. Once the decision has been made to pursue gastrostomy tube placement, it is important that the family be familiar with the type of gastrostomy tube being placed, that is, standard PEG versus low-profile gastrostomy tube, the length of time that the family can expect the initial tube to be in place, and who will perform the first change. All of these vary with institutions and specialties. An example of this is a surgically placed gastrostomy tube that could be a balloon low-profile device, a balloon replacement tube, or a mushroom-type Malecot® tube. Table 45.1 depicts the various types of gastrostomy and gastrojejunal (GJ) tubes. The personnel involved in the tube replacement procedure also varies based on who placed the original tube and the direct visualization is now recommended either through radiology or a repeat endoscopic procedure.

The initial care of the gastrostomy site may vary from institution to institution. There is also some variation in the initial care depending on the type of tubes. For all tubes, the initial gauze dressing is kept in place for 48 hours. The patient may sponge bathe during this time; after 48 hours they can shower, but emersion of the site in a tub bath is avoided for the first 2 weeks. After the initial dressing is removed, care of the site consists of simply cleaning daily with mild soap and water and avoiding any aggressive scrubbing. A small amount of serous or mucoid drainage is normal. Use of hydrogen peroxide should be avoided as it causes unnecessary drying and irritation of the skin. For initial surgically placed low profile tubes, securement of the device with tape for the first 1-2 weeks helps minimize movement in the track. For initially placed PEG/PRG tubes with a cross bar, the crossbar—not the tube—is rotated 3 times a day for the first week to avoid pressure. It is important for the tube to have a good fit and to be well stabilized. Excessive move-

ment in the tract can cause leakage, erosion of the stoma, and hypergranulation tissue formation. Similarly, excess traction on the tube can cause mucosal prolapse and erosion of the tract. Dressings should be minimized and only added as needed. A small amount of serous or mucoid drainage is normal after initial placement and should resolve over time if the tube has a good fit and is well stabilized. If the patient has a low-profile tube in place, it is important to remove the feeding extension when not in use. Keeping the feeding extension in place at all times defeats the purpose of a low-profile tube and can cause undue lateral traction on the stoma, thereby causing erosion of the tract, "buried bumper syndrome," leakage, and/or mucosal prolapse.

Complications of Gastrostomy/ Gastrojejenunostomy Tubes

Commonly encountered complications of enteral devices include infection, leakage, hypergranulation tissue, peristomal skin breakdown, stomal prolapse or erosion, tube migration, tube obstruction, and persistent fistula after removal [3–6]. Table 45.2 outlines common complications and treatment strategies.

Infection

Gastrostomy tube infections are more common in the first several weeks following percutaneous placement. It has been estimated that 25–33% of patients develop a peristomal infection [4]. Few studies have addressed the issue of peristomal infections in children. The underlying medical condition of the child may influence their risk for infection and hinder wound healing. Antibiotic prophylaxis with placement of percutaneous endoscopic gastrostomies is recommended [7].

Infection of the peristomal area can present with a variety of symptoms. Fever, spreading erythema, tenderness, pain, induration, and purulent discharge are typical. However, the yellow-brown crusty discharge that is commonly seen around the gastrostomy site is not a sign of infection, a finding that is confusing to families and caregivers. There can be mild erythema from friction at the site, which is also not indicative of infection. In case of infection, treatment with a topical antibiotic may be all that is needed, or in some cases, oral antibiotics may be necessary. Most infections respond to a first generation cephalosporin. Abscess formation adjacent to the stoma is another potential complication. These lesions have a rapid onset of a pustule or a red-purple fluid-filled lesion that is tender to the touch. When it ruptures, a punctu-

Table 45.1   Examples of types of enteral feeding devices and securement devices

Gastrostomy tubes		GJ tubes	
Initial nonsurgical G-tube	Initial PEG/PRG tube with internal bumper and external crossbar (Corpak)		Initial GJ tube with J limb threaded through G-tube
Low profile	Low-profile balloon tube		Standard replacement GJ tube
Mushroom tube secured	Standard mushroom tube (Malecot® or Pezzer®)		Low-profile balloon GJ tube
	Standard balloon tube—can be initial surgical tube (eg Kimberly Clark®)		Low-profile balloon transgastric jejunal tube
	Low-profile mushroom-type tube (eg Bard®)		"G-JET" low-profile balloon GJ tube

Table 45.1 (continued)

Gastrostomy tubes		GJ tubes	
Securement devices	Hollister Drain/Tube Attachment Device®—can be used to secure and stabilize both G-tubes and GJ tubes		Benik® enteral tube securement belt used to prevent accidental dislodgment of tube

Table 45.2 Management of common complications of percutaneous enteral tubes

Problem	Likely etiology	Prevention	Treatment
Dislodgment	Improper or inadequate securement	Adequate securement; use of products such as Griplock® or Hollister Drain Tube Attachment Device® to secure to abdominal wall; use of protective belts such as Benik Belt®; disconnect extension tubing when not in use to avoid lateral traction on tube	Replacement and securement
Leaking, peristomal irritant dermatitis	Inadequate stabilization, poorly fitting tube, inadequate balloon volume; stomal enlargement/erosion	Adequate fit of tube; securing properly; adequate balloon volume	Consider alternative types of tubes; secure well; increase balloon volume to maximum recommended; consider removing tube to allow site to contract; peristomal skin protection with silicone sealant, cyanoacrylate, or moisture barriers
Hypergranulation	Inadequate stabilization, moisture, friction	Adequate stabilization, decrease moisture, avoid moist dressings	Silver-impregnated hydrofiber or alginate; topical steroid ointment; chemical or surgical cauterization
Infection	Preoperative/preprocedure antibiotics; treatment of oral, gut, or vaginal fungal colonization; immunosuppression	Treatment of oral, gut, or vaginal fungal infection; avoid pressure injury from too tight a tube fit which can lead to cellulitis	Topical antifungal powder, sealed in with silicone liquid sealant; topical antifungal ointment or cream; topical antifungal spray; oral or systemic antibiotics
Obstruction	Inadequate flushing, buildup of residue within tube	Consistent flushing schedule before and after all feeds and medications; dilute medications; use liquid solutions whenever possible	Flushing, declogging agents (Clog-zapper®)

ate opening is apparent and may drain for several days. Treatment with warm compresses and antibiotic therapy is recommended. Although there is little prospective comparison data available, a large retrospective review of surgical versus PEG/PRG G-tube placement technique revealed surgically placed G-tubes had a lower infection rate than PEG/ PRG tubes, but PEG/PRG-placed tubes had lower costs and length of stay [8].

Feeding tubes may become colonized with microbial organisms, including fungus. There have been more than 100 different microorganisms isolated from gastrostomy tubes, with the most common being *Candida* (Fig. 45.2), *Pseudomonas, Escherichia*

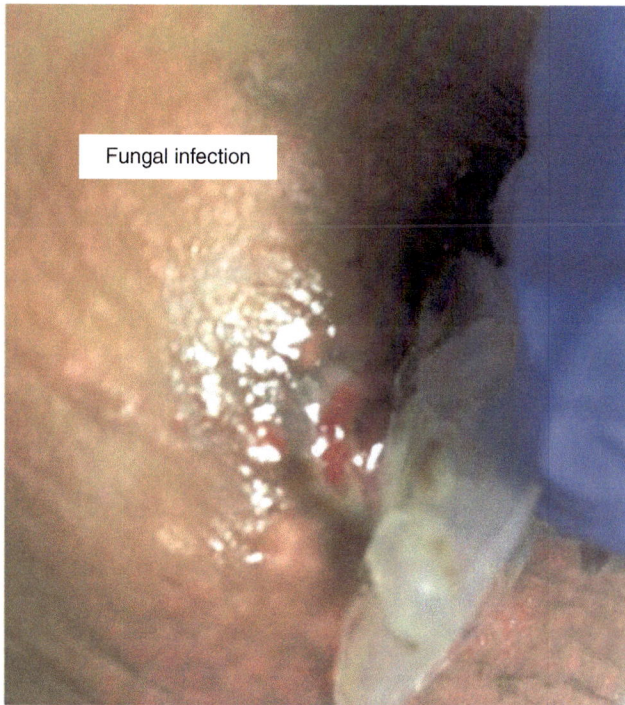

Fungal infection

Fig. 45.2 Peristomal Candida infection

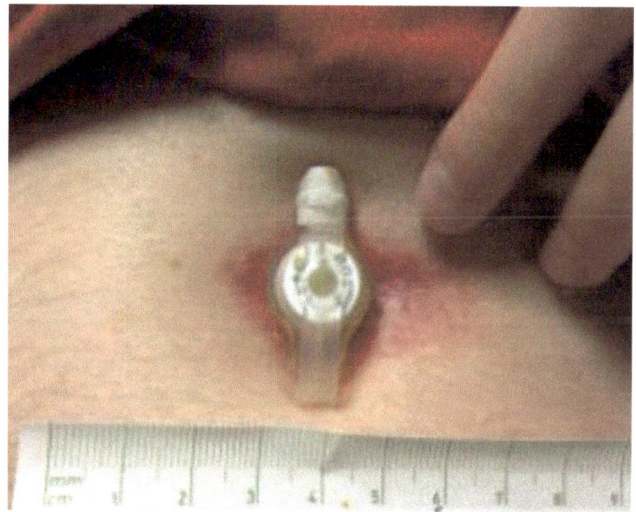

Fig. 45.3 Tight-fitting low-profile tube in patient who gained weight

coli, Enterobacter cloacae, Streptococci, Lactobacillus, Staphylococcus aureus, and *Bacteroides.* The significance of gastrostomy tube colonization is unclear; however, in the face of recurrent infections, culture of the site and treatment with the appropriately sensitive antibiotic are recommended.

Tube Migration and Dislodgment

Migration of the gastrostomy tube with aberrant tract formation has been reported. The buried bumper syndrome (retrograde migration of the gastrostomy tube's internal bumper into the abdominal wall or into the stoma tract) is well described [9]. This occurs when there is traction placed on the external portion of the gastrostomy tube that results in excessive tension on the internal bumper at the time of placement. A false tract may develop as a late complication when the shaft length of the low-profile gastrostomy tube is not resized in a growing child. Failure to remeasure the shaft length may result in a too short tube causing the balloon or internal bumper to move up into the tract. Leakage and focal abdominal discomfort may result. Long-term migration of the balloon into the tract may result in the development of a false tract or dilatation of the gastric opening. This allows for drainage of gastric contents onto the skin resulting in peristomal skin excoriation and breakdown.

It is important to remeasure the stomal tract correctly and accurately. It is best to measure with the patient in both a supine and sitting position. If the measurements significantly differ in either position, the tract length should be the average between the two measurements. It is recommended that tracts be remeasured at least annually. Patients who are gaining weight, however, will need to have the fit remeasured more frequently. Figure 45.3 depicts a teenager with Crohn's disease who initially at the time of tube placement was thin and undernourished, then gained weight while undergoing treatment, causing tightly fitting tube.

Tube migration can also occur in children with a GJ tube in place, where the jejunal limb of the tube can migrate proximally or coil backward. In the latter instance, the child may demonstrate leakage of formula from the gastric limb of the tube or leakage of formula from the stoma. A return trip to the interventional radiology suite is warranted, and the tube can then be rewired and repositioned, or replaced. If the child exhibits signs of intestinal obstruction, GJ tubes have been identified as a lead point for intussusception, and this should be investigated whenever there is concern for intestinal obstruction [10].

Leakage, Stomal Erosion, and Peristomal Skin Breakdown

Leakage, stomal erosion, and peristomal skin breakdown are all interrelated complications. Chronic leakage is a worrisome complication as it leads to chemical, irritant dermatitis (Fig. 45.4). Leakage of gastric contents often results in peristomal skin breakdown and pain, and can contribute to potential infection and proliferation of hypergranulation tissue (Fig. 45.5). The first goal is always to ascertain the cause of leakage and take steps to stop it. A good fit and proper stabilization are both crucial to preventing leakage. For low-profile balloon tubes, re-measuring the shaft length and ensuring the proper fit of the gastrostomy tube is the first

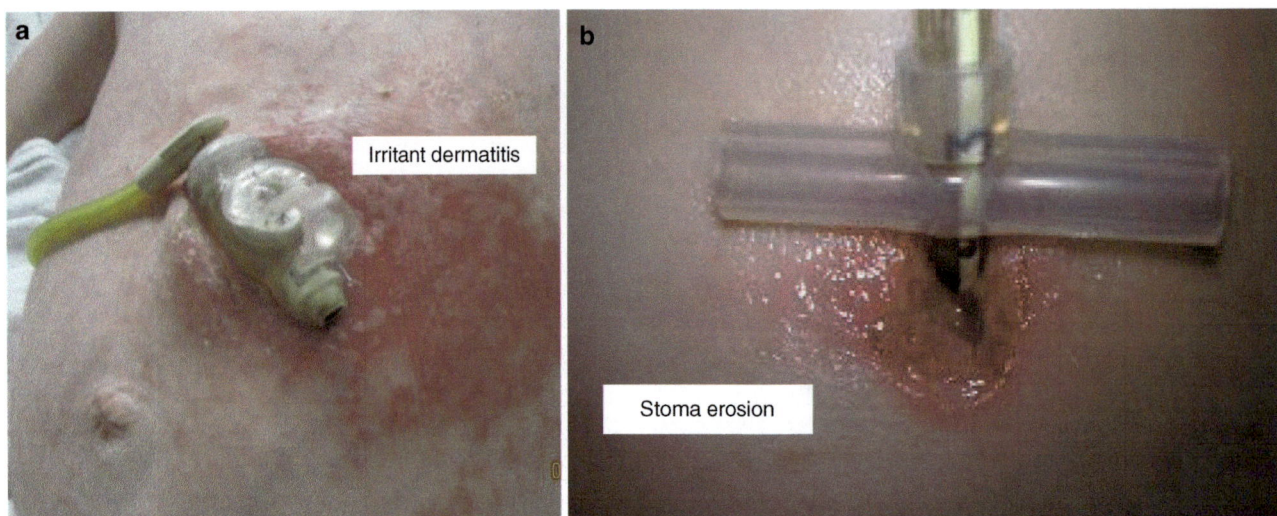

Fig. 45.4 (**a**) Skin irritation from tube leakage; (**b**) Stomal erosion

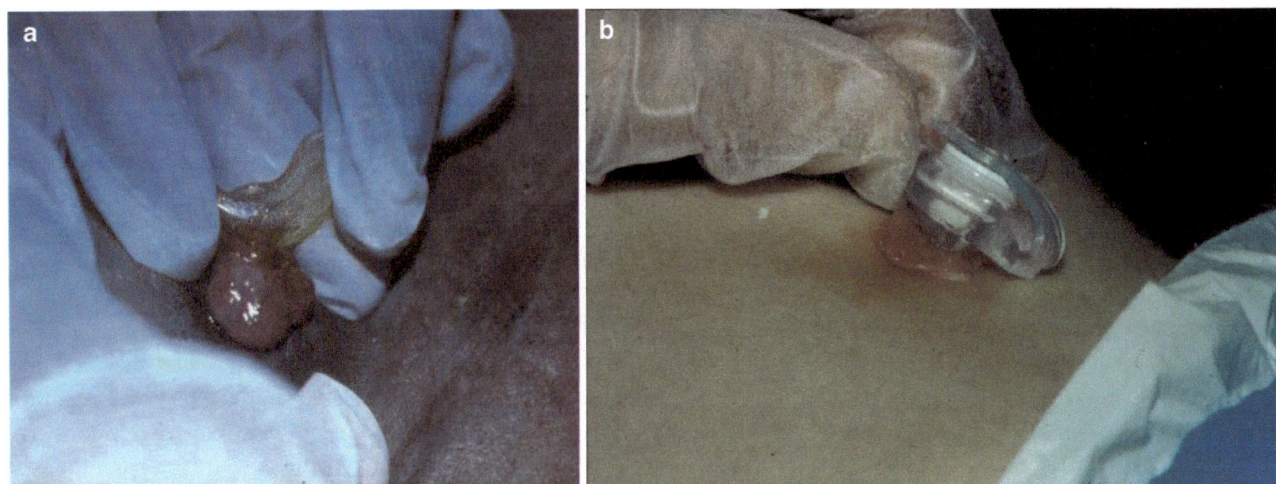

Fig. 45.5 Hypergranulation tissue

step. Ensuring that there is adequate water in the balloon is important. While most manufacturers recommend that the balloon be inflated with 4–6 ml of water, most can accommodate up to 10 ml safely. It is important to be cognizant of the size of the child and their gastric volume, to avoid exceeding gastric capacity. If the leakage is from an enlarged or eroded stoma tract, increasing the diameter of the gastrostomy tube (e.g., going from a 14 French to a 16 French) should be avoided. Increasing the lumen size of the tube only further dilates the stoma diameter. Alternatively, removing the gastrostomy tube for a short period allows the stoma to contract. If the gastrostomy is relatively recently placed, often a few hours may be enough time to allow the tract to contract. Long-standing gastrostomies may require removal of the tube overnight or even longer to get the tract to scar down.

For severe leakage and stomal erosion, more aggressive interventions may be warranted. These include temporary removal of the tube and placement of a nasojejunal tube for postpyloric feedings, while the stoma contracts and the peristomal skin heals. Placement of a small caliber balloon tube allows the site to scar down, while still utilizing the balloon to stent secretion leakage. The small-caliber balloon tube can be secured with manufactured tube stabilizers such as the Hollister Drain-Tube Attachment Device®. This type of device is often used to secure mushroom-type tubes such as Malecot® and Pezzer® tubes. Other strategies for minimizing gastric secretions include placement of an NG sump or placement of an ostomy pouch to help contain secretions while the site contracts. Many patients benefit from changing to a different type of tube if leakage is a chronic issue. If all interventions fail, surgical revision may be necessary.

Wound management of the eroded gastrostomy tube site is a challenge. While awaiting improvement in stoma contraction, the peristomal skin must be protected from caustic gastric secretions. The guidance of a wound and ostomy nurse may be necessary. Skin barriers and absorptive dressings are helpful in preventing ongoing damage from gastric secretions. Skin barriers containing zinc oxide and other topical barriers used to treat diaper dermatitis may provide comfort to the patient and protect the skin from further breakdown. Use of silicone skin sealants such as Cavilon No Sting Barrier® or cyanoacrylate skin sealant such as Marathon® (Medline) can be useful in protecting the skin. There are numerous wound dressings that can support wound healing of the stoma. Absorptive dressings include foams (e.g., Mepilex®), hydrofibers (e.g., Aquacel®), and hydroconductive (e.g., Drawtex®) dressings, and have been effective when used around gastrostomy tubes when indicated to address excessive leakage.

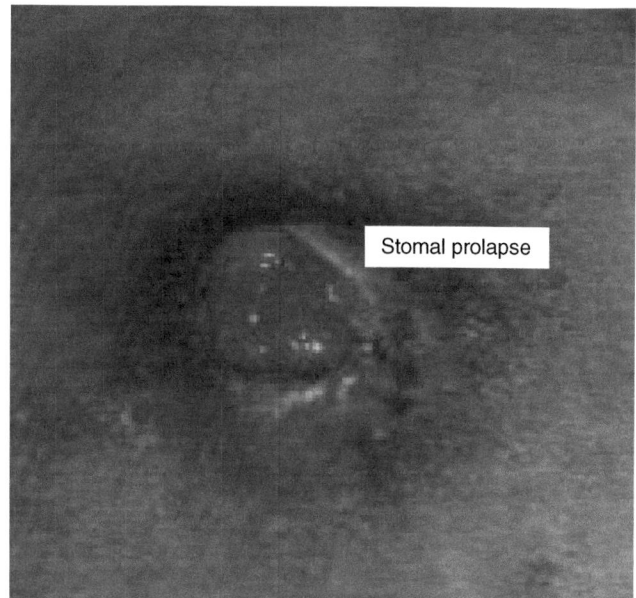

Fig. 45.6 Stomal prolapse

Hypergranulation Tissue

Hypergranulation tissue is a frequent complication of gastrostomy tube (Fig. 45.5). For some patients, it is a minor complication, but in others it results in unsightly tissue that is painful and friable, oftentimes with increased exudate and bleeding. Hypergranulation is a proliferation of capillaries that forms around the external stoma and occasionally within the gastric opening. This excessive, abnormal tissue can also harbor bacteria. Current treatment options are limited. Oftentimes, this excessive proliferation of tissue can lead to other issues such as leakage and erosion of the surrounding skin in addition to pain and bleeding. In these more severe cases, it is important to treat the condition. The usual treatment for hypergranulation consists of attempted chemical cauterization with silver nitrate, topical steroid cream, and foams or pectin-based powders. Another option is the topical cream Granulotion®. There are no randomized controlled trials investigating this particular treatment; however, there are anecdotal reports from families of a positive response in some cases.

Cauterization of hypergranulation tissue with silver nitrate has been utilized for years. It can result in significant complications if applied improperly. Burns to the surrounding skin is not uncommon, and it is essential to protect the peristomal skin. Cauterization is not ideal—it can be painful and may need to be repeated to eliminate the hypergranulation tissue. It is important to protect the healthy peristomal skin with a skin barrier or surgical lubricating jelly. In addition, chemical cautery causes trauma and inflammation to the tissue, and thus can further exacerbate proliferation of the abnormal tissue. An alternative to chemical cautery is treatment with absorbent silver-impregnated dressings such as hydrofibers or alginates [11]. The silver serves as an antimi-

crobial to treat the increased bioburden thought to occur with hypergranulation tissue.

There is little data to support the use of corticosteroid creams in the treatment of granulation tissue, however, dermatologists have for several years [12]. It is thought that the topical steroids have an antiangiogenic effect on the granulation tissue similar to that of systemic steroids in the treatment of large capillary hemangiomas. Anecdotal reports on the successful use of triamcinolone cream in the treatment of granulation tissue are available. The usual dose of 0.1% triamcinolone cream twice daily for 2 weeks has met with some success, and some centers implement a short course (2 weeks) of triamcinolone 0.5%.

Prolapsed gastric tissue (Fig. 45.6) is often confused with granulation tissue. The tissue with gastric prolapse is a deeper red, shiny, and more granular in appearance. Cautery with silver nitrate has no effect on this tissue, which is typically intermittent. Most important in treatment is proper fit of the tube, adequate securement, and avoidance of multiple layers of dressing or excessive traction on the tube.

Tube Obstruction

Obstructed tubes are an issue primarily with gastrojejunal devices. Migration or dislodgment of these tubes is common in children with gastrointestinal dysmotility. To prevent tube clogging, frequent flushing is recommended before and after bolus feeding or medication administration and every 2–4 h during continuous feedings. Families should be instructed on how to administer medication and which medications are more likely to cause tube obstruction. Water is recommended with a volume large enough to clear the tube, approximately 10 ml with each flush. Vigorous flushing with small volume syringes and warm water may help generate enough pressure to clear the tube. In addition, use of pancreatic enzyme mixed with sodium bicarbonate might help relieve tube obstruction. There is a commercially made product—Clog Zapper® (Kimberly Clark) which is effective in clearing tube obstructions.

Fistula Formation

A persistent gastrocutaneous fistula is one that does not close spontaneously in 4–6 weeks after the gastrostomy tube has been removed. Approximately 25% of all children who had an endoscopically placed gastrostomy tube will suffer this complication [13, 14]. The longer the gastrostomy tube is in place, the less likely the fistula will heal spontaneously. Oftentimes, the track becomes epithelialized which would prevent closure. A variety of techniques for promoting closure have been reported in the literature but all with limited success. Tract cauterization and use of fibrin glue have been reported in adults [15]. If the track has epithelialized, then surgical coring out of the track to create a fresh wound is warranted. Surgical consultation and closure is usually recommended if the tract has not closed within 4–6 weeks.

Gastrocolonic fistulas may develop at any time after the placement of the gastrostomy. Fecal drainage from the stoma, foul breath, or leakage of formula or medications from the rectum should raise the suspicion of a gastrocolonic fistula. Surgical closure of the fistula with a replacement of the gastrostomy tube is necessary.

Ostomy Education and Management

Children and adolescents with inflammatory bowel disease, as with many chronic illnesses, modify many aspects of their lives to gain control of their disease. Medications, dietary changes or limitations, and surgery all play a role in the management of IBD. Activities may need to be limited, and relationships are affected, all of which impact a patient's lifestyle. Many patients who undergo operative intervention ultimately feel physically better after surgery as they gain control they had previously lost. Despite feeling better after surgical intervention, oftentimes, the impact of surgery, and in particular fecal diversion, can affect their body image and self-esteem. Preoperative education should occur whenever possible. For those patients who undergo urgent fecal diversion, where preoperative education is not possible or limited, education and support postoperatively become essential in assisting the patient and family to adapt to life with an ostomy.

For the majority of children and adolescents with inflammatory bowel disease, having a surgical intervention that results in an ostomy is associated with fear. For many patients, surgery is recommended either emergently or urgently due to a complication of the disease. It is important that the patient and family be well prepared. Stressing the positives of surgery is important. Many have never heard the words stoma or ostomy, and the information they have may be incorrect. It is important that the patient and the family understand that living with an ostomy requires a lifestyle adjustment, and that new skills will be acquired and mastered. From a healthcare provider perspective, patient/family education prior to the surgery and preoperative marking of the stoma site are essential. The placement of the stoma is important for successful secure pouching and optimal patient satisfaction and outcomes. Ideally, a Certified Wound, Ostomy, Continence Nurse (CWOCN) collaborates with the surgeon to select a site that is ideal in terms of creation of the stoma. A joint position statement between the Wound Ostomy Continence Nurses Society and American Society of Colon and Rectal Surgeons outlines key points and patient characteristic factors in stoma site marking [16]. The stoma is ideally placed within the rectus muscle, but also accommodates the patient's body contour, clothing selections, and avoids creases and skin folds. Successful site marking occurs with the patient awake and interactive. The patient is assessed in lying, sitting, and standing positions with typical clothing in place. In many cases, especially in patients with Crohn's disease, ostomy surgery is done on an urgent basis. In these situations, an experienced pediatric surgeon who cares for a large volume of children with IBD can properly identify the landmarks.

It is important for the patient, with the help and support of their family, to adapt to having an ostomy. Healthcare providers can help educate the patients and family to alleviate common misconceptions. Education should take place within a developmental framework. The Wound, Ostomy Continence Nurses Society has published best practices for pediatric ostomy care, which include educational and behavioral intervention for all age groups [17]. Through education and support, clarification and reassurance can be provided regarding particular common misconceptions, including ostomies do not smell, they are not visible under clothing, and that sports participation is possible. Swimming, scuba diving and skydiving, and even professional football are all possible with an ostomy. There are a variety of "stoma guards" on the market which provide protection during contact sports. In addition, there are a number of companies who produce clothing and accessories for ostomates, including swimwear and intimacy clothing. Adolescents fear intimacy with a stoma. This too needs to be addressed up front. If the healthcare professional is uncomfortable with the topic, then a consultation with another provider or a CWOCN who can address these issues prior to surgery when possible, or at least during postoperative education in both the hospital and outpatient settings, could be arranged.

Family education and support are important. The preoperative discussion should include what the stoma will look like, how it functions, how it is managed, what the appliance or pouching system will look like. Have the pouching system available so that the patient and family can visualize how the stoma is fitted and how the pouch is emptied. Encourage the patient to wear a pouch prior to surgery so that they are familiar with the sensation of the pouch on their abdomen and to be familiar with what to expect after surgery.

One of the most common problem encountered in ostomy management is leakage from around the pouching system. It is important to be able to maintain the seal on the pouching system for a predictable period of time, for most patients, 5–7 days, minimum of 3 days. Leakage results in denuded peristomal skin, and more importantly, loss of confidence and frustration for the patient. It is important for the patient to be able to predict the timing for changing the pouching system, thus allowing them to change it on a scheduled day and avoid the worry that the system will fail in the interval.

Prevention and early recognition of peristomal complications are key to achieving patient satisfaction and positive adaptation. Table 45.3 outlines common persitomal complications and recommendations for prevention and treatment. Early intervention and treatment can minimize long-term complications. One of the most common problems encountered is irritant contact dermatitis. This often occurs with ileostomies from leakage of caustic stool on the skin under the appliance. Prevention and treatment center around appropriate appliance selection and sizing. Allergic contact der-

Table 45.3 Common peristomal complications: prevention and treatment

Problem	Likely etiology	Prevention	Treatment
Peristomal irritant contact dermatitis	Leakage of caustic effluent on peristomal skin	Proper fit of appliance and use of barrier seals as caulking to prevent leakage and undermining of wafer barrier	Alter appliance, sealants and barrier rings, or caulking as needed; protect skin with silicone or cyanoacrylate sealants
Peristomal allergic contact dermatitis	Contact/allergic dermatitis related to appliance and accessory products	Use minimal variety of products necessary for good fit and good seal	Patch testing; Switching appliance to alternative product; Topical treatment with steroid sprays or powders
Peristomal fungal infection	Colonization of mouth, gut, vagina; immunosuppression	Keep peristomal skin clean and dry; treat existing infection (oral, vaginal)	Use of antifungal powder and "seal in" with liquid silicone sealant; topical antifungal spray; oral antifungal agent if needed
Peristomal pyoderma gangrenosum	Disease process—Extraintestinal manifestation of IBD adjacent to stoma, caused by trauma, inflammation, irritation, abrasion, or pressure	Appliance with good fit Avoid pressure, abrasions, and trauma	Topical, intralesional, or systemic steroids; immunologic or biologic agents; topical dressings of silver-impregnated hydrofiber or other absorptive dressing with antimicrobial
Stoma retraction	Short length of intestine for stoma creation; stoma within crease; increased weight gain	Adequate length of stoma	Use of convex wafer and belt to assist in improving stoma profile
Stoma prolapse	Enlarged fascial opening, increased intra-abdominal pressure	Avoid convex wafers and/or belts in immediate postoperative period; avoid increased intra-abdominal pressure	Protect prolapse; can use lubricant inside pouch to prevent rubbing against prolapse; cut radial slits in wafer barrier to accommodate prolapse
Mucocutaneous separation	Poor healing, mechanical	Maximize medical treatment of IBD, maximize nutrition, whenever possible prior to surgical creation of stoma; void convex wafers in immediate postop period	Pack area with silver-impregnated hydrofiber or alginate and cover with thin hydrocolloid; obtain good seal of appliance to prevent stool coming in contact with the wound

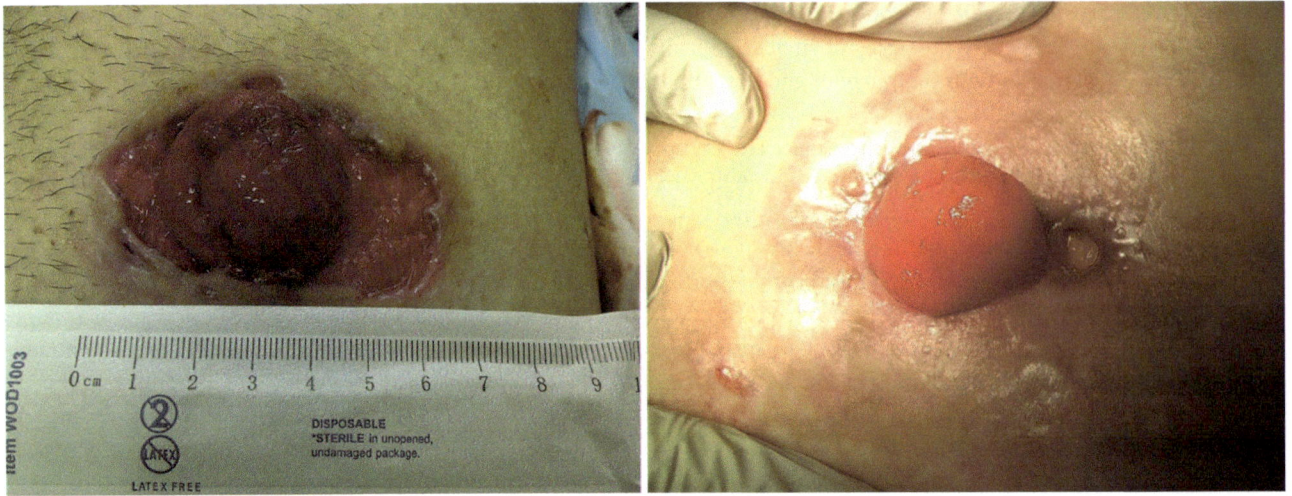

Fig. 45.7 Peristomal pyoderma gangrenosum

matitis is treated by removing the offending product and then using a topical anti-inflammatory and replacing the product. Poor wound healing contributes to mucocutaneous separation. The separated area is filled with a skin barrier powder and then covered with a solid skin barrier to protect and promote healing. Periostomal abscesses should be treated with systemic antibiotics and topically with an absorptive foam product. Candidiasis of the peristomal skin area is best treated with a topical antifungal powder that can then be "sealed in" with a silicone sealant.

Pyoderma gangrenosum (PG) may occur at or near the stoma of patients with IBD. Classically, a full thickness ulcer develops in the peristomal area with a halo of purple discoloration (Fig. 45.7). The etiology is thought to be due to pathergy-trauma such as abrasion, scratching, or pressure. The ulcers are extremely painful with significant drainage. If the ulcer is large, it may interfere with the pouch seal, resulting in leakage and further skin breakdown. Treatment of peristomal PG can be difficult and varies. Topical, intralesional, and systemic corticosteroids may be necessary and found to be effective as well as immunomodulator therapy and biologic agents [18, 19]. Absorptive dressings such as silver-impregnated hydrofiber (e.g., Aquacel AG) or a calcium alginate will absorb moisture and exudate [19]. This primary dressing is then covered with a transparent dressing or thin hydrocolloid, and then the wafer is placed over this. It is important that the PG wound be protected from stool soilage for optimal wound healing. Avoidance of peristomal trauma and pressure is key to minimizing risk of PG. This includes the use of convex wafers and ostomy belts. In addition to modifying the appliance as needed and topical dressings, maximizing medical management of disease process is integral to managing peristomal PG.

Preparing a patient and family for living with an ostomy, whether temporary or permanent, is a planned approach. They should be provided with education regarding the stoma, the skills necessary to care for the stoma, and emotional support. In addition to family preparation, the healthcare team needs to take the developmental level of the patient into consideration. A school-aged child with an ostomy has different needs and concerns than an adolescent. Adolescents may pose the most challenge regarding acceptance and adaptation, as they are not only dealing with biologic and sexual maturation, they are also striving to achieve independence and autonomy within the greater social environment [20]. A supportive healthcare team can be crucial for successful adaptation and positive self-image for the patient, and positive adjustment for the entire family.

References

1. Gauderer MW, Ponsky JL, Izant Jr RJ. Gastrostomy without laparotomy: a percutaneous endoscopic technique. J Pediatr Surg. 1980;15:872–5.
2. Preshaw RM. A percutaneous method for inserting a feeding gastrostomy tube. Surg Gynecol Obstet. 1981;152:658–60.
3. Goldberg E, Barton S, Xanthopoulos MS, Stettler N, Liacouras CA. A descriptive study of complications of gastrostomy tubes in children. J Pediatr Nurs. 2010;25:72–80.
4. Soscia J, Friedman JN. A guide to the management of common gastrostomy and gastrojejunostomy tube problems. Paediatr Child Health. 2011;16(5):281–7.
5. Rahnemai-Azar AA, Rahnemaiazar AA, Naghshizadian R, Kurtz A, Farkas DT. Percutaneous endoscopic gastrostomy: indications, technique, complications and management. World J Gastroenterol. 2014;20(24):7739–51.
6. Friedman JN, Ahmed S, Connolly B, Chait P, Mahant S. Complications associated with image-guided gastrostomy and gastrojejunostomy tubes in children. Pediatrics. 2004;114:458–61.
7. Lipp A, Lusardi G. A systematic review of prophylactic antimicrobials in PEG placement. J Clin Nurs. 2009;18:938–48.

8. Fox D, Campagna EJ, Freidlander J, Patrick DA, Rees DI, Kempe S. National trends and outcomes of pediatric gastrostomy tube placement. J Pediatr Gastroenterol Nutr. 2014;58(5):582–8.

9. Klein S, Heare BR, Soloway RD. The "buried bumper syndrome": a complication of percutaneous endoscopic gastrostomy. Am J Gastroenterol. 1990;85:448–51.

10. Hui GC, Gerstle JT, Weinstein M, Connolly B. Small bowel intussusception around a gastrojejunostomy tube resulting in ischemic necrosis of the intestine. Pediatr Radiol. 2004;34:916–8.

11. Widgerow AD, Leak K. Hypergranulation tissue: evolution, control and potential elimination. Wound Healing Southern Africa. 2010;3(2):00.

12. Mandrea E. Topical diflorasone ointment for treatment of recalcitrant, excessive granulation tissue. Dermatol Surg. 1998;24:1409–10.

13. El-Rifai N, Michaud L, Mention K, et al. Persistence of gastrocutaneous fistula after removal of gastrostomy tubes in children: prevalence and associated factors. Endoscopy. 2004;36:700–4.

14. Goldberg E, Kaye R, Yaworski J, Liacouras C. Gastrostomy tubes: facts, fallacies, fistulas, and false tracts. Gastroenterol Nurs. 2005;28:485–93. quiz 493–4

15. Gonzalez-Ojeda A, Avalos-Gonzalez J, Mucino-Hernandez MI, et al. Fibrin glue as adjuvant treatment for gastrocutaneous fistula after gastrostomy tube removal. Endoscopy. 2004;36:337–41.

16. Salvadelena G, Hendren S, MKena L, Muldoon R, Netsch D, Paquette I, Pittman J, Ramundo J, Steinberg G. WOCN Society and ASCRSS Position statement on preoperative stoma site marking for patients undergoing colostomy or ileostomy surgery. J Wound Ostomy Continence Nurs Soc. 2015;42(3):249–52.

17. Wound, ostomy, continence nurses society. Pediatric Ostomy Care: Best Practices. 2011.

18. Lyon CC, Smith A. Abdominal stomas and their skin disorders. 2nd ed. London: Informa Healthcare; 2011.

19. DeMartyn LE, Faller NA, Miller L. Treating peristomal pyoderma gangrenosum with topical crushed prednisone: a report of three cases. Ostomy Wound Manage. 2014;60(6):50–4.

20. Mohr, LD. Growth and development issues in adolescents with ostomies: a primer for WOC nurses. Journal of Wound, Ostomy Continence Nurses Society. 2012;39(5): 515–21.

Clinical Indices for Pediatric Inflammatory Bowel Disease Research

Dan Turner and Oren Ledder

Introduction

Clinical research relies on standardized markers which accurately reflect response to interventions. For both practical and ethical reasons, invasive measures are best avoided when possible, and thus clinical indices will always play some role in assessing outcomes of clinical trials. Various indices have been developed for pediatric use due to specific aspects of the disease in that population. Clinical indices were mostly initially developed for research purposes; however, they can also be of use in clinical practice by providing a standardized approach to disease evaluation and prediction of disease course.

Assessment of Instruments Used in Clinical Research

Disease activity is a concept for which no gold standard exists. Even in ulcerative colitis (UC), where colonoscopic examination is highly important in evaluating disease activity, it still cannot be regarded a gold standard because the degree of inflammation is subjective, mucosal healing lags after clinical improvement, and perhaps other measures are more important, such as histological remission. Therefore, disease activity is best measured using multi-item indices which often incorporate clinical symptoms, laboratory parameters, and, when feasible, also endoscopic findings.

According to accepted standards of health indices development [1], the introduction of a new measure for use in clinical research should follow a multistep process of item generation, reduction, grading, weighting, and evaluation [2, 3]. A list of all potentially useful items is generated by a panel of experts and then reduced to include only the most relevant items. These items are then evaluated for their ability to explain the desired attribute (e.g., signs and symptoms, disease activity, or quality of life); each item is graded and may be assigned a weight according to its ability to reflect the concept which is targeted. The final measure is then evaluated to define cutoff scores that correspond to clinically important disease states such as remission and mild to severe disease activity. For clinical indices that will be used to determine changes over time (evaluative measures), a definition of "response" (i.e., the minimal important difference) is also required.

Once the instrument has been developed, it must be evaluated for validity, reliability, responsiveness, and feasibility [4–6]. Briefly, *validity* is the degree to which the instrument measures the concept that it purports to measure [7]. The *reliability* of an instrument relates to its stability on repeated measures both over time and by different raters at one point in time [8]. *Responsiveness* refers to the instrument's ability to correctly identify change over time in the concept being measured. It is not merely sensitivity to change but rather the ability of the instrument to detect changed from unchanged patients. A highly responsive index is invaluable in clinical trials, as it allows performing the trial with a smaller sample size [9–12]. Finally, *feasibility* encompasses both respondent and administrative burden. An instrument is feasible if the participant and researcher report that the instrument is completed within reasonable limits of participant discomfort and both participant and researcher time constraints.

Outcomes for Clinical Research in Pediatric Inflammatory Bowel Disease

Crohn's Disease Activity Indices

One of the first Crohn's disease (CD) activity indices developed in adults was the Crohn's Disease Activity Index (CDAI) published in 1976 by Best and colleagues [13]. This index includes clinical symptoms, IBD-related complications,

D. Turner, MD, PhD (✉) • O. Ledder, MD
Juliet Keidan Institute of Pediatric Gastroenterology and Nutrition, The Hebrew University of Jerusalem, Shaare Zedek Medical Center, P.O.B 3235, Jerusalem 91031, Israel
e-mail: turnerd@szmc.org.il; orenl@szmc.org.il

© Springer International Publishing AG 2017
P. Mamula et al. (eds.), *Pediatric Inflammatory Bowel Disease*, DOI 10.1007/978-3-319-49215-5_46

physical examination findings, laboratory tests, weight, and use of medications to treat diarrhea (Table 46.3). Since its publication, it has been used extensively and is currently the primary outcome used in most clinical trials in adult Crohn's disease. The CDAI has been criticized for its complex calculation, potentially poor interobserver agreement [14, 15], and poor correlation with endoscopic appearance [16, 17] which is becoming an increasingly important outcome. Simpler versions have been developed, the most commonly used being the Harvey-Bradshaw Index (HBI) which incorporates only clinical symptoms and physical exam findings [18]. The respondent burden is significantly lower than the CDAI, with no need for a symptom diary or blood work (Table 46.3).

In older pediatric trials, the use of antidiarrheals in the CDAI was replaced with number of days unable to participate in normal activities, and standard weight was replaced by ideal weight in the absence of formal evaluation [19, 20]. Subsequently, the Pediatric Crohn's Disease Activity Index (PCDAI) was developed [21]. This instrument ranges from 0 to 100 points and contains patient symptoms (based on a 7 day recall), physical examination findings, laboratory parameters, and growth measures (Table 46.4). Despite its several limitations, the PCDAI performed well in multiple pediatric IBD clinical trials as a measure of disease activity. The weight variable requires a reading at an interval of at least 4 months with weight loss being quantified as a percentage ([current weight − previous weight]/ previous weight). The height variable at diagnosis is scored according to the number of channels crossed downward if prior measurement is available and, if not, according to the current centile. The height variable on follow-up visits employs height velocity, measured over a minimum period of 6–12 months [22, 23]:

$$\text{Height velocity} = \frac{2\text{nd height} - \text{baseline (cm)}}{\text{Time} \left(\text{year}\right)}$$

To compare children of different ages and gender, the height velocity is converted to a z-score:

$$z\text{-score} = \frac{\text{Observed height velocity} - \text{Mean height velocity for age and sex (cm/yr)}}{\text{SD of the mean height velocity (for age and sex)}}$$

The z-score corresponds to the standard deviation (SD) of the child's height velocity.

The PCDAI has been evaluated in seven cohorts of children with CD (Table 46.1) [21, 24–26]. In a head-to-head comparison, Otley et al. [24] showed that the PCDAI was highly correlated with physician global assessment ($r = 0.86$), higher than the CDAI ($r = 0.77$), the modified CDAI ($r = 0.76$), and the HBI ($r = 0.72$). In the largest study to date, test-retest reliability on stable patients has been shown to be good [27]. Responsiveness to change was demonstrated, and the minimal clinically important change, to define "response," was found to be at least 12.5 points [25], also in the larger study which used several methods to attain this "minimal important difference" corresponding to moderate change [27].

The optimal PCDAI cutoff score that defined remission has been open to some discussion. The initial study found that a PCDAI score of ≤10 points discriminated active from quiescent disease. Other studies found that PCDAI scores of <10 and <15 points were more sensitive and specific, respectively [24, 26]. In a more recent large study of 366 children, the best cutoff values were <10 points or <7.5 without the height item points for remission, 10–27.5 for mild disease, 30–37.5 moderate disease, and 40–100 for severe disease. This yielded the best accuracy (Table 46.1) acknowledging that the growth item is irrelevant in adolescents who passed the growing-tanner stages and that height typically improves several weeks or months after remission has been achieved (i.e., low responsiveness). The PCDAI does not differentiate well between moderate and severe disease activity and the feasibility of the PCDAI is only moderate. In the registry of a pediatric IBD collaborative research group, only 47.6% of the registered visits had a valid PCDAI score, compared to 97.6% with the Pediatric UC Activity Index (PUCAI – see below) [28]. Similarly, data to complete the PCDAI from the ImproveCareNow registry were available in the charts of only 20% of 3643 clinical visits [29]. Besides the low feasibility of the index and the limitations imposed by the growth item, the inclusion of the perianal item is debated as it reflects a different concept than luminal disease activity.

Recently, the PCDAI was subjected to a mathematical weighting on 437 children [30] (Table 46.5). The newly weighted PCDAI, termed wPCDAI, excluded three items shown to be redundant in reflecting disease activity when the other included items are in the model: height velocity, abdominal examination, and hematocrit. The score range of the wPCDAI is 0–125. In the validation cohort, it had higher correlation with PGA and ESR than the original PCDAI (0.75 vs 0.67 and 0.58 vs 0.49, respectively). The discriminant validity was better with the wPCDAI version: it differentiated those in remission from active disease (area under the ROC curve 0.95) and, unlike the original PCDAI, differentiated well between moderate and severe disease (area under the ROC curve 0.87). wPCDAI performed well as a primary outcome measure in recent studies assessing response rates to a second biological agent [31] and repeated courses of nutritional

Table 46.1 Validity, reliability, and responsiveness of Pediatric Crohn's Disease Activity Index

Instrument	Study population	Validity		Reliability	Responsiveness
PCDAI Hyams et al. [21]	n = 131 prospective cohort	PCDAI to HBImod r = 0.81		Interobserver r = 0.86	N/A
		PCDAI to PGA r = 0.80			
		Score cutoffs:			
		No disease 0–10	69% correct classification		
		Mild 11–30			
		Moderate/severe >30			
Otley et al. [24]	n = 81 prospective cohort	PCDAI to CDAI r = 0.86 PCDAI to PGA r = 0.86 PCDAI to HBI r = 0.84 Receiver operating curves to select PCDAI cut offs for no versus mild disease: Sensitivity specificity ≤10 0.75 0.905 <15 0.83 0.905		N/A	Correlation of the difference PCDAI score between the two visits was highly correlated with the difference in the CDAI in 17 patients. No other responsiveness measures are provided and time of follow-up visit not specified
Hyams et al. [26]	n = 181 from Pediatric IBD Collaborative Research Group Registry	Validation of previously defined score cutoffs: Sensitivity Specificity No disease vs mild: <10 0.81 0.68 Mod/severe vs mild: >30 0.71 0.83		N/A	Clinically significant change in PCDAI predictive of change in PGA = 12.5 points (sensitivity 0.87, specificity 0.73)
Kundhal et al. [25]	n = 25 and 63 (from 2 prospective cohorts)	N/A		N/A	Minimal clinically significant change in PCDAI predictive of PGA at 1 month follow-up = 12.5 points (sensitivity 0.83, specificity 0.92) High effect size statistics in 15 patients who responded to therapy (SES = 1.78, SRM = 1.41)
Turner et al. [67, 68]	N = 437 4 prospective cohorts	PCDAI to PGA r = 0.67 PCDAI to CRP r = 0.26 PCDAI to ESR r = 0.49 PCDAI to Alb r = −0.37 PCDAI to Hb r = −0.40 PCDAI to Plat r = 0.58		N = 90 ICC: 0.74–0.8	The PCDAI showed good responsiveness to change (r = 0.54–0.83, distributional 0.8–1.4, diagnostic utility analyses AUC ROC 0.79–0.85); minimal important difference >12 points
Turner et al.	N = 322 (from 2 prospective cohorts)	PCDAI to PGA r = 0.67 PCDAI to SES-CD r = 0.42 PCDAI to calprotectin r = 0.26		Test-retest reliability N = 25 ICC: 0.85–0.97	PCDAI showed good responsiveness to change compared to PGA (r = 0.71) and differentiated clinical improvement from those with poor response (AUC ROC 0.86–0.96)
Grover et al.	N = 24 Prospective cohort	PCDAI to SES-CD r = 0.33		N/A	PCDAI demonstrated poor responsiveness between pre- and posttreatment measures in comparison to SES-CD

DAI Crohn's Disease Activity Index, *HBI* Harvey-Bradshaw Index, *PCDAI* Pediatric Crohn's Disease Activity Index, *abPCDAI* abbreviated PCDAI, *PGA* Physician Global Assessment, *CRP* C-reactive protein, *ESR* Erythrocyte sedimentation rate, *Alb* Albumin, *Hb* Hemoglobin, *Plat* Platelets, *SES-CD* Simple Endoscopic Score – Crohn's Disease

therapy in CD [32] in which remission was defined as wPC-DAI <12.5 and response as decrease in wPCDAI >17.5.

A number of abbreviated PCDAI instruments have been proposed to increase the feasibility of the PCDAI for use in retrospective chart reviews [33, 34]. The abbreviated PCDAI (abbrPCDAI) retained the 3 history variables (abdominal pain, general well-being, and stools per day), weight variable, abdominal exam, and perirectal disease. A larger study presented a short version of the PCDAI (shPCDAI), excluding items with a low frequency of completion in a patient registry [29]. The difference between the shPCDAI from the abbrPCDAI is that the extraintestinal manifestation item has replaced the perianal item and new weights have been mathematically assigned to each item, reflecting their relative importance to physician global assessment (PGA) of disease activity. The exclusion of the lab items in both indices increased their feasibility but at the expense of reduced validity when compared head-to-head with the other PCDAI versions [35]. Nonetheless, these versions may be used in retrospective studies when not all items required for the full index are available. A third abbreviated version, a modified PCDAI (modPCDAI), aims to provide a measure of disease activity in pediatric Crohn's disease when only blood tests are available (e.g., in administrative databases) [36].

Due to the availability of improved therapeutic options in recent years and the increasing recognition of progressive intestinal damage even in the absence of clinical disease, increasing emphasis has been placed on mucosal healing as a treatment target in IBD [37–40]; PCDAI has a poor correlation with endoscopic assessment of mucosal healing both at diagnosis ($r = 0.33$) and following induction therapy ($r = 0.34$) and is an inferior marker than both CRP and fecal calprotectin [41]. Further analysis on 2 large prospectively collected cohorts (ImageKids and GROWTH studies) aimed to compare four PCDAI versions, PCDAI, wPCDAI, abbrPC-DAI, and shPCDAI, head-to-head with endoscopic degree of inflammation. All four versions had, at best, fair correlation ($r = 0.42$–0.45) and performed inadequately to provide a valid assessment of mucosal healing [35].

A validated marker of subclinical inflammation and mucosal healing is becoming an increasingly critical need for clinical trials of new therapies in CD [42]. At present all recognized clinical indices in CD fall short of fulfilling this role.

Perianal Crohn's Disease

In classification of perianal CD, a distinction should be made between the detailed anatomic description of perianal fistulas and an assessment of fistula activity [43]. There are two disease activity measures currently used in clinical trials to follow perianal CD activity: the Perianal Disease Activity Index (PDAI) and the Fistula Drainage Assessment (Table 46.6). The PDAI was developed and validated by Irvine and colleagues based on the assessment of quality of life factors [44]. It contains 5 items, each scored 0–4, with higher scores representing more severe disease. In the validation cohort, it had moderate correlation with both physician and patient assessment of perianal disease activity ($r = 0.72$ and 0.66, respectively). As expected, it correlated poorly with the CDAI and HBI ($r = 0.23$ and 0.21, respectively) implying that perianal disease can present in the absence of other CD symptoms. The PDAI scores were reproducible in patients with stable disease over 4–8 weeks, implying test-retest reliability. Although the PDAI changed in patients who improved or deteriorated on repeat visits, robust and accepted responsiveness statistics were not presented. The second instrument, the Fistula Drainage Assessment (Table 46.7), was introduced as part of a clinical trial of infliximab therapy for perianal CD [45]. A fistula was considered closed when it no longer drained despite gentle finger compression. A response was defined as a reduction of 50% or more in the number of draining fistulas, and remission was defined as absence of any draining fistulas on two consecutive visits. In this study, the Fistula Drainage Assessment was significantly lower in the treatment versus the control group, similar to the PDAI calculated simultaneously. Although these results have been replicated in other clinical trials [46–48], the PDAI has several drawbacks. "Gentle finger compression" is an investigator-dependent measure, and fistula remission is dependent on external appearance, while MRI studies demonstrate that the internal fistula tract lags behind clinical remission by a median of 12 months [49, 50].

Incorporating MRI-based scoring features in an attempt to combine anatomical fistula description with features reflecting active inflammation, van Assche et al. generated a score which, not surprisingly, correlated poorly with PDAI but in which absence of MR enhancement was found to correlate well with clinical remission [51, 52]. Of MRI features of perianal disease, recent pediatric data suggests perianal fistula length assessed by MRI was found to be the best predictor of treatment response [53].

There is no unique perianal disease activity index for children. In order for the PDAI to be considered in children, the sexual dysfunction component should be modified to reflect more age-appropriate issues. At present, the use of the Fistula Drainage Assessment definitions appears to be the preferred perianal outcome in pediatric clinical trials, as an anchor for physician assessment of disease activity; however, improved instruments to score perianal CD fistula activity are required [43].

Ulcerative Colitis Disease Activity Indices

The earliest classification of UC disease activity was a qualitative scale published by Truelove and Witts in 1955

(Table 46.8) [54]. Because of simple gradation, significant ambiguity exists in defining change in disease activity with this index. Arbitrary quantitative indices have since been introduced, including the Powell-Tuck Index [55], the Mayo Clinic score [56], Rachmilewitz Index [57], and Lichtiger Score [58] with the Mayo score currently in widespread use. The first three scores include an endoscopic evaluation of the rectosigmoid as part of the global assessment. Their validation has been largely a side product of clinical trials in which they have been used and developed. Seo and colleagues developed and evaluated a UC disease activity index [59, 60], weighted against the Truelove and Witts classification. The initial development process was biased toward severe disease since the investigators used a retrospective cohort of hospitalized patients. Walmsley and colleagues developed a Simple Clinical Colitis Activity Index that removed all laboratory parameters [61]. It correlated highly with both the Powell-Tuck Index and Seo index. The Endoscopic-Clinical Correlation Index (ECCI) was developed prospectively in 137 adults with items chosen based on their ability to predict endoscopic outcome [62]. The ECCI is highly correlated with the endoscopy colitis score ($r = 0.81$), higher than the Seo, Truelove and Witts, Powell-Tuck, and Walmsley's simple colitis index; however, separate validation is not available to assess reliability and responsiveness. In a prospective head-to-head study in adults of all noninvasive UC disease activity indices, the Walmsley index and PUCAI (see below) were best in assessing disease activity when compared to a number of parameters including the Mayo score [63] (Table 46.9).

Endoscopic evaluation of the colonic mucosa in UC is invaluable in questionable clinical cases, before major treatment changes and for cancer surveillance, but is not routinely needed to confirm mucosal healing, especially in the presence of low fecal calprotectin [64]. Unlike CD, UC has a more homogenous presentation, and thus 80–90% of patients in complete remission will also have mucosal healing or near-mucosal healing [28, 63]. Endoscopic assessment is not without limitations. It is subjective with low interobserver reliability [65]. Endoscopic appearance lags after clinical improvement, thereby underestimating response to treatment [66]. Furthermore, limited sigmoidoscopy may not reflect the entire disease burden (i.e., the product of severity and extent) especially in children in whom extensive disease is the most common phenotype. Finally, although mucosal healing has been convincingly shown to predict favorable clinical outcome in UC [67–69], it is yet to be proven that endoscopy is necessary in the presence of complete clinical remission and, separately, low fecal calprotectin. Indeed, in the combined ACT cohorts (466 adults with UC treated with either infliximab or placebo), endoscopic healing had no predictive value among the subset of patients with clinical remission after 8 weeks of therapy [67].

The PUCAI was developed with the aim of reflecting disease activity and mucosal inflammation without invasive measures, hence making it attractive for repeated use in children (Table 46.10) [70]. The feasibility and reliability of the PUCAI were demonstrated from 2503 pediatric UC patients in the ImproveCareNow registry in whom recorded data was retrospectively applied to the PUCAI model. All items in PUCAI were satisfactorily completed in 96% of visits [71]. PUCAI demonstrated good discrimination between remission, mild and moderate disease, and good correlation to PGA ($r = 0.76$) with PUCAI score changes correlating well with PGA score changes over follow-up visits.

The PUCAI is tightly correlated with endoscopic appearance of the colonic mucosa [63, 72], and the correlation with the Mayo score is as high as 0.95 [63, 72, 73]. Predictive validity of the PUCAI is high as per multiple studies. The T72 infliximab trial in children with UC showed that PUCAI-defined remission was not inferior to sigmoidoscopy in predicting 1-year steroid-free sustained remission [73], a finding recently replicated also in ambulatory UC children [74]. The PUCAI strongly predicted the need for short-term treatment escalation in pediatric UC [28] and the type of surgical intervention, when needed [75]. In two independent cohorts of children requiring admission for intravenous treatment of corticosteroids for UC exacerbations, the PUCAI has shown strong predictive validity of outcomes important to patients, accurately identifying children who will require treatment escalation to second-line medical therapy or colectomy, both by discharge and up to 1 year post discharge [76, 77]. In this setup, the PUCAI has shown to have superior predictive validity to five fecal biomarkers, including calprotectin [63, 78].

The corresponding PUCAI cutoff scores of remission (<10 points), mild (10–34 points), moderate (35–64 points), and severe (≥65) disease have been validated in several cohorts and found to have sensitivity, specificity, and area under the ROC curve of >95% [63, 72, 79]. In the regulatory T72 trial evaluating the effectiveness of infliximab in pediatric UC, the PUCAI determined week 8 remission rate was 33%, identical to the rate of complete mucosal healing found by sigmoidoscopy [80]. Similarly, the week 12 remission rate in a clinical trial evaluating beclomethasone 17,21-dipropionate (BDP) in children with UC was similar whether determined by sigmoidoscopy or the PUCAI [81] as well as when comparing sigmoidoscopy, ultrasound, and the PUCAI [82].

The PUCAI has also demonstrated predictive abilities regarding surgical management of patients with UC requiring restorative proctocolectomy with ileal pouch-anal anastomosis. A high preoperative PUCAI was significantly predictive of the likelihood of a staged procedure [75]. Beyond its use purely as a marker of disease activity, PUCAI has also been shown to correlate with both children and parents' health-related quality of life scores [83].

Future disease activity indices may possibly build on the PUCAI with additional fecal markers, microbiome, or metabolomic aspects of pediatric IBD [84].

Gastrointestinal Endoscopy Indices

Crohn's Disease

Mucosal healing in CD has been associated with better long-term outcomes [85]. Indeed, the recent ECCO/ESPGHAN position paper recommends mucosal healing, as a desired treatment target [86]. Two groups have developed standardized approaches to endoscopy findings in CD. The first designed the Crohn's Disease Endoscopic Index of Severity (CDEIS) by incorporating endoscopic findings, previously shown to have high inter-rater reliability [87], into a regression model using the physician global assessment of endoscopy severity as the dependent variable [88] (Table 46.11). The index was found to have high inter-rater reliability ($r = 0.96$) and was highly correlated with the physician endoscopy assessment in an independent cohort ($r = 0.81$). It has subsequently been used in multiple clinical trials evaluating endoscopic endpoints [89–91]. However, due to its complexity, Daperno and colleagues developed the Simplified Endoscopic Activity Score for Crohn's disease (Table 46.12) [92]. The SES-CD had high inter-rater reliability (ICC = 0.98) and was highly correlated with the CDEIS ($r = 0.92$). Lower correlations were found between both the SES-CD and CDEIS, and other parameters of disease activity including the CDAI (0.39 and 0.36, respectively) and C-reactive protein ($r = 0.47$ and 0.45, respectively) confirmed that in CD, mucosal findings do not necessarily reflect the patient's clinical status.

There is no unique endoscopic instrument for pediatric CD, but there is no evidence that endoscopic characteristics differ in children. The SES-CD seems to be a valid alternative to its more complicated counterpart also in children.

With more frequent performance of upper endoscopy (EGD) in CD, upper gastrointestinal (UGI) inflammation has become increasingly recognized. UGI CD is associated with earlier onset and more severe disease [93], and its identification may assist in predicting disease course and directing appropriate therapy. At present there exists no standardized instrument to describe UGI CD involvement. Provisional work on developing such a mechanism is currently being undertaken utilizing a modified application of the SES-CD in UGI regions. The validity and feasibility of this endoscopic score, along with its clinical relevance, are still under investigation [94].

Endoscopy is an important outcome in assessing postoperative interventions in CD [95]. Rutgeerts and colleagues [95] proposed a scoring system for recurrent endoscopic disease at the surgical anastomosis (Table 46.13). Although quite subjective, higher Rutgeerts scores consistently predicted a more severe clinical course [95]. Patients with no or mild endoscopic lesions (termed i0 and i1, respectively) at 1 year postoperative endoscopy had good long-term outcomes, as opposed to those with clearly progressive disease (i3 or i4) who developed early clinical recurrence and were more prone to a complicated disease outcome in subsequent years. Rutgeerts score i2 is a heterogeneous group defined as moderate lesions in the terminal ileum (i2a) or lesions confined to the ileocolonic anastomosis (i2b); however, recent data demonstrate equivalent rate of postoperative occurrence in both subgroups, hence calling into question the benefit of subdividing i2 [96].

Standard endoscopic indices are limited to assessment of the colon, terminal ileum, and developing indices of the upper GIT. Full small bowel assessment was made possible by the introduction of the wireless capsule endoscopy. The Lewis score was developed as a measure of mucosal inflammatory activity based on villous edema, ulcers, and stenosis [97] (see Table 46.15). The Lewis score was recently validated for the evaluation of small bowel CD, demonstrating strong interobserver agreement [98]. The Lewis score has been shown to correlate with fecal calprotectin, and CRP [99] serves as a useful clinical tool for patients with suspected CD [100] and to assess the true inflammatory burden and extent of mucosal healing in patients with clinically quiescent disease [101].

Ulcerative Colitis Endoscopic Assessment

No endoscopic index has been developed in children, but yet again, there is no reason to believe that adults are different than children in assessing the bowel mucosa. Some endoscopic assessments have shown to have low reliability [102]. Baron and colleagues found only 66% agreement on a subset of endoscopic findings in adults with proctocolitis [102]. Moderate to good agreement ($k > 0.39$) was observed among four experienced colonoscopists for 10 of 14 signs or patterns of mucosal appearance in ulcerative colitis [103]. The agreement was poor, however, for mild and moderate disease activity. Two endoscopic indices used in clinical trials are the Ulcerative Colitis Endoscopic Index of Severity (UCEIS) [65] (see Table 46.14) and the Mayo endoscopic score [104]. The UCEIS was only recently validated and demonstrated high intra-investigator and inter-investigator reliability (0.96 and 0.88, respectively) [105]. Recently a Modified Mayo Endoscopic Score (MMES) was developed which factored both severity and distribution of mucosal inflammation [106].

Patient-Reported Outcomes

Patient-reported outcomes (PROs) involve the report of health status coming directly from the patient without interpretation of the patient's response by a clinician or anyone else [107]. There has been developing interest over recent years in PRO as a tool for IBD research, led by the US Food and Drug Administration (FDA). Since PROs capture signs and symptoms of the patients not necessarily related to disease activity and endoscopic appearance, any PRO should be supplemented by an objective measure of inflammation such as fecal calprotectin or endoscopic evaluation. The accuracy of self-reported IBD medical history in comparison to medical records was shown in one study to be fairly good for major factors such as disease type and previous surgical procedures; however, it was poor when more detailed medical information was assessed [108].

An inventory PRO in adults with UC includes stool frequency, bleeding, and general well-being and was shown to correlate well with the Simple Clinical Colitis Activity Index (SCCAI) ($r = 0.71$). However, the patient-generated assessment underreported active disease in 10% of the study cohort [109].

In CD, Khanna et al. generated 3 patient-reportable clinical features which correlate with CDAI based on analysis of a previous study cohort. These PRO were validated against a second cohort, generating optimum PRO cut-points for CDAI-defined remission: stool frequency ≤ 1.5, abdominal pain score ≤ 1, and general well-being score ≤ 1. However, this PRO model only demonstrated fair-moderate responsiveness (Guyatt's 0.48) [110].

PRO in the pediatric population presents several unique challenges such as age-related vocabulary, comprehension of health concepts, unclear determination of lower age limit for which responses would be reliable and valid, and the appropriate use of parents or carers to contribute to the reportable outcomes [111]. A recent collaboration aimed to develop a PRO measure of signs and symptoms for pediatric UC, the TUMMY-UC index, by way of interviews with both pediatric UC patients and their caregivers. This preliminary work identified good correlation between children and their caregivers regarding the order of importance of various symptoms reflective of perceived disease activity [112]. No data has been published on attempts at PRO generation in pediatric CD, but the development of TUMMY-CD is also underway.

Quality of Life Instruments

Both adults and children diagnosed with IBD are at increased risk of emotional problems and decreased social functioning [113, 114]. Thus, quality of life (QOL) assessment has been increasingly recognized as an important and independent clinical outcome in IBD research. There are two types of quality of life instruments, generic and disease specific. The choice of instrument depends on the clinical question. Generic QOL instruments are preferred when comparing QOL in different diseases. However, for assessing only IBD populations, a disease-specific quality of life instrument should be used. A thorough discussion of QOL instruments available for pediatric IBD research is found in Chapter 45.

Radiographic Indices

Brief mention should be made about currently available and developing radiographic modalities which can contribute greatly to assessment of disease state and response to therapy. These modalities were described in greater detail in an earlier section of this book, but the importance of imaging in research of IBD is becoming more paramount. As research outcomes shift from clinical response and remission to mucosal healing, subtle findings of inflammation and intestinal damage may only be detected by use of various imaging techniques.

Abdominal ultrasound (US) is operator dependent, but it can be very useful to detect inflammation and assess damage including strictures, abscesses, and fistulizing disease [115]. There is currently no accepted index to objectively describe or quantify US features of CD [115].

For MRE in adults, the MaRIA and Lémann scores have been developed to assess inflammatory activity and damage, respectively [116–118]. Work is currently underway to develop and validate a radiological assessment index also in pediatric CD: the Pediatric Inflammatory Crohn's MRE Index (PICMI) and the pediatric MR Enterography-based Damage Index (pMEDIC), respectively [119].

Summary of Clinical Outcome Measures

Various instruments are available to measure clinical outcomes in pediatric IBD (Table 46.2). Valid pediatric clinical indices and quality of life measures exist for both UC and CD. Endoscopic scores, however, have not yet been evaluated in children and PRO's and MRE-related indices are being developed. The evaluation of health-related indices is an ongoing process, and therefore, the development of new indices and the reevaluation of the performance of existing indices will continue to be explored in different clinical and research settings.

Table 46.2 Clinical indices for research in pediatric inflammatory bowel disease

Clinical trial outcome	Instrument	
	Crohn's disease	Ulcerative colitis
Disease activity index	Physician global assessment PCDAI	Physician global assessment PUCAI
Perianal disease activity index	Fistula drainage assessment	N/A
Endoscopic scores	CDEIS (assessed only in adults) SES-CD (assessed only in adults)	Mayo endoscopic subscore UCEIS Modified Mayo score
Quality of life instruments Generic	Multiple (e.g., PedsQL, Child QOL questionnaire)	Multiple (e.g., PedsQL, Child QOL questionnaire)
Disease specific	IMPACT-III	IMPACT-III

Appendix A

Table 46.3 Crohn's disease activity index (CDAI) and Harvey-Bradshaw Index (HBI)

Instrument items	CDAI [13]	HBI [18]
Clinical signs and symptoms Stools Abdominal pain General well-being No. of complications	Sum of liquid/soft stools ($\times 2$) Sum of daily score of 0–3 ($\times 5$) Sum of daily score of 0–4 ($\times 7$) 1/item (6 categories) ($\times 20$)	No. of liquid/soft stools 0–3 0–4 1/item (8 categories)
Physical exam Abdominal mass Weight	0–2 ($\times 10$) 1-(wt/standard wt) $\times 100$	0–3 –
Laboratory variables	Hct ($\times 6$): 47 – Hct (male) 42 – Hct (female)	–
Other	Use of antidiarrheals: 0–1 ($\times 30$)	–
Score cutoff for disease activity	Remission <150 Mild 150–300 Moderate 300–450 Severe >450	Remission ≤4 Relapse >4
Comments	Clinical symptoms based on 7 day diary	Clinical symptoms based on previous 24 h

Table 46.4 Pediatric Crohn's disease activity index [21] history (recall, 1 week)

Abdominal pain			Score
0 = None	5 = Mild: brief, does not interfere with activities	10 = Moderate/severe: daily, longer lasting, affects activities, nocturnal	_____

Patient functioning, general well-being			Score
0 = No limitation of activities, well	5 = Occasional difficulty in maintaining age-appropriate activities, below par	10 = Frequent limitation of activity, very poor	_____

Stools (per day)			Score
0 = 0–1 liquid stools, no blood	5 = Up to 2 semiformed with small blood, or 2–5 liquid	10 = Gross bleeding, or ≥6 liquid, or nocturnal diarrhea	_____

Laboratory

Hematocrit (HCT)						Score
<10 years:			11–14 years (male):			
0 = ≥ 33%	2.5 = 28–32%	5 = < 28%	0 = ≥ 35%	2.5 = 30–34%	5 = < 30%	
11–19 years (female):			15–19 years (male):			
0 = ≥ 34%	2.5 = 29–33%	5 = < 29%	0 = ≥ 37%	2.5 = 32–36%	5 = < 32	_____

Erythrocyte sedimentation rate (ESR)						Score
0 = < 20 mm/h	2.5 = 20–50 mm/h	5 = > 50 mm/h				_____

Albumin						Score
0 = ≥ 35 g/L	5 = 31–34 g/L	10 = ≤ 30 g/L				_____

Examination

Weight			Score
0 = Weight gain or voluntary weight stable/loss	5 = Involuntary weight stable, weight loss 1–9%	10 = Weight loss ≥ 10%	_____

Height at diagnosis			Score
0 = < 1 channel decrease	5 = ≥1 to < 2 channel decrease	10 = > 2 channel decrease	_____

Height at follow-up			Score
0 = Height velocity ≥ −1SD	5 = Height velocity < −1SD, > −2SD	10 = Height velocity ≤ −2SD	_____

Abdomen			Score
0 = No tenderness, no mass	5 = Tenderness or mass without tenderness	10 = Tenderness, involuntary guarding, definite mass	_____

Perirectal disease			Score
0 = None, asymptomatic tags	5 = 1–2 indolent fistula, scant drainage, no tenderness	10 = Active fistula, drainage, tenderness, or abscess	_____

Extra-intestinal manifestations			Score
(Fever ≥38.5 °C for 3 days over past week, definite arthritis, uveitis, *E. nodosum*, *P. gangrenosum*)			
0 = None	5 = One	10 = ≥ Two	_____
Total score:			

Table 46.5 Weighted pediatric Crohn's disease activity index (wPCDAI) [68] history (recall, 1 week)

Abdominal pain			Score
0 = None	10 = Mild: brief, does not interfere with activities	20 = Moderate/severe: daily, longer lasting, affects activities, nocturnal	_____
Patient functioning, general well-being			Score
0 = No limitation of activities, well	10 = Occasional difficulty in maintaining age-appropriate activities, below par	20 = Frequent limitation of activity, very poor	_____
Stools (per day)			Score
0 = 0–1 liquid stools, no blood	7.5 = Up to 2 semiformed with small blood, or 2–5 liquid	15 = Gross bleeding, or ≥6 liquid, or nocturnal diarrhea	_____
	Laboratory		
Erythrocyte sedimentation rate			Score
0 = < 20 mm/h	7.5 = 20–50 mm/h	15 = > 50 mm/h	_____
Albumin			Score
0 = ≥ 3.5 g/dL	10 = 3.1–3.4 g/dL	20 = ≤ 3.0 g/dL	_____
Examination			
Weight			Score
0 = Weight gain or voluntary weight stable/loss	5 = Involuntary weight stable, weight loss 1–9%	10 = Weight loss ≥ 10%	_____
Perirectal disease			Score
0 = None, asymptomatic tags	7.5 = 1–2 indolent fistula, scant drainage, no tenderness	15 = Active fistula, drainage, tenderness, or abscess	_____
Extra-intestinal manifestations			Score
(fever ≥ 38.5 °C for 3 days over past week, definite arthritis, uveitis, E. nodosum, P. gangrenosum)			
0 = None		10 = One or more	_____
Total Score (0–125):			

Appendix B

Table 46.6 Perianal Crohn's disease activity index [44]

Discharge
0 No discharge
1 Minimal mucous discharge
2 Moderate mucous or purulent discharge
3 Substantial discharge
4 Gross fecal soiling
Pain/restriction of activities
0 No activity restriction
1 Mild discomfort, no restriction
2 Moderate discomfort, some limitation activities
3 Marked discomfort, marked limitation
4 severe pain, severe limitation
Restriction of sexual activity
0 No restriction sexual activity
1 Slight restriction sexual activity
2 Moderate limitation sexual activity
3 Marked limitation sexual activity
4 Unable to engage in sexual activity
Type of perianal disease
0 No perianal disease/skin tags
1 Anal fissure or mucosal tear
2 <3 perianal fistulas
3 ≥ 3 perianal fistulas
4 Anal sphincter ulceration or fistulas with significant undermining of skin
Degree of induration
0 No induration
1 Minimal induration
2 Moderate induration
3 Substantial induration
4 Gross fluctuance/abscess

Total score = sum of total score per category

Table 46.7 Fistula drainage assessment [45]

	Definition
Remission	Fistula closure or absence of any draining fistulas for at least 4 weeks
Response	≥50% decrease in draining fistulas for at least 4 weeks

Appendix C

Table 46.8 Truelove and Witts score [54]

Disease activity	Criteria
Remission	1–2 stools/day without blood No fever No tachycardia Hemoglobin normal or returning to normal ESR normal or returning to normal Gaining weight (To be in remission, must exhibit all 6 features)
Mild	≤4 stools/day with no more than small amounts of macroscopic blood No fever No tachycardia Anemia not severe ESR ≤30
Moderate	Intermediate between severe and mild
Severe	≥6 stools/day with macroscopic blood Fever >37.5 °C (mean evening temperature) or ≥37.8 °C 2 days out of 4 Tachycardia (mean HR >90/min) Anemia (Hgb 75% or less; allowance made for recent transfusion) ESR >30

Table 46.9 Ulcerative colitis disease activity indices (adult)

Instrument items	Mayo Clinic score [56, 120]	Powell-Tuck Index [55]	Rachmilewitz score [57]	Lichtiger Index [58]	Seo Index [59]	SCCAI [61]	ECCI [62]
Clinical signs and symptoms	0–6	0–6	0–7	0–9	Frequency: 1–3 (×13)	0–11	No. nocturnal × 16
Stool characteristics	–	0–2	0–3	0–3	Blood: 0–1 (×60)	–	Blood 0–4 × 17
Abdominal pain	0–3	0–3	0–3	0–5	–	0–4	–
General well-being	–	0–2	0–9	–	–	–	–
No. complications					–	1/complication	–
Physical exam	–	0–3	–	0–3	–	–	
Abdominal tenderness	–	0–2	0–3	–	–	–	0–1 × 39
Body temperature					–	–	
Laboratory variables	–	–	Hgb 0–4 ESR 0–2	–	Hgb(g/dl) × –4 ESR(mm/hr) × 0.5 Alb(g/dl) × –15	–	Alb(g/dl) × –26
Sigmoidoscopy	0–3	0–2	0–12		–	–	–
Other		Nausea, anorexia 0–2		Use of antidiarrheals 0–1	Total score added to constant = 200		
Score cutoff for disease activity	Remission: ≤2 & all subscores ≤1 Response: decrease of 3 (and 30%) from baseline and decrease in rectal bleeding score	Remission: 0 Improved: decrease ≥ 2 No change: ± 1 Worse: increase ≥ 2	Remission ≤4	Improved: 50% decrease in score (short term) and ≤4 total score (long term)	Mild <150 Moderate 150–220 Severe >220	Remission <5 Relapse ≥5	Severe endoscopic disease >5.5

SCCAI Simple clinical colitis activity index, *ECCI* Endoscopic-Clinical Correlation Index, *Hgb* Hemoglobin, *ESR* Erythrocyte sedimentation rate, *Alb* Albumin, *PGA* Physician global assessment

Table 46.10 Pediatric Ulcerative Colitis Activity Index

Item	Points
1. Abdominal pain:	
No pain	0
Pain can be ignored	5
Pain cannot be ignored	10
2. Rectal bleeding	
None	0
Small amount only, in less than 50% of stools	10
	20
Small amount with most stools	30
Large amount (>50% of the stool content)	
3. Stool consistency of most stools	
Formed	0
Partially formed	5
Completely unformed	10
4. Number of stools per 24 h	
0–2	0
3–5	5
6–8	10
>8	15
5. Nocturnal stools (any episode causing wakening)	
No	0
Yes	10
6. Activity level	
No limitation of activity	0
Occasional limitation of activity	5
Severe restricted activity	10
SUM OF PUCAI (0–85)	

Appendix D

Table 46.11 Crohn's Disease Endoscopic Index of Severity [88]

	Rectum	Sigmoid and left colon	Transverse colon	Right colon	Ileum	Total
Deep ulceration (12 present, 0 absent)						1
Superficial ulceration (6 present, 0 absent)						2
Surface involved by the disease (/10 cm)[a]						3
Ulcerated surface (/10 cm)[a]						4

Adapted from Daperno and colleagues [92]

$$\text{Total A} = \frac{\text{Total 1} + \text{Total 2} + \text{Total 3} + \text{Total 4}}{\text{No. of segments explored}(1\text{-}5)}$$

$CDEIS =$ Total A $+ 3$ (ulcerated stenosis present) $+ 3$ (nonulcerated stenosis present)

[a]Analogue scales converted to numeric values

Table 46.12 Simple endoscopic score for Crohn's disease [92]

	Score per segment			
Variable	0	1	2	3
Size of ulcers	None	Aphthous ulcers (0.1–0.5 cm[a])	Large ulcers (0.5 – 2 cm[a])	Very large ulcers (> 2 cm[a])
Ulcerated surface	None	< 10%	10–30%	> 30%
Affected surface	Unaffected segment	< 50%	50–75%	> 75%
Presence of narrowing	None	Single, can be passed	Multiple, can be passed	Cannot be passed

SES-CD = Total score from each segment (rectum, sigmoid, and left colon, transverse colon, right colon, ileum)
Final score = Total SES-CD score – 1.4 (number of affected segments)
[a]Diameter

Table 46.13 Rutgeerts score for postoperative endoscopic disease recurrence [95]

Grade	Endoscopic finding
0	No lesions in the distal ileum
1	≤5 aphthous lesions
2	>5 aphthous lesions with normal mucosa between the lesions or skip areas of larger lesions or lesions confined to the ileocolonic anastomosis
3	Diffuse aphthous ileitis with diffusely inflamed mucosa
4	Diffuse inflammation with already larger ulcers, nodules, and/or narrowing

Table 46.14 Ulcerative Colitis Endoscopic Index of Severity (UCEIS) [65]

Descriptor (score most severe lesions)	Likert scale anchor points	Definition
Vascular pattern	Normal (1)	Normal vascular pattern with arborization of capillaries clearly defined
	Patchy loss (3)	Patchy loss or blurring of vascular pattern
	Obliterated (5)	Complete loss of vascular pattern
Mucosal erythema	None (1)	The color of the mucosa is normal
	Light red (3)	Some increase in color of the mucosa that is probably abnormal but would be best compared side by side with a normal examination
	Dark red (5)	Red or crimson color of the mucosa that is similar to blood—that is, clearly abnormal even if not compared with a normal examination (does not include intramucosal hemorrhage)
Mucosal surface (Granularity)	Normal (1)	Smooth mucosa with a sharp light reflex, similar to a polished surface
	Granular (3)	Mucosal surface diffuses reflected light causing minor variation in the surface
	Nodular (5)	Evident nodular variation in mucosal surface
Mucosal edema	None (1)	Normal appearance: no white or yellow substance visible
	Probable (3)	Slight swelling and thickening of mucosa
	Definite (5)	Marked thickening and edema of the mucosa with blunting of the mucosal folds
Mucopus	None (1)	Normal appearance: no white or yellow substance visible
	Some (3)	White or yellow deposits on the mucosa unrelated to any bowel preparation
	Lots (5)	Mucopus substantially covering the mucosal surface unrelated to any bowel preparation
Bleeding	None (1)	No visible blood
	Mucosal (2)	Some spots or streaks of coagulated blood on the surface of the mucosa ahead of the scope, which can be washed away
	Luminal mild (3)	Some free liquid blood in the lumen
	Luminal moderate (4)	Frank blood in lumen ahead of endoscope or visible oozing from mucosa after washing intraluminal blood

(continued)

Table 46.14 (continued)

Descriptor (score most severe lesions)	Likert scale anchor points	Definition
	Luminal severe (5)	Frank blood in the same lumen with visible oozing from a hemorrhagic mucosa
Incidental friability	None (1)	No bleeding or intramucosal hemorrhage before or after passage of the endoscope
	Mild (2)	No bleeding at the site of assessment before, but minor bleeding or intramucosal hemorrhage after, passage of the endoscope
	Moderate (3)	Intramucosal hemorrhage without overt bleeding before passage of the endoscope
	Severe (4)	Overt bleeding after passage of the endoscope
	Very severe (5)	Overt bleeding from the mucosa
Contact friability	None (1)	No bleeding from the mucosa after light touch with closed biopsy forceps
	Probable (3)	Intramucosal hemorrhage or minor bleeding after light touch with closed biopsy forceps
	Definite (5)	Overt bleeding mucosa after light touch (within 10 s) with closed biopsy forceps
Erosions and ulcers	None (1)	Normal mucosa, no visible erosions or ulcers
	Erosions (2)	Tiny (≤5 mm) defects in the mucosa, of a white or yellow color with a flat edge
	Superficial ulcer (3)	Larger (>5 mm) defects in the mucosa, which are discrete fibrin-covered ulcers in comparison with erosions, but remain superficial
	Deep ulcer (4)	Deeper excavated defects in the mucosa, with a slightly raised edge
Extent of erosions or ulcers	None (1)	None seen during endoscopy
	Limited (2)	<10% of the affected mucosa
	Substantial (3)	10%–30% of the affected mucosa
	Extensive (4)	>30% of the affected mucosa

Table 46.15 Lewis score [97]

Parameters	Number	Longitudinal extent[a]	Descriptors
Villous appearance (worst-affected tertile)	Normal −0	Short segment–8	Single – 1
	Edematous – 1	Long segment– 12	Patchy – 14
		Whole tertile – 20	Diffuse – 17
Ulcer (worst-affected tertile)	None – 0[b]	Short segment–5	<1 /4–9[c]
	Single – 3[b]	Long segment– 10	1 /4–1 /2–12[c]
	Few– 5[b]	Whole tertile – 15	>1 /2–18[c]
	Multiple – 10[b]		
Stenosis (whole study)	None – 0	Ulcerated – 24	Traversed – 7
	Single – 14	Nonulcerated −2	Not traversed – 10
	Multiple – 20		

Lewis score: score of the worst-affected tertile [(villous parameter×extent × descriptor) + (ulcer number×extent×size)] + stenosis score (number × ulcerated × traversed)

[a]Longitudinal extent: short segment,<10% of the tertile; long segment, 11%–50% of the tertile; whole tertile, >50% of the tertile

[b]Ulcer number: single, 1; few, 2–7; multiple, ≥8

[c]Ulcer descriptor (size): proportion of the capsule picture filled by the largest ulcer

References

1. Kirshner B, Guyatt G. A methodological framework for assessing health indices. J Chronic Dis. 1985;38(1):27–36.
2. Wright JG, Feinstein AR. A comparative contrast of clinimetric and psychometric methods for constructing indexes and rating scales. J Clin Epidemiol. 1992;45(11):1201–18.
3. Marx RG, Bombardier C, Hogg-Johnson S, Wright JG. Clinimetric and psychometric strategies for development of a health measurement scale. J Clin Epidemiol. 1999;52(2):105–11.
4. Aaronson N, Alonso J, Burnam A, Lohr KN, Patrick DL, Perrin E, Stein RE. Assessing health status and quality-of-life instruments: attributes and review criteria. Qual Life Res. 2002;11(3):193–205.
5. Irvine EJ, Feagan B, Rochon J, Archambault A, Fedorak RN, Groll A, et al. Quality of life: a valid and reliable measure of therapeutic efficacy in the treatment of inflammatory bowel disease. Canadian Crohn's Relapse Prevention Trial Study Group. Gastroenterology. 1994;106(2):287–96.
6. Yoshida EM. The Crohn's Disease Activity Index, its derivatives and the Inflammatory Bowel Disease Questionnaire: a review of instruments to assess Crohn's disease. Can J Gastroenterol (Journal canadien de gastroenterologie). 1999;13(1):65–73.
7. Streiner DLN, Geoffrey R. Health measurement scales: a practical guide to their development and use. 2nd ed. Toronto: Oxford University Press; 1995.
8. Portney LW, Watkins MP. Foundations of clinical research applications to practice. 2nd ed. Upper Saddle River: Prentice Hall; 2000. p. 557–86.
9. Liang MH. Evaluating measurement responsiveness. J Rheumatol. 1995;22(6):1191–2.
10. Deyo RA, Centor RM. Assessing the responsiveness of functional scales to clinical change: an analogy to diagnostic test performance. J Chronic Dis. 1986;39(11):897–906.
11. Beaton DE. Understanding the relevance of measured change through studies of responsiveness. Spine. 2000;25(24):3192–9.
12. Beaton DE, Bombardier C, Katz JN, Wright JG. A taxonomy for responsiveness. J Clin Epidemiol. 2001;54(12):1204–17.
13. Best WR, Becktel JM, Singleton JW, Kern Jr F. Development of a Crohn's disease activity index. National Cooperative Crohn's Disease Study. Gastroenterology. 1976;70(3):439–44.
14. de Dombal FT, Softley A. IOIBD report no 1: observer variation in calculating indices of severity and activity in Crohn's disease. International Organisation for the Study of Inflammatory Bowel Disease. Gut. 1987;28(4):474–81.
15. Sands BE, Ooi CJ. A survey of methodological variation in the Crohn's disease activity index. Inflamm Bowel Dis. 2005;11(2):133–8.
16. Regueiro MKK, Schraut W, et al. Crohn's disease activity index does not correlate with endoscopic recurrence one year after ileocolonic resection. Inflamm Bowel Dis. 2011;17:118–26.
17. Schoepfer AMBC, Straumann A, et al. Fecal calprotectin correlates more closely with the simple endoscopic score for Crohn's disease (SES-CD) than CRP, blood leukocytes and the CDAI. Am J Gastroenterol. 2010;105:162–9.
18. Harvey RF, Bradshaw JM. A simple index of Crohn's-disease activity. Lancet. 1980;1(8167):514.
19. Markowitz J, Grancher K, Kohn N, Lesser M, Daum F. A multicenter trial of 6-mercaptopurine and prednisone in children with newly diagnosed Crohn's disease. Gastroenterology. 2000;119(4):895–902.
20. Escher JC. Budesonide versus prednisolone for the treatment of active Crohn's disease in children: a randomized, double-blind, controlled, multicentre trial. Eur J Gastroenterol Hepatol. 2004;16(1):47–54.
21. Hyams JS, Ferry GD, Mandel FS, Gryboski JD, Kibort PM, Kirschner BS, et al. Development and validation of a pediatric Crohn's disease activity index. J Pediatr Gastroenterol Nutr. 1991;12(4):439–47.
22. Tanner JM, Davies PS. Clinical longitudinal standards for height and height velocity for North American children. J Pediatr. 1985;107(3):317–29.
23. Tanner JM, Whitehouse RH, Takaishi M. Standards from birth to maturity for height, weight, height velocity, and weight velocity: British children, 1965. II. Arch Dis Child. 1966;41(220):613–35.
24. Otley A, Loonen H, Parekh N, Corey M, Sherman PM, Griffiths AM. Assessing activity of pediatric Crohn's disease: which index to use? Gastroenterology. 1999;116(3):527–31.
25. Kundhal PS, Critch JN, Zachos M, Otley AR, Stephens D, Griffiths AM. Pediatric Crohn Disease Activity Index: responsive to short-term change. J Pediatr Gastroenterol Nutr. 2003;36(1):83–9.
26. Hyams J, Markowitz J, Otley A, Rosh J, Mack D, Bousvaros A, et al. Evaluation of the pediatric crohn disease activity index: a prospective multicenter experience. J Pediatr Gastroenterol Nutr. 2005;41(4):416–21.
27. Turner DGA, Walters TD, et al. Appraisal of the pediatric Crohn disease activity index on four prospectively collected datasets: recommended cutoff values and clinimetric properties. Am J Gastroenterol. 2010;105:2085–92.
28. Turner D, Hyams J, Markowitz J, Lerer T, Mack DR, Evans J, et al. Appraisal of the pediatric ulcerative colitis activity index (PUCAI). Inflamm Bowel Dis. 2009;15(8):1218–23.
29. Kappelman MD, Crandall WV, Colletti RB, Goudie A, Leibowitz IH, Duffy L, Milov DE, Kim SC, Schoen BT, Patel AS, Grunow J, Larry E, Fairbrother G, Margolis P. Short pediatric Crohn disease activity index for quality improvement and observational research. Inflamm Bowel Dis. 2011;17(4):112–7.
30. Turner D, Griffiths AM, Steinhart AH, Otley AR, Beaton DE. Mathematical weighting of a clinimetric index (Pediatric Ulcerative Colitis Activity Index) was superior to the judgmental approach. J Clin Epidemiol. 2009;62(7):738–44.
31. Cozijnsen MDV, Kokke F, et al. Adalimumab therapy in children with Crohn disease previously treated with Infliximab. J Pediatr Gastroenterol Nutr. 2015;60:205–10.
32. Frivolt KST, Werkstetter KJ, et al. Repeated exclusive enteral nutrition in the treatment of pediatric Crohn's disease: predictors of efficacy and outcome. Aliment Pharmacol Ther. 2014;39:1398–407.
33. Loonen HJ, Griffiths AM, Merkus MP, Derkx HH. A critical assessment of items on the Pediatric Crohn's Disease Activity Index. J Pediatr Gastroenterol Nutr. 2003;36(1):90–5.
34. Shepanski MA, Markowitz JE, Mamula P, Hurd LB, Baldassano RN. Is an abbreviated Pediatric Crohn's Disease Activity Index better than the original? J Pediatr Gastroenterol Nutr. 2004;39(1):68–72.
35. Turner D, Levine A, Walters TD, et al.. Which PCDAI version best reflects intestinal inflammation in pediatric Crohn's disease. J Pediatr Gastroenterol Nutr. 2016. PMID: 27050050. [Epub ahead of print].
36. Leach STNL, Tilakaratne S, et al. Journal of pediatric gastroenterology and nutrition. Aug;51(2):232–673Development and assessment of a modified pediatric Crohn disease activity index. J Pediatr Gastroenterol Nutr. 2010;51(2):232–6.
37. Ruemmele FM. Mucosal healing for pediatric Crohn's disease: is it really worth the effort or just much ado about nothing? J Crohns Colitis. 2016;10(1):1–2.
38. Shah SCCJ, Sands BE, et al. Systematic review with meta-analysis: mucosal healing is associated with improved long-term outcomes in Crohn's disease. Aliment Pharmacol Ther. 2015;43(3):317–33.
39. Baert FML, Van Assche G, et al. Mucosal healing predicts sustained clinical remission in patients with early-stage Crohn's disease. Gastroenterology. 2010;138:463–8.

40. Schnitzler FFH, Ferrante M, et al. Mucosal healing predicts long-term outcome of maintenance therapy with infliximab in Crohn's disease. Inflamm Bowel Dis. 2009;15:1295–301.

41. Zubin GLP. Predicting endoscopic Crohn's disease activity before and after induction therapy in children: a comprehensive assessment of PCDAI, CRP, and fecal calprotectin. Inflamm Bowel Dis. 2015;21:1386–91.

42. Sun HPE, Hyams JS, et al. Well-defined and reliable clinical outcome assessments for pediatric Crohn's disease: a critical need for drug development. J Pediatr Gastroenterol Nutr. 2015;60:729–36.

43. Gecse KBBW, Kamm MA, et al. A global consensus on the classification, diagnosis and multidisciplinary treatment of perianal fistulising Crohn's disease. Gut. 2014;63:1381–92.

44. Irvine EJ. Usual therapy improves perianal Crohn's disease as measured by a new disease activity index. McMaster IBD Study Group. J Clin Gastroenterol. 1995;20(1):27–32.

45. Present DH, Rutgeerts P, Targan S, Hanauer SB, Mayer L, van Hogezand RA, et al. Infliximab for the treatment of fistulas in patients with Crohn's disease. N Engl J Med. 1999;340(18):1398–405.

46. Dejaco C, Harrer M, Waldhoer T, Miehsler W, Vogelsang H, Reinisch W. Antibiotics and azathioprine for the treatment of perianal fistulas in Crohn's disease. Aliment Pharmacol Ther. 2003;18(11–12):1113–20.

47. West RL, van der Woude CJ, Hansen BE, Felt-Bersma RJ, van Tilburg AJ, Drapers JA, et al. Clinical and endosonographic effect of ciprofloxacin on the treatment of perianal fistulae in Crohn's disease with infliximab: a double-blind placebo-controlled study. Aliment Pharmacol Ther. 2004;20(11–12):1329–36.

48. Colombel JF, Sandborn WJ, Rutgeerts P, Enns R, Hanauer SB, Panaccione R, et al. Adalimumab for maintenance of clinical response and remission in patients with Crohn's disease: the CHARM trial. Gastroenterology. 2007;132(1):52–65.

49. Tozer PNS, Siddiqui MR, et al. Long-term MRI-guided combined anti-TNF-alpha and thiopurine therapy for Crohn's perianal fistulas. Inflamm Bowel Dis. 2012;18:1825–34.

50. Horsthuis KZM, Bipat S, et al. Evaluation of an MRI-based score of disease activity in perianal fistulizing Crohn's disease. Clin Imaging. 2011;35:360–5.

51. Van Assche GVD, Bielen D, et al. Magnetic resonance imaging of the effects of infliximab on perianal fistulizing Crohn's disease. Am J Gastroenterol. 2003;98:332–9.

52. Savoye-Collet CSG, Koning E, et al. Fistulizing perianal Crohn's disease: contrast-enhanced magnetic resonance imaging assessment at 1 year on maintenance anti-TNF-alpha therapy. Inflamm Bowel Dis. 2011;17:1751–8.

53. Shenoy-Bhangle ANK, Goldner D, et al. MRI predictors of treatment response for perianal fistulizing Crohn disease in children and young adults. Pediatr Radiol. 2014;44:23–9.

54. Truelove SC, Witts LJ. Cortisone in ulcerative colitis; final report on a therapeutic trial. Br Med J. 1955;2(4947):1041–8.

55. Powell-Tuck J, Bown RL, Lennard-Jones JE. A comparison of oral prednisolone given as single or multiple daily doses for active proctocolitis. Scand J Gastroenterol. 1978;13(7):833–7.

56. Sutherland LR, Martin F, Greer S, Robinson M, Greenberger N, Saibil F, et al. 5-Aminosalicylic acid enema in the treatment of distal ulcerative colitis, proctosigmoiditis, and proctitis. Gastroenterology. 1987;92(6):1894–8.

57. Rachmilewitz D. Coated mesalazine (5-aminosalicylic acid) versus sulphasalazine in the treatment of active ulcerative colitis: a randomised trial. BMJ. 1989;298(6666):82.

58. Lichtiger S, Present DH. Preliminary report: cyclosporin in treatment of severe active ulcerative colitis. Lancet. 1990;336(8706):16–9.

59. Seo M, Okada M, Yao T, Ueki M, Arima S, Okumura M. An index of disease activity in patients with ulcerative colitis. Am J Gastroenterol. 1992;87(8):971–6.

60. Seo M, Okada M, Yao T, Okabe N, Maeda K, Oh K. Evaluation of disease activity in patients with moderately active ulcerative colitis: comparisons between a new activity index and Truelove and Witts' classification. Am J Gastroenterol. 1995;90(10):1759–63.

61. Walmsley RS, Ayres RC, Pounder RE, Allan RN. A simple clinical colitis activity index. Gut. 1998;43(1):29–32.

62. Azzolini F, Pagnini C, Camellini L, Scarcelli A, Merighi A, Primerano AM, et al. Proposal of a new clinical index predictive of endoscopic severity in ulcerative colitis. Dig Dis Sci. 2005;50(2):246–51.

63. Turner D, Seow CH, Greenberg GR, Griffiths AM, Silverberg MS, Steinhart AH. A systematic prospective comparison of noninvasive disease activity indices in ulcerative colitis. Clin Gastroenterol Hepatol. 2009;7(10):1081–8.

64. Turner D, Levine A, Escher JC, et al. Management of pediatric ulcerative colitis: joint ECCO and ESPGHAN evidence-based consensus guidelines. J Pediatr Gastroenterol Nutr. 2012;55(3):340–61.

65. Travis SPLSD, Krzeski P, et al. Developing an instrument to assess the endoscopic severity of ulcerative colitis: the Ulcerative Colitis Endoscopic Index of Severity (UCEIS). Gut. 2012;61:535–42.

66. Beattie RMNS, Domizio P, Williams CB, Walker-Smith JA. Endoscopic assessment of the colonic response to corticosteroids in children with ulcerative colitis. J Pediatr Gastroenterol Nutr. 1996;22(4):373–9.

67. Colombel JFRP, Reinisch W, Esser D, Wang Y, Lang Y, et al. Early mucosal healing with infliximab is associated with improved long-term clinical outcomes in ulcerative colitis. Gastroenterology. 2011;141(4):1194–201.

68. Gustavsson AJG, Hertervig E, Friis-Liby I, Blomquist L, Karlén P, et al. Clinical trial: colectomy after rescue therapy in ulcerative colitis – 3-year follow-up of the Swedish-Danish controlled infliximab study. Aliment Pharmacol Ther. 2010;32(8):984–9.

69. Froslie KFJJ, Moum BA, Vatn MH. Mucosal Healing in inflammatory bowel disease: results from a Norwegian population-based cohort. Gastroenterology. 2007;133:412–22.

70. Turner D, Otley A, deBruijne J, Mack D, Uusoue K, Zachos M, Mamula P, Hyams J, Griffiths AM. Development of a pediatric ulcerative colitis activity index (PUCAI). J Pediatr Gastroenterol Nutr. 2006;43(4):E47.

71. Dotson JL, Crandall WV, Zhang P, et al. Feasibility and validity of the pediatric ulcerative colitis activity index in routine clinical practice. J Pediatr Gastroenterol Nutr. 2014;60(2):200–4.

72. Turner D, Otley AR, Mack D, Hyams J, de Bruijne J, Uusoue K, et al. Development, validation, and evaluation of a pediatric ulcerative colitis activity index: a prospective multicenter study. Gastroenterology. 2007;133(2):423–32.

73. Turner D, Griffiths AM, Veerman G, Johanns J, Damaraju L, Blank M, et al. Endoscopic and clinical variables that predict sustained remission in children with ulcerative colitis treated with infliximab. Clin Gastroenterol Hepatol. 2013;11(11):1460–5.

74. Schechter A, Griffiths C, Gana JC, Shaoul R, Shamir R, Shteyer E, et al. Early endoscopic, laboratory and clinical predictors of poor disease course in paediatric ulcerative colitis. Gut. 2014;64(4):580–8.

75. Gray FL, Turner CG, Zurakowski D, Bousvaros A, Linden BC, Shamberger RC, et al. Predictive value of the pediatric ulcerative colitis activity index in the surgical management of ulcerative colitis. J Pediatr Surg. 2013;48(7):1540–5.

76. Turner D, Mack D, Leleiko N, Walters TD, Uusoue K, Leach ST, et al. Severe pediatric ulcerative colitis: a prospective multicenter study of outcomes and predictors of response. Gastroenterology. 2010;138(7):2282–91.

77. Turner D, Walsh CM, Benchimol EI, Mann EH, Thomas KE, Chow C, et al. Severe paediatric ulcerative colitis: incidence,

outcomes and optimal timing for second-line therapy. Gut. 2008;57(3):331–8.

78. Sylvester FA, Turner D, Draghi 2nd A, Uuosoe K, McLernon R, Koproske K, et al. Fecal osteoprotegerin may guide the introduction of second-line therapy in hospitalized children with ulcerative colitis. Inflamm Bowel Dis. 2011;17(8):1726–30.

79. Turner D, Hyams J, Markowitz J, Lerer T, Mack DR, Evans J, et al. Appraisal of the pediatric ulcerative colitis activity index (PUCAI). Inflamm Bowel Dis. 2009;15(8):1218–23.

80. Hyams J, Damaraju L, Blank M, Johanns J, Guzzo C, Winter HS, et al. Induction and maintenance therapy with infliximab for children with moderate to severe ulcerative colitis. Clin Gastroenterol Hepatol. 2012;10(4):391–9. e1

81. Romano C, Famiani A, Comito D, Rossi P, Raffa V, Fries W. Oral beclomethasone dipropionate in pediatric active ulcerative colitis: a comparison trial with mesalazine. J Pediatr Gastroenterol Nutr. 2010;50(4):385–9.

82. Civitelli F, Di Nardo G, Oliva S, Nuti F, Ferrari F, Dilillo A, et al. Ultrasonography of the colon in pediatric ulcerative colitis: a prospective, blind, comparative study with colonoscopy. J Pediatr. 2014;165(1):78–84.e2.

83. Teitelbaum JERR, Jaeger J, et al. Correlation of health-related quality of life in children with inflammatory bowel disease, their parents, and physician as measured by a visual analog scale. J Pediatr Gastroenterol Nutr. 2013;57(5):594–7.

84. Koslowe ORJ. Taking full measure of the pediatric ulcerative colitis activity index. J Pediatr Gastroenterol Nutr. 2015;60(2):148–9.

85. Travis SP, Stange EF, Lemann M, Oresland T, Chowers Y, Forbes A, et al. European evidence based consensus on the diagnosis and management of Crohn's disease: current management. Gut. 2006;55(Suppl 1):i16–35.

86. Ruemmele FMVG, Kolho KL, et al. Consensus guidelines of ECCO/ESPGHAN on the medical management of pediatric Crohn's disease. J Crohns Colitis. 2014;8(10):1179–207.

87. Reproducibility of colonoscopic findings in Crohn's disease: a prospective multicenter study of interobserver variation. Groupe d'Etudes Therapeutiques des Affections Inflammatoires du Tube Digestif (GETAID). Dig Dis Sci. 1987;32(12):1370–9.

88. Mary JY, Modigliani R. Development and validation of an endoscopic index of the severity for Crohn's disease: a prospective multicentre study. Groupe d'Etudes Therapeutiques des Affections Inflammatoires du Tube Digestif (GETAID). Gut. 1989;30(7):983–9.

89. Rutgeerts P, Diamond RH, Bala M, Olson A, Lichtenstein GR, Bao W, et al. Scheduled maintenance treatment with infliximab is superior to episodic treatment for the healing of mucosal ulceration associated with Crohn's disease. Gastrointest Endosc. 2006;63(3):433–42. quiz 64.

90. D'Haens G, Van Deventer S, Van Hogezand R, Chalmers D, Kothe C, Baert F, et al. Endoscopic and histological healing with infliximab anti-tumor necrosis factor antibodies in Crohn's disease: a European multicenter trial. Gastroenterology. 1999;116(5):1029–34.

91. Bauditz J, Haemling J, Ortner M, Lochs H, Raedler A, Schreiber S. Treatment with tumour necrosis factor inhibitor oxpentifylline does not improve corticosteroid dependent chronic active Crohn's disease. Gut. 1997;40(4):470–4.

92. Daperno M, D'Haens G, Van Assche G, Baert F, Bulois P, Maunoury V, et al. Development and validation of a new, simplified endoscopic activity score for Crohn's disease: the SES-CD. Gastrointest Endosc. 2004;60(4):505–12.

93. Crocco S, Martelossi S, Giurici N, Villanacci V, Ventura A. Upper gastrointestinal involvement in paediatric onset Crohn's disease: prevalence and clinical implications. J Crohns Colitis. 2012;6(1):51–5.

94. Ledder OCP, Griffiths A, et al. Utility of proposed modified simple endoscopic score in upper gastrointestinal Crohn's disease. United European Gastroenterol J. 2015;3(5S):A597.

95. Rutgeerts P, Geboes K, Vantrappen G, Beyls J, Kerremans R, Hiele M. Predictability of the postoperative course of Crohn's disease. Gastroenterology. 1990;99(4):956–63.

96. Bayart P DN, Nachury M, et al. Rate of postoperative clinical recurrence in Crohn's disease patients classified i2 on Rutgeerts score with lesions confined to the ileocolonic anastomosis is not different compared to patients with moderate lesions on the terminal ileum. United European Gastroenterol J. 2015;3(5S):A3.

97. Gralnek IM, Defranchis R, Seidman E, Leighton JA, Legnani P, Lewis BS. Development of a capsule endoscopy scoring index for small bowel mucosal inflammatory change. Aliment Pharmacol Ther. 2007;27(2):146–54.

98. Cotter J, Dias de Castro F, Magalhães J, Moreira MJ, Rosa B. Validation of the Lewis score for the evaluation of small-bowel Crohn's disease activity. Endoscopy. 2015;47(4):330–5.

99. Höög CM, Bark LÅ, Broström O, Sjöqvist U. Capsule endoscopic findings correlate with fecal calprotectin and C-reactive protein in patients with suspected small-bowel Crohn's disease. Scand J Gastroenterol. 2014;49:1084–90.

100. Rosa B, Moreira MJ, Rebelo A, Cotter J. Lewis Score: a useful clinical tool for patients with suspected Crohn's Disease submitted to capsule endoscopy. J Crohns Colitis. 2012;6(6):692–7.

101. Uri Kopylov DY, Lahat A, Neuman S, Levhar N, Greener T, Klang E, Rozendorn N, Amitai MM, Ben-Horin S, Eliakim R. Detection of small bowel mucosal healing and deep remission in patients with known small bowel Crohn's disease using biomarkers, capsule endoscopy, and imaging. Am J Gastroenterol. 2015;110:1316–23.

102. Baron JH, Connell AM, Lennard-Jones JE. Variation between observers in describing mucosal appearances in proctocolitis. Br Med J. 1964;1(5375):89–92.

103. Orlandi F, Brunelli E, Feliciangeli G, Svegliati-Baroni G, Di Sario A, Benedetti A, et al. Observer agreement in endoscopic assessment of ulcerative colitis. Ital J Gastroenterol Hepatol. 1998;30(5):539–41.

104. Schroeder KWTW, Ilstrup DM. Coated oral 5-aminosalicylic acid therapy for mildly to moderately active ulcerative colitis. A randomized study. N Engl J Med. 1987;317:1625–9.

105. Travis SPLSD, Krzeski P, et al. Reliability and initial validation of the Ulcerative Colitis Endoscopic Index of Severity. Gastroenterology. 2013;145:987–95.

106. Lobaton TBT, De Hertogh G, et al. The Modified Mayo Endoscopic Score (MMES): a new index for the assessment of extension and severity of endoscopic activity in ulcerative colitis patients. J Crohns Colitis. 2015;9(10):846–52.

107. Food and Drug Administration. Guideline for industry – Patient-reported outcome measures: use in medical product development to support labelling claims. Silver Spring: Food and Drug Administration; 2009.

108. Kelstrup AMJP, Korzenik J. The accuracy of self-reported medical history: a preliminary analysis of the promise of internet-based research in Inflammatory Bowel Diseases. J Crohns Colitis. 2014;8(5):349–56.

109. Bewtra MBC, Tomov VT, et al. An optimized patient-reported ulcerative colitis disease activity measure has been derived from the Mayo score and the simple clinical colitis activity index. Inflamm Bowel Dis. 2014;20(6):1070–8.

110. Khanna RZG, D'Haens G, et al. A retrospective analysis: the development of patient reported outcome measures for the assessment of Crohn's disease activity. Aliment Pharmacol Ther. 2015;41:77–86.

111. Matza LSPD, Riley AW, et al. Pediatric patient-reported outcome instruments for research to support medical product labeling: report of the ISPOR PRO good research practices for the assessment of children and adolescents task force. Value Health. 2013;16:461–79.

112. Marcovitch LNA, Mack D, et al. Item generation and reduction of the "TUMMY" index, a newly derived patient reporting outcome for pediatric ulcerative colitis (Abstract). United European Gastroenterol J. 2015;3(5S):A438.

113. Mackner LM, Crandall WV, Szigethy EM. Psychosocial functioning in pediatric inflammatory bowel disease. Inflamm Bowel Dis. 2006;12(3):239–44.

114. Sainsbury A, Heatley RV. Review article: psychosocial factors in the quality of life of patients with inflammatory bowel disease. Aliment Pharmacol Ther. 2005;21(5):499–508.

115. Kucharzik TPF, Maaser C. Bowel Ultrasonography in Inflammatory Bowel Disease. Dig Dis Sci. 2015;33(1):17–25.

116. Rimola JRS, García-Bosch O, Ordás I, Ayala E, Aceituno M, Pellisé M, Ayuso C, Ricart E, Donoso L, Panés J. Magnetic resonance for assessment of disease activity and severity in ileocolonic Crohn's disease. Gut. 2009;58(8):1113–20.

117. Rimola JOI, Rodriguez S, García-Bosch O, Aceituno M, Llach J, Ayuso C, Ricart E, Panés J. Magnetic resonance imaging for evaluation of Crohn's disease: validation of parameters of severity and quantitative index of activity. Inflamm Bowel Dis. 2011;17(8):1759–68.

118. Pariente BCJ, Danese S, Sandborn WJ, Lewin M, Fletcher JG, Chowers Y, D'Haens G, Feagan BG, Hibi T, Hommes DW, Irvine EJ, Kamm MA, Loftus Jr EV, Louis E, Michetti P, Munkholm P, Oresland T, Panés J, Peyrin-Biroulet L, Reinisch W, Sands BE, Schoelmerich J, Schreiber S, Tilg H, Travis S, van Assche G, Vecchi M, Mary JY, Colombel JF, Lémann M. Development of the Crohn's disease digestive damage score, the Lémann score. Inflamm Bowel Dis. 2011;17(6):1415–22.

119. Focht G, Traub T, Church P, Walters TD, Greer ML, Amitai M, Cytter R, Castro D, Otley A, O'Brien K, Mack D, Davila J, Griffiths AM, Turner D. Damage and inflammatory activity in pediatric Crohn's disease (CD) based on radiologist and gastroenterologist physician global assessment. J Crohns Colitis. 2014;8(S2):S410.

120. Rutgeerts P, Sandborn WJ, Feagan BG, Reinisch W, Olson A, Johanns J, et al. Infliximab for induction and maintenance therapy for ulcerative colitis. N Engl J Med. 2005;353(23):2462–76.

Clinical Trials (Clinical Perspective)

Salvatore Cucchiara and Marina Aloi

Introduction

Recent epidemiologic studies report that up to 30% of new cases of inflammatory bowel diseases (IBD) are diagnosed in childhood [1]. Pediatric IBD seem to be more extensive and severe than the adult-onset forms, with a frequent need of second-line therapies, including immunomodulators and biologics, and a more complicated disease course [2, 3]. However, excluding the very-early-onset diseases (before 5 years of age), their pathogenesis, histopathological features, and response to treatments seem to be similar to the adult-onset disease [4], and most therapeutic pediatric strategies are simply "extrapolated" from adult trials in an "off-label" use. Indeed, randomized clinical trials (RCTs) in children could be more difficult for several reasons: first of all ethical concerns, due to the natural vulnerability of this population, and then for the relative paucity of eligible patients, because of the lower number of incident and prevalent cases, compared with adults. Moreover, parents, worried about possible therapy adverse events and/or for additional invasive tests and visits, are more hesitant to have their children recruited in intervention trials, compared to adult patients. Often, the same physicians hesitate to enroll small patients to intervention studies involving invasive procedures.

However, children with IBD represent a unique cohort of patients to be explored, including the initial host immune response, the need for early "aggressive" treatment, the genotype-to-phenotype relationship, and the natural disease course which are concerned. Above all, because of the low impact of environmental factors that may influence adult-onset disease (e.g., comorbidities, disease duration, drugs, smoking), the knowledge of the pathogenetic pathways of pediatric IBD can provide insights into the initial mechanisms underlying the disease [5].

A crucial factor when evaluating the efficacy of different treatments in children with IBD is the ability to compare new drugs to known therapies in a meaningful way. Randomized clinical trials lead to gold standard evidence on the efficacy of pharmacologic and nonpharmacologic therapy of IBD. An ideal clinical trial should answer to well-defined primary research endpoints in specific study populations and should provide results that are significant both statistically and clinically. Steps that describe RCTs are clear definition of the primary (and secondary) outcomes, definition of the eligible population, randomized assignment to the treatment regimen, and standardized and well-defined interventions. Moreover, a well-defined study population is based upon clear outlined inclusion and exclusion criteria. Trial design should be sufficiently linear to fulfill the trial's questions; on the other hand, it must not be so weighty that physicians cannot complete the study. Very recently, an evidence-based, expert-driven practical statement paper of the pediatric ECCO committee on the outcome measures for clinical trials in pediatric IBD has been published [6]. Several important outcomes have been highlighted for the future RCTs on pediatric IBD, the first being the recommendation of defining steroid-free mucosal healing (MH) as assessed by endoscopy as the primary endpoint for all preauthorization trials for a new drug authorization. Mucosal healing has emerged as a specific treatment endpoint in adult IBD, both in clinical trials and in clinical practice, as it is associated with a reduced risk of disease exacerbations in the long term, treatment escalations, and colectomy [7, 8]. Sparce prospective studies in children have been performed using MH as a primary outcome so far [9]. In the case of therapies already demonstrated to induce MH in adult trials, ECCO experts recommend to use objective measures of disease activity [weighted Paediatric Crohn's Disease Activity

S. Cucchiara, MD, PhD (✉) • M. Aloi, MD, PhD
Pediatric Gastroenterology and Liver Unit, Department of Pediatrics, University of Rome "La Sapienza",
Viale Regina Elena 324, 00161 Rome, Italy
e-mail: salvatore.cucchiara@uniroma1.it

© Springer International Publishing AG 2017
P. Mamula et al. (eds.), *Pediatric Inflammatory Bowel Disease*, DOI 10.1007/978-3-319-49215-5_47

Index (wPCDAI) or Paediatric Ulcerative Colitis Activity Index (PUCAI)] as primary endpoints, although MH is always suggested as secondary outcome in subgroups of patients. Specific importance should be given to the timing of assessment of primary and secondary outcomes, being 6–12 weeks of therapy the optimal time window suggested for the induction of remission and 12 months to evaluate the maintenance of steroid-free remission. One of the main barriers to perform a pediatric RCT is the potential need of placebo arm. Indeed, although a randomized, double-blind, parallel group trial is regarded as the ideal study design for assessing the efficacy of a new drug, this can prompt ethical and feasibility problems for pediatric studies [10]. In the same guidelines, ECCO experts stated that placebo-controlled trials are hardly suitable in the design of clinical trials for the vulnerable population of children with IBD. A placebo may be considered for evaluating additional treatments, provided that both study groups (treatment and control) receive effective therapy. A recent joint position paper from ESPGHAN, ECCO, the global PIBDnet, and the Canadian pediatric IBD network further states that placebo should only be accepted in children with IBD when true equipoise exists against the active therapy, whereas it should not be used when previous adult trials have already shown the efficacy of the active treatment, supported by clinical experience in children [11].

Recently, the Food and Drug Administration (FDA) has declared that pediatric studies are not necessarily required for all new treatments; however, "extrapolation" from adult trials should always be taken into account of drug pharmacokinetics, pharmacodynamics, and evaluation of potential and real side effects/toxicities. However, it is still emphasized that the pharmaceutical industry should focus on pediatric pharmacokinetic studies for those medications with a strong potential impact in children; moreover, specific pediatric outcomes, including the impact on growth and bone-related issues, cannot be evaluated based on adult studies. Therefore, an accurate balance between the concerns of conducting a pediatric trial and the advantages of having well-defined data should always be sought for any proposed trial.

Summary

Up to now, only few RCTs in children with IBD have been performed. Although pediatric and adult IBD probably share their pathogenetic mechanisms, histopathological damage, and response to therapies, an accurate balance of the usefulness of the data collected in adult studies and those particularly required for the optimal knowledge of the efficacy and safety of new drugs suggested for pediatric IBD should always be considered. Partial extrapolation of adult data could be reasonable and tolerable, when including data on drug pharmacokinetic and pharmacodynamics, together with its potential or real adverse events; however, pediatric RCT is needed to identify specificities of treatment strategies in children, understand the long-term impact of new treatment strategies on specific outcomes (growth and bone-related issues), and ensure that children with IBD can access to new treatments in an acceptable period of time.

References

1. Benchimol EI, Fortinsky KJ, Gozdyra P, et al. Epidemiology of pediatric inflammatory bowel disease: a systematic review of international trends. Inflamm Bowel Dis. 2011;17:423–39.
2. Aloi M, Lionetti P, Barabino A, et al. Phenotype and disease course of early-onset pediatric inflammatory bowel disease. Inflamm Bowel Dis. 2014;20:597–605.
3. Jakobsen C, Bartek Jr J, Wewer V, et al. Differences in phenotype and disease course in adult and paediatric inflammatory bowel disease–a population-based study. Aliment Pharmacol Ther. 2011;34:1217–24.
4. Rigoli L, Caruso RA. Inflammatory bowel disease in pediatric and adolescent patients: a biomolecular and histopathological review. World J Gastroenterol. 2014;20:10262–78.
5. Ananthakrishnan AN. Epidemiology and risk factors for IBD. Nat Rev Gastroenterol Hepatol. 2015;12:205–17.
6. Ruemmele FM, Hyams JS, Otley A, et al. Outcome measures for clinical trials in paediatric IBD: an evidence-based, expert-driven practical statement paper of the paediatric ECCO committee. Gut. 2015;64:438–46.
7. Pineton de Chambrun G, Peyrin-Biroulet L, Lémann M, et al. Clinical implications of mucosal healing for the management of IBD. Nat Rev Gastroenterol Hepatol. 2010;7:15–29.
8. Theede K, Kiszka-Kanowitz M, Nordgaard-Lassen I, et al. The impact of endoscopic inflammation and mucosal healing on health-related quality of life in ulcerative colitis patients. J Crohns Colitis. 2015;9:625–32.
9. Nuti F, Civitelli F, Bloise S, et al. Prospective evaluation of the achievement of mucosal healing with anti-TNF-α therapy in a paediatric Crohn's disease Cohort. J Crohns Colitis. 2016;10:5–12.
10. Sands BE, Abreu MT, Ferry GD, et al. Design issues and outcomes in IBD clinical trials. Inflamm Bowel Dis. 2005;11:S22–8.
11. Turner D, Koletzko S, Griffiths AM, et al. Use of placebo in pediatric inflammatory bowel diseases: a position paper from ESPGHAN, ECCO, PIBDnet, and the Canadian children IBD network. J Pediatr Gastroenterol Nutr. 2016;62:183–7.

Clinical Trials (Industry/Regulatory Perspective)

48

Tara Altepeter, Kurt Brown, Aisha Peterson Johnson, and Andrew E. Mulberg

Key Stakeholders in Drug Development Process

Pediatric drug development presents novel challenges and opportunities. The following chapter will review relevant laws guiding drug development in the USA, provide an overview of the drug development process in general, and highlight some of the specific challenges for pediatric patients in clinical trials, utilizing inflammatory bowel disease as an example.

The drug development process in the USA is guided by relevant federal statutes and regulations. With particular respect to children, the goal of these regulations is to promote the study of therapeutic agents in pediatrics, while establishing protections for this vulnerable population. Drug development involves a collaborative effort among regulators, industry sponsors, academic researchers, and individual investigators.

Regulatory Agencies In the USA, each step in the drug development process is regulated by the Food and Drug Administration (FDA). The agency regulates a wide variety of products, including food products, drugs for human and animal use, cosmetics, biologic agents, medical devices, radiation emitting products, and animal feed. The agency's actions, under current US laws, regulate all phases of the drug development process. In recent years, efforts to standardize the drug development process across countries and promote international cooperation have been increasing. Given the difficulty in enrolling sufficient numbers of pediatric patients into trials in general, this is of particular relevance for pediatric drug development.

Industry Sponsors Industry sponsors conduct research to identify potential therapeutic targets and seek biologic or chemical agents that will affect a target to treat disease. Once a suitable target is identified, the sponsor will begin a rigorous process of preclinical, followed by clinical development, with the goal of ultimately identifying a product that can be brought to market. Close collaboration between industry sponsors and FDA is vital to expeditious development of new drugs and biologic molecules. Some sponsors will choose to utilize a contract research organization (CRO) to handle the planning and implementation of some or all of a clinical trial. This is particularly helpful for smaller companies that may not have the required experience, infrastructure, or resources to successfully run a large clinical trial.

Academic Researchers Apart from private firms, scientists and physicians at academic institutions also participate in various steps in the drug development process. Both university-based and government-funded research laboratories conduct vital basic science investigation to identify molecular mechanisms of disease, which may ultimately result in new drug target identification. Physician scientists often participate in this work and provide clinical context which allows for more direct translation of basic science concepts to clinical care. Additionally, social science research into optimal methods to measure the clinical outcomes of importance to patients (development of patient-reported outcome tools or PROs) may also be conducted by academic staff and have direct implications on clinical trials.

T. Altepeter, MD (✉)
Division of Gastroenterology and Inborn Errors Products,
US Food and Drug Administration, 10903 New Hampshire Ave,
Silver Spring, MD 20993, USA
e-mail: tara.altepeter@fda.hhs.gov

K. Brown, MD
Immuno-Inflammation Therapy Area Unit, Research and
Development, GlaxoSmithKline, 1250 S Collegeville Road,
Collegeville, PA 19426, USA
e-mail: Kurt.x.Brown@GSK.com

A.P. Johnson, MD, MPH, MBA
Division of Gastroenterology and Inborn Errors Products,
10903 New Hampshire Ave, Bldg 22, Room 5134,
Silver Spring, MD 20993, USA

A.E. Mulberg, MD
Gastroenterology and Inborn Errors Products,
Food and Drug Administration, 10903 New Hampshire Ave,
Silver Spring, MD 20993, USA
e-mail: amulberg@comcast.net

© Springer International Publishing AG 2017
P. Mamula et al. (eds.), *Pediatric Inflammatory Bowel Disease*, DOI 10.1007/978-3-319-49215-5_48

Investigators Once a proposed product has been rigorously tested in nonclinical studies and models, it must then be tested in patients. Clinical trial investigators are typically physicians treating patients with the condition of interest. They may be located in an academic or private practice setting. In collaboration with industry sponsors, individual investigators will share the responsibility for enrolling suitable patients into drug trials, monitoring the safety of those patients, and generating data that will ultimately be used to make a final determination of the safety and efficacy of a given new drug product.

Regulations Guiding Pediatric Drug Development

This section will briefly review some of the major legislation that guides the pediatric drug development process today.

In the early 1900s, regulations pertaining to the manufacturing, marketing, and distribution of drug products were minimally restrictive. The existing regulations at that time, under the Food and Drug Act of 1906, did not prohibit false therapeutic claims, nor did they provide FDA significant power to enforce the regulations that did exist [1]. Thus, the market was filled with products that lacked adequate safety or efficacy testing. The magnitude of this problem came to light with the Sulfanilamide tragedy in 1937. "Elixir of Sulfanilamide," a liquid preparation of a commonly used antibiotic, was manufactured and distributed widely without adequate safety testing. After the deaths of more than 100 people, many of them children, it was ultimately discovered that the manufacturer had utilized ethylene glycol, a poisonous substance, as a solvent [2]. It was in part this tragedy which spurred congress to pass new legislation imposing stricter regulations on the industry and providing FDA with increased authority to regulate the pharmaceutical industry. This came in the form of the Food, Drug, and Cosmetic Act (FDCA).

Food, Drug, and Cosmetic Act of 1938

President Roosevelt signed the Food, Drug, and Cosmetic Act (FDCA) into law in 1938. One of the critical provisions in the law mandated premarket approval of all new drugs. This meant that a drug manufacturer was required to prove to the FDA that its product was safe for use prior to marketing. The new law also contained provisions that extended FDA control to cosmetics and devices; provided safe tolerances be set for unavoidable poisons; authorized standards of identity, quality, and fill of container for foods; authorized factory inspections; and added penalties for those who violated these laws [1]. The passage of FDCA was an important step in improving the safety of the drugs available in the marketplace, as previously there had been no standard requiring demonstration of the safety of pharmaceutical products.

Durham-Humphrey Amendment of 1951

The Durham-Humphrey Amendment of 1951 established the need for medical supervision in the use of certain drug products and defined for the first time which drugs would be available by prescription only.

Kefauver-Harris Amendments of 1962

A major change in the history of US drug regulation occurred in 1962 with the passage of the Kefauver-Harris Amendments (KHA) to the FDCA. Passage of this amendment was spurred in part by the global tragedy of thalidomide. Thalidomide, though never approved for marketing in the USA, was widely used in Europe at this time and resulted in severe birth defects in children born to mothers who used it during pregnancy. The devastation caused by widespread use of this medication, despite a paucity of adequate safety data, in part helped to shape the reforms to the US drug approval process contained in these amendments [3].

The Kefauver-Harris Amendments first introduced into law the requirement that a drug product be proven efficacious. They led to the requirement of two adequate and well-controlled trials for demonstrating efficacy of a new drug product. Additionally, these amendments provided a number of other safeguards, including formal rules guiding good manufacturing process, provision of a 180-day period for FDA to review a new drug application, requirement of an affirmative decision by the agency to approve a drug before marketing, and requirements of drug manufacturers to report adverse events associated with drug use to FDA [4].

Orphan Drug Act of 1983

The Orphan Drug Act (ODA) is particularly relevant to the pediatric population, as it created incentives for companies to develop drugs for rare diseases. By providing significant financial incentives through tax benefits and prolonged marketing exclusivity, this statute resulted in an increased interest in conditions previously ignored by many pharmaceutical companies, due to perceived lack of financial benefit [5]. Many of the diseases covered by the ODA are conditions that affect children disproportionately, including certain cancers, cystic fibrosis, sickle cell disease, and inflammatory bowel disease.

Pediatric Labeling Rule of 1994

The Pediatric Labeling Rule was issued by FDA in 1994, to further promote access to drugs for children. The rule first introduced the concept of pediatric extrapolation – allowing the agency to label drugs for pediatric use in some limited circumstances based on less than the standard of two adequate, well-controlled clinical trials.

Food and Drug Modernization Act of 1997

The Food and Drug Modernization Act (FDAMA) reauthorized the FDCA and focused on reforming and modernizing many facets of the regulation of food, drugs, and cosmetics. One important facet was a financial incentive offered to companies for pediatric drug development. The law allowed FDA to grant 6 months marketing exclusivity to drugs which were studied appropriately in a pediatric population. However, despite companies starting to take advantage of marketing exclusivity, there remained a major deficiency in the availability of strong clinical evidence to support the safe and effective use in children of many prescription drug products [6].

Best Pharmaceuticals for Children Act of 2002/2007

Despite additional benefits for companies developing drugs for orphan indications and FDAMA incentives, the gap between high-quality evidence informing the use of many drugs for children, compared with adults, remains wide. Even when pediatric studies are conducted, there is often a lag of many years between the approval of a new drug for adults and the availability of adequate data to support labeling in children.

The Best Pharmaceuticals for Children Act (BPCA) was enacted in 2002. In addition to extending the financial incentive of 6 months of market exclusivity from FDAMA, BPCA established a program to promote pediatric drug development, through the National Institutes of Health (NIH). The act was reauthorized in 2007 and later permanently reauthorized in 2012 and provided additional measures including a process through which FDA can issue a request to a manufacturer to conduct specific trials in children, if deemed necessary by the NIH. If the manufacturer chooses not to conduct those trials, the NIH may do so [7].

Pediatric Research Equity Act of 2003/2007

The Pediatric Research Equity Act (PREA) was passed in December of 2003. The most comprehensive piece of legislation regulating pediatric drug development to date, PREA provides authority to the FDA to require sponsors to conduct studies in pediatric patients when a marketing application is first submitted to FDA for a new active ingredient, new indication, new dosage form, new dosing regimen, or new route of administration. However, under certain circumstances (e.g., if the disease for which the drug is used does not occur in children), FDA may grant a waiver for studies under PREA [8]. PREA was reauthorized in 2007 and expanded in 2012 as part of the Food and Drug Administration Safety and Innovation Act (FDASIA).

Overview of Clinical Trials

Once a pharmaceutical company has identified a compound of interest, nonclinical studies will be conducted. This typically includes animal pharmacology and toxicology studies, to assess the potential therapeutic benefit of the drug in a disease model and to permit an assessment of whether it is reasonably safe for initial testing in human subjects. Depending on the targeting of an individual new molecular entity to the pediatric population, juvenile animal toxicity studies may also be required to asses for potential effects on growth and development and assessment of effects on specific developmental systems and are especially important in the development programs for drugs that will ultimately be used in children.

Clinical trials are typically divided into four phases.

Phase I Clinical Trials

Phase I clinical trials typically involve the first exposure of humans to the new drug. Typically these studies are conducted in healthy adult volunteers and may enroll very small numbers of patients (often less than 50 patients). For ethical reasons, pediatric subjects are typically excluded from phase I clinical development programs, until the risk-benefit profile in human subjects is more clearly understood.

Phase I trials often involve the administration of a small, single dose to a small number of subjects in order to understand various aspects of its pharmacokinetics in the human body. Particular interest is paid to collecting multiple blood samples over time, in order to assess the pharmacokinetic (PK) profile of the drug. This data will be compared with PK data collected in animal models, to help direct the testing of further doses and to determine safe starting doses for use in the clinical trials. These studies may provide additional insight into the metabolism, clearance, elimination half-life, etc. of the drug in humans. Specific attention is paid to any safety concerns, including changes in vital signs, laboratory parameters, and subject symptoms [9]. Further investigation may include dose escalation strategies to test larger doses, once initial safety is confirmed. A major goal of a phase I study is to obtain sufficient understanding of pharmacokinetics to inform the design of a phase II trial which will allow safe initial evaluation of efficacy in patients.

Phase II Clinical Trials

A phase II clinical trial utilizes the background information obtained from the phase I trial to adapt the development program toward the patient population of interest. Goals of phase II studies include demonstrating proof of concept in a specific disease population, determining the optimal drug dosing regimen for a given disease, and exploring the exposure-response relationship [10].

Phase II trials are designed to be relatively short in duration and small in size and may use an early clinical response or biomarker as the endpoint of interest. They often enroll 100–200 patients, or sometimes less. The ultimate goal is to confirm that the drug will likely be successful in further development, before undertaking a large, longer-term phase III program, and to obtain the needed supportive information to inform the design of those pivotal trials.

Phase III Clinical Trials

Phase III trials are designed to utilize the previously determined effective dose to demonstrate efficacy in a specific patient population. Phase III trials are typically large (may include hundreds to thousands of patients), aim to enroll a diverse patient population, and will be statistically powered to demonstrate efficacy of the study drug in the given population. Various trial designs can be employed, including comparing the new drug to a previously approved alternative (to demonstrate non-inferiority or superiority) or to a placebo (to demonstrate initial efficacy). Apart from efficacy, safety measures are assessed carefully to determine if infrequent but serious adverse events may occur [11].

Phase IV Clinical Trials

In the USA, phase IV trials are those conducted after initial approval of a new drug. This may include studies mandated by the regulatory agency for a variety of reasons. FDA routinely issues post-marketing requirements (PMRs) for studies to obtain additional safety and efficacy data after the initial approval. This may include further studies to better assess the safety and effectiveness of the drug in various subpopulations, such as specific age groups or ethnicities that were not well represented in the original trials that supported

approval. Deferred pediatric studies required by PREA are also included. Other phase IV studies may be conducted to understand the long-term safety and/or efficacy of a product (which can be done via a long-term observational study or registry protocol). They may assist in the detection of very rare but serious adverse events. Due to the low incidence of these types of events, it may take thousands of patients and follow-up over many years to obtain the required data to fully understand the risks [12].

Key Concepts in Clinical Trial Conduct

Good clinical practice (GCP) refers to a collection of rules, regulations, and standardized procedures which are designed to protect participants in clinical trials. These standards are designed to ensure that the trial is conducted such that the credibility and accuracy of the data generated are maintained. Required components of GCP include an institutional review board (IRB), specific requirements for informed consent documents, a standardized approach to evaluation and reporting of adverse events which may occur during clinical trials, and use of a data monitoring committee. This section will describe each of these components in more detail.

Institutional Review Board (IRB)

The statutes governing the regulation of an Investigational New Drug (IND) in the USA specify that clinical investigations must be approved by an IRB. An IRB is a group of individuals designated to carry the responsibility of reviewing a proposed clinical study to ensure that it will be conducted in accordance with standard ethical principles. An IRB may be specific to one hospital or healthcare institution, or, more commonly in large multicenter trials, a centralized IRB may be utilized to oversee the study at multiple cooperating sites.

Informed Consent

A key component of good clinical practice is obtaining the research subject's informed consent to participate. As specified in the Code of Federal Regulations (21 CFR 50.2), "no investigator may involve a human being as a subject in research covered by these regulations unless the investigator has obtained the legally effective informed consent of the subject or the subject's legally authorized representative. An investigator shall seek such consent only under circumstances that provide the prospective subject or the representative sufficient opportunity to consider whether or not to participate and that minimize the possibility of coercion or undue influence. The information that is given to the subject or the representative shall be in language understandable to the subject or the representative. No informed consent, whether oral or written, may include any exculpatory language through which the subject or the representative is made to waive or appear to waive any of the subject's rights, or releases or appears to release the investigator, the sponsor, the institution, or its agents from liability for negligence."

The informed consent document (ICF) is a written form prepared by the investigator or sponsor which details the risks, benefits, and responsibilities of the research participant and the sponsor of the clinical trial. The form serves to document the discussion that the consenting investigator must have with the participant, allowing him/her the opportunity to ask questions and ensure that the subject understands what is involved in participating in the trial.

Required components of the informed consent document include (1) a statement that the study involves research, explanation of the research, and a description of the procedures involved in the study and expresses explanation of what is considered "experimental," (2) a description of known or anticipated possible risks or discomfort that a subject may experience, (3) a description of any benefit that the study may provide to the subject or to other patients in the future, (4) an explanation of other reasonable treatment options/alternatives that are available to the patient, (5) an explanation of confidentiality of the study records, and (6) an explanation of any compensation and, if more than minimal risk is involved, what remedies or treatments are available in the event of illness or injury and who to contact/how to report any injury or illness that might result from participation. The ICF should specifically detail if required care would be billed to the patient's insurance, covered directly by the sponsor, and what would occur if study participation was terminated due to an adverse event [12].

Pediatric Considerations

For pediatric patients, both parental permission and patient assent are required in most cases. The risks and benefits of proposed pediatric participation in a research study should be discussed in detail with the parent or legal guardian of the pediatric subject. The parent or guardian must provide their permission on an informed consent document, to permit their child to participate in research. Assent refers to the willingness of the child to participate. The IRB, when considering procedures for enrollment in a given study, will determine the age at which pediatric subjects' assent will be required. Typically, some degree of assent should be solicited once the child possesses the intellectual and emotional ability to

comprehend the concepts involved. The age at which this occurs varies based on the clinical situation and research in question. However, the guiding principle is that when a child is capable of understanding the nature of participation, assent must be sought. Waiving the requirement for assent should only be considered in well-defined circumstances, such as if the child's capacity for understanding is so limited that they cannot be consulted, if the intervention holds the prospect of direct benefit or well-being to the child and is only available in the context of the research, or if the research meets other conditions for waiver of informed consent for adults, as specified in the regulations [13].

Adverse Event Reporting

The clinical trial protocol should provide specific guidelines for the collection and reporting of adverse events that may occur during the trial. Adverse events will generally be reported by the investigator to the IRB, and a subset of such events must be reported promptly to the FDA. Reportable events include serious adverse events (SAEs), defined in the Code of Federal Regulations, including death, life-threatening illness, hospitalization, disability or permanent damage, congenital anomaly or birth defect, or other serious events such as those where intervention was required to prevent permanent impairment [14]. In general, events must be reported to the IRB if they are unanticipated and serious and may have implications for the continuing trial. For clinical trials conducted under an IND application, a sponsor is also required to notify the FDA in a written safety report of "any adverse experience associated with the use of the drug that is both serious and unexpected [15]."

Data Monitoring Committee

An independent data monitoring committee (DMC) may be formed to assist in the conduct and analysis of data in a clinical trial. A DMC may be appropriate for trials of long duration (when interim analysis would be appropriate and important), for trials with endpoints that include survival/mortality (where a finding of futility may require early termination of a study), in trials that involve vulnerable populations (such as elderly patients, children, or patients with disabilities), in trials involving treatment that is high risk to subjects, and in large, multicenter trials. The goal of a DMC is to evaluate incoming/cumulative data on an ongoing basis and provide feedback to the sponsor regarding the continuing safety of the trial participants, as well as the ongoing validity and benefit of continuing the trial [16].

Highlights of the Regulatory Review Process

In the USA, the first regulatory step in drug development is the submission of an Investigational New Drug (IND) application to the FDA. They are categorized as commercial (utilized for a drug that will ultimately seek marketing approval) and noncommercial research.

Current Federal law prohibits transportation or distribution of unapproved drugs across states lines. The IND provides an exemption from that legal requirement for investigational drugs. Further, the IND provides the FDA with the necessary data to ensure the potential safety of investigational products. Once an IND application is submitted, current regulations require that the applicant not commence clinical trials until 30 days of elapse; during that time the FDA makes a determination regarding the safety of the planned clinical trials. IND applications must provide animal pharmacology and toxicology data, manufacturing information, clinical protocols, and investigator information.

For the purposes of developing a new drug that will ultimately seek marketing approval, a commercial investigator IND is submitted. This type of application seeks permission to begin the first human trials of an investigational drug in the USA.

Noncommercial INDs are used to gain access to an investigational drug for research or limited treatment purposes. This may occur under a noncommercial investigator, emergency use, or treatment IND.

An investigator IND is submitted by the person who actually conducts the investigation and under whose immediate direction the investigational drug is administered or dispensed. This type of application may be utilized when an academic researcher wishes to study the effects of an investigational drug in a particular patient population, though he/she is not necessarily connected to the pharmaceutical company that is developing the drug.

An emergency use IND allows the FDA to authorize limited use of an experimental drug in an emergency clinical situation that does not allow time for submission of an IND. This situation may occur when there is no acceptable approved medical treatment for a given condition, and a prescribing physician wishes to seek permission to treat a patient or limited number of patients with an unapproved agent.

A treatment IND is submitted for experimental drugs showing promise in clinical testing for serious or immediately life-threatening conditions, while the final clinical work is conducted and the FDA review takes place. A treatment IND may be utilized to allow patients who are completing a phase III trial access to continue the drug, until final approval is obtained [17].

Once a sponsor has completed all investigations, the next step in the regulatory process is the submission of a new drug application (NDA). Utilizing the information submitted as part of the NDA, the FDA reviewer must reach the following conclusions:

- *Whether the drug is safe and effective in its proposed use(s) and whether the benefits of the drug outweigh the risks*
- *Whether the drug's proposed labeling (package insert) is truthful and not misleading and what it should contain*
- *Whether the methods used in manufacturing the drug and the controls used to maintain the drug's quality are adequate to preserve the drug's identity, strength, quality, and purity* [18]

Similar to the NDA, used for approval of drugs, a biologics license application (BLA) is a request for permission to "introduce, or deliver for introduction, a biologic product into interstate commerce [19]." The BLA should contain enough information for an FDA reviewer to reach the same conclusions (listed above) for drugs.

Regulatory Safeguards for Pediatric Patients Involved in Clinical Trials

Pediatric patients are considered a vulnerable population, and their participation in clinical trials requires specific safeguards that are detailed in regulation. For any clinical research involving pediatric patients, the Code of Federal Regulations provides specific criteria that an institutional review board (IRB) must rely upon to make decisions regarding the approval, monitoring, and review of biomedical and behavioral research. These criteria are listed below.

Criteria for IRB Approval of Pediatric Research

1. Research not involving greater than minimal risk to the children [20].
2. Research involving greater than minimal risk but presenting the prospect of direct benefit to the individual child subjects involved in the research [21].
3. Research involving greater than minimal risk and no prospect of direct benefit to the individual child subjects involved in the research, but likely to yield generalizable knowledge about the subject's disorder or condition. This type of trial must only represent a minor increase over minimal risk [22].
4. Research that the IRB believes does not meet the other conditions but finds that the research presents a reasonable opportunity to further the understanding, prevention, or alleviation of a serious problem affecting the health or welfare of children (this trial requires a special level of governmental review beyond that provided by the IRB) [23].

As a general rule, children should not be enrolled in a clinical investigation unless their enrollment is necessary to achieve important scientific and/or public health objective(s) directly benefiting children.

Pediatric Extrapolation

Given the unique challenges of conducting pediatric clinical trials, including the vulnerabilities of the pediatric population, ethical limitations on participation, and logistical challenges of studying children, the concept of pediatric extrapolation was developed. The goal of extrapolation is to leverage the available data from adult trials and to minimize the size and scope of the trials needed in pediatric patients, while still maintaining a standard of evidence to support safe use of drugs in pediatric patients.

The Pediatric Research Equity Act of 2007 states that "if the course of the disease and the effects of the drug are sufficiently similar in adults and pediatric patients, the Secretary may conclude that pediatric effectiveness can be extrapolated from adequate and well-controlled studies in adults, usually supplemented with other information obtained in pediatric patients, such as pharmacokinetic studies." It should be noted that only effectiveness (not safety) can be extrapolated.

The following algorithm illustrates the pathway used to determine if and when extrapolation may be appropriate [24].

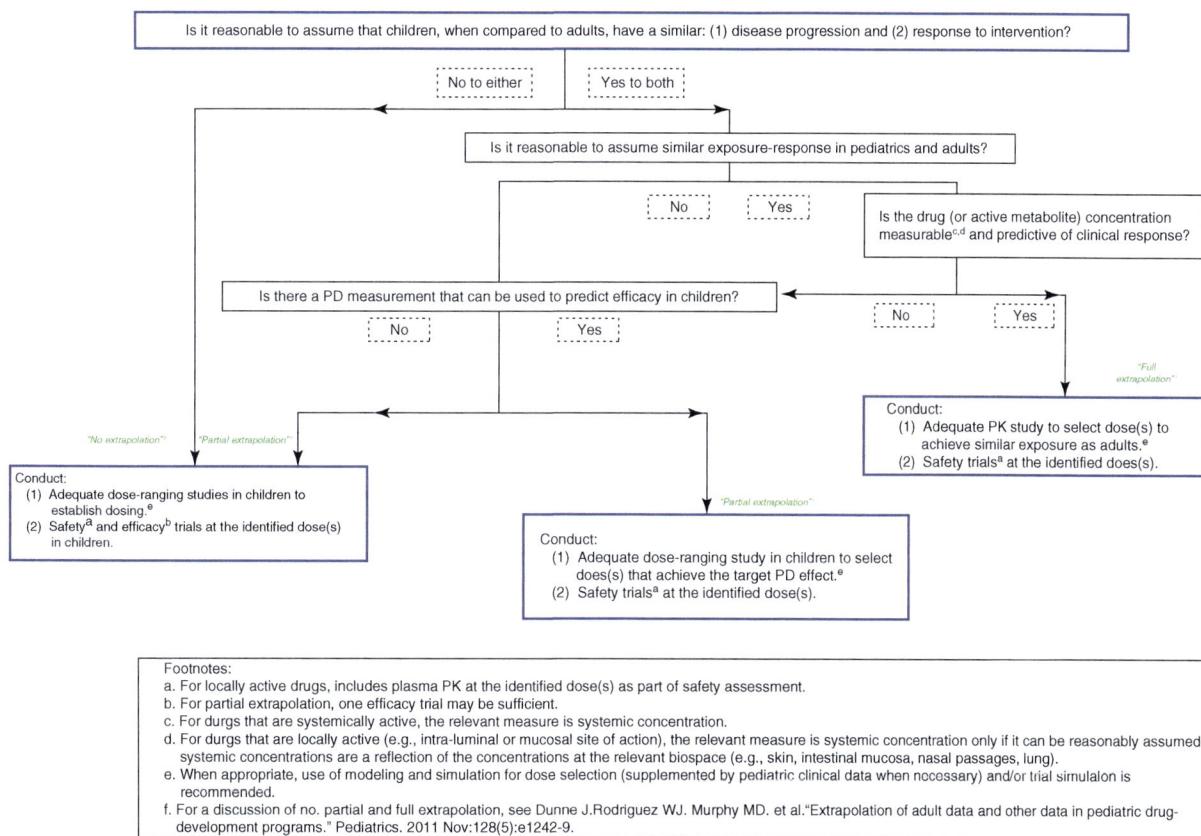

Is it reasonable to assume that children, when compared to adults, have a similar: (1) disease progression and (2) response to intervention?

No to either / Yes to both

Is it reasonable to assume similar exposure-response in pediatrics and adults?

No / Yes

Is the drug (or active metabolite) concentration measurable[c,d] and predictive of clinical response?

Is there a PD measurement that can be used to predict efficacy in children?

No / Yes

No / Yes

"Full extrapolation"

"No extrapolation" / *"Partial extrapolation"*

Conduct:
(1) Adequate dose-ranging studies in children to establish dosing.[e]
(2) Safety[a] and efficacy[b] trials at the identified dose(s) in children.

"Partial extrapolation"

Conduct:
(1) Adequate dose-ranging study in children to select does(s) that achieve the target PD effect.[e]
(2) Safety trials[a] at the identified dose(s).

Conduct:
(1) Adequate PK study to select dose(s) to achieve similar exposure as adults.[e]
(2) Safety trials[a] at the identified does(s).

Footnotes:
a. For locally active drugs, includes plasma PK at the identified dose(s) as part of safety assessment.
b. For partial extrapolation, one efficacy trial may be sufficient.
c. For durgs that are systemically active, the relevant measure is systemic concentration.
d. For durgs that are locally active (e.g., intra-luminal or mucosal site of action), the relevant measure is systemic concentration only if it can be reasonably assumed that systemic concentrations are a reflection of the concentrations at the relevant biospace (e.g., skin, intestinal mucosa, nasal passages, lung).
e. When appropriate, use of modeling and simulation for dose selection (supplemented by pediatric clinical data when necessary) and/or trial simulalon is recommended.
f. For a discussion of no. partial and full extrapolation, see Dunne J.Rodriguez WJ. Murphy MD. et al."Extrapolation of adult data and other data in pediatric drug-development programs." Pediatrics. 2011 Nov:128(5):e1242-9.

From FDA's Draft Guidance for Industry: General Clinical Pharmacology Considerations for Pediatric Studies for Drugs and Biological Products, Dec 2014

For conditions where the disease progression and response to intervention are expected to be similar between pediatric patients and adults, extrapolation may be appropriate. In this setting, depending on the degree of similarity and availability of exposure-response data in children and adults, a determination will be made as to how much additional safety and efficacy data are needed to support use of the drug in pediatric patients. Applying the extrapolation approach may reduce the burden on pediatric patients, by requiring fewer efficacy studies or smaller studies, and/or pharmacokinetic and safety studies only, depending on the disease process in question.

Pediatric-Specific Issues in IBD Trials

Using the general pediatric drug development principles described above, the development of drugs for the treatment of IBD in pediatric patients continues to evolve. In the USA, approvals for IBD products in adults continue to outnumber pediatric approvals. Pediatric approvals lag behind those for adults by a number of years, effectively restricting access to the newest advances in therapies for pediatric patients. Important pediatric IBD drug development program considerations include, but are not limited to, use of extrapolation, adequate dose selection, use of placebo arm, the burden of repeat endoscopies, and measuring outcomes that matter to patients.

A claim of efficacy requires a product demonstrate a meaningful change in a prespecified measurable endpoint. In inflammatory bowel disease, there have been a variety of different indices utilized to measure clinical response to therapy in drug trials. For example, a published review of pediatric trial data submitted to the FDA from 1950 to 2008 of products used to treat patients with ulcerative colitis (UC) identified three disease activity indices utilized as endpoint measures for the three pediatric UC products approved during that time (Colazal, Remicade, and Azulfidine). The Modified Sutherland UC Activity Index (MUCAI) was used for the Colazal pediatric trial (2006) [25]. The Mayo score and the Pediatric UC Activity Index (PUCAI) were used for the Remicade pediatric trial (2011) [26]. It should be noted that Azulfidine was initially approved for UC in 1950 and granted pediatric approval in 2009 based on full extrapolation of efficacy from adult trials; therefore, no pediatric trial was conducted. The results of this review suggest that there exists a lack of consensus on the most appropriate primary endpoint for pediatric UC trials, and the same problem exists in the study of Crohn disease [27]. Considerable debate continues in the field as to the definition of clinical response and/or remission and how best to measure it. Historically, endoscopic appearance of the mucosa was considered the gold standard for evaluating response to therapy in an IBD trial. Others have suggested that mucosal healing, as described on histology specimens (and so requiring biopsy), is the preferred endpoint of interest. Particularly in pediatric patients, where it is necessary to limit the number of endoscopies during a trial, less invasive measures of disease activity are becoming increasingly important. However, from a regulatory standpoint, the use of a noninvasive endpoint, or biomarker, introduces additional complexity. A biomarker must first be clearly demonstrated to correlate well with the outcome of interest, before it can be qualified for use in a trial that will support product labeling [27].

To quantify meaningful changes in signs and symptoms, patient-reported outcome (PRO) and observer-reported outcome (ObsRO) instruments can be used. Changes in symptoms are subjective, however, so standardization of the definitions of the symptoms of interest and carefully designed tools for their measurement are crucial. FDA has recently published guidance for industry on their development and use ("Guidance for Industry: Patient-Reported Outcome Measures: Use in Medical Product Development to Support Labeling Claims") [28].

The gold standard of evidence to support a claim of efficacy involves a double-blind, placebo-controlled clinical trial. However, inclusion of a placebo arm in a pediatric trial, particularly for patients who have a serious chronic medical condition such as inflammatory bowel disease, is controversial. Trial design is evolving over time to minimize exposure to placebo and risk from lack of treatment for patients. This may include use of an open-label induction period, followed by randomized withdrawal phase, use of an active comparator instead of placebo, or the use of randomization rates of more than 1:1, to minimize the number of subjects receiving placebo.

Given the lack of consensus across countries and regulatory agencies, international consensus regarding pediatric IBD trial outcome measures would facilitate drug development. In an attempt to develop a consensus statement regarding pediatric UC trial outcome measures, the *i*-IBD Working Group was convened in 2012 by scientists from the US Food and Drug Administration, European Medicines Agency, Health Canada, and the Pharmaceuticals and Medical Devices Agency of Japan. The *i*-IBD Working Group "concluded that outcome measurements in pediatric UC trials must account for both endoscopic disease activity of UC and improvement of signs and symptoms." The group also recommended that assessment of signs and symptoms be used as a co-primary endpoint in pediatric UC trials in conjunction with endoscopic parameters of mucosal appearance to assess disease severity [29]. A similar approach should be taken for Crohns disease.

Studying drugs to treat IBD in children presents a number of challenges, though they are not unique to this disease process. Careful assessment of study design, judicious use of placebo arm, limiting invasive procedures during the trial, consideration of patients' reported symptoms, and increasing collaboration internationally and across various regulatory agencies are all measures that will contribute toward advancing drug development in the field.

References

1. Meadows M. Promoting safe and effective drugs for 100 years. FDA Consumer magazine. Jan-Feb 2006. http://www.fda.gov/AboutFDA/WhatWeDo/History/CentennialofFDA/CentennialEditionofFDAConsumer/ucm093787.htm.

2. Ballentine C. Taste of raspberries, taste of death- the 1937 elixir sulfanilamide incident. FDA consumer magazine. June 1981. http://www.fda.gov/aboutfda/whatwedo/history/productregulation/sulfanilamidedisaster/default.htm.

3. Fintel B, Samaras A, Carias E. The thalidomide tragedy: lessons for drug safety and regulation. Helix Magazine. Jul 2009. https://helix.northwestern.edu/article/thalidomide-tragedy-lessons-drug-safety-and-regulation.

4. Kefauver-Harris Amendments Revolutionized Drug Development. FDA consumer updates. 2012. http://www.fda.gov/ForConsumers/ConsumerUpdates/ucm322856.htm.

5. Kesselheim A. Innovation and the Orphan Drug Act, 1983–2009: regulatory and clinical characteristics of approved orphan drugs. Rare diseases and orphan products: accelerating research and development. Marilyn J Field; Thomas F Boat editors. National Academies Press. 2010. http://www.ncbi.nlm.nih.gov/books/NBK56189/.
6. United States. Food and Drug Administration. *FDA backgrounder on FDAMA*. http://www.fda.gov/RegulatoryInformation/Legislation/SignificantAmendmentstotheFDCAct/FDAMA/ucm089179.htm.
7. United States. National Institutes for Health. Best pharmaceuticals for children act. http://bpca.nichd.nih.gov/Pages/Index.aspx.
8. http://blogs.fda.gov/fdavoice/index.php/tag/pediatric-research-equity-act-prea/.
9. Bigelow R. Chapter 5. Introduction to clinical experimentation. In: Lopes RD, Harrington RA, editors. Understanding clinical research. New York:McGraw-Hill; 2013. http://accessmedicine.mhmedical.com/content.aspx?bookid=674&Sectionid=45407247. Accessed 06 July 2016.
10. Guptill JT, Chiswell K. Chapter 7. Phase II clinical trials. In: Lopes RD, Harrington RA, editors. Understanding clinical research. New York: McGraw-Hill; 2013. http://accessmedicine.mhmedical.com/content.aspx?bookid=674&Sectionid=45407250. Accessed 06 July 2016.
11. Hafley GE, Leonardi S, Pieper KS. Chapter 8. Phase III and IV clinical trials. In: Lopes RD, Harrington RA, editors. Understanding clinical research. New York: McGraw-Hill; 2013. http://accessmedicine.mhmedical.com/content.aspx?bookid=674&Sectionid=45407252. Accessed 06 July 2016.
12. United States. Food and Drug Administration. A guide to informed consent- guidance for institutional review boards and clinical investigators. http://www.fda.gov/RegulatoryInformation/Guidances/ucm126431.htm#general.
13. United States. Department of Health and Human Services, Office of Human Research Protections. Research with children FAQs. http://www.hhs.gov/ohrp/regulations-and-policy/guidance/faq/children-research/index.html#.
14. Code of Federal Regulations, Investigational new drug applications, title 21, section 312.32.
15. United States. Food and Drug Administration. Guidance for clinical ynvestigators, sponsors and IRBs- adverse event reporting to IRBs, enhancing human subject protection. 2009. http://www.fda.gov/downloads/RegulatoryInformation/Guidances/UCM126572.pdf.
16. United States. Food and Drug Administration. The establishment and operation of clinical trial data monitoring committees for clinical trial sponsors- guidance for clinical trial sponsors. 2006. http://www.fda.gov/downloads/RegulatoryInformation/Guidances/ucm127073.pdf
17. United States. Food and Drug Administration. Investigational New Drug (IND) application. 2016. http://www.fda.gov/Drugs/
DevelopmentApprovalProcess/HowDrugsareDevelopedandApproved/ApprovalApplications/InvestigationalNewDrugINDApplication/default.htm.
18. United States. Food and Drug Administration. Investigational New Drug (IND) application. 2016. http://www.fda.gov/Drugs/DevelopmentApprovalProcess/HowDrugsareDevelopedandApproved/ApprovalApplications/InvestigationalNewDrugINDApplication/default.htm.
19. Code of Federal Regulations, Licensing, title 21, section 601.2.
20. Code of Federal Regulations, Protection of Human Subjects, title 45, section 46.404.
21. Code of Federal Regulations, Protection of Human Subjects, title 45, section 46.405.
22. Code of Federal Regulations, Protection of Human Subjects, title 45, section 46.406.
23. Code of Federal Regulations, Protection of Human Subjects, title 45, section 46.407.
24. United States. Food and Drug Administration. General clinical pharmacology considerations for pediatric studies for drugs and biological products. Guidance for industry. Draft guidance. 2014. http://www.fda.gov/downloads/drugs/guidancecomplianceregulatoryinformation/guidances/ucm425885.pdf.
25. Quiros JA, Heyman MB, Pohl JF, Attard TM, Pieniaszek HJ, Bortey E, Walker K, Forbes WP. Safety, efficacy, and pharmacokinetics of balsalazide in pediatric patients with mild-to-moderate active ulcerative colitis: results of a randomized, double-blind study. J Pediatr Gastroenterol Nutr. 2009;49(5):571–9.
26. Hyams J, Damaraju L, Blank M, Johanns J, Guzzo C, HS W, Kugathasan S, Cohen S, Markowitz J, JC E, Veereman-Wauters G, Crandall W, Baldassano R, Griffiths A, T72 Study Group. Induction and maintenance therapy with infliximab for children with moderate to severe ulcerative colitis. Clin Gastroenterol Hepatol. 2012;10(4):391–9. e1
27. Sun H, Lee JJ, Papadopoulos EJ, Lee CS, Nelson RM, Sachs HC, Rodriguez WJ, Mulberg AE. Alternate endpoints and clinical outcome assessments in pediatric ulcerative colitis registration trials. JPGN. 2014;58:12–7. http://www.fda.gov/downloads/Drugs/GuidanceComplianceRegulatoryInformation/Guidances/UCM230597.pdf
28. United States. Food and Drug Administration. Guidance for industry. Patient reported outcome measures: use in medical product development to support labeling claims. 2009. www.fda.gov/downloads/Drugs/Guidances/UCM193282.pdf.
29. Sun H, Vesely R, Taminiau J, Szitanyi P, Papadopoulos E, Isaac M, Klein A, et al. Steps toward harmonization for clinical development of medicines in pediatric ulcerative colitis—a global scientific discussion, part 1: efficacy endpoints and disease outcome assessments. JPGN. 2014;58(6):679–83. doi:10.1097/MPG.0000000000000306.

Monica I. Ardura and Sandra C. Kim

Introduction

The role of infections in inflammatory bowel disease (IBD) pathogenesis remains incompletely understood. Current hypotheses suggest that pathogenic or commensal gut flora act as potential cross-reactive antigens leading to a dysregulated immune response that may trigger both primary disease and relapses in IBD [1]. Animal models have demonstrated that bacterial colonization is a prerequisite for the development of intestinal inflammation in susceptible hosts, but proof of causation in humans is lacking [2, 3]. Although the exact role of microbes in causing IBD remains to be clarified, infections do play an important role in the clinical course and management of patients with IBD. Infections may be a presenting manifestation of IBD and may exacerbate disease activity. Herein, we will focus on the infections that may occur as complications of the primary inflammatory disease or secondary to therapeutic modalities including surgery and pharmacologic therapies that modulate immune system activity.

Much of the data regarding infections in patients with IBD is extrapolated from reports of clinical trials and population-based observational studies in adults; the pediatric data is limited to reported adverse events in pharmaco-epidemiological and registry studies as well case series that are specific for a pathogen or immunomodulatory therapy [4, 5, 6]. The lack of large, population-based cohort studies in the pediatric IBD population makes it difficult to reliably calculate and compare rates of infections. Factors predisposing patients with IBD to infectious complications include severity of underlying IBD, medical comorbidities, malnutrition, abdominal surgery, and immunosuppressive medications. When compared with adults with IBD, children with IBD have more extensive luminal disease, are more likely to require systemic steroids, and typically have a more severe disease course [7, 8]. These differences, coupled with a higher likelihood of acquiring primary infections during childhood and increasing use of combination immunomodulator and biologic therapies, may place pediatric patients with IBD at risk of infectious complications.

Antibiotic Use for Treatment of IBD Based on the rationale that antibiotics could potentially medically modulate and suppress the host inflammatory response to commensal or pathogenic gut flora [9], their clinical use has preceded evidence-based data. Antibiotics have been utilized broadly for the treatment of IBD luminal and fistulizing disease, maintenance of disease remission, treatment of abscesses, and as prophylactic therapy to prevent postoperative recurrences [10]. Much of the data is derived from patients with Crohn disease (CD); the presence of transmural inflammation in CD is an inherent risk factor for formation of fistulae and possible perianal disease. Indeed, the incidence of perianal CD in children is estimated to be 10–62 %, but the exact role of putative bacteria and data for therapeutic benefit for antibiotics for nonsuppurative perianal disease is unclear. Perianal fistula and abscesses may represent sterile inflammation or be infectious; small studies describing the microbiology of perianal fistulas have differing results with important antibiotic implications [11, 12, 13].

In tertiary pediatric centers in the USA, there is a wide practice variation of antibiotic prescribing for children hospitalized with IBD exacerbations, varying from 27 to 71 % [14]. This heterogeneity in antimicrobial use is likely a reflection of lack of robust efficacy data in the published literature. Systematic reviews of the available small,

M.I. Ardura, DO, MSCS (✉)
Division of Infectious Diseases and Immunology,
Host Defense Program, Nationwide Children's Hospital,
700 Children's Hospital, Columbus, OH 43205, USA
e-mail: monica.ardura@nationwidechildrens.org

S.C. Kim, MD
Division of Gastroenterology, Hepatology, and Nutrition,
Center for Pediatric and Adolescent Inflammatory Bowel Disease,
Nationwide Children's Hospital, 700 Children's Hospital,
Columbus, OH 43205, USA

randomized trials in adults evaluating the efficacy of antibiotic therapy in helping to induce remission or prevent relapse in IBD have variable results given distinct methodologies, early and differing endpoints, case definitions and disease severities, and utilization of different antibiotics (single or dual), sometimes in combination with other therapies [15, 16, 17]. When evaluating pooled antibiotic use, patients who received antibiotics, compared to placebo, were more likely to have induction of remission of active UC and CD and fewer relapses in patients with colonic but not isolated small bowel CD [15]. However, the varied antibiotics used in these trials (predominantly metronidazole and ciprofloxacin) preclude firm conclusions.

In three randomized controlled trials (RCT) evaluating antibiotics to treat perianal fistulas, the use of metronidazole or ciprofloxacin demonstrated a trend toward reducing fistula drainage in patients with CD (RR 0.8, 95 % CI 0.66–0.98, not statistically significant) [16]. Despite lack of controlled studies and conclusive efficacy data in children, pediatric treatment algorithms also recommend antibiotics for perianal fistulizing disease [18, 19]. The role of antibiotics to prevent postoperative recurrence of ileal or ileocolonic CD is unclear, though there is a trend of reduced risk for clinical and endoscopic recurrence in patients who received metronidazole over those who received placebo [20]. The optimal approach to the prevention of postoperative recurrence is unknown, and no clear prophylactic strategy is preferred [21]. There is evidence to suggest that initiation of immunomodulatory therapies for patients in higher-risk disease categories may decrease postoperative CD recurrence [22, 23].

There is even less data regarding efficacy of antibiotics for UC than CD. In clinical trials of adults who presented with severe UC, there were no differences in outcomes when intravenous empirical antibiotics were used as adjuncts to steroid therapy [24]. Therefore, in children with severe UC, empiric antibiotics are not recommended unless an infection, such as C. difficile, is suspected, pending diagnostic testing results, or in the presence of toxic megacolon. Clinical benefit of antibiotics (ciprofloxacin alone or in combination with metronidazole or rifaximin) has been observed in some trials for pouchitis, the most common complication after ileal pouch-anal anastomosis in patients with UC [25]. In addition, there is evidence to suggest that VSL#3, a probiotic preparation, decreases pouchitis in patients with UC postcolectomy [26].

To further illustrate the complex interaction of infection, the microbiome, mucosal immunity, and IBD, a recent genome-wide association study demonstrated that in a small subset of children with newly diagnosed CD, short-term (<3 months) antibiotic use prior to IBD diagnosis amplified the microbial dysbiosis associated with CD by decreasing presumed protective bacterial species [27]. Thus, at the present time, there is insufficient data to recommend universal use of antibiotics for inducing or maintaining remission in active IBD. Many of the antibiotics used may exert a potential benefit because of their immunomodulatory properties, including suppressing tumor necrosis factor alpha synthesis, and not by direct antimicrobial effects on the microbiome [28]. Altering the gut microbiome with the use of antimicrobials may indeed have a role in modulating primary IBD activity but requires further rigorous prospective, controlled investigation.

Infections Associated with Underlying IBD

Antimicrobials do however have an established role in the management of patients with IBD for microbiologically proven infectious complications of underlying disease, including intra-abdominal abscesses. Evidence-based guidelines for empirical antimicrobial therapy of intra-abdominal abscesses have been put forth by the Surgical Infection Society and Infectious Diseases Society of America [29]. In high-risk patients with complicated intra-abdominal infections, including those who are considered immunocompromised, empiric therapy with cefepime and metronidazole or piperacillin-tazobactam monotherapy is appropriate; a carbapenem (e.g., meropenem) is preferred in patients with a prior history of infection with extended spectrum beta-lactamase (ESBL)-producing Enterobacteriaceae. Targeted antimicrobial therapy should be further guided by microbiologic culture data, local epidemiology, and patient's history of bacterial colonization and resistance patterns. Visceral abscesses, frequently in the liver, have been described, particularly in patients with CD; these may occur alone and unrelated to hepatobiliary disease or as a complication of an intra-abdominal infection or cholangitis [30]. Results of aerobic and anaerobic bacterial cultures obtained from drainable abscesses help guide antimicrobial therapy. Patients with IBD may also be at higher risk for urinary stone formation leading to urinary tract infections and have a higher disease severity than patients with urinary stones who do not have underlying IBD [31]. In addition, some infections may mimic IBD lesions or occur concurrently in patients with underlying IBD. In particular, sexually transmitted infections like syphilis and lymphogranuloma venereum can cause proctocolitis and lead to rectal lesions resembling CD [32]. Thus, a high index of suspicion and appropriate diagnostic testing should be performed in sexually active adolescents with IBD who are not responding to standard therapies.

Patients with IBD may be more prone to infections of the gastrointestinal tract due to microbial dysbiosis or impaired epithelial barrier function [33]. Enteric infections may mimic, be a presenting symptom of, or lead to exacerbation of IBD; most cases of infectious colitis are caused by bacterial enteropathogens. For example, Yersinia spp. can classically cause an acute ileitis indistinguishable clinically from acute Crohn ileitis. As such, it is recommended that patients with a clinical presentation concerning for IBD or with previously diagnosed IBD presenting with diarrhea, especially if bloody, should have diagnostic testing performed for bacterial pathogens, including *C. difficile,* and receive appropriate antimicrobial therapy [19, 24].

Rates of infection in children with IBD are difficult to discern given diverse testing modalities of varied sensitivities, overall prevalence of disease, and clinical indications for testing (screening or worsening colitis symptoms). Further, there is a wide variation in diagnostic practices among gastroenterologists caring for children with IBD; a survey of pediatric gastroenterologists confirmed that 29 % of children undergoing an initial evaluation for colitis symptoms and possible CD did not have stool testing performed [34]. In a large study of US children presenting with newly diagnosed UC, the diagnostic yield of routine enteropathogenic stool testing was retrospectively evaluated; testing included bacterial stool culture including *Yersinia,* ova and parasite examination, Giardia and *Cryptosporidium* antigen, *C. difficile* toxin A/B by PCR, and viral testing (by culture, rotavirus EIA, quantitative adenovirus PCR, viral culture for adenovirus, cytomegalovirus (CMV), and enterovirus) and electron microscopic examination [35]. In 863 test samples from 152 pediatric patients with UC, *C. difficile* was the most commonly detected organism in 13.6 % of samples, followed by adenovirus (1/13, 7.7 %), non-typhoidal *Salmonella* species (4/220, 1.8 %), and parasites (2/151, 1.3 %). In other retrospective cohort studies from the USA and Europe, children with IBD and diarrheal relapse in whom stool was evaluated by a combination of microscopy, bacterial culture, and/or detection of *C. difficile* toxin, 10–20 % of relapses were associated with infections, most commonly *C. difficile* and *Campylobacter* spp. [36, 37]. When evaluating for parasitic infections in 149 children presenting with IBD flares, systematic testing detected *Cryptosporidium* by enzyme immunoassay in 4.6 % of patients (7/149) [38]. More unusual enteric infections with mycobacteria, including *Mycobacterium tuberculosis,* which has a proclivity for the terminal ileum and cecum and nontubercular mycobacteria, or fungi such as histoplasmosis, require additional diagnostic testing (culture, staining, and PCR evaluation) to distinguish the granulomatous inflammation of infection from underlying IBD. Although the diagnostic yield of testing for enteric pathogens seems to be low, a high index of suspicion and eliciting epidemiological risk factors are important to perform diagnostic testing and prescribe targeted antimicrobials.

Lack of judicious antibiotic use may also promote proliferation of resistant bacterial strains or increase the risk of other infections, such as *Clostridium difficile. C. difficile* is an important cause of antibiotic-associated diarrhea and a frequent cause of healthcare-associated infection in the United States, with a rising incidence in pediatrics [39, 40, 41]. Patients with IBD have been found to be at increased

risk of *C. difficile* infection (CDI) [42]. Risk factors for CDI in adults and children with IBD include hospitalization, previous antibiotic therapy, immunomodulatory medications, use of proton pump inhibitors, and presence of severe colonic disease. Patients with IBD receiving immunomodulators and corticosteroids may be at higher risk of CDI (corticosteroid use RR 3.4, 95 % CI 1.9–6.1); TNF-α inhibitors do not seem to increase this risk [43]. However, some patients with IBD develop CDI without any identifiable risk factors.

In children with IBD, CDI is prevalent, as documented by the disproportionate increase in *C. difficile*-associated hospitalizations. Additionally, risk factors in this pediatric subpopulation may differ [44, 45]. In addition to increased *C. difficile* detection using molecular diagnostics (e.g. *C. difficile* PCR), pediatric IBD patients with CDI were also found to have active colonic disease and a more severe disease course [46]. Currently, it is recommended that all IBD patients who require hospitalization for disease flare undergo testing for *C. difficile* and if severe colitis is present, empirically started on antimicrobial therapy; further, escalation of immunosuppression should be avoided in the setting of untreated CDI, if clinically possible [47].

Although the increasing incidence and severity of CDI has been related in part to the emergence of the North American pulsed-field type 1 (NAP1) strain that produces more toxin, some of the increase in CDI incidence may be related to changing diagnostic modalities from cell culture cytotoxicity neutralization assays to enzyme immunoassays (specific but lacking sensitivity) and most recently to highly sensitive molecular assays. Clinicians should be aware of the method and details of *C. difficile* testing performed at their institutions to improve the clinical interpretation of results in pediatric patients [48].

The detection of *C. difficile* by PCR methodology, although sensitive for infection, may not be specific for disease [49]. The majority of molecular tests detect *C. difficile* toxin genes (A, B, or both) that are present, but do not detect actual toxin production which is required for CDI disease pathogenesis. Thus, in children *C. difficile* toxin gene detection by PCR does not distinguish between *C. difficile* colonization (detection of *C. difficile* in an asymptomatic patient) and *C. difficile* disease (detection of *C. difficile* in a patient with symptoms consistent with CDI, varying from mild diarrhea to fulminant colitis). Interpretation of *C. difficile* PCR testing is even more challenging in children with IBD, in whom worsening colitis may be from underlying disease, CDI, or both. *C. difficile* colonization in the US healthy adult population has been estimated to be 3–7 %, with rates of 4–20 % for individuals that require hospitalization [50]. High *C. difficile* colonization rates are known to occur in infants <1 year of age and young children; thus, testing for CDI is discouraged. Colonization rates in children older than 3 years of age have been estimated to be <5 % [51]. However, in asymptomatic patients with IBD, *C. difficile* carriage has been detected in 8 % of adults and 17 % of children and may be higher in patients with UC versus CD [52, 53, 54]. The possibility of overdiagnosing patients with CDI through the use of molecular testing has been corroborated in a large, prospective observational study of hospitalized adults, in whom *C. difficile* detection by molecular PCR results, but a negative toxin immunoassay had outcomes similar to patients with negative *C. difficile* testing by either method [55]. This represents a clinical conundrum to clinicians faced with a child with IBD, worsening colitis symptoms, and detection of *C. difficile*, where distinguishing colonization from disease in a time-sensitive fashion may not be possible. Additional prospective studies are required in pediatric IBD patients to reliably and accurately understand CDI.

The exact role of CMV infection in patients with IBD remains poorly defined, and CMV infection (detection of CMV) must be distinguished from disease (detection of CMV in the presence of clinical signs, symptoms, and evidence of end-organ involvement). Several studies have established an association between severe IBD (in particular steroid-refractory UC) and CMV disease with reported prevalence rates of 21–36 % [56, 57]. The diagnosis of active CMV colitis in patients with IBD is challenging and requires additional testing. Histopathology continues to be the gold standard for diagnosis, but may not always reveal the enlarged viral inclusion cells that are classic of CMV infection. To improve diagnostic sensitivity, immunohistochemical staining for CMV should also be performed on tissue specimens. In patients with steroid-refractory UC with unremitting symptoms who undergo lower endoscopy with biopsy, specimens should be sent for histopathology and immunohistochemical staining for CMV [24]. Similarly, detection by NAAT alone is insufficient to confirm CMV disease. Prospective studies are required to better define disease, establish prevalence, and determine which patients may benefit from antiviral treatment.

There remain many unanswered questions regarding the interface of infection and IBD. Further research that better classifies host and microbiome immune profiles may allow for improved diagnostic and management strategies, including prognosis and therapies [58, 59]. Recent genome-wide association studies link IBD to host-microbe pathways central to sensing/signaling and mucosal-initiated effector responses [60].

Increased Risk of Infections Secondary to Therapies

The pharmacologic treatment of IBD has changed significantly in the last years, with increasing use of immunomodulators and biologic therapies. The benefits of immunosuppressive treatment for IBD should be weighed against the potential risks, including infectious complications, in each individual patient before starting immunosuppressive therapies. This may be particularly important for patients with a history of chronic, recurrent, or opportunistic infection, for those with identifiable risk factors for infection, and for patients with other comorbid medical conditions that may predispose them to infections.

Infections have been associated with all immunosuppressive therapies for IBD, most frequently with systemic corticosteroid therapies, but also with antimetabolites, purine analogues, alkylating agents, and, more recently given an increase in their use, TNF-α inhibitors [61, 62]. Serious infections are defined as infections requiring hospitalization or parenteral antimicrobial therapy and any opportunistic infections. Risk factors for severe infections in patients with IBD have included young age, severity of underlying disease, and time-dependent exposure to immunosuppressive therapies, including immunomodulators and TNF-α inhibitors. In patients with IBD, monotherapy with corticosteroids (odds ratio, OR 3.4, 95 % confidence CI 1.8–6.2), azathioprine or 6-mercaptopurine (OR 3.1, 95 % CI 1.7–5.5), and infliximab (OR 4.4, 95 % CI 1.2–17.1) was associated with increased risk for opportunistic infections in univariate analysis [63]. Multivariate analyses confirmed this finding and, importantly, noted that the risk for infection was further increased 14-fold in patients receiving two or more of these immunosuppressive medications concomitantly (OR 14.5, 95 % CI 4.9–43). An increase in adverse infectious events, including opportunistic infections, in patients receiving combination immunosuppressive therapies has been confirmed in other IBD studies [64, 65]. Pediatric patients are considered to be severely immunocompromised if they have a known primary immunodeficiency disorder that affects phagocytic, cellular, or humoral immunity or have a secondary immunodeficiency from receipt of immunosuppressive therapies including high-dose systemic corticosteroids (defined as ≥ 2 mg/kg/day of body weight or ≥ 20 mg/day of prednisone for ≥ 14 days), methotrexate > 0.4 mg/kg/week, azathioprine > 3 mg/kg/day, 6-mercaptopurine > 1.5 mg/kg/day, and biologic agents (e.g., TNF-α inhibitors, anti-CD20) or are receiving combination immunosuppressive medications [66, 67].

Purine Analogues

Mercaptopurine and azathioprine are used for maintenance of remission in IBD. Purine analogues can directly alter cell-mediated immunity, resulting in viral and fungal infections. The incidence of infections in case series of patients receiving these therapies ranges from 0.3 to 7.4 %, most frequently with viral infections, particularly herpes viruses like varicella zoster virus (VZV), herpes simplex virus (HSV), Epstein-Barr virus (EBV), and cytomegalovirus (CMV) [68,

69, 70, 63]. These agents may also cause myelosuppression; the presence of leukopenia itself, even without thiopurine use, is associated with an increased risk of infection and sepsis. The duration and severity of neutropenia can also predispose to infections with bacteria (e.g., *Pseudomonas* spp.) and fungi (*Candida* and *Aspergillus* spp.), while severe lymphopenia (<600/μL) can lead to severe primary viral infections or viral reactivations [71, 72, 73]. The highest rates of infection, and most serious infections, were reported when thiopurines were used in combination with other immunosuppressive therapies.

Corticosteroids

Corticosteroids have a broad range of anti-inflammatory activities and have historically been a mainstay in IBD treatment. However, corticosteroids have been shown to be a major independent risk factor for the development of infections and infection-related mortality (OR 2.1, 95 % CI 1.15–3.83) [74]. In one study, the relative risk of infection in IBD patients receiving corticosteroids was 1.4 (95 % CI 1.1–1.9), with increasing risk at higher corticosteroid doses (>10 mg/day of prednisone) and duration of therapy beyond 14 days [75]. Not surprisingly, infections with multiple pathogens have been reported in association with corticosteroid use. In IBD patients, the use of systemic corticosteroid therapy has also been associated with increased rates of intra-abdominal abscesses in patients with both perforating (OR 9.03, 95 % CI 2.4–33.8) and non-penetrating diseases (OR 9.31, 95 % CI 1.03–83.91); this effect seemed to be dose dependent, with increasing abscess rates in patients receiving > 20 mg of prednisone/day [76, 77]. Similarly, postoperative complications were increased in patients receiving corticosteroids (pooled analysis OR 1.68, 95 % CI 1.24–2.28) and are up to twofold higher in patients receiving greater than 40 mg of oral corticosteroids prior to surgery [78].

Worsening severity of primary viral infections or reactivations are well-described complications of systemic corticosteroid use. In IBD patients, both primary varicella and zoster infections have been reported most frequently. In pediatric IBD patients, the use of corticosteroids as monotherapy (prednisone > 10 mg/day) or in combination with other immunosuppressant medications (TNF-α inhibitors or thiopurines) was associated with an increased risk of VZV infection, including severe infection, with a case fatality rate of 25 % [79]. Ideally, patients with IBD who have not received varicella vaccine or are known to be seronegative (VZV IgG negative) should receive the two doses of vaccine (with appropriate intervals between vaccine doses) at least 4 weeks before any immunosuppressive regimen is initiated [67]. Due to the recommended time interval between the first and second VZV vaccine dose, necessary vaccinations should ideally be provided at the time of IBD diagnosis to allow sufficient time to both mount a serologic response and not interfere with timing of immunosuppressive therapies. Infection prevention by optimizing vaccine-preventable infections is discussed further in Chap. 54.

Tumor Necrosis Factor-Alpha (TNF-α) Inhibitors

TNF-α is crucial to intracellular pathogen defense, ensuring a robust cell-mediated immune response. The majority of data regarding infections in patients receiving TNF-α inhibitors has been extrapolated from adults with IBD and other autoinflammatory diseases [80, 81]. It is not surprising that granulomatous infections secondary to *Mycobacteria* spp. and fungi (e.g., endemic species; *Candida; Aspergillus* and other molds; *Pneumocystis jirovecii*) and infections with intracellular bacteria (e.g., *Bartonella; Brucella; Listeria; Salmonella; Legionella; Nocardia*) have been reported in patients receiving TNF-α inhibitors [82]. The majority of these infections occurred in the first 6 months of starting infliximab and, in the case of mycobacterial infections, likely reflected reactivation of latent infection. Infections or reactivations with viruses, including hepatitis B, hepatitis C, and herpesviruses, have also been described [79, 83, 84, 85, 86].

The TNF-α inhibitors most commonly used for the treatment of IBD in children in which there is sufficient published data related to infection are infliximab and adalimumab. When compared with adults with IBD receiving TNF-α inhibitors, the overall incidence of reported serious infections in children with IBD receiving TNF-α inhibitors was significantly lower [62]. A recent systematic literature review of infections in children with IBD receiving TNF-α inhibitors reported a predominance of mild and mostly viral infections, with incidences of 3–77 % of cases; severe infections occurred less frequently but were varied, with incidences of 0–10 % [86].

An increased risk of mycobacterial and fungal infections has been associated with TNF-α inhibitor therapy. *Mycobacterium tuberculosis* is the most frequent granulomatous infection reported in patients treated with infliximab, and the risk is further increased when the TNF-α inhibitor is combined with other immunomodulators [87, 88, 89]. Infections with *M. tuberculosis* are more common than nontubercular mycobacterial infections. However, it is unknown to what extent TNF-α inhibitor therapy increases the risk of *M. tuberculosis* disease in children. Two cases of *M. tuberculosis* presenting with disseminated disease have been reported in children with IBD during infliximab therapy despite baseline nonreactive tuberculin skin testing [90, 91]. Current guidelines recommend screening for tuberculosis prior to initiating therapy with TNF-α inhibitors, though the optimal testing strategy is unknown [92, 66, 19, 24, 93]. Immunodiagnostic screening with both a tuberculin skin test (TST) and an Interferon-Gamma Release Assay (IGRA) at the time of IBD diagnosis and before initiation of any immunomodulatory therapies, particularly steroids and TNF-α inhibitors, will increase diagnostic sensitivity and allow for more optimal patient management [94, 95].

Histoplasmosis is the most common endemic mycosis in the USA, prevalent in the Ohio and Mississippi River valleys, and is the most common fungal infection associated with TNF-α therapy in adults and children, either as a newly acquired infection or by reactivation or reinfection [96, 81]. Histoplasmosis has been described in pediatric patients with IBD receiving TNF-α inhibitors [97, 98]. Importantly, IBD patients with histoplasmosis (and similarly with other endemic fungi) most frequently presented with nonspecific symptoms indistinguishable from IBD (fever, malaise, weight loss, abdominal pain) or had a pulmonary clinical manifestation similar to community-associated pneumonia, not responding to conventional antimicrobial therapy; thus, a high index of suspicion is warranted in patients receiving TNF-α inhibitors. Diagnostic testing should involve multiple testing modalities if possible, including histopathology, fungal tissue cultures, serologic testing, and antigen detection (in both blood and urine). The sensitivity and specificity of the different tests will depend on the clinical presentation (e.g., pulmonary vs. disseminated), infection severity, and timing of infection. In a patient with compatible signs and symptoms, a high diagnostic sensitivity may be achieved when both urine and serum antigen testing are performed concomitantly as well as serology (by immunodiffusion and complement fixation) [99]. Other fungal infections in patients with IBD receiving TNF-α inhibitor therapies have also been reported [100, 82, 101].

Pneumocystis jirovecii pneumonia (PCP) has been described in patients with IBD, most commonly CD, who receive high-dose steroids (even during the tapering phase), calcineurin inhibitors, and TNF-α inhibitors [102]. The crude incidence of PCP in IBD patients was estimated to be 10.6/100,000 in a health claims database; although PCP cases have been reported in children with IBD, the overall pediatric incidence is unknown [103]. However, given the higher mortality from PCP in the non-HIV population, PCP prophylaxis should be considered in high-risk children with IBD including those receiving multiple immunosuppressive agents (TNF-α inhibitor plus a calcineurin inhibitor, TNF-α inhibitor as part of a triple immunosuppression regimen, or combination therapies that include high-dose corticosteroids), malnourished children on combination immunosuppression therapies, and in young children <6 years of age with severe IBD in whom an underlying immunodeficiency disorder is possible [104, 105, 66].

TNF-α inhibition may facilitate the risk of primary viral infection and reactivation [106]. Reactivation of hepatitis B and hepatitis C or progression of viral liver disease has been described in patients receiving TNF-α inhibitors. Therefore, it is recommended that all patients with IBD be screened for hepatitis B prior to receipt of any TNF-α inhibitor; patients with risk factors or evidence of elevated transaminases should also be screened for hepatitis C [92, 107, 85, 108, 66]. In particular, reactivation of HBV after initiation of immunosuppressive therapy has been associated with significant morbidity and mortality. High- and moderate-risk patients who require therapy with TNF-α inhibitors and are hepatitis B surface antigen positive (or hepatitis B surface antigen negative but hepatitis B core antigen positive) and do not have liver injury may be candidates for antiviral prophylaxis and viral monitoring during biologic therapy [109]. In addition, VZV infections with rates of 11.3/1000 patient-years have been reported in patients with IBD receiving TNF-α inhibitors [110]. Primary varicella seems to occur more frequently in susceptible patients with CD than those with UC, and risk of disseminated disease is increased in patients receiving highly immunosuppressive therapies, with case fatality rates of up to 25 % [79]. Similar varicella screening recommendations are recommended before starting TNF-α inhibitor therapy as described under the corticosteroid section (see above).

The use of biological agents and immunomodulatory therapy has improved IBD management. Infections, including serious infections, albeit rare, are increasingly being described in patients with IBD receiving immunosuppressive therapies. A heightened index of suspicion, timely diagnostics, and targeted therapies are needed for optimal patient management. Given the limited pediatric data, there are ample opportunities for robust pediatric studies to improve our understanding of infectious burden in this population, optimize preventative strategies, and improve patient outcomes.

References

1. Manichanh C, Borruel N, Casellas F, Guarner F. The gut microbiota in IBD. Nat Rev Gastroenterol Hepatol. 2012;9:599–608. doi:10.1038/nrgastro.2012.152.
2. Kim SC, Tonkonogy SL, Albright CA, Tsang J, Balish EJ, Braun J, Huycke MM, Sartor RB. Variable phenotypes of enterocolitis in interleukin 10-deficient mice monoassociated with two different commensal bacteria. Gastroenterology. 2005;128:891–906.
3. Kim SC, Tonkonogy SL, Karrasch T, Jobin C, Sartor RB. Dual-association of gnotobiotic IL-10−/− mice with 2 nonpathogenic commensal bacteria induces aggressive pancolitis. Inflamm Bowel Dis. 2007;13:1457–66. doi:10.1002/ibd.20246.
4. Afif W, Loftus Jr EV. Safety profile of IBD therapeutics: infectious risks. Gastroenterol Clin North Am. 2009;38:691–709. doi:10.1016/j.gtc.2009.07.005.
5. Dave M, Purohit T, Razonable R, Loftus Jr EV. Opportunistic infections due to inflammatory bowel disease therapy. Inflamm Bowel Dis. 2014;20:196–212. doi:10.1097/MIB.0b013e3182a827d2.

6. Irving PM, Gibson PR. Infections and IBD. Nat Clin Pract Gastroenterol Hepatol. 2008;5:18–27. doi:10.1038/ncpgasthep1004.

7. Jakobsen C, Bartek Jr J, Wewer V, Vind I, Munkholm P, Groen R, Paerregaard A. Differences in phenotype and disease course in adult and paediatric inflammatory bowel disease – a population-based study. Aliment Pharmacol Ther. 2011;34:1217–24. doi:10.1111/j.1365-2036.2011.04857.x.

8. Van Limbergen J, Russell RK, Drummond HE, Aldhous MC, Round NK, Nimmo ER, Smith L, Gillett PM, McGrogan P, Weaver LT, Bisset WM, Mahdi G, Arnott ID, Satsangi J, Wilson DC. Definition of phenotypic characteristics of childhood-onset inflammatory bowel disease. Gastroenterology. 2008;135:1114–22. doi:10.1053/j.gastro.2008.06.081.

9. Sartor RB. Therapeutic manipulation of the enteric microflora in inflammatory bowel diseases: antibiotics, probiotics, and prebiotics. Gastroenterology. 2004;126:1620–33.

10. Greenbloom SL, Steinhart AH, Greenberg GR. Combination ciprofloxacin and metronidazole for active Crohn's disease. Can J Gastroenterol. 1998;12:53–6.

11. Andre MF, Piette JC, Kemeny JL, Ninet J, Jego P, Delevaux I, Wechsler B, Weiller PJ, Frances C, Bletry O, Wismans PJ, Rousset H, Colombel JF, Aumaitre O. Aseptic abscesses: a study of 30 patients with or without inflammatory bowel disease and review of the literature. Medicine (Baltimore). 2007;86:145–61. doi:10.1097/md.0b013e18064f9f3.

12. Seow-Choen F, Hay AJ, Heard S, Phillips RK. Bacteriology of anal fistulae. Br J Surg. 1992;79:27–8.

13. West RL, Van der Woude CJ, Endtz HP, Hansen BE, Ouwedijk M, Boelens HA, Kusters JG, Kuipers EJ. Perianal fistulas in Crohn's disease are predominantly colonized by skin flora: implications for antibiotic treatment? Dig Dis Sci. 2005;50:1260–3.

14. Kronman MP, Gerber JS, Prasad PA, Adler AL, Bass JA, Newland JG, Shah KM, Zerr DM, Feng R, Coffin SE, Zaoutis TE. Variation in antibiotic use for children hospitalized with inflammatory bowel disease exacerbation: a multicenter validation study. J Pediatric Infect Dis Soc. 2012;1:306–13. doi:10.1093/jpids/pis053.

15. Khan KJ, Ullman TA, Ford AC, Abreu MT, Abadir A, Marshall JK, Talley NJ, Moayyedi P. Antibiotic therapy in inflammatory bowel disease: a systematic review and meta-analysis. Am J Gastroenterol. 2011;106:661–73. doi:10.1038/ajg.2011.72.

16. Talley NJ, Abreu MT, Achkar JP, Bernstein CN, Dubinsky MC, Hanauer SB, Kane SV, Sandborn WJ, Ullman TA, Moayyedi P. An evidence-based systematic review on medical therapies for inflammatory bowel disease. Am J Gastroenterol. 2011;106(Suppl 1):S2–25; quiz S26. doi:10.1038/ajg.2011.58.

17. Wang SL, Wang ZR, Yang CQ. Meta-analysis of broad-spectrum antibiotic therapy in patients with active inflammatory bowel disease. Exp Ther Med. 2012;4:1051–6. doi:10.3892/etm.2012.718.

18. de Zoeten EF, Pasternak BA, Mattei P, Kramer RE, Kader HA. Diagnosis and treatment of perianal Crohn disease: NASPGHAN clinical report and consensus statement. J Pediatr Gastroenterol Nutr. 2013;57:401–12. doi:10.1097/MPG.0b013e3182a025ee.

19. Ruemmele FM, Veres G, Kolho KL, Griffiths A, Levine A, Escher JC, Amil Dias J, Barabino A, Braegger CP, Bronsky J, Buderus S, Martin-de-Carpi J, De Ridder L, Fagerberg UL, Hugot JP, Kierkus J, Kolacek S, Koletzko S, Lionetti P, Miele E, Navas Lopez VM, Paerregaard A, Russell RK, Serban DE, Shaoul R, Van Rheenen P, Veereman G, Weiss B, Wilson D, Dignass A, Eliakim A, Winter H, Turner D. Consensus guidelines of ECCO/ESPGHAN on the medical management of pediatric Crohn's disease. J Crohns Colitis. 2014;8:1179–207. doi:10.1016/j.crohns.2014.04.005.

20. Rutgeerts P, Hiele M, Geboes K, Peeters M, Penninckx F, Aerts R, Kerremans R. Controlled trial of metronidazole treatment for prevention of Crohn's recurrence after ileal resection. Gastroenterology. 1995;108:1617–21.

21. Doherty G, Bennett G, Patil S, Cheifetz A, Moss AC. Interventions for prevention of post-operative recurrence of Crohn's disease. Cochrane Database Syst Rev. 2009;CD006873. doi:10.1002/14651858.CD006873.pub2.

22. De Cruz P, Kamm MA, Prideaux L, Allen PB, Desmond PV. Postoperative recurrent luminal Crohn's disease: a systematic review. Inflamm Bowel Dis. 2012;18:758–77. doi:10.1002/ibd.21825.

23. Regueiro M, Schraut W, Baidoo L, Kip KE, Sepulveda AR, Pesci M, Harrison J, Plevy SE. Infliximab prevents Crohn's disease recurrence after ileal resection. Gastroenterology. 2009;136:441–50.e1; quiz 716. doi:10.1053/j.gastro.2008.10.051.

24. Turner D, Travis SP, Griffiths AM, Ruemmele FM, Levine A, Benchimol EI, Dubinsky M, Alex G, Baldassano RN, Langer JC, Shamberger R, Hyams JS, Cucchiara S, Bousvaros A, Escher JC, Markowitz J, Wilson DC, van Assche G, Russell RK. Consensus for managing acute severe ulcerative colitis in children: a systematic review and joint statement from ECCO, ESPGHAN, and the Porto IBD Working Group of ESPGHAN. Am J Gastroenterol. 2011;106:574–88. doi:10.1038/ajg.2010.481.

25. Navaneethan U, Shen B. Pros and cons of antibiotic therapy for pouchitis. Expert Rev Gastroenterol Hepatol. 2009;3:547–59. doi:10.1586/egh.09.37.

26. Gionchetti P, Rizzello F, Venturi A, Brigidi P, Matteuzzi D, Bazzocchi G, Poggioli G, Miglioli M, Campieri M. Oral bacteriotherapy as maintenance treatment in patients with chronic pouchitis: a double-blind, placebo-controlled trial. Gastroenterology. 2000;119:305–9.

27. Gevers D, Kugathasan S, Denson LA, Vazquez-Baeza Y, Van Treuren W, Ren B, Schwager E, Knights D, Song SJ, Yassour M, Morgan XC, Kostic AD, Luo C, Gonzalez A, McDonald D, Haberman Y, Walters T, Baker S, Rosh J, Stephens M, Heyman M, Markowitz J, Baldassano R, Griffiths A, Sylvester F, Mack D, Kim S, Crandall W, Hyams J, Huttenhower C, Knight R, Xavier RJ. The treatment-naive microbiome in new-onset Crohn's disease. Cell Host Microbe. 2014;15:382–92. doi:10.1016/j.chom.2014.02.005.

28. Morikawa K, Watabe H, Araake M, Morikawa S. Modulatory effect of antibiotics on cytokine production by human monocytes in vitro. Antimicrob Agents Chemother. 1996;40:1366–70.

29. Solomkin JS, Mazuski JE, Bradley JS, Rodvold KA, Goldstein EJ, Baron EJ, O'Neill PJ, Chow AW, Dellinger EP, Eachempati SR, Gorbach S, Hilfiker M, May AK, Nathens AB, Sawyer RG, Bartlett JG. Diagnosis and management of complicated intra-abdominal infection in adults and children: guidelines by the Surgical Infection Society and the Infectious Diseases Society of America. Clin Infect Dis. 2010;50:133–64. doi:10.1086/649554.

30. Margalit M, Elinav H, Ilan Y, Shalit M. Liver abscess in inflammatory bowel disease: report of two cases and review of the literature. J Gastroenterol Hepatol. 2004;19:1338–42. doi:10.1111/j.1440-1746.2004.03368.x.

31. Varda BK, McNabb-Baltar J, Sood A, Ghani KR, Kibel AS, Letendre J, Menon M, Sammon JD, Schmid M, Sun M, Trinh QD, Bhojani N. Urolithiasis and urinary tract infection among patients with inflammatory bowel disease: a review of US emergency department visits between 2006 and 2009. Urology. 2015;85:764–70. doi:10.1016/j.urology.2014.12.011.

32. Arnold CA, Roth R, Arsenescu R, Harzman A, Lam-Himlin DM, Limketkai BN, Montgomery EA, Voltaggio L. Sexually transmitted infectious colitis vs inflammatory bowel disease: distinguishing features from a case-controlled study. Am J Clin Pathol. 2015;144:771–81. doi:10.1309/AJCPOID4JIJ6PISC.

33. Landsman MJ, Sultan M, Stevens M, Charabaty A, Mattar MC. Diagnosis and management of common gastrointestinal tract infectious diseases in ulcerative colitis and Crohn's disease patients. Inflamm Bowel Dis. 2014;20:2503–10. doi:10.1097/MIB.0000000000000140.

34. Colletti RB, Baldassano RN, Milov DE, Margolis PA, Bousvaros A, Crandall WV, Crissinger KD, D'Amico MA, Day AS, Denson LA, Dubinsky M, Ebach DR, Hoffenberg EJ, Kader HA, Keljo DJ, Leibowitz IH, Mamula P, Pfefferkorn MD, Qureshi MA. Variation in care in pediatric Crohn disease. J Pediatr Gastroenterol Nutr. 2009;49:297–303. doi:10.1097/MPG.0b013e3181919695.

35. Ihekweazu FD, Ajjarapu A, Kellermayer R. Diagnostic yield of routine enteropathogenic stool tests in pediatric ulcerative colitis. Ann Clin Lab Sci. 2015;45:639–42.

36. Meyer AM, Ramzan NN, Loftus Jr EV, Heigh RI, Leighton JA. The diagnostic yield of stool pathogen studies during relapses of inflammatory bowel disease. J Clin Gastroenterol. 2004;38:772–5.

37. Mylonaki M, Langmead L, Pantes A, Johnson F, Rampton DS. Enteric infection in relapse of inflammatory bowel disease: importance of microbiological examination of stool. Eur J Gastroenterol Hepatol. 2004;16:775–8.

38. Vadlamudi N, Maclin J, Dimmitt RA, Thame KA. Cryptosporidial infection in children with inflammatory bowel disease. J Crohns Colitis. 2013;7:e337–43. doi:10.1016/j.crohns.2013.01.015.

39. Kim J, Smathers SA, Prasad P, Leckerman KH, Coffin S, Zaoutis T. Epidemiological features of Clostridium difficile-associated disease among inpatients at children's hospitals in the United States, 2001-2006. Pediatrics. 2008;122:1266–70. doi:10.1542/peds.2008-0469.

40. Lessa FC, Mu Y, Bamberg WM, Beldavs ZG, Dumyati GK, Dunn JR, Farley MM, Holzbauer SM, Meek JI, Phipps EC, Wilson LE, Winston LG, Cohen JA, Limbago BM, Fridkin SK, Gerding DN, McDonald LC. Burden of Clostridium difficile infection in the United States. N Engl J Med. 2015;372:825–34. doi:10.1056/NEJMoa1408913.

41. Nylund CM, Goudie A, Garza JM, Fairbrother G, Cohen MB. Clostridium difficile infection in hospitalized children in the United States. Arch Pediatr Adolesc Med. 2011;165:451–7. doi:10.1001/archpediatrics.2010.282.

42. Rodemann JF, Dubberke ER, Reske KA, Seo da H, Stone CD. Incidence of Clostridium difficile infection in inflammatory bowel disease. Clin Gastroenterol Hepatol. 2007;5:339–44. doi:10.1016/j.cgh.2006.12.027.

43. Schneeweiss S, Korzenik J, Solomon DH, Canning C, Lee J, Bressler B. Infliximab and other immunomodulating drugs in patients with inflammatory bowel disease and the risk of serious bacterial infections. Aliment Pharmacol Ther. 2009;30:253–64. doi:10.1111/j.1365-2036.2009.04037.x.

44. Pascarella F, Martinelli M, Miele E, Del Pezzo M, Roscetto E, Staiano A. Impact of Clostridium difficile infection on pediatric inflammatory bowel disease. J Pediatr. 2009;154:854–8. doi:10.1016/j.jpeds.2008.12.039.

45. Sandberg KC, Davis MM, Gebremariam A, Adler J. Disproportionate rise in Clostridium difficile-associated hospitalizations among US youth with inflammatory bowel disease, 1997-2011. J Pediatr Gastroenterol Nutr. 2015;60:486–92. doi:10.1097/MPG.0000000000000636.

46. Martinelli M, Strisciuglio C, Veres G, Paerregaard A, Pavic AM, Aloi M, Martin-de-Carpi J, Levine A, Turner D, Del Pezzo M, Staiano A, Miele E. Clostridium difficile and pediatric inflammatory bowel disease: a prospective, comparative, multicenter, ESPGHAN study. Inflamm Bowel Dis. 2014;20:2219–25. doi:10.1097/MIB.0000000000000219.

47. Surawicz CM, Brandt LJ, Binion DG, Ananthakrishnan AN, Curry SR, Gilligan PH, McFarland LV, Mellow M, Zuckerbraun BS. Guidelines for diagnosis, treatment, and prevention of Clostridium difficile infections. Am J Gastroenterol. 2013;108:478–98; quiz 499. doi:10.1038/ajg.2013.4.

48. Sammons JS, Toltzis P. Pitfalls in Diagnosis of Pediatric Clostridium difficile Infection. Infect Dis Clin North Am. 2015;29:465–76. doi:10.1016/j.idc.2015.05.010.

49. Burnham CA, Carroll KC. Diagnosis of Clostridium difficile infection: an ongoing conundrum for clinicians and for clinical laboratories. Clin Microbiol Rev. 2013;26:604–30. doi:10.1128/CMR.00016-13.

50. Cohen SH, Gerding DN, Johnson S, Kelly CP, Loo VG, McDonald LC, Pepin J, Wilcox MH. Clinical practice guidelines for Clostridium difficile infection in adults: 2010 update by the society for healthcare epidemiology of America (SHEA) and the infectious diseases society of America (IDSA). Infect Control Hosp Epidemiol. 2010;31:431–55. doi:10.1086/651706.

51. Schutze GE, Willoughby RE. Clostridium difficile infection in infants and children. Pediatrics. 2013;131:196–200. doi:10.1542/peds.2012-2992.

52. Clayton EM, Rea MC, Shanahan F, Quigley EM, Kiely B, Hill C, Ross RP. The vexed relationship between Clostridium difficile and inflammatory bowel disease: an assessment of carriage in an outpatient setting among patients in remission. Am J Gastroenterol. 2009;104:1162–9. doi:10.1038/ajg.2009.4.

53. Hourigan SK, Chirumamilla SR, Ross T, Golub JE, Rabizadeh S, Saeed SA, Elson CO, Kelly CP, Carroll KC, Oliva-Hemker M, Sears C. Clostridium difficile carriage and serum antitoxin responses in children with inflammatory bowel disease. Inflamm Bowel Dis. 2013;19:2744–52. doi:10.1097/01.MIB.0000435434.53871.36.

54. Lamouse-Smith ES, Weber S, Rossi RF, Neinstedt LJ, Mosammaparast N, Sandora TJ, McAdam AJ, Bousvaros A. Polymerase chain reaction test for Clostridium difficile toxin B gene reveals similar prevalence rates in children with and without inflammatory bowel disease. J Pediatr Gastroenterol Nutr. 2013;57:293–7. doi:10.1097/MPG.0b013e3182999990.

55. Polage CR, Gyorke CE, Kennedy MA, Leslie JL, Chin DL, Wang S, Nguyen HH, Huang B, Tang YW, Lee LW, Kim K, Taylor S, Romano PS, Panacek EA, Goodell PB, Solnick JV, Cohen SH. Overdiagnosis of Clostridium difficile Infection in the Molecular Test Era. JAMA Intern Med. 2015;175:1792–801. doi:10.1001/jamainternmed.2015.4114.

56. Hommes DW, Sterringa G, van Deventer SJ, Tytgat GN, Weel J. The pathogenicity of cytomegalovirus in inflammatory bowel disease: a systematic review and evidence-based recommendations for future research. Inflamm Bowel Dis. 2004;10:245–50.

57. Kandiel A, Lashner B. Cytomegalovirus colitis complicating inflammatory bowel disease. Am J Gastroenterol. 2006;101:2857–65. doi:10.1111/j.1572-0241.2006.00869.x.

58. Haberman Y, Tickle TL, Dexheimer PJ, Kim MO, Tang D, Karns R, Baldassano RN, Noe JD, Rosh J, Markowitz J, Heyman MB, Griffiths AM, Crandall WV, Mack DR, Baker SS, Huttenhower C, Keljo DJ, Hyams JS, Kugathasan S, Walters TD, Aronow B, Xavier RJ, Gevers D, Denson LA. Pediatric Crohn disease patients exhibit specific ileal transcriptome and microbiome signature. J Clin Invest. 2014;124:3617–33. doi:10.1172/JCI75436.

59. Kostic AD, Xavier RJ, Gevers D. The microbiome in inflammatory bowel disease: current status and the future ahead. Gastroenterology. 2014;146:1489–99. doi:10.1053/j.gastro.2014.02.009.

60. Jostins L, Ripke S, Weersma RK, Duerr RH, McGovern DP, Hui KY, Lee JC, Schumm LP, Sharma Y, Anderson CA, Essers J, Mitrovic M, Ning K, Cleynen I, Theatre E, Spain SL, Raychaudhuri S, Goyette P, Wei Z, Abraham C, Achkar JP, Ahmad T, Amininejad L, Ananthakrishnan AN, Andersen V, Andrews JM, Baidoo L, Balschun T, Bampton PA, Bitton A, Boucher G, Brand S, Buning C, Cohain A, Cichon S, D'Amato M, De Jong D, Devaney KL, Dubinsky M, Edwards C, Ellinghaus D, Ferguson LR, Franchimont D, Fransen K, Gearry R, Georges M, Gieger C, Glas J, Haritunians T, Hart A, Hawkey C, Hedl M, Hu X, Karlsen TH, Kupcinskas L, Kugathasan S, Latiano A, Laukens D, Lawrance IC, Lees CW, Louis E, Mahy G, Mansfield J, Morgan AR, Mowat C, Newman W, Palmieri O, Ponsioen CY, Potocnik U, Prescott NJ, Regueiro M, Rotter JI, Russell RK, Sanderson JD, Sans M, Satsangi J,

Schreiber S, Simms LA, Sventoraityte J, Targan SR, Taylor KD, Tremelling M, Verspaget HW, De Vos M, Wijmenga C, Wilson DC, Winkelmann J, Xavier RJ, Zeissig S, Zhang B, Zhang CK, Zhao H, Silverberg MS, Annese V, Hakonarson H, Brant SR, Radford-Smith G, Mathew CG, Rioux JD, Schadt EE, et al. Host-microbe interactions have shaped the genetic architecture of inflammatory bowel disease. Nature. 2012;491:119–24. doi:10.1038/nature11582.

61. Aberra FN, Lichtenstein GR. Methods to avoid infections in patients with inflammatory bowel disease. Inflamm Bowel Dis. 2005;11:685–95.

62. Dulai PS, Thompson KD, Blunt HB, Dubinsky MC, Siegel CA. Risks of serious infection or lymphoma with anti-tumor necrosis factor therapy for pediatric inflammatory bowel disease: a systematic review. Clin Gastroenterol Hepatol. 2014;12:1443–51; quiz e88–9. doi: 10.1016/j.cgh.2014.01.021.

63. Toruner M, Loftus Jr EV, Harmsen WS, Zinsmeister AR, Orenstein R, Sandborn WJ, Colombel JF, Egan LJ. Risk factors for opportunistic infections in patients with inflammatory bowel disease. Gastroenterology. 2008;134:929–36. doi:10.1053/j.gastro.2008.01.012.

64. Marehbian J, Arrighi HM, Hass S, Tian H, Sandborn WJ. Adverse events associated with common therapy regimens for moderate-to-severe Crohn's disease. Am J Gastroenterol. 2009;104:2524–33. doi:10.1038/ajg.2009.322.

65. Veereman-Wauters G, de Ridder L, Veres G, Kolacek S, Fell J, Malmborg P, Koletzko S, Dias JA, Misak Z, Rahier JF, Escher JC. Risk of infection and prevention in pediatric patients with IBD: ESPGHAN IBD Porto Group commentary. J Pediatr Gastroenterol Nutr. 2012;54:830–7. doi:10.1097/MPG.0b013e31824d1438.

66. Rahier JF, Magro F, Abreu C, Armuzzi A, Ben-Horin S, Chowers Y, Cottone M, de Ridder L, Doherty G, Ehehalt R, Esteve M, Katsanos K, Lees CW, Macmahon E, Moreels T, Reinisch W, Tilg H, Tremblay L, Veereman-Wauters G, Viget N, Yazdanpanah Y, Eliakim R, Colombel JF. Second European evidence-based consensus on the prevention, diagnosis and management of opportunistic infections in inflammatory bowel disease. J Crohns Colitis. 2014;8:443–68. doi:10.1016/j.crohns.2013.12.013.

67. Rubin LG, Levin MJ, Ljungman P, Davies EG, Avery R, Tomblyn M, Bousvaros A, Dhanireddy S, Sung L, Keyserling H, Kang I; Infectious Diseases Society of A. 2013 IDSA clinical practice guideline for vaccination of the immunocompromised host. Clin Infect Dis. 2014;58:309–18. doi:10.1093/cid/cit816.

68. Gisbert JP, Gomollon F. Thiopurine-induced myelotoxicity in patients with inflammatory bowel disease: a review. Am J Gastroenterol. 2008;103:1783–800. doi:10.1111/j.1572-0241.2008.01848.x.

69. Gupta G, Lautenbach E, Lewis JD. Incidence and risk factors for herpes zoster among patients with inflammatory bowel disease. Clin Gastroenterol Hepatol. 2006;4:1483–90. doi:10.1016/j.cgh.2006.09.019.

70. Seksik P, Cosnes J, Sokol H, Nion-Larmurier I, Gendre JP, Beaugerie L. Incidence of benign upper respiratory tract infections, HSV and HPV cutaneous infections in inflammatory bowel disease patients treated with azathioprine. Aliment Pharmacol Ther. 2009;29:1106–13. doi:10.1111/j.1365-2036.2009.03973.x.

71. Connell WR, Kamm MA, Ritchie JK, Lennard-Jones JE. Bone marrow toxicity caused by azathioprine in inflammatory bowel disease: 27 years of experience. Gut. 1993;34:1081–5.

72. Gluck T, Kiefmann B, Grohmann M, Falk W, Straub RH, Scholmerich J. Immune status and risk for infection in patients receiving chronic immunosuppressive therapy. J Rheumatol. 2005;32:1473–80.

73. Present DH, Meltzer SJ, Krumholz MP, Wolke A, Korelitz BI. 6-Mercaptopurine in the management of inflammatory bowel disease: short- and long-term toxicity. Ann Intern Med. 1989;111:641–9.

74. Lichtenstein GR, Feagan BG, Cohen RD, Salzberg BA, Diamond RH, Price S, Langholff W, Londhe A, Sandborn WJ. Serious infection and mortality in patients with Crohn's disease: more than 5 years of follow-up in the TREAT registry. Am J Gastroenterol. 2012;107:1409–22. doi:10.1038/ajg.2012.218.

75. Stuck AE, Minder CE, Frey FJ. Risk of infectious complications in patients taking glucocorticosteroids. Rev Infect Dis. 1989;11:954–63.

76. Agrawal A, Durrani S, Leiper K, Ellis A, Morris AI, Rhodes JM. Effect of systemic corticosteroid therapy on risk for intra-abdominal or pelvic abscess in non-operated Crohn's disease. Clin Gastroenterol Hepatol. 2005;3:1215–20.

77. Lichtenstein GR, Abreu MT, Cohen R, Tremaine W. American Gastroenterological Association Institute medical position statement on corticosteroids, immunomodulators, and infliximab in inflammatory bowel disease. Gastroenterology. 2006;130:935–9. doi:10.1053/j.gastro.2006.01.047.

78. Subramanian V, Saxena S, Kang JY, Pollok RC. Preoperative steroid use and risk of postoperative complications in patients with inflammatory bowel disease undergoing abdominal surgery. Am J Gastroenterol. 2008;103:2373–81. doi:10.1111/j.1572-0241.2008.01942.x.

79. Cullen G, Baden RP, Cheifetz AS. Varicella zoster virus infection in inflammatory bowel disease. Inflamm Bowel Dis. 2012;18:2392–403. doi:10.1002/ibd.22950.

80. Koo S, Marty FM, Baden LR. Infectious complications associated with immunomodulating biologic agents. Infect Dis Clin North Am. 2010;24:285–306. doi:10.1016/j.idc.2010.01.006.

81. Wallis RS. Biologics and infections: lessons from tumor necrosis factor blocking agents. Infect Dis Clin North Am. 2011;25:895–910. doi:10.1016/j.idc.2011.08.002.

82. Wallis RS, Broder MS, Wong JY, Hanson ME, Beenhouwer DO. Granulomatous infectious diseases associated with tumor necrosis factor antagonists. Clin Infect Dis. 2004;38:1261–5. doi:10.1086/383317.

83. Esteve M, Saro C, Gonzalez-Huix F, Suarez F, Forne M, Viver JM. Chronic hepatitis B reactivation following infliximab therapy in Crohn's disease patients: need for primary prophylaxis. Gut. 2004;53:1363–5. doi:10.1136/gut.2004.040675.

84. Papa A, Felice C, Marzo M, Andrisani G, Armuzzi A, Covino M, Mocci G, Pugliese D, De Vitis I, Gasbarrini A, Rapaccini GL, Guidi L. Prevalence and natural history of hepatitis B and C infections in a large population of IBD patients treated with anti-tumor necrosis factor-alpha agents. J Crohns Colitis. 2013;7:113–9. doi:10.1016/j.crohns.2012.03.001.

85. Perez-Alvarez R, Diaz-Lagares C, Garcia-Hernandez F, Lopez-Roses L, Brito-Zeron P, Perez-de-Lis M, Retamozo S, Bove A, Bosch X, Sanchez-Tapias JM, Forns X, Ramos-Casals M. Hepatitis B virus (HBV) reactivation in patients receiving tumor necrosis factor (TNF)-targeted therapy: analysis of 257 cases. Medicine (Baltimore). 2011;90:359–71. doi:10.1097/MD.0b013e3182380a76.

86. Toussi SS, Pan N, Walters HM, Walsh TJ. Infections in children and adolescents with juvenile idiopathic arthritis and inflammatory bowel disease treated with tumor necrosis factor-alpha inhibitors: systematic review of the literature. Clin Infect Dis. 2013;57:1318–30. doi:10.1093/cid/cit489.

87. Lorenzetti R, Zullo A, Ridola L, Diamanti AP, Lagana B, Gatta L, Migliore A, Armuzzi A, Hassan C, Bruzzese V. Higher risk of tuberculosis reactivation when anti-TNF is combined with immunosuppressive agents: a systematic review of randomized controlled trials. Ann Med. 2014;46:547–54. doi:10.3109/07853890.2014.941919.

88. Wallis RS. Tumour necrosis factor antagonists: structure, function, and tuberculosis risks. Lancet Infect Dis. 2008;8:601–11. doi:10.1016/S1473-3099(08)70227-5.

89. Wallis RS, Broder M, Wong J, Lee A, Hoq L. Reactivation of latent granulomatous infections by infliximab. Clin Infect Dis. 2005;41(Suppl 3):S194–8. doi:10.1086/429996.

90. Cruz AT, Karam LB, Orth RC, Starke JR. Disseminated tuberculosis in 2 children with inflammatory bowel disease receiving infliximab. Pediatr Infect Dis J. 2014;33:779–81. doi:10.1097/INF.0000000000000286.

91. Jordan N, Waghmare A, Abi-Ghanem AS, Moon A, Salvatore CM. Systemic Mycobacterium avium complex infection during antitumor necrosis factor-alpha therapy in pediatric Crohn disease. J Pediatr Gastroenterol Nutr. 2012;54:294–6. doi:10.1097/MPG.0b013e31822938c3.

92. D'Haens GR, Panaccione R, Higgins PD, Vermeire S, Gassull M, Chowers Y, Hanauer SB, Herfarth H, Hommes DW, Kamm M, Lofberg R, Quary A, Sands B, Sood A, Watermeyer G, Lashner B, Lemann M, Plevy S, Reinisch W, Schreiber S, Siegel C, Targan S, Watanabe M, Feagan B, Sandborn WJ, Colombel JF, Travis S. The London Position Statement of the World Congress of Gastroenterology on Biological Therapy for IBD with the European Crohn's and Colitis Organization: when to start, when to stop, which drug to choose, and how to predict response? Am J Gastroenterol. 2011;106:199–212; quiz 213. doi:10.1038/ajg.2010.392.

93. Davies HD. Infectious Complications With the Use of Biologic Response Modifiers in Infants and Children. Pediatrics. 2016;138. doi: 10.1542/peds.2016-1209.

94. Ardura MI, Toussi SS, Siegel JD, Lu Y, Bousvaros A, Crandall W. NASPGHAN clinical report: surveillance, diagnosis, and prevention of infectious diseases in pediatric patients with inflammatory bowel disease receiving tumor necrosis actor-alpha inhibitors. J Pediatr Gastroenterol Nutr. 2016; doi:10.1097/MPG.0000000000001188.

95. Starke JR. Interferon-gamma release assays for diagnosis of tuberculosis infection and disease in children. Pediatrics 2014;134:e1763–73. doi: 10.1542/peds.2014-2983.

96. Hage CA, Bowyer S, Tarvin SE, Helper D, Kleiman MB, Wheat LJ. Recognition, diagnosis, and treatment of histoplasmosis complicating tumor necrosis factor blocker therapy. Clin Infect Dis. 2010;50:85–92. doi:10.1086/648724.

97. Dotson JL, Crandall W, Mousa H, Honegger JR, Denson L, Samson C, Cunningham D, Balint J, Dienhart M, Jaggi P, Carvalho R. Presentation and outcome of histoplasmosis in pediatric inflammatory bowel disease patients treated with antitumor necrosis factor alpha therapy: a case series. Inflamm Bowel Dis. 2011;17:56–61. doi:10.1002/ibd.21378.

98. Vergidis P, Avery RK, Wheat LJ, Dotson JL, Assi MA, Antoun SA, Hamoud KA, Burdette SD, Freifeld AG, McKinsey DS, Money ME, Myint T, Andes DR, Hoey CA, Kaul DA, Dickter JK, Liebers DE, Miller RA, Muth WE, Prakash V, Steiner FT, Walker RC, Hage CA. Histoplasmosis complicating tumor necrosis factor-alpha blocker therapy: a retrospective analysis of 98 cases. Clin Infect Dis. 2015;61:409–17. doi:10.1093/cid/civ299.

99. Hage CA, Ribes JA, Wengenack NL, Baddour LM, Assi M, McKinsey DS, Hammoud K, Alapat D, Babady NE, Parker M, Fuller D, Noor A, Davis TE, Rodgers M, Connolly PA, El Haddad B, Wheat LJ. A multicenter evaluation of tests for diagnosis of histoplasmosis. Clin Infect Dis. 2011;53:448–54. doi:10.1093/cid/cir435.

100. Ordonez ME, Farraye FA, Di Palma JA. Endemic fungal infections in inflammatory bowel disease associated with anti-TNF antibody therapy. Inflamm Bowel Dis. 2013;19:2490–500. doi:10.1097/MIB.0b013e31828f1fba.

101. Warris A, Bjorneklett A, Gaustad P. Invasive pulmonary aspergillosis associated with infliximab therapy. N Engl J Med. 2001;344:1099–100.

102. Kaur N, Mahl TC. Pneumocystis jiroveci (carinii) pneumonia after infliximab therapy: a review of 84 cases. Dig Dis Sci. 2007;52:1481–4. doi:10.1007/s10620-006-9250-x.

103. Long MD, Farraye FA, Okafor PN, Martin C, Sandler RS, Kappelman MD. Increased risk of pneumocystis jiroveci pneumonia among patients with inflammatory bowel disease. Inflamm Bowel Dis. 2013;19:1018–24. doi:10.1097/MIB.0b013e3182802a9b.

104. Green H, Paul M, Vidal L, Leibovici L. Prophylaxis of Pneumocystis pneumonia in immunocompromised non-HIV-infected patients: systematic review and meta-analysis of randomized controlled trials. Mayo Clin Proc. 2007;82:1052–9. doi:10.4065/82.9.1052.

105. Okafor PN, Nunes DP, Farraye FA. Pneumocystis jiroveci pneumonia in inflammatory bowel disease: when should prophylaxis be considered? Inflamm Bowel Dis. 2013;19:1764–71. doi:10.1097/MIB.0b013e318281f562.

106. Kim SY, Solomon DH. Tumor necrosis factor blockade and the risk of viral infection. Nat Rev Rheumatol. 2010;6:165–74. doi:10.1038/nrrheum.2009.279.

107. Hwang JP, Lok AS. Management of patients with hepatitis B who require immunosuppressive therapy. Nat Rev Gastroenterol Hepatol. 2014;11:209–19. doi:10.1038/nrgastro.2013.216.

108. Pompili M, Biolato M, Miele L, Grieco A. Tumor necrosis factor-alpha inhibitors and chronic hepatitis C: a comprehensive literature review. World J Gastroenterol. 2013;19:7867–73. doi:10.3748/wjg.v19.i44.7867.

109. Reddy KR, Beavers KL, Hammond SP, Lim JK, Falck-Ytter YT. American Gastroenterological Association Institute guideline on the prevention and treatment of hepatitis B virus reactivation during immunosuppressive drug therapy. Gastroenterology. 2015;148:215–9; quiz e16–7. doi: 10.1053/j.gastro.2014.10.039.

110. Winthrop KL, Baddley JW, Chen L, Liu L, Grijalva CG, Delzell E, Beukelman T, Patkar NM, Xie F, Saag KG, Herrinton LJ, Solomon DH, Lewis JD, Curtis JR. Association between the initiation of anti-tumor necrosis factor therapy and the risk of herpes zoster. JAMA. 2013;309:887–95. doi:10.1001/jama.2013.1099.

Psychological Aspects of Inflammatory Bowel Disease in Children and Adolescents

Bonney Reed-Knight, Laura M. Mackner, and Wallace V. Crandall

Introduction

The bidirectional brain-gut axis model is increasingly being utilized to understand how inflammatory bowel disease (IBD) presents challenges to psychological adjustment and how psychological adjustment, in turn, can impact disease course and health outcomes. Psychosocial challenges brought on by IBD have long been recognized. The disease course is unpredictable, treatment can be frustrating and intrusive, and the symptoms can be embarrassing and socially limiting. Children with IBD can be reluctant to talk about their symptoms, and their frequent visits to the bathroom can be embarrassing. They may limit their activities to those with ready access to a bathroom, or they may need to unexpectedly cancel planned activities. School attendance and engagement in age-normative activities such as camps or sleepovers may be impacted. Short stature and delayed puberty can also contribute to feeling different from peers, and this may be particularly detrimental for boys since larger and more developed boys are often favored in social and athletic settings. Furthermore, corticosteroid medication may impact psychological functioning directly via mood changes and indirectly through appearance-altering side effects. IBD clearly has the potential to affect psychosocial functioning. The purpose of this chapter is to review psychological aspects of pediatric IBD in the areas of behavioral/emotional functioning, social functioning, family functioning, quality of life, disease self-management, self-esteem, stress and coping, and academic functioning. Research on psychosocial interventions in pediatric IBD will be reviewed, and recommendations regarding psychosocial functioning will be provided.

Behavioral/Emotional Functioning

Research on behavioral/emotional functioning in pediatric IBD has investigated levels of specific symptoms as well as rates of disorders. Validated structured interviews have been developed that lead to the diagnosis of psychiatric disorders, and norm-based questionnaires typically measure specific symptoms such as depression symptoms. Since these measures are age- and gender-normed, raw scores are usually converted to a standardized score, a T score, for more meaningful comparisons. During development of these questionnaires, cutoff scores are derived that best discriminate children in the normative sample who were referred for mental health services from non-referred children. Thus, a T score above the cutoff indicates a clinically significant problem.

Some of the early work utilizing structured interviews is limited by small samples sizes ($\leq$20 participants) and inadequate description of interviewer training or reliability checks. Among studies with better methodology, rates of *current* depressive disorders range from 10 to approximately 20% [1, 2], and this rate was not significantly higher than the rate in children with cystic fibrosis (CF) in the one study that utilized a comparison group [1]. *Lifetime* prevalence of depressive disorders was significantly higher in the IBD group (25%) than the CF group (12%) [1]. For comparison, lifetime prevalence of mood disorders for US adolescents in the general population has recently been estimated at 14.3% [3].

For anxiety disorders, rates of current diagnoses in pediatric IBD patients range from 4% in a heterogeneous sample to 28% in a newly diagnosed sample [1, 4]. Lifetime

B. Reed-Knight (✉)
Children's Healthcare of Atlanta, Atlanta, GA, USA

Department of Pediatrics, Division of Gastroenterology, Hepatology, and Nutrition, Emory University School of Medicine, Atlanta, GA, USA

GI Care for Kids, Atlanta, GA, USA
e-mail: bonney.reed-knight@emory.edu

L.M. Mackner
Center for Biobehavioral Health, Nationwide Children's Hospital, Columbus, OH, USA

W.V. Crandall
Department of Pediatrics, The Ohio State University College of Medicine, Center for Pediatric and Adolescent Inflammatory Bowel Disease, Nationwide Children's Hospital, Columbus, OH, USA

prevalence was 11% and not significantly different from a CF comparison group [1]. In a retrospective chart review of patients screened for anxiety symptoms as part of regular GI care, 30% reported elevated symptoms overall, and 50% scored above the clinically significant cutoff in at least one domain [5].

Several studies have examined specific behavioral and emotional symptoms using parent-report and child self-report questionnaires. Not all studies reported the T scores that are necessary to determine clinical significance, but among the eight that did, all reported mean scores within the average range [6–13]. Rates of clinical significance for depression symptoms ranged from 7 [6] to 25% [2]. For internalizing symptoms (anxiety and depressive symptoms), rates of clinical significance ranged from 13 to 31% [7, 9, 12]. Though several studies have reported that children with IBD had significantly more behavioral and emotional symptoms overall and/or significantly more depressive symptoms than healthy children [8, 13, 14–17], other studies have not found differences [7, 18]. A meta-analysis published in 2010 found that youth with IBD had significantly more internalizing symptoms than healthy comparisons [19]. Compared to other health conditions, children with functional GI disorders had significantly more symptoms [6], but there were few differences between the IBD and other chronic illness groups [15, 16]. Sleep disturbance has been described as common for youth with IBD and increasingly problematic with increased disease activity [20].

Taken together, these results suggest that children with IBD may be at greater risk for behavioral/emotional difficulties than healthy children, particularly in the areas of depression and anxiety. Although group means typically fall in the average range, the difficulties reach clinical significance in a subset of up to 31% of youth.

Risk factors for behavioral/emotional problems have been investigated in several studies. It seems logical that a child with more severe disease may have more emotional difficulties such as depression or anxiety symptoms; however, findings have been mixed. Multiple studies have reported no significant relationship between behavioral/emotional functioning and disease factors such as validated disease activity scores, growth delay, and/or frequency of relapse [7, 8, 10, 18, 21]. Studies that have found significant relationships have typically found associations between only some disease severity indicators and specific symptoms of depression or have failed to demonstrate relationships based on both parent and child report of depressive symptoms [2, 10, 13, 22]. One study with positive findings examined 499 youth with IBD and found that disease activity as rated on the PCDAI was associated with depressive symptoms [23]. Two studies found that emotional symptoms were significantly associated with *subjective* reports of increased disease severity [10, 12], but the emotional symptoms were not associated with objective findings (laboratory values) in one of those studies [10]. Additionally, one small study reported that diagnosis of depression was significantly associated with *less* severe illness [4].

It is not surprising that disease severity has not been consistently associated with behavioral/emotional symptoms in IBD. Research in other pediatric chronic illnesses has repeatedly shown that psychosocial factors such as family functioning and stress coping strategies are better predictors of behavioral/emotional functioning than illness factors [24]. For example, a child with good family supports and stress coping skills may be less likely to develop emotional problems when faced with severe IBD than a child without these resources. Conversely, a child with poor coping skills may have difficulty with behavioral/emotional functioning even in the context of mild IBD.

Other factors associated with increased behavioral/emotional symptoms, specifically depressive symptoms, include more stressful life events, maternal depression, family dysfunction, parenting stress, and steroid treatment [2, 4, 25–27]. Two studies investigating the effects of steroids on mood and memory in children with IBD found that subjects on steroids had significantly more problems with verbal memory, working memory, and depression compared to youth not on steroids [26, 27]. Mixed results have been found for the relationships between behavioral/emotional symptoms and age at diagnosis [2, 8], as well as gender [7, 12]. Contributions of other psychosocial risk factors have not been well studied.

Health-Related Quality of Life

Health-related quality of life (QOL) is the subjective perception of the impact of a chronic medical condition on physical, psychological, and social well-being [28]. Disease-specific and generic measures are available to assess QOL [29]. Studies using generic measures have found that that youth with IBD have lower QOL than healthy youth, [19, 30–34] and a meta-analysis provided further support for this finding [19]. Although differences exist, the QOL of youth with IBD is generally high, and relatively few youth with IBD experience clinically significant impairments in QOL [19]. QOL in pediatric IBD is also comparable to that of youth with other chronic and acute conditions [19, 34].

While the findings between disease activity and anxiety and depressive symptoms have been mixed, worse disease activity is consistently associated with poorer QOL as assessed with both disease-specific [33, 35–37] and generic measures [32]. Additionally, worse disease activity predicts poorer QOL 1 year after diagnosis [36]. Findings suggest that QOL may be a more sensitive, global indicator of a patient's overall well-being compared to internalizing symptoms alone. Increased parenting stress [38] and adolescents' internalizing symptoms and parents' depressive symptoms [39] have been identified as mechanisms by which increased disease activity impacts QOL. Fatigue is an independent predictor of disease-specific QOL even when accounting for disease activity [34]. Conflicting evidence exists regarding the relationship between corticosteroid use and QOL, with one study finding lower QOL among youth prescribed steroids [30] and another study finding no relationship [36]. Similarly, one study found no differences in QOL between youth on aminosalicylates, immunomodulators, or anti-TNFα therapy [34], whereas another study found adherence to a more complex, 5-ASA medication regimen related to poorer QOL [40].

Regarding demographic factors, older age was associated with lower disease-specific QOL in one study [36]. Research on gender is mixed, with one study suggesting poorer QOL among males [31] and another suggesting poorer QOL among females with IBD [37]. In one study, adolescents with Crohn's disease reported worse QOL than those with UC [35].

Using less adaptive coping strategies (e.g., avoidance) has been associated with worse QOL, whereas higher levels of predictive control (i.e., confidence in one's ability to control situations in the future) and social support have been associated with better QOL in pediatric IBD samples [37, 41]. Similarly, family dysfunction in problem-solving, communication, and general functioning have been associated with worse disease-specific QOL among adolescents with IBD [35]. In one study, increased adolescent depressive symptoms explained the relationship between parent distress and poorer adolescent QOL [42]. Even controlling for demographic and disease factors, lower QOL has been shown to predict increased healthcare utilization among youth with IBD [43].

Social Functioning

IBD has the potential to significantly disrupt social functioning, particularly involvement in social activities such as spending the night with a friend, hanging out at the mall, and participating in many sports. Belonging to a particular social group becomes very important during adolescence, and acceptance by peers is an important part of adolescent self-identity [44, 45].

In a meta-analysis of eight studies examining social functioning, youth with IBD reported significantly worse functioning than healthy children but similar functioning compared to children with other chronic illnesses [19]. Children with IBD have been found to have fewer friends and to participate in fewer organized activities than healthy children in one study [8], but not another [46], and may be less likely to have a romantic partner as an adolescent [46].

Mean scores for social functioning typically fall in the average range, and rates of clinically significant problems in social behavior/adjustment range from 2 to 22% [7, 8]. Peer victimization has also been associated with lower medication adherence, especially for adolescents who have lower social support, highlighting the importance of social functioning [47].

A few studies have identified factors that put youth with IBD at increased risk for social difficulty. Boys with IBD have more social difficulty than girls with IBD or healthy youth, including social problems that reach clinical significance. Twenty-nine percent of boys with IBD have clinically significant social difficulty compared to girls with IBD (11%) or healthy boys (0%) or girls (5%) [48]. Onset of IBD during adolescence is also associated with worse social functioning: 35% of those diagnosed in adolescence have clinically significant social difficulty compared to 5% for childhood onset [8]. It is not yet known if diagnosis during the developmental period of adolescence confers heightened risk independently or if patients diagnosed during this time period have had less time to adjust.

Family Functioning

Having a child with a chronic illness affects the whole family, so family functioning and the behavioral/emotional functioning of parents and siblings have been investigated in families with a child with IBD. Mixed results have been reported when examining overall family functioning in those with a child with IBD compared to healthy families [8, 16]. Typically, families report healthy levels of family functioning, but many endorse clinically elevated family dysfunction with communication, family roles/responsibilities, and the degree to which family members are involved in one another's lives [35]. This pattern might reflect the course of IBD (i.e., remission and flare-ups) and its impact on family life. The demands of managing IBD may challenge families' ability to communicate with one another, and family roles/responsibilities may change to accommodate disease flares (e.g., one caregiver stays with ill child in hospital, while other caregiver cares for healthy children and household tasks). In fact, family dysfunction has been significantly related to more severe disease, increased pain/fatigue, more bowel movements, and a greater number of behavioral/emotional symptoms [49–51].

Parental functioning can also play a role in the child's psychological adjustment. Rates of depression in mothers of children with IBD were similar to mothers of children with CF (10% current diagnosis, 51% lifetime history) [52]. A small study examining specific symptoms found that mothers of children with IBD reported significantly more behavioral/emotional symptoms than mothers of healthy children [16], but T scores were not reported, which limits conclusions about clinical significance. Parents of youth with IBD also report significantly lower perceived social support, an important coping strategy, than parents of healthy children [53]. Poorer psychosocial functioning among mothers of adolescents with IBD has been linked to adolescent depressive symptoms, negative health outcomes, and IBD-related functional disability in daily activities (i.e., school, extracurricular activities) [50]. Families with greater psychosocial risk rate their children with IBD as having more emotional and behavioral problems, [54] and higher levels of parenting stress have been linked with borderline or clinically elevated internalizing symptoms in youth with IBD [55].

Finally, one study investigated behavioral and emotional functioning in healthy siblings of children with IBD. Siblings of children with Crohn disease scored significantly above the normative mean on a questionnaire, whereas the mean score of siblings of children with ulcerative colitis fell at the normative mean. No siblings of healthy children were included [56].

Body Image and Self-Esteem

In the area of body image, concerns about poor growth and appearance have been cited frequently in QOL studies [57–61], although QOL measures are not validated specifically for assessing body image, and comparison groups were not included. Using a normed questionnaire assessing self-esteem about physical appearance, one study found mean T scores in the average range and no significant differences between children with IBD and healthy children [7].

Six studies have investigated general self-esteem among children with IBD. Both studies utilizing normed questionnaires reported mean T scores in the average range [6, 7]. The studies with comparison groups reported mixed results [7, 15, 16, 30, 62]. A meta-analysis reported that the self-esteem of youth with IBD was not significantly different from that of healthy youth or children with other chronic illnesses [19].

Stress and Coping

Although stressful life events and coping strategies have been studied among adults with IBD, these areas have received little attention in pediatric IBD. In prospective, longitudinal studies of adults with IBD, stress and coping have been associated with relapse and time to relapse [63–65]. Furthermore, stress and coping were better predictors of these outcomes than disease predictors such as CRP, TNFα, baseline disease activity, and disease duration [63–65].

Surprisingly, in a small study, children with IBD have reported significantly *fewer* stressful life events than healthy children [66]. Three studies reported that children with IBD

use less effective coping strategies, such as avoidance [37, 66, 67], but another study found no differences in the coping strategies or social support of healthy children and those with IBD [7]. Few studies have investigated relationships between stress, coping, and disease outcomes. One study reported that children with IBD were more likely to have an external locus of control (i.e., believing events are out of your control rather than affected by your efforts) than healthy children, and having a stronger external locus of control was associated with worse disease severity [67]. Coping with a more passive, depressive style was associated with worse quality of life in adolescents with IBD compared to using a more positive, active coping style in another study [37]. Two studies have investigated coping with the symptom of pain specifically. In one, pain catastrophizing was associated with increased disease severity and functional disability in adolescents with IBD [68]. In the other, pain coping strategies were predictive of both depression symptoms and functional disability, particularly pain catastrophizing. For depression, social isolation and lack of social support were also predictors [69].

Education

School functioning, which includes academic performance, school attendance, educational attainment, and psychosocial functioning in the school context, is an important area of psychosocial functioning for children and a potential area of concern for children with IBD. While research on school functioning exists in pediatric IBD, many studies are limited by methodological issues such as relying on self-report of absences and academic achievement rather than school records.

Most youth with IBD perceive that their condition has adversely affected their academic performance or educational attainment altogether [70–72]. However, objective data suggest similar levels of academic performance and educational attainment of youth with IBD compared to the general population or healthy controls when using self-report [73–75] or school records [76].

Some evidence for impairments in school attendance among youth with IBD exists. In two studies, children with IBD reported absences of 12–13 weeks during a school year [71, 77]. A study using school records and a healthy comparison group found that youth with IBD had significantly more absences, an average of 12 school days [76]. Excessive school absences in the absence of active disease may reflect anxiety-based school avoidance, but this has not been studied in pediatric IBD.

Psychosocial functioning in the school context can be assessed via QOL measures. In two studies of youth with IBD, school-related QOL received the lowest subscale score on the child-report PedsQL [78], suggesting that school functioning is a concern [79]. In one study, children with

IBD reported significantly worse school QOL than normative samples of chronic illness, acute illness, and healthy comparison groups [32]. However, in a large study investigating eight chronic illness groups, children with IBD did not have significantly different school QOL [79], and their school-related QOL was not significantly different from that of healthy youth in another study [76].

Two studies have examined risk factors for difficulties in school functioning for children with IBD. Disease factors were not significantly associated with school QOL in two studies [32, 76] nor with absence or grade point average. However, demographic and psychosocial factors such as internalizing symptoms were significant predictors of achievement and attendance [76] .

Self-Management and Adherence

Psychological functioning has important implications with regard to disease self-management and adherence to medications. Poor adherence to orally administered medications is a documented problem in pediatric IBD [80]. Greater emotional and behavioral problems have been significantly related to poorer medication adherence [81]. Higher levels of attention and conduct problems have been shown to relate to poorer adherence, with higher levels of barriers explaining the relationship [82]. In one study, higher anxiety/depressive symptoms had a negative additive effect on the relationship between barriers to adherence and medication adherence, such that barriers were the most problematic for youth with anxiety/depressive symptoms [83]. In addition, family-level factors are important with regard to self-management, with poorer adherence associated with greater family dysfunction and poor child coping [84]. Accidental barriers to adherence such as forgetting are often reported, though one study found volitional nonadherence to be related to greater disease activity and poorer QOL [85]. A recent study found pediatric adherence to infliximab to be high overall, with poorer adherence related to greater acute care usage [86].

Psychotherapy and Other Resources

Interventions for depression and coping strategies have been investigated in pediatric IBD. Cognitive behavioral therapy was evaluated for depression in adolescents with IBD in two studies [87, 88]. The programs incorporated individual plus family therapy [88] or solely individual therapy [87]. Both addressed illness problem-solving, pain management, identifying and modifying negative cognitions, social problem-solving, and increasing positive individual and social activities. After treatment, depression symptoms, overall functioning, and coping skills significantly improved [89].

Improvements in global psychosocial functioning were maintained over 12 months following individual cognitive behavioral therapy [90].

Group interventions have been investigated for improving coping skills in youth with IBD [91–93]. The interventions used a cognitive behavioral framework and addressed education, problem-solving, pain management, identifying and modifying negative cognitions, social competence, and increasing social activities. They led to improvements in coping skills, quality of life, behavioral/emotional problems, and somatic symptoms.

No interventions have focused solely on social functioning, although a few interventions for other issues have briefly addressed social difficulty. Cognitive behavioral therapy in the context of both individual therapy for depression symptoms and a support group for coping skills resulted in improvements in social functioning and social QOL for youth with IBD [88, 93]. Furthermore, attending an IBD camp was also associated with improvement in social quality of life [94], but it is not unknown how long these gains continued.

Cognitive behavioral strategies have also been successful for educational difficulty such as excessive school absence or school avoidance. In research in otherwise healthy children, interventions focused on reducing anxiety and depression have been successful in increasing attendance, [95] and manualized and self-directed intervention formats are available [96]. These interventions may hold promise for school attendance in IBD as well. Phone-delivered problem-solving skills training has been shown effective for improving medication adherence [97].

For any child with IBD, psychotherapy is warranted whenever behavioral or emotional problems cause significant distress and/or significantly interfere with functioning in any area such as school, social interactions, or family relationships. Signs of distress may include lowered grades, significant school absences, social withdrawal, lack of enjoyment in social or recreational activities, increased arguments with parents and/or siblings, and significant family stressors in addition to IBD. Mental health professionals who specialize in health psychology can help children cope with the disease as well as with issues such as pain management (including biofeedback), distress with medical procedures, medication adherence, pill-swallowing training, and school attendance.

Summary

Children with IBD appear to be at increased risk for difficulties in psychological functioning in the areas of depression and anxiety, QOL, and social functioning. Evidence is mixed and/or limited in the areas of family functioning, stress and coping, and educational functioning. Self-esteem appears to be similar to that of healthy children. Typically, mean group scores fall in the average range on normed measures, although a subset of up to 35% may have clinically significant difficulty. The psychological difficulty experienced by children with IBD is generally similar to that experienced in other chronic health conditions. Greater psychological distress is related to poorer self-management and adherence.

Disease severity has not been consistently associated with behavioral/emotional functioning, and this may be due to differences in coping strategies and family/social supports. Risk factors for poor QOL include disease severity, fatigue, poor coping strategies, and family dysfunction. Onset of IBD during adolescence and male gender are risk factors for social difficulty, family dysfunction is associated with disease severity and child behavioral/emotional problems, and demographic and psychosocial factors appear to best predict educational functioning.

Cognitive behavioral therapy has been shown to be effective in improving depression symptoms, other behavioral/emotional problems, coping skills, quality of life, somatic symptoms, and social functioning in children with IBD. Individual therapy, individual plus family therapy, group therapy, and an IBD camp have all been successful in improving outcomes with these youth. Mental health professionals have expertise in treatments that can benefit children with IBD including coping skills training, evidence-based treatment for anxiety and depression, biofeedback for pain management, and behavioral techniques for improving self-management and adherence.

References

1. Burke P, Meyer V, Kocoshis S, Orenstein DM, Chandra R, Nord DJ, Sauer J, Cohen E. Depression and anxiety in pediatric inflammatory bowel disease and cystic fibrosis. J Am Acad Child Adolesc Psychiatry. 1989;28:948–51.
2. Szigethy E, Levy-Warren A, Whitton S, Bousvaros A, Gauvreau K, Leichtner AM, Beardslee WR. Depressive symptoms and inflammatory bowel disease in children and adolescents: a cross-sectional study. J Pediatr Gastroenterol Nutr. 2004;39:395–403.
3. Merikangas KR, He JP, Burstein M, Swanson SA, Avenevoli S, Cui L, Benjet C, Georgiades K, Swendsen J. Lifetime prevalence of mental disorders in U.S. adolescents: results from the National Comorbidity Survey Replication–Adolescent Supplement (NCS-A). J Am Acad Child Adolesc Psychiatry. 2010;49:980–9. doi:10.1016/j.jaac.2010.05.017.
4. Burke PM, Neigut D, Kocoshis S, Chandra R, Sauer J. Correlates of depression in new onset pediatric inflammatory bowel disease. Child Psychiatry Hum Dev. 1994;24:275–83.
5. Reigada LC, Hoogendoorn CJ, Walsh LC, Lai J, Szigethy E, Cohen BH, Bao R, Isola K, Benkov KJ. Anxiety symptoms and disease severity in children and adolescents with Crohn disease. J Pediatr Gastroenterol Nutr. 2015;60:30–5. doi:10.1097/MPG.0000000000000552.
6. Gold N, Issenman R, Roberts J, Watt S. Well-adjusted children: an alternate view of children with inflammatory bowel disease and functional gastrointestinal complaints. Inflamm Bowel Dis. 2000;6:1–7.
7. Mackner LM, Crandall WV. Long-term psychosocial outcomes reported by children and adolescents with inflammatory bowel disease. Am J Gastroenterol. 2005;100:1386–92.
8. Mackner LM, Crandall WV. Brief report: psychosocial adjustment in adolescents with inflammatory bowel disease. J Pediatr Psychol. 2006;31:281–5.
9. Odell S, Sander E, Denson LA, Baldassano RN, Hommel KA. The contributions of child behavioral functioning and parent distress to family functioning in pediatric inflammatory bowel disease. J Clin Psychol Med Settings. 2011;18:39–45. doi:10.1007/s10880-011-9228-5.
10. Ondersma SJ, Lumley MA, Corlis ME, Tojek TM, Tolia V. Adolescents with inflammatory bowel disease: the roles of negative affectivity and hostility in subjective versus objective health. J Pediatr Psychol. 1997;22:723–38.
11. Szajnberg N, Krall V, Davis P, Treem W, Hyams J. Psychopathology and relationship measures in children with inflammatory bowel disease and their parents. Child Psychiatry Hum Dev. 1993;23:215–32.
12. Väistö T, Aronen ET, Simola P, Ashorn M, Kolho KL. Psychosocial symptoms and competence among adolescents with inflammatory bowel disease and their peers. Inflamm Bowel Dis. 2010;16:27–35. doi:10.1002/ibd.21002.
13. Wood B, Watkins JB, Boyle JT, Nogueira J, Zimand E, Carroll L. Psychological functioning in children with Crohn's disease and ulcerative colitis: implications for models of psychobiological interaction. J Am Acad Child Adolesc Psychiatry. 1987;26:774–81.
14. Engstrom I. Parental distress and social interaction in families with children with inflammatory bowel disease. J Am Acad Child Adolesc Psychiatry. 1991;30:904–12.
15. Engstrom I. Mental health and psychological functioning in children and adolescents with inflammatory bowel disease: a comparison with children having other chronic illnesses and with healthy children. J Child Psychol Psychiatry Allied Disciplines. 1992;33:563–82.
16. Engstrom I. Inflammatory bowel disease in children and adolescents: mental health and family functioning. J Pediatr Gastroenterol Nutr. 1999;28:S28–33.
17. Engstrom I, Lindquist BL. Inflammatory bowel disease in children and adolescents: a somatic and psychiatric investigation. Acta Paediatr Scand. 1991;80:640–7.
18. Reed-Knight B, Lobato D, Hagin S, McQuaid EL, Seifer R, Kopel SJ, Boergers J, Nassau JH, Suorsa K, Bancroft B, Shapiro J, Leleiko NS. Depressive symptoms in youth with inflammatory bowel disease compared with a community sample. Inflamm Bowel Dis. 2014;20:614–21. doi:10.1097/01.MIB.0000442678.62674.b7.
19. Greenley RN, Hommel KA, Nebel J, Raboin T, Li SH, Simpson P, Mackner L. A meta-analytic review of the psychosocial adjustment of youth with inflammatory bowel disease. J Pediatr Psychol. 2010;35:857–69. doi:10.1093/jpepsy/jsp120.
20. Benhayon D, Youk A, McCarthy FN, Davis S, Keljo DJ, Bousvaros A, Fairclough D, Kupfer D, Buysse DJ, Szigethy EM. Characterization of relations among sleep, inflammation, and psychiatric dysfunction in depressed youth with Crohn disease. J Pediatr Gastroenterol Nutr. 2013;57:335–42. doi:10.1097/MPG.0b013e31829641df.
21. Steinhausen HC, Kies H. Comparative studies of ulcerative colitis and Crohn's disease in children and adolescents. J Child Psychol Psychiatry. 1982;23:33–42.
22. Schuman SL, Graef DM, Janicke DM, Gray WN, Hommel KA. An exploration of family problem-solving and affective involvement as moderators between disease severity and depressive symptoms in

adolescents with inflammatory bowel disease. J Clin Psychol Med Settings. 2013;20:488–96. doi:10.1007/s10880-013-9368-x.

23. Clark JG, Srinath AI, Youk AO, Kirshner MA, McCarthy FN, Keljo DJ, Bousvaros A, DeMaso DR, Szigethy EM. Predictors of depression in youth with Crohn disease. J Pediatr Gastroenterol Nutr. 2014;58:569–73. doi:10.1097/MPG.0000000000000277.

24. Thompson RJ, Gustafson KE. Adaptation to chronic childhood illness. Washington, DC: American Psychological Association; 1996.

25. Guilfoyle SM, Gray WN, Herzer-Maddux M, Hommel KA. Parenting stress predicts depressive symptoms in adolescents with inflammatory bowel disease. Eur J Gastroenterol Hepatol. 2014;26:964–71. doi:10.1097/MEG.0000000000000149.

26. Mackner LM, Crandall WV. Steroid treatment impairs memory in pediatric inflammatory bowel disease. Gastroenterology. 2005;128:A166–7.

27. Mrakotsky C, Bousvaros A, Chriki L, Kenney E, Forbes P, Szigethy E, Waber D, Grand RJ. Impact of acute steroid treatment on memory, executive function, and mood in pediatric inflammatory bowel disease. J Pediatr Gastroenterol Nutr. 2005;42:540–1.

28. Eiser C, Morse R. The measurement of quality of life in children: past and future perspectives. J Dev Behav Pediatr. 2001;22:248–56.

29. Palermo TM, Long AC, Lewandowski AS, Drotar D, Quittner AL, Walker LS. Evidence-based assessment of health-related quality of life and functional impairment in pediatric psychology. J Pediatr Psychol. 2008;33:983–96. discussion 997-8. doi: jsn038 [pii]1093/jpepsy/jsn038.

30. Cunningham C, Drotar D, Palermo T, et al. Health-related quality of life in children and adolescents with inflammatory bowel disease. Children's Health Care. 2007;36:29–43.

31. De Boer M, Grootenhuis M, Derkx B, Last B. Health-related quality of life and psychosocial functioning of adolescents with inflammatory bowel disease. Inflamm Bowel Dis. 2005;11:400–6. doi: 00054725-200504000-00012 [pii].

32. Kunz JH, Hommel KA, Greenley RN. Health-related quality of life of youth with inflammatory bowel disease: a comparison with published data using the PedsQL 4.0 generic core scales. Inflamm Bowel Dis. 2010;16:939–46. doi:10.1002/ibd.21128.

33. Loonen HJ, Grootenhuis MA, Last BF, Koopman HM, Derkx HHF. Quality of life in paediatric inflammatory bowel disease measured by a generic and a disease-specific questionnaire. Acta Paediatr. 2002;91:348–54. doi:10.1080/08035250252834049.

34. Marcus SB, Strople JA, Neighbors K, Weissberg-Benchell J, Nelson SP, Limbers C, Varni JW, Alonso EM. Fatigue and health-related quality of life in pediatric inflammatory bowel disease. Clin Gastroenterol Hepatol. 2009;7:554–61.

35. Herzer M, Denson LA, Baldassano RN, Hommel KA. Family functioning and health-related quality of life in adolescents with pediatric inflammatory bowel disease. Eur J Gastroenterol Hepatol. 2011;23:95–100. doi:10.1097/MEG.0b013e3283417abb.

36. Otley AR, Griffiths AM, Hale S, Kugathasan S, Pfefferkorn M, Mezoff A, Rosh J, Tolia V, Markowitz J, Mack D, Oliva-Hemker M, Wyllie R, Rothbaum R, Bousvaros A, Del Rosario JF, Evans J, Blanchard W, Hyams J, Group PICR. Health-related quality of life in the first year after a diagnosis of pediatric inflammatory bowel disease. Inflamm Bowel Dis. 2006;12:684–91. doi: 00054725-200608000-00003 [pii]

37. van der Zaag-Loonen HJ, Grootenhuis MA, Last BF, Derkx HH. Coping strategies and quality of life of adolescents with inflammatory bowel disease. Qual Life Res. 2004;13:1011–9.

38. Gray WN, Boyle SL, Graef DM, Janicke DM, Jolley CD, Denson LA, Baldassano RN, Hommel KA. Health-related quality of life in youth with crohn disease: role of disease activity and parenting stress. J Pediatr Gastroenterol Nutr. 2015;60:749–53. doi:10.1097/MPG.0000000000000696.

39. Reed Knight B, Lee JL, Greenley RN, Lewis J, Blount R. Disease activity doesn't explain it all: how internalizing symptoms and caregiver depressive symptoms relate to health-related quality of

life among youth with inflammatory bowel disease. Inflamm Bowel Dis. 2016;22(4):963–7.

40. Hommel KA, Davis CM, Baldassano RN. Medication adherence and quality of life in pediatric inflammatory bowel disease. J Pediatr Psychol. 2008;33:867–74. doi:10.1093/jpepsy/jsn022.

41. MacPhee M, Hoffenberg EJ, Feranchak A. Quality-of-life factors in adolescent inflammatory bowel disease. Inflamm Bowel Dis. 1998;4:6–11.

42. Herzer M, Denson LA, Baldassano RN, Hommel KA. Patient and parent psychosocial factors associated with health-related quality of life in pediatric inflammatory bowel disease. J Pediatr Gastroenterol Nutr. 2011;52:295–9. doi:10.1097/MPG.0b013e3181f5714e.

43. Ryan JL, Mellon MW, Junger KW, Hente EA, Denson LA, Saeed SA, Hommel KA. The clinical utility of health-related quality of life screening in a pediatric inflammatory bowel disease clinic. Inflamm Bowel Dis. 2013;19:2666–72. doi:10.1097/MIB.0b013e3182a82b15.

44. Brown BB. Peer groups and peer cultures. In: Feldman SS, Elliott GR, editors. At the threshold: the developing adolescent. Cambridge: Harvard University Press; 1990. p. 171–96.

45. Harter S, Bresnick S, Bouchey HA, Whitesell NR. The development of multiple role-related selves during adolescence. Dev Psychopathol. 1997;9:835–53.

46. Hummel TZ, Tak E, Maurice-Stam H, Benninga MA, Kindermann A, Grootenhuis MA. Psychosocial developmental trajectory of adolescents with inflammatory bowel disease. J Pediatr Gastroenterol Nutr. 2013;57:219–24. doi:10.1097/MPG.0b013e3182935474.

47. Janicke DM, Gray WN, Kahhan NA, Follansbee KW, Marciel KK, Storch EA, Jolley CD. Brief report: the association between peer victimization, prosocial support, and treatment adherence in children and adolescents with inflammatory bowel disease. J Pediatr Psychol. 2009;34:769–73. doi:10.1093/jpepsy/jsn116.

48. Mackner L, Vannatta K, Crandall W. Gender differences in the social functioning of adolescents with inflammatory bowel disease. J Clin Psychol Med Settings. 2012;19:270–6. doi:10.1007/s10880-011-9292-x.

49. Burke P, Kocoshis SA, Chandra R, Whiteway M, Sauer J. Determinants of depression in recent onset pediatric inflammatory bowel disease. J Am Acad Child Adolesc Psychiatry. 1990;29:608–10.

50. Tojek TM, Lumley MA, Corlis M, Ondersma S, Tolia V. Maternal correlates of health status in adolescents with inflammatory bowel disease. J Psychosom Res. 2002;52:173–9. doi: S0022399901002914 [pii]

51. Wood B, Watkins JB, Boyle JT, Nogueira J, Zimand E, Carroll L. The "psychosomatic family" model: an empirical and theoretical analysis. Fam Process. 1989;28:399–417.

52. Burke PM, Kocoshis S, Neigut D, Sauer J, Chandra R, Orenstein D. Maternal psychiatric disorders in pediatric inflammatory bowel disease and cystic firbrosis. Child Psychiatry Hum Dev. 1994;25:45–52.

53. Engström I. Parental distress and social interaction in families with children with inflammatory bowel disease. J Am Acad Child Adolesc Psychiatry. 1991;30:904–12. doi:10.1097/00004583-199111000-00007.

54. Pai AL, Tackett A, Hente EA, Ernst MM, Denson LA, Hommel KA. Assessing psychosocial risk in pediatric inflammatory bowel disease: validation of the psychosocial assessment tool 2.0_general. J Pediatr Gastroenterol Nutr. 2014;58:51–6. doi:10.1097/MPG.0b013e3182a938b7.

55. Gray WN, Graef DM, Schuman SS, Janicke DM, Hommel KA. Parenting stress in pediatric IBD: relations with child psychopathology, family functioning, and disease severity. J Dev Behav Pediatr. 2013;34:237–44. doi:10.1097/DBP.0b013e318290568a.

56. Wood B, Boyle JT, Watkins JB, Nogueira J, Zimand E, Carroll L. Sibling psychological status and style as related to the disease of their chronically ill brothers and sisters: implications for models of biopsychosocial interaction. J Dev Behav Pediatr. 1988;9:66–72.

57. Akobeng AK, Suresh-Babu MV, Firth D, Miller V, Mir P, Thomas AG. Quality of life in children with Crohn's disease: a pilot study. J Pediatr Gastroenterol Nutr. 1999;28:S37–9.

58. Griffiths AM, Nicholas D, Smith C, Munk M, Stephens D, Durno C, Sherman PM. Development of a quality-of-life index for pediatric inflammatory bowel disease: dealing with differences related to age and IBD type. J Pediatr Gastroenterol Nutr. 1999;28:S46–52.

59. Loonen HJ, Derkx BH, Koopman HM, Heymans HS. Are parents able to rate the symptoms and quality of life of their offspring with IBD? Inflamm Bowel Dis. 2002;8:270–6.

60. Loonen HJ, Grootenhuis MA, Last BF, de Haan RJ, Bouquet J, Derkx BH. Measuring quality of life in children with inflammatory bowel disease: the impact-II (NL). Qual Life Res. 2002;11:47–56.

61. Richardson G, Griffiths AM, Miller V, Thomas AG. Quality of life in inflammatory bowel disease: a cross-cultural comparison of English and Canadian children. J Pediatr Gastroenterol Nutr. 2001;32:573–8.

62. Raymer D, Weininger O, Hamilton JR. Psychological problems in children with abdominal pain. Lancet. 1984;1:439–40.

63. Bernstein CN, Singh S, Graff LA, Walker JR, Miller N, Cheang M. A prospective population-based study of triggers of symptomatic flares in IBD. Am J Gastroenterol. 2010;105:1994–2002. doi:10.1038/ajg.2010.140.

64. Bitton A, Dobkin PL, Edwardes MD, Sewitch MJ, Meddings JB, Rawal S, Cohen A, Vermeire S, Dufresne L, Franchimont D, Wild GE. Predicting relapse in Crohn's disease: a biopsychosocial model. Gut. 2008;57:1386–92. doi:10.1136/gut.2007.134817.

65. Langhorst J, Hofstetter A, Wolfe F, Häuser W. Short-term stress, but not mucosal healing nor depression was predictive for the risk of relapse in patients with ulcerative colitis: a prospective 12-month follow-up study. Inflamm Bowel Dis. 2013;19:2380–6. doi:10.1097/MIB.0b013e3182a192ba.

66. Gitlin K, Markowitz J, Pelcovitz D, Strohmayer A, Dorstein L, Klein S. Stress mediators in children with inflammatory bowel disease. In: Johnson JH, Johnson SB, editors. Advances in child health psychology. Gainesville: University of Florida Press; 1991. p. 54–62.

67. Engstrom I. Family interaction and locus of control in children and adolescents with inflammatory bowel disease. J Am Acad Child Adolesc Psychiatry. 1991;30:913–20.

68. Wojtowicz AA, Greenley RN, Gumidyala AP, Rosen A, Williams SE. Pain severity and pain catastrophizing predict functional disability in youth with inflammatory bowel disease. J Crohns Colitis. 2014;8:1118–24. doi:10.1016/j.crohns.2014.02.011.

69. van Tilburg MA, Claar RL, Romano JM, Langer SL, Walker LS, Whitehead WE, Abdullah B, Christie DL, Levy RL. Role of coping with symptoms in depression and disability: comparison between inflammatory bowel disease and abdominal pain. J Pediatr Gastroenterol Nutr. 2015;61:431–6. doi:10.1097/MPG.0000000000000841.

70. Ferguson A, Sedgwick DM, Drummond J. Morbidity of juvenile onset inflammatory bowel disease: effects on education and employment in early adult life. Gut. 1994;35:665–8.

71. Moody G, Eaden JA, Mayberry JF. Social implications of childhood Crohn's disease. J Pediatr Gastroenterol Nutr. 1999;28:S43–5.

72. Rabbett H, Elbadri A, Thwaites R, Northover H, Dady I, Firth D, Hillier VF, Miller V, Thomas AG. Quality of life in children with Crohn's disease. J Pediatr Gastroenterol Nutr. 1996;23:528–33.

73. Bernstein CN, Kraut A, Blanchard JF, Rawsthorne P, Yu N, Walld R. The relationship between inflammatory bowel disease and socioeconomic variables. Am J Gastroenterol. 2001;96:2117–25. doi:10.1111/j.1572-0241.2001.03946.x.

74. Longobardi T, Jacobs P, Bernstein CN. Work losses related to inflammatory bowel disease in the United States: results from the National Health Interview Survey. Am J Gastroenterol. 2003;98:1064–72.

75. Marri SR, Buchman AL. The education and employment status of patients with inflammatory bowel diseases. Inflamm Bowel Dis. 2005;11:171–7. doi: 00054725-200502000-00011 [pii]

76. Mackner LM, Bickmeier RM, Crandall WV. Academic achievement, attendance, and school-related quality of life in pediatric inflammatory bowel disease. J Dev Behav Pediatr. 2012;33:106–11. doi:10.1097/DBP.0b013e318240cf68.

77. Rabbett H, Elbadri A, Thwaites R, Northover H, Dady I, Firth D, Hillier VF, Miller V, Thomas AG. Quality of life in children with Crohn's disease. J Pediatr Gastroenterol Nutr. 1996;23:S28–33.

78. Varni JW, Limbers CA, Burwinkle TM. Impaired health-related quality of life in children and adolescents with chronic conditions: a comparative analysis of 10 disease clusters and 33 disease categories/severities utilizing the PedsQL 4.0 generic core scales. Health Qual Life Outcomes. 2007;5:43. doi:10.1186/1477-7525-5-43.

79. Ingerski LM, Modi AC, Hood KK, Pai AL, Zeller M, Piazza-Waggoner C, Driscoll KA, Rothenberg ME, Franciosi J, Hommel KA. Health-related quality of life across pediatric chronic conditions. J Pediatr. 2010;156:639–44. doi:10.1016/j.jpeds.2009.11.008.

80. Greenley RN, Kunz JH, Biank V, Martinez A, Miranda A, Noe J, Telega G, Tipnis NA, Werlin S, Stephens MC. Identifying youth nonadherence in clinical settings: data-based recommendations for children and adolescents with inflammatory bowel disease. Inflamm Bowel Dis. 2012;18:1254–9. doi:10.1002/ibd.21859.

81. LeLeiko NS, Lobato D, Hagin S, McQuaid E, Seifer R, Kopel SJ, Boergers J, Nassau J, Suorsa K, Shapiro J, Bancroft B. Rates and predictors of oral medication adherence in pediatric patients with IBD. Inflamm Bowel Dis. 2013;19:832–9. doi:10.1097/MIB.0b013e3182802b57.

82. Reed-Knight B, Lewis JD, Blount RL. Behavioral functioning in youth with inflammatory bowel disease: perceived barriers as mediator of medication adherence. J Pediatr Psychol. 2013;38:309–20. doi:10.1093/jpepsy/jss122.

83. Gray WN, Denson LA, Baldassano RN, Hommel KA. Treatment adherence in adolescents with inflammatory bowel disease: the collective impact of barriers to adherence and anxiety/depressive symptoms. J Pediatr Psychol. 2012;37:282–91. doi:10.1093/jpepsy/jsr092.

84. Mackner LM, Crandall WV. Oral medication adherence in pediatric inflammatory bowel disease. Inflamm Bowel Dis. 2005;11:1006–12. doi:10.1097/01.MIB.0000186409.15392.54.

85. Schurman J, Cushing C, Carpenter E, Christenson K. Volitional and accidental nonadherence to pediatric inflammatory bowel disease treatment plans: initial investigation of associations with quality of life and disease activity. J Pediatr Psychol. 2010;36:116–25. doi:10.1093/jpepsy/jsq046.

86. Vitale DS, Greenley RN, Lerner DG, Mavis AM, Werlin SL. Adherence to infliximab treatment in a pediatric inflammatory bowel disease cohort. J Pediatr Gastroenterol Nutr. 2015;61:408–10. doi:10.1097/MPG.0000000000000817.

87. Szigethy E, Kenney E, Carpenter J, Hardy DM, Fairclough D, Bousvaros A, Keljo D, Weisz J, Beardslee WR, Noll R, DeMaso DR. Cognitive-behavioral therapy for adolescents with inflammatory bowel disease and subsyndromal depression. J Am Acad Child Adolesc Psychiatry. 2007;46:1290–8. doi:10.1097/chi.0b013e3180f6341f.

88. Szigethy E, Whitton SW, Levy-Warren A, DeMaso DR, Weisz J, Beardslee WR. Cognitive-behavioral therapy for depression in adolescents with inflammatory bowel disease: a pilot study. J Am Acad Child Adolesc Psychiatry. 2004;43:1469–77.

89. Szigethy E, Carpenter J, Baum E, Kenney E, Baptista-Neto L, Beardslee WR, DeMaso DR. Case study: longitudinal treatment of adolescents with depression and inflammatory bowel disease. J Amer Acad Child Adolesc Psychiatry. 2006;45:369–400.

90. Thompson RD, Craig A, Crawford EA, Fairclough D, Gonzalez-Heydrich J, Bousvaros A, Noll RB, DeMaso DR, Szigethy E. Longitudinal results of cognitive behavioral treatment for youths with inflammatory bowel disease and depressive symptoms. J Clin Psychol Med Settings. 2012;19:329–37. doi:10.1007/s10880-012-9301-8.

91. Grootenhuis MA, Maurice-Stam H, Derkx BH, Last BF. Evaluation of a psychoeducational intervention for adolescents with inflammatory bowel disease. Eur J Gastroenterol Hepatol. 2009;21: 430–5.

92. McCormick M, Reed-Knight B, Lewis JD, Gold BD, Blount RL. Coping skills for reducing pain and somatic symptoms in adolescents with IBD. Inflamm Bowel Dis. 2010;16:2148–57. doi:10.1002/ibd.21302.

93. Szigethy E, Hardy D, Craig AE, Low C, Kukic S. Girls connect: effects of a support group for teenage girls with inflammatory bowel disease and their mothers. Inflamm Bowel Dis. 2009;15:1127–8. doi:10.1002/ibd.20775.

94. Shepanski MA, Hurd LB, Culton K, Markowitz JE, Mamula P, Baldassano RN. Health-related quality of life improves in children and adolescents with inflammatory bowel disease after attending a camp sponsored by the Crohn's and Colitis Foundation of America. Inflamm Bowel Dis. 2005;11:164–70.

95. Kearney CA. School absenteeism and school refusal behavior in youth: a contemporary review. Clin Psychol Rev. 2008;28:451–71. doi:10.1016/j.cpr.2007.07.012.

96. Kearney CA. Forms and functions of school refusal behavior in youth: an empirical analysis of absenteeism severity. J Child Psychol Psychiatry. 2007;48:53–61. doi:10.1111/j.1469-7610.2006.01634.x.

97. Greenley RN, Gumidyala AP, Nguyen E, Plevinsky JM, Poulopoulos N, Thomason MM, Walter JG, Wojtowicz AA, Blank E, Gokhale R, Kirschner BS, Miranda A, Noe JD, Stephens MC, Werlin S, Kahn SA. Can you teach a teen new tricks? Problem solving skills training improves oral medication adherence in pediatric patients with inflammatory bowel disease participating in a randomized trial. Inflamm Bowel Dis. 2015;21:2649–57. doi:10.1097/MIB.0000000000000530.

Amy Grant and Anthony Otley

Introduction

The burden of disease imposed on children and youth by Crohn disease (CD) and ulcerative colitis (UC) may be considerable, as manifested by clinical parameters such as symptoms, number of hospitalizations, growth retardation, and frequent need for surgery [1–5]. However, increasingly the psychosocial burden of inflammatory bowel disease (IBD) on young patients is being considered alongside these important clinical parameters [6–8]. One means of assessing the psychosocial burden is through evaluation of health-related quality of life (HRQOL). The purpose of this chapter is to provide the reader with an understanding of the concept of HRQOL, the approaches to its measurement in children, more specifically in pediatric patients with inflammatory bowel disease (IBD). Finally the gaps in knowledge of HRQOL in pediatric IBD and the future directions for research in this area will be discussed.

Quality of Life: Concepts/Definitions

In 1948 the World Health Organization defined health as being not only the absence of disease and infirmity but also the presence of physical, mental, and social well-being [9]. Since that time quality-of-life issues have been increasingly recognized as important parameters in determining health status. A single definition of quality of life is difficult to find [10, 11]. Without a clear definition, multiple interpretations

of what quality of life "is" have evolved. This has led to the development of a number of different measures which assess varying aspects of quality of life. This failure to achieve a unifying definition has hampered the ability to make comparisons between quality-of-life outcomes. Most recent definitions include the concept of the multidimensional nature of quality of life and incorporate domains of social, physical, and emotional functioning of the individual [12]. With HRQOL one is attempting to ascertain the impact of the disease, concentrating on the health-related aspects of quality of life. Quality-of-life outcomes have been conceptualized by viewing the domains in two dimensions: objective assessments of functioning or health status (the y axis in Fig. 51.1) and more subjective perceptions of health (the x axis) [13]. While the objective assessment is integral for describing an individual's degree of health, the individual's subjective perceptions and expectations modify the objective assessment into the real quality of life experienced (or Q, as expressed in Fig. 51.1 by the intersection of the x and y coordinates). Because perceptions and expectations may vary from individual to individual, two people with the same health status may have very different qualities of life [13].

Why Measure Health-Related Quality of Life?

Over the past several decades, a dramatic increase in the employment of quality-of-life outcome measures has been evident in the adult and pediatric clinical trials' literature. In part this is a result of the trend to expand the traditionally selected, "objective" outcome measures of morbidity (i.e., days hospitalized, number of infections) and/or mortality to include assessment of the emotional and functional status of participants. The single-minded focus on mortality and morbidity as outcomes in health is being steadily superseded by broader considerations of quality of life. This broader consideration is currently being espoused by the Food and Drug Administration (FDA) which is now mandating inclusion of patient-reported outcomes (PROs) alongside more objective

A. Grant, PhD
Division of Gastroenterology, Department of Pediatrics, Izaak Walton Killam Health Centre, 5850 University Avenue, Halifax, Nova Scotia, Canada, B3J 3G9
e-mail: amy.grant@iwk.nshealth.ca

A. Otley, MD, MSc, FRCPC (✉)
Division of Gastroenterology, Department of Pediatrics, Dalhousie University, Izaak Walton Killam Health Centre, 5850 University Avenue, Halifax, Nova Scotia, Canada, B3J 3G9
e-mail: arotley@dal.ca

© Springer International Publishing AG 2017
P. Mamula et al. (eds.), *Pediatric Inflammatory Bowel Disease*, DOI 10.1007/978-3-319-49215-5_51

Fig. 51.1 Conceptual scheme of the domains and variables involved in a quality-of-life assessment. The *x* axis represents subjective perceptions of health, the *y* axis represents objective health status, the coordinates Q(X, Y) represent the actual quality of life, and Z represents the measurement of the actual quality of life associated with a specific component (i.e., positive affect) or domain (i.e., the psychological domain) (Adapted from Testa and Simonson [13])

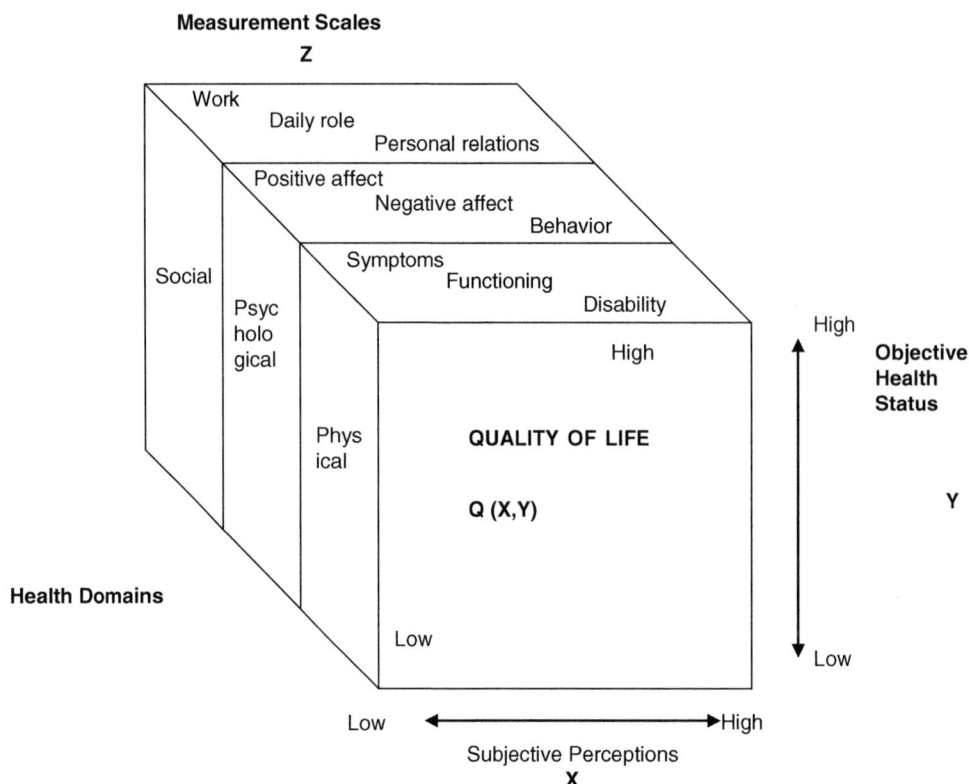

measures (i.e., endoscopic evaluation) in the design of clinical trials to evaluate new drug therapies in IBD [14].

One of the first stages in evaluating a new measure is to determine the "phenomenon of interest," to define the conceptual framework underlying the measure [15]. In IBD the primary outcome measure traditionally selected for use in clinical trials has been a multi-item disease activity index [16], such as the pediatric Crohn disease activity index (PCDAI) [17, 18]. For the disease activity measures, the concept is to use the degree of intestinal inflammatory activity as a surrogate measure of the patient's health status. This framework is based heavily on physician perceptions, with little input about the patient's perception of the disease on their health status [16]. Quality-of-life measures try to address this deficiency. Because existing measures of disease activity are not sensitive enough to assess the full impact of the disorder, HRQOL measures have been developed to do this [19].

Approaches to Health-Related Quality-of-Life Measurement

The ideal assessment of HRQOL would involve lengthy, detailed interviews between the patient and an independent interviewer, an impractical procedure in day-to-day clinical care or a clinical trial. A self-administered questionnaire that is easy to understand, complete, and covers all the important

aspects of the patient's HRQOL is a more attractive means of assessing HRQOL. The questionnaire should include all relevant elements or "domains," of HRQOL. These domains may cover physical, functional, emotional, and cognitive well-being and, in case of disease, disease-related aspects. Each domain consists of a number of "dimensions" or questions. A balance needs to be struck between including a sufficient number of dimensions so that a complete assessment of HRQOL can be made, while being careful not create too lengthy a questionnaire so that it becomes burdensome for the respondent to complete. The advantage of combining questions into domains is that interventions can be directed at these domains, attempting to ameliorate that aspect of HRQOL.

There are two basic types of HRQOL measures: generic and disease specific. A generic measure is designed to measure all aspects of health and related quality of life and can include items and domains that are broadly applicable to various diseases and populations. Although disease-specific questionnaires include some of these same issues, they also address issues specific to the particular disease. Disease-specific questionnaires are more sensitive to disease-related changes in patients' health status than generic questionnaires.

Generic measures can take several forms, from instruments with global assessments using single indicators (e.g., "What is the quality of your life on a scale of 1–10?"), utilities (e.g., standard gamble, time trade-off), or multi-item measures which give a health profile, such

Table 51.1 Four fundamental measurement characteristics to be assessed of any measure

Measurement characteristic	Definition	Examples of what to look for
Sensibility	Do the components of the instrument make sense and is it feasible to administer and complete?	Readability statistics
		Number of questions left blank
		Inappropriate inclusions or important omissions of items
Reliability	Are similar scores obtained on subsequent assessments if no change in disease status has occurred?	Test-retest reliability most commonly reported (either as intraclass correlation coefficient or Kappa value)
		Instruments with good reliability require smaller sample sizes
Validity	Is the instrument measuring what it was intended to measure?	Criterion validity testing when a gold standard exists to compare to
		Construct validity testing when no gold standard exists, and hypotheses are generated and tested on how the instrument would be expected to function
Responsiveness	Does the instrument score change with a change in disease status?	No one accepted way to evaluate
		Want to know over what time period an instrument is responsive (i.e., short term, 4 weeks, or longer term, 6 months)

as the Medical Outcomes Study Short-Form 36 (SF-36) [20]. One of the advantages of a generic measure is its generalizability. Generic measures permit comparisons between "healthy populations" and different disease groups, interventions, and demographic and cultural groups [21, 22]. Generic questionnaires, such as the SF-36 for adults [21, 23] or the Child Health Questionnaire for children [24], have been applied to groups with no defined illness, allowing normative values to be generated for these healthy populations. When such normative data is available, it offers the potential to make comparisons as to burden of illness between populations affected with and without chronic illness [25]. The chief disadvantage to generic measures is their insensitivity to important clinical change. This stems from their inherent lack of specificity, a result of the inclusion of many items which may not be relevant to the individual patient with an isolated disease. This can be addressed by the use of a disease-specific measure that focuses on concerns relevant to a particular patient group. "Specificity" is achieved by the inclusion of dimensions and domains which are targeted to the disease in question. For example, in the Pediatric Asthma Quality of Life Questionnaire, a measure developed by Juniper et al. [26], the symptom domain includes questions such as "How much did tightness in your chest bother you during the past week?" and "How often did your asthma wake you up during the night in the past week?" This specificity makes the questionnaire more sensitive to important clinical change in asthma, which is an important criterion when choosing an outcome measure in a clinical trial. In the adult literature, disease-specific questionnaires have been developed for a number of diseases, including IBD [27], rheumatoid arthritis [28], breast cancer [29, 30], and asthma [31, 32]. In comparison fewer disease-specific questionnaires have been developed for use in the pediatric population [31, 33–36].

Any measurement tool should be tested prior to use to ensure it fulfills the fundamental psychometric characteristics of a good measure. An HRQOL questionnaire would be one example of a measurement tool. The psychometric characteristics to be assessed include sensibility, reliability, validity, and responsiveness to change (Table 51.1). *Sensibility* is a measurement characteristic with many aspects and for a questionnaire should include assessment of feasibility for both the person administering and completing the questionnaire (i.e., time to complete and mark, readability), as well as a critical review of the appropriateness of items included or omitted. *Reliability* looks at whether a measure has reproducibility, i.e., if the same result is obtained when the same (unchanged) entity is measured again (17). For example, assuming that HRQOL is influenced by disease activity or medication use, one would expect a reliable HRQOL questionnaire to show very similar scores when given to a patient at time one and again at time two if no interval change in disease activity or medication has occurred. *Validity* is concerned with whether a questionnaire actually measures what it is intended to measure. Ideally one would like to measure the validity of an HRQOL measure comparing it with a gold standard. Unfortunately, HRQOL is a concept for which no gold standard exists. Thus a process of construct validity testing must be carried out. This involves generating hypotheses, called constructs, and studying whether the measure acts as one would expect. The final characteristic, *responsiveness* to change, relates to the ability of the questionnaire to detect change over time, characteristics important for use in clinical settings. A very responsive HRQOL questionnaire should be able to detect even a small change in disease status. This latter characteristic is especially important in determining the sample size for studies in which HRQOL is a main outcome, as the expected amount of change determines how many participants are needed to show a statistically significant change.

Health-Related Quality-of-Life Assessment in Pediatrics

Making quality-of-life assessments in a pediatric population requires the awareness of several key methodological issues: whether to ask children directly [37, 38] and how to allow for varying developmental level and age [10, 39]. It is not always possible to obtain the child's assessment of their quality of life, whether due to age and/or developmental or disability limits to comprehension. In these instances a proxy is sought. The proxy reporter of the child's quality of life is most often their parent/caregiver but in some cases may be another individual such as a teacher or physician [38]. Research has shown, however, that proxies tend to have a low to modest agreement with the child's reported quality-of-life self-assessment. The degree of agreement seems to relate to the objectiveness of the dimension of quality of life being assessed. Pantell et al. showed that parents and teachers agreed fairly well in reporting on child functioning but markedly less well for recent functional status, certain types of subjective feelings in regard to illness, information needs, emotional states [40], and family functioning [41]. Agreement among raters may differ as a result of factors such as child sex, age, and condition [42].

Other issues relate to the wide developmental spectrum seen across the pediatric age group. The quality of a child's self-report is highly dependent on their expressive and receptive language abilities [10]. As well, differences in time perception and memory related to their developmental stage will affect a child's ability to respond to questions based upon experiences during a specific time period [38]. Within a given culture, developmental tasks can vary by age such that some quality-of-life items may be appropriate for a specific age range but not for another. For example, perceptions on relationships with the opposite sex will vary with age. Other issues likely related to developmental age include position bias, the tendency to choose the first answer; acquiescence response bias, the tendency to agree with the interviewer; and limited understanding of negatively worded items [43]. Realizing there are low agreements for proxy ratings in some areas of response, it is unclear to what extent differences in response pattern are due to limitations in abstract reasoning or true differences in perspective or opinion.

Health-Related Quality-of-Life Assessment in Inflammatory Bowel Disease: Adult IBD Perspective

Measurement of HRQOL in IBD has received a lot of attention over the several decades, with the result that there are now validated outcome measures that have been used in clinical trials or cross-sectional studies (Table 51.2). Early

attempts at assessing HRQOL in IBD, however, were hampered by a number of methodological issues: healthy or medical comparison groups were not used, studies were done by retrospective analyses [44, 45], non-standardized instruments [45–48] and unskilled interviewers were used to obtain the data, and insensitive outcome factors (i.e., ability to work) [44, 48, 49] were used as measures of HRQOL.

The main disease-specific HRQOL instrument currently used is the Inflammatory Bowel Disease Questionnaire (IBDQ) which was developed for IBD patients and to be used in clinical trials [27, 50, 51]. It is a 32-item questionnaire, consisting of 30 items chosen most frequently and rated most important by adult IBD patients and two items added based on feedback obtained by clinicians who had practices heavily weighted with IBD patients. The four domains covered in IBDQ include bowel symptoms (10 items), systemic symptoms (5 items), emotional function (12 items), and social function (5 items). Responses are based on a seven-point Likert scale in which one represents worst function and seven represents best function. Thus, the higher the score, the better the quality of life. The questionnaire can be self-administered [52, 53] and takes approximately 15 min to complete. The IBDQ has undergone extensive testing of its measurement characteristics, including several randomized controlled trials [50, 54, 55] and cross-sectional studies [56]. From a large multicentered Canadian trial of maintenance therapy, an intraclass correlation coefficient of 0.70 was calculated for test-retest reliability in 280 patients with stable disease over an 8-week period [50]. Responsiveness testing using a modified responsiveness index developed by Guyatt et al. indicated that all IBDQ indices reflected deterioration for those patients whose condition worsened during the study [57]. Construct validity testing in the original publication of the measure, and with subsequent use of the IBDQ in trials, has shown it to be a valid measure of HRQOL in adult patients with IBD. This measure has been shown to have strong correlation with patient, relative, and physician global ratings of HRQOL and discriminate between the groups of patients who did or did not require surgery [50]. Some researchers have expressed concern about the use of a single measure to describe the HRQOL for IBD, because of the frequently disparate nature of its component diseases, Crohn disease and ulcerative colitis [58]. For example, because Crohn disease can affect variable locations in the bowel, the range of symptoms can also vary greatly, with differences exacerbated by relapsing and remitting disease activity. This is compared with ulcerative colitis in which the bowel disease is limited to the colon. Given these differences, some researchers have suggested that a different or separate approach to HRQOL evaluation for these two diseases may be required. This issue was apparently not addressed in the development of the IBDQ [27, 50]. Given the increasing number of many available

Table 51.2 Health-related quality-of-life measures for inflammatory bowel disease

Name	Scales	Comments
Adult		
Inflammatory Bowel Disease Questionnaire (IBDQ) 32-item Likert scale Interview format	Bowel symptoms, systemic symptoms, social function, emotional function	Well standardized; designed for clinical trials; developed on "sick" patients – GI referrals and inpatients
Modified IBDQ 36-item Likert scale Self-administered	Bowel symptoms, systemic symptoms, social function, emotional function, functional impairment	Derived from IBDQ; developed on "well" patients – local chapter of NFIC
Cleveland Clinic Questionnaire 47-item Likert scale Interview format	Functional/economic, social/ recreational, affect/life in general, medical/symptoms	Correlates with SIP; developed on UC/CD surgical/nonsurgical groups; quality-of-life index distinguishes groups
Rating Form of IBD Patient Concerns (RFPIC) 25-item visual analog scale Self-administered	Impact of disease, sexual intimacy, complications, body stigma	Correlates with SIP and SCL-90; developed on "well" patients – CCFA national sample
UC/CD Health Status Scales 9- or 10-item Likert scale Physician/patient scoring	Ulcerative colitis, Crohn disease	Standardized to healthcare use, function, psychological distress in CCFA national sample
Pediatric		
Computer-based animated questionnaire 35-item visual scale Children ages 5–11 years	30 generic questions, 5 disease specific (more detail not specified)	Only 16-patient pilot study reported to date. Child does not have to read
PEDIBDQ 45-item Likert scale Children ages 8–18 years	Physical, emotional, and social	Reported in abstract form, with validation and reliability data
IMPACT 35-item Likert scale Self-administered Children ages 10–17 years	Bowel, emotional, functional, tests/treatments, systemic, body image	Three versions (IMPACT-I, II, and III). Developed using several pediatric IBD cohorts; in use in clinical trials

Abbreviations used: *CCFA* Crohn's and Colitis Foundation of America, *CD* Crohn disease, *CDAI* Crohn disease activity index, *GI* gastrointestinal, *NFIC* National Foundation for Ileitis and Colitis, *SCL-90* Symptom Checklist-90, *SIP* Sickness Impact Profile, *UC* ulcerative colitis
Adapted from Drossman [58]

cross-culturally adapted versions of the IBDQ [59–65] and the development [66] and subsequent validation [67, 68] of the 10-item Short Inflammatory Bowel Disease Questionnaire (SIBDQ), it seems unlikely that other HRQOL measures for adult IBD patients will be developed, unless it is to target specific subgroups missed in the IBDQ item generation such as patients with ileostomy.

Health-Related Quality-of-Life Assessment in Pediatric Inflammatory Bowel Disease

As is the case with pediatric quality-of-life assessment in general, consideration of quality-of-life issues in pediatric IBD has lagged behind that of the adult IBD cohort. The earliest semblances of quality-of-life inquiry were from a number of centers which reported the results of long-term follow-up or cross-sectional assessments of their pediatric IBD populations [2, 3, 69–75]. In many instances, rather than actually describing the quality of life, they were describing the functional status of the patients [69–71, 74, 75].

Goel et al. [69] and Lindquist et al. [71] did not use a formal measure to describe quality of life but rather, in their description of the current status [69] or clinical course [71] of the patients, included limitations on social activities, school attendance, or occupation as descriptors. Farmer and Michener [72, 73] developed a simple measure which provided three categories of quality of life: "Good – meaning ability to function in a nearly normal manner with minimal interference from the illness and its sequelae; Poor – indicated severe effect on life style, requiring medication and often frequent hospitalization; Fair – suboptimal but adequate functioning, i.e., chronic illness and partial disability." Patients were categorized based on interviews by trained personnel. The researchers acknowledged that their view of quality of life was a composite of several elements of the patient's life and that patients might experience varying degrees of quality of life over a long period of time. Patients were asked to consider the cumulative effect of the illness and treatment and to describe their current state of health. Farmer and Michener's long-term follow-up study of 522 patients (followed from 1955 to 1974) with onset of CD under age 21 found that approximately two thirds of patients considered their functioning to be in the fair level, with only 6% rating their functioning as poor [72, 73]. Given the marked changes in management over the past five decades, it is unclear what relevance quality-of-life outcomes in such a cohort would have compared to a similar present-day cohort. More recently researchers have sought to assess quality of life in pediatric IBD using measures with domains which encompass a broader concept of quality of life [76–79]. MacPhee et al. [79] completed an assessment of 30 pediatric IBD patients using a number of generic psychological and quality-of-life questionnaires. Their study emphasized social supports and coping strategies. They used the Quality of Life for Adolescents and Parents questionnaire [80], a generic measure which gives a total satisfaction score with health status and similar scores for subscales.

Thomas et al. [76, 77] describe the early stages of development of a disease-specific quality-of-life questionnaire which they used to assess quality of life in their pediatric Crohn disease cohort. Focus group meetings were held with pediatric patients of ages from 8 to 17 years (two groups, 8–12 years and 12–17 years of age) to learn how their disease and its treatment affected their lives at school, at home, and with friends. An 88-item questionnaire was constructed based on the areas identified in the focus groups. The questionnaire contained six domains of HRQOL including symptoms and treatment, social life, emotional state, family life, education, and future aspects. No data on validity, reliability, or sensibility was provided for this questionnaire [76, 77]. The questionnaire was used in one pilot study involving 16 children from one academic IBD program in England. Acknowledging the limitations of a small sample size, they found that CD appeared to most adversely affect the HRQOL of children as manifested through school absenteeism, fatigue limiting sports activities, and difficulties in taking holidays.

Moody et al. [78] studied quality of life in pediatric Crohn disease using a questionnaire they developed in conjunction with a British national lay committee of Crohn in Childhood Research Association (CICRA) members. Limited information is provided on the questionnaire's development, and its length and exact format is unclear from the published report [78]. Results from 60 to 4 valid questionnaires were received in a pilot study. The mean age of the children in this study was 14.1 ± 2.8 years (range 6–17 years). In this cohort 60% of the children reported prolonged absences from school, with a mean 3 ± 2.8 months' absence in the previous 12 months. Eighty percent of those who had taken examinations felt that their marks had suffered due to ill health. Seventy percent of patients with CD were unable to participate in sports on a regular basis, 60% did not feel comfortable leaving their homes, and 50% did not feel they could play outside with their friends because of the illness. Forty percent of children also reported concerns about taking holidays and being able

to have sleepovers at friends' homes. This study would suggest that CD has a major impact on the QOL of pediatric patients. However, caution should be exercised in making these conclusions as there are several limitations of the published study. It is not clear if the questionnaire underwent any validity testing to ensure it was measuring what it intended to measure. Given the study design, in which a general mailing was sent to members of a society, there may be a strong response bias in favor of those whose QOL is poor. As well, the authors do not tell us the number of questionnaires distributed, nor do they clarify the response rate.

Preliminary development of the Pediatric Inflammatory Bowel Disease Questionnaire (PEDIBDQ) for children and teens [81, 82] and a computer-based animated program to assess HRQOL for young children 5–11 years of age [83] have been reported in abstract or manuscript form. Further work has not been reported using these questionnaires, however. In the mid-1990s, researchers at the Hospital for Sick Children in Toronto, Canada, began work on a disease-specific measure, the IMPACT questionnaire [84], which today is the most commonly employed disease-specific measure for assessing HRQOL in the pediatric IBD population.

Ryan et al. [85] reported on the incorporation of HRQOL screening into clinical practice and its clinical utility in predicting disease outcome and healthcare utilization. One hundred twelve IBD youth ages 7–18 years completed the Pediatric Quality of Life Inventory, Version 4.0 (PedsQL 4.0), with retrospective chart reviews conducted to examine disease outcomes and healthcare utilization for 12 months after baseline QOL assessment. They demonstrated that youth who reported lower HRQOL at baseline, on average, had increased healthcare utilization as measured by IBD-related hospital admissions, emergency department visits, use of psychological services, telephone calls to clinicians, GI clinic visits, and referral to pain management.

IMPACT

The Development of the Impact Questionnaire

There are three English iterations of the IMPACT questionnaire at present, and work is actively underway on translation of IMPACT-III into other languages. Work on IMPACT began in the mid-1990s because at that time there was no published disease-specific HRQOL instrument available for pediatric patients with IBD. Generic pediatric HRQOL questionnaires, such as the Child Health Questionnaire [24, 86], were felt to be insensitive to the disease-specific issues of IBD. Concerns about wording issues, including inappropriate omissions and inclusions for a pediatric target audience, led researchers at the Hospital for Sick Children in Toronto to seek a pediatric-derived instrument over the adult-derived

Question 10.	How often have you been bothered by diarrhea (loose or frequent bowel movements) in the past two weeks?

☐	☐	☐	☐	☐
Never	Rarely	Sometimes	Often	Very often

Fig. 51.2 Sample IMPACT-III question. As opposed to IMPACT versions I and II which used visual analog response scales, IMPACT-III uses a five-point Likert response scale

IBDQ [36]. For example, one question in the IBDQ [50] pertains to limitation of sexual activity by IBD, an issue which was felt to be of limited relevance in a pediatric cohort, except perhaps for the older adolescent. Issues not covered by the IBDQ which were felt to be of likely relevance to a pediatric cohort included growth concerns and limitations on school and extracurricular activities.

Defining how a new HRQOL tool will be used is important in guiding the development process, as this helps to ensure that the end product is addressing the underlying need. The IMPACT developers sought to create a questionnaire which would serve both as a descriptive and evaluative tool. As a descriptive tool, the measure would facilitate recognition in individual patients of disparity between apparent IBD activity and severity, organic disease-related phenomena, which the physician is accustomed to assessing, and emotional or functional disability. As an evaluative tool, it was to be incorporated as an outcome measure in clinical trials to assess change in HRQOL over time.

In the development of IMPACT, there was a focus on children aged 10–17 years. Younger patients were excluded because of concern that systematic exploration of quality of life among very young children would require significantly modified methods. Items to be included in the final questionnaire were generated chiefly from interviews of pediatric patients with IBD. Items universally of greatest importance for all IBD patients were included, as well as some items rated as very important by one subgroup of patients (CD or UC), even if not by others [84].

The original IMPACT [36], or IMPACT-I as it is currently known, consisted of 33 questions, and responses were given using a visual analog scale. Each question was scored out of seven, so that the final total score would be similar to what was seen with the adult IBDQ. Thus, the range of scores possible for IMPACT-I was 0–231. During the cross-cultural adaptation and translation process of IMPACT-I into the Dutch language, a modified version was developed [87]. This version, IMPACT-II, eliminated or modified four questions and added a new question, resulting in a 35-item questionnaire with simplified wording of the response options for the visual analog scale. IMPACT-II was available in both English [88] and Dutch [87] language versions. Some researchers preferred a Likert response scale, and IMPACT-III

Table 51.3 Cross-cultural adaptations and translations of IMPACT-III[a]

Language
Arabic
Bosnian
Bulgarian
Chinese
Croatian (male and female versions)
Czech
Danish
Dutch (Belgium, Netherlands)
English (Australia and New Zealand, Ireland, North America, UK versions)
Estonian
Farsi
French (Belgium, Canada, France, Switzerland versions)
German (Austria, Germany, Switzerland versions)
Greek
Hebrew
Hungarian
Italian (Italy, Switzerland versions)
Japanese
Lithuanian
Norwegian
Polish
Portuguese
Romanian
Russian
Slovak
Slovenian
Spanish (Argentina, Chile, Spain, US versions)
Swedish

[a]as of June 2016

[89] was created, which is identical to IMPACT-II save for the five-point Likert response scales and anchors (Fig. 51.2). IMPACT-III is available in over 40 languages (as well as culturally adapted versions in English, French, and Spanish) (see Table 51.3). IMPACT-III is the questionnaire used for ongoing cross-cultural adaptation.

Through cohort studies, and more recently in randomized controlled trials [89–91], IMPACT has demonstrated itself to be a valid measure of disease-specific HRQOL in pediatric

IBD patients 10 years of age and over. From this work, while disease activity and disease severity are two factors which have been identified as strongly correlated with HRQOL, regression modeling clearly shows that they can only explain a small part of the HRQOL "puzzle" [36, 88]. As well work to date has not shown any influence of disease type (CD or UC) or gender in influencing the performance of IMPACT. With age there remains less clarity. The original validation did not show any significant differences in perceived HRQOL across the age group studied.

Research has shown that the perceived HRQOL as assessed by IMPACT is most influenced by the current health status rather than that suffered over the previous 12 months [36]. That the IMPACT questionnaire is greatly influenced by the patient's current health status is an important feature for its use in clinical trials. If IMPACT scores continued to be influenced more by the patient's health status over the preceding year than by their current disease status, short-term responsiveness to change in clinical status would be compromised.

To date the IMPACT questionnaire has been used to evaluate HRQOL in pediatric IBD patients in a number of research studies, involving a variety of study designs [88, 91–93]. These studies provide a preliminary picture of what the HRQOL is in this population, and increasingly the data obtained from such studies will allow clinicians and researchers to develop an improved understanding of the factors which both positively and negatively influence HRQOL in older children and teenagers with IBD.

Description of the Instrument (IMPACT-III)

The IMPACT-III questionnaire takes about 10–15 minutes to complete and contains 35 questions. Each question is scored on a five-point scale (Fig. 51.2). Individual questions within IMPACT are equally weighted; hence, the scores range from a maximum of 175 to a minimum of 35, with higher scores representing better quality of life.

The 35 questions encompass six domains: bowel (7 concerns), body image (3 concerns), functional/social impairment (12 concerns), emotional impairment (7 concerns), tests/treatments (3 concerns), and systemic impairment (3 concerns) (Table 51.4). Perrin and colleagues relooked at the domain structure for IMPACT and through exploratory factor analysis proposed four factors with good to excellent reliability for IBD responses: general well-being and symptoms, emotional functioning, social interactions, and body image (two questions were dropped which did not fit well with any domain, "feel about tests/treatments" and "how condition affects family") [94]. Similarly, as part of the cross-cultural adaptation and translation of the Croatian version of IMPACT-III, Abdovic et al. used factor analysis of their cohort data to

Table 51.4 IMPACT-III: 35 questions sorted by six domains

Domain	Question
IBD symptoms	Stomachaches
	Not being able to eat what you want because of disease
	Diarrhea
	Worried about blood with bowel movement
	Being sick
	Afraid about not making to the bathroom in time
	Having to pass gas
Systemic symptoms	How much energy
	How did you feel
	How tired did you feel
Emotional functioning	Worried about having a flare-up
	Worried about having a chronic condition
	Worries about health in future
	Thinking it is unfair to have this disease
	Being angry to have this disease
	Being ashamed
	Being happy
Social functioning	The influence of the disease upon the family
	Having to miss out on hobbies
	Having rules imposed because of the disease
	Having fun
	Is it harder to make friends
	Worries not to be able to go out on dates
	Teased or bullied because of the disease or treatment
	Difficulties to travel or go on holiday
	Try and keep your disease a secret
	Able to talk to anyone about worries
	Able to play sports as much as you would like
	Able to go to school
Body image	How do you feel about height
	How do you feel about weight
	How do you feel about the way you look
Treatment/ interventions	How do you feel about taking medicines
	How do you feel about investigations
	Worries about ever having an operation

propose a five-domain structure (dropping two items) [95]. However, a major limitation of these two studies is the lack of robust representation across the spectrum of disease activity among participants, such that a vast majority had inactive or mild disease. Where disease activity has been identified as a contributor to HRQOL, restricted representation across the spectrum of disease activity limits the ability to recommend changes to the IMPACT domain structure. Future work to address this question is needed, with a balanced cohort across age, gender, disease type, and disease activity.

Readability statistics for the IMPACT-III are excellent with a Flesch-Kincaid Grade level of 4.8, a Flesch Reading ease of 74.3, and 1% passive sentences. This suggests a very appropriate level of wording given the target population of ages 10 and above.

Practical Issues for Use of IMPACT

Administration and Instructions to Respondents

The person administering IMPACT-III should verbally review the written instructions provided on the initial page of the questionnaire with the child completing the questionnaire. It is important that the responses are the child's, and parents should be specifically asked not to help their child with the answers. It is, therefore, helpful to have an assistant nearby to answer questions that the respondent might have, so that the parent(s) will not have to aid them. It should be made clear that if the child feels that the issue raised by a particular question is not a problem for them (i.e., questions mention blood in stool, but they have never had blood in stool), then the child should mark it as "best quality of life" response. This will help decrease the number of questions left blank.

Scoring

By convention, the higher the score, the better the quality of life. For IMPACT-III the "good" QOL anchors are always presented on the left, with the "poor" QOL anchors on the right. There are five Likert response options per question. For scoring purposes, from left to right, they can be numbered five through one. To obtain a total score, responses from all 35 questions are summed. Domain scores can be obtained by summing the responses for each question within a domain (Table 51.4).

Interpretation of HRQOL scores is another important area to consider. In IBD, the HRQOL outcomes from either IBDQ or IMPACT have usually been reported as the mean total score for study participants at various study time points. Other ways of reporting HRQOL outcomes would be to focus on the mean scores of a domain (i.e., the bowel domain) for study participants at various study time points. The latter may be optimal when a specific intervention would be expected to have a predominant influence on a specific domain. Work is underway to revise the scoring system for IMPACT-III to facilitate interpretation of HRQOL results reported in studies. Where scores can range from 35 to 175, understanding what an individual or cohort mean score "means" is not intuitive. Preliminary reports support moving to normalizing total and domain scores out of a range of 0–100, with a higher score still indicating better HRQOL (personal communication).

Deficiencies in Current Knowledge and Areas for Future Research

There is still much we have to learn and understand about HRQOL in pediatric IBD. Although we have a tool with which to assess disease-specific HRQOL in this population, a number of unanswered questions remain.

Identifying the Factors which Influence HRQOL

While some factors, such as disease activity and severity, are known to negatively influence HRQOL, further research is needed to elaborate other key factors which may influence HRQOL. Hommel and colleagues have begun to explore non-disease-specific factors, such as behavioral dysfunction, which may influence HRQOL [96]. They describe two main types of behavioral dysfunction: internalizing symptoms (such as anxiety and depression) and externalizing symptoms (such as aggression, disruptive behavior). In their study they demonstrated that greater disease severity, externalizing symptoms, and internalizing symptoms were all independently associated with a lower HRQOL as assessed by the IMPACT questionnaire. As well, their findings suggested that internalizing symptoms had a mediating effect on the relationship between disease activity and HRQOL.

Engelmann and colleagues [97] conducted a cross-sectional study of 47 German adolescent IBD patients where they assessed disease activity, HRQOL (using IMPACT-III), and QOL (using EQ5D, a measure of generic QOL) and whether psychopathology was present using the Clinical Assessment Scale for Child and Adolescent Psychopathology (CASCAP). The CASCAP is a tool to assess psychopathology using data derived from patient and parent interviews. Fifty-five percent of patients fulfilled DSM-IV criteria for one or more psychiatric disorders including adjustment disorders (25.6%), major depressive disorder (17.0%), anxiety disorder (6.4%), learning/developmental disorders (4.2%), and attention deficit/hyperactivity disorder (2.1%). Not surprisingly, patients with psychiatric comorbidity had significantly lower total IMPACT scores compared to those without this comorbidity. However, the effects of psychiatric comorbidity differed across categories of disease activity, where psychiatric comorbidity only affected the HRQOL and QOL scores only for patients with mild disease activity. A limitation of this study was the amalgamation of a range of psychiatric diagnoses together as one factor, where it may be that certain diagnoses have a greater or lesser influence on HRQOL/QOL.

Capturing HRQOL assessments through one moment in time, as has been done in the majority of cross-sectional studies to date, is a significant limitation. Because HRQOL is likely influenced by multiple factors, both disease-specific and non-disease-specific, ensuring a sufficient sample size and following the study population over time will be important features of future study designs to address some of these limitations. Overcoming these limitations will be important in helping us to better understand the factors which influence HRQOL. By gaining an improved understanding of factors which influence HRQOL, we can then work on developing specific interventions to target these factors, with the goal to improve HRQOL in these patients [98, 99].

Comparisons of HRQOL Between Patients with IBD, Patients with other Chronic Pediatric Illnesses, and Healthy Peers

As IMPACT is increasingly used in clinical and research settings, an improved understanding of HRQOL in patients with pediatric IBD should result. Also important, however, is understanding how these patients fare when compared to children with other chronic illnesses as well as to healthy peers. To make these comparisons, generic HRQOL tools will need to be employed. Preliminary work looking at QOL issues between patients with IBD and those with other chronic illnesses was carried out by Ingerski and colleagues [100]. They compared HRQOL across eight pediatric chronic conditions: obesity, eosinophilic gastrointestinal disorders, inflammatory bowel disease, epilepsy, type 1 diabetes, sickle cell disease, post-renal transplantation, and cystic fibrosis [100]. Using the PedsQL generic HRQOL tool, these authors showed that it was youth with obesity and eosinophilic gastrointestinal disorders who had lower HRQOL than youth with other chronic illnesses. However, limitations of this work were the small number of patients in some of the chronic illness groups (e.g., 34 of 589 patients had IBD), and considerable variation was present across disease groups in terms of demographic and disease-specific sample characteristics [100]. Thus further work needs to be done in this area but with a priori matching of participants across important demographic and disease-specific factors. Additionally, early work has also been done comparing HRQOL of pediatric IBD with healthy peers [101]. Not surprisingly they demonstrated in 55 children, ages 7–19 years, that older children with IBD had significantly lower HRQOL scores compared with age-standardized peers. Kunz and colleagues have carried out the largest study to date comparing HRQOL assessments of youth with IBD to published group data of chronically ill, acutely ill, and healthy comparison groups [102]. The one hundred thirty-six youth with IBD studied reported lower psychosocial functioning than the healthy comparison group, higher physical and social functioning than the chronically ill group, and lower school functioning than all published comparison groups. More work needs to be done to better characterize the degree and nature of any

differences in HRQOL between pediatric IBD patients and those with other chronic illnesses and healthy peers. If consistent differences are noted, and in particular if impairments in HRQOL are demonstrated, then healthcare providers will have evidence to better advocate for research to identify interventions which will target these HRQOL impairments.

Assessing Disease-Specific HRQOL in Pediatric IBD Patients not Captured by IMPACT Questionnaire

IMPACT is a tool to evaluate HRQOL in pediatric patients aged 10–17 years inclusive. The researchers who developed the questionnaire were concerned that issues of importance to younger patients with IBD may be different than the older cohort which was involved in the development of IMPACT. Also a self-administered questionnaire for these patients less than 10 years of age would be problematic given the developmental and comprehension concerns in the younger age range [11]. It is most likely that younger patients would require assistance in completing the questionnaire and/or a different method of delivery [11], such as computer-based questionnaire with video and/or audio components [83]. This is an area which requires further consideration, but it will be necessary to determine whether the relatively small population of patients with IBD who are less than 10 years of age can justify the development of a tool specifically for this age group.

During the development of IMPACT, patients with ostomies or proctitis were not included. Therefore, the applicability of IMPACT to this cohort of patients has not been established. There may be HRQOL issues unique to this population not addressed by IMPACT. As well, IMPACT development involved participants who had been diagnosed with IBD for at least 6 months. The researchers wished to have a body of "lived experiences and concerns," and it is not clear whether the perception of issues influencing HRQOL is the same when the diagnosis is more recent.

The Impact of Family on the Assessment of HRQOL in Pediatric IBD Patients

The role that family, both parents and siblings, plays in the HRQOL of pediatric IBD is just starting to be explored. There are multiple areas to be addressed. First is the whole issue of self-report and proxy-reported assessments of HRQOL. As discussed previously, in pediatrics there can be the added challenge of age or developmental status which may limit the ability to secure a self-report of HRQOL. The argument can be made regardless of whether a pediatric patient can self-report that having a parent's perspective on their child's HRQOL can add important information which impacts management decisions. A more comprehensive picture of youth HRQOL can be obtained through inclusion of the complementary perspectives of both child and parent-proxy reports of HRQOL [102]. It is not yet clear, based on some of the disparate findings of the few studies which have looked at concordance between youth with IBD and parent-proxy HRQOL reports, exactly how strong the agreement is across domains. An initial study by Loonen et al. found that parent-proxy reports of social functioning were significantly lower than youth reports, but differences were not noted across other domains [103]. Ingerski et al. reported lower parent-proxy HRQOL scores across all domains of the PedsQL compared with youth self-report [100], except for the school functioning domain, where youth self-reported HRQOL was significantly lower than parent-proxy reported HRQOL. Using the KIDSCREEN-GROUP 2004, a self-report questionnaire consisting of five domains of general QOL (physical activity, children's mood, family life, friends, and school performance), Mueller et al. compared scoring between 110 Swiss children with IBD and their parents [104]. In this study parents scored overall QOL, as well as mood, family, and friends domains, lower than the children themselves, with better concordance noted for school performance and physical activity domains.

Gallo and colleagues from Argentina concurrently assessed HRQOL using IMPACT-III in 27 patients and one of their parents (82% mothers) [105]. As a specific parent-proxy report version of IMPACT-III has not been developed, the authors used a non-validated approach, asking the parents to interpret the questions from their child's perspective. With this method they showed moderate-to-high agreement between parent-proxy and patient ratings on most IMPACT-III domains, except for the emotional functioning domain where parents underreported (compared to the child's report) their child's HRQOL. Another consideration in the interpretation of parent-proxy ratings of their child's HRQOL is the QOL of the parents themselves. Sattoe et al. suggest that assessing parents' QOL may be more useful than asking parents for a parent-proxy report [106]. Researchers have shown that parent's own QOL was significantly related to ratings of their child's QOL [107–109]. More work needs to be done to understand these differences in proxy vs. self-reported HRQOL as well as factors that influence parents' perceptions of youth's HRQOL [100]. Regardless of differences noted, the inclusion of both patients' and parents' measures of QOL can provide complementary perspectives, each of which should be respected [104].

A second area to be explored is the role that families play on an individual's perceived HRQOL. When family life is dysfunctional, there can be decreased emotional and behavioral functioning [110], while adaptive family relationships have been associated with positive psychological functioning

[111]. Building on data among youth with end-stage renal disease and diabetes showing that there is a significant relationship between family functioning and HRQOL, researchers explored these issues in a cohort of adolescents with IBD, seeking to identify which domains of family functioning may be particularly problematic [112]. After statistically controlling for known impacts of disease severity and diagnosis, their data showed that teens from families with clinically elevated difficulties in problem solving, communication, and general family functioning reported lower HRQOL. This area needs to be studied further to ascertain whether a causal link exists between family functioning and HRQOL and, additionally, in the context of a prospective study, how this may vary over time. Research has also highlighted the importance of examining maternal and paternal functioning separately, as there can be a differential impact on HRQOL outcomes [113]. As well, careful consideration of the potential interplay between the child and parent psychological status and the child's HRQOL has also been shown to be important [114]. Hommel and colleagues studied these issues, and their data suggested that adolescent depressive symptoms may serve as a mechanism by which parent distress is linked to poorer HRQOL in adolescents with IBD [114]. In a study of 99 adolescents with Crohn disease and their parents, Gray and colleagues further explored family level predictors of HRQOL by studying parenting stress as a potential mechanism through which disease activity affects HRQOL [115]. HRQOL was assessed using patient-completed IMPACT-III, while parents were given a measure of medically related parenting stress, the Pediatric Inventory for Parents. Disease activity was assessed from chart reviews. In this cohort drawn from three study sites, they demonstrated that parenting stress because of the occurrence of medical stressors partially mediated the disease severity-HRQOL relation. This study would indicate that as disease severity increases, parenting stress also increases, and patient HRQOL decreases. Better understanding of the relationship between family functioning and HRQOL may allow practitioners to better identify adolescents who are at higher risk for impaired HRQOL and to focus on families in need of support services or psychological intervention [112].

Cross-Cultural Comparisons of HRQOL in Pediatric IBD

A further gap in assessment of HRQOL in pediatric IBD is the lack of comparisons across different cultures and/or languages. Other IBD outcome measures such as the commonly employed disease activity measures can be utilized irrespective of culture or language. They collect fundamental information which are not limited by ethnicity or language. This is not true for quality-of-life assessments. While we now have the generic and disease-specific tools to evaluate HRQOL across cultures and languages, there remains no reported comparison of HRQOL across cultures or languages. There have been an increasing number of published HRQOL reports from individual countries using cross-culturally adapted versions of IMPACT-III [95, 104], but none have specifically contrasted HRQOL across cohorts of pediatric IBD patients from different countries. Cultural differences with respect to disease perception and illness experience are becoming more apparent with the increasing immigrant population residing in Western countries [116]. The exclusion from a study of a group or population, based on culture or language, could lead to a systematic bias in studies of healthcare utilization or quality of life [117].

Elaborating the Psychometric Properties of the IMPACT Questionnaire

For use in clinical trials as a key outcome measure, researchers and clinicians will need to determine the minimum clinically important difference (MCID) in IMPACT score. The MCID refers to the smallest amount of benefit that patients can perceive and value. The MCID is an important characteristic and when this is understood aids in the determination of sample size. For example, if a small MCID is determined, this limits the sample size that would be required, as compared to the scenario in which a large MCID is observed, and in which a very large sample size would be needed to show the difference (if such a difference existed).

References

1. Ferguson A, Sedgwick DM, Drummond J. Morbidity of juvenile onset inflammatory bowel disease: effects on education and employment in early adult life. Gut. 1994;35:665–8.
2. Gryboski J. Ulcerative colitis in children10 years or younger. J Pediatr Gastroenterol Nutr. 1993;17:24–31.
3. Gryboski JD. Crohn's disease in children 10 years old and younger: comparison with ulcerative colitis. J Pediatr Gastroenterol Nutr. 1994;18:174–82.
4. Barton JR, Gillon S, Ferguson A. Incidence of inflammatory bowel disease in scottish children between 1968 and 1983; marginal fall in ulcerative colitis, three-fold rise in Crohn's disease. Gut. 1989;30:618–22.
5. Mir-Madjlessi SH, Michener WM, Farmer RG. Course and prognosis of idiopathic ulcerative proctosigmoiditis in young patients. J Pediatr Gastroenterol Nutr. 1986;5(4):570–5.
6. Mackner LM, Crandall WV. Long-term psychosocial outcomes reported by children and adolescents with inflammatory bowel disease. Am J Gastroenterol. 2005;100(6):1386–92.
7. Mackner LM, Crandall WV. Oral medication adherence in pediatric inflammatory bowel disease. Inflamm Bowel Dis. 2005;11(11):1006–12.
8. Mackner LM, Crandall WV, Szigethy EM. Psychosocial functioning in pediatric inflammatory bowel disease. Inflamm Bowel Dis. 2006;12(3):239–44.
9. Constitution of the World Health Organization, in World Health Organization. Handbook of basic documents. Geneva: Palais des Nations; 1952. p. 3–20.
10. Eiser C, Morse R. Quality-of-life measures in chronic diseases of childhood. Health Technol Assess. 2001;5(4):1–168.
11. Eiser C. Children's quality of life measures. Arch Dis Child. 1997;77:347–54.
12. Jenney MEM, Campbell S. Measuring quality of life. Arch Dis Child. 1997;77:347–54.
13. Testa MA, Simonson DC. Assessment of quality-of-life outcomes. N Engl J Med. 1996;334(13):835–40.
14. Williet N, Sandborn WJ, Peyrin-Biroulet L. Patient-reported outcomes as primary end points in clinical trials of inflammatory bowel disease. Clin Gastroenterol Hepatol. 2014;12(8):1246–56. e6
15. Streiner DL, Norman GR. Health measurement scales: a practical guide to their development and use. 2nd ed. Basic Concepts. New York: Oxford University Press Inc; 1995. p. 4–14.
16. Otley AR et al. Assessing disease activity in pediatric Crohn's disease: Which index to use? Gastroenterology. 1999;116:527–31.
17. Hyams JS et al. Development and validation of a pediatric Crohn's disease activity index. J Pediatr Gastroenterol Nutr. 1991;12:439–47.
18. Hyams JS et al. Relationship of common laboratory parameters to the activity of Crohn's disease in children. J Pediatr Gastroenterol Nutr. 1992;14:216–22.
19. Ferry G. Quality of life in inflammatory bowel disease: background and definitions. J Pediatr Gastroenterol Nutr. 1999;28(4):S15–8.
20. Yacavone RF et al. Quality of life measurement in gastroenterology: what is available? Am J Gastroenterol. 2001;96(2):285–97.
21. Patrick L, Deyo RA. Generic and disease-specific measures in assessing health status and quality of life. Med Care. 1989;27:S217–32.
22. Streiner DL, Norman GR. Devising the items. In: Streiner DL, Norman GR, editors. Health measurement scales: a practical guide to their development. Basic Concepts. New York: Oxford University Press; 1995. p. 15–27.
23. Ware Jr JE, Sherbourne CD. The MOS 36-item short-form health survey (sf-36). 1. Conceptual framework and item selection. Med Care. 1992;30(6):473–83.
24. Landgraf JM, Ware J. The child health questionnaire manual. Boston: Health Institute, New England Medical Center; 1996.
25. McHorney CA et al. The MOS 36-Item short-form health survey (SF-36):III. Tests of data quality, scaling assumptions, and reliability across diverse patient groups. Med Care. 1994;32(1):40–66.
26. Juniper EF et al. Measuring quality of life in children with asthma. Qual Life Res. 1996;5:35–46.
27. Guyatt G, Mitchell A, Irvine EJ. A new measure of health status for clinical trials in inflammatory bowel disease. Gastroenterology. 1989;96:804–10.
28. DeJong Z et al. The reliability and construct validity of the RAQoL: a rheumatoid arthritis-specific quality of life instrument. Br J Rheumatol. 1997;36(8):878–83.
29. McLachlan SA, Devins GM, Goodwin PJ. Validation of the European Organization for Research and Treatment of Cancer Quality of Life Questionnaire (QlQ-C30) as a measure of psychosocial function in breast cancer patients. Eur J Cancer. 1998;34(4):510–7.
30. Carlsson M, Hamrin E. Measurement of quality of life in women with breast cancer. Development of a life satisfaction questionnaire (LSQ-32) and a comparison with the EORTC QLQ-C30. Qual Life Res. 1996;5(2):265–74.
31. Juniper EF et al. Validation of a standardized version of the asthma quality of life questionnaire. Chest. 1999;115(5):1265–70.

32. Barley EA, Quirk FH, Jones PW. Asthma health status measurement in clinical practice: validity of a new short and simple instrument. Respir Med. 1998;92(10):1207–14.

33. Duffy CM et al. The juvenile arthritis quality of life questionnaire: development of a new responsive index for juvenile rheumatoid arthritis and juvenile spondyloarthritides. J Rheumatol. 1997;24(4):738–46.

34. Eiser C et al. Development of a measure to assess the perceived illness experience after treatment for cancer. Arch Dis Child. 1995;72:302–7.

35. French DJ, Christie MJ, Sowden AJ. The reproducibility of the childhood asthma questionnaires: measures of quality of life for children with asthma aged 4-16 years. Qual Life Res. 1994;3(3):215–24.

36. Otley A et al. The IMPACT questionnaire: a valid measure of health-related quality of life in pediatric inflammatory bowel disease. J Pediatr Gastroenterol Nutr. 2002;35(4):557–63.

37. Theunissen NCM et al. The proxy problem: child report versus parent report in health-related quality of life research. Qual Life Res. 1998;7:387–97.

38. Connolly MA, Johnson JA. Measuring quality of life in paediatric patients. PharmacoEconomics. 1999;16(6):605–25.

39. Wallander JL, Schmitt M, Koot HM. Quality of life measurements in children and adolescents: issues, instruments, and applications. J Clin Psychol. 2001;57(4):571–85.

40. Achenbach TM, McConaughy SH, Howell CT. Child/adolescent behavioral and emotional problems: implications of cross-informant correlations for situational specificity. Psychol Bull. 1987;101(2):213–32.

41. Pantell RH, Lewis CC. Measuring the impact of medical care on children. J Chronic Dis. 1987;40(S1):99–108.

42. Verhulst FC, Koot HM, de Ende JV. Ifferential predictive value of parents' and teachers' reports of childrens' problem behaviors: a longitudinal study. J Abnorm Child Psychol. 1994;22:531–5.

43. Pal DK. Quality of Life assessment in children: a review of conceptual and methodological issues in multidimensional health status measures. J Epidemiol Community Health. 1996;50:391–6.

44. Nordgren SR et al. Long-term follow-up in Crohn's disease: mortality, morbidity, and functional status. Scand J Gastroenterol. 1994;29:1122–8.

45. Farmer RG, Whelan G, Fazio VW. Long-term follow-up of patients with Crohn's disease. Gastroenterology. 1985;88(6):1818–25.

46. Lind E et al. Crohn's disease: treatment and outcome. Scand J Gastroenterol. 1985;20:1014–8.

47. Sorensen VZ, Olsen BG, Binder V. Life prospects and quality of life in patients with Crohn's disease. Gut. 1987;28:382–5.

48. Munkholm P et al. Disease activity courses in a regional cohort of Crohn's disease patients. Scand J Gastroenterol. 1995;30:699–706.

49. Langholz E et al. Course of ulcerative colitis: analysis of changes in disease activity over years. Gastroenterology. 1994;107(1):3–11.

50. Irvine EJ et al. Quality of life: a valid and reliable measure of therapeutic efficacy in the treatment of inflammatory bowel disease. Gastroenterology. 1994;106(2):287–96.

51. Love JR, Irvine E, Fedorak RN. Quality of life in inflammatory bowel disease. J Clin Gastroenterol. 1992;14:15–9.

52. Irvine E, Feagan BG, Wong CJ. Does self-administration of a quality of life index for inflammatory bowel disease change the results? J Clin Epidemiol. 1996;49(10):1177–85.

53. Martin F et al. Oral 5-ASA versus prednisone in short-term treatment of Crohn's disease: a multi-centre controlled trial. Can J Gastroenterol. 1990;4:452–7.

54. Greenberg GR et al. Oral budesonide for active Crohn's disease. N Engl J Med. 1994;331(13):836–41.

55. Feagan BG et al. Methotrexate for the treatment of Crohn's disease. The North American Crohn's Study Group Investigators. N Engl J Med. 1995;332(5):292–7.

56. Casellas F et al. Influence of inflammatory bowel disease on different dimensions of quality of life. Eur J Gastroenterol Hepatol. 2001;13:567–72.

57. Guyatt G, Walter S, Norman G. Measuring change over time: assessing the usefulness of evaluative instruments. J Chronic Dis. 1987;40(2):171–8.

58. Drossman DA. Inflammatory bowel disease. In: Spilker B, editor. Quality of life and pharmacoeconomics in clinical trials. Philadelphia: Lippincott-Raven Publishers; 1996. p. 925–35.

59. deBoer AG et al. Inflammatory bowel disease questionnaire: cross-cultural adaptation and further validation. Eur J Gastroenterol Hepatol. 1995;7(11):1043–50.

60. Russel M et al. Validation of the dutch translation of the Inflammatory Bowel Disease Questionnaire (IBDQ): a health-related quality of life questionnaire in inflammatory bowel disease. Digestion. 1997;58(3):282–8.

61. Kim WH et al. Quality of life in Korean patients with inflammatory bowel diseases: ulcerative colitis, Crohn's disease and intestinal behcet's disease. Int J Color Dis. 1999;14(1):52–7.

62. Cheung WY et al. The UK IBDQ – A British version of the inflammatory bowel disease questionnaire. Development and validation. J Clin Epidemiol. 2000;53(3):297–306.

63. Hjortswang H et al. Validation of the inflammatory bowel disease questionnaire in swedish patients with ulcerative colitis. Scand J Gastroenterol. 2001;36(1):77–85.

64. Pallis AG, Vlachonikolis IG, Mouzas IA. Quality of life of greek patients with inflammatory bowel disease. validation of the greek translation of the inflammatory bowel disease questionnaire. Digestion. 2001;63(4):240–6.

65. Lopez-Vivancos J et al. Validation of the spanish version of the inflammatory bowel disease questionnaire on ulcerative colitis and Crohn's disease. Digestion. 1999;60(3):274–80.

66. Irvine E, Zhou Q, Thompson AK. The short inflammatory bowel disease questionnaire: a quality of life instrument for community physicians managing inflammatory bowel disease. CCRPT investigators. canadian Crohn's relapse prevention trial. Am J Gastroenterol. 1996;91(8):1571–8.

67. Jowett SL et al. The short inflammatory bowel disease questionnaire is reliable and responsive to clinically important change in ulcerative colitis. Am J Gastroenterol. 2001;96(10):2921–8.

68. Han SW et al. The SIBDQ: further validation in ulcerative colitis patients. Am J Gastroenterol. 2000;95(1):145–51.

69. Goel KM, Shanks RA. Long-term prognosis of children with ulcerative colitis. Arch Dis Child. 1973;48:337–42.

70. Cooke WT et al. Crohn's disease: course, treatment and long term prognosis. Q J Med. 1980;49(195):363–84.

71. Lindquist BL, Jarnerot G, Wickbom G. Clinical and epidemiological aspects of Crohn's disease in children and adolescents. Scand J Gastroenterol. 1984;19:502–6.

72. Farmer RG, Michener WM. Prognosis of Crohn's disease with onset in childhood or adolescence. Dig Dis Sci. 1979;24(10):752–7.

73. Michener WM, Farmer RG, Mortimer EA. Long-term prognosis of ulcerative colitis with onset in childhood and adolescence. J Clin Gastroenterol. 1979;1:301–5.

74. Mayberry JF. Impact of inflammatory bowel disease on educational achievements and work prospects. J Pediatr Gastroenterol Nutr. 1999;28(4):S34–6.

75. Engstrom I. Inflammatory bowel disease in children and adolescents: mental health and family functioning. J Pediatr Gastroenterol Nutr. 1999;28(4):S28–33.

76. Akobeng AK et al. Quality of life in children with Crohn's disease: A Pilot Study. J Pediatr Gastroenterol Nutr. 1999;28(4):S37–9.

77. Rabbett H et al. Quality of life in children with Crohn's disease. J Pediatr Gastroenterol Nutr. 1996;23:528–33.

78. Moody G, Eaden JA, Mayberry JF. Social implications of childhood Crohn's disease. J Pediatr Gastroenterol Nutr. 1999;28(4):S43–5.

79. MacPhee M, Hoffenberg EJ, Feranchak A. Quality-of-life factors in adolescent inflammatory bowel disease. Inflamm Bowel Dis. 1998;4(1):6–11.

80. Olson D, Barnes H. Quality of life questionnaire. St. Paul: University of Minnesota Press; 1982.

81. Forget S et al. Validation of a disease specific health-related quality of life (HRQOL) instrument for pediatric inflammatory bowel disease (IBD). Gastroenterology. 1998;114(4 (Part 2)):A978.

82. Forget S et al. Health-related quality of life in pediatric inflammatory bowel disease: a comparison of parent and child reports. Gastroenterology. 1998;114(4 (Part 2)):A977.

83. Buller H. Assessment of quality of life in the younger child: the use of an animated computer program. J Pediatr Gastroenterol Nutr. 1999;28(4):S53–5.

84. Griffiths AM et al. Development of a quality-of-life index for pediatric inflammatory bowel disease: dealing with differences related to age and IBD type. J Pediatr Gastroenterol Nutr. 1999;28:S46–52.

85. Ryan JL et al. The clinical utility of health-related quality of life screening in a pediatric inflammatory bowel disease clinic. Inflamm Bowel Dis. 2013;19(12):2666–72.

86. Piers EV, Harris DB. The piers-harris children's self-concept scale. Los Angeles: Western Psychological Services; 1996.

87. Loonen HJ et al. Quality of life in paediatric inflammatory bowel disease measured by a generic and a disease-specific questionnaire. Acta Paediatr. 2002;91(3):348–54.

88. Otley AR et al. Health-related quality of life in the first year after a diagnosis of pediatric inflammatory bowel disease. Inflamm Bowel Dis. 2006;12(8):684–91.

89. Otley A, et al. IMPACT-III is a valid, reliable and responsive measure of health-related quality of life in pediatric Crohn's disease. J Pediatr Gastroenterol Nutr. 2006. Abstract accepted for presentation at conference.

90. Otley A, et al. The effects of infliximab therapy on health-related quality of life in pediatric crohn's disease. J Pediatr Gastroenterol Nutr. 2006. Abstract accepted for presentation at conference.

91. Hyams J, et al. Safety, Tolerability, and Efficacy of Natalizumab in Adolescents with Crohn's Disease. To be submitted – should be available later in 2006. 2006.

92. Hyams J et al. Induction and maintenance infliximab therapy for the treatment of moderate-to-severe Crohn's disease in children. Gastroenterology. 2007;132(3):863–73. quiz 1165-6

93. Szabo D et al. Autoregressive cross-lagged models of impact-iii and pediatric Crohn's disease activity indexes during one year infliximab therapy in pediatric patients with Crohn's disease. J Crohns Colitis. 2014;8(8):747–55.

94. Perrin JM et al. Measuring quality of life in pediatric patients with inflammatory bowel disease: psychometric and clinical characteristics. J Pediatr Gastroenterol Nutr. 2008;46(2):164–71.

95. Abdovic S et al. The IMPACT-III (HR) questionnaire: a valid measure of health-related quality of life in Croatian children with inflammatory bowel disease. J Crohns Colitis. 2013;7(11):908–15.

96. Gray WN et al. Disease activity, behavioral dysfunction, and health-related quality of life in adolescents with inflammatory bowel disease. Inflamm Bowel Dis. 2011;17(7):1581–6.

97. Engelmann G et al. Health-related quality of life in adolescents with inflammatory bowel disease depends on disease activity and psychiatric comorbidity. Child Psychiatry Hum Dev. 2015;46(2):300–7.

98. Karwowski CA, Keljo D, Szigethy E. Strategies to improve quality of life in adolescents with inflammatory bowel disease. Inflamm Bowel Dis. 2009;15(11):1755–64.

99. Ross SC et al. Psychosocial functioning and health-related quality of life in paediatric inflammatory bowel disease. J Pediatr Gastroenterol Nutr. 2011;53(5):480–8.

100. Ingerski LM et al. Health-related quality of life across pediatric chronic conditions. J Pediatr. 2010;156(4):639–44.

101. Haapamaki J et al. Health-related quality of life in paediatric patients with inflammatory bowel disease related to disease activity. J Paediatr Child Health. 2011;47(11):832–7.

102. Kunz JH, Hommel KA, Greenley RN. Health-related quality of life of youth with inflammatory bowel disease: a comparison with published data using the PedsQL 4.0 generic core scales. Inflamm Bowel Dis. 2010;16(6):939–46.

103. Loonen HJ et al. Are parents able to rate the symptoms and quality of life of their offspring with IBD? Inflamm Bowel Dis. 2002;8(4):270–6.

104. Mueller R et al. Quality of life in swiss paediatric inflammatory bowel disease patients: do patients and their parents experience disease in the same way? J Crohns Colitis. 2016;10(3):269–76.

105. Gallo J et al. Do parents and children agree? Quality-of-life assessment of children with inflammatory bowel disease and their parents. J Pediatr Gastroenterol Nutr. 2014;58(4):481–5.

106. Sattoe JN et al. The proxy problem anatomized: child-parent disagreement in health related quality of life reports of chronically ill adolescents. Health Qual Life Outcomes. 2012;10:10.

107. Cremeens J, Eiser C, Blades M. Factors influencing agreement between child self-report and parent proxy-reports on the Pediatric Quality of Life Inventory 4.0 (PedsQL) generic core scales. Health Qual Life Outcomes. 2006;4:58.

108. Eiser C, Eiser JR, Stride CB. Quality of life in children newly diagnosed with cancer and their mothers. Health Qual Life Outcomes. 2005;3:29.

109. Goldbeck L, Melches J. Quality of life in families of children with congenital heart disease. Qual Life Res. 2005;14(8):1915–24.

110. Whittemore R et al. Correlates of depressive symptoms in adolescents with type 1 diabetes. Pediatr Diabetes. 2002;3(3):135–43.

111. Grey M et al. Personal and family factors associted with quality of life in adolescents with diabetes. Diabetes Care. 1998;21(6):909–14.

112. Herzer M et al. Family functioning and health-related quality of life in adolescents with pediatric inflammatory bowel disease. Eur J Gastroenterol Hepatol. 2010;23(1):95–100.

113. Kunz JH, Greenley RN, Howard M. Maternal, paternal, and family health-related quality of life in the context of pediatric inflammatory bowel disease. Qual Life Res. 2011;20(8):1197–204.

114. Herzer M et al. Patient and parent psychosocial factors associated with health-related quality of life in pediatric inflammatory bowel disease. J Pediatr Gastroenterol Nutr. 2011;52(3):295–9.

115. Gray WN et al. Health-related quality of life in youth with Crohn disease: role of disease activity and parenting stress. J Pediatr Gastroenterol Nutr. 2015;60(6):749–53.

116. Erbil P et al. Cancer patients psychological adjustment and perception of illness: cultural differences between belgium and turkey. Support Care Cancer. 1996;4:455–61.

117. Guillemin F, Bombardier C, Beaton D. Cross-cultural adaptation of health-related quality of life measures: literature review and proposed guidelines. J Clin Epidemiol. 1993;46:1417–32.

Irritable Bowel Syndrome and Functional GI Disorders in Inflammatory Bowel Disease

Khalil I. El-Chammas and Manu R. Sood

Irritable bowel syndrome (IBS) is a disorder characterized by altered bowel habits and abdominal pain in the absence of a detectable structural abnormality. There are no clear diagnostic markers for this illness and all definitions are based on clinical symptoms. Getting an accurate history from a child can sometimes be difficult and until recently IBS was not a common diagnosis made in children. Some pediatricians still view IBS as nothing more than a somatic manifestation of psychological stress [1]. Availability of better techniques to study bowel motility and sensory function along with advancements in functional brain imaging has improved our understanding of the pathophysiology of IBS. It is now thought that IBS symptoms result from the convergence of multiple factors including a genetic predisposition, an infectious or inflammatory injury to the gastrointestinal (GI) tract leading to altered sensory perception by the brain, and an underlying bowel dysmotility. Functional abdominal pain and visceral hypersensitivity can coexist in patients with inflammatory bowel disease (IBD). Emerging data suggest that there may be an overlap in the symptoms and etiopathogenesis of IBS and IBD. In this chapter we will discuss how to make a symptom-based diagnosis of IBS and review the pathophysiology and management of IBS. We will also discuss the sensory perception and enteric nervous system changes in patients with IBD and how these can predispose to the development of functional GI symptoms.

K.I. El-Chammas (✉)
Children's Hospital Medical Center, Cincinnati, OH, USA
e-mail: Khalil.El-Chammas@cchmc.org

M.R. Sood (✉)
Division of Pediatric Gastroenterology, Hepatology and Nutrition, Department of Pediatric, Medical College of Wisconsin, Milwaukee, WI, USA

Children's Hospital of Wisconsin, Milwaukee, WI, USA
e-mail: msood@mcw.edu

Epidemiology

A large proportion of children with IBS are still categorized under a broad umbrella of recurrent abdominal pain, and the prevalence of IBS in children is underrecognized. Subcategorizing children presenting with chronic abdominal pain into IBS, dyspepsia, and functional abdominal pain is important because it helps to narrow down the differential diagnosis, reduces the number of unnecessary investigations, and helps to better target the therapy. In a study of 478 children referred to a large gastroenterology clinic with functional abdominal pain, 26% of the subjects had symptoms of diarrhea-predominant IBS [2]. Another pediatric study of 171 subjects with chronic abdominal pain reported that 68% of subjects fulfilled the clinical criteria for the diagnosis of IBS [3]. Community-based studies from North America and China suggest that 8–17% of school children have IBS-like symptoms [4, 5].

Clinical Features

In a majority of patients, a good clinical history is sufficient to diagnose IBS and differentiate it from organic diseases that can mimic IBS symptoms (Table 52.1). To standardize the diagnosis of IBS, symptom-based criteria have been developed and amended by the Pediatric Rome Committee (Table 52.2) [6]. Specific alarm symptoms, which alert the clinicians to the increased likelihood of an underlying organic disease, can help in the management and planning of investigative workup. In a large study of 606 children, the following alarm symptoms were more likely in children with Crohn disease compared to those with pain-associated functional gastrointestinal disorders (FGIDs) including IBS, hematochezia, weight loss, and difficulty in gaining weight. Although included in the Rome criteria, nocturnal

Table 52.1 Diseases that can mimic IBS symptoms

Diarrhea-predominant IBS
GI infections
Inflammatory bowel disease
Celiac disease
Carbohydrate malabsorption (lactose, sucrose, fructose, sorbitol)
Lymphocytic and collagenous colitis
Food intolerance
Constipation-predominant IBS
Celiac disease
Hypothyroidism
Anal sphincter/pelvic floor abnormality
Tethered spinal cord
Colon motility disorder
Neoplastic disorders (rare in children)

Table 52.2 Rome III criteria for the diagnoses of irritable bowel syndrome [4]

Must include all of the following
Abdominal discomfort (an uncomfortable sensation not described as pain) or pain associated with two or more of the following at least 25% of the time
Improved with defecation
Onset associated with change in frequency of stool
Onset associated with a change in form (appearance) of the stool
No evidence of an inflammatory, anatomic/metabolic, or neoplastic process that explains the subject symptoms

The criteria should be fulfilled at least once per week for at least 2 months before diagnosis

abdominal pain and sleep disruption were not helpful in differentiating children with IBS from those with Crohn disease in this study [7].

Abdominal pain is a prerequisite for the diagnosis of IBS. The pain can vary in intensity and location but is usually restricted to the lower abdomen; it can be episodic or superimposed on a background of constant ache. It is usually relieved by the passage of stool or flatus and exacerbated by meals. Almost 50% of adults with IBS also have symptoms of dyspepsia, and overlap between other pain-associated FGIDs and IBS has been reported [8]. Urinary bladder irritability and pelvic pain have also been associated with IBS-like symptoms.

Most patients with diarrhea-predominant IBS pass liquid or semiformed stool at frequent intervals. It can be accompanied with the passage of mucus but passage of blood is rare. A majority of patients will report difficulty falling asleep, rather than sleep disruption. In patients with constipation-predominant IBS, the constipation initially can be episodic but usually becomes continuous. With time symptoms become refractory to treatment with laxatives. Stool consistency can be hard and the stool may be narrow in caliber. It can be associated with the feeling of incomplete evacuation; the child can spend a long time sitting on the toilet straining unsuccessfully to have a bowel movement. This can lead to rectal mucosal prolapse and development of solitary rectal ulcer syndrome, associated with passage of blood in the stool and tenesmus [9]. Adults with dyssynergia, a disorder where

the subject is unable to coordinate bearing down with pelvic floor relaxation during defecation, can have symptoms that mimic IBS [10]. Constipation associated with dyssynergia can improve with biofeedback training, and this should be considered in the differential diagnosis in adolescents with constipation and lower abdominal pain. Some patients have periods of constipation alternating with diarrhea. Abdominal bloating, belching, and flatulence are also common symptoms.

Pathophysiology

The pathophysiology of IBS is likely to be multifactorial, and alterations in GI sensory perception, central neuronal dysfunction, abnormal motility, stress, psychological abnormalities, and luminal factors have all been implicated. The submucosal nerve plexuses receive sensory input from the bowel lumen through the sensory receptors. The enteric nervous system communicates with the brain through neural pathways as well as by immune and endocrine systems. The pain signals are transmitted from the primary sensory afferent neurons with cell bodies in the dorsal root ganglia to the dorsal horn of the spinal cord. Spinal pathways run to the thalamus and relay messages to the limbic system and the sensory cortex. The combined functioning of the GI motor, sensory, and central nervous system activity is termed the brain-gut axis. Abnormalities along the brain-gut axis such as altered peripheral sensory perception, hypersensitivity of sensory neurons in the dorsal horn, and increased activation of brain regions associated with visceral pain sensation have been reported in IBS [11].

Visceral hyperalgesia (an exaggerated pain response to a sensory stimulus) has been reported in children with IBS [12, 13]. Visceral hyperalgesia could result from sensitization of primary sensory afferent fibers innervating the gut or the neurons receiving input from visceral afferents along the brain-gut axis (Fig. 52.1) [11]. Peripheral sensitization of nerves within the GI tract can result from noxious injury and the release of inflammatory mediators and nerve growth factor by the fibroblasts and mast cells in the bowel wall. The resulting increase in transcription of the neuropeptides, substance P, and calcitonin gene-related peptide initiates nerve

activation and the release of yet more substance P and recruitment of previously silent nociceptors [11].

Recent advances in functional brain imaging have provided a novel insight into the pathophysiology of chronic pain states and how supraspinal mechanisms of brain reorganization facilitate pain learning behavior and long-term maintenance of central sensitization. Tillisch and coworkers conducted a meta-analysis of 18 adult studies in which functional MRI or PET scans of the brain had been performed together with balloon distension of the rectum in patients with IBS and healthy controls [14]. Patients with IBS demonstrated a greater spatial extent of brain activity than controls, specifically in regions associated with pain modulation and emotional arousal. The authors concluded that published data supports a role for

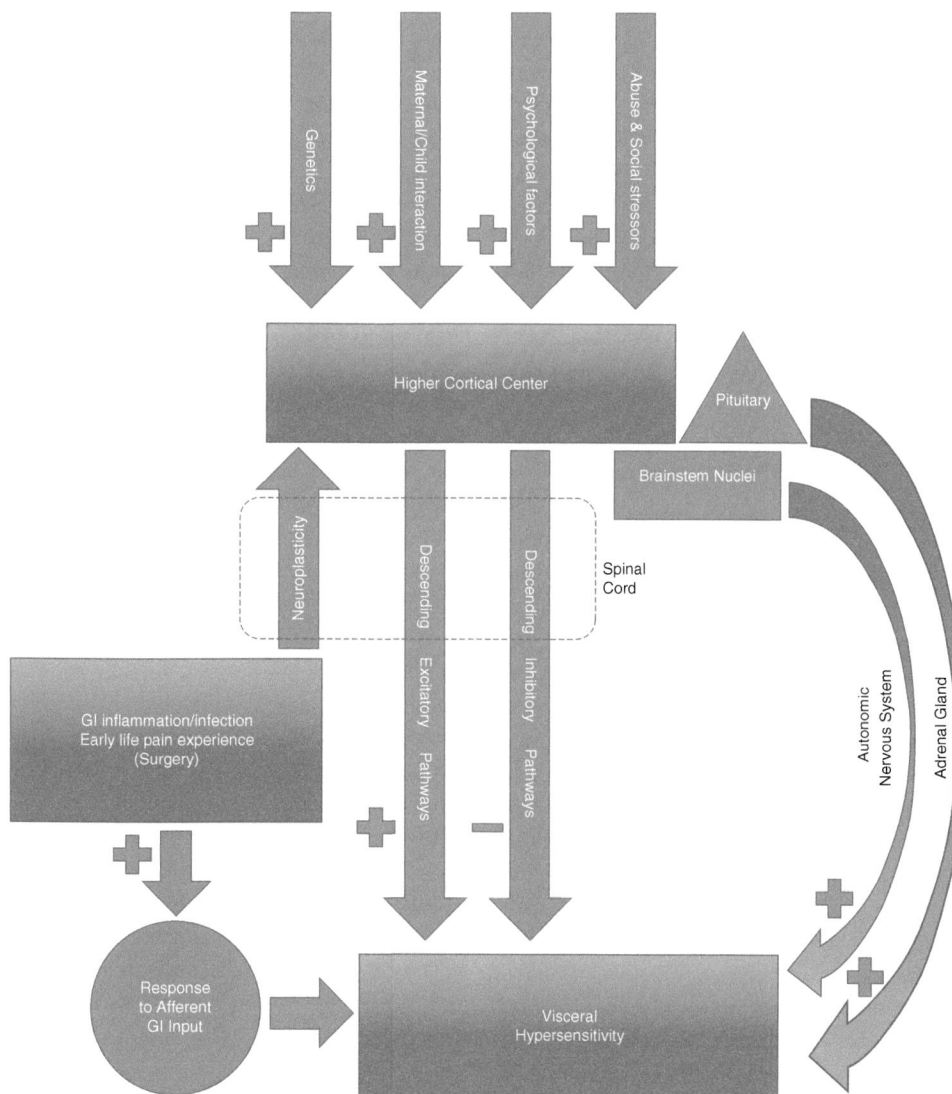

Fig. 52.1 Flowchart showing interaction between the sensory neuronal pathways and stress related activation of the hypothalamus-pituitary adrenal axis. Stress related activation of cortical and subcortical brain regions induces the release of increased quantities of corticotropin-releasing hormone (CRH) and adrenocorticotropin (ACTH) from the anterior pituitary. This in turn stimulates the release of glucocorticoids

from the adrenal glands. In response to ANS activation, cells of the adrenal medulla produce catecholamines such as adrenaline and nor-adrenaline. These have potential to modulate activity of the sensory neuronal pathways and cause visceral hypersensitivity. The cortical and subcortical brain centers can facilitate or inhibit the activation of 2nd order spinal neurons in response to visceral afferent stimulus

central nervous system dysregulation in the pathogenesis of IBS [14]. A novel functional connectivity analysis approach to functional brain imaging studies allows one to measure temporal correlation of neurophysiological events and estimate how spatially distinct brain regions coactivate or work together in a specific brain states, therefore offering a practical tool for evaluating cortical modulatory effects on brain functioning during rectal distension stimulation in health and IBS. The human brain, intrinsically, is organized into distinct functional networks supporting various sensory, motor, emotional, and cognitive functions. Of particular relevance to the understanding of visceral hypersensitivity and altered brain-gut interaction in IBS is an intrinsic brain network, the salience network [15]. The salience network plays an important role in disparate attentional, cognitive, affective, and regulatory functions. In a recent study of adolescent patients with IBS, rectal balloon distension showed greater activation of neural structures associated with homeostatic afferent and emotional networks, especially the anterior cingulate and insular cortices. Compared to healthy controls, IBS subjects also showed excessive coupling of the salience network with the default mode network and executive control network [16]. Adult IBS patients show greater engagement of cognitive and emotional brain networks including the salience network during contextual threat, suggesting that they may overestimate the likelihood and severity of future abdominal pain [17].

Low-Grade Inflammation Following gastroenteritis 7–31% of adults develop persistent low-grade inflammation and IBS-like symptoms [18–21]. A study of a large outbreak of waterborne infection with *Campylobacter jejuni* and *E. coli* O157 in Walkerton, Ontario, yielded 228 cases of postinfectious IBS and 581 controls who had fully recovered. This study found a number of single nucleotide polymorphisms that distinguished postinfectious IBS patients from infected controls who had fully recovered [22]. The relevant genes were CDH1 coding for E-cadherin, a tight junction protein controlling gut permeability, Toll-like receptor (TLR) that mediates the cellular response to bacterial DNA, and IL-6[22]. Toll-like receptors are normally downregulated to avoid inappropriate activation of the immune system by gut commensals [23]. Recently, increased expression of TLR-4 has been reported in females with IBS, predominately of mixed or diarrhea-predominant IBS [24]. Increased intraepithelial and lamina propria lymphocytic infiltration, together with an increase in enteroendocrine cells, has also been reported in bowel biopsies obtained from postinfectious IBS patients [21]. These changes can persist for up to 12 months and are associated with increased mucosal permeability [18, 21]. In children with IBS, immune cells' presence in the rectal mucosa was associated with a higher availability of 5-HT with higher 5-HT content and lower SERT mRNA compared to control subjects suggesting that mucosal inflammation may induce peripheral sensitization [25]. Bacterial gastroenteritis and Henoch-Schönlein purpura during early childhood can lead to development of IBS-like symptoms in later life [26, 27]. Bowel inflammation and pain in early childhood may lead to alteration in afferent signal processing due to neuroplasticity which can manifest in later life with functional pain during psychosocial stress.

Gut Microbiota Studies using fluorescent in situ hybridization to detect bacterial 16s RNA suggest that there is an increase in bacteria within the mucus layer in patients with IBS [28]. Recently, great advances have been made in understanding the microbiota through the development of culture-independent technologies and, in particular, metagenomics. There are great diversity and interpersonal variation in the bacterial species and strains present in the gut microbiota. Although studies of fecal microbiota in IBS are limited, a recent pediatric study reported a significantly greater percentage of the class γ-proteobacteria especially *Haemophilus parainfluenzae* in patients with IBS. A *Ruminococcus*-like microbe was also more common in IBS subjects compared to controls in this study [29]. Several adult studies have reported reduced biodiversity of gut microbiota in patients with IBS [30]. Fermentable oligosaccharides, disaccharides, monosaccharide, and polyol (FODMAP) diet which lowers the intake of several fermentable carbohydrates have been shown to decrease GI symptoms in adults and children. In one pediatric study, the baseline gut microbiome composition and microbial metabolic capacity were associated with efficacy of FODMAP diet, suggesting that evaluation of gut microbiome may be helpful in predicating response to dietary intervention [31, 32].

Altered Motility Abnormal rectal, colon, and small bowel motility has been implicated in IBS pathophysiology. Interpretation of colon motility studies in adults with IBS is hampered by a relatively primitive understanding of normal colon motility and its intrinsic variability. Abnormalities in colon motility and abnormalities in response to food and stress have been reported in patients with IBS[33]. Abnormalities in small bowel motility such as repetitive bursts of contractions or clusters, prominent high-amplitude waves in the terminal ileum, and an exaggerated jejunal motor response to a meal have also been reported in adults with IBS [33, 34].

There is also a suggestion that patients with IBS handle small bowel gas differently, and there is slow transit of gas directly infused into the small bowel in adults with IBS[33]. Abdominal bloating and flatulence can also result from higher colonic fermentation in IBS [33, 35, 36]. Some patients without evidence of small bowel bacterial overgrowth can benefit from treatment with unabsorbable antibiotics [37], which raises the question of a qualitative change in bowel bacterial flora in IBS.

Biochemical Changes Serotonin (5-hydroxytryptamine: 5-HT) is secreted in copious amounts by the gut enteroendocrine cells and serves as a critical messenger for GI fluid secretion and motility. It activates at least five different receptor types, and the 5-HT_3 and 5-HT_4 receptors are the most extensively studied in IBS [38]. The transporter of 5-HT (SERT) mediates the reuptake of 5-HT by the neurons and crypt epithelial cells and terminates its action.

Plasma 5-HT concentration is elevated in IBS patients [39], and the proportion of 5-HT secreting enteroendocrine cells is elevated in the GI tract in postinfectious patients with IBS[18]. Increased rectal mucosal 5-HT concentration has also been reported in children with IBS. The presence of low-grade inflammation was associated with higher 5-HT concentration in rectal mucosa in this study [25]. Symptom relief by serotonergic agents including 5-HT_3 antagonists and 5-HT_4 agonists provides additional support for a possible role of 5-HT in IBS pathophysiology [40].

Genetics Familial aggregation and twin studies suggest that there may be a genetic predisposition to developing IBS [41, 42]. Twin studies have shown that the concordance rate for IBS is higher in monozygotic compared to dizygotic twins [43]. However, the presence of IBS in the respondent's parents made a much larger contribution to the risk of having IBS than did the presence of IBS in one's twin, suggesting social learning may be more important than the environmental factors in determining illness behavior [43]. Family members of patients with IBS are more likely to have the condition, compared to their spouse controls. To date, nearly 60 genes involved in different pathways including serotonin, adrenergic, inflammation, and intestinal barrier function have been studied to determine whether specific genetic variants may be associated with IBS [44]. Interleukin-10 is an anti-inflammatory cytokine, and fewer patients with IBS have the high IL-10 producing (G/G) genotype compared to healthy controls [41]. Four different studies have explored the association of SERT gene polymorphism in IBS[41]. SERT is important for terminating the GI activity of 5-HT. The wild-type l/l polymorphism results in normal function, whereas the presence of the short allele (s/l or s/s) results in impaired SERT function. As a group, SERT polymorphism was similar in healthy subjects and IBS patients, but some differences were observed in subgroups of IBS patients, and these differences could be population specific.

Psychological Factors Community-based studies in adults have shown that IBS patients are indistinguishable from the rest of the population in terms of psychological comorbidities [45]. Higher psychological comorbidities have been reported in a subset of IBS patients who seek medical help [45]. Patients with psychosomatic disorders such as depression have activation of the immune system and elevated CRP [46]. Adults who develop postinfectious IBS are more likely to develop depression [47], and depressive symptoms have also been linked to relapses of colitis [48] and disease activity [49] in patients with IBD. It is not clear if the depression is the result of chronic ill health or leads to the development of IBS. In children social learning of illness behavior can also contribute to the development of IBS; children of mothers with IBS are more likely to seek medical help for functional gastrointestinal symptoms [50]. Children with IBS who have significant psychological comorbidities run a more protracted illness course and are less likely to respond to treatment [51].

Functional Pain and IBD

Bowel injury and inflammation can induce functional and structural changes in the enteric neurons and muscles. Increased numbers of ganglion cells, axonal degeneration, and a reduced number of interstitial cells of Cajal have been reported in IBD [21]. In Crohn disease there is increase in substance P and its receptors in the GI tract [21]. The bowel innervation shifts from a predominantly cholinergic to a substance P predominant innervation in ulcerative colitis (UC) [21]. Increased expression of nerve fibers expressing transient receptor potential vanilloid type 1 (TRPV1) receptor in IBD and IBS has been reported [52] as well as in quiescent IBD patients with IBS-like symptoms [53]. The expression of TRPV1 is a feature of afferent pain fiber and upregulated by inflammation [53]. These changes can cause alteration in bowel sensory perception. Patients with active UC show a decreased threshold for painful and non-painful rectal distension stimulus [54]. The hypersensitivity can be widespread, and a lower pain threshold to esophageal distension has been reported in adults with UC [55]. In contrast, patients with isolated ileal Crohn disease have an increased pain threshold following rectal distension [56]. It appears that the development of visceral hypersensitivity in IBD may depend on the disease activity, type of inflammation, and region of the GI tract involved.

There is a considerable overlap between IBS and IBD symptoms. Adults who develop IBD may have a prodrome of IBS-like symptoms that can be as long as 7 years [57]. Some of these patients could have a delayed diagnosis of IBD, but some may have GI inflammation not severe enough to make a diagnosis of IBD but sufficient to cause IBS-like symptoms. Up to 57% of adults with Crohn disease and 33% with UC have symptoms like pain and bloating when in clinical, laboratory, and endoscopic disease remission [58]. Since a few inflammatory cells located strategically near the enteric nerves or myenteric ganglion cells can alter bowel function in IBS, similar changes could be responsible for the functional symptoms in patients with Crohn disease, which cause transmural inflammation [59–61].

Evaluation of placebo response in Crohn disease provides indirect evidence to the existence of functional GI disorders in these patients. Placebo therapy can alter the natural course of Crohn disease. In a meta-analysis of 23 adult studies using Crohn's Disease Activity Index (CDAI) to measure Crohn disease activity, the pooled median remission rate with placebo was 19% (range 0–50%) [62]. Significant predictors of a placebo response were duration of participation in the study and number of clinic visits. The placebo effect increased with the increasing study duration (Fig. 52.2), suggesting that frequent contact with medical professionals relieved symptoms in some patients. A high CDAI and CRP at recruitment showed a negative correlation with the placebo response, suggesting that patients with a low or normal CRP and a comparatively mild clinical disease activity were more likely to respond to a placebo. Therefore, the obvious question is whether some of these patients with Crohn disease had functional GI symptoms to begin with and were therefore more likely to respond to a placebo.

Diagnosis

The diagnosis of IBS is based on clinical symptoms and signs (Fig. 52.3). Investigative workup and endoscopic evaluation may be necessary in a small percentage of children especially in the presence of alarm features. In one large pediatric study, anemia, hematochezia, and weight loss were most predictive of Crohn disease in children presenting with chronic abdominal pain, with a cumulative sensitivity of 94% and specificity of 62% [7]. Adult studies suggest that 5–17% of celiac disease patients have IBS-like symptoms, and in one study of 1032 adults with celiac disease, 37% were diagnosed with IBS prior to the diagnosis of celiac disease [63]. Abdominal pain is a common symptom in children with celiac disease but the prevalence of IBS is unknown. More than 90% of these adults have improvement in IBS-like symptoms after starting gluten-free diet. Lactose intolerance has been reported in 15–25% of adults with IBS. However, it is yet to be determined if lactose exclusion results in resolution of IBS symptoms.

Treatment

When evaluating children with IBS, it is important to allocate sufficient time for the consult to allow the child and family to share their concerns. One must acknowledge the presence of pain, adopt an empathic and nonjudgmental point of view, and educate and reassure the child and the parents by explaining the source of symptoms in the absence of an identifiable cause [64]. It should also be made clear that the improvement will be slow, and the focus should be on normalization of psychosocial functioning, rather than trying to identify the cause for the symptoms.

Cognitive behavioral therapy (CBT), family intervention, and guided imagery, a form of relaxed and focused concentration, have been successfully used to treat func-

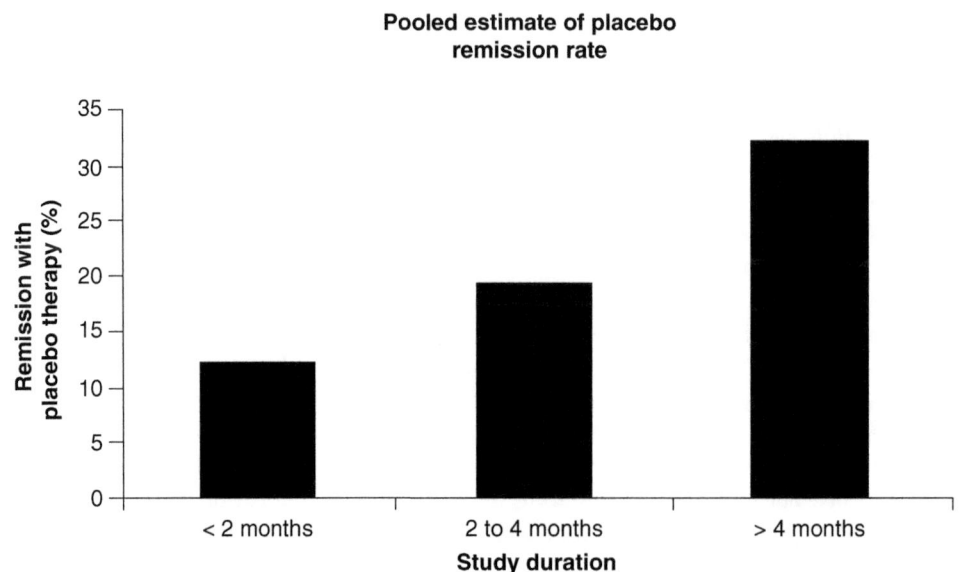

Fig. 52.2 Data from meta-analysis of 23 studies that used CDAI to measure disease activity in Crohn disease. The pooled estimate of remission with placebo therapy increased with study duration

tional abdominal pain in children and are also effective in IBS[64]. Adult studies have shown that attention management techniques such as hypnosis and mindfulness meditation are useful to treat IBS symptoms. Patients with prolonged illness and complex psychological comorbidities, which interfere with participation in a treatment plan, may require early referral to a multidisciplinary team, which includes a pain psychologist and a gastroenterologist [51]. CBT is based on the belief that our thoughts, behaviors, and feelings interact, and CBT aims to reduce or eliminate physical symptoms

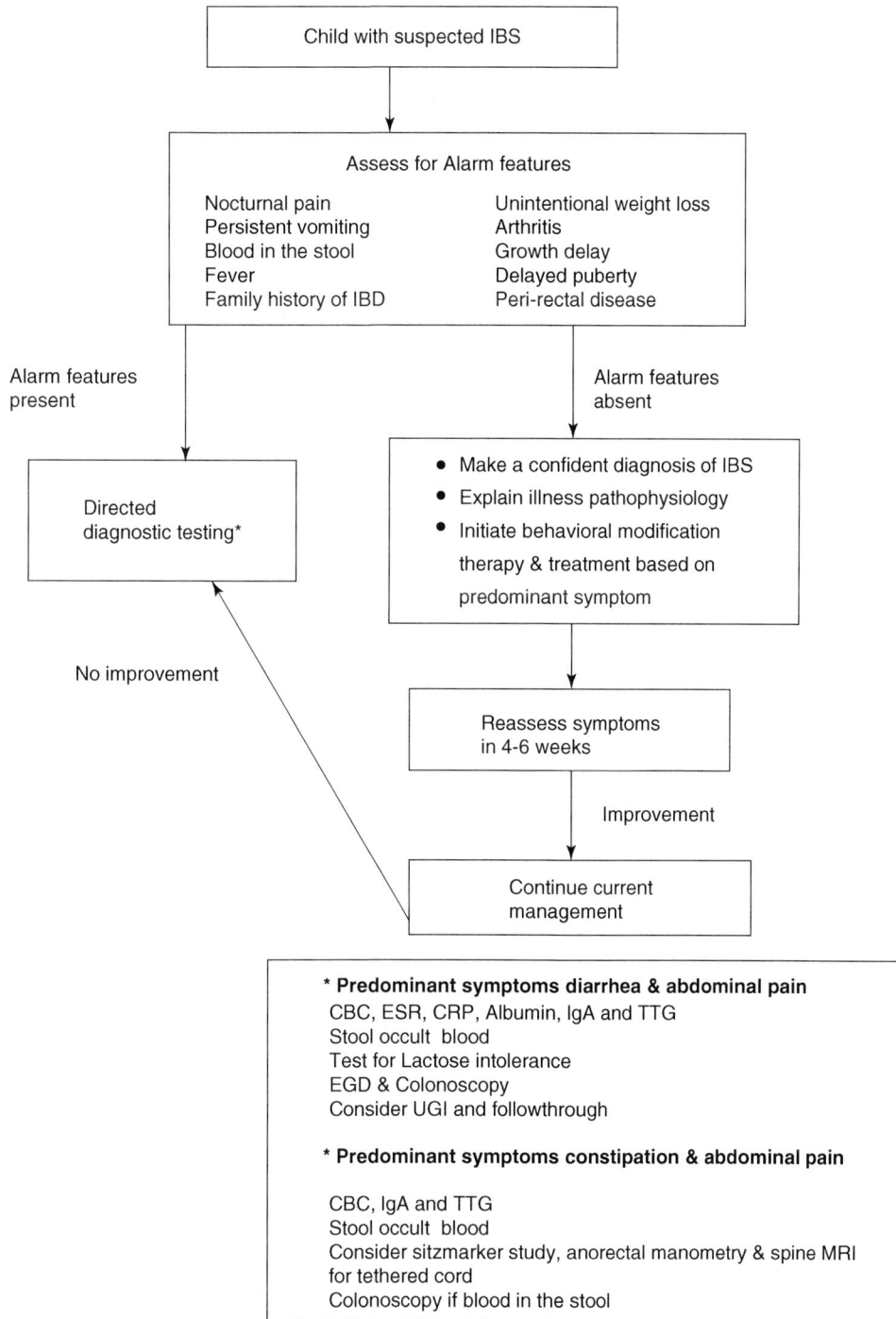

Child with suspected IBS

Assess for Alarm features

Nocturnal pain   Unintentional weight loss
Persistent vomiting   Arthritis
Blood in the stool   Growth delay
Fever   Delayed puberty
Family history of IBD   Peri-rectal disease

Alarm features
present

Alarm features
absent

Directed
diagnostic testing*

- Make a confident diagnosis of IBS
- Explain illness pathophysiology
- Initiate behavioral modification
  therapy & treatment based on
  predominant symptom

No improvement

Reassess symptoms
in 4-6 weeks

Improvement

Continue current
management

* Predominant symptoms diarrhea & abdominal pain
CBC, ESR, CRP, Albumin, IgA and TTG
Stool occult blood
Test for Lactose intolerance
EGD & Colonoscopy
Consider UGI and followthrough

* Predominant symptoms constipation & abdominal pain

CBC, IgA and TTG
Stool occult blood
Consider sitzmarker study, anorectal manometry & spine MRI
for tethered cord
Colonoscopy if blood in the stool

Fig. 52.3 Algorithm for management of children presenting with symptoms consistent with the diagnosis of IBS

through cognitive and behavioral changes. It guides the patient to modify or change cognitive distortions and negative thinking and enables the patient to substitute these with more realistic thoughts, such as that the pain is likely to subside and does not represent a terminal illness. Several randomized controlled trials to test the effectiveness of pain interventions in children with functional abdominal pain using a self-management approach that includes component of CBT have yielded encouraging results. However, methodological difficulties and different criteria used to classify patients can make interpretation difficult. Cognitive behavioral and relaxation therapy are emerging as the first-line treatment for children with functional abdominal pain and are also useful to treat children with IBS.

Dietary triggers such as caffeine, fatty meals, and carbonated soft drinks should be eliminated. A lactose-free diet can help patients with IBS symptoms associated with lactose intolerance. Increasing dietary intake of fiber can help patients with constipation-predominant IBS, but metabolism of the bulking agents by gut bacteria can produce gas, which can worsen symptoms of bloating and flatulence. A meta-analysis in adults with IBS suggested that soluble fiber sources such as psyllium, ispaghula, and calcium polycarbophil may be more effective in improving global IBS symptoms compared to insoluble fiber [65, 66]. An innovative approach for treatment of IBS in adults comprises a reduction in fermentable oligosaccharides, disaccharides, monosaccharides, and polyols (FODMAPs) in the diet [67, 68]. These short-chain carbohydrates have common functional properties in that they are poorly absorbed, osmotically active, and rapidly fermented by bacteria. A recent multicenter randomized controlled study in adults reported that FODMAP diet was not superior to traditional IBS dietary advice in adult patients [69]. In a small randomized placebo-controlled trial in children with IBS, a quarter of the study cohort reported improvement in abdominal pain and frequency of bowel movements only with FODMAP diet and another third reported improvement with FODMAP and typical American childhood diet. However, the symptom response was evaluated over a relatively short period of two days [31]. Dietary advice is an important component of symptom management in patients with IBS; however, FODMAP diet and traditional dietary advice may have similar beneficial effect on symptoms, and some experts have raised concerns about safety of FODMAP diet used over prolonged period of time.

Polyethylene glycol 3350 and milk of magnesia can be used as a stool softener in patients with constipation. Lubiprostone, a type 2 chloride channel agonist, is effective in treating constipation and constipation-predominant IBS in adults [70]. Pediatric trials documenting efficacy in pediatric age group are lacking. Menthol, the active ingredient in peppermint, inhibits smooth muscle contractions by blocking calcium channels. Enteric-coated peppermint oil capsules can help relieve abdominal pain [71]. Peppermint oil can however cause rectal burning, esophageal pain, and allergic reactions [71]. There are no controlled studies in children showing the efficacy of anticholinergics in IBS and adult trials have also produced conflicting results. In general, the anticholinergic effect in adults with IBS is comparable to a placebo [71]. The authors do not prescribe antispasmodics, but if a patient is already using them and finds them useful, then the authors do not discontinue the medication. Loperamide can be useful to reduce the stool frequency in diarrhea-predominant IBS patients.

Tricyclic antidepressants (TCAs) are useful in treating IBS symptoms in adults [71]. TCAs act primarily through noradrenergic and serotonergic pathways and have antimuscarinic and antihistaminic properties as well. TCAs facilitate descending inhibitory pain pathways and alter gastrointestinal physiology to improve IBS symptoms. Amitriptyline has sedative properties that can be used to improve sleep quality when given at bedtime. The usual dose of amitriptyline is 0.2 mg/kg once at bedtime, but higher dose can be tried if there is no improvement in 2–3 weeks. A randomized controlled trial in 83 children with pain-associated FGIDs including IBS reported no significant difference between placebo and amitriptyline group after 4 weeks of amitriptyline therapy [72]. The amitriptyline dose in this trial was fixed, and the treatment duration was relatively short and may have affected the outcome. TCAs can cause cardiac dysrhythmia in patients with prolonged QT syndrome; therefore, an electrocardiogram prior to starting the therapy is advisable.

In recent years several organisms, such as *Lactobacillus GG*, *L. plantarum*, *L. acidophilus*, *L. casei*, the probiotic cocktail VSL#3, and *Bifidobacterium animalis*, have been used to treat IBS symptoms, such as bloating, flatulence, and constipation. However, only a few products have been shown to be effective in relieving pain and global symptoms in IBS [73–77]. One organism *B. infantis* was reported to be superior to both a *Lactobacillus* and placebo in relieving abdominal pain, bloating, and difficult defecation and also improved composite score in IBS patients [77, 78]. A meta-analysis concluded that *Lactobacillus rhamnosus* GG moderately increases treatment success in children with abdominal pain-related FGIDs, particularly children with IBS [79]. The probiotic cocktail VSL#3 was reported to be superior to placebo in relieving abdominal pain and bloating and improve global symptom score in children with IBS [80]. The emerging data seems to suggest that probiotics may have a role in the treatment arsenal of pediatric IBS.

"Irritable" Pouch Syndrome

Total proctocolectomy with ileal pouch-anal anastomosis is performed in patients with fulminant colitis or ulcerative colitis refractory to medical management. The most common long-term complication of ileal pouch-anal anastomosis is pouchitis [81] and presents with increased stool frequency, urgency, abdominal cramping, and bleeding (see Chap. 44) [81]. Patients with ileal pouch-anal anastomosis who have symptoms but no identifiable structural abnormalities are thought to have irritable pouch syndrome. It resembles other pain-associated FGIDs characterized by visceral hypersensitivity in the presence of normal rectal biomechanics. In one adult study of 61 symptomatic patients with ileal pouch-anal anastomosis, 42% had no macroscopic or microscopic inflammation of the pouch [81]. Almost half of the patients with symptoms but no pouch disease responded to treatment with antidiarrheal, anticholinergic, and antidepressants, similar to what has been used in treating patients with IBS [82].

Summary

The onset of IBS symptoms most likely represents the convergence of genetic and psychosocial factors, perhaps triggered by some external stimulus such as a dramatic life event or an enteric infection or inflammatory condition. Dysmotility, hypersensitivity, and disturbed brain perception may be the consequence of these events rather than the primary abnormality. Persistent low-grade bowel inflammation may be responsible for IBS symptoms following a bacterial GI infection.

In some patients IBS symptoms may predate the development of IBD, and a subset of IBD patients can have "functional" GI symptoms. Altered bowel sensory and motor function due to inflammation-induced changes in the bowel neuromuscular apparatus may be responsible for "functional" GI symptoms in IBD. In due course we may realize that immune dysregulation plays a central role in the pathogenesis of both IBS and IBD and they are the two ends of a spectrum of GI inflammatory disorders.

Most patients with IBS have mild disease and require education, reassurance, and lifestyle changes. A smaller proportion with moderate to severe symptoms can benefit from cognitive behavioral therapy and treatment with pharmacological agents.

References

1. Sood MR, Di Lorenzo C, Hyams J, et al. Beliefs and attitudes of general pediatricians and pediatric gastroenterologists regarding functional gastrointestinal disorders: a survey study. Clin Pediatr. 2011;50(10):891–6.
2. Majeskie A, Sood MR, Miranda A. Comparison of red flags and associated factors in pediatric functional abdominal pain and Crohn's disease. Gastroenterology. 2010;138(5, Supplement 1):S-353.
3. Hyams JS, Treem WR, Justinich CJ, Davis P, Shoup M, Burke G. Characterization of symptoms in children with recurrent abdominal pain: resemblance to irritable bowel syndrome. J Pediatr Gastroenterol Nutr. 1995;20(2):209–14.
4. Dong L, Dingguo L, Xiaoxing X, Hanming L. An epidemiologic study of irritable bowel syndrome in adolescents and children in China: a school-based study. Pediatrics. 2005;116(3):e393–6.
5. Hyams JS, Burke G, Davis PM, Rzepski B, Andrulonis PA. Abdominal pain and irritable bowel syndrome in adolescents: a community-based study. J Pediatr. 1996;129(2):220–6.
6. Rasquin A, Di Lorenzo C, Forbes D, et al. Childhood functional gastrointestinal disorders: child/adolescent. Gastroenterology. 2006;130(5):1527–37.
7. El-Chammas KI, Majeskie A, Chen CC, Simpson P, Sood MR, Miranda A. Clinical predictors of Crohn's disease in pediatric patients with abdominal pain. J Pediatr Gastroenterol Nutr. 2011;53(Suppl 1):E61.
8. Locke 3rd GR, Zinsmeister AR, Fett SL, Melton 3rd LJ, Talley NJ. Overlap of gastrointestinal symptom complexes in a US community. Neurogastroenterol Motil. 2005;17(1):29–34.
9. Poon KK, Mills S, Booth IW, Murphy MS. Inflammatory cloacogenic polyp: an unrecognized cause of hematochezia and tenesmus in childhood. J Pediatr. 1997;130(2):327–9.
10. Rao SS. Constipation: evaluation and treatment of colonic and anorectal motility disorders. Gastroenterol Clin N Am. 2007;36(3):687–711. x
11. Hasler WL. Traditional thoughts on the pathophysiology of irritable bowel syndrome. Gastroenterol Clin N Am. 2011;40(1):21–43.
12. Van Ginkel R, Voskuijl WP, Benninga MA, Taminiau JA, Boeckxstaens GE. Alterations in rectal sensitivity and motility in childhood irritable bowel syndrome. Gastroenterology. 2001; 120(1):31–8.
13. Di Lorenzo C, Youssef NN, Sigurdsson L, Scharff L, Griffiths J, Wald A. Visceral hyperalgesia in children with functional abdominal pain. J Pediatr. 2001;139(6):838–43.
14. Tillisch K, Mayer EA, Labus JS. Quantitative meta-analysis identifies brain regions activated during rectal distension in irritable bowel syndrome. Gastroenterology. 2011;140(1):91–100.
15. Mayer EA, Gupta A, Kilpatrick LA, Hong JY. Imaging brain mechanisms in chronic visceral pain. Pain. 2015;156(Suppl 1):S50–63.
16. Liu X, Silverman A, Kern M, et al. Excessive coupling of the salience network with intrinsic neurocognitive brain networks during rectal distension in adolescents with irritable bowel syndrome: a preliminary report. Neurogastroenterol Motil. 2016;28(1):43–53.
17. Hong JY, Naliboff B, Labus JS, et al. Altered brain responses in subjects with irritable bowel syndrome during cued and uncued pain expectation. Neurogastroenterol Motil. 2016;28(1):127–38.
18. Spiller RC, Jenkins D, Thornley JP, et al. Increased rectal mucosal enteroendocrine cells, T lymphocytes, and increased gut permeability following acute Campylobacter enteritis and in post-dysenteric irritable bowel syndrome. Gut. 2000;47(6):804–11.
19. Gwee KA, Collins SM, Read NW, et al. Increased rectal mucosal expression of interleukin 1beta in recently acquired post-infectious irritable bowel syndrome. Gut. 2003;52(4):523–6.
20. Neal KR, Hebden J, Spiller R. Prevalence of gastrointestinal symptoms six months after bacterial gastroenteritis and risk factors for development of the irritable bowel syndrome: postal survey of patients. BMJ. 1997;314(7083):779–82.
21. Bercik P, Verdu EF, Collins SM. Is irritable bowel syndrome a low-grade inflammatory bowel disease? Gastroenterol Clin N Am. 2005;34(2):235–45. vi-vii

22. Villani AC, Lemire M, Thabane M, et al. Genetic risk factors for post-infectious irritable bowel syndrome following a waterborne outbreak of gastroenteritis. Gastroenterology. 2010;138(4):1502–13.

23. Cario E. Toll-like receptors in inflammatory bowel diseases: a decade later. Inflamm Bowel Dis. 2010;16(9):1583–97.

24. Brint EK, MacSharry J, Fanning A, Shanahan F, Quigley EM. Differential expression of toll-like receptors in patients with irritable bowel syndrome. Am J Gastroenterol. 2011;106(2):329–36.

25. Faure C, Patey N, Gauthier C, Brooks EM, Mawe GM. Serotonin signaling is altered in irritable bowel syndrome with diarrhea but not in functional dyspepsia in pediatric age patients. Gastroenterology. 2010;139(1):249–58.

26. Saps M, Pensabene L, Di Martino L, et al. Post-infectious functional gastrointestinal disorders in children. J Pediatr. 2008; 152(6):812–6. 816 e811

27. Saps M, Dhroove G, Chogle A. Henoch-Schonlein purpura leads to functional gastrointestinal disorders. Dig Dis Sci. 2011;56(6): 1789–93.

28. Moussata D, Goetz M, Gloeckner A, et al. Confocal laser endomicroscopy is a new imaging modality for recognition of intramucosal bacteria in inflammatory bowel disease in vivo. Gut. 2011;60(1): 26–33.

29. Saulnier DM, Riehle K, Mistretta TA, et al. Gastrointestinal microbiome signatures of pediatric patients with irritable bowel syndrome. Gastroenterology. 2011;141(5):1782–91.

30. Noor SO, Ridgway K, Scovell L, et al. Ulcerative colitis and irritable bowel patients exhibit distinct abnormalities of the gut microbiota. BMC Gastroenterol. 2010;10:134.

31. Chumpitazi BP, Cope JL, Hollister EB, et al. Randomised clinical trial: gut microbiome biomarkers are associated with clinical response to a low FODMAP diet in children with the irritable bowel syndrome. Aliment Pharmacol Ther. 2015;42(4):418–27.

32. Chumpitazi BP, Hollister EB, Oezguen N, et al. Gut microbiota influences low fermentable substrate diet efficacy in children with irritable bowel syndrome. Gut Microbes. 2014;5(2):165–75.

33. Quigley EM. Disturbances of motility and visceral hypersensitivity in irritable bowel syndrome: biological markers or epiphenomenon. Gastroenterol Clin N Am. 2005;34(2):221–33. vi

34. Kellow JE, Gill RC, Wingate DL. Prolonged ambulant recordings of small bowel motility demonstrate abnormalities in the irritable bowel syndrome. Gastroenterology. 1990;98(5 Pt 1):1208–18.

35. Haderstorfer B, Psycholgin D, Whitehead WE, Schuster MM. Intestinal gas production from bacterial fermentation of undigested carbohydrate in irritable bowel syndrome. Am J Gastroenterol. 1989;84(4):375–8.

36. Riordan SM, Kim R. Bacterial overgrowth as a cause of irritable bowel syndrome. Curr Opin Gastroenterol. 2006;22(6):669–73.

37. Pimentel M, Park S, Mirocha J, Kane SV, Kong Y. The effect of a nonabsorbed oral antibiotic (rifaximin) on the symptoms of the irritable bowel syndrome: a randomized trial. Ann Intern Med. 2006;145(8):557–63.

38. Tonini M, Pace F. Drugs acting on serotonin receptors for the treatment of functional GI disorders. Dig Dis. 2006;24(1–2):59–69.

39. Mawe GM, Coates MD, Moses PL. Review article: intestinal serotonin signalling in irritable bowel syndrome. Aliment Pharmacol Ther. 2006;23(8):1067–76.

40. Khoshoo V, Armstead C, Landry L. Effect of a laxative with and without tegaserod in adolescents with constipation predominant irritable bowel syndrome. Aliment Pharmacol Ther. 2006;23(1): 191–6.

41. Park MI, Camilleri M. Genetics and genotypes in irritable bowel syndrome: implications for diagnosis and treatment. Gastroenterol Clin N Am. 2005;34(2):305–17.

42. Morris-Yates A, Talley NJ, Boyce PM, Nandurkar S, Andrews G. Evidence of a genetic contribution to functional bowel disorder. Am J Gastroenterol. 1998;93(8):1311–7.

43. Levy RL, Jones KR, Whitehead WE, Feld SI, Talley NJ, Corey LA. Irritable bowel syndrome in twins: heredity and social learning both contribute to etiology. Gastroenterology. 2001;121(4): 799–804.

44. Saito YA, Mitra N, Mayer EA. Genetic approaches to functional gastrointestinal disorders. Gastroenterology. 2010;138(4): 1276–85.

45. Palsson OS, Drossman DA. Psychiatric and psychological dysfunction in irritable bowel syndrome and the role of psychological treatments. Gastroenterol Clin N Am. 2005;34(2):281–303.

46. De Berardis D, Campanella D, Gambi F, et al. The role of C-reactive protein in mood disorders. Int J Immunopathol Pharmacol. 2006;19(4):721–5.

47. Dunlop SP, Jenkins D, Neal KR, Spiller RC. Relative importance of enterochromaffin cell hyperplasia, anxiety, and depression in postinfectious IBS. Gastroenterology. 2003;125(6):1651–9.

48. Mittermaier C, Dejaco C, Waldhoer T, et al. Impact of depressive mood on relapse in patients with inflammatory bowel disease: a prospective 18-month follow-up study. Psychosom Med. 2004;66(1):79–84.

49. Mardini HE, Kip KE, Wilson JW. Crohn's disease: a two-year prospective study of the association between psychological distress and disease activity. Dig Dis Sci. 2004;49(3):492–7.

50. Levy RL, Whitehead WE, Walker LS, et al. Increased somatic complaints and health-care utilization in children: effects of parent IBS status and parent response to gastrointestinal symptoms. Am J Gastroenterol. 2004;99(12):2442–51.

51. Mulvaney S, Lambert EW, Garber J, Walker LS. Trajectories of symptoms and impairment for pediatric patients with functional abdominal pain: a 5-year longitudinal study. J Am Acad Child Adolesc Psychiatry. 2006;45(6):737–44.

52. Akbar A, Yiangou Y, Facer P, Walters JR, Anand P, Ghosh S. Increased capsaicin receptor TRPV1-expressing sensory fibres in irritable bowel syndrome and their correlation with abdominal pain. Gut. 2008;57(7):923–9.

53. Akbar A, Yiangou Y, Facer P, et al. Expression of the TRPV1 receptor differs in quiescent inflammatory bowel disease with or without abdominal pain. Gut. 2010;59(6):767–74.

54. Farthing MJ, Lennard-jones JE. Sensibility of the rectum to distension and the anorectal distension reflex in ulcerative colitis. Gut. 1978;19(1):64–9.

55. Galeazzi F, Luca MG, Lanaro D, et al. Esophageal hyperalgesia in patients with ulcerative colitis: role of experimental stress. Am J Gastroenterol. 2001;96(9):2590–5.

56. Bernstein CN, Niazi N, Robert M, et al. Rectal afferent function in patients with inflammatory and functional intestinal disorders. Pain. 1996;66(2–3):151–61.

57. Pimentel M, Chang M, Chow EJ, et al. Identification of a prodromal period in Crohn's disease but not ulcerative colitis. Am J Gastroenterol. 2000;95(12):3458–62.

58. Simren M, Axelsson J, Gillberg R, Abrahamsson H, Svedlund J, Bjornsson ES. Quality of life in inflammatory bowel disease in remission: the impact of IBS-like symptoms and associated psychological factors. Am J Gastroenterol. 2002;97(2):389–96.

59. Pardi DS. Microscopic colitis: an update. Inflamm Bowel Dis. 2004;10(6):860–70.

60. Tornblom H, Lindberg G, Nyberg B, Veress B. Full-thickness biopsy of the jejunum reveals inflammation and enteric neuropathy in irritable bowel syndrome. Gastroenterology. 2002;123(6): 1972–9.

61. Barbara G, Stanghellini V, De Giorgio R, et al. Activated mast cells in proximity to colonic nerves correlate with abdominal pain in irritable bowel syndrome. Gastroenterology. 2004;126(3):693–702.

62. Su C. Outcomes of placebo therapy in inflammatory bowel disease. Inflamm Bowel Dis. 2006;12(4):328–33.

63. Zipser RD, Patel S, Yahya KZ, Baisch DW, Monarch E. Presentations of adult celiac disease in a nationwide patient support group. Dig Dis Sci. 2003;48(4):761–4.

64. Miranda A, Sood M. Treatment options for chronic abdominal pain in children and adolescents. Curr Treat Options Gastroenterol. 2006;9(5):409–15.

65. Quartero AO, Meineche-Schmidt V, Muris J, Rubin G, de Wit N. Bulking agents, antispasmodic and antidepressant medication for the treatment of irritable bowel syndrome. Cochrane Database Syst Rev. 2005;2:CD003460.

66. Bijkerk CJ, Muris JW, Knottnerus JA, Hoes AW, de Wit NJ. Systematic review: the role of different types of fibre in the treatment of irritable bowel syndrome. Aliment Pharmacol Ther. 2004;19(3):245–51.

67. Shepherd SJ, Parker FC, Muir JG, Gibson PR. Dietary triggers of abdominal symptoms in patients with irritable bowel syndrome: randomized placebo-controlled evidence. Clin Gastroenterol Hepatol: Off Clin Pract J Am Gastroenterol Ass. 2008;6(7): 765–71.

68. Staudacher HM, Whelan K, Irving PM, Lomer MC. Comparison of symptom response following advice for a diet low in fermentable carbohydrates (FODMAPs) versus standard dietary advice in patients with irritable bowel syndrome. J Human Nutr Diet: Off J Br Diet Ass. 2011;24(5):487–95.

69. Bohn L, Storsrud S, Liljebo T, et al. Diet low in FODMAPs reduces symptoms of irritable bowel syndrome as well as traditional dietary advice: a randomized controlled trial. Gastroenterology. 2015;149(6):1399–407. e1392

70. Schey R, Rao SS. Lubiprostone for the treatment of adults with constipation and irritable bowel syndrome. Dig Dis Sci. 2011;56(6):1619–25.

71. Schoenfeld P. Efficacy of current drug therapies in irritable bowel syndrome: what works and does not work. Gastroenterol Clin N Am. 2005;34(2):319–35. viii

72. Saps M, Youssef N, Miranda A, et al. Multicenter, randomized, placebo-controlled trial of amitriptyline in children with functional gastrointestinal disorders. Gastroenterology. 2009;137(4):1261–9.

73. Nikfar S, Rahimi R, Rahimi F, Derakhshani S, Abdollahi M. Efficacy of probiotics in irritable bowel syndrome: a meta-analysis of randomized, controlled trials. Dis Colon Rectum. 2008;51(12):1775–80.

74. McFarland LV, Dublin S. Meta-analysis of probiotics for the treatment of irritable bowel syndrome. World J Gastroenterol: WJG. 2008;14(17):2650–61.

75. Hoveyda N, Heneghan C, Mahtani KR, Perera R, Roberts N, Glasziou P. A systematic review and meta-analysis: probiotics in the treatment of irritable bowel syndrome. BMC Gastroenterol. 2009;9:15.

76. Moayyedi P, Ford AC, Talley NJ, et al. The efficacy of probiotics in the treatment of irritable bowel syndrome: a systematic review. Gut. 2010;59(3):325–32.

77. Brenner DM, Moeller MJ, Chey WD, Schoenfeld PS. The utility of probiotics in the treatment of irritable bowel syndrome: a systematic review. Am J Gastroenterol. 2009;104(4):1033–49. quiz 1050

78. O'Mahony L, McCarthy J, Kelly P, et al. Lactobacillus and bifidobacterium in irritable bowel syndrome: symptom responses and relationship to cytokine profiles. Gastroenterology. 2005;128(3): 541–51.

79. Horvath A, Dziechciarz P, Szajewska H. Meta-analysis: Lactobacillus rhamnosus GG for abdominal pain-related functional gastrointestinal disorders in childhood. Aliment Pharmacol Ther. 2011;33(12):1302–10.

80. Guandalini S, Magazzu G, Chiaro A, et al. VSL#3 improves symptoms in children with irritable bowel syndrome: a multicenter, randomized, placebo-controlled, double-blind, crossover study. J Pediatr Gastroenterol Nutr. 2010;51(1):24–30.

81. Shen B, Fazio VW, Remzi FH, Lashner BA. Clinical approach to diseases of ileal pouch-anal anastomosis. Am J Gastroenterol. 2005;100(12):2796–807.

82. Shen B, Sanmiguel C, Bennett AE, et al. Irritable pouch syndrome is characterized by visceral hypersensitivity. Inflamm Bowel Dis. 2011;17(4):994–1002.

Inflammatory Bowel Disease in Pregnancy

53

Sunanda Kane

Introduction

While the incidence of ulcerative colitis has remained stable, the incidence of Crohn disease [CD] has increased over the past few decades [1]. It is not clear whether this is due to improved diagnostic techniques, an increase in smoking habits by young female patients [patients with CD tend to be smokers compared to people without CD [2]], environmental or genetic influences, or other factors not yet identified. However, the consequence of this trend is a growing population of patients in their formative and childbearing years.

Having intercourse, age of sexual debut, and pregnancy rates do not differ among adolescents with and without disability based on a study by Suris et al. [3]. Disability, defined "as a long-term reduction in ability to conduct social role activities, such as school or play, because of a chronic physical or mental condition," [4] does not interfere with sexuality of an adolescent [5]. Thus, adolescent patients with inflammatory bowel disease (IBD) may be sexually active and are at risk for pregnancy. This chapter will review how pregnancy affects the adolescent with IBD both in terms of disease and management options and how inflammatory bowel disease and its therapies may affect a pregnancy.

Contraception

The management of contraception in those female patients with IBD who do not wish to become pregnant differs from that in normal female patients. A recent study by Gawron et al. found that a quarter of women with IBD were not using any form of birth control even though they were at risk for an unintended pregnancy [6]. The most important goal still remains the selection of the most reliable method of birth control. Barrier methods of contraception are acceptable but are not as effective as alternatives. The use of intrauterine devices is not usually recommended, as any complaint of abdominal/pelvic pain could potentially delay the correct diagnosis of active IBD versus pelvic inflammatory disease. There is a single case report of a patient who experienced an exacerbation of Crohn disease after insertion of a levonorgestrel intrauterine system [7]. However, no strict contraindication exists to preclude their use in the appropriate patient.

The data regarding the safety of oral contraceptives (OCs) in IBD are conflicting. Early studies suggested an increased risk (odds ratios ranging from 1.2 to 6) for the development of Crohn disease and ulcerative colitis with OC use. Several of these studies did not, however, account for tobacco use. Reports from Europe, where contraceptives contain a higher estrogen content, continue to show modest increases in risk for the development of Crohn disease after adjusting for cigarette use (odds ratios 1.2–2.0) [8]. A meta-analysis by Cornish et al. suggests that the overall OR is significantly higher for the incidence of Crohn disease with an odds ratio of 1.46 (1.26–1.70) [9].

Other data suggest that OC use may exacerbate disease activity. Two small prospective studies have found an increased risk of disease recurrence after induction of remission in Crohn disease with OC use [8, 10]. Timmer found a hazard ratio of 3 (1.5–5.9) for increased disease activity following medical induction of remission. No information is available for a possible similar risk in ulcerative colitis. However, a more recent systematic review suggested that there was limited strong evidence for any increased risk for disease activity in women with established IBD [11]. Alternatively, Gawron et al. have demonstrated that OCP use can help with cyclical symptoms of IBD and only a small proportion of women report symptomatic worsening [12]. At this time, no standard guidelines exist for OC use, as there are many preparations available. The variable amounts of progesterone and estrogen are the factors that determine the side effect profile. The choice of which OC preparation to use has to be individualized, taking into consideration other factors including patient history, parity, and personal

S. Kane, MD, MSPH
Mayo Clinic, 200 First Street SW, Rochester, MN 55905, USA
e-mail: kane.sunanda@mayo.edu

© Springer International Publishing AG 2017
P. Mamula et al. (eds.), *Pediatric Inflammatory Bowel Disease*, DOI 10.1007/978-3-319-49215-5_53

preferences. It does appear prudent to try a formulation that contains the lowest amount of estrogen possible or the progesterone only formulations, given the additional risk factors of smoking and predilection towards thromboembolic events in patients with IBD. Hormonal contraception in the transdermal formulation may be considered because it avoids the addition of another oral pill for the adolescent patient as well as its delivery despite possible decrease in absorption during active flares in a patient with IBD. There are no data yet regarding the NuVa® ring.

Fertility

Adolescents with chronic conditions are just as likely to have sexual intercourse as their peers [3]. Even though adolescents may not be trying to get pregnant, the rising age of marriage and decreasing age of first intercourse combined with the inconsistent use of contraception has led to the continued trends of teenage motherhood [13].

Overall, the fertility rates for female patients with ulcerative colitis are essentially the same as those of the normal population [14]. Early studies suggesting lower fertility rates had not taken into account an increased voluntary childlessness rate in female patients with IBD [15]. Fear of pregnancy on disease activity and "passing it on" to offspring may also play a role in the reported reduced fertility seen in female patients with CD. Active Crohn disease, however, can reduce fertility in several ways, depending upon the location of inflammation [16]. Active inflammation in the colon and terminal ileal disease have been shown to decrease fertility. Active ileal inflammation can cause inflammation or scarring of the fallopian tubes and ovaries because of their proximity to the terminal ileum in the lower abdomen. Female patients with perianal disease may have secondary dyspareunia and decreased libido, contributing to lower fertility rates. The systemic effects of Crohn disease including fever, pain, diarrhea, and suboptimal malnutrition have also been implicated in decreased fertility. Female patients who have had any surgical resection are at risk for adhesions, which can also impair tubal function. Newer data has suggested that despite a decreased fertility rate, surgery does not affect success of in vitro fertilization in women with IBD compared to the general infertility population [17].

None of the medications used to treat IBD has an adverse effect on female fertility, but it is important to remember that sulfasalazine therapy reduces sperm motility and count in males [18]. These effects are not dose related and do not respond to supplemental folic acid. The overall reproductive capacity of men with IBD has not been found to be decreased, although male patients with CD have been noted to have small families [19]. A sperm analysis study has failed to show significant differences on count or morphology in men with exposure to 6-mercaptopurine (6-MP) compared to established WHO criteria [20]. In addition, further epidemiologic work has failed to demonstrate an effect on birth outcomes in children born to fathers on 6-MP, despite an early study that suggested this association [21, 22].

Onset and Diagnosis During Pregnancy

An early clinical series suggested that the prognosis was poor for those female patients with ulcerative colitis diagnosed during pregnancy [23]. Since that time, epidemiological data has failed to show a worse disease course than any other time [24]. There has been no large study involving de novo diagnosis of Crohn disease during pregnancy; no conclusion about its severity under these physiological conditions can be drawn.

Effect of IBD on Pregnancy

Open discussions between patient and physician are the best way to ensure a successful pregnancy outcome. If a woman is doing well and in remission, there is no evidence to suggest that her risk of a flare is greater than that of a nonpregnant patient. While there is no minimum required time period for a patient to be in remission prior to a planned conception, at least 3 months is recommended. If active disease is present, it is likely to continue through pregnancy and will place the pregnancy at greater risk for a complication [25]. This risk appears to be higher in CD than in ulcerative colitis [UC].

Female patients with inactive IBD at the time of conception appear no more likely to experience spontaneous abortion, stillbirth, or children born with a congenital abnormality [26]. Most studies suggest that babies born to female patients with IBD, regardless of disease activity, are of smaller birth weight [27] and more likely to be born preterm and small for gestational age [28].

The presence of IBD does not appear to have an impact on maternal complications related to pregnancy, including hypertension or proteinuria [29]. A recent study by Broms et al. demonstrated that women with IBD were more likely to experience venous thrombosis and hemorrhage in the setting of active disease [30].

Effect of Pregnancy on IBD

For female patients with quiescent UC at the time of conception, the rate of relapse is approximately the same in pregnant versus nonpregnant patients [24]. This is in contrast to the presence of active disease at the time of conception, which is associated with continued or worsening disease activity in approximately 70% of female patients. Comparable observations are seen in CD [25]. The older literature suggested a trend for disease to flare in the first trimester, but this was documented prior to the accepted practice of maintenance therapy, continued even during pregnancy. Some patients will have symptomatic disease only when pregnant, with quiescence between pregnancies and exacerbations during subsequent pregnancies. The clinical course or outcome of previous pregnancies cannot predict either the clinical course of IBD or the outcome of pregnancy. The activity of IBD at conception remains the primary predictor of the course of pregnancy.

One study has suggested that the course of the disease, either UC or CD, correlates with HLA maternal-fetal disparity [31]. Fifty mother-child pairs were studied for maternal disease course in relation to the amount of shared HLA alleles. Those pregnancies in which the mother had disparity at both the DR and DQ alleles tend to see an improvement in disease scores over time compared to those female patients who shared more alleles with the fetus. Subsequent pregnancies in the same female patients showed the same effect.

There are data suggesting that a history of childbearing changes the natural history of Crohn disease [32]. Female patients having been pregnant had fewer resections or longer intervals between resections as compared to female patients who had not had children but otherwise similar disease. One theory proposed is the inhibition of macrophage function by relaxin. Relaxin is a hormone produced exclusively during pregnancy which may result in less fibrosis and stricture formation by this inhibition of macrophages. In addition, a more recent population-based study of pregnancies in Copenhagen has suggested that pregnancy can change the natural history of IBD; women were less likely to experience a flare of their disease following pregnancy compared with those women who had not experienced a pregnancy [33].

Management of IBD During Pregnancy

Clinical Assessment

The main priority is to establish and maintain remission before the patient conceives. One of the problems in CD is the accurate definition of disease activity. In CD, a patient may feel fine even though she has an elevated C-reactive protein or an abnormal colonoscopy and/or x-ray. Many pregnant female patients will have intermittent abdominal discomfort related to changes in bowel habits or gastroesophageal reflux that commonly occur during pregnancy. In addition, abdominal pain in the pregnant IBD patient could be related to cholelithiasis,

pancreatitis, toxemia, or a problem with the pregnancy itself. Clinically, these processes can be distinguished from a flare of IBD by a careful history, examination, and laboratory evaluation.

It is important to remember that during pregnancy, hemoglobin and albumin levels decrease by 1 g/dl, sedimentation rate increases two- to threefold, and there is a 1.5-fold rise in serum alkaline phosphatase. Because of these normal physiologic changes, disease assessment during pregnancy should rely more on clinical symptoms than laboratory parameters. It is also important to keep in mind that a growing uterus changes normal anatomy, with the terminal ileum and appendix higher in the right upper quadrant.

In terms of radiographic testing, ultrasound exams are safe, as is magnetic resonance imaging [34] without gadolinium. Clearly, it is best to avoid exposure of the fetus to radiation from abdominal x-rays, especially early in the pregnancy. However, the absolute risk to the fetus of abdominal radiography is minimal, and clinical necessity should guide the decision making [35].

There is no evidence that, if indicated, a sigmoidoscopy or colonoscopy will induce premature labor [36]. Most patients with IBD can be evaluated with sigmoidoscopy without full colonoscopy. However, if full colonoscopy is necessary to establish diagnosis or severity of disease, sedation with propofol with close fetal monitoring is suggested [37, 38].

Medical Therapies

The key principle to management is to remember that the greatest risk to pregnancy is more likely active disease than active therapy. Since there are limited definitive data available on the safety of IBD medications in pregnancy, the focus therefore should be on establishing remission before conception and maintaining remission during pregnancy. The two fundamental issues considering medical therapy in the pregnant IBD patient are regarding the outcome of the pregnancy: whether the mother is taking medications for her IBD compared to those who are not and whether the medications used to treat the pregnant patient are safe and effective.

Early studies suggested that the rates of prematurity, spontaneous abortions, and fetal malformations among mothers with IBD undergoing medical treatment were increased [39, 40]. However, most investigators have shown that medical therapy, when analyzed as an independent variable, has no effect on pregnancy outcome [4, 14]. Those patients who have been reported to have adverse birth outcomes tend to occur more often in the setting of active disease. Table 53.1 outlines the relative safety profiles of those medications used in IBD.

Table 53.1 Safety of IBD medications during pregnancy

Safe to use when indicated	Limited data but appear safe	Contraindicated
Oral, topical mesalamine	Olsalazine	Methotrexate
Sulfasalazine	Azathioprine/6-MP	Thalidomide
Corticosteroids	Biologics	Diphenoxylate
Total parenteral nutrition	Cyclosporine	
Loperamide	Metronidazole	
	Ciprofloxacin[a]	

[a]Not safe in third trimester

Antidiarrheals

Symptomatic therapies used in IBD include the antidiarrheals and antispasmodics, as well as pain medications. Loperamide use has not been associated with an increased rate of first trimester fetal malformations, spontaneous abortion, low birth weight, or premature delivery [42] and is considered low risk. One has to keep in mind, however, that increased stool frequency may be a sign of increased activity and loperamide use should be monitored. Diphenoxylate with atropine is teratogenic in animals, and fetal malformations have been observed in infants exposed during the first trimester [43]. Antispasmodics and anticholinergics have been associated with non-life-threatening fetal malformations and are best avoided during pregnancy [44]. Codeine has been used for many years during pregnancy without reports of associated fetal abnormalities. Drug dependence and withdrawal in the newborn can occur, but fortunately is rare.

Aminosalicylates

Aminosalicylates are first-line medications for mild to moderate IBD. While the exact mechanism is unknown, it is thought that the effects result from topical action on the gastrointestinal mucosa rather than through systemic action [45]. Sulfasalazine has been used for over 50 years in the treatment of IBD. Sulfasalazine is the combination of sulfapyridine and 5-ASA, which is eventually cleaved by enteric bacteria, allowing the main anti-inflammatory effects to take place in the colon. The majority of the side effects of sulfasalazine are due to the sulfapyridine moiety; it crosses the placenta with fetal serum levels equivalent to maternal levels [46]. Multiple studies have shown that despite this phenomenon, there appears to be no increased incidence of abnormal birth outcomes [47].

Sulfasalazine has been shown to inhibit folate acid metabolism, which can cause neural tube defects in the fetus [48]. While the risk of fetal abnormalities has not been shown to increase with sulfasalazine and its derivatives, pregnant female patients taking sulfasalazine should still supplement their diet with 2 mg of folate daily.

Mesalamine is a sulfa-free aminosalicylate that is also effective in mild-moderate IBD and is widely used for acute and long-term management of IBD. 5-Aminosalicylic acid (5-ASA) and its metabolite acetyl-5-aminosaicyclic acid are found in both maternal and fetal plasma in female patients taking mesalamine; however, a meta-analysis of published studies has demonstrated its lack of effect on the incidence of adverse birth outcomes [49]. There is a single case report of renal interstitial damage in a child born to a woman taking mesalamine [50]. This finding has not been confirmed in any other studies. Use of topical 5-ASA agents during pregnancy has not been associated with any increase in adverse birth outcomes related to its use during pregnancy.

Olsalazine, another 5-ASA compound, is rated as an FDA class C based on the paucity of prospective safety data with this agent. Recently the FDA has changed the pregnancy rating of Asacol® (Warner Chilcott) from B to C secondary to the association of phthalate, an entity in the coating of Asacol®. In rodent studies, administration is association with urogenital abnormalities in male offspring [51]. However, the amount of phthalate required to replicate those animal studies in humans would equate to over 200 tablets of medication a day and thus not likely to be of clinical consequence.

Antibiotics

Currently, the most frequently used antibiotics in IBD include metronidazole and ciprofloxacin. Animal studies have not shown any evidence of teratogenicity or increased fetal loss with metronidazole. Short courses of metronidazole during the first trimester of pregnancy for *Trichomonas vaginalis* have been shown to be well tolerated and low risk [52, 53]. The most recent study of 228 female patients exposed to metronidazole during pregnancy followed female patients prospectively through their pregnancy [52]. Eighty-six percent of female patients were exposed during the first trimester. The malformation rate was 1.6% in the treatment group and 1.4% in the control group. Female patients with IBD require the use of metronidazole for longer periods of time, and there are limited data regarding prolonged use of this medication.

In animal studies, no teratogenicity has been seen with ciprofloxacin, although musculoskeletal abnormalities have been identified in immature animals [54]. Moskovitz et al. found that in 27 patients who were receiving 1 g/day, even in the first trimester, its use appeared to be safe (18 patients) [55]. Another study investigated the effects of fluoroquinolones in the first trimester and did not show an increased risk of congenital malformations, prematurity, or low birth weight [56].

While these data are comforting, this information applies to the non-IBD population, where antibiotics are used short term. These agents are more commonly used for longer durations in IBD, and the use of these two antibiotics during pregnancy should currently be restricted to short-term courses.

Corticosteroids

In moderate to severe disease, corticosteroids are a mainstay of treatment for IBD. As shown in studies for rheumatological conditions as well as for IBD, corticosteroids during pregnancy have largely been regarded as low risk [40]. Corticosteroids cross the placental barrier, but the fetal-maternal serum concentration of the steroids varies between different corticosteroid preparations. Prednisolone and prednisone are more efficiently metabolized by the placenta than dexamethasone or betamethasone, and fetal levels of this steroid are approximately eight- to tenfold lower than that of the maternal circulation [57]. Since corticosteroids are conjugated more rapidly to biologically less active sulfates in the fetus than the adult, a suppressive fetal blood concentration is not often reached with therapeutic doses used during pregnancy.

Among female patients with IBD, corticosteroids have not been found to be harmful to the fetus [25]. Mogadam et al. studied the effects of steroid use in 185 out of 531 pregnancies in female patients with IBD and did not find a statistically significant increased incidence of prematurity, spontaneous abortions, stillbirth, or development defects in the ulcerative colitis subgroup (4.6% in the treated group vs. 2.2% in the untreated group; $P > 0.10$) [58]. In the Crohn disease subgroup, patients did significantly worse in the treated group compared to the untreated group (13.5 vs. 1.9%, $P < 0.1$). Patients with CD may have more severe disease and require more medical intervention to control the activity of the disease, and it is possible that the severity of the illness in CD itself may have caused these patients to not fare as well as the ulcerative colitis patients.

Immunomodulators

Clearly as more and more patients with IBD are treated with immunomodulators, there is a growing need for information on their effects on the pregnant patient and growing fetus. There is a large body of literature on the use of these agents among pregnant transplant recipients and those patients with autoimmune diseases [59, 60]. It is generally believed by the most experienced IBD clinicians that immunomodulators such as 6-MP, azathioprine, and even cyclosporine can be used safely during pregnancy if the mother's health mandates therapy, based on the evidence from these other conditions.

Thiopurines are used for steroid-sparing and steroid-dependent inflammatory bowel disease. Azathioprine (AZA) is a prodrug of 6-mercaptopurine (6-MP) and does cross the placental barrier, but the immunomodulatory effects of azathioprine do not affect the fetus due to the lack of inosinate pyrophosphorylase in the fetus, an enzyme which converts azathioprine into the active metabolites of 6-MP and S-methyl-4-nitro-5-thioimidazole [61]. Placental concentrations of azathioprine range from 64 to 93% of the maternal blood level, while 6-MP and AZA levels in the fetal blood run about 1–5% and 1.2%, respectively [62]. Despite this, based on animal studies showing an increased risk of teratogenicity at doses significantly higher than what is used in clinical practice, thiopurines have been considered category D medications [63]. Several human studies have suggested that AZA and 6-MP are low risk during pregnancy when used for IBD [41, 64].

A large Danish cohort study used a population-based prescription registry to examine the risk of congenital malformation and perinatal mortality among patients taking azathioprine or 6-MP during pregnancy [65]. Nine pregnancies exposed to 6-MP in the first trimester and ten pregnancies exposed throughout the pregnancy were compared to 19,418 pregnancies without 6-MP exposure. Fifty-five percent of the exposed female patients had a history of IBD, and 45% had other autoimmune diseases. The adjusted odds ratios for congenital malformations, perinatal mortality, preterm birth, and low birth weight were 6.7% (95% CI, 1.4–32.4), 20.0 (95% CI, 2.5–161.4), 6.6% (95% CI, 1.7–25.9), and 3.8 (95% CI, 0.4–33.3) in female patients treated with 6-MP or AZA. The conclusion of the investigators was that a causal relationship between drug use and outcome could not be established.

Francella et al., in a retrospective cohort study, investigated the possible toxicity of 6-MP from a review of records of 485 patients who had received the drug [64]. Of the 462 female patients who were contacted, 155 had conceived at least 1 pregnancy after developing IBD. Pregnancies were analyzed based on whether the patients had taken 6-MP before or at the time of conception compared with those IBD patients who had their pregnancies before taking 6-MP. There was no statistically significant increase in spontaneous abortion rates or major congenital malformations among patients taking 6-MP compared to control subjects [RR 0.85 (95% CI, 0.47–1.55), $p = 0.59$]. The authors concluded that the use of 6-MP or AZA and its beneficial effect on maternal health outweighed any risk to the fetus and that it was not unreasonable to continue its use throughout pregnancy. Recently, results regarding pregnancy in a prospective French cohort of Crohn patients have become available. There were no observed differences in the outcome of pregnancy for patients treated with thiopurines compared to women with CD who used no medications during pregnancy [41].

In IBD, methotrexate is used in the management of steroid-dependent or steroid-resistant Crohn disease as an alternative to azathioprine and 6-MP. Methotrexate is a known abortifacient, showing increased risk of spontaneous abortions in various studies, currently used therapeutically at high doses in tubal pregnancies [66]. As a folic acid antagonist, it is a mutagenic agent known to cause neural tube defects and palatal defects. Therefore, methotrexate is a category X medication. Patients who are started on methotrexate should be strongly advised to use reliable contraception. If termination of a pregnancy is not possible, high doses of folic acid therapy are recommended to prevent CNS abnormalities, including anencephaly, meningomyelocele, and hydrocephaly. The optimum management includes careful counseling and effective contraception prior to any initiation with methotrexate therapy [67].

Biologic Agents

Infliximab was the first biologic agent FDA approved for the treatment of inflammatory and fistulizing Crohn disease. The early safety literature with infliximab includes one study by Katz et al. suggesting that infliximab exposure for CD or rheumatoid arthritis during pregnancy does not lead to a statistically significant increase in adverse outcomes compared to that of the general population, using the National Center for Health Statistics database between 1976 and 1996 for comparison [68]. Of 96 female patients who were studied, live births (67, 95% CI: 56.3–76.0 vs. 67%), miscarriages (17, 95% CI: 8.2–23.2 vs. 15%), and therapeutic terminations (16, 95% CI: 11.5–28.0 vs. 19%) were not statistically different from that of the general population. In this review, 8 of 14 miscarriages in female patients who were exposed to infliximab occurred at or before 10 weeks. It is thought that these miscarriages early in pregnancy were related more to disease activity than infliximab use. Maternal IgG is transported across the placenta as early as the late first trimester [69], but efficiency of transport is poor, so total fetal IgG levels are low until the late second or early third trimester, suggesting that it is not the infliximab exposure that would be contributing to this early miscarriage rate observation. A recent case control study from France of pregnant women treated with infliximab versus those not failed to show any increased risk in pregnancy or neonatal outcomes [70].

The second anti-TNF agent on the market is an injectable agent, adalimumab. Because it is also a full antibody, it too crosses the placenta after week 20 of pregnancy. Drug can be detected in cord blood of the newborn up to 6 months following in utero exposure [71]. The third anti-TNF to get FDA approved is certolizumab pegol. This is a pegylated Fab fragment, and early data suggest that it does not cross the placenta [72]. However, at this time there is no recommendation to switch a patient from one agent to another if she is in remission solely because of these properties as disease can be controlled with cessation of therapy after 30 weeks gestation if disease is in remission [73]. The choice of an agent still depends on multiple factors.

The anti-integrins represent a newer class of therapies and include natalizumab, a monoclonal antibody to alpha 4 integrin, and vedolizumab, a monoclonal antibody to alpha 4 beta 7 integrin. Their properties are not well characterized, but the available data suggest that while they too cross the placenta, they are low risk during pregnancy and carry a B safety rating [74, 75].

Other Immunomodulating Agents

Cyclosporine is used particularly for refractory ulcerative colitis and pyoderma gangrenosum. Cyclosporine's inhibition of interleukin-2 and its effect on cell proliferation and cell turnover make its use in pregnancy concerning. While cyclosporine is known to cross the placenta, the concentration of the drug in the newborn falls rapidly within days after birth [76]. At a dose of 10 mg/kg/day, it has not been shown to cause any fetal toxicity in rats [77]. In the renal transplant literature, cyclosporine has been associated with premature births and growth retardation, but overall, cyclosporine has not been associated with poor pregnancy outcomes or severe adverse effects to the fetus [78]. One case report in 1995 describes the successful use of cyclosporine to avoid the risk of colectomy in a pregnant patient in her 29th week of pregnancy. This woman was effectively treated with cyclosporine resulting in the delivery of a healthy baby boy at 34 weeks [79]. A retrospective review of pregnant female patients hospitalized with severe ulcerative colitis found that female patients treated with cyclosporine in addition to corticosteroids had no more of an increased risk for adverse birth outcomes than those female patients treated with steroids alone [80]. While these are encouraging, more long-term studies are required to investigate the effects of cyclosporine in the pregnant IBD population.

Recently, a variety of other therapies have been used to treat refractory IBD. Thalidomide has been found to have some efficacy in the treatment of Crohn disease [81, 82]. Thalidomide, however, is a potent teratogen and should not be given to female patients of childbearing age except those who have undergone careful counseling and strict adherence to contraceptive use. Its availability is restricted and only available to those female patients with negative serum pregnancy tests done on a monthly basis.

Some of the newer immunomodulators used in refractory Crohn disease include tacrolimus [83] and mycophenolate mofetil [84]. Again, the safety data during pregnancy comes from the transplant populations. The experience with tacrolimus has been overall favorable, with no evident increase in adverse outcomes based on case reports and National Transplant Registry data [85]. National Registry data followed 100 female patients status post solid organ transplant and reported four neonatal malformations in 68 live births.

The use of mycophenolate in CD has been recent, and to date there are no data regarding any pregnancies occurring with its use.

Nutritional Therapies

Given the poor nutrition that often accompanies IBD, it stands to reason that both total parenteral (TPN) and enteral supplementation have been used to support the pregnant IBD patient [86, 87]. Despite the theoretical concern about fat embolization to the placenta, pregnant patients receiving TPN with intravenous lipids have done well. The infants born to those mothers have been healthy, and examination of the placenta has failed to show any signs of fat emboli. Elemental diets have also been used safely during pregnancy both as primary therapy for active CD and as a source of supplemental nutrition. Because the nutritional needs of the pregnant IBD patient are quite different from the nonpregnant IBD patient, close monitoring along with a nutritional expert is necessary.

Breastfeeding

The advantages of breastfeeding in pregnancy are well known, but the effects of IBD medications on breastfeeding still remain unclear. The breastfeeding initiation rates among adolescent mothers are approximately 35–40% [88] and are significantly less than the national rate, which is 60%. In a study by Kane et al., only 44% (54/122) of female patients with IBD had breastfed their infants, the majority of whom had UC [89]. A more recent study done in Canada showed the opposite; women with IBD nursed more frequently than the background population [90]. In neither study was there an increased risk for disease activity associated with the act of nursing itself; disease activity was related to cessation of therapies to treat disease.

Table 53.2 summarizes the safety data regarding medications and their use during breastfeeding.

Sulfasalazine and other forms of 5-ASA are excreted into the breast milk with milk concentrations that are about 40–50% of the maternal serum levels with outcomes study suggesting its safety during breastfeeding [91]. There is one case report of diarrhea in a nursing infant of a mother who used mesalamine suppositories 6 weeks after childbirth with four additional challenges of breastfeeding following suppository administration leading to similar results [92].

In a case series, low concentrations of mesalamine and its metabolite were found in the breast milk of two female patients taking mesalamine at 1gram orally three times daily. Milk to plasma ratios at day 7 and 11 postpartum were 0.17 and 0.09, respectively. The mesalamine metabolite ratios were 16.5 and 6.8, respectively. The estimated intake of mesalamine and metabolites per day by the infant was 0.065 mg (0.015 mg/kg) and 10 mg (2.3 mg/kg), respectively, which are considered to be negligible amounts [93].

Data pertaining to thiopurines comes from the prospective study done by Christensen [94]. Milk concentrations were highest within the first four hours of maternal ingestion and only equated to 0.0075 mg/kg bodyweight. Thus, it seems reasonable to suggest that drug exposure is minimal and to minimize it further that a mother pump and dump any milk produced within the first four hours of thiopurine ingestion and nurse with milk produced the remainder of the day.

Cyclosporine has also been relatively contraindicated due to theoretical immunosuppression in the infant. However, a study by Nyberg et al. of transplant patients showed that breastfed infants of mothers on cyclosporine received <300 mcg/day of cyclosporine [95]. Blood cyclosporine levels ranged from 55 to 130 ng/ml in mothers (12 h trough), with a range of 50–227 ng/ml in breast milk, and were below the detection limit of 30 ng/ml in all infants. A case report of a 35-year old woman who exclusively breastfed her infant during the first 10.5 months of life while she was being treated with cyclosporine revealed mean breast milk/maternal blood level ratio of 84%, with undetectable levels in the infant [96].

Approximately 5–25% of the maternal serum concentration of corticosteroids reaches breast milk, and the amount received by the infant is considered minimal [57]. The commonly used corticosteroids, prednisone and prednisolone, result in low breast milk concentrations with doses of <20 mg of corticosteroids deemed to be safe to use during nursing [97]. Some suggest that breastfeeding is safer if delayed for 4 h after ingestion of steroids [98]. Other medications, such as metronidazole, ciprofloxacin, and methotrexate, should be discontinued in nursing mothers given their high concentrations in breast milk.

There is a small case series of women who nursed while receiving infusions of infliximab, and there was no evidence that infliximab is excreted into milk [99], and thus it is not

Table 53.2 Safety of IBD medications during breastfeeding

Safe to use when indicated	Very limited data	Contraindicated
Oral mesalamine	Olsalazine	Methotrexate
Topical mesalamine	Azathioprine	Thalidomide
Sulfasalazine	6-MP	Cyclosporine
Corticosteroids	Biologics	Ciprofloxacin
		Metronidazole
		Loperamide
		Diphenoxylate

mandated that women who receive infliximab stop nursing. There is a single case report of adalimumab use in a nursing mother [100].

Mode of Delivery

The mode of delivery should most often be an obstetrical decision and not solely based on the presence of IBD. Adolescents have lower Cesarean section rates than adult women [101]. The indications for Cesarean section for obstetrical reasons are not different in female patients with IBD. The presence of UC does not have a significant impact on the method of delivery, nor is it an indication for a section per se. However, active perianal disease in Crohn disease may worsen after a vaginal delivery. One retrospective study of female patients with CD found that 18% of those without previous perianal disease developed such disease after delivery, usually involving an extensive episiotomy [102]. A retrospective chart review from last year found that there was no difference in risk of symptomatic flares of perianal disease with a vaginal delivery versus a C-section [103]. In addition, a recent study failed to demonstrate any influence the mode of delivery on the natural history of disease [104]. General guidelines include a planned C-section for any woman with known perianal or rectal CD or if the birth appears to be more complicated than initially presumed.

Surgery and Pregnancy

In the pregnant IBD patient, elective surgical procedures are uncommon, but those that are performed in the second trimester do not appear to carry a significant increase in perinatal morality in female patients without IBD [105].

The indications for surgery during pregnancy are identical to that of nonpregnant patients. These include obstruction, perforation, abscess, and hemorrhage. The approach of continuing medical therapy may only further increase the risk to both mother and fetus. In the ill pregnant IBD patient, the greater risk to the child is continued maternal illness rather than surgical intervention [106]. In general, doing what is best for the mother results in what is ultimately best for the fetus.

Numerous case reports but only one small case series comprise the literature documenting successful surgical intervention for treatment of severe colitis in the pregnant patient. Anderson reported on the outcomes of four pregnant female patients who experience disease activity between the 28th and 37th week of gestation [107]. Three patients were treated medically and allowed to progress to labor. Two babies were stillborn and one child was healthy. All three mothers required colectomy in the weeks after delivery. The fourth patient relapsed at 28 weeks' gestation, had surgery for toxic megacolon at 31 weeks, and delivered at 34 weeks.

In patients with Crohn disease, Hill and colleagues described three pregnant patients with intraperitoneal sepsis, requiring surgery [108]. All three female patients recovered and delivered healthy infants. Most reports suggest proceeding to surgery when indicated. A variety of procedures have been performed, including proctocolectomy, subtotal colectomy with ileostomy, hemicolectomy or segmental resection, and combined subtotal colectomy and Cesarean section. Two general points should be made: (1) primary anastomosis carries a greater risk of postoperative complication rate, and thus a temporary ileostomy is generally preferred, and (2) if the fetus is significantly mature, then Cesarean section along with bowel resection is indicated.

In female patients who have a total proctocolectomy with ileal pouch-anal anastomosis (IPAA) prior to pregnancy, there is controversy regarding postoperative fertility and sexual function. An early study suggests that these are maintained [109], but most recent studies [110, 111] suggest a significant decrease in fertility following this type of surgery. The good news, however, is that there are new data to suggest that in vitro fertilization in these patients is successful [112].

There has been debate whether female patients who have had IPAA should be allowed to deliver vaginally or whether Cesarean section should be planned. In one study of 43 pregnancies in female patients' status post IPAA, pregnancy was well tolerated, with a complication rate lower than in female patients who had an ileostomy [113].

Although more Cesarean sections were performed in female patients with IPAA, the explanation was likely due to the uncertainty about the pouch function. An extended follow-up of female patients with an IPAA who delivered vaginally showed no adverse long-term effects on pouch function. During actual pregnancy, however, female patients with IPAA did note an increase in stool frequency, incontinence, and pad usage, with symptoms resolving after delivery. The authors suggest that the type of delivery in patients with an IPAA be dictated by obstetrical considerations. Other surgeons feel that the risk to permanent pouch failure is higher with a vaginal delivery and recommend any patient with surgery for UC undergo Cesarean section.

Pregnancy has not been shown to complicate stoma function. Female patients may experience some prolapse due to abdominal pressure, but no increased risk to the pregnancy is encountered.

Transition of Care

The time to transition care from a pediatric gastroenterologist to an adult gastroenterologist should be an individualized decision. Factors such as autonomy level, activity of disease, and transitioning in other phases of life all should be taken into account. When the adolescent patient becomes pregnant, there may be consideration of transitioning care to the adult provider, depending on the pediatric and adult gastroenterologist's experience and comfort level in dealing with pregnancy [114].

Summary Points

- Adolescents with IBD are at risk of pregnancy.
- Fertility is affected in postsurgical UC and in active CD.
- There is no increase in adverse outcomes with quiescent IBD.
- Active disease at conception increases the risk for adverse outcomes.
- The majority of medications for IBD are safe in pregnancy and breastfeeding—active disease is more deleterious than active therapy.

References

1. Peyrin-Biroulet L, Loftus Jr EV, Colombel JF, Sandborn WJ. Long-term complications, extraintestinal manifestations, and mortality in adult Crohn disease in population-based cohorts. Inflamm Bowel Dis. 2011;17(1):471–8.
2. Silverstein MD, Lashner BA, Hanauer SB, Evans AA, Kirsner JB. Cigarette smoking in Crohn disease. Am J Gastroenterol. 1989;84:31–3.
3. Suris JC, Resnick MD, Cassuto N, Blum RW. Sexual behavior of adolescents with chronic disease and disability. J Adolesc Health. 1996;19(2):124–31.
4. Newacheck P, Halfon N. Prevalence and impact of disabling chronic conditions in childhood. Am J Public Health. 1998;88:610–7.
5. Gittes EB, Strickland JL. Contraceptive choices for chronically Ill adolescents. Adolesc Med. 2005;16:635–44.
6. Gawron LM, Gawron AJ, Kasper A, Hammond C, Keefer L. Contraceptive method selection by women with inflammatory bowel diseases: a cross-sectional study. Contraception. 2014;89:419–25.
7. Wakeman J. Exacerbation of Crohn disease after insertion of a levonorgestrel intrauterine system: a case report. J Fam Plann Reprod Health Care. 2003;29(3):154.
8. Timmer A, Sutherland LR, Martin F. Oral contraceptive use and smoking are risk factors for relapse in Crohn disease. The Canadian Mesalamine for Remission of Crohn Disease Study Group. Gastroenterol. 1998;114(6):1143–50.
9. Cornish JA, Tan E, Simillis C, et al. The risk of oral contraceptives in the etiology of inflammatory bowel disease: a meta-analysis. Am J Gastroenterol. 2008;103(9):2394–400.
10. Cottone M, Camma C, Orlando A, et al. Oral contraceptive and recurrence in Crohn disease. Gastroenterol. 1999;116:A693.
11. Zapata LB, Paulen ME, Cansino C, Marchbanks PA, Curtis KM. Contraceptive use among women with inflammatory bowel disease: a systematic review. Contraception. 2010;82:72–85.
12. Gawron LM, Goldberger A, Gawron AJ, Hammond C, Keefer L. The impact of hormonal contraception on disease-related cyclical symptoms in women with inflammatory bowel diseases. Inflamm Bowel Dis. 2014;20:1729–33.
13. Coley RL, Chase-Lansdale PL. Adolescent pregnancy and parenthood: recent evidence and future direction. Am Psychol. 1998;53:152–66.
14. Mayberry JF, Weterman IT. European survey of fertility and pregnancy in women with Crohn disease: a case control study by European collaborative group. Gut. 1986;27:821–5.
15. Tiverneir N, Fumery M, Peyri-Biroulet L, Coumbel JF, Gower-Russen C. Systematic review: fertility in non-surgically treated inflammatory bowel disease. Aliment Pharmacol Thera. 2013;38:847–53.
16. Ban L, Tata LJ, Humes DJ, Fiaschi L, Card T. Decreased fertility rates in 639 women diagnosed with inflammatory bowel disease: a United Kingdom population-based cohort study. Aliment Pharmacol Ther. 2015;42(7):855–66.
17. Oza SS, Pabby V, Dodge LE, et al. In vitro fertilization in women with inflammatory bowel disease is as successful as in women from the general infertility population. Clin Gastroenterol Hepatol. 2015;13:1641–6.
18. Birnie GG, McLeod TI, Watkinson G. Incidence of sulphasalazine-induced male infertility. Gut. 1981;22:452–5.
19. Burnell D, Mayberry J, Calcraft BJ, Morris JS, Rhodes J. Male fertility in Crohn disease. Postgrad Med J. 1986;62:269–72.
20. Dejaco C, Mittemaier C, Reinisch W, et al. Azathioprine treatment and male fertility in inflammatory bowel disease. Gastroenterol. 2001;121:1048–53.
21. Nørgård B, Pedersen L, Jacobsen J, Rasmussen SN, Sørensen HT. The risk of congenital abnormalities in children fathered by men treated with azathioprine or mercaptopurine before conception. Aliment Pharmacol Ther. 2004;19(6):679–85.
22. Rajapakse RO, Korelitz BI, Zlatanic J, Baiocco PJ, Gleim GW. Outcome of pregnancies when fathers are treated with

6-mercaptopurine for inflammatory bowel disease. Am J Gastroenterol. 2000;95(3):684–8.

23. Banks B, Korelitz BI, Zetzel L. The course of non-specific ulcerative colitis: a review of twenty years of experience and late results. Gastroenterol. 1957;32:983–1012.

24. Miller JP. Inflammatory bowel disease in pregnancy: a review. J R Soc Med. 1986;79:221–5.

25. Willoughby CP, Truelove SC. Ulcerative colitis and pregnancy. Gut. 1980;21:469–74.

26. Fonager K, Sorensen HT, Olsen J, Dahlerup JF, Rasmussen SN. Pregnancy outcome for women with Crohn disease: a follow-up study based on linkage between national registries. Am J Gastroenterol. 1998;93:2426–30.

27. Moser MA, Okun NB, Mayes DC, Bailey RJ. Crohn disease, pregnancy, and birth weight. Am J Gastroenterol. 2000;95:1021–6.

28. Cornish J, Tan E, Teare J, et al. A meta-analysis on the influence of inflammatory bowel disease on pregnancy. Gut. 2007;56(6):830–7.

29. Porter RJ, Stirrat GM. The effects of inflammatory bowel disease on pregnancy: a case- controlled retrospective analysis. Br J Obstet Gynaecol. 1986;93:1124–31.

30. Broms G, Granath F, Linder M, Stephansson O, Elmberg M, Kieler H. Complications from inflammatory bowel disease during pregnancy and delivery. Clin Gastroenterol Hepatol. 2012;10:1246–52.

31. Kane SV, Hanauer SB, Kiesel J, Shih L, Tyan D. HLA disparity determines disease activity through pregnancy in women with IBD. Am J Gastroenterol. 2004;99(8):1523–6.

32. Nwokolo C, Tan WC, Andrews HA, Allan RN. Surgical resections in parous patients with distal ileal and colonic Crohn disease. Gut. 1994;35:220–3.

33. Riis L, Vind I, Politi P, et al. Does pregnancy change the disease course? A study in a European cohort of patients with inflammatory bowel disease. Am J Gastroenterol. 2006;101(7):1539–45.

34. Shoenut JP, Semelka RC, Silverman R, Yaffe CS, Micflikier AB. MRI in the diagnosis of Crohn disease in two pregnant women. J Clin Gastroenterol. 1993;17:244–7.

35. Brent RL. The effect of embryonic and fetal exposure to x-ray, microwaves, and ultrasound: counseling the pregnant and nonpregnant patient about these risks. Semin Oncol. 1989;16:347–68.

36. Cappell MS, Colon VJ, Sidhom OA. A study at 10 medical centers of the safety and efficacy of 48 flexible sigmoidoscopies and 8 colonoscopies during pregnancy with follow-up of fetal outcome and with comparison to control groups. Dig Dis Sci. 1996;41:2353–61.

37. Qureshi WA, Rajan E, Adler DG, et al. ASGE guideline: guidelines for endoscopy in pregnant and lactating women. Gastrointest Endosc. 2005;61(3):357–62.

38. Friedel D, Stavropoulos S, Iqbal S, Cappell MS. Gastrointestinal endoscopy in the pregnant woman. World J Gastrointest Endo. 2014;6:156–67.

39. Sachar D. Exposure to mesalamine during pregnancy increased preterm deliveries (but not birth defects) and decreased birth weight. Gut. 1998;43:316.

40. Warrell DW, Taylor R. Outcome for the foetus of mothers receiving prednisolone during pregnancy. Lancet. 1968;1:117–8.

41. Coelho J, Beaugerie L, Colombel JF. Pregnancy outcome in patients with inflammatory bowel disease treated with thiopurines: cohort from the CESAME Study. Gut. 2011;60(2):198–203.

42. Einarson A, Mastroiacovo P, Arnon J, et al. Prospective, controlled multicenter study of loperamide in pregnancy. Can J Gastroenterol. 2000;14:185–7.

43. Bonapace E, Fisher RS. Constipation and diarrhea in pregnancy. Gastroenterol Clin NA. 1998;27:197–211.

44. Briggs G, Freeman R, Yaffee S. Drugs in pregnancy and lactation: a reference guide to fetal and neonatal risk. New Jersey: Lippincott Williams & Wilkins; 2008.

45. Hanauer SB, Present DH. The state of the art in the management of inflammatory bowel disease. Rev Gastroenterol Disord. 2003;3:81–92.

46. Esbjorner E, Jarnerot G, Wranne L. Sulphasalazine and sulphapyridine levels in children to mothers treated with sulphasalazine during pregnancy and lactation. Acta Paediart Sand. 1987;76:137–42.

47. Moody GA, Probert C, Jayanthi V, Mayberry JF. The effects of chronic ill health and treatment with sulphasalazine on fertility amongst men and female patients with inflammatory bowel disease in Leicestershire. Int J Color Dis. 1997;12:220–4.

48. Hernandez-Diaz S, Werler MM, Mitchell AA, et al. Folic acid antagonists during pregnancy and the risk of birth defects. N Engl J Med. 2000;343:1608–14.

49. Rahimi R, Nikfar S, Rezaie A, Abdollahi M. Pregnancy outcome in women with inflammatory bowel disease following exposure to 5-aminosalicylic acid drugs: a meta-analysis. Reprod Toxicol. 2008;25(2):271–5.

50. Colombel JF, Brabant G, Gubler MC, et al. Renal insufficiency in infant: side-effect of prenatal exposure to mesalazine? [letter] [see comments]. Lancet. 1994;344:620–1.

51. Hernández-Díaz S, Mitchell AA, Kelley KE, Calafat AM, Hauser R. Medications as a potential source of exposure to phthalates in the U.S. population. Environ Health Perspect. 2009;117(2):185–9.

52. Diav-Citrin O, Shechtman S, Ornoy A, et al. Pregnancy outcome after gestational exposure to metronidazole: a prospective controlled cohort study. Teratology. 2001;63:186–92.

53. Piper JM, Mitchel EF, Ray WA. Prenatal use of metronidazole and birth defects: no association. Obstet Gynecol. 1993;82:348–52.

54. Linseman DA, Hampton LA, Branstetter DG. Quinolone-induced arthropathy in the neonatal mouse. Morphological analysis of articular lesions produced by pipemidic acid and ciprofloxacin. Fundam Appl Toxicol. 1995;28:59–64.

55. Moskovitz DN, Bodian C, Chapman ML, et al. The effect on the fetus of medications used to treat pregnant inflammatory bowel-disease patients. Am J Gastroenterol. 2004;99:656–61.

56. Loebstein R, Addis A, HO E, et al. Pregnancy outcome following gestational exposure to fluoroquinolones: a multicenter prospective controlled study. Antimicrob Agents Chemother. 1998;42:1336–9.

57. Beitins IZ, Bayard F, Migeon CJ, et al. The transplacental passage of prednisone and prednisolone in pregnancy near term. J Pediatr. 1972;81:936–45.

58. Mogadam M, Korelitz BI, Ahmed SW, Dobbins WD, Baiocco PJ. The course of inflammatory bowel disease during pregnancy and postpartum. Am J Gastroenterol. 1981;75:265–9.

59. Armenti V, Ahlswede KM, Ahlswede RA, et al. National transplant pregnancy registry-outcomes of 154 pregnancies in cyclosporine-treated female kidney transplant recipients. Transplantation. 1994;57(4):502–6.

60. Ramsey-Goldman RSE. Immunosuppressive drug use during pregnancy. Rheum Clin NA. 1997;23:149–67.

61. Saarikoski S, Seppala M. Immunosuppression during pregnancy: transmission of azathioprine and its metabolites from the mother to the fetus. Am J Obstet Gynecol. 1973;115:1100–6.

62. Dubinsky MC. Azathioprine, 6-mercaptopurine in inflammatory bowel disease: pharmacology, efficacy, and safety. Clin Gastroenterol Hepatol. 2004;2:731–43.

63. Matalon ST, Ornoy A, Lishner M. Review of the potential effects of three commonly used antineoplastic and immunosuppressive drugs. (cyclophosphamide, azathioprine, doxorubicin on the embryo and placenta). Reprod Toxicol. 2004;18:219–30.

64. Francella A, Dyan A, Present DH, et al. The safety of 6-mercaptopurine for childbearing patients with inflammatory bowel disease: a retrospective cohort study. Gastroenterology. 2003;124:9–17.

65. Norgard B, Pedersen L, Sorensen HT, et al. Azathioprine, mercaptopurine and birth outcome: a population-based cohort study. Aliment Pharmacol Ther. 2003;17:827–34.

66. Goldenberg M, Bider D, Oelsner G, et al. Methotrexate therapy of tubal pregnancy. Hum Reprod. 1993;8:660–6.

67. Gromnica-Ihle E, Kruger K. Use of methotrexate in young patients with regard to the reproductive system. Clin Exp Rheum. 2010;28:S80–4.

68. Katz JA, Antoni C, Lichenstein GR, et al. Outcome of pregnancy in female patients receiving infliximab for the treatment of Crohn disease and rheumatoid arthritis. Am J Gastroenterol. 2004;99:2385–92.

69. Kane SV, Acquah LA, Mahadevan U, Cucchiara S, Hyams JS, et al. The London position statement of the world congress of gastroenterology on biological therapy for IBD with the European Crohn and Colitis Organisation: pregnancy and pediatrics. Am J Gastroenterol. 2011;106(2):214–23.

70. Seirafi M, de Vroey B, Amiot A, et al. Factors associated with pregnancy outcome in anti-TNF treated women with inflammatory bowel disease. Aliment Pharmacol Thera. 2014;40:363–73.

71. Mahadevan U, Wolf DC, Dubinsky MC, et al. Placental transfer of anti tumor necrosis factor agents in pregnant patients with inflammatory bowel disease. Clin Gastroenterol Hepatol. 2013;11:286–92.

72. Pasut G. Pegylation of biological molecules and potential benefits: pharmacologic properties of certolizumab pegol. BioDrugs. 2014;28:S15–30.

73. Zelenkova Z, van der Ent C, Bruin KF, et al. Effects of discontinuing anti tumor necrosis factor therapy during pregnancy on the course of inflammatory bowel disease and neonatal exposure. Clin Gastroenterol Hepatol. 2013;11:318–21.

74. Hellwig K, Haghikia A, Gold R. Pregnancy and natalizumab: results of an observational study in 35 accidental pregnancies during natalizumab treatment. Mult Scler. 2011;17(8):958–63.

75. Vedolizumab Prescribing Information. 2014 Takeda. Accessed at www.entyvio.com on Dec 30, 2016.

76. Motta M, Ciardelli L, Marconi M, et al. Immune system development in infants born to mothers with autoimmune disease, exposed in utero to immunosuppressive agents. Am J Perinatol. 2007;24(8):441–7.

77. Khan HA. Cyclosporin-A augments respiratory burst of whole blood phagocytes in pregnant rats. Immunopharmacol Immunotoxicol. 2007;29(3–4):367–74.

78. Ramsey-Goldman R, Schilling E. Immunosuppressive drug use during pregnancy. Rheum Dis Clin N Am. 1997;23:149–67.

79. Bertschinger P, Himmelmann A, Follath F, et al. Cyclosporine treatment of severe ulcerative colitis during pregnancy. Am J Gastroenterol. 1995;90:330.

80. Kornbluth A, Reddy D. Management and outcome of severe colitis in pregnancy. Am J Gastroenterol. 2002;97:P705.

81. Ehrenpreis ED, Kane SV, Cohen LB, Cohen RD, Hanauer SB. Thalidomide therapy for patients with refractory Crohn disease: an open-label trial. Gastroenterol. 1999;117:1271–7.

82. Vasiliauskas EA, Kam LY, Abreu-Martin MT, et al. An open-label pilot study of low-dose thalidomide in chronically active, steroid-dependent Crohn disease. Gastroenterology. 1999;117:1278–87.

83. Sandborn WJ. Preliminary report on the use of oral tacrolimus (FK506) in the treatment of complicated proximal small bowel and fistulizing Crohn disease. Am J Gastroenterol. 1997;92:876–9.

84. Neurath MF, Wanitschke R, Peters M. Randomized trial of mycophenolate versus azathioprine for treatment of chronic active Crohn disease. Gut. 1999;44:625–8.

85. Kainz A, Harabacz I, Cowlrick IS, Gadgil S, Hagiwara D. Analysis of 100 pregnancy outcomes in female patients treated systemically with tacrolimus. Transpl Int. 2000;13:S299–300.

86. Jacobson L, Clapp DH. Total parenteral nutrition in pregnancy complicated by Crohn disease. JPEN. 1987;11:93–6.

87. Nugent F, Rajala M, O'Shea RA, et al. Total parenteral nutrition in pregnancy: conception to delivery. JPEN. 1987;11:424–7.

88. Park YK, Meier ER, Song WO. Characteristics of teenage mothers and predictors of breastfeeding initiation in the Michigan WIC Program in 1995. Women, infants, and children. J Hum Lact. 2003;19:50–6.

89. Kane S, Lemieux N. The role of breastfeeding in postpartum disease activity in women with inflammatory bowel disease. Am J Gastroenterol. 2005;100(1):102–5.

90. Moffatt DC, Ilnyckyj A, Bernstein CN. A population-based study of breastfeeding in inflammatory bowel disease: initiation, duration, and effect on disease in the postpartum period. Am J Gastroenterol. 2009;104(10):2517–23.

91. Klotz U, Harings-Kaim A. Negligible excretion of 5-aminosalicylic acid in breast milk. Lancet. 1993;342:618–9.

92. Nelis GF. Diarrhoea due to 5-aminosaliyclic acid in breast milk. Lancet. 1989;1:383.

93. Christensen LA. 5-Aminosalicylic acid containing drugs. Delivery, fate, and possible clinical implications in man. Dan Med Bull. 2000;47(1):20–41.

94. Christensen LA, Dahlerup JF, Nielsen MJ, Fallingborg JF, Schmiegelow K. Azathioprine treatment during lactation. Aliment Pharmacol Ther. 2008;28(10):1209–13.

95. Nyberg G, Haljamae U, Kjemeller I, et al. Breast-feeding during treatment with cyclosporine. Transplantation. 1998;65:253–5.

96. Munoz-Flores-Thiagarajan KD, Easterling T, Bond EF, et al. Breast-feeding by a cyclosporine-treated mother. Obstet Gynecol. 2001;97:816–8.

97. Ost L, Wettrell G, Rane A, et al. Prednisolone excretion in human milk. J Pediatr. 1985;106:1008–11.

98. Kane S. Breastfeeding and IBD: safety and management issues. Inflamm Bowel Dis Monit. 2004;6:50–2.

99. Kane S, Ford J, Cohen R, Wagner C. Absence of infliximab in infants and breast milk from nursing mothers receiving therapy for Crohn disease before and after delivery. J Clin Gastroenterol. 2009;43(7):613–6.

100. Ben Horin S, Yavzori M, Katz L, et al. Adalimumab level in breast milk of a nursing mother. Clin Gastroenterol Hepatol. 2010;8:475–6.

101. Gibert WM, Jandial D, Field NT, et al. Birth outcomes in teenage pregnancies. J Matern Fetal Neonatal Med. 2004;16:265–70.

102. Ilnyckyj A, Blanchard JF, Rawsthorne P, Bernstein CN. Perianal Crohn disease and pregnancy: role of the mode of delivery. Am J Gastroenterol. 1999;94:3274–8.

103. Cheng A, Oxford EC, Sauk J, et al. Impact of mode of delivery on outcomes in patients with perianal Crohn disease. Inflamm Bowel Dis. 2014;20:1391–8.

104. Ananthakrishnan A, Cheng A, Cagan A, et al. Mode of childbirth and long-term outcomes in women with inflammatory bowel diseases. Dig Dis Sci. 2015;60:471–7.

105. Levine W, Diamond B. Surgical procedures during pregnancy. Am J Obstet Gynecol. 1961;81:1046–52.

106. Kelly M, Hunt TM, Wicks ACB, et al. Fulminant ulcerative colitis and parturition: a need to alter current management? Br J Obstet Gnecol. 1994;101:166–7.

107. Anderson JB, Turner GM, Williamson RC. Fulminant ulcerative colitis in late pregnancy and the puerperium. J R Soc Med. 1987;80:492–4.

108. Hill J, Clark A, Scott NA. Surgical treatment of acute manifestations of Crohn disease during pregnancy. J R Soc Med. 1997;90:64–6.

109. Metcalf A, Dozois RR, Baert RW, et al. Pregnancy following ileal pouch-anal anastomosis. Dis Colon Rectum. 1985;28:859–61.
110. Olsen KOJS, Berndtsson I, Oresland T, Laurberg S. Ulcerative colitis: female fecundity before diagnosis, during disease, and after surgery compared with a population sample. Gastroenterol. 2002;122:15–9.
111. Waljee A, Waljee J, Morris AM, Higgins PD. Threefold increased risk of infertility: a meta-analysis of infertility after ileal pouch anal anastomosis in ulcerative colitis. Gut. 2006;55(11): 1575–80.
112. Pabby V, Oza SS, Dodge LE, et al. In vitro fertilization is successful in women with ulcerative colitis and ileal pouch anal anastomosis. Am J Gastroenterol. 2015;110:792–7.
113. Juhasz ES, Fozard B, Dozois RR, Ilstrup DM, Nelson H. Ileal pouch-anal anastomosis function following childbirth. An extended evaluation. Dis Colon Rectum. 1995;38:159–65.
114. Baldassano R, Ferry G, Griffiths A. Transition of the patient with inflammatory bowel disease from pediatric to adult care: recommendations of the North American Society for Pediatric Gastroenterology. Hepatol Nutr. 2002;34:245–8.

Immunizations in the Child with Inflammatory Bowel Disease

54

Athos Bousvaros and Ying Lu

Introduction

The vast majority of children and young adults with inflammatory bowel disease (IBD) will undergo treatment with immunosuppressive medications at some point during their lives. Such treatment may be short-lived (e.g., a brief course of corticosteroids during a colitis flare) or prolonged (e.g., combination therapy for immunomodulators and infliximab for moderate to severe Crohn disease) [1]. Treatment with immunomodulators or biologics increases the risk of opportunistic infections such as herpes zoster [2, 3], Epstein-Barr virus [4], or cytomegalovirus [5]. Some of these illnesses (especially influenza, pneumonia, and varicella) are potentially preventable by the judicious use of vaccines. While the ideal time to immunize patients with IBD is prior to the onset of any immunosuppression, for many patients, delaying treatment to "catch up on immunizations" is not possible. Papers in both adults and children have emphasized the safety of inactivated vaccines in immunocompromised IBD patients [6–8]. Most such papers also suggest withholding live vaccines in this population, despite a paucity of data on this topic [7]. The Infectious Diseases Society of America has also prepared a guideline on vaccination of the immunocompromised host which provides in-depth recommendations and also areas highly in need of future research [9].

A. Bousvaros, MD, MPH (✉)
IBD Center, Children's Hospital Boston, Boston, MA 02115, USA
e-mail: Athos.bousvaros@childrens.harvard.edu

Y. Lu, MD
Division of Pediatric Gastroenterology, Cohen Children's Medical Center of New York, 1991 Marcus Ave, M100, Lake Success, NY 11042, USA
e-mail: ylu@northwell.edu

Underimmunization

One survey of 108 adult gastroenterologists identified that the majority of adult gastroenterologists felt it was the responsibility of the primary care physician (PCP) to decide which vaccinations to give (64%) and to administer the vaccines (83%). About half of adult gastroenterologists inquired their IBD patients about vaccination history most or all of the time, citing "too busy/forgot" as the most common reason for not regularly recommending an immunization [10]. In another survey of 178 pediatric gastroenterologists, only 28% believed that PCP was solely responsible for immunizations. In contrast to their adult colleagues, the vast majority (94%) of pediatric gastroenterologists routinely assessed immunization status. Specifically, 63.5% assess at time of diagnosis, 30% at "well" visits, and 44% before starting immunosuppressive therapy. Vaccines most commonly assessed were influenza, hepatitis B, and varicella. Physicians were more likely to review immunizations if they implemented a reminder mechanism. The most common barriers to vaccination included inability to offer vaccinations in the immediate area, lack of coordination of care with PCP, and poor access to immunization records [11].

The authors of this chapter feel strongly that the pediatric subspecialist shares responsibility with the PCP in making sure their immunocompromised children are protected against vaccine-preventable diseases such as influenza. Children with IBD often have more frequent visits to their specialist than to their general pediatrician and look to the specialist to assess benefits and risks of various interventions (including immunization). The GI specialist therefore has an important role in educating patients about vaccines and in making sure that the appropriate vaccines are administered (either by the pediatrician or specialist) at the appropriate times.

The immunization rate for routine primary vaccines varies greatly among children with IBD around the world, ranging from 24% in France [12] to 90% in Canada [13]

P. Mamula et al. (eds.), *Pediatric Inflammatory Bowel Disease*, DOI 10.1007/978-3-319-49215-5_54

and Australia [14]. However, vaccination rates for influenza (8–30%) [12, 14, 15] and pneumococcus (5–32%) [12, 14] tend to be low. Factors contributing to low influenza vaccination rate include concerns that the vaccine will be ineffective, fear that patients will experience an adverse effect of the vaccine, concerns that the vaccine may cause a flare of their disease, and that the vaccine was not offered to patient [12, 15, 16]. These concerns have recently been addressed by several pediatric studies that demonstrate inactivated vaccines are generally safe and effective in children with IBD. Therefore, methods to increase vaccination rates include educating patients [17] and PCPs [11], coordinating care among the gastroenterologist, PCP, and patient, and utilizing a reminder system (by having a checklist or inclusion in electronic record template) [11].

Who and When to Immunize?

The Committee on Infectious Diseases of the American Academy of Pediatrics published an updated immunization schedule, summarized in Table 54.1. It is generally recommended by experts in the field that inactivated vaccines be given as per the recommended schedule to patients with IBD [9, 18]. There is a theoretical risk of viral dissemination with live vaccines in patients who are receiving "significant immunosuppression." Fortunately, IBD is rare in the child under 5 years, so that the majority of live vaccines [including measles/mumps/rubella (MMR), varicella] will be completed before the onset of the disease and before the onset of immunosuppressive therapy.

Patients receiving aminosalicylates as monotherapy are not considered immunosuppressed. These patients may receive all immunizations as recommended in Table 54.1. Patients considered "significantly immunosuppressed" include those who are severely malnourished or receiving high-dose steroids ($\geq$20 mg a day, or $\geq$2 mg/kg/day, for at least 14 days), thiopurines, methotrexate, cyclosporine, tacrolimus, and antitumor necrosis factor therapy. For this group of patients, live vaccines are generally not recommended [6, 7, 9]. Therefore, it is ideal to immunize prior to starting immunosuppressive therapy, especially with live vaccines. If the patient is clinically stable enough to start immunosuppressive therapy at a later time, then it is ideal to wait at least 4 weeks after varicella vaccination, and at least 6 weeks after MMR vaccination, to initiate therapy. If the patient will be taken off immunomodulators or biologics, it is recommended to wait at least 3 months prior to administering live vaccines; and for corticosteroids, at least 1 month [6, 7].

Inactivated Vaccines in Children with IBD

In general, a useful rule is that inactivated vaccines can be administered safely to IBD patients, irrespective of the degree of immunosuppression. However, patients on higher doses of immunosuppression (especially those receiving biologics) may not mount the same degree of antibody response to vaccines as patients on less immunosuppression. The best studied vaccine in children with IBD is the trivalent influenza vaccine, which is both safe and immunogenic in children and young adults. This vaccine is usually administered in the fall and protects against three strains of influenza. The trivalent influenza vaccine has generated protection against two strains of influenza A and one strain of influenza B. (In recent years, the quadrivalent influenza vaccine was developed which included a second strain of influenza B.) Three prospective studies have demonstrated that the trivalent influenza vaccine is usually well tolerated in children with IBD, including those receiving immunosuppressive therapy. However, immunogenicity may be reduced, especially in patients receiving biologic therapy. Mamula et al. performed a prospective study using the 2002–2004 vaccine, in which 51 children with IBD and 29 healthy children were immunized. Compared to the healthy controls, children with IBD receiving combination therapy (with immunomodulators and biologics) were less likely to respond to two of the three strains in the influenza vaccine [20]. In contrast, Lu et al. demonstrated a good response to the 2007–2008 influenza vaccine and a high prevalence of seroprotection to both of the influenza A strains in the vaccine. The less immunogenic influenza B strain, however, resulted in a decreased rate of seroprotection in patients receiving anti-TNF therapy [21]. DeBruyn and colleagues again demonstrated excellent safety and good response to the two A strains in the vaccine, but decreased immune response to the B strain [22]. A more recent study by deBruyn of 137 children with IBD receiving maintenance infliximab therapy demonstrated that timing of vaccination relative to infliximab infusion (immunization at time of infliximab versus midway between infusions) did not impact serological protection [23]. None of these studies demonstrated any increase in adverse events or increase in IBD flares. In summary, data from influenza vaccine studies in pediatric IBD support the recommendation that children with IBD receive annual influenza immunizations. Even patients on immunosuppressive therapies respond well to the two A strains in the vaccine, though antibody titers to the B strain may be reduced.

Hepatitis B vaccination has also been studied in children with IBD. Patients with latent hepatitis B who are treated with anti-tumor necrosis factor inhibitors are at risk for viral reactivation leading to severe viral hepatitis or even liver failure [24, 25]. Urganci et al. administered the hepatitis B

Table 54.1 Summary of immunization recommendations from the AAP Committee on Immunizations [18] and Centers for Disease Control and Prevention [19]

Immunization	Type	Route of administration	Patient age at time of recommended administration
Hepatitis B	Inactivated	Parenteral	0–1 year (three doses)
Diphtheria and tetanus toxoids and acellular pertussis	Inactivated	Parenteral	2–6 months (three doses) 15–18 months (one dose) 4–6 years (one dose)
Tetanus and diphtheria toxoids and acellular pertussis	Inactivated	Parenteral	11–12 years (one dose)
Haemophilus influenzae type b	Inactivated	Parenteral	2–6 months (three doses) 12–15 months (one dose)
Pneumococcal	Inactivated	Parenteral	2–6 months (PCV vaccine, three doses) 12–15 months (PCV vaccine, one dose) 2–18 years (in immunocompromised patients, PCV and/or PPSV depending on prior pneumococcal vaccinations, revaccinate with one dose of PPSV 5 years after first dose of PPSV)
Inactivated poliovirus	Inactivated	Parenteral	2–18 months (three doses) 4–6 years (one dose)
Influenza injection	Inactivated	Parenteral	6 months, then annually Younger than 9 years, two doses if not previously received two doses of tri- or quadrivalent influenza vaccine
Hepatitis A	Inactivated	Parenteral	1–2 years (two doses)
Meningococcal	Inactivated	Parenteral	11–12 years (first dose) 16 years (booster) 9 months and older if persistent complement deficiency
Human papillomavirus	Inactivated	Parenteral	11–12 years (three doses)
Influenza intranasal	Live attenuated	Intranasal	2 years, then annually
Rotavirus	Live attenuated	Oral	2–6 months (three doses)
Measles, mumps, rubella	Live attenuated	Parenteral	12–15 months (one dose) 4–6 years (one dose) 11–18 years (consider booster)
Varicella	Live attenuated	Parenteral	12–15 months (one dose) 4–6 years (booster)

vaccine series to children with IBD who were not previously vaccinated. Seroconversion was achieved in 70% of IBD patients compared to 90% of healthy controls ($p = 0.02$). Of children who did not achieve seroconversion, a subsequent booster dose resulted in an adequate response in 50% (7/14) of IBD patients and 60% (3/5, p = NS) of controls. There were no vaccine-associated adverse events [26]. Moses and colleagues conducted a prospective study of hepatitis B status in their pediatric IBD population on infliximab therapy and documented that 13% had never been immunized against hepatitis B and that approximately half of patients who were previously immunized did not have protective levels of anti-HBs. The investigators then administered a booster vaccine to 34 of these patients without protective titers and noted a 76% response rate. Children and young adults receiving infliximab more frequently (approximately every 5.9 weeks) were less likely to respond to the booster dose of hepatitis B [27]. In the adult IBD literature, Gisbert and colleagues found that therapy with anti-TNF was asso-

ciated with a suboptimal vaccine response, but not with immunomodulators [28]. In another study, Gisbert et al evaluated two types of hepatitis B vaccination schedules in 148 adult IBD patients with negative hepatitis B antibodies. Seventy percent of the subjects received immunosuppressive therapy (22% thiopurines, 23% anti-TNF, and 25% both). One group (46%) received the standard vaccination protocol (single dose at 0, 1 and 6 months) and other group (54%) received the double dose protocol (double dose at 0, 1 and 2 months). Anti-HBs titers were drawn 1-3 months after the last dose. The double dose group had a higher seroconversion rate (defined as anti-HBs >10 IU/L) compared to the standard dose group (75% vs 41%, $p<0.001$) [29].

Studies evaluating the immunogenicity of hepatitis A vaccine suggest that both children and adult IBD patients mount an excellent response (97–100%) after receiving two doses [26, 30, 31]. However, the rate of seroconversion was lower in adult patients on anti-TNF therapy compared to those who were not on anti-TNF therapy (92.4% vs 99.1%,

$p = 0.001$) and in patients treated with ≥ 2 immunosuppressants compared to those on <2 immunosuppressants (92.6% vs 98.4%, $p = 0.03$). There was no difference in rate of seroconversion between patients on TNF inhibitor monotherapy and those on TNF inhibitor combined with another immunosuppressant [31]. The vaccine was safe and did not exacerbate IBD [26, 30].

The theme of suboptimal immunogenicity associated with TNF inhibitor therapy extends to pneumococcal vaccine as well. Several studies within the adult IBD literature agree that the immune response to 23-valent pneumococcal polysaccharide vaccine (PPSV23) is decreased in patients receiving TNF inhibitor therapy (either as monotherapy or in combination with immunomodulators, 45–63%) compared to patients not receiving immunosuppressive therapy (78–89%) and to healthy controls (85%) [32–34]. Immunomodulator monotherapy was not associated with a hindered immune response (79%). One pediatric study immunized IBD patients aged 5–18 years with no history of pneumococcal immunization with one dose of pneumococcal conjugate vaccine (PCV13). Immunogenicity was similar between IBD patients and healthy controls (90.4% vs 96.5%, p = NS). However, the geometric mean titer was higher in patients who were not on immunosuppressive therapy compared to those who were treated with TNF inhibitors or immunomodulators [35]. The vaccine was well tolerated without serious adverse events [32, 34, 35].

In contrast, the immunogenicity of human papillomavirus vaccine (HPV) does not appear to be diminished by immunosuppressive therapy. Jacobson and colleagues administered three doses of Gardasil to girls and young women aged 9–26 years while being treated with immunomodulator or TNF inhibitor therapy for IBD. All patients developed an excellent immune response with 96–100% seropositivity to HPV types 6, 11, 16, and 18. The geometric mean titers for each serotype were similar to those of healthy historical female controls from Merck. The IBD patients did not experience serious adverse events or worsened disease activity related to the vaccine [36]. Similarly, immunosuppressive therapy does not hinder the immune response to *Haemophilus influenzae* type b vaccine. A smaller study by Dotan and colleagues concluded that thiopurine monotherapy generally does not impair the cellular or humoral response to the vaccine in adults with IBD [37].

Immunizing the Child with IBD: Practical Aspects

When a child is newly diagnosed with IBD, the ideal time to immunize is before the start of any immunosuppressive therapy. However, as many children with IBD are acutely ill, treatment can often not be withheld. Thus, the clinician is often caught between the "rock and the hard place": should the patient be immunized and treatment postponed, or should treatment be instituted with plans to immunize at a later time? Making these decisions involves a careful assessment of the risk/benefit ratio and an informed discussion with the parents.

For patients with mild to moderate ulcerative colitis who are undergoing corticosteroid induction, but in whom maintenance therapy with aminosalicylates is planned, immunizations can usually be postponed until after an initial course of corticosteroids. Once corticosteroids are weaned, and aminosalicylate therapy is started, both inactivated and live vaccines can be given. There is no consensus on how long corticosteroids need to be stopped before immunizations are given, but expert opinion suggests that 4 weeks after discontinuation of steroids is probably safe [6, 9].

More problematic is the child with moderate to severe Crohn disease or UC, who may require corticosteroid treatment and subsequent immunosuppression with thiopurines, antibody to tumor necrosis factor, or calcineurin inhibitor. In these children, obtaining immunization records from the primary care pediatrician and assessing whether the recommended immunization series have been administered are important. If children received their recommended MMR and varicella immunizations in childhood, they are probably at low risk of contracting these illnesses. Obtaining individual serum titers to measles and varicella virus may also be helpful in documenting immunity. One area of ongoing controversy is whether varicella vaccine can be safely administered to some children on immunomodulators. The American Committee on Immunization Practices does allow for the administration of zoster vaccine (which is more potent than varicella vaccine) to adults on low-dose thiopurines and methotrexate [38]. Our group published a case series of six children with IBD on 6MP or infliximab therapy who had received varicella vaccine (either inadvertently by their primary care physician or deliberately after discussion of risks and benefits), and all experienced no adverse effects. Five of the six children developed an immune response [39]. Ansari et al. vaccinated ten pediatric IBD patients with a negative or unknown varicella titer prior to starting immunosuppressive therapy. Postvaccination antibody levels were obtained in eight of these ten patients, and all eight responded [40]. Thus, in the rare situation where there is a high prevalence of wild-type varicella, the benefits of protection against the wild-type virus might outweigh the risk of the immunization. Clearly, more data are needed in this very understudied area.

Another question that frequently comes up in these patients is whether family members can receive their routine live vaccines. Once again, there is a paucity of data. Expert opinion suggests that family members can receive live vaccines (including measles, varicella, or zoster vaccine) except the oral polio vaccine, even if there is an immunosuppressed patient with IBD in the house. However, if a vaccine-associated rash develops in the affected family member, they should avoid close contact with the patient until lesions clear [9].

Women with IBD of childbearing age are often receiving immunomodulators and biologics to keep their disease in remission throughout pregnancy. Infliximab, if given in the third trimester, can pass transplacentally and enter the fetus's bloodstream. Therefore, there is the potential for infants born to women with IBD to have a reduced response to inactivated vaccines and to be at risk for complications of live vaccines. However, in a recent small study, immunoglobulin levels (IgG, IgM, and IgA) and antibodies to tetanus toxoid and *Haemophilus influenzae* type b (Hib) were drawn in infants at least 6 months old of age and born to mothers who received at least one dose of infliximab or adalimumab during the third trimester. The study found that all infants had adequate immunoglobulin levels other than IgM, which was low in half. The vast majority (92%) mounted an adequate response to both tetanus and Hib vaccines [41]. Again, this area requires further study.

Summary

Immunizations that can be given safely and should be given to children with IBD as part of the recommended immunization schedule include diphtheria and tetanus boosters, influenza, pneumococcal, meningococcal, human papillomavirus, hepatitis A, and hepatitis B. In general, the less immunosuppression a patient is receiving, the more likely they are to mount an effective immune response. Live vaccines, including measles virus and intranasal influenza vaccine, should not be given. Varicella live attenuated vaccine has been given without complication to some patients on mild immunosuppression, but is generally not recommended. Therefore, providers should ideally inquire about immunization status at time of diagnosis and vaccinate if necessary prior to starting immunosuppressive therapy, especially in the case of live vaccines. Both primary care physicians and patients need additional education on the safety and efficacy of inactivated vaccines.

References

1. Rufo PA, Bousvaros A. Current therapy of inflammatory bowel disease in children. Paediatr Drugs. 2006;8:279–302.
2. Wang X, Zhao J, Zhu S, Xia B. Herpes zoster in Crohn's disease during treatment with infliximab. Eur J Gastroenterol Hepatol. 2014;26:237–9.
3. Ma C, Walters B, Fedorak R. Varicella zoster meningitis complicating combined anti-tumor necrosis factor and corticosteroid therapy in Crohn's disease. World J Gastroenterol. 2013;19:3347–51.
4. Magro F, Santos-Antunes J, Albuquerque A, Vilas-Boas F, Macedo GN, Nazareth N, et al. Epstein-Barr virus in inflammatory bowel disease - correlation with different therapeutic regimens. Inflamm Bowel Dis. 2013;19:1710–6.
5. Sager K, Alam S, Bond A, Chinnappan L, Probert CS. Review article: cytomegalovirus and inflammatory bowel disease. Aliment Pharmacol Ther. 2015;41:725–33.
6. Wasan SK, Baker SE, Skolnik PR, Farraye FA. A practical guide to vaccinating the inflammatory bowel disease patient. Am J Gastroenterol. 2010;105:1231–8.
7. Sands BE, Cuffari C, Katz J, Kugathasan S, Onken J, Vitek C, et al. Guidelines for immunizations in patients with inflammatory bowel disease. Inflamm Bowel Dis. 2004;10:677–92.
8. Lu Y, Jacobson D, Bousvaros A. Immunizations in patients with inflammatory bowel disease. Inflamm Bowel Dis. 2009a;15:1417–23.
9. The Infectious Diseases Society of America: 2013 IDSA Clinical Practice Guideline for Vaccination of the immunocompromised host. http://cid.oxfordjournals.org/content/early/2013/11/26/cid.cit684.full. 2013. Accessed 18 Jan 2016.
10. Wasan SK, Coukos JA, Farraye FA. Vaccinating the inflammatory bowel disease patient: deficiencies in gastroenterologists knowledge. Inflamm Bowel Dis. 2011;17:2536–40.
11. Lester R, Lu Y, Tung J. Survey of immunization practices in patients with inflammatory bowel disease among pediatric gastroenterologists. J Pediatr Gastroenterol Nutr. 2015;61:47–51.
12. Longuet R, Willot S, Giniès J-L, Pélatan C, Breton E, Segura J-F, et al. Immunization status in children with inflammatory bowel disease. Eur J Pediatr. 2014;173:603–8.
13. Soon IS, deBruyn JCC, Wrobel I. Immunization history of children with inflammatory bowel disease. Can J Gastroenterol. 2013;27:213–6.
14. Crawford NW, Catto-Smith AG, Oliver MR, Cameron DJ, Buttery JP. An Australian audit of vaccination status in children and adolescents with inflammatory bowel disease. BMC Gastroenterol. 2011;11:87.
15. Peleg N, Zevit N, Shamir R, Chodick G, Levy I. Seasonal influenza vaccination rates and reasons for non-vaccination in children with gastrointestinal disorders. Vaccine. 2015;33:182–6.
16. Banaszkiewicz A, Klincewicz B, Łazowska-Przeorek I, Grzybowska-Chlebowcyzk U, Kąkol P, Mytyk A, et al. Influenza vaccination coverage in children with inflammatory bowel disease. Influenza and Other Respiratory Viruses. 2014;8:431–5.
17. Huth K, Benchimol EI, Aglipay M, Mack DR. Strategies to improve influenza vaccination in pediatric inflammatory bowel disease through education and access. Inflamm Bowel Dis. 2015;21;1761–8.
18. Committee on infectious diseases. Committee on Infectious Diseases. Recommended childhood and adolescent immunization schedules–United States. Pediatrics. 2012;129:385–6.
19. Centers for Disease Control and Prevention: Recommended immunization schedule for persons aged 0 through 18 years. http://www.cdc.gov/vaccines/schedules/hcp/imz/child-adolescent.html. 2015. Accessed 18 Jan 2016.
20. Mamula P, Markowitz JE, Piccoli DA, Klimov A, Cohen L, Baldassano RN. Immune response to influenza vaccine in pediatric patients with inflammatory bowel disease. Clin Gastroenterol Hepatol. 2007;5:851–6.
21. Lu Y, Jacobson DL, Ashworth LA, Grand RJ, Meyer AL, McNeal MM, et al. Immune response to influenza vaccine in children with inflammatory bowel disease. Am J Gastroenterol. 2009b;104:444–53.
22. de Bruyn JC, Hilsden R, Fonseca K, Russell ML, Kaplan GG, Vanderkooi O, et al. Immunogenicity and safety of influenza vaccination in children with inflammatory bowel disease. Inflamm Bowel Dis. 2012;18:25–33.

23. de Bruyn J, Fonseca K, Ghosh S, Panaccione R, Gasia MF, Ueno A, et al. Immunogenicity of influenza vaccine for patients with inflammatory bowel disease on maintenance infliximab therapy: a randomized trial. Inflamm Bowel Dis. 2015; doi:10.1097/MIB. 0000000000000615.

24. Zeitz J, Mullhaupt B, Fruehauf H, Rogler G, Vavricka SR. Hepatic failure due to hepatitis B reactivation in a patient with ulcerative colitis treated with prednisone. Hepatol. 2009;50:653–4.

25. Ojiro K, Naganuma M, Ebinuma H, Kunimoto H, Tada S, Ogata H, et al. Reactivation of hepatitis B in a patient with Crohn's disease treated using infliximab. J Gastroenterol. 2008;43:397–401.

26. Urganci N, Kalyoncu D. Immunogenicity of hepatitis A and B vaccination in pediatric patients with inflammatory bowel disease. J Pediatr Gastroenterol Nutr. 2013;56:412–5.

27. Moses J, Alkhouri N, Shannon A, Raig K, Lopez R, Danziger-Isakov L, et al. Hepatitis B immunity and response to booster vaccination in children with inflammatory bowel disease treated with infliximab. Am J Gastroenterol. 2012;107:133–8.

28. Gisbert JP, Villagrasa JR, Rodríguez-Nogueiras A, Chaparro M. Efficacy of hepatitis B vaccination and revaccination and factors impacting on response in patients with inflammatory bowel disease. Am J Gastroenterol. 2012;107:1460–6.

29. Gisbert JP, Menchén L, García-Sánchez V, Marín I, Villagrasa JR, Chaparro M. Comparison of the effectiveness of two protocols for vaccination (standard and double dosage) against hepatitis B virus in patients with inflammatory bowel disease. Aliment Pharmacol Ther. 2012;35:1379–85.

30. Radzikowski A, Banaszkiewicz A, Łazowska-Przeorek I, Grzybowska-Chlebowczyk U, Woś H, Pytrus T, et al. Immunogenecity of hepatitis A vaccine in pediatric patients with inflammatory bowel disease. Inflamm Bowel Dis. 2011;17: 1117–24.

31. Park SH, Yang SK, Park SK, Kim JW, Yang DH, Jung KW, et al. Efficacy of hepatitis A vaccination and factors impacting on seroconversion in patients with inflammatory bowel disease. Inflamm Bowel Dis. 2014;20:69–74.

32. Lee CK, Kim HS, Ye BD, Lee KM, Kim YS, Rhee SY, et al. Patients with Crohn's disease on anti-tumor necrosis factor therapy are at significant risk of inadequate response to the 23-valent pneumococcal polysaccharide vaccine. J Crohns Colitis. 2014;8:384–91.

33. Melmed GY, Agarwal N, Frenck RW, Ippoliti AF, Ibanez P, Papakakis KA, et al. Immunosuppression impairs response to pneumococcal polysaccharide vaccination in patients with inflammatory bowel disease. Am J Gastroenterol. 2010;105:148–54.

34. Fiorino G, Peyrin-Biroulet L, Naccarato P, Szabò H, Sociale OR, Vetrano S, et al. Effects of immunosuppression on immune response to pneumococcal vaccine in inflammatory bowel disease: a prospective study. Inflamm Bowel Dis. 2012;18:1042–7.

35. Banaszkiewicz A, Targońska B, Kowalska-Duplaga K, Karolewska-Bochenek K, Sieczkowska A, Gawrońska A, et al. Immunogenicity of 13-valent pneumococcal conjugate vaccine in pediatric patients with inflammatory bowel disease. Inflamm Bowel Dis. 2015;21: 1607–14.

36. Jacobson DL, Bousvaros A, Ashworth L, Carey R, Shrier LA, Burchett SK, et al. Immunogenicity and tolerability to human papillomavirus-like particle vaccine in girls and young women with inflammatory bowel disease. Inflamm Bowel Dis. 2013;19: 1441–9.

37. Dotan I, Werner L, Vigodman S, Agarwal S, Pfeffer J, Horowitz N, et al. Normal response to vaccines in inflammatory bowel disease patients treated with thiopurines. Inflamm Bowel Dis. 2012;18: 261–8.

38. Harpaz R, Ortega-Sanchez IR, Seward JF. Prevention of herpes zoster: recommendations of the Advisory Committee on Immunization Practices (ACIP). MMWR Recomm Rep. 2008;57:1–30. quiz CE2-4

39. Lu Y, Bousvaros A. Varicella vaccination in children with inflammatory bowel disease receiving immunosuppressive therapy. J Pediatr Gastroenterol Nutr. 2010;50:562–5.

40. Ansari F, Baker RD, Patel R, Baker SS. Varicella immunity in inflammatory bowel disease. J Pediatr Gastroenterol Nutr. 2011;53:386–8.

41. Sheibani S, Cohen R, Kane S, Dubinsky M, Church JA, Mahadevan U. The effect of maternal peripartum anti-TNFα use on infant immune response. Dig Dis Sci. 2016; doi:10.1007/s10620-015-3992-2.

Malignant Tumors Arising in Inflammatory Bowel Disease

55

Thomas A. Ullman and Rona Yaeger

Pathogenesis and Molecular Basis of Cancer in IBD

Drawing lessons from the molecular changes that account for colon carcinogenesis in familial adenomatous polyposis (FAP) and hereditary nonpolyposis colorectal cancer (HNPCC), now again called Lynch syndrome, the genetic and molecular basis of colon carcinogenesis have become better understood in recent years. These lessons have been directly applicable to events involved in the development of sporadic colorectal neoplasia, whose pathways mirror those of the familial cancer syndromes. It is currently believed that the vast majority (80–85%) of sporadic CRCs arise from a pathway that involves *chromosomal instability* resulting in abnormal segregation of chromosomes, aneuploidy, and altered expression of tumor suppressor genes (primarily *APC* and *p53*) and oncogenes (mainly *k-ras*) (Fig. 55.1). In this pathway, loss of *APC* function occurs as an initiating or "gatekeeper" event for subsequent molecular alterations that culminate in the development of the adenoma. Loss of p53 gene function occurs later in the sequence, typically at the transition of the adenoma to carcinoma. The remaining 15% of sporadic CRCs arise through a so-called mutator pathway that involves loss of function of DNA base mismatch repair (MMR) genes, mainly *hMLH1* and *hMSH2*. In this pathway, loss of MMR gene function results in a phenotype termed *microsatellite instability (MSI)*. Sporadic CRCs that demonstrate MSI are often diploid (as opposed to the aneuploid state of chromosomal instability pathway-related tumors), tend to occur in the proximal colon, and frequently display rather unique histological features such as a medullary or solid growth pattern, a signet-ring cell histology, a plethora of tumor infiltrating lymphocytes, and an adjacent inflammatory reaction often referred to as a "Crohn-like reaction." Another distinguishing feature of MSI-positive sporadic CRCs is the better survival of patients with those tumors compared to ones without MSI [1].

IBD-associated CRCs share several features in common with sporadic CRC. First, they both arise from a precursor dysplastic lesion. In the case of sporadic CRC, the dysplastic precursor is a discrete, polypoid growth called an adenoma, which typically progresses to cancer by enlarging in size, assuming greater degrees of dysplasia, and often assuming an increasing proportion of villous histology. In chronic colitis, while dysplasia is often polypoid, it may be flat or only slightly raised. Regardless of its growth pattern, colitis-related dysplasia progresses through increasing levels of abnormal development in its path to CRC. Second, stage-based survival of patients with CRC is similar in the two settings [2]. Third, some of same molecular alterations that contribute to the pathogenesis of sporadic CRC are found in colitis-associated neoplasms [3].

While the similarities between colitis-associated neoplasia and sporadic colorectal neoplasia are notable, they differ in several important ways. First, colitis-associated cancers affect individuals at a much younger age. Second, colitis-associated neoplasia, by definition, arises in the setting of long-standing chronic inflammation, whereas sporadic neoplasms occur in the absence of an inflammatory background. Oxidative stress or other insults may lead to earlier or more frequent genetic changes to the colon, but the precise mechanisms by which chronic inflammation leads to neoplasia remain elusive. Third, dysplasias and even cancers in colitis are often multifocal, suggesting more of a precancerous "field change" of the colitic mucosa compared to the colons of patients with sporadic adenomas and colon cancer; the clinical consequence of this difference accounts for the different surgical approach: colitis-associated neoplasms are usually treated with total proctocolectomy, whereas sporadic adenomas and cancers are treated with polypectomy or segmental resection of affected colon. Fourth, although the two

T.A. Ullman, MD (✉)
The Dr. Henry D. Janowitz Division of Gastroenterology,
The Mount Sinai School of Medicine, New York, NY, USA
e-mail: thomas.ullman@mssm.edu

R. Yaeger, MD
Memorial Sloan Kettering Cancer Center, New York, NY 10024, USA
e-mail: yaegerr@mskcc.org

© Springer International Publishing AG 2017
P. Mamula et al. (eds.), *Pediatric Inflammatory Bowel Disease*, DOI 10.1007/978-3-319-49215-5_55

Fig. 55.1 Timing in molecular
alterations in sporadic
colorectal cancer and
colitis-associated colorectal
cancer (From *Gastroenterology*,
2004) [4]

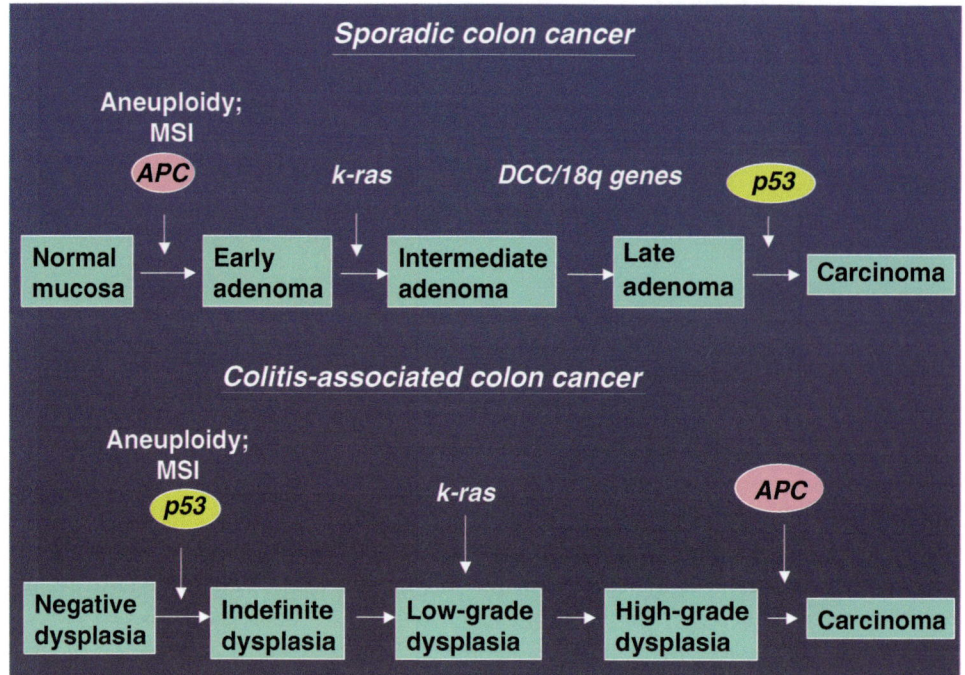

settings of colorectal neoplasia might share the several types of molecular changes, the frequency and timing with which these molecular alterations occur is different (Fig. 55.1) [4]. For example, *APC* mutations are considered to be common and initiating events in sporadic colon carcinogenesis, whereas this molecular alteration is much less frequent, affecting about one-fourth of colitis-associated CRC, and usually occurs late in the colitis-associated dysplasia-carcinoma sequence. Recent data from next-generation sequencing analysis of colitis-associated cancers suggest that *APC* mutations may be more common in Crohn's-associated cancers than in cases associated with UC [5]. Also, in colitis patients, *TP53* mutations occur early and have even been detected in mucosa that is non-dysplastic or indefinite for dysplasia [6]. Likewise, MSI has been detected in non-dysplastic mucosa from patients with ulcerative colitis, even those patients with disease of relatively short duration, but not from healthy controls or patients with other types of benign inflammatory colitis [7, 8].

TP53 alterations are nearly universal in colitis-associated CRC. The majority of these *TP53* alterations are missense mutations occurring in the DNA-binding domain of p53 [5]. Many of these missense mutations may also possess gain-of-function capacities, including enhancement of invasive properties, attenuation of apoptosis, and increased genomic instability [9]. A recent study suggests that the early presence of mutant p53 in the inflamed colon of IBD patients may actually be a driver of the subsequent progression to carcinoma by invigorating inflammation in the immediate microenvironment of the cells with mutant p53 [10]. Using a

murine model, where exposure to dextran sodium sulfate (DSS) induces an acute colitis, Cooks et al. looked at the role of mutant *TP53* versus loss of *TP53* on the development of adenomas and progression to carcinoma. The mice with mutant *TP53* developed more frequent inflammation-associated colon cancer and developed carcinoma much earlier than mice with knockout of one *TP53* allele, suggesting that mutant p53 may not only make the mice more susceptible to chronic inflammation but also accelerate the development of carcinoma on an inflammatory background.

There is emerging data of genetic differences between colitis-associated CRC and sporadic CRC. *IDH1* mutations at the R132 hotspot occur in about 10–15% of colitis-associated CRC, particularly in cases associated with CD [11]. IDH1 R132 mutations are exceedingly rare in sporadic colorectal cancer and occur in no more than 1% of cases [12, 13]. The R132 mutation in *IDH1* results in a mutant isocitrate dehydrogenase enzyme that cannot participate in the oxidative carboxylation of isocitrate, leading to dysregulated cellular metabolism, interfering with the generation of the key reducing agent (NADPH), and producing the oncometabolite 2-hydroxygluatarate, which is associated with an altered epigenetic state with the CpG island methylator phenotype (CIMP) [14, 15]. Other recurrent genetic alterations identified in colitis-associated CRC include *MYC* amplification, which occurs in both sporadic CRC and colitis-associated CRC but is significantly more common in colitis-associated CRC, and alterations in fibroblast-growth factor signaling, including FGFR1/FGFR1 amplification and translocations and ligand amplifications [5].

Colorectal Cancer in Ulcerative Colitis: Epidemiology and Clinical Practice

Epidemiology

Crohn and Rosenberg first described rectal cancer complicating UC more than 80 years ago. In their manuscript, they suggested that the malignancy was a complication of the disease [16]. Three years after Crohn and Rosenberg, Bargen, at the Mayo Clinic, reported a series of 17 patients with both chronic colitis and colorectal cancer [17]. Other cases and series followed, and the crude frequency calculations from these studies served as evidence supporting a link between UC to CRC. With the application of modern epidemiologic methods, true incidence calculations, cumulative incidence calculations, and standardized incidence rates confirmed the association between UC and CRC. Cumulative incidence rates have largely become the standard by which clinicians and public health experts assess the time-dependent risk of cancer develops in colitis. Similarly, standardized incidence rates describe the estimate of the relative risk for developing colon cancer for a segment of a colitis population (such as colitis patients with universal disease) as compared to the general population. While initial series using this more accurate epidemiologic terminology came from large referral centers in which "incident" cases were referred for evaluation and management due to a suspicion for or even the actual presence of CRC, the use of more appropriate terminology was an advance over the previously used crude rates [18–20]. Due to these now obvious referral biases, however, these first "modern" studies overestimated the true risk of CRC in UC. Subsequent studies from population-based data sources used more realistic calculations for determining the incidence of CRC in UC. Without referral and other selection biases, the cancer incidence calculated in these manuscripts was substantially lower than previously reported [21–25]. These studies, however, may have *under*estimated the true risk of cancer in long-standing UC, as they included many patients with UC who had undergone previous colectomy in the denominator of the incidence calculations. In a meta-analysis of the risk of CRC in ulcerative colitis in which 116 studies were included, Eaden and colleagues found the overall prevalence of CRC to be 3.7% and an overall incidence rate of 3 cases per 1000 person years duration (95% confidence interval ranging from 2 to 4 cases per 1000 person years duration). The rate increased with each decade of disease, leading to a calculated incidence of 12 per 1000 person years in the third decade of colitis [18]. These data corresponded to a *cumulative incidence* of CRC of 2% at 10 years, 8% at 20 years, and 18% at 30 years disease duration [26]. It is worth noting, however, that referral centers accounted for 64% of the studies included in Eaden's study; only 13 population-based reports were located by the Medline search

performed as part of the meta-analysis [26]. Based on these and older data, typical estimates of CRC incidence usually range between 0.5–1% per year after 10 years of colitis.

More recent studies, however, have raised the possibility that prior studies have overestimated the incidence and risk for CRC in this population. More recent publications from Denmark [27], Hungary [28], Canada [29], and Olmsted County, Minnesota (with its relatively small population) [30], have suggested a CRC in UC incidence of between 1 in 500 and 1 in 1600 per year, far lower than the 1 in 300 rate calculated in Eaden's meta-analysis [26]. These have corresponded to relative risk calculations ranging from 1.1 to 2.7 times the general population. While some have argued that these more "modern" calculations support a declining incidence over calendar time, as seen by Rutter and colleagues [31], no definitive analysis has been performed to support this hypothesis. To what extent such reductions in incidence (if they exist) are a function of colonoscopic surveillance (see below), chemoprevention with mesalamine-based agents or other medicines (also below), or other factors remains unknown.

Risk Factors

A number of clinical variables have been demonstrated to modify the risk for colorectal cancer in UC patients. These variables include duration of UC, anatomic extent of disease, age at UC diagnosis, concomitant primary sclerosing cholangitis (PSC), a family history of colorectal cancer, and inflammatory activity. The use of certain medications may lessen the risk of developing CRC, but the impact of these potentially chemopreventive agents is modest. Table 55.1 classifies these different risk modifiers.

Duration of Ulcerative Colitis

A number of investigators have demonstrated that the duration of ulcerative colitis correlates with the risk of cancer [18, 32–34]. Duration of disease, however, can be a rather subjective measurement. Most studies have used the date of UC diagnosis as the point at which the clock starts, but others have argued that the time of symptom onset is a better measure of disease duration. Whichever point is chosen, a number of distortions can be imagined that would impact the findings in any individual study. If *date of diagnosis* is used as a starting point, then patients with long-standing, subclinical disease would appear to have relatively shorter duration of disease, and such subjects would contribute less to any calculation of the effect of disease duration. Conversely, by using *date of first symptoms*, subjects who were without colitis might mistakenly contribute years of disease-free time

Table 55.1 Risk modifiers of colorectal cancer in ulcerative colitis

Accepted risk modifiers	
Disease duration	*Longer duration increases risk*
Extent of disease	*Greater extent increases risk*
PSC	*Presence of PSC increases risk*
Age of onset	*Early age of onset increases risk*
Family history of carcinoma	*Positive family history increases risk*
Probable risk modifiers	
Inflammation	*Increased inflammation increases risk*
Possible risk modifiers	
Sulfasalazine/5-ASA	*Use reduces risk*
Folic acid	*Supplementation reduces risk*
Ursodeoxycholic acid	*Use reduces risk in UC patients with PSC*
Unlikely risk modifier	
Glucocorticoid use	
6-MP/AZA use	

PSC primary sclerosing cholangitis

to calculations of duration. This distinction in the definition of disease duration may be particularly problematic for patients with primary sclerosing cholangitis (PSC) who frequently have clinically quiescent colitis. Without unanimity in definition, there is variability in the estimate of this factor's effect on subsequent CRC development. In Eaden's meta-analysis, the effect of duration was made clear as the passage of each successive decade resulted in an increase in incidence. Incidence was calculated to be 2 per 1000 patient years (95% C.I. 1–4/1000) at 10 years and 11 per 1000 (95% C.I. 4–28/1000) at 30 years; the rate at 20 years was intermediate [26]. As the overall curve for cumulative CRC risk starts to meaningfully exceed that of the general population by 8–10 years, most clinicians will initiate surveillance colonoscopy once this threshold has been reached. Because many of the studies that were entered in to Eaden's meta-analysis antedated the widespread application of colonoscopic dysplasia surveillance, it remains unclear whether duration of colitis exerts a seeming exponential effect, as Eaden found, or a linear effect, which might result if highest-risk patients are serially removed from the denominator via colectomy from surveillance-identified dysplasia.

Anatomic Extent of Ulcerative Colitis

The length of involved colon also correlates with cancer risk: the greater the surface area of colitis, the greater the cancer risk. Defining the anatomic extent of ulcerative colitis, as with duration of disease, can vary from study to study. In initial reports documenting this independent risk factor, anatomic extent was defined by a barium enema at diagnosis.

Flexible endoscopy long ago replaced barium radiography for diagnosing colitis and its extent, but there is no consensus as to whether naked eye findings at colonoscopy or microscopic extent determined histologically should be the gold standard for measuring extent. Additionally, definitions of "pancolitis," "universal colitis," and "extensive colitis" vary within studies, although they are all typically used to describe disease proximal to the splenic flexure. Another feature that invites confusion into the definition of anatomic extent is the timing of the measurement. As extent can change over time [35], should we take the extent at diagnosis or at some point in follow-up? Like other questions surrounding the issue of extent, this question has been left unresolved, although the majority of studies have used the terms "extent" and "extent at diagnosis" interchangeably. Extent at follow-up has not been well studied as an independent risk factor.

A population-based investigation of a cohort of more than 3000 patients with UC defined extent of UC by barium enema exam at diagnosis and demonstrated an impressive gradient of risk as one moves from proctitis (standardized incidence ratio of 1.7, 95% confidence interval 0.8–3.2) to left-sided colitis (SIR=2.8, 95% C.I. 1.6–4.4) to pancolitis (SIR=14.8, 95% C.I. 11.4 to 18.9) [22]. Devroede [18], Greenstein [34], Gyde [33], Katzka [36], Mir-Madjlessi [37], and Gilat [23] all reported similar gradients in their studies. This finding was confirmed, though not directly studied, in Eaden's meta-analysis [26]. In terms of "how" extent should be defined, it is worth noting that a group from University of California San Francisco found CRC in areas proximal to the endoscopically perceived margin of colitis that turned out to have microscopic disease in that region [38]. On this basis, clinicians should consider the most proximal extent of disease *microscopically* as the proximal extent of disease and plan any prevention strategy accordingly.

Age of Ulcerative Colitis Onset

Important to pediatricians, age of colitis onset, as a variable independent of disease duration, has been implicated in some studies to modify the risk of IBD-related colon cancer. This hypothesis, however, remains in question. Reporting one of the highest published cumulative rates of CRC in colitis, Devroede and colleagues found that at 35 years of follow-up, 43% of subjects with documented UC prior to age 15 had developed CRC [18]. This study, however, reflected pediatric patients seen at a large referral center; additionally, the number of patients available to analyze after 35 years of follow-up was quite small, with the error surrounding this point estimate correspondingly quite wide. While some investigators have failed to demonstrate a link between age of colitis onset and the subsequent development of CRC [23, 36], others have confirmed the direction if not the magnitude of

Devroede's findings [22, 33]. In the previously mentioned study by Ekbom, for example, the authors found that the relative risk of cancer in colitis decreased with advancing age—younger patients have a higher risk [22]. This overall gradient was confirmed by Eaden, who found that cumulative rates of CRC were greater than the pooled estimates for CRC among adult colitis patients, though this difference did not meet conventional thresholds for statistical significance [26]. Although neither the precise nature nor the precise magnitude of CRC risk for younger patients with UC has been determined, extra caution should be applied to pediatric patients given both the suggestion of an increased risk from the medical literature and the obvious increased lifetime risk given a longer life expectancy.

Primary Sclerosing Cholangitis

Primary sclerosing cholangitis is a chronic cholestatic liver disease in which there is progressive inflammatory fibrosis of the biliary tree. It is an infrequent complication of IBD, affecting 2–8% of patients with ulcerative colitis. However, among patients with PSC, 62–72% have underlying IBD. Since the intersection of CRC *and* PSC would be expected to occur in small absolute numbers in patients with UC, it is largely through case-control studies and referral center-based cohort studies that the majority of data have been generated to support an association between PSC and CRC in UC. Although a positive association has not always been noted [39–41], most studies do support such an association, with derived odds ratios from these "positive" studies ranging from 9 to 16 [42–46]. In a population-based study from Sweden, Kornfeld and colleagues found a substantially elevated cumulative incidence of CRC in UC/PSC patients: 33% at 20 years [47]. As noted above, since colitis activity in PSC is often mild or even subclinical, PSC patients in these studies might well have had a longer duration of disease than was appreciated, making it difficult to tease out the precise, independent contribution of PSC to the development of CRC.

Family History of Colorectal Cancer

Family history of CRC has long been recognized as a risk factor for the development of sporadic colorectal cancer. This risk increases according to the number of relatives affected with CRC [48]. In UC, only a few clinical studies have been performed to investigate the independent contribution of a positive family history for colorectal cancer. An early study from Lashner's group at the University of Chicago supported family history of CRC as a potential risk factor for CRC in colitis, although the association did not

reach statistical significance [49]. A second report from the Cleveland Clinic documented a *lower* rate of positive family history of CRC among UC patients with cancer or dysplasia compared to UC controls without colonic neoplasia, though this finding, too, failed to exclude the null hypothesis [50]. Both of these studies, however, were designed to test hypotheses concerning the association between folic acid supplementation and colorectal cancer in colitis. Testing for family history as a risk factor was performed as part of a secondary analysis, and these studies did not specify the rigor with which a family history was obtained.

More recently, a handful of studies have suggested an increased risk for CRC in UC when a positive family history of CRC was documented. Nuako and colleagues at the Mayo Clinic were the first to clearly demonstrate this increased risk, calculating an odds ratio of 2.3 (95% CI 1.1–5.1) in their case-control study [51]. In a population-based study from Scandinavia, Askling and colleagues found a similar elevated risk of 2.5 (95% C.I. 1.4–4.4) [52], while Eaden (in the UK) found an even greater risk (OR 5.0, 95% CI 1.1–22.8) in a multivariable model using case-control derived data [53]. Whatever the absolute magnitude, it appears quite likely that a positive family history confers an increased risk of CRC in UC.

Inflammation

Curiously, although inflammation has been assumed to be a key factor contributing to higher risk of colonic neoplasia in UC, few studies have examined this issue. One well-conducted retrospective case-control study recently reported that histologic inflammation was indeed associated with an increased risk of neoplastic progression based on a retrospective case-control analysis of patients followed at a specialized center [54]. A retrospective cohort study from Mount Sinai, New York, has also demonstrated a link between histologic inflammation on dysplasia and cancer risk, with a two-fold risk increase for each unit of inflammation derived from a 4-point scale [54, 55].

Pharmacotherapy and Chemoprevention

As with sporadic colorectal cancer and interest in cyclooxygenase-inhibiting compounds, investigators, clinicians, and patients are actively seeking medications that might *decrease* the risk of developing CRC in UC. Retrospective studies have been performed examining a number of potential chemopreventive agents with mixed results. As is often the case in retrospectively performed studies of medication use, the dose and duration of use that defines exposure can be arbitrarily chosen. Nevertheless, a number of studies have been performed looking at different hypothesized chemopreventive medication with exposure defined in a number of different ways.

Sulfasalazine/5-Aminosalicylates

Sulfasalazine and the newer 5-aminosalicylic acid (5-ASA) products have been investigated for their chemopreventive effect, mainly by post hoc secondary analyses, yielding conflicting results. In a study designed to investigate the effect of supplemental folic acid on CRC risk, sulfasalazine use was found to have a positive (i.e., predisposing) effect on the development of CRC (slightly but not significantly higher rates of CRC in the exposed group); sulfasalazine allergic patients, however, were noted to have a substantially lower risk of developing CRC [49]. Subsequently, Pinczowski and Eaden were able to demonstrate a protective effect for sulfasalazine or mesalazine [53, 56], when dose and duration were considered. Tung [57] failed to demonstrate a meaningful protective effect, but this study was limited to high-risk PSC patients. A number of additional studies with a variety of definitions for exposure have now been performed with conflicting results. Some have shown benefit with exposure to mesalamine-based agents [58, 59], while others have been less optimistic [60, 61]. A systematic review reviewed a number of these studies, but its conclusion that mesalamine is chemopreventive with nearly a 50% reduction in cancer incidence must be taken with some caution owing to the heterogeneity of the included studies as well as the different designs that were used (case-control, retrospective cohort, secondary analyses, population-based and tertiary centers) [62]. Given the lack of unanimity of these studies, it remains in question whether mesalamine-based medications constitute truly chemopreventive agents. Asking a related question as to whether mesalamines are chemopreventive among patients undergoing dysplasia surveillance, a center-based cohort study that was able to account for changes in exposure over time found no such effect [63]. Given their utility at preventing flares in patients in remission, however, their use should be advocated in all UC patients.

Folic Acid

Folic acid, which has been demonstrated to have a protective effect in sporadic colorectal cancer, was twice studied by Lashner, once at the University of Chicago [49] and again at the Cleveland Clinic [50]. In neither study was a significant protective effect noted, although the point estimates of risk (0.38 and 0.45) suggested the possibility of a chemopreventive effect. Given the low cost and the low risk of adverse events at conventional doses of 400 ug per day and 1 mg per day, the administration of folic acid as a chemopreventive drug should be strongly considered for all at risk patients.

Ursodeoxycholic Acid

Ursodeoxycholic acid, an exogenous bile acid used in the treatment of PSC, has also been studied. In UC-PSC patients, an impressive chemopreventive effect has been demonstrated, with a 40 percent difference in neoplasia noted between the ursodeoxycholic acid-treated group (32%) and the untreated group (72%) [57]. This was additionally demonstrated in a randomized clinical trial of ursodeoxycholic acid in which a 74% reduction in dysplasia or CRC was noted [64]. Newer data, however, from the same group that studied it in the earlier trial, demonstrated that high-dose ursodeoxycholic acid at 28–30 mg/kg per day actually gave rise to *more* colorectal neoplasia [65]. As the benefits of ursodeoxycholic acid on PSC are questionable at best, it is uncertain whether low-dose administration should be given as a chemopreventive agent.

Methods to Reduce Risk/Mortality

Until we discover or develop a meaningful chemopreventive agent and effective strategies to identify a minimal risk subgroup, only two acceptable forms of CRC prophylaxis exist: surgery and dysplasia surveillance. In dysplasia surveillance, high-risk patients are identified by the identification of neoplasia (either dysplasia or cancer) at colonoscopy and are subsequently referred to surgery, while cancer and dysplasia-free patients continue with periodic colonoscopy [66]. The presumption is that only the highest-risk patients will undergo a colectomy, and lower-risk patients will be able to maintain a higher quality of life with their colons intact. A third option, watch and wait, with colonoscopy performed only for symptoms, is available but due to the available evidence that symptomatic cancers are associated with a worse survival than asymptomatic ones [67, 68] never used in clinical practice.

Surgery

Without question, the most effective method for minimizing CRC risk in UC patients is to perform a total proctocolectomy. This nearly eliminates the risk of colon or rectal cancer, and, while cancers have been reported in case reports and series in patients who have undergone either hand-sewn or stapled anastomoses, the risk of such an event is quite small. In the pre-endoscopic era, this strategy of cancer prevention was often advocated for patients with long-standing colitis, and should still be considered, particularly for patients with medically refractory or difficult disease. As surgery is not without its potential complications and change in quality of life, however, and as the absolute risk of developing a lethal colon cancer may not be sufficiently high to warrant such a radical approach in *all* colitis patients, surgical prophylaxis in asymptomatic patients with long-standing colitis is now viewed with skepticism by both patients and clinicians. At present, surgical options (for colorectal cancer prophylaxis *or* as primary treatment for colitis-related dysplasia or cancer) include total proctocolectomy with creation of an ileal pouch-anal anastomosis (often referred to as a restorative proctocolectomy) or total proctocolectomy with end ileostomy. Subtotal colectomy with ileorectal anastomosis is to be avoided, although there are no studies comparing this procedure to either of the other conventional choices. Pouch surgery is generally reserved for younger patients, as it requires sufficient anal sphincter tone. Following pouch surgery, patients may expect to have five or more bowel movements per day due to pouch size and ileal flow. Possible complications include sexual and bladder dysfunction, incontinence, pouchitis (which usually responds to short courses of antibiotics but may become chronic and refractory), fistula formation, stricture formation, anastomotic leakage, and pouch failure. The overall failure rate (the proportion of patients eventually converted to end ileostomy) is approximately 5% [69]. It should also be noted that the malignant potential of ileal pouch mucosa in colitis patients remains unknown. Initial reports of pouch dysplasia have been reported, and there have been reports of cancer in the cuff of rectal mucosa to which the pouch is anastomosed [70, 71]. While cancer risk following proctocolectomy with Brooke ileostomy is close to nil, the loss of anorectal function and attendant stoma make this option less appealing to most patients who would otherwise be candidates for pouch surgery. Potential complications of total proctocolectomy with end ileostomy include sexual and bladder dysfunction, stomal fistula, parastomal hernia, and small bowel obstruction [69].

Dysplasia Surveillance

As it results in too many colectomies in patients who would otherwise be unaffected by CRC, prophylactic total proctocolectomy is seldom performed. Even if limited to the high-risk groups of patients with long-standing and extensive UC, with or without PSC or a family history of CRC, a large number of colectomies would be performed in patients who would never develop CRC. What is needed is a tissue marker that better determines the highest-risk patients, those with an imminent risk of colorectal cancer. While imperfect on many levels, mucosal dysplasia serves as such a marker.

In 1967 Morson and Pang first reported the association between mucosal dysplasia and CRC in patients with UC [72]. In their seminal report, they noted that rectal dysplasia, then termed "precancer" and identified by blind rectal biopsy of colitis mucosa, heralded the presence of an invasive adenocarcinoma *elsewhere* in the colon. If appropriately discriminating, mucosal dysplasia, it was hypothesized, could be used as a diagnostic test to identify the highest-risk patients to whom surgery would be offered.

Subsequent studies revealed that, although by no means a perfect test, dysplasia was discriminating enough to be tested in clinical practice. Retrospective studies confirmed Morson and Pang's findings, noting the presence of dysplasia either adjacent to or remote from cancer in colitis [73–75]. Additionally, cancer foci were discovered in colons resected for the indication of dysplasia [76]. These data, along with the advent of flexible fiber-optic instruments with their ability to deliver multiple mucosal samples to the pathologist's microscope, led to the development of protocol-based surveillance programs. Unfortunately, no randomized, controlled trials of surveillance were performed. (This may have been a function of difficulty in defining suitable control patients: would patients allow themselves to be randomized to a "no surgery" or "no endoscopy" arm of a surveillance study? Or to a "prophylactic surgery" arm?) Nevertheless, based on the clinical characteristics of dysplasia and the results of numerous surveillance programs, as well as the very limited acceptability of other prevention strategies, namely, surgery for all long-standing colitis or waiting for cancer symptoms, periodic colonoscopy with biopsy for dysplasia became an accepted form of cancer prevention in UC. In addition to its widespread use in clinical practice, it has been advocated in guidelines statements for colon cancer prevention [77] and ulcerative colitis care [78].

Single-armed surveillance programs have demonstrated the feasibility, though not the efficacy, of conventional surveillance [24, 76, 79–89]. When "control" arms were used in these studies, they included patients in whom surveillance at another institution or referral to the institution for malignancy could be considered as "no surveillance." Nevertheless, the finding that cancers found during surveillance were more often at earlier stages than cancers found in a "watch and wait" strategy contributed to the acceptance of dysplasia surveillance as a form of cancer prevention [67, 68]. Other key features about surveillance programs worth noting include the presence of advanced stage cancers despite inclusion in a surveillance program (some due to patient dropout and some due to progression while under surveillance) [86, 89, 79] the variable intervals used for surveillance, the variable rates of patient dropout, and the substantially varied rates of dysplasia incidence across studies. For surveillance to be effective, it should reduce CRC mortality in IBD patients. In the absence of prospective controlled studies, a well-designed population-based case-control study sheds light on this issue. Karlen and colleagues compared the exposure to colonoscopy among cases with CRC deaths and alive controls matched for age, gender, disease duration, and disease extent [90]. The point estimate of cancer mortality reduction from either one or only two previous colonoscopic exams was a threefold decrease. Although the odds ratio of 0.3 did not reach statistical significance, (95% CI: 0.1 to 1.3), this is certainly a clinically impressive result. A recent case-control study from the Mayo Clinic confirmed these findings and even crossed the threshold of statistical significance with an odds ratio of 0.4 for 1–2 surveillance examination (95% CI: 0.2 to 0.7) [91]. While these data were not population-based in their orientation, they nevertheless support the notion that surveillance is likely effective. Additional support comes from decision analysis models [92–94] that demonstrate improved outcomes for a population in surveillance compared to no surveillance. As with all such modeled data, there are many assumptions that lack real-world support, such as a lack of dropout while under surveillance and an orderly progression from no dysplasia to low-grade dysplasia to high-grade dysplasia to colorectal cancer [92, 93, 95]. Cost-effectiveness analyses have similarly predicted that surveillance was a superior strategy to no surveillance (although prophylactic colectomy, while unacceptable to patients, was the preferred strategy vis-à-vis life-years saved over time).

What then might limit the effectiveness of dysplasia surveillance in UC in practice? One factor may be difficulties in histologic interpretation among pathologists. Indeed this was thought to be so substantial a problem after the initial reports of surveillance studies that in 1983, an international group of experts convened to establish true definitions for the evaluation of dysplasia surveillance specimens: no dysplasia, indefinite for dysplasia (with three subtypes), low-grade dysplasia, high-grade dysplasia, and colorectal cancer [96]. Unfortunately, despite these codified definitions, substantial rates of disagreement, even among expert GI pathologists, have been noted [96–99]. Rates of disagreement among community pathologists, not surprisingly, have been substantial, too [97]. In these studies, crude rates of agreement have been as low as 40% and as high as 72%, with best agreement when no dysplasia was present; kappa values, which can account for chance agreement, were fair to good. Clearly, this system needs less subjectivity and overall improvement.

Lack of perfection from practicing pathologists is not the only reason for surveillance not to reach its potential. Gastroenterologists also fall short of ideal practices. One variable that contributes to lack of uniform clinician practices stems from the uncertainty that surrounds the predictive value of dysplasia. While there is near-universal agreement that patients found to have high-grade dysplasia should undergo colectomy due to rates of concurrent adenocarcinoma near 50% [74], considerable controversy surrounds the management of low-grade dysplasia. Adding to the controversy is the fact that LGD can be flat or polypoid, unifocal or multifocal, or not repeatedly found on sequential colono-

scopic exams. Few studies have directly addressed these variables in patients with LGD.

How to best manage LGD depends in large part on how likely patients with this finding are to either already harbor or progress to more advanced neoplasia (HGD or cancer). More specifically, the essential unanswered question is whether failure to perform a colectomy in patients with LGD results in a poor outcome. In a landmark study from St. Marks Hospital in which the Inflammatory Bowel Disease Morphology Study Group's 1983 definitions were used [96], the rate of progression to advanced dysplasia from LGD was 54% at 5 years [100]. In the same year as the St. Mark's publication, a systematic review of surveillance programs by Bernstein and colleagues noted a 19% rate of cancer at "immediate colectomy" following the discovery of LGD. These results were confirmed by studies from the Mayo Clinic [101] and Mount Sinai in New York [102], in which the rates of progression for flat LGD were 33% (95% CI 9 to 56%) and 53% (95% CI 29 to 77%), respectively. Furthermore, in the Mount Sinai study, 19% of patients who underwent colectomy within 6 months of their initial flat LGD finding were found to have CRC in their resection specimens. Of those who progressed, cases of node-positive cancer without intervening HGD were found. Neither the number of biopsies positive for LGD nor any other clinical variable were found to be predictive of subsequent progression, with unifocal flat LGD carrying a 5-year rate of progression of 53% [102]. Investigators from the University of Washington where an aggressive biopsy protocol is followed [103] and from the Karolinska Institute, Sweden [104], however, discovered less frequent progression and no cancers. Not all investigators have discovered the same high risk for LGD as that noted by St. Mark's, Mayo Clinic, and Mount Sinai in New York. A group from Karolinska in Sweden noticed a near-total lack of progression following discovery of LGD, but this group's pathologists did not use the full panoply of IBD Morphology Study Group definitions, as readings of "indefinite" for dysplasia were not allowed. Additionally, a number of patients were included whose discovery of LGD occurred prior to establishment of the Riddell criteria [105]. Additionally, the Leeds, UK, group led by Lim found little progression from LGD, leading him and his coauthors to conclude that continued surveillance with satisfactory biopsy practices was a safe alternative to surgery [106]. Finally, the University of Chicago group found a low actuarial rate of progression among patients with both flat and polypoid low-grade dysplasia [107]. While the variable rates of progression (perhaps secondary to variable biopsy practices, observer variation in the interpretation of dysplasia, or imperfect follow-up) make it difficult to draw absolute conclusions for the management of patients with flat LGD, early colectomy for LGD that is histologically confirmed by two expert pathologists should be strongly considered at the least. For patients who defer or refuse colectomy for LGD, gastroenterologists must make certain that patients return for follow-up examinations and that surveillance is appropriately performed with an adequate number of biopsies taken to exclude dysplasia.

It should be noted that a negative exam following LGD can occur for a number of reasons: (1) the previous examination was a false positive due to pathologic interpretation error; (2) the present examination is a false negative due to sampling or interpretation error; or (3) both exams were accurate. Not finding dysplasia on a repeat colonoscopy following one that detected LGD is no reassurance that dysplasia has regressed or will not "recur" [89]. It was estimated that to exclude dysplasia with 95% confidence, 56 biopsies must be performed, and to exclude 90% confidence, 33 biopsies should be taken [108]. This number of biopsies is rarely performed even in academic centers [109, 110]. Eaden noted that 57% of UK gastroenterologists take fewer than 10 biopsies in a surveillance exam based on their response to a questionnaire [109]. In a study examining actual gastroenterologists' practices, Ullman and colleagues found that the mean number of evaluable biopsies in patients with LGD was only 17.5 [102]. Such undersampling represents another limitation for dysplasia surveillance among gastroenterologists. Whether such practices truly limit the effectiveness of surveillance remains unknown.

The appropriate management of polypoid LGD, like that of flat LGD, is equally challenging. Polypoid dysplastic lesions in UC were labeled DALMs (dysplasia-associated lesions or masses) by Blackstone and colleagues in 1981 [80]. In this study, in which the pond was effectively stocked with patients referred for a suspicion of CRC and many lesions were noted to be > 2 cm in diameter, DALMs were noted to harbor a 58% (7 of 12) risk of cancer [80]. Despite the impressive cancer risk of DALMs in the Blackstone report, astute clinicians hypothesized that smaller, adenoma-like lesions might present a lesser risk. Two simultaneously published studies reported on their experience of treating smaller, sessile lesions with endoscopic resection (without surgery). Rubin and colleagues from Mount Sinai, New York, followed 48 patients with ulcerative or Crohn's colitis in whom dysplastic polyps were detected at colonoscopy [111]. In those patients in whom polyps were endoscopically resected and the remaining colon was dysplasia-free, no patients progressed to colorectal cancer after a mean follow-up of 4.1 years [111]. In Engelsgjerd's study from the Brigham and Women's Hospital in Boston, none of the 24 colitis patients with adenoma-like polyps treated with polypectomy developed adenocarcinoma after a mean follow-up of 42.4 months [112]. Odze reported on the continued follow-up of the Brigham group 5 years later, and only one case of CRC developed, this in a patient 7.5 years after her initial polypoid lesion had been resected [113]. Similar results were noted in a recent publication by Rutter and colleagues [31]. And both Goldstone [114] and Pekow [107] have documented a more favorable outcome for polypoid LGD as compared to patients with nontargeted LGD findings, likely a function of the success of polypectomy as in sporadic CRC. The need for complete resection of polypoid lesions was underlined in a publication by Vieth, in which 10 of 60 patients in whom residual neoplasia was left behind progressed to CRC [115]. These data seem to indicate the relative safety of endoscopic polypectomy in colitis provided that the lesions are small and completely resected and that the rest of the surveillance run is dysplasia-free. When removing a suspicious polyp in a colitic colon, it is important to separately biopsy the mucosa immediately adjacent to the polyp base because if the polyp resides in a bed of dysplasia, colectomy is warranted.

The colitic colon with numerous inflammatory pseudopolyps presents another challenge to the endoscopist. It is wise to remove any polyp that has unusual features. Molecular studies using global gene expression arrays suggest that DALMs can be distinguished from apparently sporadic adenomas [116] holding promise for managing these difficult lesions. Finding a dysplastic lesion in a sea of inflammatory polyps, however, poses a substantial challenge to the endoscopist. It is not surprising that a recent publication found that the presence of inflammatory pseudopolyps carries a substantial (2.5-fold) risk for subsequent colorectal cancer [91].

In addition to a lack of certainty among experts as to how to manage flat, low-grade dysplasia and polypoid dysplasia, other impediments to the success of surveillance exist within the GI community. Poor understanding of dysplasia and surveillance practices exist among trained gastroenterologists [109, 110, 117]. Indeed, only 19% of respondents correctly identified dysplasia as neoplastic tissue in Bernstein's two-decade's old questionnaire study [117]. Whether gastroenterologists' understanding has improved since that time remains uncertain.

Patient factors have also limited the effectiveness colonoscopic surveillance in colitis. Patient dropout or noncompliance with surveillance programs has been demonstrated to be a substantial source of colorectal cancer mortality [68, 84, 86, 89].

Despite the limitations of surveillance based on the difficulties of dysplasia interpretation, poor agreement on dysplasia management, suboptimal surveillance performance, and risks of patient dropout, no other acceptable method for cancer prevention in colitis exists. As such, dysplasia surveillance will remain with us until a superior substitute is found. Current recommendations for how surveillance should be performed have been published in a number of different formats [4, 118, 119]. All of these publications agree that 4-quadrant biopsies, with each quartet of biopsies in a separate jar, should be taken every 10 cm, with suspicious lesions labeled and placed in a separate jar; examinations should be performed every 1–2 years for patients with disease involving 1/3 or more of their colon after 8 years of disease. Surveillance should begin at diagnosis for all patients with UC and PSC. A recent position statement in *Gastroenterology* summarizes these findings [120].

Alternatives to Surveillance

Augmentation of white light surveillance has been proposed using *chromoendoscopy* using the dye stains methylene blue or indigo carmine to better highlight subtle and "flat" lesions. These procedures have demonstrated higher detection rates for dysplasia in head-to-head comparisons [121] with conventional dysplasia surveillance and in back-to-back surveillance in which each patient serves as his/her own control [122, 123]. While an increased yield in the detection of dysplasia is a worthy finding, whether the introduction and application of chromoendoscopic surveillance will alter *outcome* for colitis patients remains untested: potential benefits may come in the form of reduced intensity of surveillance for patients with dysplasia-free chromoendoscopic examinations, decreased nontargeted biopsies, decreased cost per examination, and potentially others. Other types of advanced endoscopy have been proposed as well, including narrowband imaging and various forms of spectroscopy. To date, none have been demonstrated a benefit to patients. Molecular markers, whether from serum, RNA, or stool, may also hold promise for complementing or replacing dysplasia surveillance, but as yet, they have not been incorporated into surveillance protocols.

Colorectal Cancer in Crohn's Disease

Like UC, colitis in Crohn's disease carries a risk for colorectal cancer greater than that of the general population. This was not always appreciated, however, as initial reports noted only a small, and sometimes not statistically significant, increase in colorectal cancer among patients with Crohn's disease [124, 125]. A number of factors likely contributed to the dilution of the true effect of Crohn's disease on colorectal carcinogenesis. First, patients with disease limited to the small bowel were included in some calculations of incidence. Second, patients who had undergone surgery, particularly colectomy, were often included. And finally, a number of investigators performed their analyses without taking into account the duration of disease or, more importantly, the extent of colonic involvement for this often segmental disease. Together, these factors resulted in a long-held belief

that Crohn's disease carried a *lower* risk for colon cancer than ulcerative colitis. Other studies [126–129] and even reanalysis of original data in which only subjects with long-standing and anatomically substantial Crohn's colitis were examined [130] demonstrated that Crohn's *colitis* harbored a CRC risk increase similar to that of ulcerative colitis and that both greater duration of colitis and greater length of involved colon increased the risk. As with UC, earlier disease onset resulted in even greater increases in relative risk of CRC, likely as a function decreased risk in the rate of sporadic CRC used in the denominator of these calculations. Population-based studies from separate continents have demonstrated a clear increase in CRC rates not only when limited to cases of Crohn's colitis, but even when all patients with Crohn's disease are considered [29, 131]. A recent meta-analysis by Canavan and colleagues calculated a pooled estimate of CRC relative risk to be 2.5 (95% CI: 1.3 to 4.7) for all patients with Crohn's disease, culled from 12 published manuscripts; for patients with colonic disease (in the 4 reports where it was available), the pooled RR was 4.5 (95% CI: 1.3 to 14.9) [132]. Clearly patients with Crohn's have a higher risk than the general population.

Similarities Between CRC in Crohn and UC and Rationale Behind Recommendation for Surveillance

In addition to the greater rate and earlier appearance of CRC in Crohn's colitis when compared to the general population, investigators have noted other important similarities between Crohn's-related CRC and UC-related CRC [133]. These include:

- A higher proportion of mucinous and signet-ring histology
- A greater proportion of synchronous lesions compared to sporadic CRC
- Similar survival rates once detected (also true of sporadic CRC)
- Presence of tumor in areas of macroscopic disease (although this point remains in question for Crohn's disease)
- Presence of dysplasia adjacent to and distant from tumor suggesting a field effect

This latter feature has led a number of experts to recommend a strategy of serial surveillance colonoscopy for patients with long-standing, extensive Crohn's colitis as is performed and recommended for UC patients. To date, only one single-practice-based retrospective Crohn's surveillance program has been reported in the literature [134]. In this study, Friedman and colleagues demonstrated both the feasibility and practicality of surveillance in Crohn's patients with colitis affecting at least 1/3 of their colon for a minimum of 8 years. The authors detected dysplasia or cancer in 16% of their 259 patients over a 16-year period, in which 663 examinations were performed; there were no cancer deaths [134]. As this is the only available study describing a surveillance program in Crohn's disease and there is no available control arm (i.e., no surveillance) against which to compare mortality rates, the efficacy of surveillance in Crohn's disease is not yet established. Nevertheless, it has been recommended that all patients with extensive Crohn's colitis (greater than one-third of colon involved) undergo periodic surveillance or be recommended prophylactic surgery after 8 years of disease, as is done with extensive ulcerative colitis. Guidelines have suggested that practices used in surveillance should be similar to those demonstrated to be able to rule out dysplasia in ulcerative colitis [4]. The effects of agents thought to be chemopreventive in UC are untested in Crohn's disease.

Crohn's Disease and Adenocarcinoma of the Small Intestine

As with colonic adenocarcinoma in Crohn's colitis, an increased risk of small intestine adenocarcinoma has been demonstrated in patients with small bowel Crohn's. Unlike colorectal cancer, the second most common lethal malignancy in the USA, adenocarcinoma of the small intestine is uncommon. Even when evaluated in population-based reports, absolute numbers are quite small, with the largest such series having only 5 patients with small bowel adenocarcinoma [29]. A summary of these studies is presented in Table 55.2. Since the absolute rate for these cancers is so small and the best means of prevention is uncertain if a preclinical, precancerous finding were detected, it would be impractical to perform screening and surveillance in all patients with small bowel Crohn's disease. When there is a change in clinical symptoms or a change in barium exams, however, the possibility of a small bowel malignancy should be entertained, particularly in a patient with long-standing disease.

Table 55.2 Small intestinal cancer and Crohn's disease

Year	Author	Subjects	Cases	Risk/odds	95% CI
1992	Ekbom [131]	1655	1	3.4	0.1–18.6
1993	Munkholm [125]	373	2	50	37.1–65.9
1994	Persson [135]	1251	4	15.6	4.7–40.1
2001	Bernstein [29]	2857	5	17.4	4.2–72.9

95% CI = 95 percent confidence interval

Other Malignancies

Following case reports and series of extraintestinal malignancies, investigators questioned whether certain neoplasms might be related to either the presence or treatment of IBD. Greenstein and colleagues performed one of the first studies in which relative risks were calculated [136]. Using patients hospitalized for IBD at a tertiary care hospital, the authors determined that there was an increased incidence of leukemias, lymphomas, and squamous cell cancers when compared to published population-based controls [136]. Given the source of their sampling, a likelihood of selection and detection biases must be considered. Other referral-based studies examining this issue have demonstrated increased incidence of leukemias [137, 138] as well as bile duct [37] and endometrial cancers [37]. Despite the large number of Crohn's and ulcerative colitis patients, low absolute numbers of extraintestinal malignancies with broad confidence intervals have resulted in claims of "significance," when one less case would have resulted in "no significance." Ultimately, population-based analyses of cancer incidence in IBD have replaced the center-specific studies with their inherent biases. One such population-based study came from Ekbom and colleagues who determined that in a cohort from Uppsala, Sweden, there was no increase in the incidence of leukemias, lymphomas, bile duct cancers, or uterine cancers [131]. However, an increase was noted in connective tissue cancers and squamous cell cancers of the skin as well as brain cancers among patients with extensive ulcerative colitis [131]. It is worth noting, however, that no adjustments were made for the multiple comparisons in Ekbom's studies. Other population-based studies have also failed to detect an increased number of extraintestinal malignancies. These include another Swedish study in which Crohn's patients from Stockholm county were analyzed [135]—only a slight increase in bladder cancer was found, and no increase in leukemias, lymphomas, bile duct cancers, or endometrial cancers was demonstrated—and one from North America [29]. In this latter population-based study from Manitoba, Canada, that included over 6000 IBD subjects, Bernstein and colleagues found an increase in liver and biliary tumors in both Crohn's and ulcerative colitis (with only five such cases) and a small increase in lymphomas only among men with Crohn's disease. As increased rates of lymphoma and other hematologic malignancies have been raised as possible adverse effects of either azathioprine or 6-mercaptopurine use in other conditions [139–141] and rates of these malignancies have been calculated in series from large referral practices and centers [142, 143], it is notable that Bernstein and colleagues demonstrated *no* relation to an increased risk of hematologic malignancies and purine analogue use, the first population-based data set to do so [29]. More recently, rare lymphomas (hepatosplenic T-cell lymphomas), particularly in younger patients, have been noted with anti-TNF therapy particularly in combination with purine analogue immunomodulators [144]. This topic is reviewed elsewhere in this volume.

Summary

Colorectal cancer remains a major threat to patients with long-standing ulcerative colitis and Crohn's colitis. Due to patients' and physicians' desires to avoid unnecessary surgery, prophylactic colectomies are rarely performed in these patients. Instead, caregivers and IBD patients tend to elect a program of dysplasia surveillance in an effort to simultaneously minimize cancer mortality and unnecessary colectomies. Although only circumstantial evidence supports the use of such a strategy as a means of reducing CRC-related mortality, dysplasia surveillance will remain the standard of care until better tests are available. Extra caution should be given to pediatric patients whose relative risk and lifetime risk of cancer is increased. Small intestinal cancer occurs at an increased rate in patients with Crohn's enteritis, but the absolute risk remains small. Extraintestinal malignancies are uncommon in IBD but lymphomas, biliary tract cancers, and squamous cell cancers of the skin may occur at an increased rate in IBD patients. The mechanisms for all of these processes remain elusive, but it is hoped that advances in molecular medicine will help to unravel these issues in the future.

References

1. Itzkowitz SH, Yio X. Inflammation and cancer IV. Colorectal cancer in inflammatory bowel disease: the role of inflammation. Am J Physiol Gastrointest Liver Physiol. 2004;287:G7–17.
2. Leowardi C, Schneider ML, Hinz U, Harnoss JM, Taratino I, Lasitschka F, Ulrich A, Büchler MW, Kadmon M. Prognosis of ulcerative colitis-associated colorectal carcinoma compared to sporadic colorectal carcinoma: a matched pair analysis. Ann Surg Oncol. 2016;23(3):870–6.
3. Itzkowitz SH. Inflammatory bowel disease and cancer. Gastroenterol Clin North Am. 1997;26:129–39.
4. Itzkowitz SH, Harpaz N. Diagnosis and management of dysplasia in patients with inflammatory bowel diseases. Gastroenterology. 2004;126:1634–48.
5. Yaeger R, Shah MA et al. Gastroenterology, 2016 – PMID 27063727.
6. Brentnall TA, Crispin DA, Rabinovitch PS, Haggitt RC, Rubin CE, Stevens AC, Burmer GC. Mutations in the p53 gene: an early marker of neoplastic progression in ulcerative colitis. Gastroenterology. 1994;107:369–78.
7. Brentnall TA, Crispin DA, Bronner MP, Cherian SP, Hueffed M, Rabinovitch PS, Rubin CE, Haggitt RC, Boland CR. Microsatellite instability in nonneoplastic mucosa from patients with chronic ulcerative colitis. Cancer Res. 1996;56:1237–40.
8. Suzuki H, Harpaz N, Tarmin L, Yin J, Jiang HY, Bell JD, Hontanosas M, Groisman GM, Abraham JM, Meltzer SJ. Microsatellite instability in ulcerative colitis-associated colorectal dysplasias and cancers. Cancer Res. 1994;54:4841–4.
9. Muller PA, Vousden KH. Mutant p53 in cancer: new functions and therapeutic opportunities. Cancer Cell. 2014;25:304–17.
10. Cooks T, Pateras IS, Tarcic O, et al. Mutant p53 prolongs NF-kappaB activation and promotes chronic inflammation and inflammation-associated colorectal cancer. Cancer Cell. 2013;23:634–46.
11. Hartman DJ, Binion D, Regueiro M, et al. Isocitrate dehydrogenase-1 is mutated in inflammatory bowel disease-associated intestinal adenocarcinoma with low-grade tubuloglandular histology but not in sporadic intestinal adenocarcinoma. Am J Surg Pathol. 2014;38:1147–56.
12. Cancer Genome Atlas N. Comprehensive molecular characterization of human colon and rectal cancer. Nature. 2012;487:330–7.
13. Ross JS, Wang K, Khaira D, et al. Comprehensive genomic profiling of clinically advanced colorectal carcinoma to reveal frequent opportunities for targeted therapies. J Clin Oncol. 2015; 33:abstr 3553
14. Dang L, White DW, Gross S, et al. Cancer-associated IDH1 mutations produce 2-hydroxyglutarate. Nature. 2009;462(7274):739–44.
15. Turcan S, Rohle D, Goenka A, et al. IDH1 mutation is sufficient to establish the glioma hypermethylator phenotype. Nature. 2012;483(7390):479–83. doi:10.1038/nature10866.
16. Crohn BB, Rosenberg H. The sigmoidoscopic picture of chronic ulcerative colitis. Am J Med Sci. 1925;170:220–8.
17. Bargen TA. Chronic ulcerative colitis associated with malignant disease. Arch Surg. 1928;17:862–8.
18. Devroede GJ, Taylor WF, Sauer WG, Jackman RJ, Stickler GB. Cancer risk and life expectancy of children with ulcerative colitis. N Engl J Med. 1971;285:17–21.
19. Bargen JA, Gage RP. Carcinoma and ulcerative colitis: prognosis. Gastroenterology. 1960;39:385–92.
20. Slaney G, Brooke BN. Cancer in ulcerative colitis. Lancet. 1959;2:694–8.
21. Rozen P et al. Low incidence of significant dysplasia in a successful endoscopic surveillance program of patients with ulcerative colitis. Gastroenterology. 1995;108:1361–70.
22. Ekbom A, Helmick C, Zack M, Adami HO. Ulcerative colitis and colorectal cancer. A population-based study. N Engl J Med. 1990;323:1228–33.
23. Gilat T, Fireman Z, Grossman A, Hacohen D, Kadish U, Ron E, Rozen P, Lilos P. Colorectal cancer in patients with ulcerative colitis. A population study in central Israel. Gastroenterology. 1988;94:870–7.
24. Leidenius M, Kellokumpu I, Husa A, Riihela M, Sipponen P. Dysplasia and carcinoma in longstanding ulcerative colitis: an endoscopic and histological surveillance programme. Gut. 1991;32:1521–5.
25. Langholz E, Munkholm P, Davidsen M, Binder V. Colorectal cancer risk and mortality in patients with ulcerative colitis. Gastroenterology. 1992;103:1444–51.
26. Eaden JA, Abrams KR, Mayberry JF. The risk of colorectal cancer in ulcerative colitis: a meta-analysis. Gut. 2001;48:526–35.
27. Winther KV, Jess T, Langholz E, Munkholm P, Binder V. Long-term risk of cancer in ulcerative colitis: a population-based cohort study from Copenhagen County. Clin Gastroenterol Hepatol. 2004;2:1088–95.
28. Lakatos L, Mester G, Erdelyi Z, David G, Pandur T, Balogh M, Fischer S, Vargha P, Lakatos PL. Risk factors for ulcerative colitis-associated colorectal cancer in a Hungarian cohort of patients with ulcerative colitis: results of a population-based study. Inflamm Bowel Dis. 2006;12:205–11.
29. Bernstein CN, Blanchard JF, Kliewer E, Wajda A. Cancer risk in patients with inflammatory bowel disease: a population-based study. Cancer. 2001;91:854–62.

30. Jess T, Loftus Jr EV, Velayos FS, Harmsen WS, Zinsmeister AR, Smyrk TC, Schleck CD, Tremaine WJ, Melton LJ, Munkholm P, Sandborn WJ. Risk of intestinal cancer in inflammatory bowel disease: a population-based study from olmsted county, Minnesota. Gastroenterology. 2006;130:1039–46.

31. Rutter MD, Saunders BP, Wilkinson KH, Rumbles S, Schofield G, Kamm MA, Williams CB, Price AB, Talbot IC, Forbes A. Thirty-year analysis of a colonoscopic surveillance program for neoplasia in ulcerative colitis. Gastroenterology. 2006;130:1030–8.

32. Edwards F, Truelove S. The course and prognosis of ulcerative colitis III and IV. Gut. 1964;5:1.

33. Gyde SN, Prior P, Allan RN, Stevens A, Jewell DP, Truelove SC, Lofberg R, Brostrom O, Hellers G. Colorectal cancer in ulcerative colitis: a cohort study of primary referrals from three centres. Gut. 1988;29:206–17.

34. Greenstein AJ, Sachar DB, Smith H, Pucillo A, Papatestas AE, Kreel I, Geller SA, Janowitz HD, Aufses Jr AH. Cancer in universal and left-sided ulcerative colitis: factors determining risk. Gastroenterology. 1979;77:290–4.

35. Langholz E, Munkholm P, Davidsen M, Nielsen OH, Binder V. Changes in extent of ulcerative colitis: a study on the course and prognostic factors. Scand J Gastroenterol. 1996;31:260–6.

36. Katzka I, Brody RS, Morris E, Katz S. Assessment of colorectal cancer risk in patients with ulcerative colitis: experience from a private practice. Gastroenterology. 1983;85:22–9.

37. Mir-Madjlessi SH, Farmer RG, Easley KA, Beck GJ. Colorectal and extracolonic malignancy in ulcerative colitis. Cancer. 1986;58:1569–74.

38. Mathy C, Schneider K, Chen YY, Varma M, Terdiman JP, Mahadevan U. Gross versus microscopic pancolitis and the occurrence of neoplasia in ulcerative colitis. Inflamm Bowel Dis. 2003;9:351–5.

39. Gurbuz AK, Giardiello FM, Bayless TM. Colorectal neoplasia in patients with ulcerative colitis and primary sclerosing cholangitis. Dis Colon Rectum. 1995;38:37–41.

40. Loftus Jr EV, Sandborn WJ, Tremaine WJ, Mahoney DW, Zinsmeister AR, Offord KP, Melton LJ. Risk of colorectal neoplasia in patients with primary sclerosing cholangitis. Gastroenterology. 1996;110:432–40.

41. Nuako KW, Ahlquist DA, Sandborn WJ, Mahoney DW, Siems DM, Zinsmeister AR. Primary sclerosing cholangitis and colorectal carcinoma in patients with chronic ulcerative colitis: a case-control study. Cancer. 1998;82:822–6.

42. Brentnall TA, Haggitt RC, Rabinovitch PS, Kimmey MB, Bronner MP, Levine DS, Kowdley KV, Stevens AC, Crispin DA, Emond M, Rubin CE. Risk and natural history of colonic neoplasia in patients with primary sclerosing cholangitis and ulcerative colitis. Gastroenterology. 1996;110:331–8.

43. Broome U, Lindberg G, Lofberg R. Primary sclerosing cholangitis in ulcerative colitis – a risk factor for the development of dysplasia and DNA aneuploidy? Gastroenterology. 1992;102:1877–80.

44. Broome U, Lofberg R, Veress B, Eriksson LS. Primary sclerosing cholangitis and ulcerative colitis: evidence for increased neoplastic potential. Hepatology. 1995;22:1404–8.

45. D'Haens GR, Lashner BA, Hanauer SB. Pericholangitis and sclerosing cholangitis are risk factors for dysplasia and cancer in ulcerative colitis. Am J Gastroenterol. 1993;88:1174–8.

46. Marchesa P, Lashner BA, Lavery IC, Milsom J, Hull TL, Strong SA, Church JM, Navarro G, Fazio VW. The risk of cancer and dysplasia among ulcerative colitis patients with primary sclerosing cholangitis. Am J Gastroenterol. 1997;92:1285–8.

47. Kornfeld D, Ekbom A, Ihre T. Is there an excess risk for colorectal cancer in patients with ulcerative colitis and concomitant primary sclerosing cholangitis? A population based study. Gut. 1997;41:522–5.

48. Burt RW. Familial risk and colorectal cancer. Gastroenterol Clin North Am. 1996;25:793–803.

49. Lashner BA, Heidenreich PA, Su GL, Kane SV, Hanauer SB. Effect of folate supplementation on the incidence of dysplasia and cancer in chronic ulcerative colitis. A case-control study. Gastroenterology. 1989;97:255–9.

50. Lashner BA, Provencher KS, Seidner DL, Knesebeck A, Brzezinski A. The effect of folic acid supplementation on the risk for cancer or dysplasia in ulcerative colitis. Gastroenterology. 1997;112:29–32.

51. Nuako KW, Ahlquist DA, Mahoney DW, Schaid DJ, Siems DM, Lindor NM. Familial predisposition for colorectal cancer in chronic ulcerative colitis: a case-control study. Gastroenterology. 1998;115:1079–83.

52. Askling J, Dickman PW, Karlen P, Brostrom O, Lapidus A, Lofberg R, Ekbom A. Family history as a risk factor for colorectal cancer in inflammatory bowel disease. Gastroenterology. 2001;120:1356–62.

53. Eaden J, Abrams K, Ekbom A, Jackson E, Mayberry J. Colorectal cancer prevention in ulcerative colitis: a case-control study. Aliment Pharmacol Ther. 2000;14:145–53.

54. Rutter M, Saunders B, Wilkinson K, et al. Severity of inflammation is a risk factor for colorectal neoplasia in ulcerative colitis. Gastroenterology. 2004;126:451–9.

55. Gupta RB, Harpaz N, Itzkowitz S, et al. Histologic inflammation is a risk factor for progression to colorectal neoplasia in ulcerative colitis: a cohort study. Gastroenterology. 2007;133:1099–105.

56. Pinczowski D, Ekbom A, Baron J, Yuen J, Adami HO. Risk factors for colorectal cancer in patients with ulcerative colitis: a case-control study. Gastroenterology. 1994;107:117–20.

57. Tung BY, Emond MJ, Haggitt RC, Bronner MP, Kimmey MB, Kowdley KV, Brentnall TA. Ursodiol use is associated with lower prevalence of colonic neoplasia in patients with ulcerative colitis and primary sclerosing cholangitis. Ann Intern Med. 2001;134:89–95.

58. van Staa TP, Card T, Logan RF, Leufkens HG. 5-Aminosalicylate use and colorectal cancer risk in inflammatory bowel disease: a large epidemiological study. Gut. 2005;54:1573–8.

59. Rubin DT, LoSavio A, Yadron N, Huo D, Hanauer SB. Aminosalicylate therapy in the prevention of dysplasia and colorectal cancer in ulcerative colitis. Clin Gastroenterol Hepatol. 2006;4:1346–50.

60. Bernstein CN, Blanchard JF, Metge C, Yogendran M. Does the use of 5-aminosalicylates in inflammatory bowel disease prevent the development of colorectal cancer? Am J Gastroenterol. 2003;98:2784–8.

61. Terdiman JP, Steinbuch M, Blumentals WA, Ullman TA, Rubin DT. 5-Aminosalicylic acid therapy and the risk of colorectal cancer among patients with inflammatory bowel disease. Inflamm Bowel Dis. 2007;13:367–71.

62. Velayos FS, Terdiman JP, Walsh JM. Effect of 5-aminosalicylate use on colorectal cancer and dysplasia risk: a systematic review and metaanalysis of observational studies. Am J Gastroenterol. 2005;100:1345–53.

63. Ullman T, Croog V, Harpaz N, et al. Progression to colorectal neoplasia in ulcerative colitis: effect of mesalamine. Clin Gastroenterol Hepatol. 2008;6:1225–30.

64. Pardi DS, Loftus Jr EV, Kremers WK, Keach J, Lindor KD. Ursodeoxycholic acid as a chemopreventive agent in patients with ulcerative colitis and primary sclerosing cholangitis. Gastroenterology. 2003;124:889–93.

65. Eaton JE, Silveira MG, Pardi DS, Sinakos E, Kowdley KV, Luketic VA, Harrison ME, McCashland T, Befeler AS, Harnois D, Jorgensen R, Petz J, Lindor KD. High-dose ursodeoxycholic acid is associated with the development of colorectal neoplasia in

patients with ulcerative colitis and primary sclerosing cholangitis. Am J Gastroenterol. 2011;106(9):1638–45.

66. Laine L, Kaltenbach T, Barkun A, et al. SCENIC international consensus statement on surveillance and management of dysplasia in inflammatory bowel disease. Gastroenterology. 2015;148(3):639–51. e628

67. Choi PM, Nugent FW, Schoetz Jr DJ, Silverman ML, Haggitt RC. Colonoscopic surveillance reduces mortality from colorectal cancer in ulcerative colitis. Gastroenterology. 1993;105:418–24.

68. Connell WR, Lennard-Jones JE, Williams CB, Talbot IC, Price AB, Wilkinson KH. Factors affecting the outcome of endoscopic surveillance for cancer in ulcerative colitis. Gastroenterology. 1994;107:934–44.

69. Becker JM. Surgical therapy for ulcerative colitis and Crohn's disease. Gastroenterol Clin North Am. 1999;28:371–90. viii-ix

70. Stern H, Walfisch S, Mullen B, McLeod R, Cohen Z. Cancer in an ileoanal reservoir: a new late complication? Gut. 1990;31:473–5.

71. Thompson-Fawcett MW, Marcus V, Redston M, Cohen Z, McLeod RS. Risk of dysplasia in long-term ileal pouches and pouches with chronic pouchitis. Gastroenterology. 2001;121:275–81.

72. Morson BC, Pang LS. Rectal biopsy as an aid to cancer control in ulcerative colitis. Gut. 1967;8:423–34.

73. Cook MG, Goligher JC. Carcinoma and epithelial dysplasia complicating ulcerative colitis. Gastroenterology. 1975;68:1127–36.

74. Ransohoff DF, Riddell RH, Levin B. Ulcerative colitis and colonic cancer. Problems in assessing the diagnostic usefulness of mucosal dysplasia. Dis Colon Rectum. 1985;28:383–8.

75. Taylor BA, Pemberton JH, Carpenter HA, Levin KE, Schroeder KW, Welling DR, Spencer MP, Zinsmeister AR. Dysplasia in chronic ulcerative colitis: implications for colonoscopic surveillance. Dis Colon Rectum. 1992;35:950–6.

76. Dickinson RJ, Dixon MF, Axon AT. Colonoscopy and the detection of dysplasia in patients with longstanding ulcerative colitis. Lancet. 1980;2:620–2.

77. Levin B, Lennard-Jones J, Riddell RH, Sachar D, Winawer SJ. Surveillance of patients with chronic ulcerative colitis. WHO Collaborating Centre for the Prevention of Colorectal Cancer. Bull World Health Organ. 1991;69:121–6.

78. Kornbluth A, Sachar DB. Ulcerative colitis practice guidelines in adults. American College of Gastroenterology, Practice Parameters Committee. Am J Gastroenterol. 1997;92:204–11.

79. Brostrom O, Lofberg R, Ost A, Reichard H. Cancer surveillance of patients with longstanding ulcerative colitis: a clinical, endoscopical, and histological study. Gut. 1986;27:1408–13.

80. Blackstone MO, Riddell RH, Rogers BH, Levin B. Dysplasia-associated lesion or mass (DALM) detected by colonoscopy in long-standing ulcerative colitis: an indication for colectomy. Gastroenterology. 1981;80:366–74.

81. Lashner BA, Silverstein MD, Hanauer SB. Hazard rates for dysplasia and cancer in ulcerative colitis. Results from a surveillance program. Dig Dis Sci. 1989;34:1536–41.

82. Lashner BA, Kane SV, Hanauer SB. Colon cancer surveillance in chronic ulcerative colitis: historical cohort study. Am J Gastroenterol. 1990;85:1083–7.

83. Lennard-Jones JE, Morson BC, Ritchie JK, Shove DC, Williams CB. Cancer in colitis: assessment of the individual risk by clinical and histological criteria. Gastroenterology. 1977;73:1280–9.

84. Lennard-Jones JE, Melville DM, Morson BC, Ritchie JK, Williams CB. Precancer and cancer in extensive ulcerative colitis: findings among 401 patients over 22 years. Gut. 1990;31:800–6.

85. Lofberg R, Brostrom O, Karlen P, Tribukait B, Ost A. Colonoscopic surveillance in long-standing total ulcerative colitis – a 15-year follow-up study. Gastroenterology. 1990;99:1021–31.

86. Lynch DA, Lobo AJ, Sobala GM, Dixon MF, Axon AT. Failure of colonoscopic surveillance in ulcerative colitis. Gut. 1993;34:1075–80.

87. Nugent FW, Haggitt RC, Gilpin PA. Cancer surveillance in ulcerative colitis. Gastroenterology. 1991;100:1241–8.

88. Rutegard J, Ahsgren L, Stenling R, Janunger KG. Ulcerative colitis. Cancer surveillance in an unselected population. Scand J Gastroenterol. 1988;23:139–45.

89. Woolrich AJ, DaSilva MD, Korelitz BI. Surveillance in the routine management of ulcerative colitis: the predictive value of low-grade dysplasia. Gastroenterology. 1992;103:431–8.

90. Karlen P, Kornfeld D, Brostrom O, Lofberg R, Persson PG, Ekbom A. Is colonoscopic surveillance reducing colorectal cancer mortality in ulcerative colitis? A population based case control study. Gut. 1998;42:711–4.

91. Velayos FS, Loftus Jr EV, Jess T, Harmsen WS, Bida J, Zinsmeister AR, Tremaine WJ, Sandborn WJ. Predictive and protective factors associated with colorectal cancer in ulcerative colitis: a case-control study. Gastroenterology. 2006;130:1941–9.

92. Gage TP. Managing the cancer risk in chronic ulcerative colitis. A decision- analytic approach. J Clin Gastroenterol. 1986;8:50–7.

93. Delco F, Sonnenberg A. A decision analysis of surveillance for colorectal cancer in ulcerative colitis. Gut. 2000;46:500–6.

94. Inadomi JM. Cost-effectiveness of colorectal cancer surveillance in ulcerative colitis. Scand J Gastroenterol Suppl. 2003;237: 17–21.

95. Provenzale D, Kowdley KV, Arora S, Wong JB. Prophylactic colectomy or surveillance for chronic ulcerative colitis? A decision analysis. Gastroenterology. 1995;109:1188–96.

96. Riddell RH, Goldman H, Ransohoff DF, Appelman HD, Fenoglio CM, Haggitt RC, Ahren C, Correa P, Hamilton SR, Morson BC, et al. Dysplasia in inflammatory bowel disease: standardized classification with provisional clinical applications. Hum Pathol. 1983;14:931–68.

97. Eaden J, Abrams K, McKay H, Denley H, Mayberry J. Inter-observer variation between general and specialist gastrointestinal pathologists when grading dysplasia in ulcerative colitis. J Pathol. 2001;194:152–7.

98. Dixon MF, Brown LJ, Gilmour HM, Price AB, Smeeton NC, Talbot IC, Williams GT. Observer variation in the assessment of dysplasia in ulcerative colitis. Histopathology. 1988;13:385–97.

99. Melville DM, Jass JR, Morson BC, Pollock DJ, Richman PI, Shepherd NA, Ritchie JK, Love SB, Lennard-Jones JE. Observer study of the grading of dysplasia in ulcerative colitis: comparison with clinical outcome. Hum Pathol. 1989;20:1008–14.

100. Connell WR, Talbot IC, Harpaz N, Britto N, Wilkinson KH, Kamm MA, Lennard-Jones JE. Clinicopathological characteristics of colorectal carcinoma complicating ulcerative colitis. Gut. 1994;35:1419–23.

101. Ullman TA, Loftus Jr EV, Kakar S, Burgart LJ, Sandborn WJ, Tremaine WJ. The fate of low grade dysplasia in ulcerative colitis. Am J Gastroenterol. 2002;97:922–7.

102. Ullman T, Croog V, Harpaz N, Sachar D, Itzkowitz S. Progression of flat low-grade dysplasia to advanced neoplasia in patients with ulcerative colitis. Gastroenterology. 2003;125:1311–9.

103. Brentnall T, Bronner M, Rubin C, Rabinovitch P, Kimmey M, Kowdley K, Edmond M, Haggitt R. Natural history and management of low-grade dysplasia in ulcerative colitis. Gastroenterology. 1999;116:A382.

104. Befrits R, Ljung T, Jaramillo E, Rubio C. Low grade dysplasia in flat colonic mucosa in patients with extensive longstanding inflammatory bowel disease - a follow-up study. Gastroenterology. 1999;116:A376.

105. Befrits R, Ljung T, Jaramillo E, Rubio C. Low-grade dysplasia in extensive, long-standing inflammatory bowel disease: a follow-up study. Dis Colon Rectum. 2002;45:615–20.

106. Lim CH, Dixon MF, Vail A, Forman D, Lynch DA, Axon AT. Ten year follow up of ulcerative colitis patients with and without low grade dysplasia. Gut. 2003;52:1127–32.

107. Pekow JR, Hetzel JT, Rothe JA, Hanauer SB, Turner JR, Hart J, Noffsinger A, Huo D, Rubin DT. Outcome after surveillance of low-grade and indefinite dysplasia in patients with ulcerative colitis. Inflamm Bowel Dis. 2010;16(8):1352–6.
108. Rubin CE, Haggitt RC, Burmer GC, Brentnall TA, Stevens AC, Levine DS, Dean PJ, Kimmey M, Perera DR, Rabinovitch PS. DNA aneuploidy in colonic biopsies predicts future development of dysplasia in ulcerative colitis. Gastroenterology. 1992;103:1611–20.
109. Eaden JA, Ward BA, Mayberry JF. How gastroenterologists screen for colonic cancer in ulcerative colitis: an analysis of performance. Gastrointest Endosc. 2000;51:123–8.
110. Ullman T, White J, Harpaz N, Itzkowitz S. Assessment of biopsy practices in colonoscopic surveillance in ulcerative colitis. Gastroenterology. 2001;120:A-446.
111. Rubin PH et al. Colonoscopic polypectomy in chronic colitis: conservative management after endoscopic resection of dysplastic polyps. Gastroenterology. 1999;117:1295–300.
112. Engelsgjerd M, Farraye FA, Odze RD. Polypectomy may be adequate treatment for adenoma-like dysplastic lesions in chronic ulcerative colitis. Gastroenterology. 1999;117:1288–94. discussion 1488-91
113. Odze RD, Farraye FA, Hecht JL, Hornick JL. Long-term follow-up after polypectomy treatment for adenoma-like dysplastic lesions in ulcerative colitis. Clin Gastroenterol Hepatol. 2004;2:534–41.
114. Goldstone R, Itzkowitz S, Harpaz N, Ullman T. Progression of low-grade dysplasia in ulcerative colitis: effect of colonic location. Gastrointest Endosc. 2011;74(5):1087–93.
115. Vieth M, Behrens H, Stolte M. Sporadic adenoma in ulcerative colitis: endoscopic resection is an adequate treatment. Gut. 2006;55:1151–5.
116. Selaru FM, Xu Y, Yin J, Zou T, Liu TC, Mori Y, Abraham JM, Sato F, Wang S, Twigg C, Olaru A, Shustova V, Leytin A, Hytiroglou P, Shibata D, Harpaz N, Meltzer SJ. Artificial neural networks distinguish among subtypes of neoplastic colorectal lesions. Gastro. 2002;122:606–13.
117. Bernstein CN, Weinstein WM, Levine DS, Shanahan F. Physicians' perceptions of dysplasia and approaches to surveillance colonoscopy in ulcerative colitis. Am J Gastroenterol. 1995;90:2106–14.
118. Rubin DT, Turner JR. Surveillance of dysplasia in inflammatory bowel disease: The gastroenterologist-pathologist partnership. Clin Gastroenterol Hepatol. 2006;4:1309–13.
119. Itzkowitz SH, Present DH. Consensus conference: colorectal cancer screening and surveillance in inflammatory bowel disease. Inflamm Bowel Dis. 2005;11:314–21.
120. Farraye FA, Odze RD, Eaden J, Itzkowitz SH, McCabe RP, Dassopoulos T, Lewis JD, Ullman TA, James T, McLeod R, Burgart LJ, Allen J, Brill JV, AGA Institute Medical Position Panel on Diagnosis and Management of Colorectal Neoplasia in Inflammatory Bowel Disease. AGA medical position statement on the diagnosis and management of colorectal neoplasia in inflammatory bowel disease. Gastroenterology. 2010;138(2):738–45.
121. Kiesslich R, Fritsch J, Holtmann M, Koehler HH, Stolte M, Kanzler S, Nafe B, Jung M, Galle PR, Neurath MF. Methylene blue-aided chromoendoscopy for the detection of intraepithelial neoplasia and colon cancer in ulcerative colitis. Gastroenterology. 2003;124:880–8.
122. Rutter MD, Saunders BP, Schofield G, Forbes A, Price AB, Talbot IC. Pancolonic indigo carmine dye spraying for the detection of dysplasia in ulcerative colitis. Gut. 2004;53:256–60.
123. Marion JF, Waye JD, Present DH, Israel Y, Bodian C, Harpaz N, Chapman M, Itzkowitz S, Steinlauf AF, Abreu MT, Ullman TA, Aisenberg J, Mayer L. Chromoendoscopy-targeted biopsies are superior to standard colonoscopic surveillance for detecting dysplasia in inflammatory bowel disease patients: a prospective endoscopic trial. Am J Gastroenterol. 2008;103(9):2342–9.
124. Gollop JH, Phillips SF, Melton LJ, Zinsmeister AR. Epidemiologic aspects of Crohn's disease: a population based study in Olmsted County, Minnesota, 1943-1982. Gut. 1988;29:49–56.
125. Munkholm P, Langholz E, Davidsen M, Binder V. Intestinal cancer risk and mortality in patients with Crohn's disease. Gastroenterology. 1993;105:1716–23.
126. Weedon DD, Shorter RG, Ilstrup DM, Huizenga KA, Taylor WF. Crohn's disease and cancer. N Engl J Med. 1973;289:1099–103.
127. Greenstein AJ, Sachar DB, Smith H, Janowitz HD, Aufses Jr AH. A comparison of cancer risk in Crohn's disease and ulcerative colitis. Cancer. 1981;48:2742–5.
128. Gillen CD, Walmsley RS, Prior P, Andrews HA, Allan RN. Ulcerative colitis and Crohn's disease: a comparison of the colorectal cancer risk in extensive colitis. Gut. 1994;35:1590–2.
129. Ekbom A, Helmick C, Zack M, Adami HO. Increased risk of large-bowel cancer in Crohn's disease with colonic involvement. Lancet. 1990;336:357–9.
130. Sachar DB. Cancer in Crohn's disease: dispelling the myths. Gut. 1994;35:1507–8.
131. Ekbom A, Helmick C, Zack M, Adami HO. Extracolonic malignancies in inflammatory bowel disease. Cancer. 1991;67:2015–9.
132. Canavan C, Abrams KR, Mayberry J. Meta-analysis: colorectal and small bowel cancer risk in patients with Crohn's disease. Aliment Pharmacol Ther. 2006;23:1097–104.
133. Choi PM, Zelig MP. Similarity of colorectal cancer in Crohn's disease and ulcerative colitis: implications for carcinogenesis and prevention. Gut. 1994;35:950–4.
134. Friedman S, Rubin PH, Bodian C, Goldstein E, Harpaz N, Present DH. Screening and surveillance colonoscopy in chronic Crohn's colitis. Gastroenterology. 2001;120:820–6.
135. Persson PG, Karlen P, Bernell O, Leijonmarck CE, Brostrom O, Ahlbom A, Hellers G. Crohn's disease and cancer: a population-based cohort study. Gastroenterology. 1994;107:1675–9.
136. Greenstein AJ, Gennuso R, Sachar DB, Heimann T, Smith H, Janowitz HD, Aufses Jr AH. Extraintestinal cancers in inflammatory bowel disease. Cancer. 1985;56:2914–21.
137. Mir Madjlessi SH, Farmer RG, Weick JK. Inflammatory bowel disease and leukemia. A report of seven cases of leukemia in ulcerative colitis and Crohn's disease and review of the literature. Dig Dis Sci. 1986;31:1025–31.
138. Cuttner J. Increased incidence of acute promyelocytic leukemia in patients with ulcerative colitis. Ann Intern Med. 1982;97:864–5.
139. Wilkinson AH, Smith JL, Hunsicker LG, Tobacman J, Kapelanski DP, Johnson M, Wright FH, Behrendt DM, Corry RJ. Increased frequency of posttransplant lymphomas in patients treated with cyclosporine, azathioprine, and prednisone. Transplantation. 1989;47:293–6.
140. Opelz G, Henderson R. Incidence of non-Hodgkin lymphoma in kidney and heart transplant recipients. Lancet. 1993;342:1514–6.
141. Silman AJ, Petrie J, Hazleman B, Evans SJ. Lymphoproliferative cancer and other malignancy in patients with rheumatoid arthritis treated with azathioprine: a 20 year follow up study. Ann Rheum Dis. 1988;47:988–92.
142. Loftus Jr EV, Tremaine WJ, Habermann TM, Harmsen WS, Zinsmeister AR, Sandborn WJ. Risk of lymphoma in inflammatory bowel disease. Am J Gastroenterol. 2000;95:2308–12.
143. Korelitz BI, Mirsky FJ, Fleisher MR, Warman JI, Wisch N, Gleim GW. Malignant neoplasms subsequent to treatment of inflammatory bowel disease with 6-mercaptopurine. Am J Gastroenterol. 1999;94:3248–53.
144. Mackey AC, Green L, Liang LC, Dinndorf P, Avigan M. Hepatosplenic T cell lymphoma associated with infliximab use in young patients treated for inflammatory bowel disease. J Pediatr Gastroenterol Nutr. 2007;44:265–7.

Quality Improvement in Inflammatory Bowel Disease

56

Jeremy Adler, Richard B. Colletti, Wallace V. Crandall, and Peter A. Margolis

Introduction

In recent decades, research has generated an enormous growth of medical science, technology, and therapeutics. Knowledge from basic research, translational research, randomized clinical trials, and outcomes research has enabled experts in many fields to develop and disseminate evidence-based clinical practice guidelines with recommendations for medical practitioners. Yet health services research suggests that health care could perform a great deal better than it does today. For example, an audit of medical records of 4000 adults in 12 cities in the USA showed that only 55% of recommended preventive, acute, and chronic care was being received [1]. Similar deficits have been observed in ambulatory pediatrics [2]. A study of 3000 hospitals found that for only 5 of 10 measures were recommended care provided to a large majority of patients [3]. A report of the Institute of Medicine, Crossing the Quality Chasm, calls for improvements in six dimensions of health-care performance: safety, timeliness, efficiency, effectiveness, equity, and patient-centeredness (STEEEP) [4]. The National Scorecard on US Health System Performance, an assessment of health-care outcomes, quality, access, equity, and efficiency, found that the USA achieves an average score of only 66%. If the USA improved performance in key areas, an estimated 100,000–150,000 lives and 50–100 billion dollars could be saved annually [5].

To improve the care of patients requires more than knowledge; achievement of improvements requires the application of the principles of continuous quality improvement [6, 7]. Quality improvement in health care is the application of knowledge to make changes that result in better care and outcomes.

One of the barriers to quality improvement is unnecessary variation in care. Unnecessary variation, which erodes quality and reliability and adds to costs, is derived in part from habitual differences in practice style that are not grounded in knowledge or reason [8]. Variation makes it impossible to determine if a change in practice results in change in care because small improvements are frequently obscured by the background noise of variation. Quality improvement efforts can reduce unnecessary variation; reducing variation is a necessary prerequisite to improving quality. To attain continuous quality improvement in health care, it is necessary to repeatedly measure the processes and outcomes of care, design and implement interventions to improve the processes of care, and remeasure to determine the effect of the interventions [9]. In this chapter, we present an introduction to quality improvement and how it has been applied to pediatric inflammatory bowel disease, with brief discussions of variation in care, the chronic illness care model, the need for quality improvement, the improvement model, the improvement collaborative, and the ImproveCareNow (ICN) Network.

J. Adler, MD, MSc (✉)
Department of Pediatrics and Communicable Diseases, Pediatric Inflammatory Bowel Disease Program, C.S. Mott Children's Hospital, University of Michigan Health System
Ann Arbor, MI, USA
e-mail: jeradler@med.umich.edu

R.B. Colletti, MD
Department of Pediatrics, University of Vermont College of Medicine, Burlington, VT, USA

ImproveCareNow, Burlington, VT, USA
e-mail: Richard.Colletti@UVM.edu

W.V. Crandall, MD
Department of Pediatrics, The Ohio State University College of Medicine, Center for Pediatric and Adolescent Inflammatory Bowel Disease, Nationwide Children's Hospital, Columbus, OH, USA
e-mail: Wallace.Crandall@nationwidechildrens.org

P.A. Margolis, MD, PhD
James M. Anderson Center for Health System Excellence, Cincinnati Children's Hospital Medical Center, Cincinnati, OH, USA
e-mail: peter.margolis@cchmc.org

Variation in Care

Inflammatory bowel disease (IBD) is the most common serious chronic gastrointestinal disease afflicting children and adolescents in North America. Yet there is currently considerable variation in the way gastroenterologists diagnose and treat IBD [10, 11]. Variation in care can be due to underuse, overuse, or misuse of diagnostic and therapeutic interventions. An example of underuse is failure to obtain small bowel imaging or neglecting to identify and treat growth failure; an example of overuse is unnecessary prolonged prednisone treatment; and an example of misuse is prescribing infliximab to a patient with tuberculosis. While some variations are due to patient needs or preferences, many variations are due to a lack of adherence by practitioners to best practices. Other variations are due to lack of data to guide practice, leading to different practice strategies based on anecdotal experience or other non-evidence-based reasons [10]. Standardization of care occurs when physicians and other practitioners agree to provide care in a uniform manner of care appropriate for each patient. This can be evidence based or, in the absence of evidence, can be based on expert opinion or consensus. Standardization of care reduces unnecessary variation and, when combined with systematic studies of planned variations (including randomized studies), can lead to increased knowledge and improved outcomes.

Figure 56.1a is a theoretical example of a wide variation in the number of diagnostic tests performed prior to initiating treatment (labeled Before). Performance of larger number of tests than average could indicate the overuse of some tests, while a smaller number than average could indicate underuse. In this example, after a successful quality improvement project leading to less unnecessary variation in care, there is less overuse and less underuse than before, although the average number of tests is the same. Figure 56.1b is a theoretical example of a wide variation and a low percentage of patients at most sites having a skin test for tuberculosis before initiating infliximab therapy (labeled Before). After a successful improve-

ment project, there is less variation and a higher rate of skin testing.

Variation in care has been demonstrated in pediatric IBD [10–12]. In one study, pediatric gastroenterologists enrolled patients with Crohn disease who were starting treatment with a thiopurine (6-mercaptopurine or azathioprine) or infliximab [11]. Data from 250 patients at 80 sites were examined for variation in diagnostic and therapeutic interventions. Diagnostic studies in which care was uniform included complete blood count, performed in 100% of patients, erythrocyte sedimentation rate and colonoscopy in 96%, and upper endoscopy in 89%. However, imaging of the small bowel had not been performed in 19%, and a stool test for pathogens had not been performed in 29%. Thiopurine methyltransferase (TPMT) had been measured in 61% of patients before treatment with a thiopurine; in 85%, TPMT was normal. Nonetheless, even when TPMT was normal, 40% of patients received an initial dose of thiopurine that was lower than recommended. Testing for tuberculosis before initiating treatment with infliximab was not documented in 30%. In addition, 36% of severely underweight patients were not receiving a multivitamin supplement, supplemental formula, or tube feeding [12]. Another study demonstrated widespread intercenter variation in the treatment of newly diagnosed children with Crohn disease, even after adjusting for possible differences in case mix between institutions [12]. Variation in the use of immunomodulators and infliximab in patients with Crohn disease has also been reported [10, 13]. Thus, there is clear documentation of considerable variation in diagnostic and therapeutic care in pediatric IBD, suggesting the presence of underuse, overuse, and potentially misuse of interventions that may lead to unintended differences in health-care costs and outcomes.

Documentation of variation in care has been important in efforts to standardize and improve care in other fields of

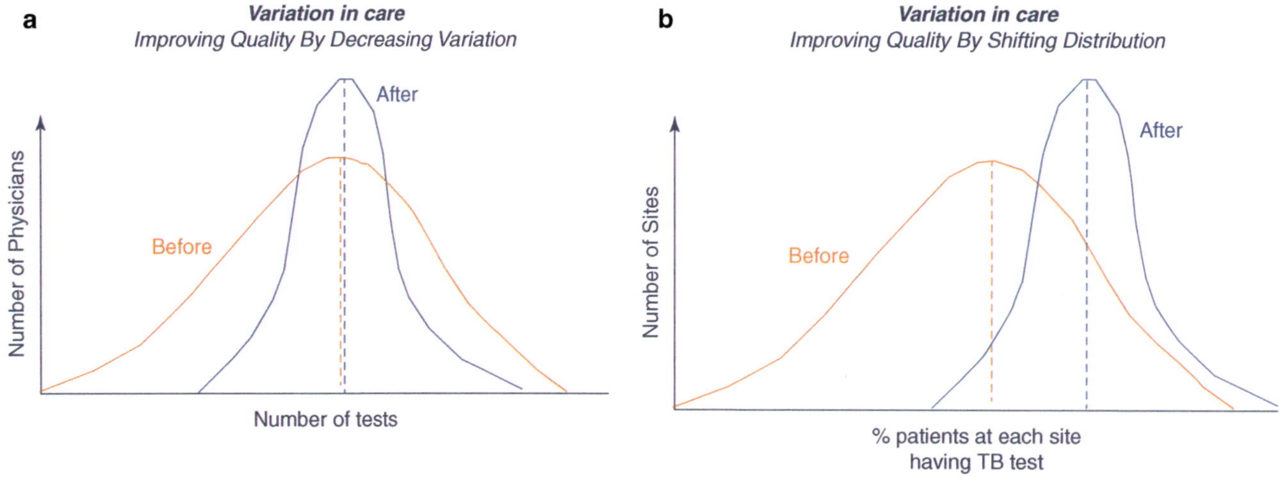

Fig. 56.1 Variation in care. (**a**) Improving quality by decreasing variation. (**b**) Improving quality by shifting distribution

medicine [3]. For example, the Epidemiologic Study of Cystic Fibrosis demonstrated large variations in practice patterns regarding the prescription of various therapies as well as the fact that a significant proportion of cystic fibrosis (CF) patients are not monitored as recommended by the Cystic Fibrosis Foundation (CFF) [14, 15]. In this study, only 58% of patients had quarterly visits to their CF Care Center, 76% had biannual spirometry, 79% had annual airway cultures, and 68% had annual chest radiographs [16]. CF Registry reports are now presented in such a way as to reveal practice variation among practice sites, partly in order to motivate an evaluation of this variation and to promote standardization where indicated.

The Chronic Illness Care Model

The chronic illness care model provides a useful framework for developing changes to the system of IBD care [17, 18]. Wagner and colleagues conducted an exhaustive literature review and program assessment to identify the key components of systems of health-care delivery that result in improved outcomes for patients with chronic illness. Wagner's model includes the following components: family and patient self-management support, decision support, delivery system design, clinical information systems, community resources, and health-care organization (Fig. 56.2). Family and patient self-management support includes the methods used by the clinic to increase families' participation in care. Decision support includes the use of care protocols that are integrated into practice systems. The delivery system design component includes the use of planned encounters,

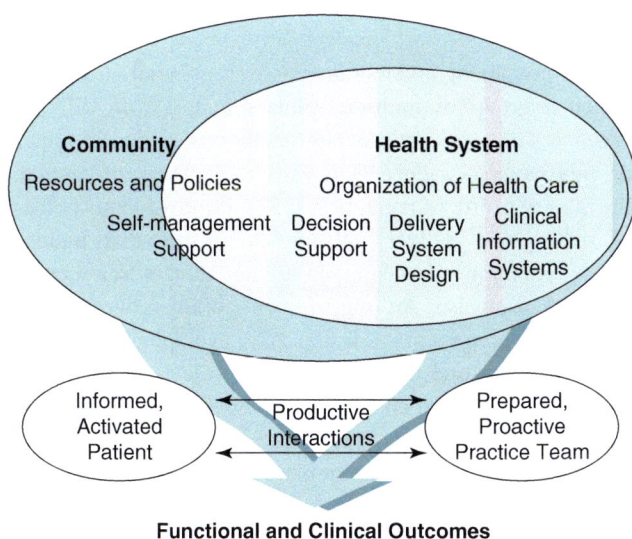

Functional and Clinical Outcomes

Fig. 56.2 The chronic illness care model (Adapted from EH Wagner, Joint Commission Journal on Quality Improvement 2001;27:65, by permission)

clarity in the roles and responsibilities of team members with appropriate training, and the use of regular meetings of the care team to review performance. The clinical information system refers to the ability of caregivers to access data and use registries for care and to provide regular feedback to the team and also information technology to facilitate scheduling and patient tracking. A prepared proactive practice team interacts with an informed activated patient to improve functional and clinical outcomes.

Improvement science is broadly defined as the science of implementing and testing change. There are many different ways in which improvement science is applied in practice. Each involves the common theme of methodically implementing and testing small changes and then adopting or rejecting the changes based on the findings of testing [19]. Improvement interventions can range from prospective randomized controlled trials to observational studies [20]. The application of improvement science has led to major advances in quality in the automobile, microchip, and other industries [21–23]. Does quality improvement work in health care? Quality improvement interventions utilizing the chronic care illness model have improved clinical outcomes, processes of care, and quality of life in asthma, congestive heart failure, depression, and diabetes [24]. Studies of controlled trials of interventions that contain at least one element of the chronic care illness model have demonstrated significant improvements in care [25]. In a cohort study to determine the effect of a specialist nurse on the outcome of 340 patients with IBD, intervention was associated with a 38% reduction in hospital visits, a 19% reduction in hospital length of stay, and a 10% increase in patients in remission and improvement in patient satisfaction [26]. A multicenter randomized controlled trial of a quality improvement project in IBD showed similar results [27]. In the UK, development of a pediatric IBD service has improved provision of services and access to care for patients [28]. In Australia, the implementation of a dedicated IBD service was associated with a reduction in the use of steroids and opiates as well as a reduction in hospitalizations for IBD [29].

The Need for Quality Improvement in IBD

Have Crohn disease outcomes improved during the last four decades? In a report published in 2004, a structured systematic literature review was performed to evaluate measurable outcomes in Crohn disease. Evaluation of mortality, cancer, disease recurrence, extraintestinal manifestations, and medication use failed to show hard evidence for the improvement in disease outcome in Crohn disease during the last four decades [30]. Despite advances in research and therapy, the application of knowledge to the improvement of health outcomes and quality of life has lagged. Hospitalization rates for IBD, particularly Crohn disease, increased from 1988–2011, incurring a substantial rise in inflation-adjusted economic burden [31, 32]. Further, even in the era of biologics, the proportion of patients with inflammatory bowel disease not entering remission remains high [33].

Are patients with IBD receiving optimal care? A study found that adults with IBD referred for a second opinion often were not receiving optimal medical therapy [34]. There was prolonged use of corticosteroids, failure to use steroid-sparing agents, suboptimal dosing of mesalamine and immunomodulatory medications, inadequate measures to prevent metabolic bone disease, and inadequate screening for colorectal cancer.

A study of the diagnostic evaluation of pediatric patients diagnosed with IBD also identified substantial gaps in small bowel imaging, though this was found to improve over the 5-year course of study [35]. Many pediatric patients diagnosed with Crohn disease had not been tested for intestinal pathogens, had not had imaging of the small intestine, were not receiving a multivitamin supplement, had not been tested for TPMT prior to treatment with a thiopurine, had not been tested for tuberculosis prior to treatment with infliximab, and were receiving suboptimal dosage of medications [11].

Quality improvement in adult gastroenterology has previously focused on endoscopic procedures [36–44]. More recently, there has been an emphasis on reducing venous thromboembolic events in hospitalized IBD patients [45, 46]. However, the American Gastroenterological Association (AGA) Task Force on Quality in Practice issued a report recommending the formation of an AGA Quality Center to assure uniform documentable excellence in quality of clinical care and GI practice, to support the aims for quality health care set forth by the Institute of Medicine, to identify key quality of care indicators in the treatment of digestive diseases and how they will be measured, to develop programs and tools to assist in implementing evidence-based guidelines and measuring and reporting adherence to quality indicators, and to develop patient education materials to ensure that patients have appropriate expectations regarding high-quality, patient-centered, evidence-based care [47]. In 2011 the AGA developed a set of IBD process measures, approved by the American Medical Association's Physician Consortium for Performance Improvement, which focus on transitioning patients to corticosteroid-sparing therapy and preventive care. The AGA subsequently developed a series of quality improvement measures called the Physician Quality Reporting System (PQRS) [48]. The North American Society for Pediatric Gastroenterology, Hepatology and Nutrition (NASPGHAN) has also developed a set of process measures. In conjunction with measure development, the AGA has also developed the Digestive Health Outcome Registry (DHOR) to help practices develop benchmarking, outcomes measurement, and population management capabilities for patients with IBD [49].

The Improvement Model

The improvement model is the foundation of a system for innovation and a framework for developing, testing, and implementing incremental change [50]. The model is based on three questions (Fig. 56.3): What are we trying to accomplish? How will we know that a change is an improvement? What change can we make that will result in improvement? Any approach to improvement must be based on building and applying knowledge. Within the overall framework, the plan-do-study-act (PDSA) cycle is a structured application of the scientific method that provides a means to learn rapidly in complex organizational settings. The plan phase consists of stating the objective of the test, making predictions, and developing a plan to carry out the test. The do phase consists of carrying out the test, documenting problems and unexpected observations, and beginning an analysis of the data. The study phase consists of completing the analysis of the data, comparing the test data to predictions, and summarizing what was learned. The act phase consists of deciding upon and carrying out the changes to be made and considering what will be the objective of the next cycle. The improvement model means applying the principles of using data; developing, testing, and implementing changes; and working collaboratively to bring about improvement in the outcomes of health care (Fig. 56.4). The improvement model can be applied to any aspect of health care.

The Improvement Collaborative

An improvement collaborative is a sequential process in which a group of multidisciplinary teams from different practice sites work intensively together using the principals of improvement science to improve the delivery of care and the quality of life of patients [51, 52]. Improvements consist of redesigning delivery systems to ensure that patients receive recommended care and are not subject to underuse, overuse, or misuse. An improvement collaborative includes three main phases: (1) a design and development phase, in which the aim and measures for the project are developed (see Table 56.1) and changes to be tested are identified and summarized using formal methods for the design of new processes and systems; (2) an implementation phase, in which practice sites work together to test and adapt changes in care delivery; and (3) a dissemination phase, where, as changes in the processes of care delivery are tested and reliably achieve desired goals, they are disseminated to other and eventually all pediatric gastroenterology practice sites. Participating

Fig. 56.3 The improvement model (Adapted from Langley, Nolan, Nolan, Norman and Provost [37], page 10, by permission of Jossey Bass)

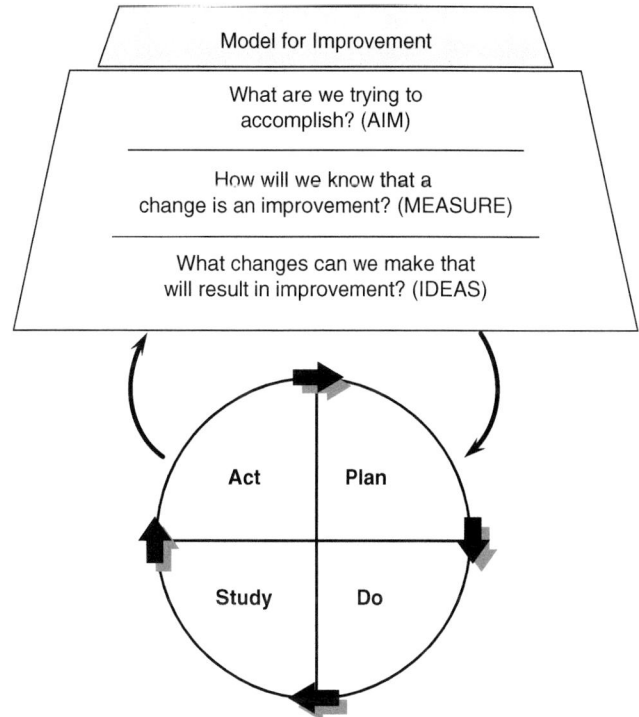

Fig. 56.4 Repeated use of the plan-do-study-act cycle. (Adapted from Langley, Nolan, Nolan, Norman and Provost [37], page 9, by permission of Jossey Bass)

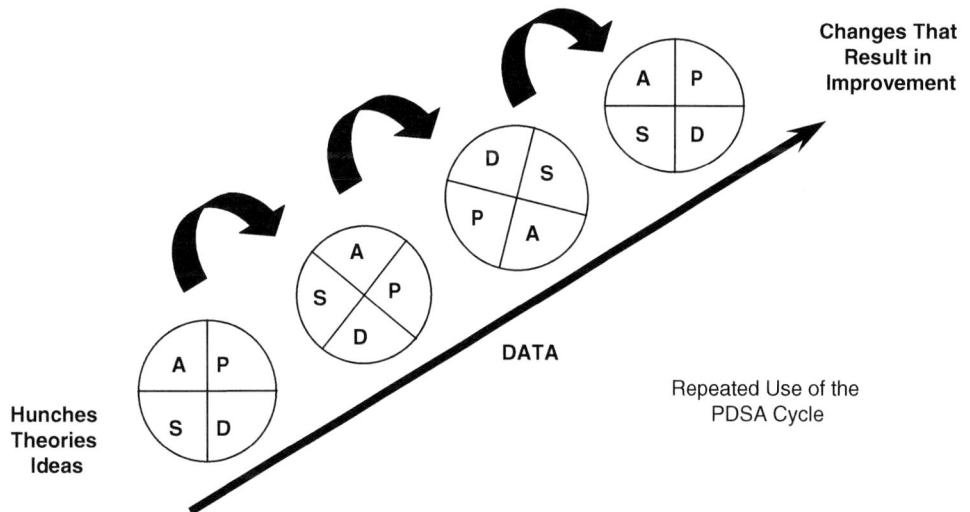

sites collect data about their patients' care, share data about the outcomes of care with all of the other sites, identify sites that are performing better, examine reasons for the better performance, set benchmarks for outcomes, and share ideas to enable the other sites to improve their outcomes. Participating sites gather together for conferences to share data and ideas and then return to their sites to perform PDSA improvement projects there, gathering and sharing new data in an incremental process (Fig. 56.5).

An IBD improvement collaborative is intended to encourage practices to adopt a more organized approach to IBD care. It is based on models of behavior change and diffusion of innovations in medical practice including involvement of

opinion leaders in the medical community, recognition of a performance gap, involving physicians and staff in developing a strategy to make changes to close the gap, compatibility of the intervention with current practice, and reinforcement of positive change [53]. It is designed to identify and address barriers in the way care is delivered in IBD clinics.

This type of systems intervention is especially important in pediatric IBD clinics because many pediatric IBD practice sites operate within large tertiary medical centers with relatively rigid infrastructures requiring significant and determined effort to change. IBD care is characterized by a complex mixture of preventive and chronic therapeutic interventions; distance and other factors make frequent return

Table 56.1 Measurable outcomes of treatment of pediatric IBD

Disease activity
Remission rate
Interval between relapses
Complication rates (e.g., fistula)
Nutritional status
Growth, final adult height
Days missed from school
Emergency department visits
Hospitalization rate
Hospital length of stay
Surgery
Patient and family satisfaction
Patient quality of life
Adverse drug events (e.g., infusion reactions)
Surgical complication rate

Fig. 56.5 A schematic drawing of the sequence of events in an improvement collaborative. (Adapted from a presentation of the Institute for Healthcare Improvement)

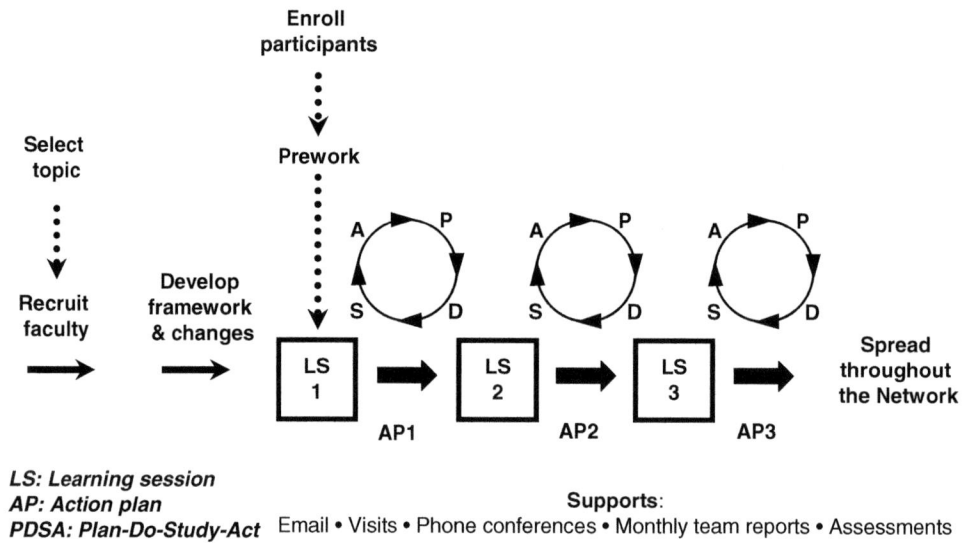

LS: Learning session
AP: Action plan
PDSA: Plan-Do-Study-Act
Supports: Email • Visits • Phone conferences • Monthly team reports • Assessments

visits difficult for many patients, so accidental omission of services and other missed opportunities for care are difficult to recognize and are harder to correct. Also, the responsibility for care is shared by multidisciplinary teams and multiple physicians with diverse responsibilities who may overestimate the consistency with which they deliver specific services [54].

The ImproveCareNow Network

The first improvement collaborative in IBD, called ImproveCareNow, was established in early 2007; its global aim is to build a sustainable network of all pediatric gastroenterologists in the USA to improve the care and outcomes of children with Crohn disease and ulcerative colitis [55]. In its first five years, it grew from 8 to 34 centers, with approximately 300 pediatric gastroenterologists and 10,000

pediatric IBD patients. By 2015, the ImproveCareNow Network grew to 85 centers, across 36 states in the US and in England, which include approximately 750 pediatric gastroenterologists and 24,000 patients. The six primary drivers of the ImproveCareNow Network are (1) a prepared proactive practice team, (2) accurate diagnosis and disease classification, (3) appropriate drug selection and dosage, (4) adequate nutritional intake, (5) adequate growth monitoring, and (6) informed, activated, and engaged patients and families.

ImproveCareNow developed and implemented five major interventions: (1) enrollment and data quality, (2) consistent reliable care, (3) population management, (4) pre-visit planning, and (5) self-management support. The centers aimed to identify and enroll all of their IBD patient population, collect data from all visits using a standardized template for data elements, and provide complete and accurate data in a timely fashion. ImproveCareNow developed a Model IBD Care

Guideline for Consistent Reliable Care, based on an integration of evidence and consensus, and key clinical measures, and process and outcome measures, to monitor the performance at each center and the collaborative as a whole [56]. In addition, an algorithm for nutrition and growth was developed.

A population management tool was developed and used to ensure patients were being seen regularly and to identify patients who were not receiving model IBD care and who could benefit from a proactive change in their management. A pre-visit planning checklist was developed and implemented at centers to review important clinical data, identify and highlight variables that fall outside of protocol guidelines (e.g., drug dosages and results of previous laboratory tests), identify and arrange for needed resources at the time of visit (e.g., preordering laboratory tests, scheduling a dietician), and assist the clinician in preparing an agenda of important issues requiring attention at the visit. In 2011, a systematic program was undertaken to develop tools for patient and family self-management support, including providing patient education, eliciting patient and family priorities for visits, confirming patient understanding of new information, setting and monitoring patient goals collaboratively, and improving adherence.

One of the primary strengths of ImproveCareNow is a focus on learning from data. Each participating center receives monthly reports with tables and longitudinal graphs of their performance on the key clinical and data quality measures and twice-monthly population management reports. These electronic reports provide both aggregate and individual patient- and visit-level data that can be used to monitor populations of patients and identify subgroups of patients in need of attention or intervention. The reports are used to identify subpopulations of patients with medical issues in need of attention, such as patients who are on systemic steroids or patients with suboptimal nutritional status. They also are used to identify patients who have outgrown the doses of their medications. The reports can also facilitate failure mode and effects analyses to study problems and gain insights to inform improvement efforts. The reports also include run charts and control charts to help identify special cause variation when a significant change from baseline has occurred. Centers also have the ability to compare their performance to that of other centers and of the entire network [57].

The data that inform these reports are collected from each patient at each outpatient visit. ImproveCareNow has developed processes by which automated data transfer can be done from electronic medical record systems to populate the data registry. This has reduced the burden of data collection and errors associated with duplicate data entry for many of the participating network sites. For sites without the capability of electronic data transfer, manual data entry is performed. There are numerous quality checks to minimize errors in manual data entry. Data collection includes all the data necessary for calculating the short pediatric Crohn disease activity index (sPCDAI) and the pediatric ulcerative colitis activity index (PUCAI) [58–60].

The ImproveCareNow Network has implemented a process for generating automated pre-visit planning forms that can be automatically generated on demand for each patient (Fig. 56.6). These forms are one-page summary sheets that are pre-populated with patient-specific historical data pulled from the registry. These forms served to streamline the pre-visit planning process for each practice. The automation was part of a larger emphasis on improving the digital architecture of the ImproveCareNow network registry [57].

The first ImproveCareNow report of outcomes was based on a 3-year follow-up of six of the initial centers with 1188 patients [61]. Changes in care delivery were associated with an increase in the proportion of visits with complete disease classification, measurement of thiopurine methyltransferase (TPMT) prior to initiation of thiopurines, and patients receiving an initial thiopurine dose appropriate to their TPMT status. There were significant increases in the proportion of Crohn disease (55–68%) and ulcerative colitis (61–72%) patients with quiescent disease (Fig. 56.7). There was also a significant increase in the proportion of Crohn disease patients not taking prednisone (86–90%). These findings suggest that improvements in the outcomes of patients with Crohn disease and ulcerative colitis were associated with improvements in the process of chronic illness care. Variation in the success of implementing changes suggests the importance of overcoming organizational factors related to quality improvement success. As ImproveCareNow grew and sustained its improvements, the network was recognized as an exemplar of pediatric collaborative improvement network [62]. After 7 years, in addition to these improvements, the ImproveCareNow network quality improvement efforts have led to further increase in the remission rate for children with IBD to 77% [63, 64]. To further improve outcomes, ImproveCareNow is creating a learning health network in which patients and parents play an integral role in participation and governance of the network and work together with network clinicians and researchers [63].

Conclusion

Whereas the fundamental purpose of research is to gain knowledge, the goal of quality improvement is to improve care and outcomes. Ultimately knowledge gained through research can be applied to clinical care, and quality improvement depends on research to advance care, so both research and quality improvement are necessary to improve outcomes [65, 66]. The road map of translational research begins with basic biomedical science and advances to clinical efficacy knowledge, to

IBD PRE-VISIT ASSESSMENT

Patient Name:	Birth Date:	Primary Provider:
Patient Num: 21	Current Age: 22.1	Secondary Provider:

Diagnosis: Crohn's Disease - 10/2003	Last Visit:	Last PPD & Date:
Phenotype: Inflammatory, non-penetrating, non-stricturing	Wt (kg): 53.80	Not Recorded
Lower: Ileocolonic	Ht (cm): 164.00	Last CXR:
Upper Proximal: No	BSA: 1.566	Negative 12/21/2006
Upper Distal: No	Date of last hospitalization:	Last Gold Test & Date:
Perianal Phenotype: Yes	Not Recorded	Not Done

>> Visits:	01/16/2012	07/23/2012	09/04/2012	10/15/2012	06/25/2013	07/30/2013	11/12/2013	05/29/2014	Age of Result
sPCDAI		10	20				5	5	
PGA	Mild	Mild	Moderate	Mild	Moderate	Quiescent	Quiescent	Mild	
Nutritional Status	Satisfactory	Satisfactory	Satisfactory	Satisfactory	Satisfactory	Satisfactory	Satisfactory	Satisfactory	
Growth Status	N/A, > 14 YOF	N/A, > 14 YOF	N/A, > 14 YOF	N/A, > 14 YOF	N/A, > 14 YOF	N/A, > 14 YOF	N/A, > 14 YOF	N/A, > 14 YOF	
Albumin	4.2	4.2	4.3	4.3	4.1	4.4	4.5	3.9	5 mo ⓘ
CRP	0.10	0.10	0.20	0.20	0.10	0.10	0.10	0.10	5 mo ⓘ
ESR	17.0	8.0	36.0	36.0	8.0	12.0	12.0	17.0	5 mo ⓘ
Hematocrit	38.3	38.9	38.7	38.7	42.5	42.2	43.5	43.0	5 mo ⓘ

*Result date may differ from visit date   ⓘ Lab ordering guidelines: 5-ASA:q6mo   6mp/ASA/MTX:q3-4mo   Biologics:q2-3mo

Care Stratification

CS Score	CSS Group	Current Disease Activity	12 Month Disease Activity	BMI Z-Score	Ht Velocity	Hosp Adm within 3 months	Currently on Cortico	Cortico last 12 months	Psychosocial Risk Factors
2	0-3 (Low)	1 (Mild)	1 (Mild/Moderate/Severe)	0 (BMIZscore >=-1 or Missing)	0 (HtvelocityZscore >=-1 or Missing or N/A)	0 (No or Unknown)	0 (No or Unknown)	0 (No or Unknown)	No

>> Treatments	Dose (mg)	mg/kg (last wt)	Guideline		Attention Needed
Biologics					
Remicade/Infliximab Last Infusion:	500.0	9.3	Consideration: If active (moderate/severe) dz, consider trough/HACA at least q 180 days		
Interval (weeks)	5				
Other Labs	Levels	Dates	Levels	Dates	Notes
Infliximab Patients	Trough: 7.6	6/25/2013	Antibodies: -BQL	6/25/2013	

Fig. 56.6 Automated pre-visit planning form for one patient pre-populated with data drawn from the ImproveCareNow registry specific to the individual patient. The form includes summary information about the patient's disease phenotype as well as longitudinal data from the last several visits including weight, height, and laboratory information

clinical effectiveness knowledge, and finally to improved health-care quality and value [67]. Measurement and accountability of health-care quality and cost, implementation of interventions and health-care system redesign, and scaling and spread of effective interventions are necessary to transform the health-care system.

There has been a growing interest in the quality of care, particularly in the era of health-care reform and the emphasis on performance, accountability, and value in health care [68]. Multiple stakeholders have emerged with strong interests in defining what quality is, how it should be measured, and how the results should be used. These include patients and patient advocacy groups; pro-

viders and their professional societies; Medicare, Medicaid, and commercial payers focused not only on quality but also value; foundations; certifying boards and credentialing bodies; various not-for-profit organizations, notably the National Quality Forum, as well as the National Committee for Quality Assurance; and business consortia such as The Leapfrog Group, an organization which fosters public reporting of health-care quality and outcomes (hospital quality ratings). The Patient Protection and Affordable Care Act emphasizes quality measurement and requires Medicare to develop mechanisms for Accountable Care Organizations, a new delivery model that rewards groups of providers with payments if they

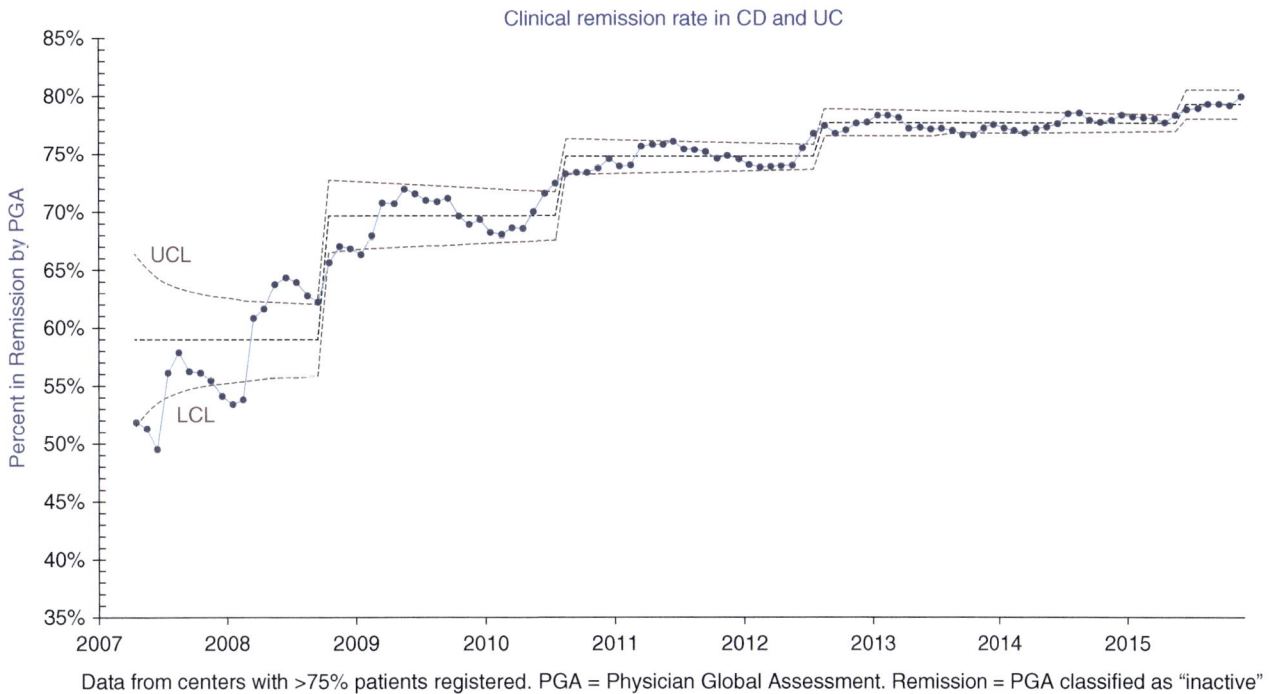

Clinical remission rate in CD and UC

Data from centers with >75% patients registered. PGA = Physician Global Assessment. Remission = PGA classified as "inactive"

Fig. 56.7 Improvement in remission rate, based on physician global assessment, of a cohort of patients with Crohn disease in the ImproveCareNow Network from 2007 to 2015. Monthly results for all centers combined are presented as a control chart (Shewhart chart). The center line represents the mean proportion; the dashed upper and lower control limits reflect the inherent variation in the data and were calculated as ± 3 standard deviations of the center line proportion. The shift in center line indicates a special cause variation in remission rate. *UCL* upper control limit, *LCL* lower control limit

can contain costs, improve quality, and assume financial risk for their outcomes. In sum, issues related to quality of care have permeated all areas of health-care delivery, including training, credentialing, clinical care, documentation, cost, and reimbursement [69]. As the quality landscape continues to change, so too will its impact on the practicing clinician [70].

References

1. McGlynn EA, Asch SM, Adams J, et al. The quality of health care delivered to adults in the United States. N Engl J Med. 2003;348:2635–45.
2. Mangione-Smith R, DeCristofaro AH, Setodji CM, et al. The quality of ambulatory care delivered to children in the United States. N Engl J Med. 2007;357:1515–23.
3. Jha AK, Li Z, Orav EJ, et al. Care in U.S. hospitals – the Hospital Quality Alliance program. N Engl J Med. 2005;353:265–74.
4. Institute of Medicine (U.S.) Committee on Quality of Health Care in America. Crossing the quality chasm: a new health system for the 21st century. Washington,(DC): National Academy Press; 2001.
5. Berwick DM, Hackbarth AD. Eliminating waste in US health care. JAMA. 2012;307:1513–6.
6. Berwick DM, Nolan TW. Physicians as leaders in improving health care: a new series in Annals of Internal Medicine. Ann Intern Med. 1998;128:289–92.
7. Clemmer TP, Spuhler VJ, Berwick DM, et al. Cooperation: the foundation of improvement. Ann Intern Med. 1998;128:1004–9.

8. Berwick DM. Controlling variation in health care: a consultation from Walter Shewhart. Med Care. 1991;29:1212–25.
9. Ferguson Jr TB, Peterson ED, Coombs LP, et al. Use of continuous quality improvement to increase use of process measures in patients undergoing coronary artery bypass graft surgery: a randomized controlled trial. JAMA. 2003;290:49–56.
10. Adler J, Sandberg KC, Shpeen BH, et al. Variation in infliximab administration practices in the treatment of pediatric inflammatory bowel disease. J Pediatr Gastroenterol Nutr. 2013;57:35–8.
11. Colletti RB, Baldassano RN, Milov DE, et al. Variation in care in pediatric Crohn disease. J Pediatr Gastroenterol Nutr. 2009;49:297–303.
12. Kappelman MD, Bousvaros A, Hyams J, et al. Intercenter variation in initial management of children with Crohn's disease. Inflamm Bowel Dis. 2007;13:890–5.
13. Donovan M, Lunney K, Carter-Pokras O, et al. Prescribing patterns and awareness of adverse effects of infliximab: a health survey of gastroenterologists. Dig Dis Sci. 2007;52:1798–805.
14. Konstan MW, Butler SM, Schidlow DV, et al. Patterns of medical practice in cystic fibrosis: part II. Use of therapies. Investigators and Coordinators of the Epidemiologic Study of Cystic Fibrosis. Pediatr Pulmonol. 1999;28:248–54.
15. Morgan WJ, Butler SM, Johnson CA, et al. Epidemiologic study of cystic fibrosis: design and implementation of a prospective, multicenter, observational study of patients with cystic fibrosis in the U.S. and Canada. Pediatr Pulmonol. 1999;28:231–241
16. Konstan MW, Butler SM, Schidlow DV, et al. Patterns of medical practice in cystic fibrosis: part I. Evaluation and monitoring of health status of patients. Investigators and Coordinators of the Epidemiologic Study of Cystic Fibrosis. Pediatr Pulmonol. 1999;28:242–7.
17. Bodenheimer T, Wagner EH, Grumbach K. Improving primary care for patients with chronic illness. JAMA. 2002;288:1775–9.

18. Available at: http://www.improvingchroniccare.org.
19. Provost LP. Analytical studies: a framework for quality improvement design and analysis. BMJ Qual Saf. 2011;20(Suppl 1):i92–6.
20. Portela MC, Pronovost PJ, Woodcock T, et al. How to study improvement interventions: a brief overview of possible study types. BMJ Qual Saf. 2015;24:325–36.
21. Deming WE. Out of the Crisis. Cambridge: MIT Center for Advanced Engineering Study; 1982.
22. Grove AS. Efficiency in the health care industries: a view from the outside. JAMA. 2005;294:490–2.
23. Imai M. The key to Japan's competitive success. New York: McGraw-Hill Publishing Company; 1986.
24. Schouten LM, Hulscher ME, van Everdingen JJ, et al. Evidence for the impact of quality improvement collaboratives: systematic review. BMJ. 2008;336:1491–4.
25. Tsai AC, Morton SC, Mangione CM, et al. A meta-analysis of interventions to improve care for chronic illnesses. Am J Manag Care. 2005;11:478–88.
26. Nightingale AJ, Middleton W, Middleton SJ, et al. Evaluation of the effectiveness of a specialist nurse in the management of inflammatory bowel disease (IBD). Eur J Gastroenterol Hepatol. 2000;12:967–73.
27. Kennedy AP, Nelson E, Reeves D, et al. A randomised controlled trial to assess the effectiveness and cost of a patient orientated self management approach to chronic inflammatory bowel disease. Gut. 2004;53:1639–45.
28. Fitzgerald MF, Mitton SG, Protheroe A, et al. The organisation and structure of inflammatory bowel disease services for children and young people in the UK in 2010: significant progress but still room for improvement. Frontline Gastroenterol. 2012;4:25–31.
29. Phan VA, Langenberg D, Grafton R, et al. A dedicated inflammatory bowel disease service quantitatively and qualitatively improves outcomes in less than 18 months: a prospective cohort study in a large metropolitan centre. Frontline Gastroenterol. 2012;3:137–42.
30. Wolters FL, Russel MG, Stockbrugger RW. Systematic review: has disease outcome in Crohn's disease changed during the last four decades? Aliment Pharmacol Ther. 2004;20:483–96.
31. Nguyen GC, Tuskey A, Dassopoulos T, et al. Rising hospitalization rates for inflammatory bowel disease in the United States between 1998 and 2004. Inflamm Bowel Dis. 2007;13:1529–35.
32. Sandberg KC, Davis MM, Gebremariam A, et al. Increasing hospitalizations in inflammatory bowel disease among children in the United States, 1988-2011. Inflamm Bowel Dis. 2014;20:1754–60.
33. Peyrin-Biroulet L, Lemann M. Review article: remission rates achievable by current therapies for inflammatory bowel disease. Aliment Pharmacol Ther. 2011;33:870–9.
34. Reddy SI, Friedman S, Telford JJ, et al. Are patients with inflammatory bowel disease receiving optimal care? Am J Gastroenterol. 2005;100:1357–61.
35. de Bie CI, Buderus S, Sandhu BK, et al. Diagnostic workup of paediatric patients with inflammatory bowel disease in Europe: results of a 5-year audit of the EUROKIDS registry. J Pediatr Gastroenterol Nutr. 2012;54:374–80.
36. Ball JE, Osbourne J, Jowett S, et al. Quality improvement programme to achieve acceptable colonoscopy completion rates: prospective before and after study. BMJ. 2004;329:665–7.
37. de Lange T, Moum BA, Tholfsen JK, et al. Standardization and quality of endoscopy text reports in ulcerative colitis. Endoscopy. 2003;35:835–40.
38. Johanson JF. Continuous quality improvement in the ambulatory endoscopy center. Gastrointest Endosc Clin N Am. 2002;12:351–65.
39. O'Connor JB, Sondhi SS, Mullen KD, et al. A continuous quality improvement initiative reduces inappropriate prescribing of prophylactic antibiotics for endoscopic procedures. Am J Gastroenterol. 1999;94:2115–21.
40. Robertson DJ, Lawrence LB, Shaheen NJ, et al. Quality of colonoscopy reporting: a process of care study. Am J Gastroenterol. 2002;97:2651–6.
41. Rogers A, Kennedy A, Nelson E, et al. Patients' experiences of an open access follow up arrangement in managing inflammatory bowel disease. Qual Saf Health Care. 2004;13:374–8.
42. Seematter-Bagnoud L, Vader JP, Wietlisbach V, et al. Overuse and underuse of diagnostic upper gastrointestinal endoscopy in various clinical settings. Int J Qual Health Care J Int Soc Qual Health Care / ISQua. 1999;11:301–8.
43. Zebris J, Maurer W. Quality assurance in the endoscopy suite: sedation and monitoring. Gastrointest Endosc Clin N Am. 2004;14:415–29.
44. Matharoo M, Thomas-Gibson S, Haycock A, et al. Implementation of an endoscopy safety checklist. Frontline Gastroenterol. 2014;5:260–5.
45. Wallaert JB, De Martino RR, Marsicovetere PS, et al. Venous thromboembolism after surgery for inflammatory bowel disease: are there modifiable risk factors? Data from ACS NSQIP. Dis Colon rectum. 2012;55:1138–44.
46. Gross ME, Vogler SA, Mone MC, et al. The importance of extended postoperative venous thromboembolism prophylaxis in IBD: a National Surgical Quality Improvement Program analysis. Dis Colon rectum. 2014;57:482–9.
47. Brotman M, Allen JI, Bickston SJ, et al. AGA Task Force on Quality in Practice: a national overview and implications for GI practice. Gastroenterology. 2005;129:361–9.
48. Siegel CA, Allen JI, Melmed GY. Translating improved quality of care into an improved quality of life for patients with inflammatory bowel disease. Clin Gastroenterol Hepatol : Off Clin Practice J Am Gastroenterol Ass. 2013;11:908–12.
49. Melmed GY, Siegel CA. Quality improvement in inflammatory bowel disease. Gastroenterol Hepatol. 2013;9:286–92.
50. Langley GJ. The improvement guide : a practical approach to enhancing organizational performance. 2nd ed. San Francisco: Jossey-Bass; 2009.
51. Vos L, Duckers ML, Wagner C, et al. Applying the quality improvement collaborative method to process redesign: a multiple case study. Implement Sci : IS. 2010;5:19.
52. Institute for Healthcare Improvement. The Breakthrough Series: IHI's Collaborative Model for Achieving Breakthrough Improvement, IHI Innovation Series white paper. Boston: Institute for Healthcare Improvement; 2003.
53. Rogers EM. Diffusion of innovations. 5th ed. New York: Free Press; 2003.
54. Travaglia JF, Nugus PI, Greenfield D, et al. Visualising differences in professionals' perspectives on quality and safety. BMJ Qual Saf. 2012;21:778–83.
55. Crandall W, Kappelman MD, Colletti RB, et al. ImproveCareNow: The development of a pediatric inflammatory bowel disease improvement network. Inflamm Bowel Dis. 2011;17:450–7.
56. Crandall WV, Boyle BM, Colletti RB, et al. Development of process and outcome measures for improvement: lessons learned in a quality improvement collaborative for pediatric inflammatory bowel disease. Inflamm Bowel Dis. 2011;17:2184–91.
57. Marsolo K, Margolis PA, Forrest CB, et al. A Digital Architecture for a Network-Based Learning Health System: Integrating Chronic Care Management, Quality Improvement, and Research. EGEMS. 2015;3:1168.
58. Kappelman MD, Crandall WV, Colletti RB, et al. Short pediatric Crohn's disease activity index for quality improvement and observational research. Inflamm Bowel Dis. 2011;17:112–7.

59. Dotson JL, Crandall WV, Zhang P, et al. Feasibility and validity of the pediatric ulcerative colitis activity index in routine clinical practice. J Pediatr Gastroenterol Nutr. 2015;60:200–4.
60. Turner D, Hyams J, Markowitz J, et al. Appraisal of the pediatric ulcerative colitis activity index (PUCAI). Inflamm Bowel Dis. 2009;15:1218–23.
61. Crandall WV, Margolis PA, Kappelman MD, et al. Improved outcomes in a quality improvement collaborative for pediatric inflammatory bowel disease. Pediatrics. 2012;129:e1030–41.
62. Billett AL, Colletti RB, Mandel KE, et al. Exemplar pediatric collaborative improvement networks: achieving results. Pediatrics. 2013;131(Suppl 4):S196–203.
63. Forrest CB, Margolis P, Seid M, et al. PEDSnet: how a prototype pediatric learning health system is being expanded into a national network. Health Aff. 2014;33:1171–7.
64. Lee GJ, Kappelman MD, Boyle B, et al. Role of sex in the treatment and clinical outcomes of pediatric patients with inflammatory bowel disease. J Pediatr Gastroenterol Nutr. 2012;55:701–6.
65. Boyle BM, Palmer L, Kappelman MD. Quality of health care in the United States: implications for pediatric inflammatory bowel disease. J Pediatr Gastroenterol Nutr. 2009;49:272–82.
66. Margolis P, Provost LP, Schoettker PJ, et al. Quality improvement, clinical research, and quality improvement research--opportunities for integration. Pediatr Clin North Am. 2009;56:831–41.
67. Dougherty D, Conway PH. The "3 T's" road map to transform US health care: the "how" of high-quality care. JAMA. 2008;299:2319–21.
68. Porter ME, Long Jr JH. Vertebrae in compression: Mechanical behavior of arches and centra in the gray smooth-hound shark (Mustelus californicus). J Morphol. 2010;271:366–75.
69. Park KT, Crandall WV, Fridge J, et al. Implementable strategies and exploratory considerations to reduce costs associated with anti-TNF therapy in inflammatory bowel disease. Inflamm Bowel Dis. 2014;20:946–51.
70. Kappelman MD, Dorn SD, Peterson E, et al. Quality of care for gastrointestinal conditions: a primer for gastroenterologists. Am J Gastroenterol. 2011;106:1182–7.

Fostering Self-Management and Patient Activation

57

David Alain Wohl and Justin Vandergrift

Introduction

As chronic medical conditions, such as inflammatory bowel disease (IBD), predominate as a reason for seeking medical care, both patients and their healthcare providers have increasingly recognized the importance of their forging a long-term partnership in which both take actions to achieve clinical goals. In this model, the provider provides guidance, advice, and feedback, while the patient engages in behaviors aimed at achieving and maintaining health – and there is a degree of shared responsibility for outcomes. The patient side of this bargain is often described as *self-management*.

Below, we outline what self-management is, highlight evidence that self-management can improve clinical outcomes, and provide guidance on how healthcare providers can cultivate strong self-management of children living with IBD – all from the perspective of parents of young patients with Crohn disease.

Defining Self-Management

Although often equated with adherence to medication and clinic visits, self-management entails a number of complex, evolving, and lifelong activities, of which adherence is but one part. Therefore, successful self-management of chronic disease is not pegged to any one action but is characterized by the cultivation of a number of behaviors and strategies that lead to a better quality of life and increased likelihood for improved disease-related outcomes.

A concise and useful conceptualization of self-management includes *tasks* that need to be undertaken and the set of *skills* that are required to help achieve them (Fig. 57.1) [1].

Clinicians can help patients identify unfulfilled tasks and work to help develop the skills that may be lacking.

Self-Management Tasks

The model calls for three major tasks: *medical management, role management, and emotional management*. *Medical management* addresses some of the most obvious elements of taking care of one's self including adhering to medication or a specific diet or nutritional intervention. *Role management* involves the patient making minor or major lifestyle and activity adjustments in response to disease – for example, having specific accommodations at school or avoiding certain sports for those with colostomies. In *emotional management*, the many fears, anxieties, and frustrations that accompany a chronic illness are acknowledged and addressed as part of handling life with the disease.

For each task there are obvious leverage points that clinicians can use to make the patient aware of the problem and work together to arrive at a solution. Importantly, though, efforts to successfully develop these self-management tasks will require cognizance of a patient's perceptions and priorities. For example, in the case of a child living with IBD for whom avoiding abdominal cramps is a primary focus, the medical, role, and emotional management has to be conducted largely within the stated context of reducing pain and discomfort – even if the clinician's priority is ensuring control of inflammation and promoting proper growth. Therefore, clinician recommendations regarding the need to take daily oral medication (medical), eliminating trigger foods (role), and referral to a clinical psychologist (emotional) are, in the case above, all couched as being part of the plan to keep the pain away.

© Springer International Publishing AG 2017
P. Mamula et al. (eds.), *Pediatric Inflammatory Bowel Disease*, DOI 10.1007/978-3-319-49215-5_57

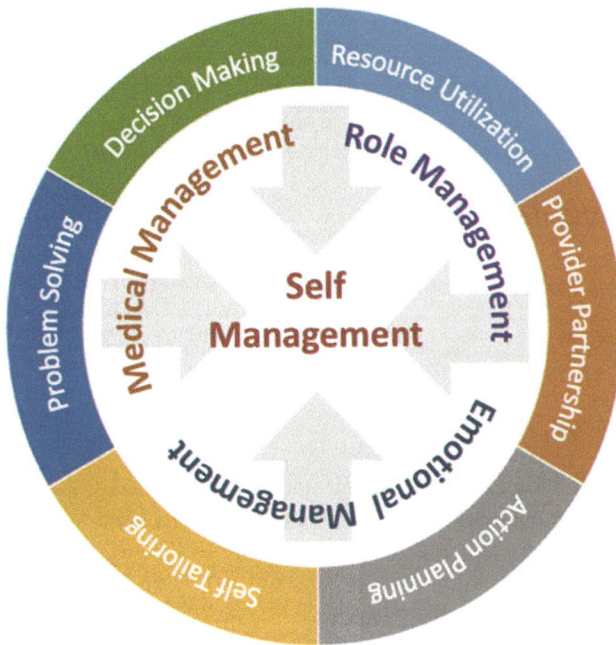

Fig. 57.1 Tasks (*outer circle*) and skills (*inner circle*) that support disease self-management [1, 2]

Self-Management Skills

These key tasks can be achieved through developing a set of six skills that *Loring and Holman* recently added and which provide a greater sense of the work involved in self-management [2]. These skills include *problem-solving, decision-making, resource utilization, patient-provider partnership, action planning,* and *self-tailoring.* As described below, each skill can call on innate resources of the patient and family and/or be fostered and supported through intervention.

Problem-solving is a core self-management skill. Obstacles to well-being and quality of life are inevitable, and being able to tackle them is critical to managing chronic illness. To do this, patients need to be capable of defining the problem, developing potential solutions, implementing these solutions, and evaluating the results. Advice and support from family, providers, and community may be necessary. For example, an 11-year-old with indeterminate colitis dreads going to the clinic to get his anti-TNF infusion. He finds it boring, and "not fun," and he hates feeling sedated by the premedication. His parents discuss the problem with the physician, and she considers infusion without premedication. His parents suggest that they download favorite TV shows for him to watch during the infusion and then go out to his favorite pizza shop afterward.

Decision-making can follow problem-solving and is enhanced by education and training. When a 15-year-old

with Crohn disease receiving weekly methotrexate injections developed a fever of 101 degrees Fahrenheit on the day of his shot, based on instructions they had received at the clinic, he and his parents decide to hold the injection and contact the on-call clinician the next day.

Resource utilization is becoming an increasingly important element of disease management. Paradoxically, as more information becomes available and accessible to patients regarding their condition, particularly online, there is less clarity as to which sources provide the most relevant and valuable advice. In pediatric IBD, the Crohn's and Colitis Foundation of America (CCFA) website (www.ccfa.org) is a trove of reliable information in written and video format. ImproveCareNow (ICN), a large network of pediatric IBD programs dedicated to quality improvement, supports blogs and patient/parent discussion forums (www.improvecarenow.org). The North American Society for Pediatric Gastroenterology, Hepatology and Nutrition (NASPGHAN) also has a site for families to learn more about digestive diseases including IBD (www.gikids.org). Teaching patients and families to access these and other reliable resources has become integral to successful self-management.

Patient-provider partnering can be considered the keystone skill for managing a chronic disease – one on which all other self-management skills rely – but is also the most complex. The doctor-patient relationship model has traditionally been "vertical," with the healthcare provider issuing orders that the patient was expected to dutifully follow. While this model may be more applicable to the management of acute medical problems (e.g., appendicitis), it is ill-suited for longer-term care. In recent years, patients have advocated for a more "horizontal" or level relationship with their healthcare providers – clinics and hospitals, vying for healthcare dollars, have obliged. Strong partnerships between children with IBD, their families, and the clinician lead to greater trust, adherence, and engagement.

Action planning can be thought of as a next step to problem-solving and decision-making and entails skills for making a behavior change and sticking with it. A college freshman at an out-of-state school has been using nightly tube feeds to help keep her Crohn disease in remission since she was 12 years old. Now living in a single-room dorm, she often feels like not "dropping the tube," especially on weekends, and is missing feeds. During her clinic visit, she is able to discuss the problem with the clinician and nutritionist, and together they develop an action plan to take weekends off from the tube and use oral supplements these days instead. The patient feels she can do this and implements the plan.

Self-tailoring calls for a practical approach to using the self-management skills. Not every self-management skill is needed at all times, and there must be some adaptation of response to fit the current demand. However, this tailoring is conducted by the patient/family. Therefore, the high school senior learning how to reorder his own medications from a specialty pharmacy calls on problem-solving and action-planning skills to keep his refills from running out.

Self-Management for Kids

Together these skills and the core tasks are intended to provide a path toward minimizing the deleterious effects of a chronic illness while maximizing opportunities to maintain well-being and quality of life. It should be recognized that this self-management framework was developed following work with adult patients. For children, particularly those who are younger, much of the self-management heavy lifting is done by parents. The "self" in self-management, therefore, is not "myself" but is "my child living with IBD" and perhaps "my other family members affected by my child's illness." This is an important distinction and the literature speaks even less to this self-management-by-proxy model than it does to traditional self-management.

That said, the principles of self-management can be applied to and adopted by the parent of a child living with IBD. Naturally, over time, there is a shift from parent management to self-management by the patient. This transition process can be smooth, or not, as discussed in Chap. 60 and below.

For the healthcare provider, supporting and motivating health-promoting behaviors for a parent or caregiver is going to look different than it will for a child.

Does Self-Management Really Matter?

Intuitively, good self-management could be expected to produce better health outcomes. While this is a reasonable assumption, medicine is replete with examples where good sense did not translate into good results. An evidence-based approach to the incorporation of self-management into medical care in general has been challenged by its complexity and a lack of uniformity in its definition. Most of the work in this area has focused on medication adherence, which via self-report, pill count, and pharmacy refill can be more readily estimated and quantified.

For children living with IBD, risks for suboptimal medication adherence that have been identified include predictable treatment-specific factors such as patient perceptions regarding the side effects and the complexity of the regimen [3, 4], as well as pill size and taste [4, 5]. Among the patient-level factors linked to suboptimal IBD medication adherence, it will come as no surprise to the parent of a teenager that none are as potent as adolescence [5, 6]. During this period of childhood development, there is a desire for autonomy, a strong interest in peer relationships, and more challenging school and social demands – all developmentally appropriate but potential barriers to adherence for all but those with the most well-developed self-management skills. Additionally, perceptions that the IBD medication is not necessary or not working can lead to missed doses [3, 6]. Family-level barriers to adherence include conflict and dysfunction, while high parent involvement in IBD care facilitates adherence and models self-management skills [5, 7–9]. Lastly, provider-level factors also can influence medication adherence in children. Satisfaction with the provider, provider trust, continuity of care with same provider, and verbal support by the provider are each associated with higher adherence in children across different disease states [10].

Overall, these studies describe a spectrum of a behavior (adherence) influenced by multiple factors across different levels. These associations are instructive insomuch as they can guide interventions, most of which have had modest effects on medication taking.

Even less is known about what works best to foster strong true self-management behaviors more broadly. A recent meta-analysis looked at published randomized controlled trials of self-management interventions for IBD in adults [11]. Only six studies met the researchers' criteria for inclusion. The studies had disparate populations, sample sizes, primary outcomes, and interventions. One, a psychologist-delivered intervention, had all of the self-management skills proposed by Lorig and Holman, while most included two skills (*decision-making* and *patient-provider partnering*). Overall, there was an emphasis of the interventions on disease management with less attention paid to dealing with symptoms, education, and lifestyle accommodations. There was a generally favorable effect on disease activity in four of the six studies and positive quality of life impact in three. This analysis provides a signal for the benefits of self-management in IBD while making plain the severe limitations of the research that has been conducted thus far. Again, much less is understood about this approach in children with chronic diseases such as IBD.

How to Cultivate Self-Management

Given the potential benefits of self-management in pediatric IBD, the question that arises is how to foster these skills. As mentioned above, for some, self-management comes naturally. These patients and families are engaged in the care being provided, are proactive and adherent, and work closely with the medical team. For others, self-management skills have to be cultivated. Unfortunately, most clinics are not well equipped to evaluate and support self-management among their patients. Training and education take time which is generally not reimbursed.

However, there are opportunities to promote self-management that are low-intensity and inexpensive. Foremost is development of a trusting patient-provider relationship or ideally a trusting patient-*clinic* relationship. As mentioned above, a lack of connection between child (or parent) and provider can have consequences including poor adherence to medication and care. Additionally, electronic record systems (EMRs) are providing patients more direct access to their records and to their providers. Many support electronic communication portals for reporting of issues between visits – a boon to those, like us, who "lean in" hard to self-management for our children. Increasingly, there are technological innovations that facilitate self-management including applications that send reminders to take medication or track stool frequency and devices that measure physical activity.

Lastly, an aspect of self-management that has not been explicitly mentioned by those who have conceptualized it is community connectivity. Like *resource utilization*, community connectivity involves tapping into a source of information and support, but here the resource is obtained on a human-to-human level and is reciprocal. In the existing model of self-management described above, skills are present or, ideally, developed by patients and professionals. Increasingly, patients are learning from other patients how to best manage their disease. This can occur face-to-face during support groups or educational forums or virtually on the Internet.

In pediatric IBD, ImproveCareNow has created a network of clinics with the mission of raising the quality of medical care and services. An intentional by-product has been the creation of a community of parents of children with IBD. These "parent-leaders" work with their clinics to achieve better self-management and ultimately better outcomes for families at their centers by rapidly sharing and distributing advances and knowledge to other families. The connectivity of patients, families, and providers through technology adds an entirely new and novel tool to bolster self-management awareness and skills.

Parent and Patient Activation

Through interactions with patients and their families, clinicians can find those who are willing to go the extra step to learn, educate, and participate. Often these "activated" patients and families are eager to help the clinic to understand what life with IBD is really like between the clinic visits, and these insights can create solutions for self-

management issues which can be shared and applied to other patients.

The core of this activation is the understanding that patients and families are experts in the care of IBD. Their experiences are tangible, personal, and value-rich because their child's disease is forefront to daily activities. Often a family will develop a simple solution at home that solves common problems faced by many patients. These "silent solutions" can dramatically change outcomes for 100 of families but will remain silent if the clinic does not engage the patient and their family.

Clinicians can discover such pearls where they may least expect it. A simple question asking the patient *if* they are taking their medication often gets a simple answer. Probes for *how* and *when* they take medication, what they do to not forget a dose, or how they overcome side effects deliver richer information and will encourage greater interaction between the family and provider.

Clinic parent-leaders are parents of children with IBD who are willing to work with families at the clinic to distribute advances and knowledge. The parent-leader might organize events with other parents to share ideas about treatment or answer questions from newly diagnosed parents. Other examples include quarterly newsletters prepared by the parent-leader and distributed to other clinic IBD families; at some centers mentoring programs have been established where newly diagnosed families or those facing invasive interventions such as initiation of nasogastric tube feeds, or major events such as surgery, speak with a "veteran" family that has been through the experience.

Co-production

Following patient activation is co-production. Co-production is best summed as an environment where clinicians and patients share decision-making and work in harmony to create a better healthcare experience. At its core, co-production requires trust between patients (parents) and providers. The benefit of co-production is a better system of treatment for all patients.

According to Ruth Dineen, founder and co-director of Co-Production Wales, *co-production is an approach to public services which enables citizens and professionals to share power and work together in equal partnership, creating opportunities for people to access support when they need it and to contribute to social change* [12]. She outlines four key features of co-production:

- Values all participants as equals and assets
- Develops and supports peer networks
- Reciprocity so that benefits accrue to all involved

- Outcomes focus such that the outcome of interest is that which matters most to the individuals rather than process

Co-production only occurs when clinicians value parents and patients as partners and experts in their disease. This trust is essential in developing a bi-directional communication where clinicians provide advice to patients and patients provide feedback to clinicians. Co-production will bloom where communication flow is open, honest, and nonjudgmental.

Below are four examples of co-production from IBD clinics that work with a parent-leader. Each problem and solution was created through a foundation of open communication, valuing of opinions, and with the goal of producing better outcomes for other families at the clinic.

Pill Cases

During a routine call with a parent-leader, a nurse practitioner described the difficulties another family was having while their child was tapering off of prednisone. Careful not to share identifying details, the nurse practitioner related how the child's family incorrectly followed the taper sequence three times and was putting him at risk for complications.

The parent-leader came up with a simple solution to solve the issue. If the taper sequence was pre-loaded into pill cases, then patients would have less difficulty in following the schedule. The parent-leader raised funds and bought pill cases for the entire clinic. This clinic has an on-site a pharmacy. Now when a prednisone taper is prescribed, the medication is pre-loaded into pill cases before the family leaves the clinic. This simple solution costs less than $2 per patient, is easy to implement, and can change the outcomes for countless patients.

This solution presented itself because of trust between the clinic and their parent-leader. No confidential information was shared, just a simple exchange of ideas and solutions.

Shot Anxiety

A parent-leader in another clinic identified a simple solution to help children who receive injections at home. This parent saw that "shot time" was often met with anxiety and was creating a difficult family life for many patients. Through research, this parent identified a device which uses sensory confusion to make shot administration easier. She purchased the device (less than $25) and used it at home with great success. Adherence improved, anxiety was lessened, and both the child and her family were less tense around injection time.

During a clinic visit the parent-leader mentioned their success with the device to the physician. Later, she helped the clinic obtain grant funding to purchase additional devices so that all patients at the clinic who received injections at home could benefit.

Spanish Language Educational Videos

One parent-leader met a Latino family sitting in the IBD waiting room while waiting for their own appointment and noticed that the hospital provided an interpreter for them during the visit. However, at the end of the visit, the after visit summary and disease information given to them was in English, not Spanish. The parent-leader saw the family throw all printed material into the trash can as they left the clinic.

In response, this parent proposed that the clinic show short educational videos in English and Spanish. These videos featured children asking providers common questions about IBD, covering treatment and how will it interfere with their daily life. In one version a Spanish-speaking physician answered the young patient's questions. During the filming, the parent-leader noticed the interest of the patient's father peaked. After filming the child, the father and mother asked if they would participate in the video. The result is a rich video where the parents asked questions at the forefront of their child's care (https://youtu.be/fton8Vx95K4?t=6m31s). The questions asked were perfect and familiar to many IBD families. This example, in particular, demonstrates that most people will help and educate others if provided the opportunity to do so.

Empowered by Kids (www.empoweredbykids.com)

Another example of co-production involved 20 parent-leaders across ImproveCareNow's network of IBD care centers. A feeling of isolation is reported by many parents and patients during and just after the diagnosis of IBD. Many of these families do not know much about IBD and most do not know anyone else who has the disease. The parent-leaders at ImproveCareNow felt this was an area where they could provide assistance.

In 2013 these parents collaborated to create the *Book of Hope*, a colorful collection of inspirational stories of hope written by family members and pediatric IBD patients. Their messages of hope are expressed in their own words, often with kid-created artwork. The *Book of Hope* is given to newly diagnosed IBD families across the ImproveCareNow network; more than 8000 copies have been distributed to families across over 40 IBD facilities in the United States.

The Need for Reliable Education

As described above in the description of the *resource utilization* skill, parents and patients need quality information to better manage IBD. This need for reliable data and guidance is at its peak during three phases of treatment: diagnosis, before procedures and surgery, and during medication changes. Although the Internet can be a useful tool for finding information, it is recommended that clinicians steer patients toward sites which contain unbiased and useful information as early in the relationship as possible.

The CCFA, ImproveCareNow, and NASPGHAN (http://www.naspghan.org/ and www.gikids.org) all have websites that are content-rich and unbiased. Information is presented in written and video formats.

Self-education can be supplemented with interactive events. Several major IBD clinics, including the Center for Pediatric IBD at The Children's Hospital of Philadelphia, hold annual education sessions for patients and their families. Educational events can even be facilitated by a parent-leader. Parents have also established resource libraries for patients, quarterly newsletters, and monthly educational seminars or "Q&A" nights. Each of these is designed with the aim of steepening the learning curve for patients and families so that with knowledge they will be more confident in their treatment decisions and self-management.

Conclusions

Self-management of a chronic illness like IBD seems easy as following medical advice and taking medication as directed. However, the successful navigation of a lifelong condition that can be quiescent and then flare is anything but simple. Each child living with IBD and each of their families need to develop strategies that will optimize well-being and minimize the risk of adverse outcomes.

These strategies allow the patient to take on tasks that encompass therapeutics, lifestyle adjustment, and coping while leveraging a set of necessary skills. Clinicians can facilitate such self-management by becoming familiar with their patients and understanding where they are on the spectrum of self-management. Opportunities for intervention must be identified and then acted on.

Patient/parent activation can be a powerful self-management tool that enhances empowerment and engagement in care while also providing lessons that can be shared and applied to help others. Considering parents and patients as partners, who can co-produce solutions, will allow clinicians to better care for their patients and address commonly encountered problems.

References

1. Corbin J, Strauss A. Unending work and care: managing chronic illness at home. San Francisco: Jossey-Bass; 1988.
2. Lorig KR, Holman H. Self-management education: history, definition, outcomes, and mechanisms. Ann Behav Med. 2003;26(1):1–7.
3. Greenley RN, Stephens M, Doughty A, Raboin T, Kugathasan S. Barriers to adherence among adolescents with inflammatory bowel disease. Inflamm Bowel Dis. 2010;16(1):36–41.
4. Schurman JV, Cushing CC, Carpenter E, Christenson K. Volitional and accidental nonadherence to pediatric inflammatory bowel disease treatment plans: initial investigation of associations with quality of life and disease activity. J Pediatr Psychol. 2011;36(1):116–25. 2011
5. Hommel KA, Baldassano RN. Brief report: barriers to treatment adherence in pediatric inflammatory bowel disease. J Pediatr Psychol. 2010;35(9):1005–10.
6. Ingerski LM, Baldassano RN, Denson LA, Hommel KA. Barriers to oral medication adherence for adolescents with inflammatory bowel disease. J Pediatr Psychol. 2010;35(6):683–91.
7. Mackner LM, Crandall WV. Oral medication adherence in pediatric inflammatory bowel disease. Inflamm Bowel Dis. 2005;11(11):1006–12.
8. Greenley RN, Kunz JH, Biank V, et al. Identifying youth nonadherence in clinical settings: data-based recommendations for children and adolescents with inflammatory bowel disease. Inflamm Bowel Dis. 2012;18:1254–9.
9. Reed-Knight B, Lewis JD, Blount RL. Association of disease, adolescent, and family factors with medication adherence in pediatric inflammatory bowel disease. J Pediatr Psychol. 2010;36(3):308–17.
10. Hazzard A, Hutchinson SJ, Krawiecki N. Factors related to adherence to medication regimens in pediatric seizure patients. J Pediatr Psychol. 1990;15(4):543–55.
11. Conley S, Redeker N. A systematic review of self-management interventions for inflammatory bowel disease. J Nurs Scholarsh. 2016;48(2):118–27.
12. Ruth Dineen. Co-producing prudent healthcare: putting people in the picture at www.prudenthealthcare.org.uk/coproduction/. Accessed 23 June 2016.

Advocacy for Pediatric Patients with IBD

58

Janis Arnold and Athos Bousvaros

Introduction

Physicians who treat patients with chronic illnesses know that the practice of medicine has come to involve the practice of patient advocacy. Whether it be justifying a prescription for a non-formulary medication or trying to help a child obtain necessary accommodations from a school, physicians who treat children with IBD have to learn to be advocates. Although this is not something we are taught in medical school, it has become an integral facet of practicing collaborative medicine in the United States in the twenty first century. Use of a medical team approach is most important to meet the advocacy needs of patients. The medical team may involve the physician, nurses, social workers, nutritionists, psychologists, and administrative staff.

In smaller centers, providers may find themselves taking on multiple roles. We will discuss the following four substantive areas in which advocacy for patients is necessary:

1. Navigating school administrative requirements to enable optimal academic plans for ill children with IBD to attend school
2. Insurance company denials of a needed therapy, including mental health services
3. Social Security disability assistance for children and adolescents
4. Family and medical leave for caretakers of children with IBD

Advocacy Directed at Schools

Children with IBD are often embarrassed to attend school because of their digestive symptoms. For example, we cared for a child who had not been in school for a year and one-half because his parents did not understand that they could request accommodations for him that would have allowed him to stay in school. They essentially hoped his symptoms would resolve or that he would learn to adjust on his own. The family was unaware of where to go for help or what legal recourse they had. When the school district sent them forms to fill out to begin the process of evaluating the child for accommodations, the family did not understand what the purpose of the forms or the evaluation was, so the child stayed absent from school for nearly 18 months. Ultimately, intervention by an attorney with expertise in school advocacy resulted in resolution of the problem and the return of the child to school.

There are two related statutes that provide protection for students with IBD: the Individuals with Disabilities Education Act ("IDEA")[1] and Section 504 of the Rehabilitation Act of 1973 ("Section 504").[2] The IDEA applies to state and local education agencies, whereas Section 504 applies to educational institutions that are recipients of federal funds. The two statutes are related, but they are not identical.

Whereas the IDEA applies only to grade and secondary schools, Section 504 pertains to all levels of education – grade school to college to graduate schools that accept federal funding. The IDEA is geared toward students who need special education services related to a learning disability as opposed to students with a physical condition like IBD, whereas Section 504 is broader and includes physical disabilities as

J. Arnold, LICSW (✉) • A. Bousvaros, MD, MPH
Inflammatory Bowel Disease Center, Children's Hospital Boston,
300 Longwood Avenue, Boston, MA 02115, USA

---

[1] 20 U.S.C. § 1400, *et seq.*
[2] 29 U.S.C. § 794(a).

© Springer International Publishing AG 2017
P. Mamula et al. (eds.), *Pediatric Inflammatory Bowel Disease*, DOI 10.1007/978-3-319-49215-5_58

well as learning disabilities (although special education services are available only under the IDEA). Patients with IBD usually do not have a lifelong learning disability that requires placement in special education classes. However, they may require some accommodations due to school absence during periods of illness or because their illness sometimes limits their participation. Thus, patients with IBD are more likely to be eligible for accommodations under Section 504 than they are for accommodations under IDEA.

The IDEA provides that a child with a disability who needs special education is entitled to a free appropriate public education. The IDEA defines a child with a disability to include children with a number of specific types of disabilities, including visual and hearing impairments, speech and language impairments, autism, traumatic brain injury, and emotional disturbances. While inflammatory bowel disease is not explicitly stated in the IDEA, the law does include a proviso providing assistance to children with "other health impairments." However, children who qualify for assistance under IDEA must have a physical or mental disability that affects their ability to fully participate in school without some form of assistance, whereas children who qualify for accommodations under Section 504 need only to show that they have a medical condition that substantially impairs one or more major life activities, regardless of how they perform in school.

Under the IDEA, the first requirement imposed on the states is to "identify, locate, and evaluate" children in need of special education services (called "child find"). Once children are located, the IDEA requires states to meet the needs of those children. The core of the IDEA is the "individualized education program" or "IEP." Under the IDEA, states are required to conduct an evaluation before special education benefits are granted. The evaluation determines whether the child is, in fact, a "child with a disability" and has special educational needs. The process should be initiated by the school, which should provide notice of the evaluation to the parents. The child may be tested and evaluated using a variety of tools; after this evaluation is completed, the actual IEP is formulated.

The IEP should be a separate written statement for each qualifying student that includes a statement of the child's level of educational performance; a statement of goals; a statement of the special education and related services to be provided; an explanation of the extent, if any, of the child's participation in mainstream programs; a statement of any individual modifications; the projected date for commencement of these services; and the duration of the services. In fashioning the IEP, the strengths of the child, the parents' concerns, and the results of the most recent evaluation of the child must be considered.

The IEP "team" includes the parents, at least one non-special education teacher, at least one special education teacher, a representative of the local agency who is qualified to assist in formulating IEPs, other experts brought in at the request of the parents or the state, and, if appropriate, the child. The IDEA provides safeguards to ensure parental involvement at all stages of the child's education, and parents may challenge any aspect of an IEP by requesting a hearing, and if they remain dissatisfied, they may file a lawsuit in federal court. Schools that provide services under the IDEA are also eligible for financial support through the state and federal government.

In contrast, Section 504 of the Rehabilitation Act was enacted to promote the inclusion and integration of people with disabilities into the mainstream. Section 504 provides that disabled children cannot be denied the benefits of any program that receives federal financial assistance, including public education. In general, a child is disabled if he or she has a "physical or mental impairment" that "substantially limits" one or more "major life activities" as those terms are used in the Americans with Disabilities Act.[3] Major life activities include bodily functions, such as the bowel, digestion, and immune functions.

Once the student's medical disability is established, the next step is to determine what accommodations (under Section 504) or special services (under the IDEA) must be provided. While section 504 is a more inclusive statute than IDEA, school districts providing services under 504 plans are not reimbursed for their expenses by the federal government. Because Section 504's definition of disability is broader than the IDEA's, many IBD patients will qualify under Section 504 but not under the IDEA. These are called "504-only students." For some patients, accommodations are minimal (e.g., providing medication during school hours or being excused from physical education class), whereas for other students, accommodations are more extensive (including limiting homework loads and home tutoring). Under the IDEA, a child may be eligible for speech therapy, special education services, and even nursing care. Any assistance a student receives from a school must be provided for free.

Any child who needs accommodation under IDEA or Section 504 must be the subject of an evaluation *before* taking any action with respect to placement. Once testing is concluded, schools use the results, as well as teacher recommendations, physical condition, social or cultural background, and adaptive behavior in designing the plan for the student. Parents must have notice and opportunity to examine the evaluation records, there must be a hearing at which the parents and/or other guardian can appear, and there must be a procedure for review of the decision.

There are at least two issues that face IBD patients that are not well addressed by the law. First, children who do well in school are presumed not to need help. The IDEA defines

---

[3] 42 U.S.C. § 12,101, *et seq.*

"child with a disability" to mean a child with health problems "who, by reason thereof, needs special education and related services." A student who does not need special education because she is performing well academically is not a "child with a disability" under the IDEA. Therefore, only children with IBD who have neurologic or developmental conditions that impair learning are covered under the IDEA. However, this is not the case under Section 504, which provides reasonable accommodations to any student who is substantially impaired by a major life activity, regardless of the effect – or lack thereof – on the ability to learn.

Second, the IDEA does not provide explicit guidance for children with a chronic disease that remits and relapses. However, as of January 2009, Section 504 provides that an episodic illness that is disabling when active also is considered to be disabling when in remission. This presents a challenge for both the parents and the school, because even though Section 504 now recognizes chronic illness, it is difficult to write an IEP or Section 504 plan that is intended to apply only intermittently. Because chronic illness is cyclical in nature, there will be times when a student needs home schooling or temporary access to typed handouts and other times when the student has no need for help. The waxing and waning course of IBD and the unpredictability of the illness necessitate that the Section 504 plan for an IBD patient be flexible and change depending on whether the patient is ill or in remission.

Generally, it is the child's parents in conjunction with members of the health-care team that realize that educational accommodations may be needed for their chronically ill child. In patients with IBD, this need is often recognized during a period of prolonged illness (such as in a hospitalization for intravenous medication or surgery). At this point, parents and members of the health-care team should list the child's needs in writing and discuss with school officials to develop a written plan. A plan under either the IDEA or Section 504 may include accommodations such as seating chart placement, extended time for testing, adjustment of class schedules, use of aids such as tape recorders, permission to photocopy a classmate's handwritten notes, class and/or homework assistance, administration of medication, behavioral support, initiation of tutoring prior to the standard 14 consecutive day absence, access to bathroom without required hall passes, permission to have a water bottle in class, or multiple sets of textbooks. For chronically ill patients with IBD, parents and school officials should have this integrated academic plan for IBD students in place.[4]

The IBD Center at Boston's Children's Hospital had the opportunity to work with a high school student who experienced her first severe flare-up of her ulcerative colitis, which had been well-controlled for many years. Her symptoms were initially unresponsive to various medications. She ultimately was placed on tacrolimus, which led her to develop the side effects of hand tingling, joint pain, and hand tremors. Though her medication regimen decreased her GI symptoms enough to allow school reentry, the side effects from the necessary medication left her unable to fully participate in the classroom requirements, including note-taking. Consequently, this interfered with her ability to have the adequate review materials to study for tests. We collaborated with the patient's mother and the school to develop a Section 504 plan for the patient. Among other plan provisions, relevant accommodations included allowing her to identify a classmate in each course whose notes she had permission to photocopy. It also was detailed that the teacher would, when appropriate, provide the student with typed copies of the class notes and outlines. An additional item was written into her Section 504 plan that stated that if she had to be absent unpredictably, the plan coordinator would be responsible for getting the student a copy of the classmates' notes and teacher outlines within 48 h of missed school days. This protected the student's academic performance and reduced the anticipatory anxiety regarding not being able to keep up with the class notes – anxiety that could lead to exacerbation and prolonging of her disease's symptoms.

Although a Section 504 plan can be implemented during periods of illness, many families and patients find it helpful to coordinate and delineate these educational adaptations prior to what may be experienced as a medical crisis or complications, given our awareness that this disease process is unpredictable and can change quickly. It is often difficult and burdensome to try to arrange these meetings and plan at times when families are simultaneously focusing on acute medical demands and the family reorganization that must accommodate them. Nonetheless, it is critical that normal school attendance, curriculum participation, and activity should be encouraged during periods of remission (see Appendix 1).

While written advocacy through letters supporting a Section 504 plan is helpful, sometimes a direct phone call from the physician to the principal or vice-principal is even more effective. For example, we had a patient who could not complete tests in a timely manner because the stress of the test would cause her intestinal symptoms to flare. While written documentation was sent, and most teachers responded adequately to the written documentation, one teacher remained resistant to implementing "stop the clock testing." A call from the patient's physician to the school authorities resulted in a more detailed discussion between the principal and the teacher, which enabled the student to receive appropriate accommodations.

---

[4]Ketlak D. Advocating for your chronically ill child within the school setting. *Pediatric Crohn's and Colitis Association* Website http://pcca.hypermart.net/advocating.html 2002.

Advocacy Directed at Insurance Companies

Inflammatory bowel disease is a costly illness; one 1992 study estimated the per capita annual costs of Crohn disease ("CD") to be approximately $6,500 dollars, though a small number of patients account for the bulk of that cost.[5] Charges for a hospitalization may approach $30,000, especially when that hospitalization involves surgery.[6] In addition, the increasing utilization of highly expensive biologic therapies (including infliximab, adalimumab, and vedolizumab) means that annual costs of medications may be tens of thousands of dollars. For these reasons, coverage by third-party payors is essential for most patients.

Insurance company denials of prescribed therapies are exceedingly common. Often, pediatric prescriptions are automatically denied simply because the patient is under the age of 18, and the drug has only been approved by the FDA for individuals over 18 years. When coverage for a therapy is denied by an insurance company, the patient in all likelihood will not be able to pay for it him- or herself. Thus, appealing the decision may be necessary. Nationally, approximately 70% of health insurance appeals are granted.[7] That means that, in most cases, appealing is not a waste of the patient's time. However, without the physician's help and advocacy, appeals are difficult, if not impossible.

Yet, not all physicians know what to say to an insurance company. For example, when one physician was sent a denial of coverage for a 30-day supply of ondansetron (Zofran), and the patient asked her to call her insurance company and appeal the denial, the physician's response was "what do you want me to say?" In this case, the patient was also a patient advocate and could coach her doctor through the appeal by telling her to explain that everything else had been tried and failed and that intractable nausea required this medication. But what happens to a patient whose physician does not know how to be an advocate?

There are at least two main categories of appeals: *medical necessity appeals* and *experimental/investigational appeals* due to the nature of the medicine, device, or other treatments. For medical necessity appeals, the physician and patient must highlight the particulars of the patient's medical condition and why a given condition requires a specific medication. As an example of a *medical necessity appeal*, a patient who develops nausea from generic sulfasalazine but tolerates enteric-coated brand name sulfasalazine may initially have the brand name drug denied. However, a brief letter from the physician describing the precise adverse event to the generic medication and the need for the brand name drug will usually result in approval by the insurance company. Here, both forms of the medication have similar proven efficacy, but one form is medically necessary because it is better tolerated by the patient.

The second category, *experimental/investigational appeals*,[8] typically occurs with a newer, more expensive therapy that is beginning to enter the armamentarium of accepted treatments, or perhaps a medication that is being used off-label, including medications that are approved for adults but not yet for the pediatric population. Typically, in this circumstance, the physician has access to published literature that supports a claim that a given medication or treatment will help their patient. "However, the insurance company or other payor is either unaware of the published literature or does not feel the evidence in support of this new treatment is sufficient to provide reimbursement." For this reason, the payor denies coverage and refuses to reimburse for therapy. This type of appeal (appeal of coverage denial) is more difficult. The physician and patient must demonstrate that the patient has failed other conventional treatments, highlight the patient's specific need for the novel therapy requested, and provide published, peer-reviewed literature and supportive information that support the novel treatment's safety and efficacy.

When writing a letter of appeal to an insurance company, it is very important to not let the insurer equate "off-label use" with "investigational" use. When the FDA approves a medication for use, they typically approve it for one very narrow indication. An "indication" implies a specific disease, condition, or age group. For example, The FDA may approve a medication for patients with ulcerative colitis over 18 years of age. However, that does not mean the medication should be restricted to that population. According to the American Academy of Pediatrics, "the term off label does not imply an improper, illegal, contraindicated or investigational use. Therapeutic decision-making must always rely on the best available evidence and the importance of the benefit for the individual patient" (AAP committee on Drugs, "Off Label use of drugs in Children." Pediatrics 2014; 133:563–7).

When appealing the denial of coverage of a treatment that the insurer states is off-label, experimental, or investigational, the essential tool for obtaining approval is the appeal letter/letter of medical necessity. In summary, the physician

[5] Hay JW, Hay AR. Inflammatory bowel disease: costs-of-illness. *J Clin Gastroenterol* 1992; 14:309–17.

[6] Cohen RD, Larson LR, Roth JM, Becker RV, Mummert LL. The cost of hospitalization in Crohn's disease. *Am J Gastroenterol* 2000; 95:524–30.

[7] Block S. Don't take it lying down if your insurer refuses to pay. USA Today Sept 1, 2005 2005; State of Connecticut's Office of the Health-Care Advocate. Connecticut survey of managed care. Available online at http://www.ct.gov/oha/cwp/view.asp?a=2277&q=299978 2002.

[8] Some insurers characterize these as medical necessity appeals. However, regardless of the label the insurer places on the denial, when an insurer denies coverage on the ground that a service has not been studied adequately, our advice regarding the content of the appeal is the same.

should first describe the patient's illness in detail. The history should include the approximate date of diagnosis and the effects on the patient's life (including a history of prior hospitalizations and surgeries). Other more conventional medications that have been utilized should be described and why they are not being used now (e.g., lack of efficacy, adverse effects). Peer-reviewed literature supporting the medication the patient now needs should be attached to the appeal. Insurers tend to appreciate longitudinal trials in which patients are followed for a significant period of time and which involve placebos. This may well be impossible in all cases; for example, if a patient or physician is seeking coverage for a medical device, there may not be a functional equivalent of a placebo that ethically could be used. However, the best literature will be peer-reviewed articles published in medical journals documenting randomized trials in which the treatment is compared to a control group of some kind. Other evidence, including open-label trial data or recent proceedings from medical meetings may also be useful, but will not carry the same weight.

If feasible, the physician also should obtain a letter of support from experts in the field stating that the proposed treatment plan is appropriate. In one instance, a physician prescribed adalimumab for ulcerative colitis, and coverage initially was denied as "experimental, investigational, or unproven." In this case, once the payor was provided with sufficient information regarding the patient's ulcerative colitis, the failure of other treatments, and the medical literature supporting the efficacy of adalimumab for this condition, they agreed to reimburse for the necessary treatment.

A third type of denial by insurers is an *administrative denial*. Administrative denials do not involve a medical necessity determination. This type of denial occurs when there is a coverage request for a treatment that is expressly excluded from coverage. For example, if an insurance policy expressly excludes abdominoplasty as a cosmetic surgery, a coverage request for abdominoplasty will be denied without regard for medical necessity. Even in this type of case, though, it is possible to force an insurer to conduct a medical necessity review. For example, if a patient requires a medically necessary stoma revision and hernia repair that cannot be performed without the abdominoplasty, the physician may be able to convince the insurance company to consider the medical necessity of the abdominoplasty as long as the insurer agrees that the stoma revision and hernia repair are medically necessary.

Regardless of the type of appeal, there are some general considerations. Insurers will not grant benefits solely based on a patient's subjective report of symptoms. The physician and patient in describing the indication for the appeal must provide "objective medical evidence" (i.e., evidence that can be measured scientifically). In addition to describing the patient's current symptoms (e.g., abdominal pain, diarrhea,

fatigue), the physician should provide results of recent blood tests, radiographs, and endoscopic examinations that demonstrate ongoing intestinal inflammation. In addition, if a patient develops an adverse event (AE) to a conventional therapy, the AE should be described in detail (e.g., not simply "infusion reaction to infliximab" but "chest pain and hives with infliximab, which recurred on rechallenge"). While the provider should not ignore the patient's subjective reports of symptoms, subjective evidence of ongoing disease activity may not be sufficient to prove medical necessity. A physician who writes a letter of medical necessity according to the above guidelines (summarized in Appendix 2) stands a good chance of getting the needed treatment covered. Appendix 3 includes a recent letter from our program requesting a peer-to-peer review on a child who repeatedly had ustekinumab (Stelara) denied by insurance, despite multiple phone calls from the office to the company and specialty pharmacy. This letter resulted in a successful appeal and provision of the medication.

Another area in which letters of medical necessity may be necessary is in obtaining mental health referrals for patients with IBD. Given the stress of IBD and the social stigma associated with its symptoms (rectal bleeding and diarrhea), the risk for exacerbations of IBD during periods of stress, and the mood-altering effects of medications, patients with CD and ulcerative colitis ("UC") often derive significant benefit from psychological support. We are aware that there are often significant associated psychological and social effects resulting from both short- and long-term steroid use, including mood lability, mania, anxiety, and symptoms mirroring those of depression. Many children with IBD not only have to cope with the unpredictable impact of these emotional ramifications but also the body image issues that are often secondary to side effects of the unavoidable and recurrent steroid administration necessary to keep the disease process controlled. Studies have demonstrated that a significant proportion of adolescents and young adults with IBD have symptoms of depression, which in turn contribute to decreased quality of life.[5 6 9] Most payors are receptive to the concept that treatment of a chronic illness in childhood requires psychological as well as medical support. On occasion, however, payors will deny mental health services on the ground that coping with IBD does not warrant formal treatment by a psychologist or psychiatrist. Health-care providers caring for children with IBD are acutely aware that anxiety

---

[9] Szigethy E, Levy-Warren A, Whitton S, et al. Depressive Symptoms and Inflammatory Bowel Disease in Children and Adolescents: A Cross-Sectional Study. *J Pediatr Gastroenterol Nutr* 2004; 39:395–403; Engstrom I. Mental health and psychological functioning in children and adolescents with inflammatory bowel disease: a comparison with children having other chronic illnesses and with health children. *Journal of Child Psychology and Psychiatry and Allied Disciplines* 1992; 33:563–582.

and depression may impact both disease activity and compliance with the medical regimen. Thus, properly timed psychological or psychosocial intervention often is a crucial factor in the overall treatment success and likelihood of a prolonged remission.

Appealing a denial of psychological support is similar to appealing a denial of any other medically necessary therapy. A letter from the medical team should summarize relevant literature that describes the psychological needs in patients with IBD. The letter also can emphasize the complex relationship between a patient's GI condition, mental health, compliance, and quality of life. It should be emphasized that a patient who is psychologically sound is less likely to undergo recurrent testing and hospitalization for a symptom related to stress and anxiety, all of which would be more costly for the insurance company. This usually is a sufficient reason for insurers to grant limited benefits. While a limited series of sessions is not ideal, these sessions at least allow the patient to gain entrance into the mental health system. At that point, a mental health provider can then determine further indications for ongoing treatment (see Appendix 4).

In one instance, a 14-year-old patient with Crohn disease had a complicated course of her illness, having been hospitalized twice for unpredictable flares of her disease and a blood clot in the venous portion of her brain, both times leading to lengthy admissions followed by intensive outpatient follow-up. Her illness' sporadic and inconsistent response to her treatment plan led to periods of intense stress and pressure, thereby exacerbating symptoms of her disease. The family lived in a small town in a different state from the one in which her gastroenterologist practiced, and the only local mental health providers available practiced from a more psychotherapeutic framework. Her insurance company would not cover services at the urban hospital's specialized medical coping clinic, which was out-of-network for mental health services, yet provided the specific cognitive behavioral approach that the medical team and family felt would be the best fit for her targeted goals of learning relaxation strategies and coping with the present medical demands. The social worker and physician composed a letter to the insurance company outlining the patient's specific circumstances, the physical and psychological complications, and the importance of the patient obtaining mental health services that were based in a framework specific to her needs at that time. The letter detailed that the clinic specialized in treating children and teenagers with treatment specifically geared toward management of comorbid medical and emotional issues related to IBD. The appeal highlighted that the patient's access to particular cognitive behavioral strategies could reduce the risk factors for a necessary and more costly medical or psychological hospitalization and the unavailability of access to these services through local providers covered under the plan. Her insurance company ultimately authorized coverage for ten treatment sessions, allowing her to learn biofeedback and other concrete mechanisms to help her best cope with the concurrent medical challenges, and provided a forum for ongoing formal assessment and treatment of depression or an anxiety disorder related to the disease process.

Although a good result was achieved in this case, what happens if denials continue to occur? At that point, it may be appropriate to have your patient enlist the assistance of an individual with expertise in conducting health insurance appeals, such as a patient advocate or an attorney. Under the Patient Protection and Affordable Care Act (ACA), all insurance plans must now offer what is called an external appeal. External appeals involve an independent review of the noncoverage decision. All decisions involving the exercise of medical judgment – and, in some states, even administrative denials – are subject to external appeal. The independent reviewer, who will be a medical professional with the relevant expertise, has the authority to overturn the insurer's denial of coverage. Thus, do not give up if your first level appeal is denied. Many of the more complex cases – especially those deemed experimental/investigational by the insurer – will be won at the external appeal stage.

Also under the ACA, every state has a Consumer Assistance Program (CAP) to help consumers with insurance appeals. The CAP in your state may be in your state's Insurance Department, or it may be a separate entity. These CAPs are funded largely by federal grant funds.

Finally, under the ACA, as well as under pre-existing law, the insurer must offer to provide a free copy of the materials upon which they relied in denying coverage. In addition, upon request, they have to provide diagnosis and procedure codes so that you can ensure that the denial is not due to a billing error. If you have any question about the reason for the denial of coverage, you or your patient should request a copy of the insurer's file.

Many insurers maintain their clinical policy bulletins on the "provider" section of their website; if not, you are entitled to a copy by mail. If you have a denial based on the fact that the insurer does not believe the treatment you have prescribed is medically necessary or experimental/investigational, you should search the insurer's website for the clinical policy bulletin on point, which will explain exactly when the insurer believes the treatment is or is not medically necessary or experimental/investigational. Note the date on which the clinical policy bulletin was reviewed last, as well as the medical literature on which the insurer relied in formulating its coverage policy. This will suggest the points that you will need to address in your appeal.

If a physician and patient are both frustrated by repeated denials of a treatment thought to be medically necessary, consider three steps:

1. Have your patient discuss the difficulty with the human resources department at their employer, especially if they work for a large employer that self-insures. The employee can ask the employer to grant what is called an "extra-contractual benefit," providing coverage for something that otherwise would not be covered.

2. Request a copy of the insurance company's file, which is guaranteed by law. This information may be valuable in the future.

3. Consider referral to an attorney or patient advocate.

Health insurance appeals can be labor intensive. In addition to the patient's physician, a team of professionals (including nurses, social workers, therapists, and attorneys) may need to assist in preparing the appeal. However, in the United States, effective advocacy to explain medical needs to third-party payors has become an essential element of care of complex patients.

Social Security Disability

Many people do not realize that children may be eligible for Supplemental Security Income ("SSI"), one of two forms of Social Security disability benefits.[10] However, medically impaired children up to the age of 18 may receive benefits if the income and resources of the parents and child are within allowed limits, as long as the parent worked long enough to be insured under the Social Security system (typically, 40 quarters, or a total of 10 years, with 20 of those quarters occurring in the last 10 years). The child must not be doing any substantial work and must have a medical condition that has lasted or is expected to last for at least 12 months. A child eligible for SSI will qualify for Medicaid.

Whether a child is considered disabled depends on whether he or she has a physical or mental condition that can be medically proven and which results in marked and severe functional limitations that last or are expected to last at least 12 months. A physical or mental condition that results in marked and severe functional limitations might be one that meets the applicable listing of impairments (see Appendix 5), or it might involve a combination of impairments (e.g., inflammatory bowel disease and attention deficit hyperactivity disorder or IBD and depression).

Although both the income and the benefit levels for SSI are low, the value of Medicaid is great for children with IBD. While some physicians do not accept Medicaid assignments, Medicaid coverage for children under the Early and

Periodic Screening, Diagnostic, and Treatment ("EPSDT") services is extraordinarily broad – broader than most commercial insurance, especially for children with mental health and even dental needs.

In order to assist a family to apply for SSI, the health-care provider should consult the listings of impairments set forth in Appendix 4 and write a letter that addresses each element of the listing. The listing itself tells you what sorts of evidence the Social Security Administration ("SSA") will need. For all intents and purposes, this is the same as the "objective evidence" needed in commercial insurance appeals; the listings may require specific testing. For example, the listing for malnutrition associated with a gastrointestinal problem requires a measure of stool fat excretion, even though the current medical standard may be other diagnostics, such as blood tests. Therefore, while the physician can include any diagnostic testing relevant to the patient's case, he/she should expressly include the diagnostic testing required by the SSA.

Although the SSA will ask you for your medical records, a letter of support that culls the records and explains the child's condition in the terms set forth in the listings of impairments may well be the key to obtaining these benefits. A physician who is asked to write a letter in support of an application for SSI should track the listings of impairments as closely as possible and attach the evidence that the listings mention. The physician or provider who facilitates this process, and who helps successfully obtain SSI benefits for a patient who needs such assistance, is playing a critical role in improving the likelihood of the success of the prescribed treatment plan.

In addition, an integral part of living with any chronic illness is helping maintain self-identity, so that self-esteem and feeling victimized by the disease demands do not disempower the patient. As health-care providers, we want to attempt to help the patient preserve that sense of control and self-esteem and, thus, avoid an internalized notion of a "disabled" self-concept. This is another reason to help make the process of securing entitlement from these state programs as efficient and seamless as possible. The burden of having to go to such lengths to prove disability can often take on a life of its own in the pursuit, and this would be counterproductive to the message we reinforce – the child as a whole person, who is more than the disease. Health-care providers, who can facilitate the SSI application to prevent a lengthy proof process, can be doing their part to help preserve this message.

Family and Medical Leave for Caregivers

Caregivers of children with IBD risk losing their jobs when they take time off to care for their children. Providers may be able to spare them this crisis by educating them on the

---

[10] The other form of Social Security disability is called Social Security Disability Income or SSDI. This benefit is available only to patients who have worked and paid into the Social Security system for 40 credits, or 40 quarters (10 years). As such, this benefit is available only to adults.

availability of and helping them to obtain leave and maintain employment security under the Family and Medical Leave Act ("FMLA").[11] Covered employers must grant an eligible employee up to a total of 12 workweeks of unpaid leave during a 12-month period to care for an immediate family member (spouse, child, or parent) with a serious health condition. The FMLA applies only to an employee who has been working for the same employer for at least 12 months, for at least 1,250 h during the previous 12 months, and at a location where at least 50 individuals are employed by the employer within a 75-mile area.

A child has a "serious health condition" if he or she is "incapable of self-care" due to a mental or physical disability that limits one or more of the "major life activities." Just as is the case under the Americans with Disabilities Act, processing of bodily waste is a "major life activity," so children with active IBD have a "serious health condition" under the FMLA.[9] Even if symptoms are inactive, children with an IBD diagnosis have the potential to require this care, due to the cyclical nature of chronic illness. The FMLA does not provide for paid leave. In addition, an employer may permit an employee to use all available accrued but unused vacation, sick, or PTO time during such leave. The use of other such leaves does not extend the time off beyond 12 weeks.

One of the lesser-known aspects of the FMLA is that the 12 weeks of leave need not be consecutive. For example, a parent of a child who is on infliximab treatments can take a day or two of leave every few weeks under FMLA.

Primary caregivers of children with IBD should ask for FMLA leave at the beginning of every year, whether or not they use it, so that they are protected if the child's disease becomes active. In order to obtain FMLA leave, the employee must request it in writing, and the physician often must complete paperwork that employers give the employee and provide a medical certification establishing the need or potential need for FMLA leave. An FMLA medical certification can describe IBD as a serious health condition falling into various descriptive categories. Depending on the symptom severity, demonstrating need for FMLA leave may best be accomplished by the physician. The medical certification supporting the need for FMLA leave is in some ways similar to a letter of medical necessity one prepares for a health insurance appeal (see Appendix 6).

If a physician anticipates a child will require increased parental care because of the worsening of illness, this should be discussed with the family. Parents who may need to take time off from work should request FMLA leave before the crisis occurs. Parents who do so will protect their jobs as long as they do not take more than the maximum 12 weeks

of leave during the year. This job security can go far in helping ease caregiver's anxiety, allowing them to better focus on coping with the child's acute needs and the impact on the family.

Summary

Inflammatory bowel disease affects more than a patient's intestines; it affects their life, including otherwise routine functions of school and work. In addition, IBD affects families, not just individual patients. Therefore, physicians should become familiar with the ways they can help patients and their families overcome the varied hurdles facing children with IBD. In particular, providers should train themselves, or be trained, in how to appeal insurance company denials, assist in the development of a plan of accommodation for a school-aged child, support an application for Social Security benefits, and point out the availability of family and medical leave to caregiver parents. Collaboration with other members of the medical team such as nurses and social workers to address these issues is essential, as is the ability to identify advocacy resources in the community, such as Advocacy for Patients with Chronic Illness. By providing such services, the physician may alleviate some of the financial, educational, and social complications that can turn a flare of IBD into a more serious family crisis. The provider who is an effective advocate will derive gratification from the knowledge that they have helped their patient have a better quality of life.

Acknowledgment We would like to acknowledge the contributions of two individuals who are no longer with us. Jennifer Jaff (deceased) was the principal author of the first two published versions of this chapter. She founded and ran Advocacy for Patients with Chronic Illness, a legal advocacy group that fought vigorously against insurance company denials and got chronically ill patients access to needed therapies. Suzanne Rosenthal wrote the first two versions of chapter 59 on legislative advocacy. She was one of the original founders of the Crohn's and Colitis Foundation of America and a strong force on Capitol Hill to raise awareness of this disease among legislators and the lay public.

Appendix 1. Sample Letter for Patient's Student File Regarding Educational Accommodations Needed for an IBD Diagnosis

To whom it may concern:

This letter is being written on behalf of our patient, *XXXXX (DOB: XX/XX/XX)*, who recently was diagnosed with Crohn's Disease, a chronic inflammatory bowel disease of the intestines. As chronic illness is cyclical in nature, XXX can face gastrointestinal symptoms in a recurrent

---

[11]29 U.S.C. § 2601, *et seq.* Many states have their own, more liberal version of family and medical leave. You should consult your State's Department of Labor for more information.

pattern, with periods of symptom inactivity in between active flare-ups and complications. Cramps may be severe and may be worse when there is a need to use the toilet; symptoms may worsen in an unpredictable manner and conversely, may go into remission for varying lengths of time. During a flare-up, this illness will substantially impair the major life activities of bowel and digestive functions. The medical team is currently working to coordinate the long-term treatment plan as the team explores the impact of these symptoms on her body and her body's response to the medication regimen.

Even if a patient no longer requires an inpatient hospitalization, we could expect the patient still to experience ongoing symptoms until the medical team is able to arrange her maintenance treatment regimen. XXX has been seen for her first outpatient follow-up appointment since diagnosis, and the medical team continues to monitor her symptoms, which continue to intermittently interfere with her ability to attend school for a full day.

In the long-term, however, with the understanding and support of her teachers and other school personnel, we expect XXX to participate in school activities. When the medical team better determines the best course of maintenance treatment for her, we have no reason to expect that it should routinely interfere with her academic plan or performance. In addition, XXX may be tardy or absent from school from time to time if her condition is flaring. The disease process can affect many aspects of a person's life; depending on the current symptoms, patients can find it difficult to cope as there is an interference with their physical and social functioning.

We feel it would be helpful for XXX's school re-entry to begin in a partial day format, as her body continues to adjust. In the immediate, short-term, we believe it is in XXX's best interest that she be eligible for home tutorial services so that her academic studies are not compromised by this acute period of her condition. These services would also be recommended to have in place, should flare-ups occur in the future, causing her to intermittently and unpredictably miss schoolwork.

We know that the emotional and physical pieces are interrelated in complex ways, and patients can experience flare-ups during times of emotional tensions and stress. This can relate to changes in the physiologic functioning of the gastrointestinal tract. While periods of intense stress and pressure can exacerbate symptoms, it is important to note that they do not cause the disease and are not responsible for the development of the illness.

Please understand the extenuating circumstances facing XXX, should the physical or emotional adjustment to the demands of her chronic illness intermittently impact her ability to carry out her academic responsibilities. Please contact XXX with further questions. Thank you for your time and understanding. We look forward to being able to collabo-

rate with the school in any manner that will optimize her future academic and medical plans.

Appendix 2. Preparing an Effective Insurance Company Letter of Medical Necessity

- Patient's name (and name of insured if not the patient).
- Patient's Insurance ID number, Social Security number, and date of birth.
- The treatment requested and denied.
- Your specialty and years of experience.
- Your experience with the particular device, medication, or treatment.
- The patient's diagnosis, including both subjective and objective support for the diagnosis (patient's subjective complaints **plus** weight loss, recent barium study, endoscopy reports with pathology, etc.).
- What treatments have been tried over what period of time (go back to the date of diagnosis and describe all that has been tried and failed, explain the reason for the failure, i.e., failure to control disease, allergic reaction, and adverse event such as pancreatitis).
- If device, medication, or other treatment is considered by the insurance company to be experimental, investigational, or unproven, summary of the medical literature, preferably including copies of the literature (both summary and copies of literature are enclosed).
- Why you believe this therapy or service is clinically indicated for this patient at this time.
- Describe your plan to assess treatment efficacy (whether your therapy will help this patient). For example, in a patient with CD involving the ascending colon, state you will follow the patient monthly and monitor exam, hematocrit, and C-reactive protein and perform a colonoscopy after 6 months to assess mucosal healing.
- Summarize your medically necessary request again, and offer to talk to any health-care professional from the insurance company if additional information is needed.

Appendix 3. Letter of Medical Necessity for Ustekinumab

Dear sirs:

I am writing this letter to request a formal outside peer to peer review from a pediatric gastroenterologist for the approval of ustekinumab for my patient _____ Using this medication is medically essential in order to treat her severe, refractory Crohn disease, which remains active despite multiple medications and two surgeries, the most recent being a diverting ileostomy.

To summarize her course, _____ developed her Crohn disease at the age of 9. Her disease involves her ileum, colon, and perianal region. She has been treated with mercaptopurine (disease remained active), infliximab (did well initially but developed antibodies in 2010), adalimumab (no response), certolizumab (no response), thalidomide (partial control of her disease but triggered ovarian failure), methotrexate (disease flared), and vedolizumab (no response). She underwent an ileal resection in 2009, and because of her refractory disease underwent a diverting ileostomy in March 2015.

Unfortunately, the patient's disease has recurred, both at her ileostomy and in her perianal region. We admitted her for intravenous corticosteroids, and administered ustekinumab, a monoclonal antibody that has proven efficacy in Crohn disease, based on randomized phase 2 and 3 clinical trials (papers attached). For some reason, while the initial doses of this medication were approved, we recently had a denial by a physician reviewer who has no expertise in pediatric gastroenterology.

_____'s insurance has been very supportive in the past, and understands of the severity of this child's illness and the need for treatment. Our medical options are limited, and a panel of experts in this division supports the use of ustekinumab. The patient has also received an outside second opinion by Dr. _____ (another Crohn expert in the region) who supports this approach. If _____ is not treated, her Crohn disease will progress, resulting in additional hospitalizations and surgeries.

I am a pediatric gastroenterologist who is considered a national authority in the treatment of pediatric Crohn disease (see attached CV). I would be happy to speak with anyone from the insurance or any physician reviewer to describe _____'s clinical situation.

Sincerely,

Athos Bousvaros MD, MPH

Appendix 4. Sample Letter for Appeal of Denial of Mental Health Benefits

To whom it may concern:

This letter is being written on behalf of our patient, *XXX (DOB:)*, whom we follow for her diagnosis of Crohn's Disease, a chronic inflammatory bowel disease of the colon and small intestine. We submit this letter in support of her being permitted to receive out-of-network mental health benefits at/through *(agency name/private provider)* as a clinical case exception. XXX has had a complicated course of her illness, having been hospitalized several times for unpredictable flares of her disease, both times leading to lengthy admissions followed by intensive outpatient follow-up. Her illness' response to our treatment plan has been sporadic and inconsistent, causing great stress on both her mind and body. We know that the emotional and physical pieces are interrelated in complex ways, and patients can experience flare-ups during times of emotional tensions and stress. This can relate to changes in the physiologic functioning of the gastrointestinal tract; we have seen this occur with XXX. Her medical complications have led to periods of intense stress and pressure, thereby exacerbating symptoms. XXX's specific circumstances are physically and psychologically complicated, and it is crucial to be able to integrate the medical and psychiatric services; this will be critical to providing the most comprehensive and cost-effective care.

(agency name/private provider) specializes in diagnosing and treating children and teenagers with comorbid physical and psychiatric/psychological issues. (Agency) provides and coordinates integrated plans of treatment, including psychopharmacology, cognitive behavioral therapies, and family work specifically geared toward helping manage these comorbid populations. Studies have shown that this type of integration of medical and psychiatric services can decrease both medical and psychiatric morbidity, and thus medical costs.

XXX's ability to access these services could be essential in reducing the risk factors for a necessary medical or psychological hospitalization. A hospitalization would be much more costly, both financially and in terms of the missed developmental learning opportunities in the social and academic realms.

It is in XXX's best interest to receive ongoing psychological care in a formal clinical model. However, we would request authorization for at least a two–session evaluation so that the formulation and treatment recommendations can be passed on to community psychiatric providers in their network. We feel strongly that the optimal coordinated care plan would include your insurance plan's willingness to authorize 12–14 treatment sessions so that XXX and her family can have access to the specialized skills of (agency/provider), thereby reducing the chances of an emergent, and perhaps more costly, hospitalization.

Please understand the extenuating circumstances impacting XXX. Thank you very much for your time and consideration in this urgent matter. Feel free to contact XXX with further questions. We look forward to hearing your response.

Appendix 5. Social Security Listing of Impairments for Children with IBD

Section 105.00, Digestive Impairments in Children

A. *Disorders of the digestive system* which result in disability usually do so because of interference with nutrition and growth, multiple recurrent inflammatory lesions, or other complications of the disease. Such lesions or complications usually respond to treatment. To constitute a listed impairment, these must be shown to have persisted or be expected to persist despite prescribed therapy for a continuous period of at least 12 months.

B. *Documentation of gastrointestinal impairments* should include pertinent operative findings, appropriate medically acceptable imaging studies, endoscopy, and biopsy reports. Where a liver biopsy has been performed in chronic liver disease, documentation should include the report of the biopsy. Medically acceptable imaging includes, but is not limited to, x-ray imaging, computerized axial tomography (CAT scan) or magnetic resonance imaging (MRI), with or without contrast material, myelography, and radionuclear bone scans. "Appropriate" means that the technique used is the proper one to support the evaluation and diagnosis of the impairment.

C. *Growth retardation and malnutrition.* When the primary disorder of the digestive tract has been documented, evaluate resultant malnutrition under the criteria described in 105.08. Evaluate resultant growth impairment under the criteria described in 100.03. Intestinal disorders, including surgical diversions and potentially correctable congenital lesions, do not represent a severe impairment if the individual is able to maintain adequate nutrition, growth and development.

D. *Multiple congenital anomalies.* See related criteria, and consider as a combination of impairments.

105.07 Chronic inflammatory bowel disease (such as ulcerative colitis, regional enteritis), as documented in 105.00. With one of the following:

A. Intestinal manifestations or complications, such as obstruction, abscess, or fistula formation which has lasted or is expected to last 12 months; or
B. Malnutrition as described under the criteria in 105.08; or
C. Growth impairment as described under the criteria in 100.03.

105.08 Malnutrition, due to demonstrable gastrointestinal disease causing either a fall of 15 percentiles of weight which persists or the persistence of weight which is less than the third percentile (on standard growth charts). And one of the following:

A. Stool fat excretion per 24 h:

1. More than 15% in infants less than 6 months.
2. More than 10% in infants 6–18 months.
3. More than 6% in children more than 18 months; or

B. Persistent hematocrit of 30% or less despite prescribed therapy; or
C. Serum carotene of 40 mcg./100 ml. or less; or
D. Serum albumin of 3.0 g./100 ml. or less.

Appendix 6. Preparing an Effective Letter for Family Medical Leave Act Provisions

• Caregiver's/parent's name (employee).
• Patient's name.
• Patient's diagnosis, date of diagnosis, length of treatment – chronic illness requires lifelong medical attention of some level.
• If relevant, recent or upcoming overnight stay in a hospital including estimation of incapacity after discharge home.
• Explain incapacitation as inability to attend school or perform other regular daily activities during the times of hospitalization, recovery, or scheduled outpatient medical procedures.
• All occasions and specifics of ongoing and continued treatment by a health-care provider as an outpatient, specifically outlining caregiver's responsibility for medication administration, monitoring and reporting of bowel habits at home, and coordination with other subspecialty providers, as applicable.
• Phrases indicating episodic, intermittent, unpredictable, and cyclical nature of the IBD disease process, with the need for ongoing, periodic outpatient visits.
• Emphasis of importance of the caregiver being present at these visits for active and ongoing discussion with the medical team to be able to participate in progressive treatment plan decisions that impact the child.
• Explanation that child's intermittent incapacity may cause the caregiver to work intermittently or on less than a full schedule.
• Identification of any potential future treatment or collateral providers in the child's care, including medication infusion at a Day Hospital Center, routine exploratory procedures, and imaging studies.
• Anticipate the potential involvement of radiologists, laboratory technicians, infusion center staff, physical therapists, dieticians, and mental health professionals, so that if a caregiver has to accompany a child to an appointment with one of these providers, without your presence, it can still be validated by the employer as qualifying for FMLA hours.
• Specification that a child requires basic medical assistance for medical decision making, transportation to appointments, and psychological comfort to assist in the management of the impact of the treatment regimen, given the interruption to daily functioning and the invasive nature of portions of the treatment plan.

Legislative Advocacy

Sarah Buchanan

Introduction

The Crohn's & Colitis Foundation of America (CCFA) has long encouraged medical professionals to champion quality care and research in health policy making on behalf of their patients. The medical community's participation in public policy advocacy is especially important now as policies implemented by federal and state governments, insurance companies, pharmaceutical companies, and medical industries increasingly affect the delivery of care and patient outcomes. In coordination with patients and like-minded organizations, medical practitioners and researchers can – and should – leverage their expertise and firsthand experiences to advise and advocate for the adoption of healthcare policies that best serve patients.

From the earliest days of its founding in 1967, CCFA has led efforts to raise awareness among the public and Members of Congress concerning the significant impact of inflammatory bowel diseases (IBD) in the United States. Initially, the goal of CCFA's advocacy program was to dramatically increase IBD research supported by CCFA and federal agencies like the National Institutes of Health. As improved treatments were approved by the Food and Drug Administration (FDA), and with the passage and implementation of the *Affordable Care Act,* CCFA expanded its focus on patient access to quality care. CCFA became and remains the largest national voluntary health agency dedicated to seeking the cause and cure of Crohn's disease and ulcerative colitis while improving the quality of life of people with these diseases.

Previous versions authored by Suzanne Rosenthal, Co-founder, Crohn's and Colitis Foundation of America

S. Buchanan
Crohn's & Colitis Foundation of America,
733 Third Avenue, Suite 510, New York, NY 10017, USA
e-mail: advocacy@ccfa.org

Advocacy

Advocacy is the means by which citizens affect policy change. It entails raising awareness of an issue among decision-makers, proposing a solution, and providing compelling justification for decision-makers to enact change or maintain a popular policy. Advocacy can take place on the local, state, and federal levels with several access points including legislatures, agencies, and other stakeholders. Advocacy is most successful when citizens coalesce together on an agreed-upon priority with an agreed-upon recommendation. For this reason, the partnership of patients, physicians, and voluntary health organizations has been effective in championing the interests of patients and sustaining medical research funding through both friendly and tumultuous political eras.

Medical professionals can play a leadership role in advocating on behalf of their patients. CCFA works with members of its National Scientific Advisory Council to analyze key issues experienced by the community and develop position statements that outline and explain subsequent policy recommendations. Researchers and practitioners are highly respected witnesses and CCFA coordinates with professional members to testify in hearings held by legislatures and agencies and submit written testimony. Medical experts also frequently accompany patients in meetings with legislative representatives or agency officials in order to provide technical information and complement the patient's personal story.

Popular legislative initiatives championed by CCFA and other voluntary health organizations fall into two main categories: medical research and patient access to care. Several entities support medical research including industry, foundations like CCFA, and universities. Federal agencies also support medical research with a focus on research that will advance a concept until it is attractive for industry investment, or research that will address a problem impacting the nation. The agency that leads the United States' health research portfolio is the National Institutes of Health (NIH). Other agencies include the Centers for Disease Control and

© Springer International Publishing AG 2017
P. Mamula et al. (eds.), *Pediatric Inflammatory Bowel Disease*, DOI 10.1007/978-3-319-49215-5_59

Prevention (CDC), the Department of Defense (DOD), and the Department of Veterans Affairs (VA).

The ability for patients to access the care they need directly affects their health outcomes and quality of life. The *Affordable Care Act (ACA)* provided significant patient protections including prohibiting discrimination against preexisting conditions, establishing out of pocket maximums, allowing young adults to stay on their parents' insurance until age 26, and eliminating lifetime caps on insurance. As a result of the ACA, many patients with IBD found it easier to obtain coverage and experienced less catastrophic costs that led to bankruptcy. However, the ACA did not eliminate all barriers to care. Persons with chronic conditions like IBD are especially vulnerable to prevalent cost-sharing and cost-control strategies like high out-of-pocket costs and step therapy. High cost-sharing renders biologics and other expensive medications grossly unaffordable for many Americans. As prices for sophisticated medications skyrocket, insurers increase the cost burden imposed on patients by requiring high copays or even coinsurance, a percentage copay rather than a fixed copay. Many patients subject to this kind of cost-sharing reach their out of pocket maximum of covered services within the first month of their plan year. Step therapy is a management protocol in which insurers require patients to fail first on preferred therapies before providing coverage for the physician-prescribed therapy. Both high out-of-pocket costs and step therapy bar patients from accessing needed medications and negatively impact patient outcomes. A balanced look at these issues raises questions about drug pricing, insurer coverage policies, and the delivery of affordable, high-quality care.

Whether advocating for medical research or championing patient access to care, the perspective of medical professionals is a critical component of the advocacy strategy. Medical expertise is highly valued for issues analysis, the development of recommended policies, testimony and other correspondence with decision-makers, and supplementing patient stories. Physicians, researchers, and other practitioners can team with like-minded patients and organizations to strengthen their message. Many voluntary health organizations including CCFA have advocacy departments, medical advisory committees, and/or professional memberships that can provide an entry point for medical experts to join their cause.

Legislative History

Under the leadership of Suzanne Rosenthal, Co-Founder of CCFA, CCFA's advocacy led to significant strides in expanding federal research on digestive diseases, creating informational resources for patients available at federal agencies, and advancing policies that make it easier for patients to get the care they need. CCFA recognized in the mid-1970s that it was important to have a professional presence in Washington, DC, to recommend and represent advocacy efforts affecting patients with IBD. Since 1978, the Health & Medicine Counsel of Washington (HMCW) has assisted CCFA on IBD advocacy programs by coordinating both the Foundation's own IBD-specific efforts and more encompassing efforts through the Digestive Disease National Coalition (DDNC). The DDNC was founded by CCFA leadership in 1978 and is currently comprised of over 40 lay and medical member organizations. The combined efforts of CCFA, HMCW, DDNC, and the leading national gastrointestinal professional societies added to the effectiveness and success of several important IBD legislative initiatives, described below.

Research Funding at the National Institutes of Health

The IBD research portfolio at NIH started in the early 1960s with $25,000. From 1999 to 2003, CCFA actively participated in the successful effort to double the budget of NIH. During this period, NIH support for IBD research grew to $63 million. Funding for NIH has continued to grow from $27 billion in fiscal year 2003 (FY03) to $32 billion in FY16. This steady increase can be credited in part to consistent advocacy from the health community to educate legislators on the need for better treatments. In FY15, NIH support for IBD research exceeded $120 million – primarily targeted to the IBD programs at the National Institute of Diabetes, Digestive & Kidney Diseases (NIDDK) and the National Institute of Allergy and Infectious Diseases (NIAID). NIH supports several pediatric IBD research initiatives, including the Predicting Response to Standardized Pediatric Colitis Therapy (PROTECT) study which is reviewing how children that have been newly diagnosed with ulcerative colitis respond to the standard initial therapies, mesalamine and prednisone (corticosteroid). Current advocacy initiatives for NIH focus on continuing to grow the NIH budget and improving the pace of therapy development by advancing translational science.

IBD Bill Signed by President George W. Bush and Enacted into Law on November 30, 2004

CCFA's most important initiatives included the creation of IBD-specific legislation. The "Inflammatory Bowel Disease Research Act" was introduced in the House in January 2003 by original cosponsors – Rep. Sue Kelly (R-NY) and Rep. Jesse Jackson, Jr. (D-IL). In February 2003, original cosponsors Senators Harry Reid (D-NV) and Thad Cochran (R-MS) introduced the same bill in the Senate, and CCFA launched a national effort to advance the bill in both chambers of Congress. Web email and daily Internet announcements, letter campaigns, and telephone calls from the national and chapter offices and from hundreds of volunteers helped to secure the cosponsorship of 183 Representatives and 37 Senators. With the large number of bipartisan cosponsors supporting the bill, it passed quickly through Congress and President Bush signed it into law. The bill was enacted as the "Research Review Act" on November 30, 2004 – just short of 2 years after the introduction of the legislation in early 2003. Professional and lay organizations that added support to CCFA's effort to seek passage of the Bill included the DDNC, the North American Society for Pediatric Gastroenterology Hepatology and Nutrition (NASPGHAN), the American Gastroenterological Association (AGA), the American College of Gastroenterology (ACG), the United Ostomy Association (UOA), the American Society for Gastrointestinal Endoscopy (ASGE), the International Foundation for Functional Gastrointestinal Disorders (IFFGD), and the Hepatitis Foundation International (HFI).

The "Research Review Act" provided two major benefits for patients with IBD:

A. Studies by the General Accountability Office (GAO): Social Security Disability Report and Medicare and Medicaid Coverage Report. In 2005, as mandated by the "Research Review Act," GAO undertook the first federal studies specific to patients with IBD. The first study investigated the challenges patients with IBD patients are facing when applying for Social Security Disability. The second study focused on Medicare and Medicaid coverage of IBD therapies including FDA-approved therapies for Crohn's disease and ulcerative colitis, ostomy supplies, medical necessary foods, enteral nutrition formula, and parenteral nutrition.

CCFA and the United Ostomy Association (UOA) leaders met with GAO researchers in Washington in January of 2005 to discuss both issues. The GAO released the Social Security Disability study (*GAO-05-495*) in May of 2005. The report made several recommendations for improving the disability process for patients with IBD and has proven to be a beneficial resource when pursuing disability claims with the Social Security Administration.

The Medicare/Medicaid study (*GAO-06-63*) was issued in December of 2005 and provided a comprehensive analysis of national Medicare coverage of IBD therapies and state-based Medicaid policies (including analysis of Medicaid coverage in all 50 states and the District of Columbia). The report served as a guide for advocacy efforts to address gaps in coverage for Medicare and Medicaid beneficiaries.

B. The Establishment of Centers for Disease Control Inflammatory Bowel Disease Epidemiology Study. In 2002, CCFA prioritized the need to financially support a National IBD Epidemiology Study to determine the true prevalence of the disease and the unique demographic characteristics of the IBD patient population. It sought a proposal from CDC to be underwritten by CCFA in the amount of $750,000 to create and monitor the study. In 2005, with the passage of the "Research Review Act," CCFA secured support from Congress to continue the IBD Epidemiology Study. Through competitively awarded cooperative agreements, CCFA helps administer the epidemiology study and directs research activities in partnership with CDC utilizing the funds provided by the Congress. Although challenged by shrinking federal budgets, the IBD Epidemiology Study has been maintained at the CDC due to proactive advocacy efforts from the IBD community since 2004. In FY16, the program received an annual appropriation of $750,000. This research is critical to providing accurate data on disease incidence, which will inform targeted interventions.

Other IBD-Specific Legislations

Since the passage of the "Research Review Act" in the 108th Congress, it has been necessary to continue to raise the profile of IBD in Congress and to encourage NIH and CDC to expand support for IBD research, particularly in pediatrics. Legislation that built on the progress of the "Research Review Act" was introduced in 109th, 110th, and 111th Congress with the support by many of the same digestive disease organizations. This kind of disease-specific legislation has become unpopular in favor of bills that broadly affect a number of communities. Nonetheless, the key elements of the legislation remain worthwhile goals to pursue through congressional oversight and partnerships with federal agencies. The components of the subsequent IBD research legislation are characterized by the following:

A. Expand the IBD research portfolio at NIH. In 2007, specific recommendations were made on research areas of focus:
   1. Pediatric-related research
   2. Genetic and environmental research into the cause and progression of IBD
   3. Clinical research, including translational studies and treatment trials
   4. Support for the training of new investigators specializing in IBD with an emphasis on pediatric care
B. Establish a "Pediatric IBD Patient Registry" through CDC. This registry would collect and analyze data on the incidence and prevalence of the diseases in children,

genetic and environmental factors associated with pediatric disease, and treatment approaches and outcomes for pediatric IBD patients.

C. Require CDC to develop a "National Inflammatory Bowel Disease Action Plan." This plan would detail a comprehensive strategy for addressing the burden of IBD in both pediatric and adult populations. Specifically, the plan would create mechanisms for increasing awareness of IBD and preventing its progression and related complications, such as colorectal cancer.

Healthcare Reform

The *Affordable Care Act*, signed by President Obama in March 2010, demonstrated the effectiveness of CCFA's advocacy on several counts. The Foundation articulated and published a Statement of Principles of Healthcare Reform. The majority of its objectives were reflected in the new legislation. Phased-in over time, the legislation provides chronic disease patients with relief from pre-existing coverage exclusions, annual and lifetime benefit caps, medical underwriting, policy rescissions, and extended waiting periods for coverage. Additionally, the bill requires insurers to cover young adults on their parents' policies until age 26. It also covers routine medical costs associated with participation in clinical trials. The dynamics of implementation have had many implications for IBD patients, particularly in third-party payer efforts to share and/or control the cost of care. CCFA is dedicated to protecting the physician-patient health decision-making relationship and remains vigilant in educating stakeholders and activating on health policy changes that affect access and affordability of care for IBD patients.

Department of Defense Medical Research Program Eligibility

In FY08, IBD became one of only twenty-nine diseases eligible to compete for $50 million in funding available through the DOD Peer-Reviewed Medical Research Program. CCFA continues to advocate for annual funding and inclusion of IBD as a disease eligible for study. The funding for the Peer-Reviewed Medical Research Program has since grown to $278.7 million in FY16. CCFA members serve on a consumer advisory committee to the DOD for this program.

The Launch of a Congressional Crohn's and Colitis Caucus in 2011

In March of 2011, a major milestone for IBD advocacy was reached with the launch of the Congressional Crohn's and Colitis Caucus. A congressional caucus is a group of members of the US Congress that coalesce to champion legislative issues of mutual interest. By caucusing, legislators can multiply their power to advance priority policies. The founding Representatives of the Congressional Crohn's and Colitis Caucus were Jesse L. Jackson, Jr. (D-IL) and Ander Crenshaw (R-FL). The Caucus creates a congressional locus of support for expanding investment in IBD research at a national level – through NIH, DOD, and CDC – as well as for issues of healthcare access, most crucial in these times. The Caucus has grown from 27 members by the end of 2011 to 67 members at the end of 2015. This growth is important for strengthening the initiatives of the Caucus.

Crohn's and Colitis Awareness Week

December 2011 marked the inauguration of the national Crohn's and Colitis Awareness Week from December 1 to December 7. This event reflects the awareness that has been created in the US Congress of the plight of patients and caregivers who face up to IBD every day. In May 2011, Resolution 199 was introduced in the US Senate by Senator Reid and Senator Cochran. The Resolution states:

- Crohn's disease (CD) and ulcerative colitis (UC) are serious, chronic inflammatory diseases of the gastrointestinal tract.
- The cause of CD and UC are unknown and no medical cure exists.
- CD and UC are at high risk for developing colorectal cancer.
- Lack of awareness among health professionals and the general public may contribute to the misdiagnosis and mismanagement of CD and UC.
- The annual direct cost of CD and UC in this country is estimated to be $6.1 billion.
- The goals of "Crohn's and Colitis Awareness Week" are
  - To invite and encourage all people in the United States to join the effort to find a cure for CD and UC
  - To engage in activities aimed at raising awareness of CD and UC among the general public and healthcare providers
  - To promote and support biomedical research needed to find better treatments and a cure for CD and UC

The First National Digestive Disease Commission

CCFA advocated with national GI professional associations to rename the NIH National Institute of Arthritis and Metabolic Diseases (NIAMD) to the National Institute of

Arthritis, Metabolism, and Digestive Diseases (NIAMDD) (May, 1972; PL 92–305), thus securing a separate digestive disease division at NIH. CCFA worked in the 1970s with GI professional and lay associations to create the first National Digestive Disease Commission (NDDC) and to have key elements of its findings and conclusions implemented. The Arthritis, Diabetes, and Digestive Disease Amendments of 1976 (Oct, 1976, PL 94–562) created the first National Commission on Digestive Diseases with the goal of establishing a long-term plan for digestive disease research in the United States, last published in 2009. CCFA represented the digestive disease lay community as Chair of the NDDC's Patient and Public Education Work Group. CCFA-affiliated physicians served as commissioners.

Silvio O. Conte Digestive Disease Research Centers

In December of 1980, the Commission's efforts led to Congress enacting Public Law 96–541, which changed the NIAMDD to the National Institute of Arthritis, Diabetes, and Digestive and Kidney Diseases (NIADDK). This Public Law also created the statutory authority for the Digestive Disease Research Centers Program (DDRC), the National Digestive Diseases Information Clearinghouse, and an intramural NIDDK digestive disease epidemiology data program. CCFA worked with the late Congressman Silvio O. Conte (R-MA) and Congressman William Natcher (D-KY) to support the creation and funding for the Conte Digestive Disease Research Centers Program within the NIDDK. The first grants, six of them, were awarded in November of 1984. Currently there are 21 Digestive Disease Research Centers, several of which have a primary focus on inflammatory bowel disease. The DDRCC Program provides a mechanism for funding shared resources (core facilities) that serve to integrate, coordinate, and foster interdisciplinary cooperation between groups of established investigators who conduct programs of high-quality research that are related to a common theme in digestive diseases research. An existing base of high-quality digestive disease-related research is a prerequisite for the establishment of a center.

National Digestive Disease Information Clearinghouse

CCFA and other lay organizations sought for years the creation and funding of an important digestive diseases education resource. Finally, the National Digestive Diseases Information Clearinghouse (NDDIC) was formed in 1980 through PL 96–541 which established an Executive Committee and an Advisory Board that meets annually.

Digestive Disease National Coalition

CCFA was the founding organization of the Digestive Disease National Coalition (DDNC) created in 1978 to provide a forum for all professional and voluntary organizations interested in digestive diseases to work together to address national issues related to research, patient care, and public/professional awareness of digestive diseases. The collective number of patients and lay and medical members represented by over 40 DDNC member organizations was formidable. Founding organizations included CCFA, NASPGHAN, AGA, ACG, ASGE, the American Liver Foundation, IFFGD, as well as a number of Celiac Disease groups. The DDNC has been successful in advocating for additional funding for digestive disease research, improving patient access to preventive and diagnostic GI care, and serving as the collective voice of the digestive disease community on all matters related to national health policy and digestive diseases. Consistently, the DDNC has had high-quality representation from the IBD patient and scientific and medical community.

National Colorectal Cancer Roundtable

CCFA, as a founding member of the National Colorectal Cancer Roundtable (NCCRT), sought the originating legislation to create and fund the NCCRT. It was authorized in 1997 and funded in FY98. The NCCRT is supported through a cooperative agreement by CDC and the American Cancer Society. The NIH National Cancer Institute (NCI) is also a lead organization. The NCCRT meets annually with work done in several committees throughout the year. It has grown to over 60 member organizations and has the major goal of increasing the safe and effective use of proven colorectal cancer screening tests among appropriate populations. A major accomplishment of the NCCRT was to develop consensus CRC screening guidelines among all professional and voluntary organizations concerned with colorectal cancer. Important medical publications arising out of NCCRT have advanced the knowledge of prevention of colorectal cancer. NCCRT has also created many attractive public awareness programs for radio and television and produced educational materials for different ethnic and age populations at high risk of colon cancer.

Crohn's & Colitis Foundation of America: Government Affairs Committee

In the 1970s, CCFA created a Government Affairs Committee (GAC) of the Board of Trustees to monitor, recommend actions, and implement activities to advance IBD research at NIH and other federal entities including:

(a) Activity targeted to seek the cosponsorship of members of the relevant House and Senate health subcommittees that consider and recommend to their full committees authorization legislation and its associated appropriations. Cosponsorship is simultaneously sought from the rest of the members of Congress. Letter writing, faxes, and emails are encouraged to promote CCFA's agenda before all federal legislators.

(b) Organizing "IBD Days on the Hill" starting in 2002. Cumulatively through March 2015, over 1300 men, women, and children have made pilgrimages to Washington, DC, to participate in CCFA's advocacy effort. They meet and educate legislators about IBD and its impact on patients and their families and urge support of important NIH and CDC initiatives through cosponsorship of IBD legislation, increasing IBD appropriations, and other IBD-related matters. This is an annual effort maintained to keep legislators and legislative aides aware of CCFA's mission and to seek increased funding for the NIH, DOD, and CDC IBD programs.

(c) In 2004, the GAC created its National IBD Advocacy Network, which has a current enrollment of several thousands of people with IBD and their families who are provided with the opportunity to engage in advocacy efforts from their homes and offices and go to Washington, DC, on CCFA's annual IBD Days on the Hill.

Advocacy and the Future of IBD Research and Care

The forty-eight-year history of CCFA has demonstrated the necessity of investment in the search for better treatments and quality of life for those affected by inflammatory bowel diseases. Private and government research funding, as well as healthcare policies that benefit patients, are as crucial today as they were in the 1960s. The formula followed by CCFA has advocacy at its core. It has changed the landscape for the healthcare profession, research science, and patient resources related to Crohn's disease and ulcerative colitis. However, the landscape continues to change and requires a redoubling of efforts with every year that passes. Legislation and public awareness work hand-in-hand to create real progress.

Transition from Pediatric to Adult Care

Stacy A. Kahn and Sandra C. Kim

60

Introduction

Transition of care is emerging as an increasingly important area of care in patients with chronic conditions including inflammatory bowel diseases (IBD). Transition from pediatric to adult care is not simply a transfer of patient care from one provider to another. It is a dynamic process defined as the purposeful planned movement of adolescents and young adults with chronic physical and medical conditions from child-centered to adult-oriented health-care systems [1]. Education, communication, and preparation promote self-management skills, confidence, and independence, which help ensure a successful transition. Effective transition requires a multidisciplinary and coordinated approach to ensure successful "graduation" which is marked by independence, effective self-management, and establishment of care with an adult gastroenterologist and adult medical care team. Several medical societies and groups have issued consensus statements regarding the need for coordinated and well-planned transition for adolescents and young adults with chronic medical conditions [2, 3], [4, 5]. According to the American Academy of Pediatrics (AAP), transition should address the following: (1) Ensure that all young people with special health-care needs have an identified health-care professional who attends to the unique challenges of transition and assumes responsibility for current health care, care coordination, and future health-care planning. (2) Identify the core knowledge and skills required to provide developmentally appropriate health-care transition services to young

people with special health-care needs and make them part of training and certification requirements for primary care residents and physicians in practice. (3) Prepare and maintain an up-to-date medical summary that is portable and accessible. (4) Create a written health-care transition plan by age 14 together with the young adult and family. At a minimum, this plan should include what services need to be provided, who will provide them, and how they will be financed. This plan should be reviewed and updated annually and whenever there is a transfer of care. (5) Apply the same guidelines for primary and preventive care for all adolescents and young adults, including those with special health-care needs, recognizing that young people with special health-care needs may require more resources and services than other young people to optimize their health. (6) Ensure affordable, continuous health insurance coverage for all young people with special health-care needs throughout adolescence and adulthood [3].

Similarly, the North American Society for Pediatric Gastroenterology, Hepatology and Nutrition (NASPGHAN) and the Crohn's and Colitis Foundation of America (CCFA) have issued specific statements regarding the transition of care for adolescents with IBD [6, 7]. NASPGHAN recommendations for the practitioner suggest the following: (1) The pediatric gastroenterologist should begin seeing adolescent IBD patients without their parents to build a relationship promoting independence. (2) Introduce the patient and family to the concept and benefits of transition. (3) Identify a skilled gastroenterologist who cares for young adults and recognizes the different set of expectations that young adults with childhood-onset IBD have versus those recently diagnosed with IBD. (4) Prepare a detailed medical letter and brief medical summary for the new adult gastroenterologist. (5) Recognition that the timing of transition requires flexibility due to individual special circumstances. These guidelines addressed a number of issues that adolescents with IBD encounter, including the process of moving from parental oversight to independence and self-reliance and transferring care from the nurturing medical care approach commonly seen in pediatric care practices. Other

S.A. Kahn, MD
Transitional IBD Clinic, The University of Chicago Medicine, 5841 S. Maryland Avenue, MC 4065, Chicago, IL 60637, USA

S.C. Kim, MD (✉)
Gastroenterology, The Ohio State University College of Medicine, Department of Pediatrics and Center for Pediatric and Adolescent IBD, Nationwide Children's Hospital, 700 Children's Drive, Columbus, OH 43205, USA
e-mail: Sandra.Kim@chp.edu

© Springer International Publishing AG 2017
P. Mamula et al. (eds.), *Pediatric Inflammatory Bowel Disease*, DOI 10.1007/978-3-319-49215-5_60

factors that should be incorporated into the transition process include the need of both parents/guardians and pediatric health-care providers (including physicians, nurses, and many other health-care providers) to relinquish caregiver roles of young adults living with a chronic illness and to facilitate successful transfer of care to an adult subspecialist.

Despite these useful guidelines, there is still no "gold standard" or defined best practices for transition of care in IBD, highlighting the need for more research on this vulnerable population [8]. In this chapter, we will outline the recommendations for transition of care in IBD, unique features of the adolescent IBD population, barriers to transition of care, and approaches, skills, and tools that can facilitate a successful transition to adult IBD care.

Background

Although there is growing emphasis on transition of care for adolescents with chronic medical conditions, there is a relative lack of data about which approaches and models work best in adolescents and young adults (AYA) with IBD [9]. This gap in our knowledge is due in part to a dearth of research on this topic, as well as the high degree of variability between health-care systems on a regional, national, and international level, therefore limiting the generalizability of a given approach. Despite these limitations, transition of care for young adults with IBD is important for several reasons. First, up to one-third of parents and one-fourth of teens are apprehensive about transition to an adult provider [10]. Second, youth with IBD have diminished health-related quality of life (HRQOL) [11] that can dramatically increase during adolescence when they are especially vulnerable to psychological stress [12]. HRQOL is a vital aspect of patient care, patient-physician communication, and shared decision-making. Finally, a well-planned and coordinated transition to adult care has been shown to improve outcomes in patients with other chronic disease [13]. Factors associated with successful health-care transition include starting the process early, having family members and health-care providers foster personal and medical independence, and confirming that the young adult verbalizes the desire to function in the adult medical world [14].

The ultimate goal is a prepared, proactive health-care team and an informed, active patient – a concept particularly applicable to patients with IBD. Evidence supports the idea that pediatric and adult-oriented medical practices represent two different medical subcultures. If young adults and family members are not well prepared for participation in the adult health-care system, they will have trouble with this transition and may not receive the care they need [14].

Challenges and Barriers to Transition for Adolescent IBD Patients

Researchers have begun to identify specific barriers to transition in teens and young adults with IBD. These barriers include differences in pediatric-onset versus adult-onset IBD, differences between pediatric and adult care, psychosocial factors, treatment adherence and poorly developed self-management skills, attachment to pediatric providers, individual maturity, and readiness for transition. Recently, two different groups found that patient and parent/guardian attachment to pediatric providers was among the most significant barriers to transition [15, 16]. Not surprisingly, Bensen et al. also found that patients with emotional and cognitive delay faced additional challenges in the transition process [15].

Differences between pediatric- or adolescent-onset IBD and adult IBD can also have a significant impact on the transition process. Although pediatric- and adolescent-onset IBD is common, occurring in roughly 20–30% of all cases [17, 18], there are significant differences in pediatric and adolescent disease presentation and severity; most notably, pediatric/adolescent IBD is more aggressive and extensive [19, 20, 21]. A recent study by Van Limbergen and colleagues found patients with pediatric-onset disease were almost twice as likely to have extensive ulcerative colitis (UC) compared to those with adult-onset disease. Similarly, among those children with Crohn's disease, 40% had extensive disease compared to 3% of their adult counterparts. Surgery within 10 years of diagnosis was twice as common in pediatric-onset UC. Although there was less surgery in pediatric-onset CD, more than one-third required surgical intervention within 10 years of diagnosis [21].

Goodhand et al. have demonstrated that compared to adults, teens have more severe disease. Adolescents were more likely to be on azathioprine (46% vs. 17%, $P < 0.0001$) or infliximab (20% vs. 8%, $P < 0.05$). Furthermore, teens were more likely to require hospitalization (46% vs. 14%, $P < 0.0001$). This is further complicated by the fact that teens were significantly more likely to miss medical appointments than adults (median appointments missed: adolescents 20% vs. adults 0%; $P < 0.0001$). The authors concluded that earlier-onset IBD is more complex, and, therefore, specific adolescent transitioning clinics should be established [19]. This highlights the need for additional research to better understand outcomes and the natural history of IBD in this unique group that spans both the pediatric and adult populations.

Treatment adherence and self-management are key skills that teens must master during the transition process but are often difficult for AYA [22, 23, 24]. Several studies have identified barriers to adherence in adolescents that include the following: forgetting to take medications [25], lack of time, feeling well, medication side effects [26], and therapeutic regimen complexity [27]. These barriers can be further exacerbated by the patients' underlying anxiety and depression [25]. In addition to adherence, teens must develop a wide range of self-management skills often lacking in teens with IBD prior to "graduation" from their pediatric provider. Fishman et al. surveyed teenagers aged 16–18 years and found that only 43% confidently knew their medication name and dose and even fewer knew about important side effects. In addition AYA relied heavily on parents to schedule appointments (85%), request refills (75%), and contact providers between visits (74%) [22]. In a follow-up study, Fishman and colleagues surveyed 294 youth, 10 years and older, and found that although 95% could name their medication, just over half knew the correct dose and less than one-third could report a single major side effect [28]. Although self-management skills and independence have been shown to increase with age, they do not necessarily correlate with disease duration, reinforcing the complex nature of teaching skills to teens with IBD [24].

Differences in approaches to pediatric and adult medical care can have a profound impact on the transition process as well. Hait and colleagues point out that pediatric care tends to be multidisciplinary and family focused and requires parental direction and consent. On the other hand, a single physician often provides care in adult medicine; the relationship involves shared decision-making exclusively between the patient and provider rather than the entire family. The adult health-care clinic visit is patient focused, and the provider expects the patient to be autonomous and independent [29].

A survey of adult gastroenterologists in 2009 reported that 51% had received an inadequate medical history from pediatric providers, 55% of young adults with IBD demonstrated deficits in knowledge of their medical history, and 69% did not know their medication regimens [29]. The authors suggested that educating the young adult IBD patient is essential but not a substitute for delivering an accurate medical history to the adult provider. In contrast to this survey of adult gastroenterologists, a French survey of 48 young patients with IBD (and their parents) who had transitioned from pediatric to adult care revealed that the majority (85% of patients and 74% of parents) felt they were ready for transition to adult care [10]. Only 22% of patients and 32% of parents were apprehensive of the process. Of the 57% that attended a joint medical visit with the pediatric and adult providers, all considered it beneficial for transmitting records and most (93% of patients and 100% of parents) considered it beneficial for building confidence in the new gastroenterologist, highlighting the benefit and need for more transition clinics.

Transition Steps

The appropriate age to begin teaching these skill sets will vary with each patient's level of maturity and interest. However, starting by age 12–14 years gives the patient and family adequate time for the process and allows each patient the opportunity to gradually assume more responsibility for taking care of their own unique problems. The skill sets involve accruing knowledge (education), developing self-management skills based on that knowledge (focus on independence), and understanding the mutual impact of inflammatory bowel disease and lifestyle decisions on future health and well-being. This process should be tailored to the individual patient based on their needs.

NASPGHAN, the National Alliance to Advance Adolescent Health, and others have made useful planning and readiness checklists to help facilitate the successful transition to adult care (GotTransition.org [30]; [31]; NASPGHAN [32]).

Overview of the Transition Process

A number of tools, checklists, and planners to facilitate the transition process and transfer of care are described in Table 60.1. It is important to remember that the process should be tailored to the individual patient and family and may need to be adapted according to factors such as insurance, location, and post-high school plans.

Patients (Age 12–14)

At this age, the patients should be introduced and educated on the idea of transition and begin steps to prepare themselves toward this goal. There are two skill sets that should be attained for this age group.

Skill set 1 Knowledge related to their illness: This first step is designed to help patients learn about their specific disease, either Crohn's disease or ulcerative colitis. The patient should be able to articulate that they have IBD, including both gastrointestinal and extraintestinal symptoms, and recognize when they are having a flare and what might be precipitating the flare (diet, stress, other medications, etc.) and when they should visit their physician. The child should be able to express the impact of his/her disease on daily functioning at school, socially, and at home. Providing handouts with these key points and specific age-appropriate websites can help patients develop resources for ongoing education and new information (e.g., http://www.ccfa.org/kids-teens).

Skill set 2 Knowledge related to medications: This step includes information about specific medications they are

Table 60.1 Transition resources and tools

Educational resources and transition guidelines for providers
"A case-based monograph focusing on IBD: Improving health supervision in pediatric and young adult patients with IBD" (NASPGHAN)
"Educate, communicate, anticipate: Practical recommendations for transitioning adolescents with IBD to adult health care" [31]
Transition of the patient with inflammatory bowel disease from pediatric to adult care: Recommendations of the North American Society for Pediatric Gastroenterology, Hepatology and Nutrition" [6]
"Transitioning the adolescent inflammatory bowel disease patient: Guidelines for the adult and pediatric gastroenterologist" [7]
Transition readiness assessment and tools
For patients
Patient checklist for preparing to transition from a pediatric to adult care practitioner [33]
"Preparing to transition from a pediatric to adult care practitioner": http://www.gikids.org/files/documents/resources/IBD-TransitionTeenIBD.pdf
For providers
Healthcare provider checklist for transitioning a patient with IBD from pediatric to adult care [32]
"Transitioning a patient with IBD from pediatric to adult care": http://www.gikids.org/files/documents/resources/Checklist_ONLYHealthcareProdiver_TransitionfromPedtoAdult.pdf
TRxANSITION scale and STARx transition readiness questionnaire [34, 35]
Health passports, self-management tools, and symptom trackers
GI Buddy (symptom tracker): http://www.ibdetermined.org/Tracker.aspx
Good 2 Go Transition Program – MyHealth Passport: https://www.sickkids.ca/myhealthpassport/
Gut Check app (symptom tracker): https://www.gutcheckapp.com
myIBD (symptom tracker): http://www.sickkids.ca/IBDacademy/IBD-Mobile-App/
Resources for adolescents and parents
American Academy of Pediatrics: "How to help your teen transition to adult health care": http://www.healthychildren.org/English/family-life/health-management/Pages/How-to-Help-Your-Teen-Transition-to-Adult-Health-Care-Video.aspx
CCFA Campus Connection: http://www.ccfa.org/campus-connection/
CCFA IBDetermined: http://www.ibdetermined.org/
IBD University (IBD U): http://www.ibdu.org/
ImproveCareNow: https://improvecarenow.org
Just Like Me: http://www.justlikemeibd.org
Transition advocacy and support for patients, parents, and providers
"Got Transition/Center for Health Care Transition": http://gottransition.org/
The Society of Adolescent Health and Medicine: http://www.adolescenthealth.org/Home.aspx

taking (name, dose, why they are taking the medication, timing of each dose, possible side effects) and, finally, establishing a plan to take medications on their own without being reminded. This step is also crucial as a first step in preventing the lapses in adherence to medication, which occurs quite frequently at this age and throughout adolescence [23]. Bell has also noted that adolescent risk taking, magical thinking, and denial can all contribute to poor treatment adherence [36]. Patient education and problem-solving skills training are key approaches to overcome these issues, as is having a positive relationship with health-care providers and family members ([37]; [38]). Because increased authority from parents and professionals, overprotection, and sick role in teens with chronic disease may lead to learned dependency ([36]), this is a good time to begin to promote independence by setting a date when the patient will visit with their provider alone, starting by performing the physical exam without the parents/guardians in the room.

Parents/Family (Age 12–14)

Reiss and colleagues have found that parents often feel excluded when their child transitions to an adult provider, especially after they have dedicated many years of supporting and being involved in their children's health care [14]. Parents may also have concerns about "letting go," and family resistance can be a major barrier to successful transition. In order to prevent these negative feelings, parents should also be informed and educated regarding the eventual need for transition – the process of "letting go," so that their child can function independently as they leave home for work or college. The main role of the family at this time is to support the child through the disease symptoms and exacerbations and to provide a comfortable and protective atmosphere for this transitioning period. Since parents are actively involved in the daily care of their young adult children, they are the key personnel to reinforce the list of items needed at each visit for a successful transition. They should be notified that future clinic visits might include an established period of time for the young adult patient to meet with the health-care provider on their own. As part of the process, the parents can be provided the opportunity and a primary role in making their child independent through each step, as they help educate their son/daughter on crucial topic areas including insurance coverage, refilling medications, and scheduling appointments independently. Another important role for parents is to observe and confirm to the pediatric GI team that their child is making progress mastering the skills required for independence prior to the transfer of their care to adult providers.

Pediatric Team (Age 12–14)

The pediatric team often includes the pediatric gastroenterologist, nurse, psychologist, dietitian, and other pediatric subspecialists involved in managing the patient's care. The pediatric gastroenterologist, who is usually the primary provider, will establish the parameters for the support staff in promoting this transition period. Teaching of transition skills (those chosen as most important by each practice or institution) may be directed by a nurse, nurse practitioner, or the gastroenterologist, depending on staffing and availability. It is critically important for the physician to convey the importance of the process to the patient and family so that they understand, recognize, and accept the benefits of increasing the patient's self-management of their disease.

The pediatric gastroenterologist should address the concept of independent clinic visits for the patient with the family. This should start by including the parents for the initial portion of the visit, followed by the gastroenterologist performing the physical exam without parents/guardians in the examination room. Topics the pediatric gastroenterologist should address include information and guidance regarding drugs, alcohol, dating/sexuality, and health maintenance issues (i.e., diet, exercise). It is also important to address the medication adherence and compliance, which can impact future health and can be a significant issue in young adults with IBD [39]. Furthermore, potential psychological issues should be screened and identified so that referrals can be placed with mental health professionals. This helps address anxiety disorder/depression which, when left untreated, can hinder the transition process and successful attainment of the necessary self-management skills [25].

Focus on Independence

Patients (Age 14–17)

Patients in this age group should acquire the following two major skill sets that focus on increasing their independence:

Skill set 3 Knowledge related to procedures and tests: This would include laboratory tests, diagnostic imaging, and endoscopic procedures used in managing the patient with IBD. The goal is for patients to not only be comfortable with the different tests and procedures but also to recognize their importance and purpose in managing their disease long term.

Skill set 4 Basic medical knowledge: This step emphasizes basic medical knowledge that all patients should know, regardless of the presence or absence of a chronic illness. This includes knowing how to measure their weight, take their temperature, and read a thermometer. It also includes learning or knowing where to find telephone numbers and locations for their health-care provider, their clinic, and the hospital. They should be able to articulate their medical history and to identify names of community-based social support groups and organizations (e.g., Crohn's and Colitis Foundation of America, CCFA). Patients should be able to articulate the medical risk of nonadherence, and they should understand the impact of illicit drugs and alcohol on their illness as well as the interactions with their ongoing medications. This may take a little time in the office demonstrating some of these skills, and it will require some work from the family to help set up their own system for reinforcing this information. In addition, patients might be asked to prepare questions ahead of time for the doctor and nurse or dietician.

The patients should begin filling their own prescriptions, scheduling their own appointments, and keeping medical information and insurance information. The patient should also develop a method of tracking symptoms and issues related to their IBD. This makes their clinic visit with their physician effective and centered on the patient while helping the patient to demonstrate the ability to be more independent with their health care. During the visit, the patient can privately address questions they have regarding adolescent issues and discuss future plans upon the completion of high school. Patients should be educated, however, that the parent or guardian must legally be informed about the overall condition and high-risk behaviors more common in teens and young adults that could seriously affect their disease.

Parents (Age 14–17)

Since the main focus at this age is to promote independence, the family/parents/guardians should teach their child the intricacies of medical care as if they were out on their own. Examples include the following: maintaining a current medication list, filling and refilling prescriptions, and scheduling clinic appointments. They can provide guidance on organizing medical information in a dynamic fashion, which is crucial. Parents should also provide all information regarding insurance (insurance card, relevant contact numbers). Most importantly, the parents should continue to reinforce the skill sets that the patients need at this developmental stage outside routine clinic visits and to update the pediatric health-care team on their child's progress during the transitioning process.

Pediatric Team (Age 14–17)

The pediatric gastroenterologist as well as the pediatric health-care team should start and continue to focus on the patient instead of the parents or guardians when providing explanations and when obtaining the history. This includes making sure part of the visit occurs without parents in the room and allowing the patient to decide on the appropriate timing. This allows the physician to directly interact with the patient and is essential in the progression toward independence the young adult needs prior to transfer of care. The physician should explain to the patient what the parent or guardian must legally be informed about regarding their condition. During this process, the physician and patient should develop goals and timelines for specific skills required during the transitioning process (i.e., filling prescriptions and scheduling appointments). These visits should also address sensitive topics including drug and alcohol usage, as well as the impact of disease on sexuality and fertility. Future work and school timelines need to be considered during this transitioning process to optimize effective timing for the transfer of care as well as identifying future adult providers. Psychosocial monitoring including screens for anxiety, depression, and quality of life as well as transition readiness is recommended given the impact of ongoing psychosocial comorbidities on medication adherence and effective transfer of care.

Self-Management: Health and Lifestyles

Patients (Age 17–18)

This is the crucial period before the actual transfer of care to an adult provider. The two skill sets they need at this stage include the following:

Skill set 5 General self-management skills: Skills attained in this set put the knowledge acquired in the other skill sets to practical use and help patients move toward independence. The patient should receive an outline or plan for managing their disease, especially as they may leave home for work or school. They should be familiar with their medications and their medical history, learn to call in their own prescriptions, make their own clinic appointments, begin to collect copies of their health records/medical summary for work/school, and learn about adult providers, based on the location of where they will be in the near future (adult gastroenterologists near their new home/school/work). They should carry an insurance card and understand the concept of medical

insurance as well as more specific details including eligibility requirements, co-pays, and other potential resources for coverage such as Social Security Disability Insurance (SSDI).

Skill set 6 Health and lifestyle decisions: The acquisition of skills from this skill set includes the patient gaining a general understanding of the importance of health maintenance and the potential interplay of their disease and lifestyle decisions. General knowledge includes the beneficial effects of exercise and an appropriate diet as well as the adverse effects of drugs, alcohol, and smoking. They should know the specific impact of disease activity on fertility and sexuality and the consequences of nonadherence. Patients should understand that at age 18, they are considered autonomous adults in terms of their health care; they have the right to make their own health choices, and their health information cannot be shared with others including parents or guardians without permission.

Parents (Age 17–18)

Several studies in other chronic diseases have shown that parents may feel relegated to the sidelines as their children transfer to adult care. If the transition process has been implemented from an earlier age, and the parents have been educated, this should not occur. Parents can have concerns about their sons' or daughters' limitations in self-advocacy or cognitive function, and thus, can be justifiably worried about their ability to cope. These issues should be addressed at this visit, so everyone involved (the parents, the pediatric team, and the patient) in conjunction can find a solution to overcome any obstacles. Ultimately, at this age, the parents should show less and less responsibility for the patient's care as the patient assumes more responsibility. This is the time where the parents need to officially practice letting go. They should encourage their child to go to their follow-up visit alone or at least allow them to visit with the doctor alone for at least part of their visit. To address concerns most parents could have of missing critical information, it is helpful to address a list of questions addressing their concerns and to have the young adult patient ask the questions (or let the parents ask separately after the visit but generally with the patient present). They should also understand that once their child turns 18, HIPAA regulations come into play, and the parent cannot obtain medical information unless the patient provides approval. This becomes an issue as parents often call the adult clinic asking for results and medication refills, appointments, and management decisions/plans.

Pediatric Team (Age 17–18)

At this stage, the pediatric team should prepare for the final clinic visits prior to transfer of care. The pediatric health-care

Table 60.2 Medical summary letter

Medical summary letter for transitioning IBD patients
Disease information: date of diagnosis, location, severity
Findings: labs, endoscopy, histology, radiology results, and dates
Medical therapies: dose, duration, adverse reactions, reasons for discontinuation
Surgical history
Psychosocial, developmental, and educational issues

Adapted from Hait et al. [31]

team should remind the patient and the parents that at age 18, patients have the right to make their own decisions. The pediatric team should help identify potential adult IBD providers and encourage and facilitate an initial visit. Ideally, a transition clinic setup is optimal; however, few clinical centers/hospitals have one. A return visit after they have seen the adult provider may be helpful to discuss their experience and troubleshoot any remaining concerns. Plans for insurance coverage should be discussed with the patient and parents. Identifying any insurance coverage is important as this may impact who they may be able to see as they transition. The patient should be provided a summary of their medical history for school or work and obtain any consent for health information in order to provide to the new adult gastroenterologist. In addition, the team should complete a medical summary of the patient to provide to the adult provider. Hait and colleagues have suggested the following to be included in this letter (Table 60.2).

Before the last visit, the provider should confirm that psychosocial needs are addressed to ease the transitioning process as well as any other potential barriers to transfer of care, including financial issues, attitudes, access, and family resistance. The medical team should discuss differences in the cultures of pediatric and adult medicine. It is important whenever possible to refer the patient in times of disease quiescence and social stability when the transition is most likely to be successful. This may occur at different ages for various patients. For those who attend college, the transfer may be after graduation and after a job is secured or graduate education has begun. For those who choose not to attend college, the transfer of care should occur when housing and employment arrangements are stabilized.

Adult Team (Age 18+)

The adult gastroenterologist's role in the early transition process is minimal as the patient only arrives to them at the end of this process around the age of 18; however, his/her role in accepting and facilitating transfer of care is a key. In general, the adult gastroenterologist should only accept the transfer after he or she has been given an adequate medical history of this patient from the pediatric provider. This will help provide the most optimal care as medications, and prior medical and surgical history will be important in ongoing medical

care. Since the adult gastroenterologist can potentially have an even longer role in the patient's chronic care, the transition is crucial in establishing a physician-patient relationship that fosters independence as well as confidence, trust, and communication in both parties.

The adult gastroenterologist's role is to continue to foster this independence with the patient. The patient should continue to be the main focus and should be seen independently from the parents, especially if over-concerned parents tend to drive the visit interactions. At this time, legal implications of health care can also play a role. The patient is solely responsible for their medical information. It will be up to him or her to decide if, and to what extent, the parents should be involved. HIPAA regulations will come into play as parents, once used to obtaining and providing information, now legally do not have a role without the patient's consent. The adult gastroenterologist and the adult care team (nurses, medical assistants) should be aware of this when parents of transitioned patients call for information. However, if the transition process is successful, the patients will contact the office themselves for medical information.

The adult gastroenterologist should acknowledge the parents and work jointly to continue to allow for the patient to remain independent and communicate any issues they have at the first visit. There should be mutual understanding of everyone's role. Since the parents have been a key player in their child's chronic illness, it is understandable that the parents will have concerns and questions, as well as some resistance toward the transition. However, with the understanding and acknowledgement that the adult gastroenterologist's goal is to provide optimal care for the patient, then the family, patient, and physician can work together toward the same goals.

The adult gastroenterologist should confirm that the patient has established a relationship with an adult primary care physician, especially if the patient has been seeing a pediatrician for their general health care. Specialists often take on the role of "generalist" due to their frequent interaction related to IBD visits. However, obtaining a primary care provider (PCP) is important to provide optimal care regarding other illnesses such as general health care, immunizations, and screening for other diseases such as breast and prostate cancer and for preventive care for other diseases such as hyperlipidemia, diabetes, and hypertension.

The adult team should confirm that all relevant medical records are obtained, including any outstanding information that may still be needed. This may warrant a phone conversation with the pediatric health-care providers to include specific social history, developmental issues, and family dynamics that may not have been fully explained in the records. The importance of adherence to therapy should continue to be addressed at this time as well as any parental concerns. The adult provider should anticipate and answer any questions about smoking, alcohol, substance abuse, and sexuality as well as the psychosocial impacts their disease may have. They should also educate the patient regarding the adult chronic care model.

Monitoring the Process

Some system should be established to monitor both the teaching of the above skills and what has been learned and retained. This might be done through pop-up messages on an electronic medical record, where objectives and follow-up learning must be recorded by date, or a special form could be kept in the patient's chart to check off each set once taught and then mastered. The patient could also be given a copy of this checklist so they know what the entire skill set contains. A member of the health-care team should be dedicated to documenting this process to ensure patients are making progress in becoming independent. Having set questions at follow-up visits to document what has been learned is also important. Typical questions that patients might be expected to answer at a follow-up visit are as follows: (1) Can you describe your disease? (2) What are your symptoms of IBD? (3) What situations should you avoid? (4) When should you call or see the doctor? (5) What is your doctor's or nurse's phone number? (6) Did you make this appointment? (7) Have you called in one of your prescriptions for refill? (8) What health records have you collected (i.e. endoscopy reports; laboratory test results)? (9) Who is your insurance carrier? Before final transition, time should be set up to do a final review of their competence in all areas, and then when the patient is ready, preparations can be made to transition care to an adult provider. At this point, the patient should already be taking care of his or her health issues, and a successful outcome for transition is likely.

Conclusion

The transition process can be a challenging time period for adolescents living with IBD as they move toward adulthood. However, a successful transition can be implemented if steps are taken early in the process with the combined effort from the patient, the parents/guardians, and the pediatric gastroenterology team. The key is to provide sufficient and early training around the process so that the young adult patient, their family, and their providers can progress through the process together ensuring adequate time to adapt and prepare for a successful transition and graduation to adult gastroenterology care. A dynamic and supportive process will help young adult IBD patients effectively self-manage their health-care needs and become independent young adults who can manage their own complex medical needs.

References

1. Blum RW, Garell D, Hodgman CH, Jorissen TW, Okinow NA, Orr DP, Slap GB. Transition from child-centered to adult health-care systems for adolescents with chronic conditions. A position paper of the Society for Adolescent Medicine. J Adolesc Health. 1993;14:570–6.
2. American Academy of P, American Academy of Family P, American College of P, Transitions Clinical Report Authoring G, Cooley WC, Sagerman PJ. Supporting the health care transition from adolescence to adulthood in the medical home. Pediatrics. 2011;128:182–200. doi: 10.1542/peds.2011-0969.
3. American Academy of P, American Academy of Family P, American College of Physicians-American Society of Internal M. A consensus statement on health care transitions for young adults with special health care needs. Pediatrics. 2002;110:1304–6.
4. McPheeters M, Davis AM, Taylor JL, Brown RF, Potter SA, Epstein Jr RA. Transition care for children with special health needs. Rockville: Agency for Healthcare Research and Quality; 2014.
5. Rosen DS, Blum RW, Britto M, Sawyer SM, Siegel DM, Society for Adolescent M. Transition to adult health care for adolescents and young adults with chronic conditions: position paper of the Society for Adolescent Medicine. J Adolesc Health. 2003;33:309–11.
6. Baldassano R, Ferry G, Griffiths A, Mack D, Markowitz J, Winter H. Transition of the patient with inflammatory bowel disease from pediatric to adult care: recommendations of the North American Society for Pediatric Gastroenterology, Hepatology and Nutrition. J Pediatr Gastroenterol Nutr. 2002;34:245–8.
7. Leung Y, Heyman MB, Mahadevan U. Transitioning the adolescent inflammatory bowel disease patient: guidelines for the adult and pediatric gastroenterologist. Inflamm Bowel Dis. 2011;17:2169–73. doi:10.1002/ibd.21576.
8. Kahn SA. Transition of care for adolescents and young adults with IBD: the more we learn, the less we know. J Pediatr Gastroenterol Nutr. 2016 doi:10.1097/MPG.0000000000001285.
9. El-Matary W. Transition of children with inflammatory bowel disease: big task, little evidence. World J Gastroenterol. 2009;15:3744–7.
10. Dabadie A, Troadec F, Heresbach D, Siproudhis L, Pagenault M, Bretagne JF. Transition of patients with inflammatory bowel disease from pediatric to adult care. Gastroenterol Clin Biol. 2008;32:451–9. doi:10.1016/j.gcb.2008.01.044.
11. Marcus SB, Strople JA, Neighbors K, Weissberg-Benchell J, Nelson SP, Limbers C, Varni JW, Alonso EM. Fatigue and health-related quality of life in pediatric inflammatory bowel disease. Clin Gastroenterol Hepatol. 2009;7:554–61.
12. Karwowski CA, Keljo D, Szigethy E. Strategies to improve quality of life in adolescents with inflammatory bowel disease. Inflamm Bowel Dis. 2009;15:1755–64. doi:10.1002/ibd.20919.
13. Crowley R, Wolfe I, Lock K, McKee M. Improving the transition between paediatric and adult healthcare: a systematic review. Arch Dis Child. 2011;96:548–53. doi:10.1136/adc.2010.202473.
14. Reiss JG, Gibson RW, Walker LR. Health care transition: youth, family, and provider perspectives. Pediatrics. 2005;115:112–20. doi:10.1542/peds.2004-1321.
15. Bensen R, McKenzie R, Fernandes S, Fishman L. Transitions in pediatric gastroenterology: results of a National Provider Survey. J Pediatr Gastroenterol Nutr. 2016;63(5):488–93. doi:10.1097/MPG.0000000000001199.
16. Gray WN, Maddux MH. Current transition practices in pediatric IBD: findings from a National Survey of Pediatric Providers. Inflamm Bowel Dis. 2016;22:372–9. doi:10.1097/MIB.0000000000000642.

17. Adamiak T, Walkiewicz-Jedrzejczak D, Fish D, Brown C, Tung J, Khan K, Faubion Jr W, Park R, Heikenen J, Yaffee M, Rivera-Bennett MT, Wiedkamp M, Stephens M, Noel R, Nugent M, Nebel J, Simpson P, Kappelman MD, Kugathasan S. Incidence, clinical characteristics, and natural history of pediatric IBD in Wisconsin: a population-based epidemiological study. Inflamm Bowel Dis. 2013;19:1218–23. doi:10.1097/MIB.0b013e318280b13e.

18. Kugathasan S, Judd RH, Hoffmann RG, Heikenen J, Telega G, Khan F, Weisdorf-Schindele S, San Pablo Jr W, Perrault J, Park R, Yaffe M, Brown C, Rivera-Bennett MT, Halabi I, Martinez A, Blank E, Werlin SL, Rudolph CD, Binion DG. Epidemiologic and clinical characteristics of children with newly diagnosed inflammatory bowel disease in Wisconsin: a statewide population-based study. J Pediatr. 2003;143:525–31.

19. Goodhand J, Dawson R, Hefferon M, Tshuma N, Swanson G, Wahed M, Croft NM, Lindsay JO. Inflammatory bowel disease in young people: the case for transitional clinics. Inflamm Bowel Dis. 2010;16:947–52. doi:10.1002/ibd.21145.

20. Turunen P, Kolho KL, Auvinen A, Iltanen S, Huhtala H, Ashorn M. Incidence of inflammatory bowel disease in Finnish children, 1987–2003. Inflamm Bowel Dis. 2006;12:677–83.

21. Van Limbergen J, Russell RK, Drummond HE, Aldhous MC, Round NK, Nimmo ER, Smith L, Gillett PM, McGrogan P, Weaver LT, Bisset WM, Mahdi G, Arnott ID, Satsangi J, Wilson DC. Definition of phenotypic characteristics of childhood-onset inflammatory bowel disease. Gastroenterology. 2008;135:1114–22. doi:10.1053/j.gastro.2008.06.081.

22. Fishman LN, Barendse RM, Hait E, Burdick C, Arnold J. Self-management of older adolescents with inflammatory bowel disease: a pilot study of behavior and knowledge as prelude to transition. Clin Pediatr (Phila). 2010;49:1129–33. doi:10.1177/0009922810379042.

23. Greenley RN, Kunz JH, Biank V, Martinez A, Miranda A, Noe J, Telega G, Tipnis NA, Werlin S, Stephens MC. Identifying youth nonadherence in clinical settings: data-based recommendations for children and adolescents with inflammatory bowel disease. Inflamm Bowel Dis. 2012;18:1254–9. doi:10.1002/ibd.21859.

24. Whitfield EP, Fredericks EM, Eder SJ, Shpeen BH, Adler J. Transition readiness in pediatric patients with inflammatory bowel disease: a patient survey of self-management skills. J Pediatr Gastroenterol Nutr. 2015;60:36–41. doi:10.1097/MPG.0000000000000555.

25. Gray WN, Denson LA, Baldassano RN, Hommel KA. Treatment adherence in adolescents with inflammatory bowel disease: the collective impact of barriers to adherence and anxiety/depressive symptoms. J Pediatr Psychol. 2012;37:282–91. doi:10.1093/jpepsy/jsr092.

26. Greenley RN, Stephens M, Doughty A, Raboin T, Kugathasan S. Barriers to adherence among adolescents with inflammatory bowel disease. Inflamm Bowel Dis. 2010;16:36–41. doi:10.1002/ibd.20988.

27. Greenley RN, Karazsia B, Schurman JV, Gumidyala AP, Nguyen EU, Thomason MM, Walter JG, Noe J, Werlin S, Kahn SA. Trajectories of oral medication adherence in youth with inflammatory bowel disease. Health Psychol. 2015b;34:514–21. doi:10.1037/hea0000149.

28. Fishman LN, Houtman D, van Groningen J, Arnold J, Ziniel S. Medication knowledge: an initial step in self-management for youth with inflammatory bowel disease. J Pediatr Gastroenterol Nutr. 2011;53:641–5. doi:10.1097/MPG.0b013e3182285316.

29. Hait EJ, Barendse RM, Arnold JH, Valim C, Sands BE, Korzenik JR, Fishman LN. Transition of adolescents with inflammatory bowel disease from pediatric to adult care: a survey of adult gastroenterologists. J Pediatr Gastroenterol Nutr. 2009;48:61–5. doi:10.1097/MPG.0b013e31816d71d8.

30. GotTransition.org. Sample Transition Readiness Assessment for Youth.

31. Hait E, Arnold JH, Fishman LN. Educate, communicate, anticipate-practical recommendations for transitioning adolescents with IBD to adult health care. Inflamm Bowel Dis. 2006;12:70–3. doi:10.1097/01.MIB.0000194182.85047.6a.

32. NASPGHAN. Transitioning a patient with IBD from pediatric to adult care.

33. CDHNF. Preparing to transition from a pediatric to adult care practitioner: transitioning to adulthood with IBD.

34. Ferris ME, Harward DH, Bickford K, Layton JB, Ferris MT, Hogan SL, Gipson DS, McCoy LP, Hooper SR. A clinical tool to measure the components of health-care transition from pediatric care to adult care: the UNC TR(x)ANSITION scale. Ren Fail. 2012;34(6):744–753. doi:10.3109/0886022X.2012.678171. Epub 2012 May 14. PMID: 22583152.

35. Ferris M, Cohen S, Haberman C, Javalkar K, Massengill S, Mahan JD, Kim S, Bickford K, Cantu G, Medeiros M, Phillips A, Ferris MT, Hooper SR. Self-management and transition readiness assessment: development, reliability, and factor structure of the STARx questionnaire. J Pediatr Nurs. 2015;30(5):691–699. doi:10.1016/j.pedn.2015.05.009. Epub 2015 Jul 22. PMID: 26209873.

36. Bell L. Adolescents with renal disease in an adult world: meeting the challenge of transition of care. Nephrol Dial Transplant. 2007;22:988–91. doi:10.1093/ndt/gfl770.

37. Desir B, Seidman EG. Transitioning the paediatric IBD patient to adult care. Best Pract Res Clin Gastroenterol. 2003;17:197–212.

38. Greenley RN, Gumidyala AP, Nguyen E, Plevinsky JM, Poulopoulos N, Thomason MM, Walter JG, Wojtowicz AA, Blank E, Gokhale R, Kirschner BS, Miranda A, Noe JD, Stephens MC, Werlin S, Kahn SA. Can you teach a teen new tricks? Problem solving skills training improves oral medication adherence in pediatric patients with inflammatory bowel disease participating in a randomized trial. Inflamm BowelDis.2015a;21:2649–57.doi:10.1097/MIB.0000000000000530.

39. Spekhorst LM, Hummel TZ, Benninga MA, van Rheenen PF, Kindermann A. Adherence to oral maintenance treatment in adolescents with inflammatory bowel disease. J Pediatr Gastroenterol Nutr. 2016;62:264–70. doi:10.1097/MPG.0000000000000924.

Index

© Springer International Publishing AG 2017
P. Mamula et al. (eds.), *Pediatric Inflammatory Bowel Disease*, DOI 10.1007/978-3-319-49215-5